Textbook of Cultural Psychiatry

Second Edition

Textbook of Cultural Psychiatry

Second Edition

Edited by

Dinesh Bhugra
Emeritus Professor of Mental Health and Cultural Diversity, Institute of Psychiatry, Psychology and Neuroscience, King's College London, UK

Kamaldeep Bhui
Professor of Cultural Psychiatry and Epidemiology, Queen Mary University of London, UK

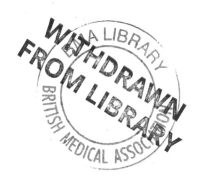

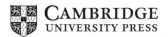

CAMBRIDGE
UNIVERSITY PRESS

CAMBRIDGE
UNIVERSITY PRESS

University Printing House, Cambridge CB2 8BS, United Kingdom

One Liberty Plaza, 20th Floor, New York, NY 10006, USA

477 Williamstown Road, Port Melbourne, VIC 3207, Australia

314–321, 3rd Floor, Plot 3, Splendor Forum, Jasola District Centre, New Delhi – 110025, India

79 Anson Road, #06–04/06, Singapore 079906

Cambridge University Press is part of the University of Cambridge.

It furthers the University's mission by disseminating knowledge in the pursuit of education, learning and research at the highest international levels of excellence.

www.cambridge.org
Information on this title: www.cambridge.org/9781316628508
DOI: 10.1017/9781316810057

© Cambridge University Press (2007) 2018

First published 2007
Second edition 2018

Printed in the United Kingdom by Clays, St Ives plc

A catalogue record for this publication is available from the British Library

Library of Congress Cataloging in Publication data
Names: Bhugra, Dinesh, editor. | Bhui, Kamaldeep, editor.
Title: Textbook of cultural psychiatry / edited by Dinesh Bhugra, Kamaldeep Bhui.
Description: Second edition. | Cambridge ; New York, NY : Cambridge University Press, 2018. | Includes bibliographical references and index.
Identifiers: LCCN 2018003582 | ISBN 9781316628508 (paperback)
Subjects: | MESH: Mental Disorders – ethnology | Ethnic Groups – psychology | Ethnopsychology – methods | Cultural Diversity | Cultural Characteristics | Cross-Cultural Comparison
Classification: LCC RC455.4.E8 | NLM WM 140 | DDC 616.89–dc23
LC record available at https://lccn.loc.gov/2018003582

ISBN 978-1-316-62850-8 Paperback

....

Every effort has been made in preparing this book to provide accurate and up-to-date information which is in accord with accepted standards and practice at the time of publication. Although case histories are drawn from actual cases, every effort has been made to disguise the identities of the individuals involved. Nevertheless, the authors, editors and publishers can make no warranties that the information contained herein is totally free from error, not least because clinical standards are constantly changing through research and regulation. The authors, editors and publishers therefore disclaim all liability for direct or consequential damages resulting from the use of material contained in this book. Readers are strongly advised to pay careful attention to information provided by the manufacturer of any drugs or equipment that they plan to use.

This volume is dedicated to the memory of

Richard Marley (1963–2016)

Publishing Director of Life Sciences and Medicine at
Cambridge University Press

with thanks for all his support and friendship over the years

Contents

Section 4: Theoretical Aspects of Management

Section 5: Management with Special Groups

Section 6: Cultural Research and Training

Contributors

Iqbal Ahmed
Department of Behavioral Health
Tripler Army Medical Center
Honolulu, Hawaii
USA

Anne E. Becker
Department of Global Health and Social Medicine
Harvard Medical School
Department of Psychiatry and Massachusetts General
Hospital
Boston, Massachusetts
USA

John W. Berry
Psychology Department
Queen's University
Kingston, Ontario, Canada
and National Research University
Higher School of Economics
Moscow
Russian Federation

Sabyasachi Bhaumik
University of Leicester and Leicestershire Partnership
NHS Trust
Leicester
UK

Dinesh Bhugra
Institute of Psychiatry, Psychology
and Neuroscience
King's College London
London
UK

Kamaldeep Bhui
Centre for Psychiatry
Wolfson Institute of Preventive Medicine Barts
and The London, Queen Mary University
of London
London
UK

Chad A. Bousman
Departments of Medical Genetics, Psychiatry, and
Physiology and Pharmacology
Cumming School of Medicine
University of Calgary
Calgary, Alberta
Canada

Yulisha Byrow
Department of Psychiatry
Sydney Medical School
University of Sydney
Sydney
Australia

Santosh K. Chaturvedi
Department of Psychiatry
National Institute of Mental Health and
Neurosciences
Bangalore
India

Margaret S. Chisolm
Johns Hopkins University School
of Medicine
Baltimore, Maryland
USA

Carl I. Cohen
SUNY Downstate Medical Center
Brooklyn, New York
USA

Christopher C. H. Cook
Department of Theology and Religion
Durham University
Durham
UK

Rubens Dantas
Medical Student, Fundação do ABC
Santo André
Brazil

Joop T. V. M. de Jong
Faculty of Social and Behavioural Sciences
University of Amsterdam
Amsterdam
The Netherlands

Geetha Desai
Department of Psychiatry
National Institute of Mental Health and
Neurosciences
Bangalore
India

Nisha Dogra
Greenwood Institute of Child Health
Department of Neuroscience, Psychology and Behaviour
University of Leicester
Leicester
UK

William W. Dressler
Department of Anthropology
The University of Alabama
Tuscaloosa, Alabama
USA

Mehdi Elmouchtari
SUNY Downstate Medical Center
Brooklyn, New York
USA

Horacio Fabrega Jr
Department of Psychiatry
School of Medicine
University of Pittsburgh
Pittsburgh, Pennsylvania
USA

Sarah A. Fortune
Department of Psychological Medicine
University of Otago
Dunedin
New Zealand

Satheesh Kumar Gangadharan
Leicestershire Partnership NHS Trust
Leicester
UK

Shweta Gangavati
Leicestershire Partnership NHS Trust
Leicester
UK

Angela Glover
Department of Psychiatry
Rush University Medical Center
Chicago, Illinois
USA

Rohit Gumber
Leicestershire Partnership NHS Trust
Leicester
UK

Keith Hawton
Centre for Suicide Research
Department of Psychiatry
University of Oxford
Warneford Hospital
Oxford
UK

Devon Hinton
Department of Global Health and Social Medicine
Harvard Medical School
Cambridge, Massachusetts
USA

Heidi Hjelmeland
Department of Mental Health Faculty of Medicine
and Health Sciences
Norwegian University of Science and Technology
Trondheim
Norway

Pamela Hoffman
Warren Alpert Medical School of Brown University
Providence, Rhode Island
USA

David Holzer
Psychiatry University Clinic Vienna
Vienna
Austria

Assen Jablensky
Centre of Clinical Research in Neuropsychiatry
School of Psychiatry and Clinical Neuroscience
University of Western Australia
Perth, Western Australia
Australia

Janis H. Jenkins
Departments of Anthropology and Psychiatry
University of California, San Diego
La Jolla, California
USA

Gurvinder Kalra
Latrobe Regional Hospital (LRH)
LRH Mental Health Services
Traralgon, Victoria
Australia

Niranjan Karnik
Department of Psychiatry
Rush University Medical Center
Chicago, Illinois
USA

Brendan D. Kelly
Department of Psychiatry
Trinity College Dublin
Trinity Centre for Health Sciences
Tallaght Hospital
Dublin
Ireland

Matthew Kelly
St Andrew's Healthcare
Northampton
UK

Laurence J. Kirmayer
Division of Social and Transcultural Psychiatry
McGill University
Montreal, Quebec H3T 1E4
Canada

Robert Kohn
Warren Alpert Medical School
Brown University
Providence, Rhode Island
USA

Arlene Laliberté
Centre for Research and Intervention on Suicide and Euthanasia
Université of Québec in Montréal
Montreal, Quebec H3 C 3P8
Canada

Fiona Larkan
School of Medicine and Centre for Global Health

Institute of Population Health
Trinity College
University of Dublin
Ireland

Kate M. Loewenthal
Psychology Department
Royal Holloway
University of London
Egham, Surrey
UK

Sieglinde McGee
Independent Consultant
Portlaoise
Ireland

Malcolm MacLachlan
Assisted Living and Learning (ALL) Institute &
Department of Psychology
Maynooth University
Maynooth, Co Kildare
Ireland

Gin S. Malhi
Department of Psychiatry
Sydney Medical School
University of Sydney
Sydney
Australia

Harry Minas
Global and Cultural Mental Health Unit
Centre for Mental Health
Melbourne School of Population and Global Health
University of Melbourne
Melbourne
Australia

Driss Moussaoui
Department of Psychiatry
Ibn Rushd University Psychiatric Centre
Casablanca
Morocco

Chee H. Ng
The Melbourne Clinic Professorial Unit
Department of Psychiatry
University of Melbourne
Richmond
Australia

Albert Persaud
Centre for Applied Research and Evaluation
International Foundation (Careif)
Wolfson Institute of Preventive Medicine
Barts and The London, Queen Mary University
of London
London
UK

Gayatri Saraf
Department of Psychiatry
Maharashtra Institute of Mental Health
Pune
India

Jerome Sarris
NICM
Western Sydney University
Campbelltown
The Melbourne Clinic Professorial Unit
Department of Psychiatry
University of Melbourne
Richmond
Australia

Kemal Sayar
Marmara University Medical School
Istanbul
Turkey

Ajit Shah
School of Health
University of Central Lancashire
Preston
UK

Jay H. Shore
University of Colorado Anschutz
Medical Campus
Helen and Arthur E. Johnson
Depression Center
Denver, Colorado
USA

Andrew Sims
Formerly Department of Psychiatry
University of Leeds
Leeds
UK

Stephanie Solazzo
Johns Hopkins University School of Medicine
Baltimore, Maryland
USA

Thomas Stompe
Psychiatry University Clinic Vienna
Vienna
Austria

John Strang
Addictions Department
Institute of Psychiatry, Psychology
and Neuroscience
King's College London
London
UK

Digby Tantam
Existential Academy
London
UK

Michel Tousignant
Centre for Research and Intervention on Suicide and
Euthanasia
Université of Québec in Montréal
Montreal, Quebec H3 C 3P8
Canada

Rachel Tribe
School of Psychology
University of East London
London
UK

Aneta D. Tunariu
School of Psychology
College of Applied Heath and Communities
University of East London
London
UK

Antonio Ventriglio
Department of Mental Health and
Department of Clinical and Experimental Medicine
University of Foggia
Foggia
Italy

Panos Vostanis
School of Neuroscience, Psychology and Behaviour
University of Leicester
Leicester
UK

Shamil Wanigaratne
National Rehabilitation Center
Abu Dhabi
United Arab Emirates

Maryann Waugh
University of Colorado Anschutz Medical Campus
School of Medicine
Helen and Arthur E. Johnson

Depression Center
Denver, Colorado
USA

Mitchell G. Weiss
Swiss Tropical and Public Health Institute and
University of Basel
Basel
Switzerland

Joseph Westermeyer
University of Minnesota Hospital
Department of Psychiatry
Minneapolis, Minnesota
USA

Foreword

Most of us live today in multiethnic environments, in which cultural variations in the expression of psychopathology can be directly observed by the average practitioner, and in which problems in communication and diagnostic approach to persons with different ethnic and cultural backgrounds are being experienced on a daily basis.

The diversity of idioms of distress and explanatory models of disease related to different cultural backgrounds is today something that a large proportion of psychiatrists can increasingly witness in their ordinary clinical practice rather than just discovering, as in the past, through articles or textbooks.

Increasingly widespread is also the awareness of the ethnic and cultural variations in the response to the most common psychotropic medications, which is certainly to some extent a matter of genetic polymorphisms, but also a consequence of the impact of a variety of environmental factors.

Nowadays, most trials of psychotropic drugs are multicentric, and an increasing number of them are carried out in various regions of the world. However, ethnic variations in response to the tested medications are rarely a focus of attention in these trials. Moreover, treatment guidelines produced in North America and Europe are often regarded as universally valid, and rarely adapted to other cultural contexts or to ethnic minorities.

There is also an emerging evidence that the most common psychotherapeutic techniques may be not equally adaptable to the needs of all cultures. Cognitive-behavioural interventions, for instance, may prove to be more flexible than psychodynamic psychotherapies. On the other hand, psychosocial interventions may pose special problems if the patient belongs to an ethnic minority, although this issue has been relatively neglected by research up to now.

On the scientific side, findings such as the increased prevalence of psychotic disorders among some (but not all) groups of migrants (for instance, among black Caribbean and African migrants in the UK, but not among people of Turkish origin in the Netherlands or of Hispanic descent in the United States) still remain without a convincing explanation, and are likely not to be just a consequence of misdiagnosis or different access to services.

Still, a culturally informed approach to psychiatric training, clinical practice and research is uncommon in the vast majority of regions of the world, and the attempts that have been made by some major diagnostic systems to include a cultural component do not seem to have generated an extensive effort to explore their feasibility and practical usefulness.

This book is probably the best response currently available in the psychiatric literature to this complex array of unmet needs. Its first edition received a commendation in the 2008 British Medical Association Awards and was the recipient of the 2012 Creative Scholarship Award from the Society for the Study of Psychiatry and Culture.

The current second edition contains several completely new chapters (those on lifestyle medicine in psychiatry, social media, telepsychiatry and globalization), while all other chapters have been extensively revised and updated.

I recommend the book not only to an élite of researchers and scholars, but also to all responsible clinicians who feel today the motivation and the duty to adapt their ordinary practice to a social context which is rapidly changing.

Mario Maj
Past President, World Psychiatric Association

Preface to the Second Edition

In the decade since the first edition of this book was published, cultural psychiatry has come into its own. For the first time, DSM-5 now takes into account the cultural formulation leading to embedding of cultural factors in diagnosis of psychiatric disorders. As more people migrate for educational and economic reasons – as well those who are seeking refuge – clinicians and researchers alike need to be aware of the cultural needs of individuals. Cultural values expand as well as shrink in response to movement into a new culture. Cultural competency is essential but it also needs to be recognized that it is good clinical practice for the patient to be seen in a holistic manner in the context of their social proximal factors related to family and kinship and distal factors related to society and culture.

All the chapters in this edition have been updated and a majority have been completely rewritten and revised. We are immensely grateful to all our authors for their commitment and delivery of manuscripts on time in spite of their busy schedules. We are thankful to the staff at Cambridge University Press for their encouragement and support, and especially to Richard Marley, who sadly passed away before final publication of the book.

Immense thanks are due to Andrea Livingstone, who has been a pillar of strength in organizing, re-organizing and supporting the work of the editors, from initial invitations to authors to the final versions of the chapters.

Dinesh Bhugra
Kamaldeep Bhui

Chapter

1

Cultural Psychiatry in Historical Perspective

Laurence J. Kirmayer

Editors' Introduction

The evolution of cultural psychiatry over the last few decades has been an interesting phenomenon to observe. Psychiatry is perhaps one of the younger disciplines of medicine. The coming of age of psychiatry as a profession was clearly linked with the development of training and laying claim to a knowledge base which gradually has become more evidence based. The period between the two World Wars led to greater questioning of social factors in the aetiology and management of psychiatric disorders. In the UK at least, social psychiatry as a discipline became clearly established and produced impressive studies on life events and their impact on phenomenology, attachment and other social factors. In the last two decades, it would appear that social psychiatry has transmogrified into cultural psychiatry.

Kirmayer, in this chapter, maps out the history of cultural psychiatry as a discipline. In addition, he raises concerns related to this discipline, especially to universality of psychopathology and healing practices, development of diverse service needs of black and ethnic minority groups and analysis of psychiatric theory and practice as products of a particular cultural history. Culture has been defined as a civilizing process which, in European history, Kirmayer asserts, had to do with the transformations from migratory groups to agrarian societies to city states and, eventually, nation states. The definition of culture in this context was related to standards of refinement and sophistication. The second definition of culture has to do with collective identity, which is based on historical lineage, language, religion, genetics or ethnicity. Kirmayer suggests that these two definitions have become conflated. The historical development of comparative psychiatry in colonial times and until the 1960s, when research across cultures used dimensions of distress, ignored local cultural practices and interpretation of these experiences. The role of racism in diagnosis and management of individuals with psychiatric illnesses has not entirely gone away. Large-scale migrations from east to west and north to south across the globe have raised questions about ethnocultural diversity. An organized and relative newcomer within the larger discipline of psychiatry, cultural psychiatry is becoming mainstream and beginning to influence health-service delivery and research.

Introduction

Cultural psychiatry stands at the crossroads of disciplines concerned with the impact of culture on behaviour and experience. It emerges from a history of encounters between people of different backgrounds, struggling to understand and respond to human suffering in contexts that confound the alien qualities of psychopathology with the strangeness of the cultural 'other'. The construct of culture offers one way to conceptualize such differences, allowing us to bring together race, ethnicity and ways of life under one broad rubric to examine the impact of social knowledge, institutions and practices on health, illness and healing. Cultural psychiatry differs from the social sciences of medicine, however, in being driven primarily not by theoretical problems but by clinical imperatives. The choice of research questions and methods, no less than the interpretation of findings and the framing of professional practice, is shaped by this clinical agenda, which emphasizes the quest for therapeutic efficacy.

Over the course of its history, cultural psychiatry has been driven by three major sets of concerns: questions about the universality or relativity of psychopathology and healing practices; the dilemmas of providing services to ethnically diverse populations; and, most recently, the analysis of psychiatric theory and practice as products of a particular cultural history and as vehicles of globalization. These concerns correspond to three successive waves of development of the field from colonialist and comparative psychiatry, to the mental health of ethnocultural communities and indigenous peoples in settler societies, and the post-colonial anthropology of psychiatry.

The emergence and development of each of these themes in cultural psychiatry can be tied to major historical events, especially to global patterns of migration and their associated social, political and economic consequences (Castles *et al.*, 2013; Papastergiadis, 2000). From the mid 1700s onwards, colonialist expansion of European powers led to observations relevant to psychiatry and to occasional efforts to provide healthcare in distant lands. Large-scale migrations of Europeans to North America, Australia and other regions in the nineteenth and twentieth centuries prompted attention to the impact of ethnicity on mental health and illness. Successive wars made psychological reactions to stress and trauma a salient concern for psychiatry. The Great Depression and the emergence of the welfare state highlighted the impact of social class and poverty as causes of illness. The promulgation of scientific racism forced researchers and clinicians to clarify their thinking about ethnocultural difference. The flight of refugees and displaced peoples following World War II and later conflicts, led to renewed work both on trauma-related disorders and the adaptation of migrants (Murphy, 1955). The UN Universal Declaration of Human Rights in 1948 and emerging anti-colonialist struggles around the world challenged the hegemony of Western versions of history and opened up the consideration of alternative systems of knowledge on both ethical and epistemological grounds.

Most recently, new waves of migration from east to west and south to north have challenged models of culture and ethnicity developed for earlier groups of immigrants from relatively similar European countries (Castles *et al.*, 2013). At the same time, increasing recognition of the historical injustices suffered by indigenous peoples has made their cultures a focus of attention both in terms of the damaging effects of forced assimilation and the potential for resilience in indigenous identity, community and healing practices (Cohen, 1999; Kirmayer *et al.*, 2003). The growth of the Hispanic, Asian and other non-European populations in the USA, and the corresponding increase in the numbers of mental health professionals from diverse ethnocultural backgrounds, pressed for change both from without and within the profession, and this has been reflected in the attention to culture in official psychiatric nosology, with inclusion of an Outline for Cultural Formulation in DSM-IV and the Cultural Formulation Interview in DSM-5 (Alarcon, 2001; American Psychiatric Association, 2013; Mezzich *et al.*, 1996; Lewis-Fernández *et al.*, 2015). Similar demographic changes are affecting most societies, and will continue to make cultural issues a matter of central concern for psychiatry in the years to come. At the same time, backlash against globalization and the dynamics of migration, the Internet and social media will continue to give new meanings to cultural identity and community.

The Uses of Culture

There are three broad but distinct uses of the term culture that are often conflated (Eagleton, 2000; Kuper, 1999) and each has its reflection in the history of cultural psychiatry. Originally, 'culture' meant 'cultivation': the civilizing process which, in European history, had to do first with the move from migratory groups to agrarian societies (cultivating crops) and then to city states and larger political entities including nations and empires. Throughout this history, there was a progressive elaboration of codes of conduct and civility and the cultivation of specialized knowledge and power, initially the possession of elite social classes, but gradually accessible to others through formal education (Elias, 1982; Gellner, 1988). Culture in this sense represents a standard of refinement or sophistication, measured against the cosmopolitan life of urban centres, the achievements of those with higher education, and the 'high culture' (with a capital 'C') of arts and letters. The view of culture as civilization has influenced thinking about psychopathology from Vico's Renaissance views of culture as a civilizing force (Bergin and Fisch, 1984). Early versions of this critiqued European society by contrasting it with the 'natural' qualities of the noble savage (Ellingson, 2001); this took more dynamic form in Freud's tragic view of the ego wrestling with conflicts of 'instinctual' desire and sociomoral constraint in *Civilization and its Discontents* (Freud, 1962). Western European civilization has tended to view itself myopically as the singular standard against which other traditions can be measured, and this hierarchical view of culture persists in characterizations of the contemporary world as a contest of great civilizations with incommensurable values and epistemologies (Huntington, 1996; Bettiza, 2014).

A second meaning of culture has to do with collective identity, the setting apart of one group of people from another on the basis of historical lineage, language, religion, gender or ethnicity which may include membership in a community, regional group, nation or other historical people (Banks, 1996). While the notion of culture as cultivation may be presented in terms of a universal system of values that can be attained by anyone allowed the opportunity to become 'civilized' (even if, in most instances, it depends on racialized or essentialized notions of identity that subvert this possibility), ethnocultural identity is local and particular, the property of groups that regulate its distribution along lines of historical descent, kinship, citizenship or other social markers of identity. Ethnicity is differently constructed in each society, and may merge with local notions of 'race', national identity or other invented traditions (Hobsbawm and Ranger, 1983). While ethnicity has been a source of positive identity, self-esteem and group cohesion, it has also fuelled discrimination, inter-group conflicts, social exclusion and genocidal violence.

The third notion of culture corresponds to its current use in anthropology as a way of life: the values, customs, beliefs, knowledge, institutions and practices that form a complex system (Kuper, 1999). As such, culture encompasses all of the humanly constructed and socially transmitted aspects of the environment. Cultural systems involve many levels of social organization including institutions, communities, families and local practices that cannot be reduced to the cultural models internalized by individuals. Much of culture resides in what might be called 'affordances', structured environments that provide opportunities for cooperative action (Kirmayer and Ramstead, 2017). In the contemporary world, cultural affordances may be constituted both by local communities or 'subcultures' and transnational flows of knowledge and practice shared by groups of experts and professionals (Hannerz, 1992, 1996). Psychiatry itself is one such transnational cultural institution with national variants and subcultures (Ernst and Mueller, 2010).

Comparative Psychiatry and the Legacy of Colonialism

The roots of cultural psychiatry can be traced to the very beginnings of modern psychiatry. Indeed, long before psychiatry emerged as a distinct medical specialty, examples of odd or deviant behaviour among distant peoples stimulated philosophical reflections on the uniqueness of humankind and the impact of the 'civilizing process' on human nature (Jahoda, 1993). These early commentaries drew on travellers' observations of foreign peoples who were culturally different, whether viewed as members of a different civilization or simply as undeveloped 'barbarians'. This literature reveals an aesthetic fascination with the strangeness of the other that was often both morally and erotically charged (Segalen, 2002). European explorers and colonizers generally took their own traditions to be the zenith of civilization, while others were seen as backward, primitive and uncivilized (Jahoda, 1999; Gilman, 1985; Lucas and Barrett, 1995; Todorov, 1993).

The taken-for-granted superiority of European civilization demanded that its institutions be established in the colonies, and asylum psychiatry was one of these exports. While attempting to care for suffering individuals, colonial psychiatry also served to justify and maintain the social order of colonial regimes (Bhugra and Littlewood, 2001; Keller, 2001, 2005; McCulloch, 1995; Sadowsky, 1999; Vaughan, 1991). Colonial asylums became important sites for comparative studies of psychopathology. However, their status as colonizers and limited access to the everyday life of people outside hospitals and asylums made it difficult for the practitioners of colonial psychiatry to recognize the social and cultural context of patients' afflictions. As local psychiatrists were trained and took over these institutions, possibilities emerged for innovative approaches to care based on local cultural values. The work of Thomas Adeoye Lambo at Aro village in Abeokuta, Nigeria was an important example of this 'post-colonial' turn, and his integration of traditional healers influenced international views of culture and community mental health through his tenure as Deputy Director General at the World Health Organization (Heaton, 2013).

In general, colonizers and alienists did not see large numbers of mentally ill persons and this prompted speculation about the protective effects of 'primitive' ways of life. The idea that insanity was rare among primitive or uncivilized peoples, as claimed by Jean-Jacques Rousseau, was popular among early writers in psychiatry including Esquirol, Moreau de Tours, Griesinger and Krafft-Ebing (Raimundo Oda *et al.*, 2005). Sometimes this notion of the 'healthy savage' was framed in terms of the protective effects of living a simple life with few demands, in contrast to the increasing expectations for productivity and consumption in the complex, urbanized, industrialized environment of Europe. An increase in nervousness was associated with the over-stimulation of modern civilization, especially for those required to do 'brain work', and hence the upper classes were seen as particularly prone to maladies like neurasthenia or nervous weakness – a diagnosis introduced by the American neurologist George Beard and taken up widely throughout Europe and East Asia (Beard, 1869; Rabinbach, 1990). Over time, the living conditions of the poor in large cities, along with the impact of alcohol and a general erosion of traditional moral and religious values, were invoked to explain the apparent increase in mental disorders in urban settings.

Early studies in comparative psychiatry focused on the exotic in order to examine the universality of major psychiatric disorders. The psychiatric literature of the late 1800s and early 1900s was peppered with reports of 'culture-bound syndromes', e.g. *pibloktoq*, *latah*, *amok*, thought to be uniquely linked to cultural beliefs and practices (Simons and Hughes, 1985). These reports seemed to indicate the malleability of expression of psychopathology, captured in the distinction between *pathoplasticity* and *pathogenesis* (Yap, 1952, 1974). Major psychiatric textbooks usually devoted a chapter to exotic and culture-bound conditions. Unfortunately, early observers paid relatively little attention to the social context of the syndromes they were observing and describing.

For example, *pibloktoq* or 'Arctic hysteria', which was described in early accounts by explorers among the polar Inuit, became a stock example of a culture-bound syndrome. Anthropologists and psychiatrists have sought to link *pibloktoq* to specific features of Inuit child-rearing, social structure, religious practice, environment and nutrition (Brill, 1913; Foulks, 1974; Gussow, 1960; Landy, 1985; Wallace and Ackerman, 1960). Historian Lyle Dick (1995, 2002) reviewed all available accounts of *pibloktoq* and found that the few detailed case descriptions came from Admiral Robert E. Peary's visits to Greenland (c. 1982). There, on a few occasions, Inuit women were observed to become agitated and run out on the ice, stripping off their clothes, prompting others to restrain them until their agitation eventually subsided some hours later. This 'hysterical' behaviour seemed entirely inexplicable until Dick provided the missing context: Admiral Peary had sent these women's menfolk out on exploratory missions at a time before

solid ice, exposing them to great risk. The women presumably engaged in shamanistic prayer and magic to ensure the men's safety. Peary also thought it important for the well-being of his crew that they have sexual companions and encouraged his men to take Inuit partners with little regard for existing relationships. Alcohol also played a role in these episodes. The women's 'erratic' behaviour – watched with amusement by Peary's men (as can be seen in a photograph reproduced as figure 6 in Dick 1995: 21) – now seems less like evidence of a discrete culture-bound syndrome than a grimly familiar story of exploitation.

In another historical analysis, Marano (1983) showed how the culture-bound syndrome *windigo*, described among the Ojibway as the fear that one is possessed by a spirit that is turning one into a cannibal, probably never occurred as a behavioural syndrome, but was a part of a legend or mythological belief that could be used as an accusation to attack others. This accusation was effective not only in traditional society but served to mobilize the Royal Canadian Mounted Police as well, invoking a new form of social control available as a result of colonization. Once again, a phenomenon better understood in terms of power, conflict and social change was reified as a psychopathological entity located within individuals (Waldram, 2004). Similar historical accounts of behaviours like *amok* or *latah* suggest that adequate description of culture bound syndromes requires attention to the social context of power and the dynamics of protest and resistance (Kua, 1991; Winzeler, 1990, 1995). Recognition of the importance of context, has led to a de-emphasis of culture bound syndromes in recent cultural psychiatry in favour of concepts (including idioms of distress and explanatory models) that focus on the pragmatic, social and communicative functions of local terminology (Lewis-Fernández, *et al.*, 2015).

This tendency to ignore social context also was characteristic of the comparative psychiatry (*Vergleichende Psychiatrie*) advanced by Emil Kraepelin (1856–1926), who visited Southeast Asia and Indonesia to study *amok* and examine the universality of major psychoses (Jilek, 1995). Kraepelin's conclusion was that clinical phenomenology justified a qualified universalism. However, the differences he did find, he explained in terms of a developmental hierarchy:

> based on a comparison between the phenomena of disease which I found there and those with which I was familiar at home, the overall similarity far outweighed the deviant features ... In particular, the

relative absence of delusions among the Javanese might be related to the lower stage of intellectual development attained and the rarity of auditory hallucinations might reflect the fact that speech counts for far less than it does with us and that thoughts tend to be governed more by sensory images.

(Kraepelin, 1904)

Kraepelin viewed cultural differences as reflections of biological differences in races or peoples and effectively elided the social context of psychiatric illness (Roelcke, 1997). His advocacy of theories of biological degeneration as a cause of mental disorder contributed to the rise of eugenic policies in Germany that culminated in the Nazi genocides.

While not adhering to Kraepelin's biological essentialism, H. B. M. Murphy (1915–1987) at McGill University and Julian Leff at the Institute of Psychiatry in the UK identified themselves as heirs to the tradition of comparative psychiatry and used both clinical observations and epidemiological methods to make systematic cross-cultural comparisons. Although they eschewed the sort of colonialist thinking and social Darwinism that plagued earlier writing, both invoked developmental hierarchies in their explanations of certain cultural differences. Murphy (1982) contrasted 'traditional' and 'modern' societies and Leff (1981) argued for a progressive differentiation of the emotion lexicon in Indo-European languages with contemporary British English as the most differentiated (for a critique, see Beeman, 1985).

Much of the innovative work of Alexander Leighton and Jane Murphy (Leighton, 1981; Murphy and Leighton, 1965) in Africa, Alaska and rural Nova Scotia also falls under the rubric of comparative psychiatry, although they employed dimensional measures of distress and, owing to their anthropological training, were interested in the impact of social and cultural context on mental health and illness. Despite this ethnographic orientation, Jane Murphy's (1976) influential paper arguing for the universal recognition of psychotic symptoms across diverse cultures did not consider the impact of colonial history on attitudes toward psychosis in the African and Alaskan communities she studied (Sadowsky, 1999).

The 'neo-Kraepelinian' revolution of DSM-III in 1980 introduced operationally defined discrete diagnostic categories in place of dimensional or narrative descriptions of psychiatric disorders (Wilson, 1993). With this new nosology and the accompanying technology of highly structured diagnostic interviews,

comparative psychiatry followed the rest of the discipline, abandoning in-depth ethnographically informed studies in favour of research organized around discrete diagnostic categories. This line of research has culminated in a series of important cross-national studies of the prevalence, course and outcome of major psychiatric disorders including the International Pilot Study of Schizophrenia (IPSS; World Health Organization, 1973; Leff et al. 1992), the Determinants of Outcome Study (Sartorius et al., 1986), the WHO Collaborative Study on Standardized Assessment of Depressive Disorders (World Health Organization, 1983), and the International Consortium of Psychiatric Epidemiology (e.g. Andrade et al., 2003). Successive generations of studies have used more refined measures, particularly standardized diagnostic interviews, most recently the Composite International Diagnostic Interview (Robins et al., 1989). However, these instruments continue to have limitations when used across cultures and methodological artifacts have not been eliminated (Hicks, 2002; van Ommeren et al., 2000). As well, most epidemiological studies have made little provision to identify culture-specific symptoms not included in the core definitions of disorders. In this way, the diagnostic categories of psychiatry bury the traces of their origins in European and American cultural history and become self-confirming 'culture-free' commodities ready for export.

Another important line of work in comparative psychiatry has centred on the effectiveness of traditional or indigenous healing practices (Kiev, 1969; Marsella and White, 1982; Rivers, 1924). Drawing from a rich ethnographic literature on healing rituals, Jerome Frank (1961), Raymond Prince (1980) and others argued that psychotherapy shares essential features with traditional healing and that both could be understood in terms of symbolic action at social, psychological and physiological levels. This work has become increasingly important as efforts are made to integrate or coordinate the activity of mental health practitioners and traditional or indigenous healers in many societies.

Cultural Essentialism and Racism in Psychiatry

A central feature of most colonial enterprises was the use of racist concepts and ideologies to justify the subordination and exploitation of colonized peoples

(Fredrickson, 2002). Though they have no clear foundation in biology, notions of race serve to mark off particular groups as intrinsically different and less than other human beings (Lock, 1993). Psychiatry itself has been used to buttress racist perspectives (Littlewood, 1993). The notion that southern or non-Western peoples had underdeveloped frontal lobes and hence were prone to disinhibited behaviours was promoted by several generations of neuropsychiatrists, both to explain cross-national differences and to account for inequalities within colonized nations that actually reflected the legacy of racism, slavery and economic marginalization. For example, influenced by Lucien Lévy-Bruhl's notion of primitive mentality, Antoine Porot, the head of the École d'Alger, argued that the native Algerian's mind was structurally different from that of the civilized European (Lévy-Bruhl, 1923; Porot 1918; Begue, 1996). This biological essentialism was matched by a complete disregard of social, cultural and political context that served colonial interests. This sort of essentialism persisted into the 1950s in the work of J. C. Carothers on the African mind. For Carothers, the African was developmentally child-like owing to underdeveloped frontal lobes that result in an effective leucotomy (Carothers, 1953; McCulloch, 1993, 1995). A whole generation of African psychiatrists was educated with texts containing this tendentious account.

Of course, there were also essentializing accounts of cultural difference presented in psychological terms. In *Prospero and Caliban* (1990; originally published in French in 1948), French intellectual Octave Mannoni described the people of Madagascar as primitive, and uncivilized, with a fundamentally different mentality based on a 'dependency complex' that protected them from the neurotic conflicts that were the burden of Europeans. Although Mannoni later developed a more nuanced account of the psychology of colonization, with Lacan displacing Adler in his psychodynamic theorizing, his earlier portrait remained a provocation to others seeking to understand and escape from the colonization of the psyche that accompanied political domination (Lane, 2002).

The migration of North African workers to France after 1945 stimulated French psychiatrists' interest in cultural difference and gave rise to the field of ethnopsychiatry (Fassin and Rechtman, 2005). Thus, the study of ethnic diversity in colonizing societies was closely linked with the history of colonial comparative psychiatry. At the same time, there was the growing recognition that the colonial context itself was one of exploitation and stress that could account for some of the suffering and symptomatology seen in clinical contexts.

Frantz Fanon (1925–1961) was an important voice in this critique of the colonial origins of psychopathology (Gordon, 2015; Macey, 1996; Razanajao *et al.*, 1996). Fanon denounced the theories of the École d'Alger, which he saw as based on a colonial perspective with racist devaluing of the values, traditions and autonomy of others. In *Peau noire, masques blancs* (1982; originally published in 1952), Fanon powerfully portrayed the self-alienating effects of racism and colonialism. Fanon's account of the psychopathology of colonialism echoed the earlier account by the sociologist W. E. B. Du Bois (1868–1963) in *The Souls of Black Folk* on the 'double consciousness' of African Americans (Du Bois, 1989). Fanon worked in the space between the political and the psychological – insisting on the primacy of politics and power, but showing how it was inscribed in the psychological and how change could come from within and without (Vergès, 1996). Ultimately, however, Fanon was less interested in the dynamics of culture and colonialism than in the struggle for political revolution and fell prey to the same tendency to essentialize cultural difference that plagued writers less aware than he was to the violence of racial stereotypes.

The process of unpacking the impact of racism and colonialism on the psychology of the colonizer and colonized is far from complete, the more so because the forms that oppression takes continue to mutate. This has been one focus of post-colonial theory, which offers a rich array of ideas about identity and alterity in the contemporary world that has as yet had little impact on cultural psychiatry (Bhabha, 1994; Chakrabarty, 2000; Gunew, 2003; Lazarus, 2011; Said, 1994).

Ethnocultural Diversity: Settler Societies and Indigenous Peoples

The large migrations of Europeans to North America, Australia and other countries from the 1700s onwards created settler societies with high levels of ethnocultural diversity. This experience of people from many different national and regional backgrounds living side by side made ethnicity salient (Banks, 1996). Epidemiological studies conducted from the 1930s onwards documented differential rates of psychiatric hospitalization for ethnocultural groups (Westermeyer, 1989). Of course, this difference reflected help-seeking and pathways to care more than population base rates. Subsequent waves of migration following World War II and other conflicts made the mental health needs of immigrants and refugees increasingly important in most psychiatric settings and led to a substantial literature on ethnic differences in illness behaviour.

The response to ethnic diversity has followed different trajectories in different countries owing to the history of colonization and migration but also following local ideologies of citizenship and dominant theories within psychiatry itself (Kirmayer and Minas, 2000; see for example, Bäärnhielm et al., 2005; Beneduce and Martelli, 2005; Fassin and Rechtman, 2005; Fernando, 2005). Thus, the US and France share republican values of egalitarianism that imply that all citizens should be treated the same, with no regard to their cultural background (Todorov, 1993). Along with this came the assumption that, over time, ethnic groups would assimilate and acquire the cultural identity and practices of the dominant society. In fact, ethnicity has persisted in most settler societies despite pressure to assimilate. In the US, the egalitarian ideal has been complicated by the history of slavery and racial discrimination against African Americans and other groups. The current language of culture refers to 'diversity', defined in terms of ethno-racial blocs (Hollinger, 1995), but this diversity is recognized mainly insofar as it is associated with health disparities (Smedley et al., 2003). In Canada and Australia, the ideology of multiculturalism has encouraged explicit attention to ethnic difference as a positive social value that warrants direct support by the state (Kivisto, 2002). At other moments, and in other societies, ethnicity has been profoundly divisive and, along with biologically essentialized notions of race, served as an incitement to violence and genocide (Fredrickson, 2002; wa Wamwere, 2003).

In Britain, cultural psychiatry has focused more on issues of race than on culture or ethnicity because of the conviction that racism is a crucial determinant of mental health and of the adequacy of psychiatric services (Fernando, 1988; Littlewood and Lipsedge, 1982). African Caribbean immigrants have been observed to have high rates of schizophrenia. This phenomenon, which affects some other migrant groups in other countries as well, does not appear to be due to diagnostic biases but may result from the stresses of marginalization, discrimination and social exclusion (Hutchinson and Haasen, 2004; Kelly, 2005; Veling, 2013).

Recognition of the importance of culture, ethnicity and race has been prompted by demographic and political changes in settler countries, sometimes crystallized by specific confrontations or violent events that have commanded public attention. In the UK the death of Stephen Lawrence increased public awareness of issues of racism and social exclusion and prompted a government inquiry that led to changes in policy, with attention being directed to counter racism in institutions including health services (Fernando, 2003). In Canada, the Oka Crisis of 1990 (York and Pindera, 1991) led to the reports of the Royal Commission on Aboriginal Peoples and the establishment of the Aboriginal Healing Foundation to provide support for projects to address the legacy of the residential school system (Kirmayer, Simpson and Cargo, 2003). A Truth and Reconciliation Commission concluded that Canada had committed cultural genocide and called for wide ranging efforts to acknowledge and support indigenous peoples' identity and communities.[1] However, much of the response to cultural diversity has been at the grassroots level with minimal governmental support (Fernando, 2005). At the same time, subtler forms of racism and social exclusion continue to go unmarked and unchallenged (Gilroy, 2005; Holt, 2000).

Anthropology of Psychiatry

The revolution in philosophy of science provoked by the work of Thomas Kuhn made biomedicine and psychiatry appear not so much universal truths as culturally constructed bodies of knowledge. Postcolonial writing challenged the taken-for-grantedness of Euroamerican values. The antipsychiatry 'movement' of the 1960s (Boyers, 1974) and the labelling theory of mental illness (Rosenhan, 1973; Scheff, 1974) drew attention to the social and political dimensions of psychiatric diagnosis. Historical accounts showed the ways in which psychiatric notions of madness emerged from and helped to maintain core cultural values (Ellenberger, 1970; Foucault, 1965; Micale and Porter, 1994; Porter, 1988). Within mainstream psychiatry itself, the US–UK Diagnostic Project

---

[1] See www.trc.ca.

(Cooper *et al.*, 1972) revealed important differences in the practice of British and American psychiatrists, with overdiagnosis of schizophrenia and underdiagnosis of bipolar disorder in the US. Subsequent efforts to improve the reliability of diagnostic practice in the US contributed to the emergence of DSM-III (Wilson, 1993). These and other social changes encouraged a more self-reflective stance and led anthropologists to consider biomedicine and psychiatry as cultural institutions (Good, 1994; Kleinman, 1988; Lock and Gordon, 1988). The anthropology of psychiatry developed a substantial body of literature showing how psychiatric practices draw from and contribute to cultural concepts of the person and experiences of the self (Gaines, 1992; Kleinman, 1995; Young, 1995). The third phase in the history of cultural psychiatry is strongly influenced by this turn toward cultural analysis and critique of the institutions and practices of psychiatry itself.

The seminal figure in this body of work has been Arthur Kleinman (1977, 1980, 1986, 1988, 1995), who, through his incisive writing, vision and leadership, has stimulated a whole generation of scholars. The 'new cross-cultural psychiatry' introduced by Kleinman (1977) argued for a renewed emphasis on ethnographic research. Rather than assuming the universality of psychiatric categories and psychological modes of expressing distress, Kleinman insisted on paying close attention to the social and cultural context of suffering and healing. This approach could be applied equally well across cultures and within the institutional and community settings of Western psychiatry.

Kleinman introduced the notion of the category fallacy, the erroneous assumption that conceptual categories that work well in one cultural context will have the same meaning and utility in another. In cultural psychiatry this is most obvious in questions about the meaning of psychiatric diagnostic categories. A further epistemological complexity arises from what the philosopher Ian Hacking (1999) has called 'the looping effect of human kinds' – that is, the tendency for the ways we categorize the world to become reified and institutionalized as cognitive and social facts.

The importance of these ideas for cultural psychiatry can be seen in the history of the emergence of diagnostic categories like post-traumatic stress disorder (Young, 1995) and dissociative disorders like multiple personality or fugue (Hacking, 1995,

1998). Psychiatric knowledge and practice reflect and reshape folk psychologies (Gaines, 1992; Littlewood, 2002; Nuckolls, 1992). For example, the reception and evolution of psychoanalysis and other forms of psychotherapy in different countries provides a window onto cultural concepts of the person (Cushman, 1995; Ellenberger, 1970; Rose, 1996; Shamdasani, 2003; Zaretsky, 2004). The broad shift away from psychoanalysis and toward biological accounts in the US in the 1980s reflects tensions within the discipline of psychiatry as well as larger political and economic forces (Luhrmann, 2000). Psychopharmacology has played a crucial role in the development of psychiatry, driving diagnostic nosology and clinical practice (Healy, 2002). A growing body of research shows the role of the pharmaceutical industry in controlling the production of clinical 'evidence', establishing clinical guidelines, and influencing popular conceptions of mental illness, which now extends to marketing new disorders (Lakoff, 2005; Metzl, 2003; Petryna *et al.*, 2006; Cosgrove and Wheeler, 2013).

Psychiatric theory and practice are embedded in larger social and cultural systems. Understanding the impact of these systems on patients' lives and psychiatric practice demands critical and social science perspectives. A growing body of work in critical neuroscience examines the social origins and implications of the increasing reliance on neurobiology in psychiatry (Choudhury and Slaby, 2011; Rose and Abi-Rached, 2013). Of course, the attempt to apply social science perspectives to analysing psychiatric practice raises the problem of self-reflexivity, since social science theory itself is a product of the society it seeks to critique. Indeed, the notion of culture is also a cultural construction that changes with new configurations of society and geopolitical concerns.

The Contribution of Psychological Anthropology

Cultural psychiatry derived some of its early theoretical models from the various schools and approaches of psychological anthropology that link individual personality with broader social processes, particularly culturally shaped child-rearing practices (Bock, 1999; Spindler, 1978). Franz Boas (1858–1942), often called the father of American anthropology, argued that culture could affect personality and behaviour by amplifying or suppressing certain traits, thus creating conflicts for different individuals. In the 1930s, 'culture and personality' researchers (notably Ruth Benedict and Margaret Mead) attempted to relate social structure, child-rearing and other cultural lifeways to modal national characters and specific patterns of psychopathology within groups (Spindler, 1978; Stocking, 1986). They used mainly ethnographic observations and borrowed psychodynamic theory or learning theory to explain the links between individual and culture.

For Benedict, Mead and later contributors to the field of culture and personality, psychopathology could be understood in part as an exaggeration of cultural traits or as a mismatch between individual personality and overarching cultural norms and values. This tradition enjoyed a period of prominence during and after World War II when studies of 'nations at a distance', based on interviews with small numbers of emigrés and analysis of media, were used as a form of military intelligence (e.g. Benedict, 1934).

Benedict (1934) saw culture as personality writ large. Anthropologist Edward Sapir rejected this view, arguing that culture had no reality beyond the actions and representations of individuals, each of whom responds differently to social exigencies. Sapir was a close colleague of psychiatrist Harry Stack Sullivan and looked to psychiatry to provide a way of understanding culture through the vicissitudes of individual biographies (Sapir, 1938; Kirmayer, 2001). This approach led to more theoretically sophisticated accounts of the interplay of culture, social structure and character, notably in the work of A. I. Hallowell (1955), but the field of culture and personality waned in the late 1950s owing to the failure to develop more rigorous methodology and a tendency to caricature whole societies with broad strokes (Levine, 2001).

A parallel tradition in psychological anthropology has used clinical psychoanalytic methods and perspectives to study individuals cross-culturally (Devereux, 1961, 1979; Kardiner and Linton, 1939; Delille, 2016). In these various forms of 'ethnopsychoanalysis', the emphasis has been on examining the universality of psychodynamics and considering the ways in which these psychological mechanisms might resolve dynamic tensions created by particular social systems. In-depth interviews, prolonged relationships with subjects and attention to 'clinical material' including psychopathological symptoms, dreams, fantasies and 'transference' distortions, all contributed to the effort to characterize the psychic interior cross-culturally. A nuanced attempt to integrate cultural identity and psychoanalytic ideas was developed in the work of the Department of Psychiatry at the Fann Hospital of the University of Dakar in Senegal in the 1960s. Under the direction of Dr Henri Collomb (who remained chief until 1978), a group of clinicians and researchers undertook careful empirical studies on the interface of Senegalese culture and Western psychiatry (Bullard, 2005; Collignon, 1978). There is a rich literature based on clinical experiences with psychoanalytic theory and methods that offers insights into the cultural logic of diverse traditions, increasingly conducted by clinicians who can integrate psychodynamic perspectives with their own intimate cultural knowledge (e.g. Crapanzano, 1973; Doi, 1973; Kakar, 1978; Levy, 1978; Obeyesekere, 1981, 1991).

In contrast to the case study approach of ethnopsychoanalysis, the field of cross-cultural psychology has employed quantitative statistical methods to compare personality and psychopathology in different cultural or national groups. Despite its origins in German social psychology (Hogan and Tartaglini, 1994; Jahoda, 1993), cross-cultural psychology has been dominated methodologically by Anglo-American empiricism and conceptually by an individualistic cultural concept of the person (Kim and Berry, 1993; Marsella et al., 1985). This cultural concept is taken over from American folk psychology and supports a large body of research that is generally presented as universal truths about the human psyche. The recent movement for indigenous psychologies attempts to reformulate basic models of personality from alternative perspectives, emphasizing, for example, the centrality of relationships with others in the dynamics of the self (Ho et al., 2001).

Another strand in the development of psychological anthropology relevant to cultural psychiatry has its roots in the early ethnographic work of W. H. R. Rivers (1864–1922), who emphasized the rationality and potential efficacy of healing practices in the Melanesian and other societies he studied (Rivers, 1924). As a leading figure in both anthropology and psychiatry, Rivers used a variety of models to understand psychopathology and healing, but was most invested in psychological explanations that could be connected to an evolutionary biology (Young, 1993; 1999). Gregory Bateson (1904–1980) followed the direction of Rivers' work, incorporating psychological notions from Benedict and Mead, but approaching mind with biological metaphors (Bateson, 1972). Bateson challenged the static view of culture in early British social anthropology by developing a 'cybernetic' approach to culture as a dynamical system (Stagoll, 2005; Wardle, 1999). In the 1950s and 1960s, Bateson's ideas about communication, interaction and the 'ecology of mind' had tremendous influence on the emerging field of family therapy.

Psychological anthropology has had a renaissance in recent decades with an increasingly eclectic range of theories brought to bear on understanding personality, identity, and psychopathology (Good, 1992). Most recently, contemporary versions of cognitive, social and developmental psychology, and social neuroscience have provided models for the interplay of culture and psychology (Casey and Edgerton, 2005; Hinton, 1999; Shore, 1996; Shweder, 1991; Sperber, 1996; Stigler et al., 1990; Strauss and Quinn, 1997). This work is concerned with understanding culture in terms of discourse, interpersonal interaction and socially distributed knowledge, and makes links with cognitive science and discursive psychology (Kirmayer, 2006; Kirmayer and Ramstead, 2017).

A Fourth Wave? Cultural Psychiatry in the Anthropocene

Recent events suggest we are on the cusp of a fourth wave in the history of cultural psychiatry. In part, this reflects the changing meanings of culture brought on by globalization and the pervasive impact of the Internet and social media. Information and telecommunication media made new forms of community possible by linking distant individuals in real time. This can give rise to new forms of pathology (like 'Internet addiction'), forms of social support and networks that may help or exacerbate particular mental health problems as well as pointing toward new strategies for prevention and intervention (Kirmayer et al., 2013).

Globalization has reduced some economic inequalities but amplified others – and we now face a world in which inequalities within and between countries are likely to accelerate (Milanovic, 2016). Recognition of the enormous disparities in mental health across the globe has given new impetus to efforts to make mental health a higher priority in global development, as advocated by the Movement for Global Mental Health (Patel, 2014). Efforts to provide mental health services for the majority of the world population acknowledges the importance of cultural and contextual adaptation but usually assume that current diagnostic and treatment methods of psychiatry are adequate to the task. The history of cultural psychiatry provides some reasons for caution and urges on us a more serious engagement with diversity and with the power structures that privilege the interests of wealthy countries and corporations (Kirmayer and Pedersen, 2014).

Finally, theories of globalization have emphasized the role of economic systems but a broader perspective would approach health in terms of our planetary ecosystems (Whitmee et al., 2015). Geologists have proposed that we have entered the Anthropocene, a new epoch characterized by the human reshaping of our planet on a large scale (Davies, 2016). In the years to come, urbanization, climate change, and forced migration will challenge our concepts of culture, community and mental health in ways that will demand rethinking the concepts of cultural psychiatry (Kirmayer et al., 2015).

Conclusion: a World in Flux

As an organized field within the larger discipline, cultural psychiatry has a relatively short institutional history. A section of transcultural psychiatry was established in 1955 at McGill University by Eric Wittkower and Jacob Fried (1959). At the Second International Psychiatric Congress in Zurich in 1957, Wittkower organized a meeting attended by psychiatrists from 20 countries, including many who became major contributors to the field: Tsung-Yi Lin (Taiwan), Thomas A. Lambo (Nigeria), Morris Carstairs (Britain), Carlos Alberto Seguin (Peru) and Pow-Meng Yap (Hong Kong) (Prince, 2000). The American Psychiatric Association established a Committee on Transcultural Psychiatry in 1964, as did the Canadian Psychiatric Association in 1967. H. B. M. Murphy of McGill founded the World Psychiatric Association Section on Transcultural Psychiatry in 1970. By the mid 1970s transcultural psychiatry societies were set up in England, France, Italy and Cuba (Cox, 1986). The World Association for Cultural Psychiatry was founded in 2005. The major journals in the field, Transcultural Psychiatry (formerly Transcultural Psychiatric Research Review), Psychopathologie Africaine, Culture Medicine and Psychiatry and Curare, began in 1956, 1965, 1977 and 1978, respectively.

Over the last 60 years, the discipline has grown from a marginal field, concerned mainly with folklore, exotica and the distant cultural 'other', to a dynamic research and clinical enterprise of crucial importance in the light of increasing migration, globalization, cultural intermixing and new insights from social and cultural neuroscience (Seligman *et al.*, 2015). Over this same period of time, both the meanings of culture and the dominant theory and modes of practice of psychiatry have changed substantially in ways that have reshaped the field of cultural psychiatry.

Despite this progress, there is a persistent legacy of colonialism in contemporary cultural psychiatry that can be seen in the continuing romance with exoticism, the de-contextualized view of mental health problems and focus on culture-bound syndromes, efforts to reify and essentialize culture as individual traits, and the tendency to employ developmental hierarchies contrasting traditional and modern societies. The corrective to these biases requires thinking about culture as a dynamic process of creativity and contestation among individuals participating in different ways of life, with issues of power and agency always at stake.

Wittkower adopted the term 'transcultural' to imply moving through and beyond cultural barriers (Wittkower and Rin, 1965). Others have preferred to call the field 'cultural psychiatry' to indicate that all human experience is culturally constituted and that we can examine cultural meanings in a single society as well as comparatively (Prince, 1997). In the context of globalization, 'transcultural' takes on new meaning based on the recognition that cultures are always mixed or creolized, giving rise to new forms (Glissant, 1997; Kraidy, 2005). Many urban settings now present a sort of 'hyperdiversity' in which many different groups co-exist and hybrid forms of identity abound. Transcultural psychiatry must explore the significance for mental health and illness of various forms of cultural hybridity at both social and individual levels (Bibeau, 1997).

Among the central questions for contemporary cultural psychiatry are the nature of the interaction of psychopathological processes and cultural idioms of distress in the genesis and course of disorders; the specific mechanisms of action of socio-cultural factors on the course of schizophrenia and other disorders; the range of cross-cultural applicability of psycho-pharmacological, psychotherapeutic and psychosocial interventions – both those derived from biomedicine and those of indigenous origin; and the impact of emerging practice models and healthcare systems that aim to provide culturally sensitive or responsive care across cultures and within culturally diverse settings. To do this, cultural psychiatry must consider how local clinical and research practices reproduce larger gender, class and other social differences of the dominant society.

In addition to these enduring concerns, new issues are emerging. Psychiatry has been enjoined to play a role in conflict resolution and rebuilding communities torn apart by ethnic violence (Kirmayer, 2010). Cultural psychiatry itself has been co-opted by pharmaceutical companies seeking strategies to open up new markets for their products (Kirmayer, 2006). Clinical trials for new drugs are now taking place in the developing economies of Eastern Europe and South Asia, raising important questions about the role of culture in psychopharmacology. At the same time, the changing configurations of the world system – through migration, ethnic nationalism, ethnogenesis, globalization, telecommunications and the growing web of the Internet with its communities and identities forged in cyberspace – require us to rethink the nature of culture. These social changes directly impact on health and raise fundamental questions, not only of a scientific nature but also with an ethical or sociomoral dimension that concerns the value of diversity versus integration, of sameness and difference, and the implications for mental health and illness of cultural pluralism and the dramatically enlarged scale of community and malleability of identity made possible by new technologies. The creative potential of cultural pluralism will be an essential resource in the years to come as we face the challenges of the growth of political extremism and the crisis of climate change.

Acknowledgements

Preparation of this chapter was supported by a Senior Investigator Award from the Canadian Institutes of Health Research (MSS-55123). An earlier version was presented at the Annual Meeting of the Society for the Study of Psychiatry and Culture, Asilomar, CA, 7 October, 1994. I thank Elizabeth Anthony and Eric Jarvis for their helpful comments. Address correspondence to the author at: Institute of Community and Family Psychiatry, Sir Mortimer B. Davis – Jewish General Hospital, 4333 Côte Ste-Catherine Road, Montréal, Québec H3 T 1E4.

References

Alarcon, R. (2001). Hispanic psychiatry: from margin to mainstream. *Transcultural Psychiatry*, **38**(1), 5–25.

American Psychiatric Association (2013). *Diagnostic and Statistical Manual of Mental Disorders (DSM-5®)*. Washington, DC: American Psychiatric Pub.

Andrade, L., Caraveo-Anduaga, J. J., Berglund, P. *et al.* (2003). The epidemiology of major depressive episodes: results from the International Consortium of Psychiatric Epidemiology (ICPE) Surveys. *International Journal of Methods in Psychiatric Research*, **12**(1), 3–21.

Bäärnhielm, S., Ekblad, S., Ekberg, J. and Ginsburg, B. E. (2005). Historical reflections on mental health care in Sweden: the welfare state and cultural diversity. *Transcultural Psychiatry*, **42**(3), 394–419.

Banks, M. (1996). *Ethnicity: Anthropological Constructions*. London: Routledge.

Bateson, G. (1972). *Steps to an Ecology of Mind*. New York: Ballantine Books.

Beard, G. (1869). Neurasthenia, or nervous exhaustion. *Boston Medical and Surgical Journal*, **3**(13), 217–221.

Beeman, W. O. (1985). Dimensions of dysphoria: the view from linguistic anthropology. In *Culture and Depression* ed. A. M. Kleinman and B. Good. Berkeley: University of California Press, pp. 216–243.

Begue, J. M. (1996). French psychiatry in Algeria (1830–1962): from colonial to transcultural. *History of Psychiatry*, 7(28 pt 4), 533–548.

Benedict, R. (1934). *Patterns of Culture*. Boston: Houghton Mifflin.

Beneduce, R. and Martelli, P. (2005). Politics of healing and politics of culture: ethnopsychiatry, identities and migration. *Transcultural Psychiatry*, **42**(3), 367–393.

Bergin, T. G. and Fisch, M. H. (1984). *The New Science of Giambattista Vico*, 3rd edn. Ithaca: Cornell University Press.

Bettiza, G. (2014). Civilizational analysis in international relations: mapping the field and advancing a 'civilizational politics' line of research. *International Studies Review*, **16**(1), 1–28.

Bhabha, H. K. (1994). *The Location of Culture*. London, New York: Routledge.

Bhugra, D. and Littlewood, R. (eds) (2001). *Colonialism and Psychiatry*. New Delhi: Oxford University Press.

Bibeau, G. (1997). Cultural psychiatry in a creolizing world: questions for a new research agenda. *Transcultural Psychiatry*, **34**(1), 9–41.

Bock, P. K. (1999). *Rethinking Psychological Anthropology: Continuity and Change in the Study of Human Action*, 2nd edn. Prospect Heights, IL: Waveland Press.

Boyers, R. (1974). *R. D. Laing and Anti-psychiatry*. New York: Octagon Books.

Brill, A. A. (1913). Piblokto or hysteria among Peary's Eskimos. *Journal of Nervous and Mental Disease*, **40**, 514–520.

Bullard, A. (2005). *L'Oedipe Africain*: a retrospective. *Transcultural Psychiatry*, **42**(2), 171–203.

Carothers, J. C. (1953). *The African Mind in Health and Disease: A Study in Ethnopsychiatry*. Geneva: World Health Organization.

Casey, C. C. and Edgerton, R. B. (2005). *A Companion to Psychological Anthropology: Modernity and Psycho-cultural Change*. Malden, MA: Blackwell Publishing.

Castles, S., de Haas, H. and Miller, M. J. (2013). *The Age of Migration: International Population Movements in the Modern World*, 5th edn. New York: Guilford.

Chakrabarty, D. (2000). *Provincializing Europe: Postcolonial Thought and Historical Difference*. Princeton, NJ: Princeton University Press.

Choudhury, S., and Slaby, J. (eds)(2011). *Critical Neuroscience: A Handbook of the Social and Cultural Contexts of Neuroscience*. New York: John Wiley and Sons.

Cohen, A. (1999). *The Mental Health of Indigenous Peoples: An International Overview*. Geneva: World Health Organization.

Collignon, R. (1978). Vingt ans de travaux à la clinique psychiatrique de Fann-Dakar. *Psychopathologie Africaine*, **XXIII**(2–3), 133–323.

Cooper, J. E., Kendell, R. E., Gurland, B. J., Sharpe, L., Copeland, J. R. M. and Simon, R. (1972). *Psychiatric Diagnosis in New York and London*. London: Oxford University Press.

Cosgrove, L. and Wheeler, E. E. (2013). Drug firms, the codification of diagnostic categories, and bias in clinical guidelines. *The Journal of Law, Medicine and Ethics*, **41**(3), 644–653.

Cox, J. L. (ed.) (1986). *Transcultural Psychiatry*. London: Croon Helm.

Crapanzano, V. (1973). *The Hamadsha: A Study in Moroccan Ethnopsychiatry*. Berkeley: University of California Press.

Cushman, P. (1995). *Constructing the Self, Constructing America: A Cultural History of Psychotherapy*. Boston, MA: Addison-Wesley Publishing.

Davies, J. (2016). *The Birth of the Anthropocene*. Berkeley, CA: Univerity of California Press.

Delille, E. (2016). On the history of cultural psychiatry: Georges Devereux, Henri Ellenberger, and the psychological treatment of Native Americans in the 1950s. *Transcultural Psychiatry*, **53**(3), 392–411.

Devereux, G. (1961). *Mohave Ethnopsychiatry and Suicide: The Psychiatric Knowledge and the Psychic Disturbances of an Indian Tribe*. Washington, DC: US Government Printing Office.

Devereux, G. (1979). *Basic Problems of Ethnopsychiatry*. Chicago: University of Chicago Press.

Dick, L. (1995). 'Pibloktoq' (Arctic hysteria): a construction of European–Inuit relations. *Arctic Anthropology*, **32**(2), 1–42.

Dick, L. (2002). Aboriginal–European relations during the great age of North Polar exploration. *Polar Geography*, **26**(1), 66–86.

Doi, T. (1973). *The Anatomy of Dependence*. Tokyo: Kodansha International.

Du Bois, W. E. B. (1989). *The Souls of Black Folk*. New York: Penguin Books.

Eagleton, T. (2000). *The Idea of Culture*. Oxford: Blackwell.

Elias, N. (1982). *The Civilizing Process*. Oxford: B. Blackwell.

Ellenberger, H. F. (1970). *The Discovery of the Unconscious: the History and Evolution of Dynamic Psychiatry*. New York: Basic Books.

Ellingson, T. (2001). *The Myth of the Noble Savage*. Berkeley: University of California Press.

Ernst, W., and Mueller, T. (eds) (2010). *Transnational Psychiatries: Social and Cultural Histories of Psychiatry in Comparative Perspective c. 1800–2000*. Newcastle upon Tyne, UK: Cambridge Scholars Publishing.

Fanon, F. (1982). *Black Skin, White Masks*. New York: Grove Press. (Originally published in French in 1952.)

Fassin, D. and Rechtman, R. (2005). An anthropological hybrid: the pragmatic arrangement of universalism and culturalism in French mental health. *Transcultural Psychiatry*, **42**(3), 347–366.

Fernando, S. (1988). *Race and Culture in Psychiatry*. London: Tavistock/Routledge.

Fernando, S. (2003). *Cultural Diversity, Mental Health and Psychiatry: the Struggle Against Racism*. New York: Brunner/Routledge.

Fernando, S. (2005). Multicultural mental health services: projects for minority ethnic communities in England. *Transcultural Psychiatry*, **42**(3), 420–436.

Foucault, M. (1965). *Madness and Civilization: A History of Insanity in the Age of Reason*. New York: Pantheon Books.

Foulks, E. F. (1974). *The Arctic Hysterias*. Seattle: University of Washington Press.

Frank, J. D. (1961). *Persuasion and Healing: A Comparative Study of Psychotherapy*. Baltimore: Johns Hopkins University Press.

Fredrickson, G. M. (2002). *Racism: A Short History*. Princeton, NJ: Princeton University Press.

Freud, S. (1962). *Civilization and its Discontents*, trans. and ed. J. Strachey. New York: W. W. Norton.

Gaines, A. (1992). *Ethnopsychiatry: The Cultural Construction of Professional and Folk Psychiatries*. Albany: State University of New York Press.

Gellner, E. (1988). *Plough, Sword and Book: The Structure of Human History*. Chicago: University of Chicago Press.

Gilman, S. L. (1985). *Difference and Pathology: Stereotypes, Race and Madness*. Ithaca: Comell University.

Gilroy, P. (2005). *Postcolonial Melancholia*. New York: Columbia University Press.

Glissant, E. (1997). *Poetics of Relation*, trans. B. Wing. Ann Arbor: University of Michigan Press.

Good, B. J. (1992). Culture and psychopathology: directions for psychiatric anthropology. In *The Social Life of the Self: New Directions in Psychological Anthropology*, ed. T. Schwartz, G. M. White and C. A. Lutz. Cambridge: Cambridge University Press, pp. 181–205.

Good, B. J. (1994). *Medicine, Rationality, and Experience: An Anthropological Perspective*. Cambridge: Cambridge University Press.

Gordon, L. R. (2015). *What Fanon Said: A Philosophical Introduction to his Life and Thought*. New York, NY: Fordham University Press.

Gunew, S. M. (2003). *Haunted Nations: The Colonial Dimensions of Multiculturalisms*. New York: Routledge.

Gussow, Z. (1960). Pibloktoq (hysteria) among the polar Eskimo. *The Psychoanalytic Study of Society*, **1**, 218–236.

Hacking, I. (1995). *Rewriting the Soul*. Princeton: Princeton University Press.

Hacking, I. (1998). *Mad Travelers: Reflections on the Reality of Transient Mental Ilnesses*. Charlottesville: University Press of Virginia.

Hacking, I. (1999). *The Social Construction of What*. Cambridge, MA: Harvard University Press.

Hallowell, A. I. (1955). *Culture and Experience*. Philadelphia: University of Pennsylvania Press.

Hannerz, U. (1992). *Cultural Complexity: Studies in the Social Organization of Meaning*. New York: Columbia University Press.

Hannerz, U. (1996). *Transnational Connections: Culture, People, Places*. New York: Routledge.

Healy, D. (2002). *The Creation of Psychopharmacology*. Cambridge, MA: Harvard University Press.

Heaton, M. M. (2013). *Black Skin, White Coats: Nigerian Psychiatrists, Decolonization, and the Globalization of Psychiatry*. Athens, OH: Ohio University Press.

Hicks, M. (2002). Validity of the CIDI probe flow chart for depression in Chinese-American women. *Transcultural Psychiatry*, **39**, 434–451.

Hinton, A. L. (1999). *Biocultural Approaches to the Emotions*. Cambridge: Cambridge University Press.

Ho, D. Y., Peng, S., Lai, A. C. and Chan, S. F. (2001). Indigenization and beyond: methodological relationalism in the study of personality across cultural traditions. *Journal of Personality*, **69**(6), 925–953.

Hobsbawm, E. J. and Ranger, T. (eds)(1983). *The Invention of Tradition*. Cambridge: Cambridge University Press.

Hogan, J. D. and Tartaglini, A. (1994). A brief history of cross-cultural psychology. In *Cross-Cultural Topics in Psychology*, ed. L. L. Adler and U. P. Gielen. Westport, CT: Praeger, pp. 15–23.

Hollinger, D. A. (1995). *Postethnic America: Beyond Multiculturalism*. New York: Basic Books.

Holt, T. C. (2000). *The Problem of Race in the Twenty-First Century*. Cambridge, MA: Harvard University Press.

Huntington, S. P. (1996). *The Clash of Civilizations and the Remaking of World Order*. New York: Simon and Schuster.

Hutchinson, G. and Haasen, C. (2004). Migration and schizophrenia: the challenges for European psychiatry and implications for the future. *Social Psychiatry and Psychiatric Epidemiology*, **39**(5), 350–357.

Jahoda, G. (1993). *Crossroads between Culture and Mind*. Cambridge, MA: Harvard University Press.

Jahoda, G. (1999). *Images of Savages: Ancient Roots of Modern Prejudice in Western Culture*. London: Routledge.

Jilek, W. G. (1995). Emil Kraepelin and comparative socio-cultural psychiatry. *European Archives for Psychiatry and Clinical Neurosciences*, **245**, 231–238.

Kakar, S. (1978). *The Inner World: A Psycho-analytic Study of Childhood and Society in India*. Delhi: Oxford University Press.

Kardiner, A. and Linton, R. (1939). *The Individual and his Society: The Psychodynamics of Primitive Social Organization*. New York: Columbia University Press.

Keller, R. C. (2001). Madness and colonialism: psychiatry in the British and French empires, 1800–1962. *Journal of Social History*, **35**, 295–326.

Keller, R. C. (2005). Pinel in the Maghreb: liberation, confinement, and psychiatric reform in French North Africa. *Bulletin of the History of Medicine*, **79**(3), 459–499.

Kelly, B. D. (2005). Structural violence and schizophrenia. *Social Science and Medicine*, **61**(3), 721–730.

Kiev, A. (ed.) (1969). *Magic, Faith and Healing*. New York: Free Press.

Kim, V. and Berry, J. W. (eds) (1993). *Indigenous Psychologies: Research and Experience in Cultural Context*. Newbury Park: Sage Publications.

Kirmayer, L. J. (2001). Sapir's vision of culture and personality. *Psychiatry*, **64**(1), 23–30.

Kirmayer, L. J. (2006). Beyond the 'new cross-cultural psychiatry': cultural biology, discursive psychology, and the ironies of globalization. *Transcultural Psychiatry*, **43**(1), 126–144.

Kirmayer, L. (2010). Peace, conflict, and reconciliation: contributions of cultural psychiatry. *Transcultural Psychiatry*, **47**(1), 5.

Kirmayer, L. J. and Minas, H. (2000). The future of cultural psychiatry: an international perspective. *Canadian Journal of Psychiatry*, **45**(5), 438–446.

Kirmayer, L. J. and Pedersen, D. (2014). Toward a new architecture for global mental health. *Transcultural Psychiatry*, **51**(6), 759–776.

Kirmayer, L. J. and Ramstead, M. J. D. (2017). Embodiment and enactment in cultural psychiatry. In *Embodiment, Enactment and Culture: Investigating the Constitution of the Shared World*, ed. C. Durt, T. Fuchs and C. Tewes. Cambridge, MA: MIT Press, pp. 397–422.

Kirmayer, L. J., Simpson, C. and Cargo, M. (2003). Healing traditions: culture, community and mental health promotion with Canadian Aboriginal peoples. *Australasian Psychiatry*, **11**, S15–S23.

Kirmayer, L. J., Raikhel, E. and Rahimi, S. (2013). Cultures of the Internet: identity, community and mental health. *Transcultural Psychiatry*, **50**(2), 165–191.

Kirmayer, L. J., Lemelson, R. and Cummings, C. (eds) (2015). *Re-visioning Psychiatry: Cultural Phenomenology, Critical Neuroscience and Global Mental Health*, Cambridge: Cambridge University Press.

Kivisto, P. (2002). *Multiculturalism in a Global Society*. Oxford: Blackwell.

Kleinman, A. M. (1977). Depression, somatization and the 'new cross-cultural psychiatry'. *Social Science and Medicine*, **11**, 3–10.

Kleinman, A. M. (1980). *Patients and Healers in the Context of Culture*. Berkeley: University of California Press.

Kleinman, A. (1986). *Social Origins of Distress and Disease*. New Haven: Yale University Press.

Kleinman, A. (1988). *Rethinking Psychiatry*. New York: Free Press.

Kleinman, A. (1995). *Writing at the Margin: Discourse between Anthropology and Medicine*. Berkeley: University of California Press.

Kraepelin, E. (1904). Vergeichende psychiatrie. *Zentralblatt fur Nervenherlkande und Psychiatrie*, **15**, 433–437.

Kraidy, M. (2005). *Hybridity, or the Cultural Logic of Globalization*. Philadelphia: Temple University Press.

Kua, E. H. (1991). *Amok* in nineteenth-century British Malaya history. *History of Psychiatry*, **3**, 429–436.

Kuper, A. (1999). *Culture: The Anthropologists' Account*. Cambridge, MA: Harvard University Press.

Lakoff, A. (2005). *Pharmaceutical Reason: Knowledge and Value in Global Psychiatry*. Cambridge: Cambridge University Press.

Landy, D. (1985). Pibloktoq (hysteria) and Inuit nutrition: possible implication of hypervitaminosis A. *Social Science and Medicine*, **21**(2), 173–186.

Lane, C. (2002). Psychoanalysis and colonialism redux: why Mannoni's 'Prospero complex' still haunts us. *Journal of Modern Literature*, **25**(3/4), 127–150.

Lazarus, N. (2011). *The Postcolonial Unconscious*. Cambridge: Cambridge University Press.

Leighton, A. H. (1981). Culture and psychiatry. *Canadian Journal of Psychiatry*, **26**, 522–530.

Leff, J. (1981). *Psychiatry around the Globe: A Transcultural View*. London: Gaskell.

Leff, J., Sartorius, N., Jablensky, A., Korten, A. and Ernberg, G. (1992). The International Pilot Study of Schizophrenia: five-year follow-up findings. *Psychological Medicine*, **22**, 131–145.

Levine, R. A. (2001). Culture and personality studies, 1918–1960: myth and history. *Journal of Personality*, **69**(6), 803–818.

Levy, R. I. (1978). *Tahitians: Mind and Experience in the Society Islands*. Chicago: University of Chicago Press.

Lévy-Bruhl, L. (1923). *Primitive Mentality*. London: George Allen and Unwin.

Lewis-Fernández, R., Aggarwal, N. K., Hinton, L., Hinton, D. E. and Kirmayer, L. J. (eds) (2015). *DSM-5 Handbook on the Cultural Formulation Interview*. Washington, DC: American Psychiatric Press.

Littlewood, R. (1993). Ideology, camouflage or contingency: racism in British psychiatry. *Transcultural Psychiatric Research Review*, **30**(3), 243–291.

Littlewood, R. (2002). *Pathologies of the West: An Anthropology of Mental Illness in Europe and America*. Ithaca: Cornell University Press.

Littlewood, R. and Lipsedge, M. (1982). *Aliens and Alienists*. New York: Penguin.

Lock, M. (1993). The concept of race: an ideological concept. *Transcultural Psychiatric Research Review*, **30**(3), 203–227.

Lock, M. and Gordon, D. (eds) (1988). *Biomedicine Examined*. Dordrecht: Kluwer.

Lucas, R. H. and Barrett, R. J. (1995). Interpreting culture and psychopathology: primitivist themes in cross-cultural debate. *Culture, Medicine and Psychiatry*, **19**(3), 287–326.

Luhrmann, T. M. (2000). *Of Two Minds: The Growing Disorder in American Psychiatry*. New York: Knopf.

Macey, D. (1996). Frantz Fanon 1925–1961. *History of Psychiatry*, 7(28 pt 4), 489–497.

Mannoni, D. O. (1990). *Prospero and Caliban: The Psychology of Colonization*. New York: Praeger. (Originally published in French in 1948.)

Marano, L. (1983). On Windigo psychosis. *Current Anthropology*, **24**(1), 121–125.

Marsella, A. J. and White, G. M. (eds) (1982). *Cultural Conceptions of Mental Health and Therapy*, vol. **4**. Dordrecht, Holland: D. Reidel Publishing Company.

Marsella, A. J., DeVos, G. and Hsu, F. L. K. (eds) (1985). *Culture and Self: Asian and Western Perspectives*. New York: Tavistock.

McCulloch, J. (1993). The empire's new clothes: ethnopsychiatry in colonial Africa. *History of the Human Sciences*, **6**(2), 35–52.

McCulloch, J. (1995). *Colonial Psychiatry and 'the African Mind'*. Cambridge: Cambridge University Press.

Metzl, J. (2003). *Prozac on the Couch: Prescribing Gender in the Era of Wonder Drugs*. Durham: Duke University Press.

Mezzich, J., Kleinman, A., Fabrega, H., Jr and Parron, D. (eds) (1996). *Culture and Psychiatric Diagnosis*. Washington, DC: American Psychiatric Press.

Micale, M. S. and Porter, R. (1994). *Discovering the History of Psychiatry*. New York: Oxford University Press.

Milanovic, B. (2016). *Global Inequality: A New Approach for the Age of Globalization*. Cambridge, MA: Harvard University Press.

Murphy, H. B. M. (ed.) (1955). *Flight and Resettlement*. Paris: UNESCO.

Murphy, H. B. M. (1982). *Comparative Psychiatry: The International and Intercultural Distribution of Mental Illness*. New York: Springer-Verlag.

Murphy, J. M. (1976). Psychiatric labeling in cross-cultural perspective. *Science*, **191**, 1019–1028.

Murphy, J. M. and Leighton, A. H. (eds) (1965). *Approaches to Cross-Cultural Psychiatry*. Ithaca: Cornell University Press.

Nuckolls, C. W. (1992). Toward a cultural history of the personality disorders. *Social Science and Medicine*, **35**(1), 37–47.

Obeyesekere, G. (1981). *Medusa's Hair: An Essay on Personal Symbols and Religious Experience*. Chicago: University of Chicago Press.

Obeyesekere, G. (1991). *The Work of Culture: Symbolic Transformation in Psychoanalysis and Anthropology*. Chicago: University of Chicago Press.

Papastergiadis, N. (2000). *The Turbulence of Migration*. Cambridge: Polity Press.

Petryna, A., Lakoff, A. and Kleinman, A. (eds) (2006). *Global Pharmaceuticals: Ethics, Markets, Practices*. Durham: Duke University Press.

Porot, A. (1918). Notes de psychiatrie musulmane. *Annales Médico-Psychologiques*, **4**, 225–240.

Porter, R. (1988). *A Social History of Madness: The World through the Eyes of the Insane*. New York: Weidenfeld and Nicolson.

Prince, R. (1980). Variations in psychotherapeutic procedures. In *Handbook of Cross-Cultural Psychology*, vol. **6**, ed. H. C. Triandis and J. G. Draguns. Boston: Allyn and Bacon, pp. 291–349.

Prince, R. (1997). What's in a name? *Transcultural Psychiatry*, **34**(1), 151–154.

Prince, R. H. (2000). Transcultural psychiatry: personal experiences and Canadian perspectives. *Canadian Journal of Psychiatry*, **45**(5), 431–437.

Rabinbach, A. (1990). *The Human Motor: Energy, Fatigue and the Origins of Modernity*. New York: Basic Books.

Raimundo Oda, A. M., Banzato, C. E. M. and Dalgalarrondo, P. (2005). Some origins of cross-cultural psychiatry. *History of Psychiatry*, **16**(2), 155–169.

Razanajao, C., Postel, J. and Allen, D. F. (1996). The life and psychiatric work of Frantz Fanon. *History of Psychiatry*, 7(28 pt 4), 499–524.

Rivers, W. H. R. (1924). *Medicine, Magic and Religion*. London: Kegan Paul.

Robins, L. N., Wing, J., Wittchen, H.-U. *et al.* (1989). The Composite International Diagnostic Interview: an epidemiologic instrument suitable for use in conjunction with different diagnostic systems and in different cultures. *Archives of General Psychiatry*, **45**, 1069–1077.

Roelcke, V. (1997). Biologizing social facts: an early 20th century debate on Kraepelin's concepts of culture, neurasthenia, and degeneration. *Culture, Medicine and Psychiatry*, **21**(4), 383–403.

Rose, N. (1996). *Inventing Our Selves: Psychology, Power, and Personhood*. Cambridge: Cambridge University Press.

Rose, N. S. and Abi-Rached, J. M. (2013). *Neuro: The New Brain Sciences and the Management of the Mind*. Princeton, NJ: Princeton University Press.

Rosenhan, D. L. (1973). On being sane in insane places. *Science*, **179**, 250–258.

Sadowsky, J. H. (1999). *Imperial Bedlam: Institutions of Madness in Colonial Southwest Nigeria*. Berkeley: University of California Press.

Said, E. W. (1994). *Culture and Imperialism*. New York: Vintage Books.

Sapir, E. (1938). Why cultural anthropology needs the psychiatrist. *Psychiatry*, **1**(1), 7–12.

Sartorius, N., Jablensky, A., Korten, A. *et al.* (1986). Early manifestations and first-contact incidence of schizophrenia in different cultures. A preliminary report on the initial evaluation phase of the WHO Collaborative Study on determinants of outcome of severe mental disorders. *Psychological Medicine*, **16**(4), 909–928.

Scheff, T. J. (1974). The labelling theory of mental illness. *American Sociological Review*, **39**, 444–452.

Segalen, V. (2002). *Essay on Exoticism: An Aesthetics of Diversity*, trans. Y. R. Schlick. Durham: Duke University Press.

Seligman, R., Choudhury, S. and Kirmayer, L. J. (2015). Locating culture in the brain and in the world: from social categories to the ecology of mind. In *Handbook of Cultural Neuroscience* ed. J. Y. Chiao, R. Turner, S. Li and R. Seligman. Oxford: Oxford University Press, pp. 3–20.

Shamdasani, S. (2003). *C. G. Jung and the Making of Modern Psychology: The Dream of a Science*. Cambridge: Cambridge University Press.

Shore, B. (1996). *Culture in Mind: Cognition, Culture, and the Problem of Meaning*. Oxford: Oxford University Press.

Shweder, R. (1991). *Thinking Through Culture: Expeditions in Cultural Psychology*. Cambridge, MA: Harvard University Press.

Simons, R. C. and Hughes, C. C. (eds) (1985). *The Culture-Bound Syndromes: Folk Illnesses of Psychiatric and Anthropological Interest*. Dordrecht: D. Reidel.

Smedley, B. D., Stith, A. Y. and Nelson, A. R. (2003). *Unequal Treatment: Confronting Racial and Ethnic Disparities in Health Care*. Washington, DC: National Academy Press.

Sperber, D. (1996). *Explaining Culture: A Naturalistic Approach*. Oxford: Blackwell Publishers.

Spindler, G. D. (ed.) (1978). *The Making of Psychological Anthropology*. Berkeley: University of California Press.

Stagoll, B. (2005). Gregory Bateson (1904–1980): a reappraisal. *Australia and New Zealand Journal of Psychiatry*, **39**(11–12), 1036–1045.

Stigler, J. A., Shweder, R. A. and Herdt, G. (eds) (1990). *Cultural Psychology: Essays on Comparative Human Development*. New York: Cambridge University Press.

Stocking, G. W. (1986). *Malinowski, Rivers, Benedict, and Others: Essays on Culture and Personality*. Madison, WI: University of Wisconsin Press.

Strauss, C. and Quinn, N. (1997). *A Cognitive Theory of Cultural Meaning*. Cambridge: Cambridge University Press.

Todorov, T. (1993). *On Human Diversity: Nationalism, Racism, and Exoticism in French Thought*. Cambridge, MA: Harvard University Press.

Van Ommeren, M., Sharma, B., Makaju, R., Thapa, S. and de Jong, J. (2000). Limited cultural validity of the Composite International Diagnostic Interview's probe flow chart. *Transcultural Psychiatry*, **37**(1), 119–129.

Vaughan, M. (1991). *Curing their Ills: Colonial Power and African Illness*. Stanford, CA: Stanford University Press.

Veling, W. (2013). Ethnic minority position and risk for psychotic disorders. *Current Opinion in Psychiatry*, **26**(2), 166–171.

Vergès, F. (1996). To cure and to free: the Fanonian Project of 'decolonized psychiatry'. In *Fanon: A Critical Reader*, ed. L. R. Gordon, T. D. Sharpley-Whiting and R. T. White. Oxford: Blackwell, pp. 85–99.

wa Wamwere, K. (2003). *Negative Ethnicity: From Bias to Genocide*. New York: Seven Stories Press.

Waldram, J. (2004). *Revenge of the Windigo: The Construction of the Mind and Mental Health of North American Aboriginal Peoples*. Toronto: University of Toronto Press.

Wallace, A. F. C. and Ackerman, R. E. (1960). An interdisciplinary approach to mental disorders among the polar Eskimos of northwest Greenland. *Anthropologica*, II(2), 1–12.

Wardle, H. (1999). Gregory Bateson's lost world: the anthropology of Haddon and Rivers continued and deflected. *Journal of the History of the Behavioral Sciences*, **35**(4), 379–389.

Westermeyer, J. (1989). Psychiatric epidemiology across cultures: current issues and trends. *Transcultural Psychiatric Research Review*, **26**(1), 5–25.

Whitmee, S., Haines, A., Beyrer, C. *et al.* (2015). Safeguarding human health in the Anthropocene epoch: report of the Rockefeller Foundation–Lancet Commission on planetary health. *The Lancet*, **386**(10007), 1973–2028.

Wilson, M. (1993). DSM-III and the transformation of American psychiatry: a history. *American Journal of Psychiatry*, **150**(3), 399–410.

Winzeler, R. (1990). *Amok*: historical, psychological, and cultural perspectives. In *Emotions of Culture: A Malay Perspective*, ed. W. J. Karim. New York: Oxford University Press, pp. 96–122.

Winzeler, R. L. (1995). *Latah in Southeast Asia: The History and Ethnography of a Culture-Bound Syndrome*. Cambridge: Cambridge University Press.

Wittkower, E. D. and Fried, J. (1959). A cross-cultural approach to mental health problems. *American Journal of Psychiatry*, **116**, 423–428.

Wittkower, E. D. and Rin, H. (1965). Transcultural psychiatry. *Archives of General Psychiatry*, **13**(5), 387–394.

World Health Organization (1973). *Report of the International Pilot Study of Schizophrenia*, vol. **1**. Geneva: World Health Organization.

World Health Organization (ed.) (1983). *Depressive Disorders in Different Cultures, Report on the WHO Collaborative Study on Standardized Assessment of Depressive Disorders*. Geneva: World Health Organization.

Yap, P. M. (1952). The latah reaction: its pathodynamics and nosological position. *Journal of Mental Science*, **98**(413), 515–564.

Yap, P. M. (1974). *Comparative Psychiatry: A Theoretical Framework*. Toronto: University of Toronto.

York, G. and Pindera, L. (1991). *People of the Pines*. Toronto: Little, Brown and Company (Canada) Ltd.

Young, A. (1993). W. H. R. Rivers and the anthropology of psychiatry. *Social Science and Medicine*, **36**, iii–vii.

Young, A. (1995). *Harmony of Illusions: Inventing Posttraumatic Stress Disorder*. Princeton, NJ: Princeton University Press.

Young, A. (1999). W. H. R. Rivers and the war neuroses. *Journal of the History of the Behavioral Sciences*, **35**(4), 359–378.

Zaretsky, E. (2004). *Secrets of the Soul: A Social and Cultural History of Psychoanalysis*. New York: Alfred A. Knopf.

Anthropology and Psychiatry
A Contemporary Convergence for Global Mental Health

Janis H. Jenkins

Editors' Introduction

Anthropology and psychiatry have long shared common intellectual and scientific ground. Both are interested in human beings, the societies within which they live and their behaviours. A key starting difference between the two is anthropology's interest in relativism, whereas psychiatry has been interested in universalism. Also, both anthropology and psychiatry have a long history of common interest in phenomenology and the qualitative dimensions of human experience, as well as a broader comparative and epidemiological approach. Jenkins illustrates the common ground by emphasizing that both disciplines contribute to the philosophical questions of meaning and experience raised by cultural diversity in mental illness and healing. Both disciplines also contribute to the practical problems of identifying and treating distress of patients from diverse ethnic, gender, class and religious backgrounds. Psychiatry focuses on individual biography and pathology, thereby giving it a unique relevance and transformation. Patient narratives thus become of great interest to clinicians and anthropologists. Development of specializations such as medical or clinical anthropology puts medicine in general and psychiatry in particular under a magnifying glass. Using Jungian psychology as an exemplar could lead to a clearer identification of convergence between the two disciplines. The nexus between anthropology of emotion and the study of psychopathology identified in her own work by Jenkins looks at normality and abnormality, feeling and emotion, variability of course and outcome, among others. She ends the chapter on an optimistic note, highlighting the fact that the convergence between these two disciplines remains a very fertile ground for generating ideas and issues with the potential to stimulate both disciplines.

Introduction

Contemporary emphasis on global mental health can benefit greatly by a well-informed understanding of the long-standing interface of anthropology and psychiatry. Indeed, such knowledge is a prerequisite for transnational inquiry into specific aspects of mental health as well as broader questions of human being. Nineteenth century eugenic notions of the inferiority of then-considered 'primitive' minds were scientifically critiqued and denounced by anthropologist Franz Boaz (1911), but in comparative psychiatry implicit or explicit presumptions regarding the similarity or difference in 'primitive' or 'modern' minds dates back at least as far as the early twentieth century with psychiatrist Emil Kraepelin (1904) and subsequent challenges by anthropologist–psychiatrist W. H. R. Rivers (1918). Psychiatrists since Freud have been fascinated with the experiential diversity of ethnographic data, and anthropologists such as Margaret Mead (1930, 1935), Ruth Benedict (1934) and Edward Sapir (1932, 1938), all students of Boaz, produced pioneering works which actively engaged the methods and data of psychiatry. All were concerned with the vexing problem of differentiating the normal and the abnormal, whether conceived dichotomously or on a continuum. Such collaborations led to highly productive exchanges, including that of Sapir and psychiatrist Harry Stack Sullivan (1940, 1964), whose scholarly interchange has been documented by Helen Swick Perry (1982). Psychiatric anthropologist Cora Du Bois (1944) and Georges Devereux (1980) wrote convincingly about the unreliable boundary between normal and abnormal, as did, in 1943, philosopher of medicine Georges Canguilhem (1991) and anthropologist Claude Levi-Strauss (1962). In addition to the issues surrounding the normal and the abnormal in defining forms of psychopathology, anthropologists and psychiatrists have struggled together with the question of relativity in debates surrounding the a priori presumption of the universality of core symptoms of particular types of disorder in the absence of empirical demonstration. Although the expertise of the two disciplines is distinct, both contribute to the conceptual questions and experiential questions of meaning in mental illness and healing. Likewise, both contribute to the immediate and significant problems of how best to treat the distress of patients across domains of diversity prominently to include gender, ethnicity, religion and marginalization by virtue of intolerance, discrimination, warfare and political violence. Productive work on these questions has been accomplished by the foregoing scholars not only through interdisciplinary scholarship but also by their close transnational relations; in 1942, while giving a speech at the Columbia University Faculty Club during which he attacked the Nazis, Franz Boaz died from a stroke in the arms of Levi-Strauss.

In this chapter, I outline a series of topics of common interest for psychiatry and anthropology by highlighting areas of mutual interest concerning the relation between culture and mental illness, and healing. In doing so, I also organize the material in such a way as to call attention to conceptual contrasts that transcend or lie outside the disciplinary distinctions between anthropology and psychiatry. How, for example, is it different to examine the cultural factors affecting the use of psychopharmaceuticals and those affecting the use of alcohol and social drugs? What is the consequence of adopting the different perspectives implied by the study of psychiatric treatment and services? How to conceptualize and classify psychiatric disorder in successive revisions of the *Diagnostic and Statistical Manual* (DSM) or International Classification of Diseases (ICD) nosology? How to compare indigenous ritual healing and psychotherapy, as undertaken by psychiatrist Jerome Frank (1973), the potential efficacy of distinct cultural genres of treatment? What is the difference in views of human variability that seek out the existence of culturally peculiar syndromes and those that recognize cultural variations in psychiatric disorders defined essentially by researchers and clinicians from the global north or the global south? How much in common is there among the perspectives of psychiatric anthropology, (trans)cultural psychiatry, ethnopsychiatry, and the burgeoning field of global mental health?

Delineating the Convergence

Diverse formulations both synthetic and programmatic have defined the convergence between anthropology and psychiatry since the early essay by Kraepelin on 'Comparative Psychiatry' in 1904. A useful collection of seminal works from 1880 to 1971 edited by Littlewood and Dein (2000) traces a repertoire of interests ranging across definitions of the normal and the abnormal, family structure, cultural symbolism, suicide, anxiety, intoxicants and controversially conceived 'culture-bound syndromes'. Current thought among contemporary psychiatric anthropologists places less stock in the existence of such 'exotic' and 'rare' occurrences and more attention to the way in which culturally and historically defined conditions of mental illness or distress *typically* have culturally distinct features worldwide. Cultural psychiatrists and psychiatric anthropologists share common interest in epidemiological variation of disorders across populations, potential aetiological variation in relation to cultural, biogenetic and structural-institutional features, and the cultural puzzle of significant variations in the course and outcome of disorders transnationally.

Raimundo *et al.* (2005) have traced the convergence of psychiatry and anthropology to the historical precursors of cross-cultural psychiatry from nineteenth century alienists who proposed evolutionary notions of insanity as supposedly rare among 'primitive' peoples and increased with 'civilization' that were imagined to require increasing levels of cognitive organization and demands for mental production. While the colonial legacy of racist thinking seemed 'apparent' during that historical epoch, it is worth noting that the notion of 'non-Western' (non-European) populations as being relatively less 'sophisticated' has not entirely disappeared in contemporary discourse. Developments in transcultural psychiatry following World War II served to delineate a specific identity of transcultural psychiatry as a field concerned with replacing racist evolutionary frameworks with cross-cultural empirical data. At the same time, existential and meaning-centred approaches began to appear. A powerful voice from this post-war period was Ernest Becker (1962, 1963), whose concern with meaning resonates more than five decades later. The 1970s and 1980s was a period of rapid development and reformulation, in the midst of which a 'new cross-cultural psychiatry' that emerged from a synthesis of interpretive approaches from anthropology and an increasingly sophisticated academic psychiatry (Martins, 1969; Wittkower and Wintrob, 1969; Galdston, 1971; Kiev, 1972; Kennedy, 1974; Cox, 1977; Kleinman, 1977, 1980; Miller, 1977; Padilla and Padilla, 1977; Estroff, 1978; Murphy, 1984).

Summarizing the decade of work since Kleinman's (1977) watershed definition of the revitalized inter-disciplinary field, Littlewood (1990) contrasted the new cross-cultural psychiatry's anthropological emphasis on psychiatric epistemology and clinical practice to assess the universality of psychopathology with earlier attempts in cross-cultural psychiatry to apply psychoanalytic concepts to non-European societies. Within several years Lewis-Fernandez and Kleinman (1995) hailed cross-cultural psychiatry as a mature discipline addressing the complexities of sociosomatics and clinically relevant cultural pro-cesses, while decrying the limited impact of the field with respect to cultural validation of the DSM-IV, persistent misdiagnosis of minority patients, contin-ued presence of racial bias in treatment, and inatten-tion to ethnic issues in medical ethics. This claim to maturity of the field has been reiterated by Lopez and Guarnaccia (2005) with reference to the study of cultural psychopathology as the study of culture and the definition, experience, distribution and course of psychological disorders. An important synthesis of the discipline in textbook form has been contributed by Helman (2000).

Contemporary analysis of practices in psychiatry can be shown to be entangled in what was classically formulated in anthropology several decades ago, that is, the conceptual triad of magic, science and religion (Rivers, 1924). In Malinowski's (1954: 35) terms, problems arise over how to reduce a 'complex and unwieldy bit of reality into a simple and handy form'. Applying this to the global field of mental health, we have recently seen the circulation of public-health cam-paigns that are culturally formulated under banners such as 'A Flaw in Chemistry, not Character' in the US, or 'Defeat Depression, Spread Happiness' in India, 'Silence is not Health' in Argentina, or 'Chains Free' in Indonesia (Jenkins, 2015a). As set forth by Jenkins (2010), the conceptual mélange of magic/science/reli-gion can also help to illuminate applied contemporary developments with respect to pharmaceutical practices, markets and global capitalism. Multivalent symbols of pharmaceuticals as 'magic bullets', 'awakenings', 'pla-cebo', 'gold standard' or 'God's miracle' are suffused across cultural domains of magic, religion and science. Strategic areas for investigation in anthropology and

psychiatry concern the increasingly widespread distri-bution of psychopharmacological drugs worldwide and raises the question of whether we are *all* becoming *pharmaceutical selves* (Jenkins, 2010). Specific domains of inquiry are:

> . . . how are culturally constituted selves transformed by regular ingestion of these drugs – for therapeutic, non-therapeutic, or recreational reasons; whether to allevi-ate suffering or enhance performance; whether awake or asleep? To what extent are *Homo sapiens* transform-ing themselves into pharmaceutical selves on a scale previously unknown? Does the meaning of being human increasingly come to mean not only *oriented* to drugs but also *produced* and *regulated* by them?
>
> (Jenkins, 2010: 4)

Further, 'how unequal distribution and access to these drugs reproduce social inequalities in health and sub-jective states of suffering?' (Jenkins, 2010: 4).

In sum, the mutual relevance of anthropology and psychiatry thus remains an important concern for scholars and clinicians in the field (Stix, 1996; Skultans and Cox, 2000; Mihanovic *et al.*, 2005). Even so, Skultans (1991) examines the uneasy alliance between anthropology and psychiatry historically and with respect to the way differences in orientation between the two disciplines have led to conflicting ideas about the nature of cross-cultural research, par-ticularly anthropological fieldwork. On the one hand, Kleinman (1987, 1988) has highlighted the contribu-tion of anthropology to cross-cultural psychiatry with respect to issues such as translation, the category fallacy in defining psychiatric disorder, and patho-plasticity/pathogenicity, emphasizing anthropology's attention to cultural validity in addition to reliability, and to the relevance of cultural analysis to psychiatry's own taxonomies and methods. On the other hand, Kirmayer (2001) has reprised Edward Sapir's argu-ment that psychiatry's focus on individual biography and pathology gives it a unique relevance for anthro-pology's concern with cultural transmission, suggest-ing that recent work focused on illness narratives helps to position individuals in a social world.

Expanding and Refining the Scope of this Convergence

A serious challenge concerns the gap between the established research in cultural psychiatry and psy-chiatric anthropology and the aims of the burgeoning field of global mental health (GMH) with calls to 'scale

2 Anthropology and Psychiatry

up' mental health services worldwide (Patel *et al.*, 2007, 2009; Andreoli *et al.*, 2009; Eaton *et al.*, 2011; Campion *et al.*, 2012; Becker and Kleinman, 2013). Recently, Jenkins and Kozelka (2017) have argued that while proponents of GMH advocate mental health as a matter of urgent need and human rights, the evidence-based approaches that are advocated are typically restricted to psychopharmaceuticals with little or no actual psychosocial intervention (Patel *et al.*, 2007, 2009; Patel, 2014). Typically, only the former is offered, with psychosocial interventions understood as requiring adaptation as a matter of cultural validity. This is a serious misconception since psychopharmaceutical practices are substantially shaped by cultural processes (Whyte *et al.*, 2002; Metzl, 2003; Jain and Jadhov, 2009; Read, 2012; Ecks, 2013; Ecks and Kupfer, 2015). We argue that what currently counts as 'evidence-based' treatment typically does not adequately take into account both structural and ecological constraints (Kleinman, 1986; Jenkins, 1991b; Jadhav and Littlewood, 1994; Farmer, 2004a, b, 2015; Jain and Jadhav, 2009; Metzl and Hansen, 2014; Jenkins, 2015b). Broadening the scope of global mental health holds 'enormous potential to contribute to [these] challenges by exploring cultural feasibility and acceptability of interventions, understanding the impact of health services on the daily lives of providers and patients, and uncovering institutional processes that lead to inadequate and disproportionate commitment to mental health' (Kohrt *et al.*, 2015: 341).

Effective efforts to advance the newly emerging field of global mental health can only be accomplished through serious and sustained engagement with the aforementioned summary of the decades of substantial scholarship that has been accomplished at the intersection of anthropology and psychiatry. Toward this end, this chapter identifies specific problems with respect to illness experience, cultural interpretation and local provision of care in relation to psychopharmaceuticals. This is vital to avoid shortcomings of earlier pioneering efforts such as the WHO International Pilot Studies of Schizophrenia (IPSS), which found significant differences in course and outcome. Because these investigators did not collect ethnographic data for the sites, the findings of cultural variation have been difficult to interpret (although see theoretical model of empirical variation provided by Jenkins and Karno, 1992). The IPSS could have averted much of the difficulty of interpreting their important findings by incorporating an

interdisciplinary team for the research at the outset. Key issues concern the cultural validity and meanings of particular conditions, and ethnographic understandings of local interpretations and healing practices. By working from a foundation of ethnographic knowledge, along with perspectives of health practitioners from other disciplines such as nursing, public health, clinical psychology, health policy, social work and intervention implementation sciences) in collaboration with local indigenous non-medically oriented practitioners, the psychiatry–anthropology interface is considerably enhanced. Anthropologists can work toward these collaborative efforts not only by providing ethnographic techniques to observe, interpret and assess the mental-health landscape both 'up close' (through experience-near, person-centred ethnographies) but also to provide an overall integration of perspectives (through holistic, multilevel analysis that incorporates institutional and structural arrangements). We further suggest the need for attention to the perspectives of first-person experience should be foregrounded in research agendas and clinical approaches, to include partnerships with increasingly popular approaches among 'voice hearing/voice hearer' groups (see Woods and colleagues (2013). Such movements embody the fundamental anthropological insistence on the primacy of subjective experience, the personal and cultural meanings of illness experience, and the legitimacy of defining problems and strategies in accord with the lived realities from those with first-person experience. Insistence that capacities to hear voices, and so forth, are entirely real for those experiencing such, meaningful (vs random or little more than rubbish to be discarded), and not necessarily to be pathologized (even if often experienced as distressing).

Specific Issues of Common Interest: Theoretical, Methodological and Clinical Considerations

Emphasizing the critical importance of the patient's understanding of illness episodes, Kleinman (1980) inspired a substantial body of research (Bhui *et al.*, 2002, 2004, 2015; Dein, 2002). Recent illustrations that take an integrated approach to theory, method and clinical relevance are set forth here with respect to four issues: (1) cultural meaning; (2) methodological advances; (3) psychiatric–anthropological research constructs of enduring relevance; and (4) approaches that seek to move 'beyond' culture.

The Centrality and Magnitude of Cultural Meaning

Byron Good (1994) places meaning squarely at the conceptual centre of the convergence between anthropology and psychiatry, with a hermeneutic critique of rationality that flows into a celebration of experience. Good's (1994) incisive critique of the notion of 'belief' in anthropology and psychiatry is essential reading for any informed approach. In the context of a critical examination of how we interpret psychiatric symptoms, Martinez-Hernaez (2000) elaborates the complementarity of psychiatric observation and anthropological understanding. Equally important as the theoretical and philosophical bridge between disciplines of anthropology and psychiatry is the pragmatic bridge from the conceptual work to its clinical relevance. Alarcon *et al.* (1999) describe five interrelated dimensions that specify the clinical relevance of culture as (1) an interpretive/explanatory tool in understanding psychopathology; (2) a pathogenic or pathoplastic agent; (3) a diagnostic/nosological factor; (4) a therapeutic or protective element; (5) a service/management instrument (see also Emsley *et al.*, 2000). Good and Good (1981) argue cogently for a cultural hermeneutic model for understanding patient experience in clinical practice. Moldavsky (2003) points out that contemporary transcultural psychiatry focuses more on the illness experience than the disease process, while distancing itself from the absolute relativism of antipsychiatry, focusing on clinical issues that aid clinicians in their primary task of alleviating suffering. DiNicola (1985a, b) has offered a synthesis between family therapy and transcultural psychiatry, and Castillo (1997) elaborates a client-centred approach to culture and mental illness. Okpaku (1998) offered a global compendium of case studies and clinical experience to provide practising clinicians with a basic foundation of culturally informed psychiatry. Ponce (1998) advocates a value-orientations model of culture for use in clinical practice, the rationale and internal logic of which is predicated on the concepts of paradigm and epistemology. Most recently, the outline for a cultural formulation for the *Diagnostic and Statistical Manual-5* which has been reviewed and updated in light of myriad cultural factors and the diagnostic process and how best to assess these (Lewis-Fernandez *et al.*, 2014).

Productive Methodological Advances

Guarnaccia (2003) has outlined methodological advances that will likely help define research in cross-cultural psychiatry in the early twenty-first century. Hollan (1997) advocates person-centred ethnography as a method ideally compatible with the goals of cross-cultural psychiatry. Experiments have been made with focus-group methods in order to enhance the contextual basis for making culturally sensitive interpretations (Ekblad and Bäärnhielm, 2002). Rogier (1999) offers a methodological critique of the procedural norms that lead to cultural insensitivity in mental health research, highlighting the development of content validity based on experts' rational analysis of concepts, linguistic translations that conform rigidly to the literal terms of standardized instruments, and the uncritical transferring of concepts across cultures. The methodological contribution of cognitive neuroscience is discussed by Henningsen and Kirmayer (2000), comparing the two orders of higher level explanation constituted by intentional vs dynamical systems theory and the sub-personal explanation of cognitive psychology and neurobiology.

Yet another productive avenue comes from interdisciplinary research collaboration by anthropologist Thomas Csordas and child psychiatrist Michael Storck (Csordas *et al.*, 2008, 2010). Their research team, working longitudinally on religious healing among First Nation Navajo people, demonstrated that methodological approaches which combined ethnographic methods with 'gold standard' research-reliable clinical instruments produced a rich context for 'double dialogue' that could reciprocally reveal dimensions of depression that, in isolation, neither approach could singly achieve. Ethnography vitally enhanced clinical understandings and revealed information not available to the psychiatrist; conversely, the psychiatrist was able to determine and to interpret a great deal of experience that the anthropologist could not (Csordas *et al.*, 2010). Together, their research team pioneered an integrated approach that can usefully serve as a model for future studies (Storck *et al.*, 2000). Additional interdisciplinary collaborations (with relatively large sample sizes) are of value because they were designed to combine specific research clinical diagnostic instruments (requiring months of methodological training for administration and scoring to achieve research reliability) along with intensive anthropological techniques of ethnographic interviews, observations, and participation in everyday settings

(Karno *et al.*, 1987; Jenkins and Schumacher, 1999; Nasser *et al.*, 2002; Lopez *et al.*, 2004; Hollifield *et al.*, 2005; Sajatovic *et al.*, 2005; Jenkins and Hollifield, 2008; Floersch *et al.*, 2009; Jenkins and Haas, 2015).

Vital and Enduring Research Constructs

For present purposes, we restrict ourselves to two vital and enduring research constructs that are indispensable. The first of these (noted earlier) is that of an 'explanatory model' (EM) as formulated by Arthur Kleinman (1980). The formulation of an EM is fundamental and thus crucial to obtain initially and to continue to engage over time (since EMs are hardly static or immutable) for all clinical and research endeavours. The second research construct remains as the most robust and thoroughly investigated of psychosocial research constructs for several decades now, that of 'expressed emotion' (EE), initially developed in London by Brown *et al.* (1972) and replicated by Vaughn and Leff (1976). The early British studies were later replicated by Vaughn and colleagues (1984) among English-speaking Euro-Americans in California and led by psychiatrist Marvin Karno and colleagues (1987) among Spanish-speaking families of Mexican descent. These research projects utilized the same methodologies (for research diagnostic reliability, to ascertain EE according to research-reliable methods for administration and scoring of the Camberwell Family Interview (CFI). The Mexican–American study was only begun following a 1-year period of pilot testing to ensure cultural and linguistic validity (see Jenkins, 1991a). Having done so, Karno and colleagues (1987) found the same statistically significant relationship with respect to relapse among families of Mexican descent in southern California, that is, persons living in high EE (critical, hostile) environments were far more likely to relapse than their counterparts. Also notable were significant differences in levels and qualitative types of EE, that is, families of Mexican descent were less likely to be critical, more likely to be sympathetic and to display warmth toward their afflicted relative. Further, kin were likely to conceptualize the problem (diagnosed as schizophrenia) as *nervios* (a culturally specific, normative problem that anyone can suffer but varies as a matter of degree (Jenkins, 1988a, b). These early collaborations for British, Euro-American, and Mexican–American studies thus provided data that revealed that EE was culturally distinct in a variety of ways. While the dimensions of 'expressed emotion' varied, with Mexican-origin families significantly less critical or hostile and far more likely to express sympathy and warmth, the significant relationship of EE for statistical prediction of the course and outcome was nonetheless replicated (Jenkins, 1991a). This Mexican–American research, carried out through a psychiatric–anthropological partnership in close collaboration with colleagues from the original studies, draws us back to earlier anthropological research on conceptions of mental illness. Anthropologist Robert Edgerton, in his classic 1966 article in the flagship journal *American Anthropologist*, examined conceptions of psychosis in four East African societies. This seminal work is clearly a forerunner to what anthropologist–psychiatrist Kleinman (1980) later formulated as 'explanatory models'. These two constructs, EMs and EE, are central to shaping social and emotional response of kin that is of significance for who will improve and who will not. Additional overviews of the clinical relevance of attitudes toward mental illness, including 'explanatory models', have been provided (Bhugra, 1989; Bhugra and Bhui, 2002), demonstrating the continuing relevance of understanding patients' perspectives, particularly among minority or marginalized groups, and particular types of clinical distress that receive little attention among such groups (Fernández de la Cruz *et al.*, 2015).

Beyond Culture: Nation State, Structural Ecology, Political Economy and Globalization

While a deep understanding of culture in accord with contemporary anthropological formulations (see Jenkins, 2015a: 9) is requisite, it is also clear that more than culture need be considered. While economic and social determinants are undeniably involved, so too are variations across nation states, as pioneered through the work of DelVecchio Good and colleagues (1985). This research drew attention beyond culture and toward understandings of the ways in which emotion and sentiment are formulated nationally and transnationally. Further, it is possible to extend the work of Gregory Bateson (1936) through his formulation of the notion of 'ethos' in micro-social settings (such as English society), as a patterning of social sentiment, Jenkins (1991b) extended Bateson's notion by formulating the concept of a specifically 'political ethos' for its relation to the mental health of a population, including those plagued by political violence and warfare. This concept provides a bridge between the analysis of the state construction of affect, on the one hand, and the phenomenology of those affects in the mental health sequelae of warfare, political violence and dislocation, on the other. In other works that link anthropology and psychiatry, there has been an examination of the nexus between the anthropology of emotion and the psychiatric study of psychopathology with respect to distinctions between normal and pathological emotion, feeling and emotion, interpersonal and intrapsychic accounts of distress and disorder, variability of course and outcome, mind–body dualism, and the conceptualization of psychopathology as biologically natural event or socio-politically produced response (Jenkins, 1991a, 1994a, b, 1996). Finally, we have influential collaborative studies of the forces of globalization in relation to mental status, treatment and social stigma (Bhugra and Mastrogianni, 2004; Jadhav et al., 2007; Korszun et al., 2012: Klineberg et al., 2013; Trani et al., 2015; Keown et al., 2016).

Shared Research Agendas

The research agenda for this continuing hybrid field continues to be dynamically defined and redefined. At the current moment, the field has been given a certain degree of coherence and consistency by a collective mobilization to address the strengths and weaknesses of the attempt to integrate cultural factors into the professional psychiatric nosology institutionalized in the DSM-IV. Good (1992) has made a cogent argument mediating between cultural relativists who consider the DSM nosology as culture-bound and ethnocentric, and universalists who understand the nosology to reflect a priori presumed invariant characteristics of psychopathology, pointing out that the psychiatric nosology is a valuable ready-made comparative framework while at the same time being vulnerable to cross-cultural critique by demonstration of variability in psychiatric syndromes. A substantial body of experts collaborated in the effort to incorporate cultural issues into DSM-IV. Eventually included were an introductory cultural statement, cultural considerations for the use of diagnostic categories, a glossary of culture-bound syndromes and idioms of distress, and an outline for a cultural formulation of diagnoses in individual cases (Mezzich et al., 1999). In the aftermath, these same experts collaborated in an analysis and critique of what was

proposed in comparison to what was excluded (Mezzich et al., 1996; Kirmayer, 1997). Meanwhile, the ongoing development and testing of psychiatric categories in the eleventh revision of the International Classification of Diseases (due 2018) has proceeded significantly in the wake of sustained attention by Sartorius and colleagues (1988, 1991, 1993, 1995). For the DSM-5, attention has continued to focus on the challenge of further enhancing the role of culture in DSM-5 (Alarcon et al., 2002; Lewis-Fernandez et al., 2014).

An important tool for furthering the integration of culture into DSM-IV and DSM-5 has been its inclusion of an outline for cultural formulation (Lewis-Fernandez and Diaz, 2002; Lewis-Fernandez et al., 2014). The cultural formulation is perhaps the most concrete expression of the contemporary convergence of anthropology and psychiatry. It is also at the same time a clinical tool in that it is a comprehensive summation of cultural factors in an individual case, and an ethnographic document in which cultural context and themes are elaborated from a person-centred standpoint. It is unclear the extent to which the cultural formulation is currently being used in clinical practice, but it has a strong presence in the research arena as a regular feature in the journal Culture, Medicine, and Psychiatry, which for more than two decades has published cultural formulations in the form of articles of value to both clinicians and ethnographers. Novins et al. (1997) take a step toward using the DSM-IV outline to develop comprehensive cultural formulations for children and adolescents, critically reviewing the use of the outline in the context of preparing cultural formulations of Native American 6–13 year olds. Sethi et al. (2003) suggest that the cultural formulation can be useful for bridging the gap between understandings of form and content in the understanding of psychiatric signs and symptoms.

The traditional North American conceptualization of ethnopsychiatry focuses on the study of indigenous forms of healing understood as analogous to what in European terms is broadly defined as psychotherapy (Frank and Frank, 1991). Renewing and updating this agenda, cultural variants of healing and therapeutic process emphasizing modulations in bodily experience, transformation of self, aesthetics and religion have been contributed by Csordas (1994, 2002), Desjarlais (1992) and Mullings (1984). The case for the untenable separation of studies of psychiatry and studies of religion has been argued by Bhugra

(1997). At the same time, the distinction between ethnopsychiatry as traditional, religious or indigenous healing and biomedical psychiatry as a cosmopolitan and scientific clinical enterprise has broken down insofar as professional psychiatries from many countries have been subjected to analysis as ethnopsychiatries (Fabrega, 1993; Hughes, 1996). This was already evident in Kleinman's (1980) juxtaposition of Taiwanese psychiatry and shamanism in his seminal examination of depression and neurasthenia in Taiwan.

Also important for investigation, from a variety of psychiatric-anthropological approaches, is the analysis of professional psychiatry, which can be culturally heterogeneous (Gaines, 1992). Sartorius (1990) has compared diagnostic traditions and the classification of psychiatric disorders in French, Russian, American, British, German, Scandinavian, Spanish and Third World psychiatric traditions. Al-Sabaie (1989) has examined the situation in Saudi Arabia, and Angermeyer et al. (2005) have compared the situation in the Slovak Republic, Russia and Germany. In the United States, Luhrmann (2000) documents a watershed moment in contemporary psychiatry as cultural meanings and social movements across the entire field from a clinical culture in which psychoanalysis was prominent to one in which biological psychiatry and neuropsychiatry are dominant. Significant works in clinical ethnography in the United States include Angrosino's (1998) study of a home for the mentally retarded, Estroff's (1981, 1982) study of an outpatient psychiatric facility, Desjarlais' (1997, 1999) work on a shelter for the homeless mentally ill and Joao Biehl (2005) has contributed an examination of an asylum for the socially abandoned mentally ill in Brazil. Anthropologist–psychiatrist Robert Barrett (1996) conducted a close analysis of how psychiatrists in Australia construct schizophrenia through social interaction and discursive practices. A volume edited by Meadows and Singh (2001) examines mental health in Australia, though it pays little attention to cultural psychiatry and care for indigenous and migrant groups. This shortcoming has been addressed, however, as recently formulated by Ventriglio and Bhugra (2015).

An early discussion of ethnopsychiatry in Africa by Margetts (1968) emphasizes the importance of investigating topics such as conceptions of normality and abnormality, magic and religion, social hierarchy, life-cycle rituals, symbolism, demonology, secret societies, death and burial customs, politics, suicide

and cannibalism. More recently, the state of psychiatry in Africa has been discussed by Ilechukwu (1991), who observes that colonial era notions about the rarity of major mental disorder in Africa have been disproven, leading to changes in the healthcare system, with particular mention of the Aro village system which integrates indigenous and psychiatric care developed in the global north. Swartz (1996, 1998) examined the changing notion of culture in South African psychiatry, from a de-emphasis of difference in order to avoid the use of relativism as a justification of oppression to an interest in diversity with a post-apartheid society, and the potential contribution of this change to developing community-based care, understanding indigenous healing, and nation-building.

In counterpoint to this trend toward analytically indigenizing professional psychiatry are observations about international intercommunication and globalization as processes affecting institutional psychiatry (Belkin and Fricchione, 2005). Kirmayer and Minas (2000) observe that globalization has influenced psychiatry through socio-economic effects on the prevalence and course of mental disorders, changing notions of ethnocultural identity, and the production of psychiatric knowledge. Crises in the global world system in the context of development create a truly global challenge and an urgency in understanding links between culture and mental disorders (Kleinman and Cohen, 1997). Fernando (2002, 2003) argues that global psychiatric imperialism and individual racial/cultural insensitivity must be surmounted in order to achieve legitimately universal concepts of mental health. In this domain, theoretical and clinical appear especially clearly as sides of the same coin. For example, thinking about the effects of racism in psychiatry is parallel to viewing psychiatry as an arena in which to analyze and understand racism (Bhugra and Bhui, 2002; Bhui et al., 2015). In a postmodern, postcolonial and creolizing world, argues Miyaji (2002), attention must be given to clinicians' shifting identities and fluid cultures, as well as to positionality in local and global dynamics of power.

Cultural competence has proliferated as a catch-word in parallel with a shift in focus from 'treatment' development and efficacy to 'service' provision and delivery (Cunningham et al., 2002). Distinctive clinical training has been developed in dozens of residency programmes in the United States (Jeffress, 1968), such as one for residents treating Hispanic patients and emphasizing the availability of cultural

25

experts in supervision, skills in cultural formulation of psychiatric distress, and culturally distinct family dynamics (Garza-Trevino *et al.*, 1997). Yager *et al.* (1989) describe training programmes in transcultural psychiatry for medical students, residents and fellows at UCLA. Rousseau *et al.* (1995) show that psychiatry residents' perceptions of transcultural practice varies in relation to their own cultural origin rather than with respect to their degree of exposure to patients from different cultures or their training in cultural psychiatry. International videoconferencing has been introduced to the training of medical students in transcultural psychiatry, in one case linking Sweden, Australia and the United States (Ekblad *et al.*, 2004). Beyond the training of clinicians, insofar as social and cultural factors can impact treatment modalities and outcomes, managed and rationed healthcare must take this into account to ensure the availability of cost-effective treatment within an integrated system of services to patients of all cultural and economic backgrounds (Moffic and Kinzie, 1996).

An extensive review of empirical work on the perennial topic of cultural variability in psychopathology would require at least as much space as I have devoted to general theoretical, methodological, topical and clinical considerations. I mention here only the most comprehensive and definitive edited collections as a pointer toward three critical issues: on culture-bound syndromes see the volume by Simons and Hughes (1985); on depression see the volume by Kleinman and Good (1985); and on schizophrenia see the volume by Jenkins and Barrett (2004). The relation of culture to trauma, violence and memory has been taken up in a series of critical works by Antze and Lambek (1996), Bracken (2002), Breslau (2000), Robben and Suarez-Orozco (2000), Young (1995), Kinzie (2001a, b) and Rousseau (1995). Related to the literature of trauma, the experience of geographical dislocation has become of increasing concern as researchers and clinicians address the mental health of immigrants and refugees (Boehnlein and Kinzie, 1995; Azima and Grizenko, 1996; Bhugra, 2000; Kinzie, 2001a, b; Hodes 2002; Hollifield *et al.*, 2002; Kirmayer, 2002; Lustig *et al.*, 2004; Ingleby and Watters, 2005). The specific vulnerability of girls and women in relation to mental health problems, particularly depression, has been documented globally; the 2:1 epidemiological ratio of depression among females is to be accounted for in significant part by gender inequality, discrimination, misogyny and sexism (Jenkins and DelVecchio Good 2014).

The cultural analysis of psychopharmacology both from the standpoint of subjective experience and global political economy is attracting increasing attention (Metzl, 2003; Lakoff, 2005; Jenkins, 2010; Petryna *et al.*, 2006). Significantly more attention should be paid to the consequences of distinguishing studies oriented by the therapeutic discourse of 'treatment' (Seeley, 2000; Tseng and Streltzer, 2001) and studies oriented by the economic discourse of 'services' (Kirmayer *et al.*, 2003) in mental healthcare, particularly since the discourse on services has grown increasingly dominant in the arena of research and funding. Finally, although my concern has been with the convergence between anthropology and psychiatry, some acknowledgment must be made of a third discipline that operates in the sphere of mental illness and psychiatric disorder. Psychiatric epidemiology makes an important contribution regardless of the fact that epidemiology shares neither the methodological disposition nor the intellectual temperament that renders the dialogue between anthropology and psychiatry so natural. These issues do not exhaust the evolving research agenda that continues to take shape in the convergence of anthropology and psychiatry. The underlying comparative approach of this field has led to the recognition of variations in the practice of cultural psychiatry itself across national boundaries (Alarcon and Ruiz, 1995).

Summary and Concluding Considerations: Psychiatry, Anthropology and Global Mental Health

To summarize, we now have several decades of research at the interface of psychiatric anthropology and cultural psychiatry which have provided empirical evidence that demonstrates the inextricability of culture and mental disorder. As Jenkins (2015a: 14) recently set forth, 'from onset to recovery, culture matters vitally in understanding the experience of mental illness'. Indeed, the range and depth of cultural factors and processes that shape mental illness are compelling, and include (Jenkins, 2015a: 14):

1. risk/vulnerability factors;
2. type of onset (sudden or gradual);
3. symptom content, form, constellation;
4. clinical diagnostic process;

5. subjective experience and meaning of problem/illness;
6. kin identification and conception of and social-emotional response ('expressed emotion') to problem/illness;
7. community social response (support, stigma);
8. healing modalities and healthcare utilization;
9. experience, meaning, and utilization of healthcare/healing modalities (including psychotropic drugs);
10. resources for resilience and recovery; and
11. most significantly, course and outcome.

At this juncture, it is worth emphasizing the particularly productive research paradigm that should neither be neglected nor forgotten in light of the volume of transcontinental research on 'expressed emotion' that has empirically demonstrated (1) significance for clinical outcomes, and (2) substantial cultural differences in the features of social and emotional response by kin toward relatives who experience distressing disorders (psychiatric and stress-related non-psychiatric alike; see Jenkins (2015a) for an updated overall summary of this literature). Given the importance of 'expressed emotion' for the onset, course and outcome of mental illnesses, there had been a notable theoretical gap in formulations to identify precisely what a research index as significant as EE is actually 'tapping'. Working from conjoined anthropological and psychiatric perspectives, ten specific features of this research construct have been identified (Jenkins and Karno, 1992). Nevertheless, future studies are needed to flesh out features that could be particularly vital for the course and outcome of disorders transnationally. This is an important charge since Hopper (1991) has critically examined the validity of the WHO cross-cultural studies of schizophrenia longitudinally over a 25 year period, seeking to address various aspects of methodological critiques registered by critics of the WHO and EE studies. Following systematic analysis and re-analysis of the original data sets, Hopper (2004: 71) concluded that the findings of 'consistent outcome differential favoring the developing centres is remarkably robust' pointing to WHO investigators who themselves had urged the examination of cultural and social factors (Sartorius et al., 1977). Clearly, we have considerably more work ahead of us to identify precise pathways and mechanisms, including the subjective experience of persons living with such conditions (individuals and their kin).

Currently, it is disconcerting that such research has taken a back seat to the identification of 'neuro-signatures' that are elusive at best and as a matter of urgency hold little to no relevance for the immediacy of needed care. The World Health Organization (2014), the United States National Institute of Mental Health, and several other institutional bodies have increasingly de-emphasized funding for cultural psychiatry and psychiatric anthropology in imbalanced favour of neuroscience. We cannot fail to observe the gaps, silences and erasures of decades of research that has been accomplished despite the productive convergence between anthropology and psychiatry thus far, and the need for more in the future with calls to 'scale up' in the field of global mental health. In the final analysis, the convergence between anthropology and psychiatry remains an exceedingly fertile ground for generating ideas and issues with the potential to stimulate both parent disciplines. With respect to theory and clinical practice, global political economy and intimate subjective experience, the nature of pathology and the process of therapy, this hybrid field is a critical locus for addressing the question of what it means to be human, whole and healthy or suffering and afflicted.

References

Alarcon, R. D. and Ruiz, P. (1995). Theory and practice of cultural psychiatry in the United States and abroad. *American Psychiatric Press Review of Psychiatry*, **14**, 599–626.

Alarcon, R. D., Westermeyer, J., Foulks, E. F. *et al.* (1999). Clinical relevance of contemporary cultural psychiatry. *Journal of Nervous and Mental Disease*, **187**(8), 465–471.

Alarcon, R. D., Bell, C. C. Kirimayer, L. J., Lin, K. M., Ustun, B. and Wisner, K. (2002). Beyond the funhouse mirrors: research agenda on culture and psychiatric diagnosis. In *A Research Agenda for DSM-5*, ed. D. J. Kupfer, M. B. First and D. A. Regier. Washington DC: American Psychiatric Press, Inc., pp. 219–281.

Al-Sabaie, A. (1989). Psychiatry in Saudi Arabia: cultural perspectives. *Transcultural Psychiatric Research Review*, **26**(4), 245–262.

Andreoli S., Ribeiro, W., Quintana, M. *et al.* (2009). Violence and post-traumatic stress disorder in Sao Paulo and Rio de Janeiro, Brazil: the protocol for an epidemiological and genetic survey. *BMC Psychiatry*, **9**(1), 34.

Angermeyer, M. C., Breier, P., Dietrich, S. *et al.* (2005). Public attitudes toward psychiatric treatment: an international comparison. *Society for Psychiatry and Epidemiology*, **40**(11), 855–864.

Angrosino, M. V. (1998). *Opportunity House: Ethnographic Stories of Mental Retardation*. Walnut Creek, CA: AltaMira Press.

Antze, P. and Lambek, M. (eds) (1996). *Tense Past: Cultural Essays in Trauma and Memory*. New York: Routledge.

Azima, F. and Grizenko, N. (eds) (1996). *Immigrant and Refugee Children and their Families: The Role of Culture in Assessment and Treatment*. Madison, CT: International University Press.

Barrett, R. (1996). *The Psychiatric Team and the Social Definition of Schizophrenia: An Anthropological Study of Person and Illness*. Cambridge: Cambridge University Press.

Bateson, G. (1936). *Naven: A Survey of the Problems Suggested by a Composite Picture of the Culture of a New Guinea Tribe Drawn from Three Points of View*, vol. **21**. Stanford: Stanford University Press.

Becker, A. and Kleinman, A. (2013). Mental health and the global agenda. *The New England Journal of Medicine*, **369**(1), 66–73.

Becker, E. (1962). *The Birth and Death of Meaning: A Perspective in Psychiatry and Anthropology*. New York: Free Press of Glencoe.

Becker, E. (1963). Social science and psychiatry: the coming challenge. *The Antioch Review*, **23**(3), 353–366.

Belkin, G. S. and Fricchione, G. L. (2005). Internationalism and the future of academic psychiatry. *Academic Psychiatry*, **29**(3), 240–243.

Benedict, R. (1934). *Patterns of Culture*, vol. **8**. New York: Houghton Mifflin Harcourt.

Bhugra, D. (1989). Attitudes towards mental illness. *Acta Psychiatrica Scandinavica*, **80**(1), 1–12.

Bhugra, D. (1997). *Psychiatry and Religion: Context, Consensus and Controversies*. London: Routledge.

Bhugra, D. (2000). Migration and schizophrenia. *Acta Psychiatrica Scandinavica*, **102**(s407), 68–73.

Bhugra, D. and Bhui, K. (2002). Racism in psychiatry: paradigm lost–paradigm regained. In *Racism and Mental Health: Prejudice and Suffering*, ed. K. Bhui. London: Jessica Kingsley, pp. 111–128.

Bhugra, D. and Mastrogianni, A. (2004). Globalisation and mental disorders. *The British Journal of Psychiatry*, **184**(1), 10–20.

Bhui, K., Bhugra, D. and Goldberg. D. (2002). Causal explanations of distress and general practitioners' assessments of common mental disorder among Punjabi and English attendees. *Social Psychiatry and Psychiatric Epidemiology*, **37**(1), 38–45.

Bhui, K., Bhugra, D., Goldberg, D. *et al.* (2004). Assessing the prevalence of depression in Punjabi and English primary care attenders: the role of culture, physical illness and somatic symptoms. *Transcultural Psychiatry*, **41**(3), 307–322.

Bhui, K., Aslam, R. W., Palinski, A. *et al.* (2015). Interventions to improve therapeutic communications between black and minority ethnic patients and professionals in psychiatric services: systematic review. *The British Journal of Psychiatry*, **207**(2), 95–103.

Biehl, J. (2005). *Vita: Life in a Zone of Social Abandonment*. Berkeley: University of California Press.

Boaz, Franz (1911). *The Mind of Primitive Man*. New York: The Macmillan Company.

Boehnlein, J. K. and Kinzie, D. (1995). Refugee trauma. *Transcultural Psychiatric Research Review*, **32**(3), 223–252.

Bracken, P. (2002). *Trauma: Culture, Meaning and Philosophy*. London/Philadelphia: Whurr.

Breslau, J. (2000). Globalizing disaster trauma: psychiatry, science, and culture after the Kobe earthquake. *Ethos*, **28**(2), 174–197.

Brown, G. W., Birley, J. L., and Wing, J. K. (1972). Influence of family life on the course of schizophrenic disorders: a replication. *The British Journal of Psychiatry*, **121**(562), 241–258.

Campion, J., Bhui, K., and Bhugra, D. (2012). European Psychiatric Association (EPA) guidance on prevention of mental disorders. *European Psychiatry*, **27**(2), 68–80.

Canguilhem, G. (1991). *The Normal and the Pathological*, trans. Carolyn R. Fawcett and Robert S. Cohen. New York: Zone Books.

Castillo, R. J. (1997). *Culture and Mental Illness: A Client-Centered Approach*. Pacific Grove: Brooks/Cole Publications.

Cox, J. L. (1977). Aspects of transcultural psychiatry. *British Journal of Psychiatry*, **130**, 211–221.

Csordas, T. J. (1994). *The Sacred Self: A Cultural Phenomenology of Charismatic Healing*. Berkeley: University of California Press.

Csordas, T. J. (2002). *Body/Meaning/Healing*. New York: Palgrave.

Csordas, T. J., Storck, M. J. and Strauss, M. (2008). Diagnosis and distress in Navajo healing. *The Journal of Nervous and Mental Disease*, **196**(8), 585–596.

Csordas, T. J., Dole, C., Tran, A., Strickland, M. and Storck, M. G. (2010). Ways of asking, ways of telling. *Culture, Medicine, and Psychiatry*, **34**(1), 29–55.

Cunningham, P. B., Foster, S. L. and Henggeler, S. W. (2002). The elusive concept of cultural competence. *Children's Services: Social Policy, Research, and Practice*, **5**(3), 231–243.

Dein, S. (2002). Transcultural psychiatry. *British Journal of Psychiatry*, **181**(6), 535–536.

DelVecchio Good, M. J., Good, B. J. and Moradi, R. (1985). The interpretation of Iranian depressive illness and dysphoric affect. In *Culture and Depression: Studies in the Anthropology and Cross-Cultural Psychiatry of Affect and Disorder*, ed. Arthur Kleinman and Byron J. Good. Berkeley: University of California Press, pp. 369–428.

Desjarlais, R. (1992). *Body and Emotion: The Aesthetics of Illness and Healing in the Nepal Himalayas*. Philadelphia: University of Pennsylvania Press.

Desjarlais, R. (1997). *Shelter Blues: Sanity and Selfhood among the Homeless*. Philadelphia: University of Pennsylvania Press.

Desjarlais, R. (1999). The makings of personhood in a shelter for people considered homeless and mentally ill. *Ethos*, **27**(4), 466.

Devereux, G. (1980). *Basic Problems of Ethnopsychiatry*. Chicago: University of Chicago Press.

DiNicola, V. F. (1985a). Family therapy and transcultural psychiatry: an emerging synthesis. Part I: the conceptual basis. *Transcultural Psychiatric Research Review*, **22**, 81–113.

DiNicola, V. F. (1985b). Family therapy and transcultural psychiatry: an emerging synthesis. Part II: portability and culture change. *Transcultural Psychiatric Review*, **22**, 151–180.

Du Bois, C. A. (1944). *The People of Alor: A Social-Psychological Study of an East Indian Island*. Minneapolis, MN: University of Minnesota Press.

Eaton, J., McCay, L., Semrau, M. *et al.* (2011). Scale up of services for mental health in low-income and middle-income countries. *The Lancet*, **378** (9802), 1592–1603.

Ecks, S. (2013). *Eating Drugs: Psychopharmaceutical Pluralism in India*. New York: New York University Press.

Ecks, S. and Kupfer, C. (2015). 'What is strange is that we don't have more children coming to us': a habitography of psychiatrists and Scholastic pressure is Kolkata, India. *Social Science & Medicine*, **143**, 336–342.

Edgerton, R. (1966). Conceptions of psychosis in four East African societies. *American Anthologists*, **68**(2), 408–425.

Ekblad, S. and Bäärnhielm, S. (2002). Focus group view research in transcultural psychiatry: reflections on research experiences. *Transcultural Psychiatry*, **39**(4), 484–500.

Ekblad, S., Manicavasagar, V., Silove, D. *et al.* (2004). The use of international videoconferencing as a strategy for teaching medical students about transcultural psychiatry. *Transcultural Psychiatry*, **41**(1), 120–129.

Emsley, R. A., Waterdrinker, A., Pienaar, W. P. and Hawkridge, S. M. (2000). Cultural aspects of psychiatry. *Primary Care Psychiatry*, **6**(1), 29–32.

Estroff, S. E. (1978). The anthropological psychiatry fantasy: can we make it a reality? *Transcultural Psychiatric Research Review*, **15**, 209–213.

Estroff, S. (1981). *Making It Crazy*. Berkeley: University of California Press.

Estroff, S. (1982). Long-term psychiatric clients in an American community: some socio-cultural factors in chronic mental illness. In *Clinically Applied Anthropology. Anthropology in Health Science Settings*, ed. N. J. Chrisman and T. W. Maretzki. Dordrecht: Reidel, pp. 369–393.

Fabrega, H. J. (1993). Biomedical psychiatry as an object for a critical medical anthropology. In *Knowledge, Power, and Practice: The Anthropology of Medicine and Everyday Life*, ed. S. Lindenbaum and M. Lock, Berkeley, CA: University of California Press.

Farmer, P. (2004a). An anthropology of structural violence. *Current Anthropology*, **45**(3), 305–325.

Farmer, P. (2004b). *Pathologies of Power: Health, Human Rights, and the New War on the Poor*. Berkeley: University of California Press.

Farmer, P. (2015) Who lives and who dies. *London Review of Books*, **37**(3), 17–20.

Fernández de la Cruz, Lorena, Kolvenbach, Sarah, Vidal-Ribas, Pablo *et al.* (2015). Illness perception, help-seeking attitudes, and knowledge related to obsessive–compulsive disorder across different ethnic groups: a community survey. *Social Psychiatry and Psychiatric Epidemiology*, **51**(3), 455–464.

Fernando, S. (2002). *Mental Health, Race, and Culture*, 2nd edn. New York: St. Martin's.

Fernando, S. (2003). *Cultural Diversity, Mental Health and Psychiatry: The Struggle against Racism*. East Sussex and New York, NY: Brunner-Routledge.

Floersch, J., Townsend, L., Longhofer, J., *et al.* (2009). Adolescent experience of psychotropic treatment. *Transcultural Psychiatry* **46**, 157–179.

Frank, J. D. (1973). *Persuasion and Healing: A Comparative Study of Psychotherapy*. Baltimore and London: Johns Hopkins University Press.

Frank, J. D. and Frank, J. B. (1991) *Persuasion and Healing: A Comparative Study of Psychotherapy*, revised edn. Baltimore and London: Johns Hopkins University Press.

Gaines, A. D. (1992). *Ethnopsychiatry: The Cultural Construction of Professional and Folk Psychiatries*. Albany, NY: State University of New York Press.

Galdston, I. (ed.) (1971). *The Interface between Psychiatry and Anthropology*. New York: Brunner/Mazel.

Garza-Trevino, E., Ruiz, P. and Venegas-Samuels, K. (1997). A psychiatric curriculum directed to the care of the Hispanic patient. *Academic Psychiatry*, **21**(1), 1–10.

Good, B. J. (1992). Culture and psychopathology: directions for psychiatric anthropology. In *New Directions in Psychological Anthropology*, ed. T. Schwartz, G. M. White and C. A. Lutz. Cambridge: Cambridge University Press, pp. 181–205.

Good, B. J. (1994). *Medicine, Rationality, and Experience: An Anthropological Perspective*. Cambridge: Cambridge University Press.

Good, B. J. and Good, M. J. (1981). The meaning of symptoms: a cultural hermeneutic model for clinical practice. In *The Relevance of Social Science for Medicine*, ed. L. Eisenberg and A. Kleinman. Dordrecht: Reidel, pp. 165–196.

Guarnaccia, P. (2003). Editorial. Methodological advances in cross-cultural study of mental health: setting new standards. *Cultural Medical Psychiatry*, 27(3), 249–257.

Helman, C. G. (2000). *Culture, Health, and Illness*. Oxford: Butterworth-Heinemann.

Henningsen, P. and Kirmayer, L. J. (2000). Mind beyond the net: implications of cognitive neuroscience for cultural psychiatry. *Transcultural Psychiatry*, 37(4), 467–494.

Hodes, M. (2002). Three key issues for young refugees' mental health. *Transcultural Psychiatry*, 39(2), 196–213.

Hollan, D. (1997). The relevance of person-centered ethnography to cross-cultural psychiatry. *Transcultural Psychiatry*, 34(2), 219.

Hollifield, M., Warner, T. D., Lian, N., *et al.* (2002). Measuring trauna and health status in refugees: a critical review. *JAMA*, 288(5), 611–621.

Hollifield, M., Eckert, V., Warner, T., *et al.* (2005). Development of an inventory for measuring war-related events in refugees. *Comprehensive Psychiatry*, 46, 67–80.

Hopper, K. (1991). Some old questions for the new crosscultural psychiatry. *Medical Anthropology Quarterly*, 5(4), 299–330.

Hopper, K. (2004). Interrogating the meaning of 'culture' in the WHO International Studies of Schizophrenia. In *Schizophrenia, Culture, and Subjectivity: The Edge of Experience*, ed. Janis H. Jenkins and Robert J. Barrett. New York: Cambridge University Press, pp. 62–86.

Hughes, C. C. (1996). Ethnopsychiatry. In *Medical Anthropology: Contemporary Theory and Method* (revised edn), ed. C. F. Saragent and T. M. Johnson. Westport, CT: Praeger Publishers, pp. 131–150.

Ilechukwu, S. T. (1991). Psychiatry in Africa: special problems and unique features. *Transcultural Psychiatric Research Review*, 28(3), 169–218.

Ingleby, D., and Watters, C. (2005). Mental health and social care for asylum seekers and refugees. In *Forced Migration and Mental Health*. Springer US, pp. 193–212.

Jadhav, S., and Littlewood, R. (1994). Defeat Depression Campaign. *The Psychiatrist*, 18(9), 572–573.

Jadhav, S., Littlewood, R., Ryder, A. G. *et al.* (2007). Stigmatization of severe mental illness in India: against the simple industrialization hypothesis. *Indian Journal of Psychiatry* 49(3), 189–194.

Jain, S. and Jadhov, S. (2009). Pills that swallow policy: clinical ethnography of a community mental health program in Northern India. *Transcultural Psychiatry*, 46(1), 60–85.

Jeffress, J. E. (1968). Training in transcultural psychiatry in the United States: a 1968 survey. *International Journal of Social Psychiatry*, 15(1), 69–72.

Jenkins, Janis H. (1988a). Ethnopsychiatric interpretations of schizophrenic illness: the problem of *nervios* within Mexican-American families. *Culture, Medicine, and Psychiatry*, 12, 303–331.

Jenkins, Janis H. (1988b). Conceptions of schizophrenic illness as a problem of nerves: a comparative analysis of Mexican-Americans and Anglo-Americans. *Social Science and Medicine*, 26, 1233–1243.

Jenkins, J. H. (1991a). Anthropology, expressed emotion, and schizophrenia. *Ethos*, 19, 387–431.

Jenkins, J. H. (1991b). The state construction of affect: political ethos and mental health among Salvadoran refugees. *Culture, Medicine and Psychiatry*, 15(2), 139–165.

Jenkins, J. H. (1994a). Culture, emotion, and psychopathology. In *Emotion and Culture: Empirical Studies of Mutual Influence*, ed. S. Kitayama and H. R. Markus. Washington, DC: American Psychological Association Press, pp. 309–335.

Jenkins, J. H. (1994b). The psychocultural study of emotion and mental disorder. In *Psychological Anthropology*, ed. P. K. Bock. Westport, CT: Praeger Publishers, pp. 97–120.

Jenkins, J. H. (1996). Culture, emotion, and psychiatric disorder. In *Medical Anthropology: Contemporary Theory and Method* (revised edn), ed. C. F. Sargent and T. M. Johnson. Westport, CT: Praeger Publishers, pp. 71–87.

Jenkins, J. H. (2010). Introduction. In *Pharmaceutical Self: The Global Shaping of Experience in an Age of Psychopharmacology*, ed. J. H. Jenkins. School of Advanced Research Press, pp. 3–16.

Jenkins, J. H. (2015a). *Extraordinary Conditions: Mental Illness as Experience*. Berkeley: University of California Press.

Jenkins, J. H. (2015b). Psychic and social sinew: life conditions of trauma among youths in New Mexico. *Medical Anthropology Quarterly*, 29(1), 42–60.

Jenkins, J. H. and Barrett, R. J. (eds) (2004). *Schizophrenia, Culture, and Subjectivity. The Edge of Experience*. Cambridge/New York: Cambridge University Press.

Jenkins, J. H. and DelVecchio Good, M.-J. (2014). Women and global mental health: vulnerability and empowerment. In *Essentials of Global Mental Health*, ed. S. O. Opakpu. Cambridge: Cambridge University Press.

Jenkins, J. H. and Haas, B. M. (2015). Trauma in the lifeworlds of adolescents: hard luck and trouble in the land of enchantment. In *Culture and PTSD*, ed. Devon Hinton and Byron Good. Philadelphia: University of Pennsylvania Press, pp. 215–245.

Jenkins, J. H. and Hollifield, M. A. (2008). Postcoloniality as the aftermath of terror between Vietnamese refugees. In *Postcolonial Disorders*, ed. M. J. D. Good, S. T. Hyde, S. Pinto and B. J. Good. Berkeley and Los Angeles: University of California Press.

Jenkins, J. H. and Karno, M. (1992). The meaning of expressed emotion: theoretical issues raised by crosscultural research. *American Journal of Psychiatry*, **149**(1), 9–21.

Jenkins, J. H. and Kozelka, E. E. (2017). Global mental health and psychopharmacology in precarious ecologies: anthropological considerations for engagement and efficacy. In *Handbook of Sociocultural Perspectives on Global Mental Health*, ed. Ross White, Ursula Read, Sumeet Jain, David Orr. London: Palgrave Press.

Jenkins, J. H. and Schumacher, J. (1999). Family burden of schizophrenia and depressive illness: specifying the effects of ethnicity, gender and social ecology. *British Journal of Psychiatry*, **174**, 31–38.

Karno, M., Jenkins, J. H., de la Selva, A. *et al.* (1987). Expressed emotion and schizophrenic outcome among Mexican-American families. *Journal of Nervous and Mental Disease*, **175**, 143–151.

Kennedy, J. G. (1974). Cultural psychiatry. In *Handbook of Social and Cultural Anthropology*, ed. J. J., Honigmann. Chicago: Rand McNally.

Keown, P., McBride, O., Twigg, L., *et al.* (2016). Rates of voluntary and compulsory psychiatric in-patient treatment in England: an ecological study investigating associations with deprivation and demographics. *The British Journal of Psychiatry*, **209**(2), 157–161.

Kiev, A. (1972). *Transcultural Psychiatry*. New York: Free Press.

Kinzie, J. D. (2001a). Psychotherapy for massively traumatized refugees: the therapist variable. *American Journal of Psychotherapy*, **55**(4), 475–490.

Kinzie, J. D. (2001b). The Southeast Asian refugee: the legacy of severe trauma. In *Culture and Psychotherapy: A Guide to Clinical Practice*, ed. W.-S. Tseng and J. Streltzer. Washington, DC: American Psychiatric Press, pp. 173–191.

Kirmayer, L. (ed.) (1997). Culture in DSM-IV. *Transcultural Psychiatry*, **35**(3). Special Theme Issue.

Kirmayer, L. J. (2001). Commentary on 'Why cultural anthropology needs the psychiatrist': Sapir's vision of culture and personality. *Psychiatry: Interpersonal and Biological Processes*, **64**(1), 23–31.

Kirmayer, L. J. (2002). The refugee's predicament. *Evolution Psychiatrique*, **67**(4), 724–742.

Kirmayer, L. J. and Minas, H. (2000). The future of cultural psychiatry: an international perspective. *Canadian Journal of Psychiatry*, **45**(5), 438–446.

Kirmayer, L. J., Groleau, D., Guzder, J., Blake, C. and Jarvis, E. (2003). Cultural consultation: a model of mental health service for multicultural societies. *Special issue: Transcultural Psychiatry*, **48**(3), 145–153.

Kleinman, A. (1977). Depression, somatization, and the new cross-cultural psychiatry. *Social Science and Medicine*, **11**(1), 3–10.

Kleinman, A. (1980). *Patients and Healers in the Context of Culture: An Exploration of the Borderland between Anthropology, Medicine and Psychiatry*. Berkeley: University of California Press.

Kleinman, A. (1986). *Social Origins of Distress and Disease: Depression, Neurasthenia, and Pain in Modern China*. New Haven: Yale University Press.

Kleinman, A. (1987). Anthropology and psychiatry: the role of culture in cross-cultural research on illness. *British Journal of Psychiatry*, **151**, 447–454.

Kleinman, A. (1988). *Rethinking Psychiatry: From Cultural Category to Personal Experience*. New York: Free Press.

Kleinman, A. and Cohen, A. (1997). Psychiatry's global challenge: an evolving crisis in the developing world signals the need for a better understanding of the links between culture and mental disorders. *Scientific American*, March, 86–89.

Kleinman, A. and Good, B. (eds) (1985). *Culture and Depression. Studies in the Anthropology and Crosscultural Psychiatry of Affect and Disorder*. Berkeley: California University Press.

Klineberg, E., Kelly, M. J., Stansfeld, S. A. and Bhui, K. S. (2013). How do adolescents talk about self-harm: a qualitative study of disclosure in an ethnically diverse urban population in England. *BMC Public Health*, **13**(1), 572.

Kohrt, B., Mendenhall, E. and Brown, P. J. (2015). A road map for anthropology and global mental health. In *Global Mental Health: Anthropological Perspectives*, ed. Brandon Kohrt and Emily Mendenhall. Walnut Creek, CA: Left Coast Press, pp. 341–363.

Korszun, A., Dinos, S., Ahmed, K. and Bhui, K. (2012). Medical student attitudes about mental illness: does medical-school education reduce stigma? *Academic Psychiatry*, **36**(3), 197–204.

Kraepelin, E. (1904). Comparative psychiatry. In *Cultural Psychiatry and Medical Anthropology: An Introduction and Reader*, ed. R. littlewood and S. Dein. London: Athlone Press, pp. 38–42.

Lakoff, A. (2005). *Pharmaceutical Reason: Knowledge and Value in Global Psychiatry*. Cambridge: Cambridge University Press.

Levi-Strauss, C. (1962). *Savage Mind*. University of Chicago.

Lewis-Fernandez, R. and Diaz, N. (2002). The cultural formulation: a method for assessing cultural factors affecting the clinical encounter. *Special Issue: The Fourteenth Annual New York State Office of Mental Health Research Conference*, **73**(4). 271–295.

Lewis-Fernandez, R. and Kleinman, A. (1995). Cultural psychiatry: theoretical, clinical, and research issues. *Psychiatric Clinics of North America*, **18**(3), 433–448.

Lewis-Fernández, R., Aggarwal, N. K., Bäärnhielm, S. *et al.* (2014). Culture and psychiatric evaluation:

operationalizing cultural formulation for DSM-5. *Psychiatry*, **77**(2), 130–154.

Littlewood, R. (1990). From categories to contexts: a decade of the 'new cross-cultural psychiatry'. *Special Issue: Cross-Cultural Psychiatry*, **156**, 308–327.

Littlewood, R. and Dein, S. (eds) (2000). *Cultural Psychiatry and Medical Anthropology: An Introduction and Reader*. London: Athlone Press.

Lopez, S. R. and Guarnaccia, P. J. (2005). Cultural dimensions of psychopathology: the social world's impact on mental illness. In *Psychopathology: Foundations for a Contemporary Understanding*, ed. J. E. Maddux and B. A. Winstead. Mahwah, NJ: Lawrence Erlbaum Associates Publishers, pp. 19–37.

López, S. R., Nelson, K. A., Polo, A. J., Jenkins, J. H., Karno, M., Snyder, K. (2004). Ethnicity, expressed emotion, attributions and course of schizophrenia: family warmth matters. *Journal of Abnormal Psychology*, **113**, 428–439.

Luhrmann, T. M. (2000). *Of Two Minds: The Growing Disorder in American Psychiatry*. New York: Knopf.

Lustig, S. L., Kia-Keating, M., Knight, W. G. *et al.* (2004). Review of child and adolescent refugee mental health. *Journal of the American Academy of Child and Adolescent Psychiatry*, **43**(1), 24–36.

Malinowski, B. (1954). *Magic, Science and Religion: and Other Essays*. Garden City, NY: Doubleday.

Margetts, E. L. (1968). African ethnopsychiatry in the field. *Canadian Psychiatric Association Journal*, **13**(6), 521–538.

Martinez-Hernaez, A. (2000). *What's Behind the Symptom? On Psychiatric Observation and Anthropological Understanding*, translated by S. M. DiGiacomo and J. Bates, foreword by A. Kleinman. Amsterdam: Harwood Academic Publishers.

Martins, C. (1969). Transcultural psychiatry: some concepts. *ArquiPos de Neuro-Psiquiatria*, **27**(2), 141–144.

Mead, M. (1930). *Growing Up in New Guinea: A Comparative Study of Primitive Education*. New York: New American Library.

Mead, M. (1935). *Sex and Temperament in Three Primitive Societies*. New York: William Morrow Publishers.

Meadows, G. N. and Singh, B. S. (eds) (2001). *Mental Health in Australia*. South Melbourne, Australia: Oxford University Press.

Metzl, J. M. (2003). Selling sanity through gender: the psychodynamics of psychotropic advertising. *Journal of Medical Humanities*, **24**(1–2), 79–103.

Metzl, J. M. and Hansen, H. (2014). Structural competency: theorizing a new medical engagement with stigma and inequality. *Social Science and Medicine* **103**, 126–133.

Mezzich, J. E., Kleinman, A. Fabrega, H. and Parron, D. L. (eds) (1996). *Culture and Psychiatric Diagnosis: A DSM-IV Perspective*. Washington, DC: American Psychiatric Association Press.

Mezzich, J. E., Kirmayer, L. J., Kleinman, A., Fabrega, H., Parron, D. and Good, B. (1999). The place of culture in DSM-IV. *Journal of Nervous and Mental Disease*, **187**(18), 457–464.

Mihanovic, M., Babic, G., Kezic, S., Sain, I. and Loncar, C. (2005). Anthropology and psychiatry. *College of Anthropology*, **29**(2), 747–751.

Miller, L. (1977). Transcultural psychiatry. In Proceedings of the International Congress on Transcultural Psychiatry, Bradford, July 1976. *Mental Health and Society*, **4**(3-supp-4), 121–244.

Miyaji, N. T. (2002). Shifting identities and transcultural psychiatry. *Transcultural Psychiatry*, **39**(2), 173–195.

Moffic, H. S. and Kinzie, J. D. (1996). The history and future of cross-cultural psychiatric services. *Community Mental Health Journal*, **32**(6), 581–592.

Moldavsky, D. (2003). The implication of transcultural psychiatry for clinical practice. *Israel Journal of Psychiatry and Related Sciences*, **40**(1), 47–56.

Mullings, L. (1984). *Therapy, Ideology, and Social Change: Mental Healing in Ghana*. Berkeley: University of California Press.

Murphy, H. B. M. (1984). Handling the cultural dimension in psychiatric research. In *Culture and Psychopathology*, ed. J. E. Mezzich and C. E. Berganza. New York: Columbia University Press, pp. 113–123.

Nasser, L., Walders, N. and Jenkins, J. H. (2002). The experience of schizophrenia: what's gender got to do with it? A critical review of the current status of research on schizophrenia. *Schizophrenia Bulletin*, **28**, 351–362.

Novins, D. K., Bechtold, D. W., Sack, W. H., Thompson, J., Carter, D. R. and Manson, S. M. (1997). The DSM-IV outline for cultural formulation: a critical demonstration with American Indian children. *Journal of the American Academy of Child and Adolescent Psychiatry*, **36**(9), 1244–1251.

Okpaku, S. (ed.) (1998). *Clinical Methods in Transcultural Psychiatry*. Washington, DC: American Psychiatric Press.

Padilla, E. R. and Padilla, A. M. (1977). Transcultural psychiatry: an Hispanic perspective. *Spanish Speaking Mental Health Research Center Monograph Series*, **4**, 110.

Patel, V. (2014). Why mental health matters to global health. *Transcultural Psychiatry*, **51**(6), 777–789.

Patel, V., Araya, Ricardo, Chatterjee, Sudipto *et al.* (2007). Treatment and prevention of mental disorders in low-income and middle-income countries. *The Lancet*, **370**(4), 991–1005.

Patel, V., Simon, G., Chowdhary, N., *et al.* (2009). Packages of care for depression in low- and middle-income countries. *PLoS Medicine*, **6**(10), e1000159. doi:1000110.1001371/journal.pmed.1000159.

Perry, H. S. (1982). *Psychiatrist of America: The Life of Harry Stack Sullivan*. Cambridge, MA: Belknap Press.

Petryna, A., Lakoff, A. and Kleinman, A. (eds) (2006). *Global Pharmaceuticals: Ethics, Markets, Practices*. Durham: Duke University Press.

Ponce, D. E. (1998). Cultural epistemology and value orientations: clinical applications in transcultural psychiatry. In *Clinical Methods in Transcultural Psychiatry*, ed. S. O. Okpaku. Washington, DC: American Psychiatric Press, pp. 69–87.

Raimundo Oda, A. M., Banzato, C. E. and Dalgalarrondo, P. (2005). Some origins of cross-cultural psychiatry. *Historical Psychiatry*, **16**(62 Pt 2), 155–169.

Read, U. (2012). 'I want the one that will heal me completely so it won't come back again': the limits of antipsychotic medication in rural Ghana. *Transcultural Psychiatry*, **49**(3–4), 438–460.

Rivers, W. H. R. (1918). The repression of war experience. Proceedings of the Royal Society of Medicine 11. Section on Psychiatry.

Rivers, W. H. R. (1924). *Medicine, Magic, and Religion*. New York: Harcourt, Brace.

Robben, A. C. G. M. and Suarez-Orozco, M. M. (eds) (2000). *Cultures under Siege: Collective Violence and Trauma*. Cambridge/New York: Cambridge University Press.

Rogier, L. H. (1999). Methodological sources of cultural insensitivity in mental health research. *American Psychologist*, **54**(6), 424–433.

Rousseau, C. (1995). The mental health of refugee children. *Psychiatric Research Review*, **32**(3), 299–331.

Rousseau, C., Perreault, M. and Leichner, P. (1995). Residents' perceptions of transcultural psychiatric practice. *Special Issue: International Perspectives in the Care of the Severely Mentally Ill*, **31**(1), 73–85.

Sajatovic, M., Davies, M., Bauer, M. *et al.* (2005). Attitudes regarding the collaborative practice model and treatment adherence among individuals with bipolar disorder. *Comprehensive Psychiatry*, **46**, 272–277.

Sapir, E. (1932). Cultural anthropology and psychiatry. *The Journal of Abnormal and Social Psychology*, **27**(3), 229.

Sapir, E. (1938). Why cultural anthropology needs the psychiatrist. *Psychiatry*, **1**(1), 7–12.

Sartorius, N. (1988). International perspectives of psychiatric classification. *British Journal of Psychiatry*, **152**(Supplement 1), 9–14.

Sartorius, N. (1990). *Sources and Traditions of Classification in Psychiatry*. Toronto: Hogrefe & Huber.

Sartorius, N. (1991). The classification of mental disorders in the Tenth Revision of the International Classification of Diseases. *European Psychiatry*, **6**(6), 315–322.

Sartorius, N., Jablensky, A. and Shapiro, R. (1977). Two-year follow-up of the patients included in the WHO International Pilot Study of Schizophrenia. *Psychological Medicine*, **7**(03), 529–541.

Sartorius, N., Kaelber, C. T., Cooper, J. E. *et al.* (1993). Progress toward achieving a common language in psychiatry: results from the field trial of the clinical guidelines accompanying the WHO classification of mental and behavioral disorders in ICD-10. *Archives of General Psychiatry*, **50**(2), 115–124.

Sartorius, N., Ustun, T. B., Korten, A., Cooper, J. E. and Van Drimmelen, J. (1995). Progress toward achieving a common language in psychiatry: II. Results from the international field trials of the ICD-10 Diagnostic Criteria for Research for mental and behavioral disorders. *American Journal of Psychiatry*, **152**(10), 1427–1437.

Seeley, K. M. (2000). *Cultural Psychotherapy: Working with Culture in the Clinical Encounter*. Lanham, MD: Jason Aronson (a division of Rowman and Littlefield Publishing Group).

Sethi, S., Bhargava, S. C. and Shirpa, V. (2003). Cross-cultural psychiatry at cross-roads. *Journal of Personality and Clinical Studies*, **19**(1), 103–106.

Simons, R. C. and Hughes, C. (eds) (1985). *The Culture-Bound Syndromes: Folk Illnesses of Psychiatric and Anthropological Interest*. Dordrecht: Reidel.

Skultans, V. (1991). Anthropology and psychiatry: the uneasy alliance. *Transcultural Psychiatric Research Review*, **28**(1), 5–24.

Skultans, V. and Cox, J. (eds) (2000). *Anthropological Approaches to Psychological Medicine: Crossing Bridges*. London, Jessica Kingsley Publishers.

Stix, G. (1996). Listening to culture: psychiatry takes a leaf from anthropology. *Scientific American*, January, 16–21.

Storck, M., Csordas, T. J. and Strauss, M. (2000). Depressive illness and Navajo healing. *Medical Anthropology Quarterly*, **14**(4), 571–597.

Sullivan, H. S. (1940). Conceptions of modern psychiatry: the first William Alanson White memorial lectures. *Psychiatry* 3(1), 1–117.

Sullivan, H. S. (1964). *The Fusion of Psychiatry and Social Science*, vol. **603**. New York: Norton.

Swartz, L. (1996). Culture and mental health in the Rainbow Nation: transcultural psychiatry in a changing South Africa. *Transcultural Psychiatric Research Review*, **33**(2), 119–136.

Swartz, L. (1998). *Culture and Mental Health. A Southern African View*. Cape Town: Oxford University Press.

Trani, J.-F., Bakhshi, P. and Kuhlberg, J. (2015). Mental illness, poverty and stigma in India: a case–control study. *BMJ Open*, 5(2), e006355.

Tseng, W.-S. and Streltzer, J. (eds) (2001). *Culture and Psychotherapy: A Guide to Clinical Practice*. Washington, DC: American Psychiatric Press.

Vaughn, C. E. and Leff, J. (1976). The influence of family and social factors on the course of psychiatric illness: a comparison of schizophrenic and depressed neurotic patients. *British Journal of Psychiatry* 129, 125–137.

Vaughn, C. E., Snyder, K. S., Jones, S., Freeman, W. B. and Falloon, I. R. (1984). Family factors in schizophrenic relapse: replication in California of British research on expressed emotion. *Archives of General Psychiatry*, 41(12), 1169–1177.

Ventriglio, A. and Bhugra, D. (2015). Migration, trauma and resilience. In *Trauma and Migration*, ed.

M. Schouler-Ocak. Cham: Springer International Publishing, pp. 69–79.

Whyte, S. R., van der Geest, S. and Hardon, A. (2002). *Social Lives of Medicines*. Cambridge: Cambridge University Press.

Wittkower, E. D. and Wintrob, R. (1969). Developments in Canadian transcultural psychiatry. *Canada's Mental Health*, 17(3–4), 21–27.

Woods, A., Romme, M., McCarthy-Jones, S., Escher, S. and Dillon, J. (2013). Special edition: voices in a positive light. *Psychosis* 5(3), 213–215.

World Health Organization (2014). *Social Determinants of Mental Health*. Geneva, Switzerland.

Yager, J., Chang, C. and Karno, M. (1989). Teaching transcultural psychiatry. *Academic Psychiatry*, 13(3), 164–171.

Young, A. (1995). *The Harmony of Illusions: Inventing Posttraumatic Stress Disorder*. Princeton, NJ: Princeton University Press.

Suicide, Violence and Culture

Michel Tousignant and Arlene Laliberté

Editors' Introduction

Suicide and violence are both culturally determined and influenced. There is considerable evidence that rates of suicide vary dramatically across nations, and cultures deal with these acts in different manners. There is debate that the variations may well be a result of biological causes. The relationship between mental illness and suicide also varies. In some cultures, such as China and Sri Lanka, the rates of suicide are very high, but the rates of mental illness among those committing suicide are not. This variation has been noted across different aboriginal groups within the same country indicating that social and cultural factors may be important. Social factors such as education, employment, high aspirations and poverty, along with stressors such as life events, may play a role. In some societies, the act of suicide remains illegal; therefore it is impossible to get accurate rates of suicide. Violence is related to a number of similar factors and globalization and urbanization may play an important role. Gender differences in suicide and violence vary too.

In this chapter, Tousignant and Laliberté propose that the national and gender differences in suicide and violence are culturally determined. Marital conflicts and relationship problems with in-laws are common causes of domestic violence and dowry deaths are sometimes passed off as suicide or accidental deaths. Embedded within these acts are the gender role and gender-role expectations. The socio-cultural model these authors put forward is important in understanding vulnerability factors, which are more likely to be specific for specific groups; for example, the symbolic violence towards vulnerable individuals, especially in the underclass, who are often denied their rights, face prejudice and rejection, and thus get into a downward spiral of self-destruction. The lessons for policy makers are many, and empowering vulnerable individuals is an important first step.

Introduction

The analysis of suicide brings new challenges to cross-cultural studies of mental health. Suicide is not, as such, a mental illness, despite the fact that some of its related behaviours are considered symptoms of depression and borderline personality disorder. All the studies based on the psychological autopsy method around the world report a high association between suicide and psychiatric morbidity or comorbidity (Pouliot and DeLeo, 2006). Before generalizing on the extent of the association, we need more conclusive studies, especially from India and China. In countries with a high rate of suicide such as China (Zhang *et al.*, 2002) or Sri Lanka (Marecek, 1998), local psychiatrists are not ready to corroborate that suicide is as highly related to mental illness as is the case in Western countries.

If suicide is related to known factors of mental illness such as poverty, recent life events, alcohol and drug abuse, impulsivity and hopelessness, to name the main ones only, there are central questions raised by the important variations found between countries and, within a single country, between different ethnic groups. There are also wide differences between countries. Many Muslim countries report rates near zero per 100,000 population, whereas other countries present rates for both sexes near or above 30 such as the Republic of Korea (36.8), Lithuania (33.5) and Sri Lanka (29.2) (WHO, 2016).

National Differences

Hypotheses are needed to explain the wide national differences. Durkheim's theory (1897) is still a basic reference in the field but is unsatisfactory to account for the numerous data collected during the century after his work. The main limitation of this theory, beyond its lack of operationalization, is the aggregate approach which is now accepted as a good preliminary tool for exploring new ideas but as a less valid one than the study of individual records, especially in the form of the psychological autopsy as proposed by Shneidman (2004). A good cultural explanation should also go beyond archived information and be based on more clinical and ethnological data. Unfortunately, there are few such studies. Mental health investigators have generally been reluctant to invest in ethnological studies or been insufficiently trained in this area, whereas anthropologists have been rarely involved in epidemiological studies of suicide.

There is certainly no unique model able to explain suicide in general or the cultural variations of suicide across the planet. A good methodological starting point is not to concentrate on national data but to focus attention on these high-risk groups within a nation which account for a large part of the variance of suicide. To paraphrase H. B. M. Murphy (1982), the important question is to identify which groups have higher rates and under which circumstances. Whenever possible, the comparative approach should be completed with a historical study of trends. Many groups with high rates of suicide today were relatively immune one generation ago. Children may take their life, but not their parents; the husbands but not the wives; or relatively more young women in some countries.

The thesis proposed in this chapter is that a sub-group with a high suicide rate within a culture is often a category with a declining or low status, or getting more aware that its rights are thwarted, and unable to build a social identity of outcasts or otherwise. The members of the category committing suicide are also likely to be the object of internal aggression or rejection within the clan or the family and, at the same time, unable to externally express their frustration through legitimate cultural channels or through marginal organizations. This model can throw some light on some of the most spectacular variations noticed in the recent literature. In order to illustrate this model, we will restrict the overview to in-depth analyses of cases where there is information on cultural changes and family dynamics of individual suicides.

Canadian and South American Aboriginals

Many aboriginal communities of Northern Canada harbour some of the highest suicide rates in the world. Suicide among the aboriginal people of Canada is higher among the populations of the north, having been put more recently in contact with the shock of *deculturation* as opposed to acculturation. The age group of 15–25 is generally the most vulnerable. For instance, the youth suicide rate of aboriginals from British Columbia was five times higher than among the non-aboriginals during the years 1987–1992 and this trend was similar in many areas of Canada (Royal Commission on Aboriginal Peoples, 1995). In the United States, the suicide rate among aboriginals of 19 years old and younger in 1997–1998 was 9.1/100,000 compared to a rate of 2.9/100,000 for Caucasian Americans (CDC, 2003).

When older members of the aboriginal tribe of Central Quebec were asked why their generation had very rarely witnessed suicide while the phenomenon had reached an epidemic level among the youth generation, they responded that, in the old times, violence mainly came from outside, from the 'white' society, whereas now violence is a component of family and village life. This appears as a leading thread to understanding suicide in that community and, likely, in other parts of the world (Coloma, 1999).

In one aboriginal village of Central Quebec with a population of around 2,000, there has been more than one suicide per year (Laliberté and Tousignant, 2009). Most people committing suicide were below the age of 35 and one recent series was started by a young girl of only 12 years old. In the year 2003, three teenage girls committed suicide and a fourth one was saved *in extremis* by her sister while hanging in a closet. A long list of males in their late teens and their twenties has died after being imprisoned, or rejected by a girlfriend. Sometimes suicide is made in the presence of other people as when a man rolled under the wheels of a lorry in front of a children's playground. The phenomenon of violence is not restricted to suicide in this environment. There is a case of *amok* where a driver rushed into a crowd during a ritual celebration, causing many serious injuries. Fights with injuries are common among young men and the situation reached a climax after one homicide when the entire local police force quit and was replaced by an emergency unit.

A study of 30 suicide cases, mostly young adult males, with the psychological autopsy method using a member of the family as informant, provided the following results. Most cases (80%), predominantly males, had a serious problem of alcohol or drug abuse, a fact not far different from young suicides in the rest of Quebec. A majority of these men had also suffered from chronic neglect during their childhood, mainly while both parents used to go on a drinking bout and leave the home with the children unattended. Discipline was generally inconsistent with a laisser-faire attitude interspersed with outbursts of violence. Suicides were for the most part triggered by two situations. The first was the rejection by the girlfriend or wife. The peculiarity of this community was that the girlfriend was abusing the man in three cases, was pregnant in a few cases, or had been cheating with another man. At least in this sub-group, women appeared to wield a significant emotional leverage over men. Some of the men were living in the girl's parental home and had nowhere to go after being rejected. The other situation related to suicide was to be in police custody or being imprisoned and not visited by family or friends.

These individual observations have to be put in a more socio-historical background in order to understand how the situation has worsened to reach this level. What characterizes these aboriginal communities is first of all a long history of exploitation and discrimination by the 'white' society through invasion of the territory for the purpose of logging or building dams, of treaties signed under ignorance or submission, plus the christening by priests prohibiting the ancestral beliefs and rituals such as the use of drums and sweatlodges. Despite this power imbalance and the introduction of alcohol as a means of payment for furs, suicide was almost unheard of until the forced settlement in villages with Western style houses and home appliances. The goal was well intentioned: children had to be schooled. The dramatic changes in the means of production and income provoked a rupture between the generations. Besides, school brought other values possessed only by the younger generation but with little means by which to translate this learning into market jobs still lacking on the reserves.

Witnessing the rapid decline of their status as providers and of their ancestral culture, some fathers started to exert a desperate form of control over their children, at least in many families where suicide was observed. This took the form of domestic violence and, in some extreme instances, in incest gestures, either with their daughters or with their sons' girlfriends. In one village, the repeated transgressions of a paedophilic priest also acted as a negative model.

Altogether, many important social changes happened at the same time and contributed each in their own way to demoralization and internal aggression within these villages. They are self-evident and easy to document: high levels of unemployment and lack of a structured daily life cycle; introduction of hard drugs; presence of multichannel television programmes around which daily life is organized; disintegration of communal family life in the form of sharing cooked food; and overcrowding with an average of seven residents per house.

What many of these young people who committed suicide have in common is a history of family negligence and violence. At the same time, they belong to a new generation with rising expectations through the schooling process. But social promotion is at the same time hindered by a lack of jobs, most suicide cases being unemployed at the time of their death. Being the object of negligence and rejection during childhood, these youths are later under the influence of the rejecting girlfriends or in-laws. Besides, they have no institution or marginal group with a minimal structure to reorient their frustrations and energies. So, when under the pressure of a sudden shock, they cannot contain their rage and they tend to kill themselves within only hours of the triggering event.

There are, however, important regional variations in the aboriginal suicide rates. For instance, in a survey of British Columbia, 8 of the 29 Aboriginal groups had no suicide or very low rates whereas one-third of them had rates over 100/100,000, or approximately seven times the Canadian average (Chandler et al., 2003; see also Westlake and May, 1986).

Their hypothesis is that the protected villages have a much higher control over their local administration. Meanwhile, the Inuit of Nunavut have still to find a way to tackle the problem of youth suicide many years after being granted an important degree of autonomy in administering their territory. The political capital has to be transformed into social capital in order to tackle the internal problems of the communities.

A similar observation about variable suicide rates has been made in three regions of South America. In French Guyana, the isolated villages of the forest, mostly of Wayana origin, are much more concerned by suicide than the Kali'na villages on the littoral which have been progressively integrated to urban life (Géry et al., 2014). Wayana children have to leave home and migrate after primary school to complete upper levels of education. The villages have also to live in the proximity of the illegal gold miners from Brazil and to face the pollution of their rivers and sources of food from mercury. In Southern Brazil, the Guaranis-Kaiowa and Nandeva present much higher rates of suicide than other neighbouring Guarani groups (Coloma *et al.*, 2006). The destruction of the traditional family, poverty and the violence of the landholders, documented by assassination of local leaders in recent years as well as the invasion of their ancestral territories, have put a high stress on these communities, especially on young people. Another example of highly variable rates of suicide is found in the Aguaruna or Awajun community in the Jivaro territory of Peru (Guevara, 2006). These people, described as proud and with a long tradition of warrior life that allowed them to resist the conquest of the Inca empire, is much more affected by suicide than the surrounding groups. One likely source is the destruction of the way of life by what is called biopiracy, by the foreign oil companies, causing the radical transformation of the territory and the villages.

Aboriginals of the South Pacific

In the South Pacific Islands, many communities have also experienced a sudden rise of suicide among young men, originating during the period 1975–1980 (Rubinstein, 1983, 1987). The rate for Micronesia during the early 1980s was 48/100,000 and suicides were mainly among the 15- to 29-year-old group. Western Samoa had a rate half that size, but many suicides were apparently hidden by the family due to the subsequent shame, because the family was thought to have been incompetent and unable to cope with its internal conflicts (MacPherson and MacPherson, 1987). Cases of suicide were reported from before the modern period as a means to repair damage done to the family and restore its reputation by avoiding a public trial. More recent suicides by young people tend to take the form of revenge on the parents following frustrations by the most educated portion of youth. For a while, young educated men could immigrate more freely to New Zealand, but policy restrictions forced them to stay on the island and to confront a new generation of senior citizens created by the rise in life expectancy. To express their resentment, some of these young took poison in the form of herbicides in the presence of older people.

A similar phenomenon of rising youth suicide took place in the islands of Guam, Ponape, Gilbert and Truk during the same period, recalling an epidemic reported in the schools during the early colonial period (Hezel, 1984). Again, contagions had been reported in the schools of this area during the early colonial period. Hezel (1984) conducted an in-depth analysis of 129 cases in the Truk territory where he estimated that the rate of suicides reached the level of 30/100,000 during a 30-year period. Eleven cases were in children less than 14 years old, suicide at this age being a very frequent occurrence in comparison to Western countries. Interviewing kin, Hezel concluded that more than 60 per cent of the cases were provoked by repressed anger. The highest rates were found in the population with a middle level of acculturation and were not closely related with evident signs of psychopathology or alcoholism. A 10-year analysis of a community of 1,500 identified 100 persons with a registered suicide attempt and a key informant was of the opinion that half the adult population had in reality attempted to commit suicide.

Many of these suicides are triggered by apparently innocuous incidents such as a reprimand for singing too loud or the refusal by the parents to buy a shirt. The act of dying was not seemingly made with an intention of revenge as in Samoa, though there was a history of chronic conflicts with the family. The attitude was rather one of self-pity epitomized by the emotion called *amwunumwun*, to express abasement.

According to Hezel (1987), the modernization of this region provoked the break of the matrilineal structure organized around the authority of maternal uncles to replace it with the nuclear type of family (see also Hezel, 1984; Rubinstein, 1983, 1987). The wage economy had transferred the authority to the biological father, but these fathers had not learned to behave as fathers but rather as uncles. As the authority structure was cracked, children started to use suicide threats as a means to blackmail and control their parents.

Women in Asia

Men in most countries die two to four times more often from suicide than women. There are two notorious exceptions in Asia: India and China where suicide is more evenly distributed among genders. This should not be considered as an exception to the rule when these two countries amount to one-third of the world population and report more than half the total number of suicides (also see the chapters by Fortune and Hawton in this volume and by Portzky and van Heeringen in the previous edition).

The phenomenon of high female suicide rates is not new in India and Thakur (1963) quotes Shri Dhebar, a local congress president in the region of Calcutta, lamenting the situation in a newspaper release of 1955. A survey we conducted in Bangalore in 1997 with police officers making suicide investigations, nurses in emergency departments and focus groups showed that women had to bear more often than men the responsibility for their own suicide except in the case where they were persecuted by their in-laws (Tousignant *et al.*, 1998). Even when their suffering derived from their husband's bad behaviour, they were expected to suffer the pain and to patiently change their mate's behaviour. In the case of a male chauffeur who committed suicide while dependent on alcohol, his wife was thought to have failed in making him happy. A sociologist, analysing data from Pondicherry where men have a rate double that of women, underlined the general moral strength of women but blamed them nevertheless for divorcing their husbands and pushing them towards death (Aleem, 1994).

The case of dowry death is an important issue which has raised a long debate in the media as well as among experts. This type of suicide is found among young married women below the age of 30, and happens when the bride or her parents are pressured after marriage to continue to pay a dowry exceeding the family's financial capacity. According to one forensic enquiry, it accounts for one out of six female suicides (Khan and Ramji, 1984). Statistics from the Indian Parliament (Desjarlais *et al.*, 1995) point out that there were 4,000 dowry suicides in India in the years 1980–1990. Because this type of death is usually spectacular, the woman burning herself with kerosene or being so attacked, the popular press is prompt to report on the case. Two field studies quoted by Desjarlais *et al.* (1995) also concluded that around 40 per cent of female suicides were connected with domestic conflicts in the form of harassment, beating and even torture of the wife by the husband or the in-laws. In Pune, a large hospital with a burn ward admits numerous female burn victims daily with a survival rate of 20 per cent (Waters, 1999). There is a female police officer permanently on the ward to take the 'dying declaration' in case of future court litigation by the woman's family. In the population of Durban with Indian ancestry in South Africa, a statistical report included a rate of suicide of 40 per 100,000 among married women between the ages of 15 and 19 (Meer, 1976). A crime reporter from Bangalore mentioned to us the story of four daughters

in Agra who had committed suicide because their family was too poor to pay for a dowry. The problem is sufficiently prevalent in this country to have brought the Indian penal code to include a law preventing incitement to suicide. Waters (1999) reports three long stories of female suicide or suspected suicide in Pune where a conflict with the in-laws was seen as the source of the suffering. As the tie between the son and his mother is usually very strong, husbands often side with their mother or are shy to oppose their will when she is wrong. Sometimes, the dejected woman acquires more power after her death than before. For instance, a village woman drowned herself in a local well after receiving a threat from her mother-in-law and her suicide made later marriage arrangements among the in-laws more difficult to arrange (Minturn, 1992).

One pattern of dowry suicide in India fits a scenario where the poverty of the bride's family frustrates the expectations of the in-laws. Another likely scenario is the clash between the bride's assertive personality and the mother-in-law's bad character, as women are increasingly fighting for their rights as in the case of Ashwini in Pune (Waters, 1999). In this example, there was a march of militant women from Ashwini's natal home to her marital home. We are here in the presence of a case of protracted anger following harassment with little outlet to express the bad feelings and hopelessness to redress the wrong. In this regard, Bhugra *et al.* (1999), in a study in west London, found that Asian females who attempted suicide or other acts of self-harm held more liberal views than non-attempters and were probably more frustrated.

China offers a different picture to that of India. There are three times more suicides in rural areas in contrast to urban ones, and female rates are 20 per cent higher than male rates (Phillips *et al.*, 2002; Phillips *et al.*, 1999). The rate is 30 per 100,000 even in the absence of alcoholism or evident psychopathology in many cases. Altogether, 93 per cent of all suicides in China take place in the countryside. Certainly, the use of pesticides instead of drug prescriptions and the lack of emergency medicine contribute to this high rate. Though the phenomenon is epidemiologically very important, both the national authorities and even the local population were unaware of its extent until recently. An enquiry by a journalist in a village where many older women had committed suicide found that local people were not aware of the extent of the problem. It was not sheer denial of a secret, but the fact that these women had already lost their status and were quickly left to oblivion after their death.

The dynamic of power in the family structure in China is somewhat different from India. Men exert a patriarchal dominance both in external and domestic business and women still have a second-rate status as documented by the surplus of male babies at birth. Traditionally, wives and concubines were encouraged to commit suicide to show their loyalty when their man died. In the modern period, causes leading to suicide seem to be similar to the ones found in India. Conflict between in-laws is the major factor for young married women to commit suicide (Pearson, 1995).

The following case may not be representative but it opens a window on some cultural dimensions of suicide in China (Pearson and Liu, 2002). The material was collected during a series of ethnographic interviews and it happened in a family after the programme had started. A conflict quickly arose between Ling and her mother-in-law because her marriage was a love marriage against the family wishes. The tension went up and Ling insulted her mother-in-law seriously using the term 'whore'. The reason for the tension was that not only that Ling was not chosen by the family, but that she came from a village considered 'foreign', cultivating tea instead of rice and wheat. Ling tried her best at first but she soon became rebellious because of the lack of sympathy. The fact that she had been slapped by her husband after he heard about the insult contributed to isolate Ling even more. To make things worse, Ling coped by converting to Christianity and tried to free herself from the family by having a job outside home. In this case, the suicide was at a great cost to the in-law family, both in terms of its social reputation and the high cost of the funeral to avoid persecution by her biological family. As pointed out by the authors, this case is far from being representative, but it illustrates the power that excluded women can achieve through their death. This suicide is also a case of thwarted anger with no social or personal channel of expression.

Phillips *et al.* (1999) have been considering if recent social changes in China brought about by the economic revolution have had an effect on the high rates of suicide. The answer can only be hypothetical because valid data on suicide from before that period are not available. With regard to the theme of suicide among young women, the economic gap between rich and poor and the awareness of this gap through television may have had a major impact in the rural areas. Also, the weakening of family ties and increasing marital problems related to infidelity are changes with more impact on women. A case study quoted from a report described how Mrs Huan, a 38-year-old woman and her daughter, 17, both killed themselves because the father started to have an affair with another woman in another village and neglected his family. This transgression would have been met with strong community action and sanction in the pre-reform period, whereas nowadays the victims are left with their frustrated feelings. Another young woman of 19 experienced the abuse of her sister-in-law after her own father had died, and decided to find domestic work in the city and she likely became depressed. Finally, another young woman had violent arguments with her husband over her workload in the field before she unexpectedly took a very large dose of insecticides. Some of these suicides may be related to social change, but what seems to come out is the decreasing pressure of social norms in daily life, the lack of reference values in case of conflict, and the population movement towards cities. As men still maintain a higher status, women may be relatively disadvantaged.

One of the first published psychological autopsies in China (Zhang *et al.*, 2004) provided a more systematic analysis of suicide in rural areas. Despite targeting the total population and obtaining a 100 per cent rate of acceptance, only 18 of the 66 cases were female. Family dispute was the major triggering factor as perceived by the close kin. The social analysis revealed that these young women had a more constricted social life and had to heavily rely on the family for support. When the family failed them, there was little way out. A similar conclusion had been reached in a Chinese report quoted by Zhang *et al.* (2004). In an analysis of 260 suicides by young women, nearly half (121) followed a confrontation with the husband or abuse by him; another 13 per cent were related to arranged marriage and 30 per cent were consecutive to quarrels with in-laws, claims about chastity and other related issues. Numerous authors also recalled the Confucian attitude toward death and the possibility of starting a new life to avoid the miseries of this one.

The Period of Colonial Slavery

With a few exceptions for South Africa, Ghana and Uganda, there has been little information originating from Africa. The comparative work of Bohannan (1960) with the collaboration of anthropologists working in the field has concluded that suicide was extremely rare in traditional rural Africa. Two important historical publications have illustrated, however, that, under the rapid expansion of slavery in North America and the Caribbean islands suicide has been the object of much attention among the groups of African origin during the eighteenth and nineteen centuries. This historical overview helps, however, to better understand the contemporary period.

In her book *The Power to Die*, Snyder (2015) analysed suicide among slaves in America. Her sources were mainly the reports from European mariners transporting slaves overseas, the memoirs of the plantation owners and court documents. The Akan people from Ghana were reputed for their fearlessness and they considered the suicide of war prisoners as admirable while the Igbo from Nigeria were repulsed by the idea. But even those groups who had a negative view of suicide had their perception eroded consecutive to the depredations of slave trade.

It is difficult to prove that slavery was the cause of suicide because the material originates from the masters. Nevertheless, these testimonies served to promote the anti-slave movement of the nineteenth century. Even in the absence of reliable statistics, the evidence points to a causal relationship and to a complex picture. Added to the high rate of mortality from epidemics, the loss of slaves by suicide represented a heavy loss for the traders. It was sufficient for some of them to install safety nets around their boats or to devise an instrument, the speculum oris, well documented by the abolitionist Thomas Clarkson in 1786, to force feed those who refused to eat. There are also reports of slave owners mutilating the corpses of those committing suicide, by severing the head for instance, so as to prevent the contagion of the behaviour.

Suicide could be perceived as an act of rebellion because it deprived masters of their property. There is enough evidence, however, to think that the hardships of the slavery process were involved. Many women took their lives following rape or sexual assault, some slaves jumped into the sea while witnessing the bodies of victims of epidemics being thrown into the water. There was also a fear of cannibalism from the Europeans, a view confirmed by the observation that they drank a red liquid, in reality wine, confused in their mind with human blood.

Suicide was certainly facilitated by the belief that death could bring the slaves back to their land of origin or could reunite them with their ancestors. Slaves also envied the freedom of the dead.

There is some strong evidence from individual and collective stories that the violence of slavery was the motive for suicide. After a man was separated from his wife during the sales on boat at the arrival port, he killed himself the day after. A log book from a boat mentioned that, of the initial load of 602 slaves, 155 had died during the transatlantic trip, two-thirds of them from melancholy according to the author, because they had refused food or treatment. In 1786, nearly 20 slaves jumped from the *Enterprise*. When, in 1737, Captain Japhet Bird released the slaves from their chains upon arrival to disembark at St Kitts, 100 immediately jumped overboard, only two-thirds of whom could be saved by the mariners.

Suicide and suicide threats were common during the period of seasoning or adaptation to the routine of forced work on the farms. Conditions were so harsh that from one-fourth to one-third of slaves died during the first year of settlement. According to a West Indian planter, suicide was one of the six main sources of mortality. A nineteenth century report of a House of Commons investigation corroborated the problem of suicide of unseasoned slaves. One important source of suffering was being torn away from kin, friends and the land of the ancestors and this kind of alienation is recognized as an important risk factor for suicide. There were reports of collective hanging from North Carolina and Georgia as well as from the Caribbean islands where an owner found all his slaves hanging on trees when returning to a small island where he had left them. In the United States, numerous bodies of slaves during the nineteenth century were found without life lying in the woods, floating on rivers or otherwise dead from unknown causes.

It seems reasonable to conclude that the status of slavery was as important as the conditions of life in precipitating suicide. Slave owners had a different view, and for them the culprit was the personality of the Africans. But it appears from the reports that depriving human beings of what makes them human, their liberty, their homeland and their immediate network leads to a symbolic death that increases the will to die and therefore to take action to fulfil this desire.

Another historical monography from Luis Pérez (2012) vividly describes the ordeals of slavery in Cuba and the circumstances surrounding suicide in that population. He quotes a medical treatise by Francisco Barrera y Domingo providing a detailed picture of the experience of suffering and sadness leading to the will to die. There are also numerous reports in Cuba from plantation owners. An estimate dating from around 1850 concluded that as many as 20 per cent of all African slaves on the island committed suicide during the first year after arrival. The shock of adaptation seemed more instrumental than the extremely harsh conditions experienced on the farms. Few of those who died in this manner died after a period of 'seasoning'. There were also differences in the propensity to suicide found throughout Africa. For instance, it was among the Carabalî and especially the Lucumi of Yoruban origin that the toll was highest, and they were described as 'very proud and haughty'. They also accounted for a large proportion of the slave population.

Conclusions

At the end of this review, we can present suggestions to build a socio-cultural model of suicide. The purpose of this exercise is not to arrive at a universal model of suicide, but to understand some types of suicide specific to certain cultures. The only way to improve this understanding is to accumulate as much information as possible on individual cases of suicide within a specific sub-group and to understand what the vulnerability factors are which lead to suicidal behaviour. We also need to know about the presence of resilience factors in the community. The model should also apply to a variety of cultural settings including Western countries. In the reality of the large metropolis, those who commit suicide are mostly men on the margins of society. There are drug addicts and alcoholic males in powerless situations trying to regain their lost status by projecting themselves into a universe of fantasies; they are the mentally ill people who are without meaning in a world of values centred on self-determination and competitiveness. We also find them among men in jail or gay youth; in this last group the rate of suicide attempts is extremely high. Whole cultures are also submitted to a similar process as is the case for Inuit and aboriginal communities. Elsewhere, we find women in poor districts of China and India sharing an underclass status. In all these cases, we find a symbolic violence toward these individuals in the

form of denial of their needs and rights, prejudices, rejection, and a process of self-fulfilling prophecy. Exclusion and rejection in these marginalized groups will provoke rage, free-floating aggression and a deep feeling of lack of equity, leading to despair. Without support and compassion, or the possibility of channelling this aggression into a collective action by such means as structured activities for youth, political action, spiritual movements, which provide a collective identity to replace the fledging ego, isolation and meaninglessness will reinforce the temptation of suicide.

This mode of thinking brings a new challenge to suicide prevention. There is the imperative to heal and not only to treat the illness. There is also the requirement to listen to the suffering, with an attitude going against the social dynamic of exclusion and oppression. In general, suicidal persons are more in need of self-respect than emotional catharsis, not only as individuals but also as part of a collective self. If medication in the form of anti-depressants doubled with psychotherapy can be a useful strategy to cope with despair, this solution is not enough when a significant minority within a culture is alienated from the mainstream of society. A real prevention will start with the empowerment of these groups and a call for radical social change. This may not be regarded as the mission of the mental health professionals, but these have a responsibility to promote a collective form of assistance.

References

Aleem, S. (1994). *The Suicide: Problems and Remedies*. New Delhi: Ashish.

Bhugra, D., Desai, M. and Baldwin, D. (1999). Attempted suicide in West London: inception rates. *Psychological Medicine*, **29**, 1125–1130.

Bohannan, P. (1960). *African Homicide and Suicide*. Princeton, NJ: Princeton University Press.

Center for Disease Control and Prevention (CDC) (2003). Injury mortality among American Indian and Alaska Native children and youth – United States 1989–1998. *Morbidity and Mortality Weekly Report*, **52**(30), 697–701.

Chandler, M. J., Lalonde, C. E., Sokol, B. W. and Hallett, D. (2003). Personal persistence, identity development, and suicide: a study of Native and non-Native North American adolescents. *Monographs of the Society for Research in Child Development*, **68**(2), 1–130.

Coloma, C. (1999). Programme Mikon: La mortalité dans les communautés Atikamekw [The Mikon programme: mortality in the Atikamekw communities]. Unpublished research report.

Coloma, C., Hoffman, J. S. and Crosby, A. (2006). Suicide among Guaraní Kaiowá and Nandeva youth in Mato Grosso do Sul, Brazil. *Archives of Suicide Research*, **10**(2), 191–207.

Desjarlais, R., Eisenberg, N., Good, B. and Kleinman, A. (1995). *World Mental Health: Problems and Priorities in Low-Income Countries*. New York: Oxford University Press.

Durkheim, E. (1897). *Le Suicide: étude de sociologie*. Paris: F. Alcan.

Géry, Y, Mathieu, A. and Gruner, C. (2014). *Les Abandonnés de la république. Vie et mort des Amérindiens de Guyane Française*. Paris: Albin Michel.

Guevara, W. (2006). *El suicidio femenino Aguaruna*. [Female Aguaruna suicide]. Lima, Peru: Organización Panamericana de la Salud.

Hezel, F. X. (1984). Cultural patterns in Trukese suicide. *Ethnology*, **23**(3), 193–206.

Hezel, F. X. (1987). Truk suicide epidemic and social change. *Human Organization*, **46**(4), 283–291.

Kahn, M. Z. and Ramji, R. (1984). Dowry death. *Indian Journal of Social Work*, **45**, 303–315.

Laliberté, A. and Tousignant, M. (2009). Alcohol and other contextual factors of suicide in four aboriginal communities of Quebec, Canada. *Crisis*, **30**(4), 215–221.

Macpherson, C. and Macpherson, L. (1987). Towards an explanation of recent trends in suicide in Western Samoa. *Man*, **22**, 305–330.

Marecek, J. (1998). Culture, gender, and suicidal behavior in Sri Lanka. *Suicide and Life-Threatening Behavior*, **28**, 69–81.

Meer, F. (1976). *Race and Suicide in South Africa*. International Library of Sociology Series. London: Routledge and Kegan Paul.

Minturn, L. (1992). *Sita's Daughters: Coming out of Purdah*. New York: Oxford.

Murphy, H. B. M. (1982). *Comparative Psychiatry*. Berlin: Springer.

Pearson, V. (1995). Goods on which one loses: women and mental health in China. *Social Science and Medicine*, **41**, 1159–1193.

Pearson, V. and Liu, M. (2002). Ling's death: an ethnography of a Chinese woman's suicide. *Suicide and Life-Threatening Behavior*, **32**(4), 347–358.

Phillips, M. R., Liu, H. and Zhang, Y. P. (1999). Suicide and social change in China. *Culture, Medicine and Psychiatry*, **23**, 25–50.

Phillips, M. R., Li, X. and Zhang, Y. (2002). Suicide rates in China, 1995–99. *The Lancet*, **359**(9309), 835–840.

Pérez, L. A., Jr. (2012). *To Die in Cuba: Suicide and Society*. UNC Press Books.

Pouliot, L. and DeLeo, D. (2006). Critical issues in psychological autopsy studies: the need for a standardisation. *Suicide and Life-Threatening Behavior*, **36**(5), 491–510.

Royal Commission on Aboriginal Peoples (1995). *Choosing Life: Special Report on Suicide among Aboriginal People*. Ottawa: Canada Communication Group.

Rubinstein, D. H. (1983). Epidemic suicide among Micronesian adolescents. *Social Science and Medicine*, **10**, 657–665.

Rubinstein, D. H. (1987). Cultural patterns and contagion: epidemic suicide among Micronesian youth. In *Culture, Youth and Suicide in the Pacific: Papers from the East–West Center Conference*, ed. F. X. Hezel, D. H. Rubenstein and G. H. White. Honolulu, HI: East–West Center, pp. 127–148.

Shneidman, E. S. (2004). *Autopsy of a Suicidal Mind*. New York: Oxford University Press.

Snyder, T. L. (2015). *The Power to Die: Slavery and Suicide in British North America*. Chicago: University of Chicago Press.

Thakur, U. (1963). *The History of Suicide in India: An Introduction*. Delhi: Munshi Ram Manohar Lal.

Tousignant, M., Seshadri, S. and Raj, A. (1998). Suicide and gender in India: a multiperspective approach. *Suicide and Life-Threatening Behavior*, **28**(1), 50–61.

Waters, A. B. (1999). Domestic dangers: approaches to women's suicide in contemporary Maharashtra, India. *Violence Against Women*, **5**, 525–547.

Westlake, V. W. N. and May, P. A. (1986) Native American suicide in New Mexico, 1957–1979: a comparative study. *Human Organization*, **45**(4), 296–309.

World Health Organization (2016). World Health Statistics 2016: Monitoring health for the SDGs. Annex A: Summaries of the SDG health and health-related targets, Table A.10.1, available online at www.who.int/gho/publications/world_health_statistics/2016/EN_WHS2016_AnnexA.pdf?ua=1

Zhang, J., Jia, S., Wieczorek, W. F. and Jiang, C. (2002). An overview of suicide research in China. *Archives of Suicide Research*, **6**(2), 167–184.

Zhang, J., Conwell, Y., Zhou, L. and Jiang, C. (2004). Culture, risk factors and suicide in rural China: a psychological autopsy case control study. *Acta Psychiatrica Scandinavica*, **110**(6), 430–437.

Psychology and Cultural Psychiatry

Malcolm MacLachlan, Sieglinde McGee, Brendan D. Kelly
and Fiona Larkan

Editors' Introduction

Psychology as a discipline focuses on the study of human behaviour in different settings; its relationship with psychiatry in general has been one of healthy tension, even though biopsychosocial models of aetiology and management emphasize psychological factors as one of the three prongs along with biological and social factors. Psychology emerged in the Eurocentric tradition, even though mental illnesses and abnormal behaviours had been described for centuries across cultures. The relationship between psychology and cultural psychiatry has been infected by mutual suspicion. The suspicion is due to several reasons, including political imperatives on both sides. Cross-cultural psychology as a discipline aims to provide localized cultural perspective and comparative cultural perspectives, and is a relatively recent development. Psychology focuses on both the individual and their development, and the consequences in response to their actions.

MacLachlan, McGee, Larkan and Kelly emphasize that psychology focuses on the smallest unit in society – the individual – and on how the individual's life experiences and characteristics influence health, and the experience is seen as central to but not independent of cultural factors. The relationship between medical anthropology, medical sociology and clinical/health psychology is of great interest in trying to make sense of the practice of cultural psychiatry. Describing the development of problem portrait technique, which seeks to convey a likeness of a person's presenting problems through both words and images, is one way of trying to understand a person's inner experience. Some of these questions are fairly similar to questions asked while exploring explanatory models, and this technique gives the clinician a complete outline of causal factors that a more conventional approach to assessment may have overlooked. MacLachlan, McGee, Larkan and Kelly argue that the distinction between

disease and illness seems a useful one, and indeed one that bridges cultural psychiatry and psychology. Using depression as an exemplar, they raise the question of biology as a mediating factor. The relationship between psychology and cultural psychiatry has to be seen in the context of changing social and cultural nuances, both at macro- and micro-levels; and they suggest that both disciplines need to contribute at both of these levels.

Introduction

This chapter explores the relationship between psychology and cultural psychiatry. In so doing it focuses particularly on those areas of psychology most salient to cultural psychiatry. We begin with some definitions to try to present some clarity to the plethora of social science and psychology sub-disciplines in this area, as they relate to cultural psychiatry.

Kirmayer and Minas (2000: 438) state that 'cultural psychiatry is concerned with understanding the impact of social and cultural difference on mental illness and its treatment'. They identify three lines along which cultural psychiatry has evolved: (1) cross-cultural comparative studies of psychiatric disorders and traditional healing; (2) efforts to respond to the mental health needs of culturally diverse populations that include indigenous peoples, immigrants and refugees; and (3) the ethnographic study of psychiatry itself as the product of a specific cultural history. These paths reflect broader perspectives in the social sciences, to which we shall return shortly, but now we consider which aspects of psychology are particularly relevant to cultural psychiatry.

Psychology is often defined as the study of human behaviour. However, such a bland definition fails to acknowledge that 'psychology' has been understood to be synonymous with a predominantly Anglo-American perspective on human behaviour; characterized by a rationalist, reductionist and individualist approach to truth seeking. However, this is problematic, for such a psychology is, in itself, a cultural construction. Other psychologies, curiously referred to as 'indigenous', relate different conceptions of how human behaviour ought to be accounted for. Thus we need to acknowledge that there are different – culturally constructed – conceptions of just what psychology is, and how it should study human behaviour (MacLachlan and Mulatu, 2004).

Areas of psychology which might be considered to be of particular relevance to cultural psychiatry include social psychology, clinical psychology and health psychology, with each contributing to a broader understanding of how human behaviour influences health, broadly defined. In our understanding, 'health' here refers to well-being in general, and is not confined to either physical complaints or mental complaints. 'Cross-cultural' psychology (a perspective within social psychology) must always first be 'cultural' psychology in order for it to be meaningful. Cultural psychology seeks to understand how behaviour is influenced by the social context in which it occurs. It further acknowledges that this context is woven through particular customs, rituals, beliefs, ways of understanding and communicating and so on, so that distinctive patterns of behaviour are *cultivated*. Only by understanding how a culture patterns meaning can we be sure to know that the sort of things we might want to compare between different cultures actually have some similarity. Having established a meaningful similarity in the structure or function of aspects of human behaviour, it may then be enlightening to compare such behaviour in different cultural contexts, that is, across cultures. Thus good cross-cultural psychology should incorporate both the localized cultural perspective, and the comparative cultural perspective (Berry *et al.*, 2002).

Cultural Psychiatry and the Social Health Sciences

Already, it may be easy to confuse the distinctive contribution of psychology to the understanding of mental health, not alone in comparison to cultural psychiatry, but also in relation to medical sociology and medical anthropology. Figure 4.1 schematically represents the relationship between these three social health sciences. Psychology focuses on the smallest unit in society, the individual, and how the individual's life experience and characteristics influence health. This experience is seen

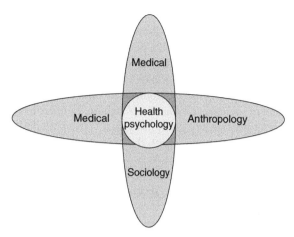

Figure 4.1 A schematic representation of the relationship between health psychology, medical anthropology and medical sociology.

as central to, but not independent of, structural and cultural factors. Medical sociology provides a wider, societal frame of reference, one that addresses why certain groups are more vulnerable and less well treated than others in a given social system. As a result of medical sociology's interest in the structure and inequalities of a society's health system, this is represented as a 'vertical' oval, which indicates that a particular health culture may be stratified at different levels.

Medical anthropology's perspective allows for comparison of the cultural systems that construct differing social and health systems, and therefore this is represented as a 'horizontal' oval, looking across societies. Although some might question the centrality that we have given to psychology, we feel that it is justified on the grounds that, whatever one's structural or cultural context, individuals operate according to their own health psychology. In fact, to put it more emphatically – everybody is entitled to their own health psychology (MacLachlan, 2006)!

Kirmayer and Minas's (2000) description of the three paths that cultural psychiatry has followed, noted earlier, may be seen to have approximate mappings onto the three social health sciences: (1) cross-cultural comparative studies of psychiatric disorders and traditional healing (medical anthropology); (2) efforts to respond to the mental health needs of culturally diverse populations that include indigenous peoples, immigrants and refugees (clinical/health psychology); and (3) the ethnographic study of psychiatry itself as the product of a specific cultural history (medical sociology). Of course, this mapping is only approximate and in reality many aspects of cultural health are relevant across these three domains.

Culture, which is itself a process, forms the implicit backdrop to many of the variables studied in psychiatry, psychology, sociology and anthropology. However, the clinician requires an understanding of them in some sort of 'joined-up' fashion. In order to be able to provide any given individual – from whatever cultural background – with the optimal care, we have not only to appreciate this backdrop but also to embrace it in the most conducive manner – from the perspective of the person seeking healthcare.

Figure and Ground

As long ago as 1935 Dollard was grappling with the problem of how clinicians ought to incorporate an awareness of culture into their practice. Dollard (1935) describes the individual seeking help as a palpable, concrete and real entity. The immediacy of the individual stands out against the abstractness and generalities of his or her culture. Thus Dollard notes that the individual always remains 'figure' while the culture is 'ground'. In other words the individual is seen as the foreground and the cultural context as the background. The difficulty is to appreciate the contribution of each at the same time. One can think of this problem as being similar to that of a reversing figure, where only the foreground or background can be focused on at one time, but both exist together and depend on each other in order to define their own existence. What we really need therefore is a way to see both – foreground and background – at once. Next, we outline how the cultural perspective can be understood, from the perspective of the individual patient/client presenting with a distressing problem. Understanding the cultural braiding of somatic complaints is an important challenge for cultural psychiatry. We now discuss the case of a man presenting with what might be diagnosed as irritable bowel syndrome, and we do this to illustrate use of the problem portrait technique.

The Problem Portrait Technique

According to Chambers' *Twentieth Century Dictionary* a portrait is 'the likeness of a real person'; it is also 'a vivid description in words'. The problem portrait technique (PPT) seeks to convey a likeness of a person's presenting problems through both words and images. First of all, we will consider the use of this technique

with words. The PPT is simply one way of trying to understand a person's inner experience.

The problem portrait begins with the person's description of his or her own distress, be it a broken leg, a broken marriage or a broken heart. Perhaps the first obvious question is how and/or why has the problem occurred? What is the cause of the problem? The problem portrait is intended to give an impression of the ecocultural context in which the person is living and in which the problem occurs. This means that we need to know the range of causes, which possibly relate to the problem at hand (Figure 4.2).

Clearly, the list of causes can be long and their excavation requires careful and sensitive interviewing. For some people, explanations for their problems, which arise though consideration of their ecocultural framework, will be easily discussed. In terms of a 'clinician as archaeologist' analogy, their 'social artefacts' are buried just below the surface. Yet for others their social constructions of reality may be much further below the surface, lodged in various strata of uncertainties or unwillingness to speak about things that you and I may not understand and may possibly even ridicule.

To conclude the investigation of possible causes and to appreciate something of the client's expectations of the consultation, he is asked: 'What do you think that most GPs would say about the cause of your problem?' (Note that the client is not being asked to predict what his own GP is going to say – referring to 'most GPs' retains some 'distance'.) This gives us a range of possible alternative causes to work with. The PPT presents the clinician with a complex outline of causal factors that a more conventional approach to assessment would have overlooked. However, those tempted towards a 'simpler' form of assessment – identifying the 'main' or 'real' cause – will simply be operating out of ignorance. If such complexity exists, it is always better to know about it, even if it does not make your job any easier! For each cause given, it is important that the clinician understands its rationale.

Although we now have a sort of 'word map', or picture, of the ecocultural context in which the client is experiencing his problems, we have yet to identify what is 'figure' (foreground) and what is 'ground' (background) from his own perspective. The ease with which he discusses different causal beliefs may be no indication of this. We can, however, now ask the client to rate the causes that he has mentioned. This could be done in many ways but the recommended way is as

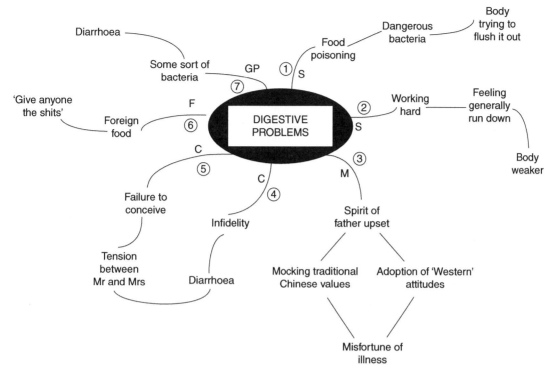

Figure 4.2 The problem portrait technique illustrating different causes identified by Mr Lim for his 'digestive problems'. (S, self; M, mother; C, Community; F, friend; GP, most GPs.)

follows. A brief description of each cause is written at the end of lines radiating from a circle (Figure 4.3). Each of these lines is the same length. Each line now becomes a scale of measurement (a visual analogue scale) wherein the strength of belief in each possible cause can be rated.

The further one moves along the radiating arms, away from the centre, the stronger is one's belief in that particular causal factor. The scale may be made clearer by the use of statements 'anchoring' each end of one of the radiating lines.

The client could now rate each of the beliefs described previously. We can also establish some measure of how tolerant of different beliefs he is. If each of the lines radiating from the centre is made the same length (say, 5 cm) then where the 'X' is placed on each line constitutes a relative ranking of the different causal factors. However, most importantly this ranking is not presented in a linear context but in the context of multiple comparisons. There are significant advantages of the attributes of measurement when it comes to statistical analysis. Statistical analysis will not be necessary for the majority of clinicians, however, who simply wish to use the PPT to gain an impression of the range of causal factors and their relative importance.

What we have described here is the 'Rolls Royce' version of the PPT. Sometimes it will be possible to use the technique in its entirety, whereas at other times simplifications and perhaps dilutions of it will be necessary. Constraints of language, translation and time, to mention just a few, may prohibit the power of the technique. However, whether the version used is the 'Rolls Royce' or the 'Mini', the orientation adopted through using the technique should enhance the quality of clinical assessment and therefore the efficacy of the treatment.

Some may feel that, if we study one illness or problem in many different cultures, it is as if we see the problem from many different angles. Thus by taking away the cultural 'noise' we can reveal the true nature of the illness or problem outside its cultural context. This 'sterilizing' view sees the cross-cultural perspective affording us with a sort of psychological X-ray, penetrating more deeply to a common bedrock

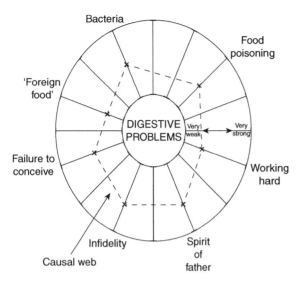

Figure 4.3 The problem portrait technique for Mr Lim's 'digestive problems' with the strength of different causal factors rated along visual analogue scales.

of human processes. Culture in this view is a problem to be overcome, a social construction to be deconstructed and outwitted, something that clouds the essential objective truth. An alternative view developed here draws on the argument that culture shapes social reality and individual experience, and that different cultures create different causes, experiences, expressions and consequences of suffering, be it physical and/or mental. A complaint makes no sense in a cultural vacuum, because its meaning cannot be accurately communicated.

Depression: A Classic Debate in Cultural Psychiatry

Depression is dealt with in detail elsewhere in this volume (see Chapters, 15, 17 and 19). Our discussion of it here is intended only to highlight the interaction between cultural psychiatric aspects and broader social science – and particularly psychological – issues. According to DSM (*Diagnostic and Statistical Manual* of the American Psychiatric Association) an episode of major depressive disorder ('depression' from here on) is said to exist when a person experiences either markedly depressed mood or a marked loss of interest in pleasurable activities for most of the day, every day for at least two weeks. In addition to this, the person must simultaneously experience at least four or more of the

following symptoms: significant weight loss (when not dieting) or weight gain, or a decrease or increase in appetite; under sleeping (insomnia) or oversleeping (hypersomnia); slowing down (psychomotor retardation) or speeding up (psychomotor agitation) of mental and physical activity; fatigue or loss of energy; feelings of worthlessness or excessive or inappropriate guilt; diminished ability to think or concentrate or indecisiveness; and recurrent thoughts of death or suicide.

Kleinman (1980) has suggested that the way in which people experience distress – such as depression – varies across cultures and at different times within the same culture. He uses the word 'illness' to refer to a person's experience of a disease. Of course, most of the diseases which affect the body are not observed at their source of action. Instead it is the consequences of the disease's actions, the rash, the limp, the lethargy, etc. which are observed. This 'illness behaviour' includes our physical and mental responses to a disease. For the moment it is the psychological component of this response to disease which is of interest to us. A key point in Kleinman's argument is that illness behaviour is the result of an underlying disease process and that this disease process may be expressed in different forms of illness behaviour.

This distinction between disease and illness seems a useful one and indeed one that bridges cultural psychiatry and psychology. It helps us to account for the admittedly vast array of symptoms associated with a diagnosis (of the disease) depression. According to the diagnostic criteria described here, two people may be depressed, but their experience of being depressed may be quite different. For instance, one person may have depressed mood, weight loss, poor appetite, difficulty sleeping and behave in a very slow and withdrawn manner. Another person, with the same diagnosis, may not experience depressed mood at all. Instead, they may show a loss of interest or pleasure in many different activities, gain weight, feel constantly hungry, over-sleep and appear very agitated. However, according to the DSM criteria their very different 'illness behaviours' are explained by the presence of the same underlying disease process.

The experience of depression within an individual can vary over time – commonly referred to as the disease course – and, as already noted, it can vary between individuals of the same culture – commonly referred to as a disease syndrome. Kleinman's suggestion that depression can also vary across cultures and across different historical epochs is quite consistent with a biological view of depression. He has also studied a condition known as neurasthenia (Kleinman, 1982). This condition, commonly reported in China, is characterized by a lack of energy and physical complaints such as a sore stomach. Kleinman has suggested that while depression and neurasthenia are different illness experiences, they are both products of the same underlying disease processes – depression. In other words neurasthenia is the Chinese version of the 'Western' depression.

Shweder (1991) suggests that this interpretation 'privileges' a biological understanding of how depression occurs. He points out a range of factors which can theoretically cause depression, including biological ones. Table 4.1 illustrates the different factors in what he calls biomedical, moral, socio-political, interpersonal and psychological 'causal ontologies'.

Kleinman believes that the ultimate cause of depression and neurasthenia is the same. This ultimate cause concerns the experiences of defeat, loss, vexation and oppression by local hierarchies of power. In Kleinman's view such 'socio-political' experiences produce a biological disease process. However, the way in which this disease is expressed is influenced by the culture within which one lives. Some forms of suffering – because they can be understood to provide a message, a communication – are more acceptable than others. In North America, for instance, there is a great emphasis on individualism, competitiveness, slogging it out in the market place, achieving, personal growth, realizing one's own (amazing!) potential, and so on. There is also a great emphasis on 'letting it out', on the right of the individual to openly express what she or he feels. This allows for the expression of depression as a demonstration of the individual's disillusionment with not 'succeeding'. On the other hand, in China, or so it can be argued, depression is not the 'right' form of suffering. In China, demoralization and hopelessness may be stigmatized as losing faith in the political ideals of 'the system'. Such a public display of disengagement is not welcome. Instead, a variety of symptoms consistent with fatigue, with being physically run-down, with being exhausted by the pressures of work may be seen as an acceptable reason for failure.

In summary then, Kleinman (1980, 1982) suggested that depression and neurasthenia have similar

Table 4.1 Different types of causes for depression

Domain	Factors
Biomedical	Organ pathology
	Physiological impairment
	Hormone imbalance
Moral	Transgression
	Sin
	Karma
Socio-political	Oppression
	Injustice
	Loss
Interpersonal	Envy
	Hatred
	Sorcery
Psychological	Anger
	Desire
	Intrapsychic conflict
	Defence

Based on Shweder (1991).

socio-political origins, which produce a similar biological disease process, which expresses itself differently in North America and China because the different cultural conditions favour different forms of expression. However, Shweder (1991) suggests that there is no need to say that among the Chinese neurasthenia is somatized depression. We might just as well say that North American depression is emotionalized neurasthenia and that neurasthenia is the underlying disease process, not depression. More important – and more challenging for cultural psychiatry – is, however, Shweder's questioning of the value of talking about disease processes at all. For him, the concepts of 'illness' and 'disease' do not add any value to our understanding of the relationship between neurasthenia and depression. While these two conditions may have similar origins in socio-political adversity, we are able to distinguish between the two forms of suffering. If there is therefore no need to think in terms of a biological 'middle man', then there is no need for either neurasthenia or depression to be the primary disorder.

Under contention then is the mediating role of biology in a causal chain that recognizes an ultimate (social) causal origin that culminates in a proximate personal psychological experience (depression) or proximate personal biological experience (neurasthenia). While the thinking of both Kleinman and Shweder may well have moved on, the dilemmas described previously are still central to the interplay between cultural psychiatry and psychology. For more on this topic see Kleinman and Good (1985), Kleinman (2004), and Lee, Kleinman and Kleinman (2007)

This assumed primacy of depression over somatic symptoms has also been explored in Banglagore, India. Weiss and colleagues (1995) sought to explore the relationship between depressive, anxious and somatoform experiences, not only from the 'Western' diagnostic perspective of the DSM classification systems, but also from the perspective of an individual's own illness experience. Their study used established structured interview schedules to glean both types of information from their interviewees who were all first time presenting psychiatric outpatients attending a clinic in Bangalore. When the same 'symptom' presentation was interpreted by the patient and by the DSM system, generally patients preferred to describe their problems in terms of somatic symptoms while the DSM system described them in terms of depression.

Weiss *et al.* (1995), commenting on their results, write:

> These limitations of the diagnostic system identified here appear to reside more with the professional construction of categories than with the inability of patients and professionals to comprehend each other's concepts of distress and disorder ... *Personal meanings* and other aspects of phenomenological and subjective experience should be incorporated into psychiatric evaluation and practice ... facilitating an empathic clinical alliance and enabling a therapist to work with patients' beliefs over the course of treatment ...

This seems to chime with our enthusiasm to explore individuals' own health psychology – their personal understanding of the relationship between their thoughts, actions and health, and how their social and cultural context influence these. Thus, whatever the presenting complaint, the belief system of the person who 'owns' the complaint has to be the medium for working through. The context of the presentation – not an abstracted diagnostic system – is what gives the complaint meaning. Without taking the context into account, clinically we can misinterpret the meaning of somatic complaints to be the

'masked' presence of cognitive distortions, low self-esteem, and low mood, and so on. However, we wish to acknowledge that our own views are not in agreement with some others. In a recent review of the literature on somatization, neurasthenia and depression in China, Parker, Gladstone and Tsee Chee (2001) concluded that the 'Chinese do tend to deny depression or express it somatically', a conclusion all the more remarkable for their acknowledgement that the literature is fraught with interpretative difficulties due to:

> the heterogeneity of people described as 'the Chinese' and due to factors affecting collection of data, including issues of illness definition, sampling and case finding; differences in help seeking behaviour; idiomatic expression of emotional distress; and the stigma of mental illness.   (Parker *et al.*, 2001: 857)

Lee (2001) claims that the Chinese Classification of Mental Disorders (CCMD) instrument has resolved differences between international classification systems and Chinese 'culture-related' disorders. However, in an article curiously entitled 'From diversity to unity: the classification of mental disorder in 21st century China', Lee concludes that 'Personality disorders are not common diagnoses or popular research topics in China because personality disorders are perceived as *moral rather than medical problems*' (emphasis added). Such a conclusion again seems to resonate with Kleinman and Shweder's debate on depression.

Ultimately, because all the categories in classification systems such as DSM are based entirely on symptoms rather than demonstrated biological abnormalities, the value-defining question for any given diagnostic category is: How does making this diagnosis help? What is the utility of reaching this particular diagnosis in this specific case at this time? Does applying this diagnosis deepen understanding for the person or their community, assist with the interpretation or navigation of reported symptoms, or indicate a course of action or treatment likely to alleviate suffering? All of these possible utilities are deeply rooted in the individual's own psychology and cultural context, and underline the wisdom of interpretative paradigms that incorporate both the health psychology of the individual and the evolving cultural context in which the person develops symptoms, interprets them, seeks assistance or support, and – later – defines their own 'recovery'.

The Psychology of Transition

Psychologists have a long-standing interest in how people adapt to stressful situations, and the stressful situation of cross-cultural transition has been a focus of much concern. The model outlined in Ward, Bochner and Furnham (2001) distinguishes an affective (how people feel), a behavioural (what people do) and a cognitive (what people think and how they perceive their situation) response to culture change. In this model the affective reaction is thought of as a response to trying to cope with a stressful situation, and an individual's personal coping characteristics are stressed as being important in their adjustment. The behavioural component relates to the notion of cultural learning, essentially that people need to have the opportunity of learning culturally relevant knowledge and social skills in order to be able to navigate their way through a socially quite different environment to that into which they were socialized. The behavioural and affective components of the 'culture shock' reaction are seen to be often mutually reinforcing, with positive affective reactions encouraging socially skilled behaviour and negative affective reactions increasing social anxiety. The third component of the 'culture shock' reaction, the cognitive component, is concerned with psychological processes involved in 'looking outward', e.g. stereotyping, prejudice and discrimination towards out groups (those not like me), and those involved in 'looking inward' such as identity formation and transition (see later). This overall affect–behaviour–cognitions, or ABC, model of 'culture shock' continues to be influential.

Ward *et al.* (2001) use the concept of cultural distance to account for different reactions to encountering new cultures, and to different degrees of 'culture shock'. Cultural distance refers to the extent of the 'cultural gap' between participants. For example, there is less of a cultural gap between people from Australia and New Zealand/Aotearoa than between people from Malaysia and Mexico, because in the former there are more customs and beliefs in common, than in the latter. Interestingly, one can actually have more 'cultural commonality' between people from elsewhere than between people from one's own country, e.g. those whose ancestors migrated to Australia or New Zealand/Aotearoa from Britain probably have much more in common with each other than with those who are 'native' to those lands, the Aboriginal people of Australia or the Māori people of New Zealand/Aotearoa. Thus 'culture

shock' can apply as much to getting to know your 'neighbours' as it can to migrants getting to know a new country. As much of the research on cultural adaptation has concerned migrants, we now consider this case in more detail.

Acculturation

'Acculturation', a related term to culture shock, refers to the process of transition that is brought about by the meeting of peoples from two different cultures. Such transition may occur in either one, or both, of the cultures. Increasing internationalism and multi-culturalism have produced a hive of activity in research and thinking on the effects of people from different cultures coming together. Berry and colleagues (see Berry, 1997, 2003a, and in this volume for a review) have been researching a framework of acculturation that considers to what extent the new-comer modifies his or her cultural identity and characteristics when coming to a new country. The framework is shown in Figure 4.4. It fits the situation of an immigrant well. Although this acculturation framework expresses the degree of cultural identity as a dichotomized choice, it should be thought of as, in fact, lying along a continuum. The framework (Berry and Kim, 1988; Berry, 1997, 2003a) has been very influential and can provide some valuable insights into cross-cultural experiences. According to the framework, a person decides whether or not to keep his or her original cultural identity and characteristics, and also whether or not to acquire the host culture's identity and characteristics (taking the case of an immigrant).

More recently Berry has developed the frame-work to take account of an important third dimension – the acculturation attitudes of the – usually much more powerful – receiving society. As illustrated in Figure 4.4 the same two choices concerning identification with 'own' or 'other' identity produces four dichotomized options (which again are in reality located along continua). When the dominant receiving society seeks assimilation, this 'mixing in' to the receiving society is termed the 'melting pot' (or 'pressure cooker', in extremes!). When the dominant group seeks separation from immigrants this constitutes their segregation. When the dominant group seeks to marginalize the migrant group, by not wishing them to identify with either their heritage culture or the receiving culture, this is termed 'exclusion'. Finally, when the

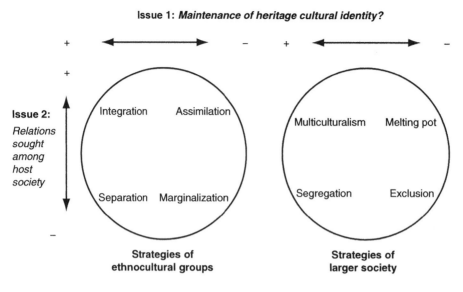

Issue 1: *Maintenance of heritage cultural identity?*

Figure 4.4 Acculturation strategies among immigrant groups and the receiving society. Adapted from Berry, 1997. (Also see Figure 16.1.)

Issue 2:

Relations sought among host society

Integration   Assimilation

Separation   Marginalization

Multiculturalism   Melting pot

Segregation   Exclusion

Strategies of ethnocultural groups

Strategies of larger society

receiving society seeks to become a culturally diverse society and recognize the cultural heritage of immigrants while also promoting their own cultural heritage, this is termed 'multiculturalism'. It is important to note that the two-dimensional model of acculturation developed by Berry and his colleagues has been challenged and continues to be a matter of lively debate (see, for example, Berry and Sam, 2003; Rudmin, 2003).

Health and Acculturation

Especially interesting from the point of view of health professionals is that Berry also suggests that the four different types of acculturation have implications for physical, psychological and social aspects of health, through the experience of 'acculturative stress'. Cultural norms for authority, civility and welfare may break down. Individuals' sense of uncertainty and confusion may result in identity confusion and associated symptoms of distress. In fact Berry and Kim (1988), reviewing the literature on acculturative stress and mental health, have identified a hierarchy of acculturation strategies: marginalization is considered the most stressful, followed by separation, which is also associated with high levels of stress. Assimilation leads to intermediate levels of stress, with integration having the lowest levels of stress associated with it (Berry, 1994; Ward *et al.*, 2001). The greatest relevance for this sort of 'background' psychological analysis is in the possible interaction of these factors with what

might be considered to be psychiatric symptoms. Furthermore, the presence of psychiatric symptoms may push individuals away from preferred modes of acculturation and towards more stressful experiences. The consequences of interactions between acculturative skills and symptomatology, however, can be quite complex and sometimes counterintuitive. For instance, Bhugra's (2003) review of the literature on migration and depression – using language as a proxy measure of acculturation – found that 'acculturated individuals' are more likely to be depressed, than those with poorer 'host' language skills. Treating psychiatric symptoms without taking into account the broader acculturation experience may therefore be overlooking factors that are crucial in producing or maintaining these symptoms. Of course, individual therapy will not be able to adequately address the realities of economic segregation, prejudice and so on. In such circumstances cultural psychiatry should seek to engage with advocacy opportunities in order to influence the broader cultural determinants of mental health.

It is important to acknowledge that migration, and the adoption of new lifestyles and diets, as well as many other types of transition, need not necessarily be stressful experiences that interfere with health; in fact, they can be quite positive experiences. It is also important to note that 'acculturation is not everything'. Lazarus (1997) has argued that migrants, for example, experience a range of stressful demands that have more to do with changing contexts than changing cultures. Lazarus and Folkman (1984) see their own 'stress-coping' model accounting for such factors as loss of social support, the need to find new employment, etc., as an equally valid account of migrants' experience. Of course, the stress coping and acculturation accounts interact, the cultural backdrop constructing the meaning of stress-coping difficulties, and perhaps the ways in which these occur and the resources that may be accessible for dealing with them. The general point is, however, that perhaps, at times, migration can be over-culturalized (Ryan, 2005) and that culture therefore may be 'over-cooked' as the primary analytical perspective. It should also be noted that 'cultural identity' may be nested within ethnic, civic and/or national identities (Berry, 2003b).

There is a particular issue in relation to human rights, sometimes criticized as a concept imposed by Western countries on non-Western ones, and of limited applicability or usefulness in other cultural settings (Osiatyński, 2009). This area is a complex one (Kelly, 2016), but Kirmayer (2012), writing in the context of human rights, cultural relativism and psychiatry, argues convincingly that human rights provide a language for the oppressed to speak back to power in political and social struggles that cut across cultures, and that dialogue about the relevance of culture to human rights provides a way of addressing cultural difference as an element within the political project of extending the reach of rights to diverse peoples and societies. Cultural difference is, then, a tool for deepening rights discourse, rather than a factor undermining it.

We are also aware that the discourse around culture and rights should extend to other aspects of diversity and that both psychology and cultural psychiatry need to extend their reach into influencing policy in order to inform priorities and resource allocation. Based on the simple premise that 'There is nothing more unequal than the equal treatment of unequal people' (Thomas Jefferson) we have developed two policy instruments that seek to assess the extent to which vulnerable/marginalized groups and core concepts of human rights are incorporated in existing health and welfare policies: EquiFrame (Amin et al., 2011; Mannan et al., 2011) assesses this in terms of what is actually written in the policies; while EquIPP (Huss and MacLachlan, 2016) assesses the extent to which vulnerable and marginalized groups are actually included in the development and evaluation of the policies that affect them. For different people to have the opportunity of equivalent outcomes (for instance

from health services) they require inputs that are arranged equitably (to take account of specific barriers they may confront). We have used these instruments in a range of countries, contexts and cultures (see MacLachlan et al., 2012), including in the assessment of mental health policy in Namibia, Malawi and Sudan (Mannan et al., 2013). This last study found that while all three countries incorporated at least two-thirds of EquiFrame's 21 core concepts of human rights in their policies; Malawi included only a third of the 12 vulnerable groups in EquiFrame; Namibia included seven; while Sudan included all but one. Even though culture and context play important roles in shaping mental health, the stigma against the social difference that is apparent in many types of disability, including mental health problems, appear omnipresent (MacLachlan and Swartz, 2009). The social construction of difference and stigma are clearly important areas for both psychology and cultural psychiatry.

Practitioner–Client Communication

Any brief consideration of the relationship between cultural psychiatry and psychology is going to be necessarily selective and restricted, but should at least consider the nature of therapeutic communication, as this is such a culturally saturated medium. Radley's (1994) review of the importance of the healing relationship highlights the neglected area of the influence of faith in healing. We may talk of faith in the practitioner, and faith in the treatment, or the 'placebo effect'. The role of faith in practitioners is no less important than it is in the medicines. The actions of a clinician can be seen as having a placebo effect: the doctor's reassurance may make you feel better. Similarly the doctor's involvement in prescribing some treatment may give you greater faith in the treatment. However, without faith in your doctor, treatment or no treatment, your health may continue to be compromised. This presents us with a rather tantalizing notion, that of the 'placebo practitioner'.

What exactly would a placebo practitioner be? It would be somebody who looks like and perhaps acts like a competent practitioner but who does not have access to truly therapeutic tools (e.g. effective medicines, techniques or procedures). The theme of placebos and faith is highly relevant to health practices across different cultures. Within one culture the idea of the placebo practitioner is at the root of much professional rivalry. Alternative, or complementary, practitioners are often castigated as presenting themselves as having therapeutic knowledge but are in fact being inert. When we consider practitioners from a different culture, the situation becomes even more complex. We may well accept that people from their own culture have some faith in them but we dismiss the efficacy of their methods, e.g. we may not believe that the amalgam of various herbs presented by an Indian traditional healer has any intrinsic value in alleviating an illness, but we may acknowledge that the way in which it is prescribed does have a therapeutic effect.

Frank and Frank (1991: 19) have argued that 'psychotherapy's practitioners are almost as varied as its recipients' and that 'extensive research efforts have produced little conclusive knowledge about the relative efficacy of its different forms'. Furthermore, they state 'features common to all types of psychotherapy contribute as much, if not more, to the effectiveness of those therapies than do the characteristics that differentiate them' (Frank and Frank, 1991: 20). According to Frank and Frank, people are drawn to psychotherapy because of their persistent failures to cope, resulting from 'maladaptive assumptive systems' (or, how they understand their world), and consequently producing demoralization – *then people seek therapy.*

The shared characteristics of different forms of psychotherapy may include an emotionally charged, confiding relationship with a helpful person (or group); a healing setting; a rationale, conceptual scheme, or myth that provides a plausible explanation for the patient's symptoms along with a prescribed ritual or procedure for resolving them. The ritual or procedure requires the active participation of both patient and therapist, with this shared belief in the ritual being the means of restoring the patient's health (Frank and Frank, 1991).

These therapeutic elements pervade cultural psychiatry, psychology, traditional forms of healing and perhaps even the more biomedically mediated forms of intervention, such as IVF treatment. Frank and Frank emphasize that myth and ritual have important functions in therapeutic relationships. These include combating the patient's sense of alienation and strengthening the therapeutic relationship; inspiring and strengthening the patient's expectation of help; providing new learning experiences; arousing emotions; enhancing the patient's sense of mastery or self-efficacy; and providing opportunities for practice.

Frank and Frank do not set out to undermine psychotherapy in any way, rather they highlight that it is a culturally constructed system of healing which, in fact, has much in common with other systems of healing, not necessarily in its content, but in the processes it adopts. All healing is comprised of myths and rituals, and it is these elements that often mobilize the 'recipient's' expectations, hopes and commitment. In cultural psychiatry the possibility of distinguishing complaints from their cultural context, and the effects of interventions from cultural expectations, can be daunting and perhaps even counterproductive. Although the scientific method seeks to distinguish the 'active' agents in treatment from more 'common' factors across interventions, or from straight out-and-out placebo effects, the appropriateness of this is increasingly being questioned. Paterson and Dieppe (2005) have in fact argued that it is not meaningful to split complex interventions into the 'characteristic' (particular) and the 'incidental' (more general in the sense of occurring because of the mode of intervention rather than the intrinsic aspect of the treatment). They argue that elements classed as incidental in drug trials may in fact be integral to non-pharmacological treatments. Taking the example of acupuncture and Chinese medicine they note that the simple additive model of the RCTs (randomized control trials) is too simplistic and that therapeutic effects interact on multiple levels. They state that

> treatment factors characteristic of acupuncture include, in addition to needling, the diagnostic process and aspects of talking and listening. Within the treatment sessions these characteristic factors are distinctive *but not dividable from incidental elements,* such as empathy and focused attention.
> (Paterson and Dieppe 2005: 1204; italics added for emphasis)

They concluded that it is the underlying theory of a therapeutic intervention that should determine which elements are 'active' and which may be considered 'placebo', rather than a simple biomedical common denominator of therapeutics. This perspective has quite profound implications for cultural psychiatry as it is clear that in many healing processes (including non-Western ones) the healing agents, and the beliefs that surround them, may be distinct, but not necessarily divisible.

Returning to Frank and Frank's argument, such a perspective helps to shine a light on our own practices. Hubble, Duncan and Miller (1999: xxii), in their review of 'what works in psychotherapy', state

> ... we found that the effectiveness of therapies resides not in the many variables that ostensibly distinguish one approach from another. Instead, it is principally found in the factors that all therapies share in common.

These factors are the so-called 'common' factors. Importantly, however, Hubble *et al.* (1999) are at pains to point out – unlike some previous critics – that psychotherapy works!

Hubble *et al.* (1999) stress that different components of the psychotherapeutic process contribute to different extents to positive outcomes: extra therapeutic change (or what happens outside the consulting room), the therapeutic relationship (the common factors), expectancy or placebo effects, and specific techniques (e.g. empty chair, thought record sheets, dream analysis). They also stress that different sorts of psychotherapy work equally well for the vast majority of problems. These arguments are quite challenging for disciplines such as psychology or cultural psychiatry, which, while theoretically being open to relativists' positions also drive towards the pragmatic need to identify essential therapeutic elements.

Rethinking Culture and Pathology

Just what culture 'is', is becoming increasingly contested, as the notion of 'culture' is being used to explain an increasingly diverse array of social phenomena. MacLachlan (2015) has described a variety of ways in which 'culture' can affect people, in terms of both their health and their broader sense of empowerment. A taxonomy, that is intended to be neither comprehensive nor mutually exclusive, is summarized in Table 4.2; and serves to highlight the scope of cultural influences on health. To conclude, we briefly consider just one of these themes: cultural evolution.

Cultural evolution refers to the situation where values, attitudes and customs change within the same social system, over time. Thus different historical epochs, although being characteristic of the same 'national' culture (e.g. Victorian England compared to contemporary England), actually constitute very different social environments – cultures. Peltzer (1995,

Table 4.2 A typology of themes relating culture, empowerment and health

Cultural colonialism

Rooted in the nineteenth century when Europeans sought to compare a God-given superior 'us' with an inferior 'them' and to determine the most advantageous way of managing 'them' in order to further European elites.

Cultural sensitivity

Being aware of the minorities among 'us' and seeking to make the benefits enjoyed by mainstream society more accessible and modifiable for 'them'.

Cultural migration

Taking account of how the difficulties of adapting to a new culture influence the opportunities and well-being of geographical migrants.

Cultural alternativism

Different approaches to healthcare offer people alternative ways of being understood and of understanding their own experiences.

Cultural empowerment

As many problems are associated with the marginalization and oppression of minority groups, a process of cultural reawakening offers a form of increasing self and community respect.

Cultural globalization

Increasing (primarily) North American political, economic and corporate power reduces local uniqueness, and reinforces and creates systems of exploitation and dependency among the poor, throughout the world.

Cultural evolution

As social values change within cultures, adaptation and identity can become problematic with familiar support systems diminishing and cherished goals being replaced by alternatives.

Adapted from MacLachlan (2015).

2002), working in the African context, has described people who live primarily traditional lives, those who live primarily modern lives, and those who are caught between the two – transitional people. However, these 'transitional' people can be found throughout the world, including in its most 'advanced' industrial societies. Inglehart and Baker (2000) examined three waves of the World Values Survey (1981–1982, 1990–1991 and 1995–1998), encompassing 65 societies on six continents. Their results provide strong support for both massive cultural change and the persistence of distinctive traditional values with different world views, rather than converging, moving on parallel trajectories shaped by their cultural heritages. We doubt that the forces of modernization will produce a homogenized world culture in the foreseeable future (Inglehart and Baker, 2000: 49). Cultural differences may change, but are unlikely, it seems, to go away.

Use of the term 'cultural evolution' does not necessarily imply biological evolution in the sense that the fittest for the changing environmental niche will prosper at the expense of those less adaptive. Yet adapting to culture change within one's own culture may be every bit as demanding as adapting to cultural change across geographical boundaries, even when the changes within a culture are broadly welcomed (see for instance, Gibson and Swartz's 2001 account of the difficulties some people in South Africa have faced in making sense of their past experience under apartheid in the context of their current democratized experience). As regards the problem of suicide, this sort of analysis is not new, but is still not widely accepted. One of the four 'types' of suicide delineated by Durkheim (1897) included so-called anomic suicide, which was understood as resulting from the state of (the then, i.e. 1900s) 'modern' economies, and the effect they might have on individuals. In particular, dramatic and rapid changes in social structures (such as may accompany sudden increases in a country's wealth) may broaden an individual's horizons beyond what they can cope with, especially when such changes are accompanied by diminishing forms of traditional support structures.

This cultural evolution argument, along with aspects of cultural globalization and several other cultural themes noted in Table 4.2 have been incorporated into discussions of why Ireland has experienced such a rapid rise in suicide over the past 10 years, why it has such a high male:female suicide ratio (compared to other European countries), and its strong correlation with increased gross national product (GNP; Smyth, MacLachlan and Clare, 2003). There was a particularly strong relationship between male suicides (with most of these being accounted for by young men) and increased economic growth, as indexed by GNP, with an associated correlation of $r = 0.82$. Thus changes in the Irish economy, which were surely a hallmark of the 'Celtic Tiger', seem to be in some ways associated with changes in the rate of suicide, particularly among young men. This idea is supported by the subsequent stabilization of suicide rates following the economic recession that commenced in 2008, as Ireland's annual suicide rate fell from 12.2 per 100,000 population in 2004 to 10 per 100,000 in 2014 (National Office for Suicide Prevention, 2015).

The challenge for cultural psychiatry is to recognize, as Berman (1997: 6) states, that:

> culture is the nutrient medium within which the organism is cultivated. Suicidality grows, as well, when that culture is pathological … Suicidal behaviour can be designed to protect, to rescue the self from otherwise certain annihilation.

The interface between cultural psychiatry and psychology is in the domain of the individual's interaction with broader social identities, values and customs. To articulate this interaction requires not just recognition of the interplay between psychology and cultural psychiatry but also that with medical sociology and medical anthropology. Culture is not, however, simply a cloak which a person dons and which then determines their behaviour. Individuals are active agents who sift through their culture, not passive receptacles of it. Cultural psychiatry and psychology have to develop ways of working with people which recognizes this complexity, engages with individuals' right to their own health psychology and embraces the broader social and cultural context in which they live. However, both disciplines should also seek to not simply respond to the 'ills of society'; but to shape society through influencing pro-social policies that promote human rights and social inclusion, particularly for vulnerable and marginalized groups (MacLachlan, 2014).

References

Amin, M., MacLachlan, M., Mannan, H., *et al.* (2011). EquiFrame: a framework for analysis of the inclusion of human rights and vulnerable groups in health policies. *Health and Human Rights*, **13**(2), 1–20.

Berman, A. L. (1997). The adolescent: the individual in cultural perspective. *Suicide and Life-Threatening Behaviour*, **27**, 5–14.

Berry, J. W. (1994). Cross-cultural health psychology. Paper presented at International Congress of Applied Psychology, Madrid, 17–22 July.

Berry, J. W. (1997). Immigration, acculturation and adaptation. *Applied Psychology: An International Review*, **46**, 5–68.

Berry, J. W. (2003a). Conceptual approaches to acculturation. In *Acculturation: Advances in Theory, Measurement, and Applied Research*, ed. K. M. Chun, P. B. Organista and G. Marin. Washington, DC: American Psychological Association.

Berry, J. W. (2003b). How shall we all live together? In *Multicultural Estonia*, ed. M. Luik. Tallin: Estonian Integration Foundation, pp. 3–11.

Berry, J. W. and Kim, U. (1988). Acculturation and mental health. *Health and Cross-Cultural Psychology*, ed. P. Dasen, J. W. Berry and N. Sartorius. London: Sage.

Berry, J. W. and Sam, D. L. (2003). Accuracy in scientific discourse. *Scandinavian Journal of Psychology*, **44**, 65–68.

Berry, J. W., Poortinga, Y. H., Segall, M. H. and Dasen, P. R. (2002). *Cross-Cultural Psychology*. Cambridge: Cambridge University Press.

Bhugra, D. (2003). Migration and depression. *Acta Psychiatrica Scandinavica*, **108** (Supplement 4), 67–72.

Dollard, J. (1935). *Criteria for the Life History: With Analysis of Six Notable Documents*. New Haven, CT: Yale University Press.

Durkheim, E. (1897). *Le Suicide*. (Translated by J. A. Spaulding and C. Simpson, 1952 as *Suicide: a Study of Sociology*.) London: Routledge and Kegan Paul.

Frank, J. D. and Frank, J. B. (1991). *Persuasion and Healing: A Comparative Study of Psychotherapy*, 3rd edn. Baltimore, MD: Johns Hopkins University Press.

Gibson, K. and Swartz, L. (2001). Psychology, social transition and organisational life in South Africa: 'I can't change the past – but I can try'. *Psychoanalytic Studies*, 3, 381–392.

Hubble, M. A., Duncan, B. L. and Miller, S. D. (1999). *The Heart and Soul of Change: What Works in Therapy*. Washington, DC: American Psychological Association.

Huss, T. and MacLachlan, M. (2016) *EquIPP: Equity and Inclusion in Policy Processes*. Dublin: Global Health Press.

Inglehart, R. and Baker, W. E. (2000). Modernization, cultural change and the persistence of traditional values. *American Sociological Review*, **65**, 19–51.

Kelly, B. D. (2016). *Mental Illness, Human Rights and the Law*. London: RCPsych Publications.

Kirmayer, L. J. (2012). Culture and context in human rights. In *Mental Health and Human Rights: Vision, Praxis and Courage*, ed. M. Dudley, D. Silove and F. Gale. Oxford: Oxford University Press, pp. 95–112.

Kirmayer, L. J. and Minas, H. (2000). The future of cultural psychiatry: an international perspective. *Canadian Journal of Psychiatry*, **45**(5), 438–446.

Kleinman, A. (1980). *Patients and Healers in the Context of Culture*. Berkeley, CA: University of California Press.

Kleinman, A. (1982). Neurasthenia and depression: a study of somatization and culture in China. *Culture, Medicine and Psychiatry*, **6**(2), 117–90.

Kleinman, A. (2004). Culture and depression. *New England Journal of Medicine*, **351**(10), 951–953.

Kleinman, A. and Good, B. (eds) (1985). *Culture and Depression: Studies in the Anthropology and Cross-Cultural Psychiatry of Affect and Disorder*. Berkeley: University of California Press.

Lazarus, R. S. (1997). Acculturation isn't everything: commentary on immigration, acculturation, and adaptation by J. Berry. *Applied Psychology: An International Review*, **46**, 39–43.

Lazarus, R. S. and Folkman, S. (1984). *Stress, Appraisal and Coping*. New York: Springer.

Lee, D., Kleinman J., and Kleinman, A. (2007). Rethinking depression: an ethnographic study of the experiences of depression among Chinese. *Harvard Review of Psychiatry*, **15**, 1–8.

Lee, S. (2001). From diversity to unity: the classification of mental disorder in 21st century China. *Psychiatric Clinics of North America*, **24**, 421–431.

MacLachlan, M. (2006). *Culture and Health*, 2nd edn. Chichester: Wiley.

MacLachlan, M. (2014). Macropsychology, policy and global health. *American Psychologist*, **69**, 851–863.

MacLachlan, M. (2015). Health, empowerment and culture. In *Critical Health Psychology*, 2nd edn, ed. M. Murray. London: Sage.

MacLachlan M. and Mulatu, M. (2004). Cross-cultural health psychology. In *Encyclopaedia of Applied Psychology: Volume II*, ed. N. Speilberger. New York: Academic Press.

MacLachlan, M. and Swartz, L. (2009). *Disability and International Development: Towards Inclusive Global Health*. New York: Springer.

MacLachlan, M., Amin., M., Mannan, H., El Tayeb, S., El Khatim, A., Swartz, L., Munthal, A. and Van Rooy, G. (2012). Inclusion and human rights in African health policies: using EquiFrame for comparative and benchmarking analysis of 51 policies from Malawi, Sudan, South Africa and Namibia. *PLoS One*, 7(5), e35864.

Mannan, H., Amin, M., MacLachlan, M. and The EquitAble Consortium (2011). *The EquiFrame Manual: An analytical tool for evaluating and facilitating the inclusion of core concepts of human rights and vulnerable groups in policy documents*. Dublin: The Global Health Press.

Mannan, H., El Tayeb, S., MacLachlan, M., Amin, M., McVeigh, J., Munthali, A. and Van Rooy, G. (2013). Core concepts of human rights and inclusion of vulnerable groups in the mental health policies of Malawi, Namibia, and Sudan. *International Journal of Mental Health Systems*, 7(7), 1–13.

National Office for Suicide Prevention (2015). *Annual Report: 2014*. Dublin: Mental Health Division, Health Service Executive.

Osiatyński, W. (2009). *Human Rights and their Limits*. Cambridge: Cambridge University Press.

Parker, G., Gladstone, G. and Tsee Chee, K. (2001). Depression in the planet's largest ethnic group: the Chinese. *American Journal of Psychiatry*, **158**, 857–864.

Paterson, C. and Dieppe, P. (2005). Characteristic and incidental (placebo) effects in complex interventions such as acupuncture. *British Medical Journal*, **330**, 1202–1204.

Peltzer, K. (1995). *Psychology and Health in African Cultures: Examples of Ethnopsychotherapeutic Practice*. Frankfurt: IKO Verlag.

Peltzer, K. (2002). Personality and person perception in Africa. *Social Behavior and Personality*, **30**(1), 83–94.

Radley, A. (1994). *Making Sense of Illness: The Social Psychology of Health and Disease*. London: Sage.

Rudmin, F. W. (2003). Critical history of the acculturation psychology of assimilation, separation, integration and marginalization. *Review of General Psychology*, 7, 3–37.

Ryan, D. (2005). Psychological stress and the asylum process in Ireland. Unpublished doctoral thesis. Dublin: University College Dublin.

Shweder, R. A. (1991). *Thinking through Cultures: Expeditions in Cultural Psychology*. Cambridge, MA: Harvard University Press.

Smyth, C., MacLachlan, M. and Clare, A. (2003). *Cultivating Suicide? Destruction of Self in a Changing Ireland*. Dublin: The Liffey Press.

Ward, C., Bochner, S. and Furnham, A. (2001). *The Psychology of Culture Shock*, 2nd edn. London: Routledge.

Weiss, M. G., Raguram, R. and Channabasavanna, S. M. (1995). Cultural dimensions of psychiatric diagnosis: a comparison of DSM-III-R and illness explanatory models in South India. *British Journal of Psychiatry*, **166**, 353–359.

Spirituality and Cultural Psychiatry

Kate M. Loewenthal

Editors' Introduction

Religion and spiritual factors form a core of cultures and cultural identity of individuals. Religious taboos, rituals and religious cognitions affect individual functioning and this may well influence adjustment in other cultures. Religion/spirituality (RS) is a core aspect of self-concept and of coping. This determines social networks and social support systems. These values play an important role shaping not only identity but also underlying beliefs and behaviours. Religious and spiritual beliefs form an integral part of a cultural group and moving away from often unacceptable norms. The individual who develops mental illness may well change religion or may become more religious compared with others around them. It is entirely possible that in many low- and middle-income countries due to lack of resources the individuals and their families may seek help from religious healers. These religious and shamanistic interventions may well be more popular in traditional countries. This chapter looks at the place of religious and spiritual (RS) factors in cultural psychiatry. It looks at whether spirituality and religiosity need to be distinguished, at the role of spirituality in cultural psychiatry, at the distinction between RS and cultural factors in psychiatric illness, and whether we can generalize from the findings of Western, Christian studies on RS factors in relation to mental health, to other cultures. The chapter then examines how RS factors, in the context of cultural psychiatry, affect the prevalence of psychiatric illnesses – depressive disorders, anxiety and OCD, and psychosis. Gender differences in prevalence are discussed, and the role of RS factors in help-seeking, compliance, diagnosis, clinical management and therapy.

Introduction

The examples that follow here are paraphrased (and greatly abbreviated) from the original sources.

Indonesia: Belo's behaviour was difficult to live with. He beat up the children in his village, claiming they were 'bad', and he destroyed his neighbours' precious banana plants. He said Allah (Tuhan) had commanded him to teach the right ways of Islam, that he could see through objects, and he could see the future. Sometimes he said his deceased uncle Om was directing him. His neighbours sometimes found his bouts of craziness unbearable and dangerous, and sent him away or locked him up. On one occasion it was agreed to sacrifice to a Jinn, who some neighbours believed was really controlling Belo. The villagers accepted that many people go through periods of craziness, for example, children when distressed, or young people in love, and there was always hope that Belo would settle down.

(Broch, 2001)

Israel: Jonah's behaviour was also difficult to live with. As in other orthodox Jewish homes, dairy and meat meals are eaten separately, and separate utensils are used. But Jonah worries that packs of 'neutral' food, which may be eaten with either meat or dairy, may have become contaminated. Jonah's rabbi has been consulted frequently, and has tried tactfully to convince Jonah that he is going to unnecessary lengths. Jonah's family feel they are being driven crazy, but Jonah insisted that his actions are religiously appropriate and he does not need help. Finally, he was persuaded to seek professional advice.

(Greenberg and Witztum, 2001)

England: Ellen, a Pentecostalist Christian, was working as a psychiatric nursing auxiliary. She is a religious enthusiast: patients and colleagues tolerate her attempts to convert them, and to persuade them that Jesus will help them more than the doctors can. One day, she starts rolling on the floor, babbling incoherently. The psychiatrist who witnessed this wondered if she was practicing glossolalia – speaking in tongues – encouraged in Pentecostalism. When consulted, Ellen's fellow church member said that this was not genuine speaking in tongues: she was ill and needed medication.

(Littlewood and Lipsedge, 1997)

These examples throw up several important themes in considering spirituality in the context of cultural psychiatry:

- Religion/spirituality (RS) is an essential premise, and a core aspect of self-concept and of coping.
- Religious and spiritual (RS) forces are seen to play a key role in shaping beliefs and behaviours – including unacceptable ones.
- RS beliefs are an intrinsic feature of the cultural group, therefore difficult to distinguish from cultural factors.
- However, the sufferer and his or her social circle may have different views on precisely which RS factors are important, for example, whether Belo's actions were being controlled by a Jinn, Tuhan (Allah) or Om, or whether Jonah had gone too far with his religious scruples.
- RS beliefs influence the kinds of help believed to be effective and acceptable.

These themes lead to questions, and this chapter will discuss some of these.

Aims

In this chapter we will first consider several aspects of the relations between cultural psychiatry, and RS issues. In particular, we ask:

- Do spirituality and religiosity need to be distinguished?
- What role does spirituality play in cultural psychiatry?
- Can we distinguish spiritual and cultural factors affecting mental illness?
- Can we generalize from Western, Christian studies on RS factors in relation to mental health to other cultures?

Then we examine, in the context of cultural psychiatry how RS factors affect:

- the prevalence of psychiatric illnesses, including gender differences in prevalence;
- help-seeking and compliance;
- diagnosis, and decisions about clinical management and therapy.

Psychiatry and Spirituality: Some Issues

Psychiatry and the related mental health professions have had a long and sometimes difficult relationship with RS issues, and cultural factors are often deeply embedded in these difficulties.

We consider here the four previously mentioned particular issues.

Do Spirituality and Religiosity Need to Be Distinguished?

Religiosity is in itself difficult to define, given the many factors involved. Am I religious because I identify myself as an orthodox Jew? Because I believe in G-d? Because I am aware of G-d's presence? G-d's unity? G-d's support? Most authors would accept that religion involves affiliation and identification with a religious group, cognitive factors – beliefs, and emotional and experiential factors (e.g. Loewenthal, 2000). In recent decades, there has been growing emphasis on spirituality, as different or separable from religion (Zinnbauer *et al.*, 1997; King *et al.*, 2013). King and Dein (1998) argued that using spirituality as a variable in psychiatric research encompasses a broader range of both people and experiences than does the religious variable: spirituality is 'a person's experience of, or a belief in, a power apart from their own existence', a power is revered and sacred. Spirituality might be what all religious–cultural traditions have in common, and, contemporary commentators say, is an aspect of human experience open to those who do not identify with a specific religious tradition. Zinnbauer *et al.* (1997) found a number of features that distinguished adults who defined themselves as religious, from adults who defined themselves as spiritual but not religious. The latter were more likely to engage in New Age religious beliefs and practices, but were less likely to be engaged with the beliefs and practices of traditional religions. While levels of religiosity may be associated with higher levels of well-being (Koenig *et al.*, 2012) spirituality as distinct from religiosity may not be so reliably associated with well-being. For example, King *et al.* (2013) found that spirituality among those self-identified as spiritual but not religious (SBNR) was not associated with well-being.

This indicates support for the view that spirituality is possible outside the context of organized or traditional religion, but it is also a common feature of different religious traditions. When the term 'religious' is used in this chapter, this has the implication that spirituality is an essential feature. There are, additionally, practices and beliefs specific to a given cultural–religious group.

What Role does Spirituality Play in Cultural Psychiatry?

Spirituality has been problematic for psychiatry for two reasons. First, the 'demon problem':

> J has violent abdominal pains and insists that these are caused by bad spirits unleashed by a former friend, whose boyfriend has left her and taken up with J.

The person who believes that s/he is being persecuted by malign spiritual forces presents dilemmas for the clinician. How helpful is it to think of this as delusory? Would s/he be better off without a spiritual belief system, or is the belief system simply affecting the shaping of symptoms? Should spiritually based remedies be deployed? Is the person in fact suffering from psychiatric illness? A somatic symptom disorder?

Belief in possession by malign spiritual forces has been a long-standing problem in psychiatry. Lipsedge (1996) and others have concluded that, in the past, demons were not invariably regarded as the only possible causes of psychiatric illness: stress, fever and malnutrition were more likely to be seen as causal factors. Nevertheless, belief in malign spiritual forces as possible causes of psychiatric illness is probably culturally and historically universal, though stress and other factors are also seen as important (e.g. Pfeifer, 1994; Srinivasan and Thara, 2001; Wilkens, 2009).

There are two factors making diagnosis and treatment difficult: the conviction that illness may be caused by malign spiritual forces, and second, the positive symptoms of schizophrenia, particularly hallucinations and delusions, may be common among non-disordered people.

The 'demon' problem is only one way in which spiritual issues obtrude in psychiatry. The second set of difficulties is the debate over whether religion is consoling or harmful. The consolations of religion have been recognized by the provision of chaplaincies in psychiatric hospitals. Towards the end of the eighteenth century there were attempts to treat the insane humanely, and spiritual issues were important. But attitudes were as mixed as they were strong. In the 1790s, Tuke, a Quaker merchant, founded the York retreat, where prayer and religious devotion were seen as central to the healing process. In Britain, the Lunacy Act of 1890 ordered a church in every asylum, which the inmates had to attend twice a day. In France, by contrast, Pinel – who abolished chains for the insane in the Bicetre – insisted that the mentally ill should not be exposed to religious practices: it was felt that these might encourage delusions and hallucinations.

These contrasting attitudes and practices appear elsewhere. Thus Freud (e.g. 1927) spearheaded a movement which viewed religion as possibly crippling for psychological health. Recently, at a meeting involving mental health service users, one user complained that, although she and her fellow Christians on their psychiatric ward found prayer and Bible study very helpful (and indeed as we shall see there is scientific support for this), they were not permitted to organize ward prayer meetings or Bible-study sessions. The Christian patients believed that the ward staff feared that this would 'make some patients worse'.

There is some mutual mistrust, with religious authority figures suggesting that the 'psych' professions – psychiatrists, psychoanalysts, psychotherapists, clinical psychologists – are not to be trusted. For example: 'Psychoanalysis has effected no cures. Freud and his cohorts are charlatans and vampires that prey upon society' (Miller, 1984).

Neeleman and Persaud (1995), treading cautiously, suggest that RS issues are indeed outside the clinician's area of competence, and therefore best left alone in negotiating treatments. Recent years have seen less reticence. There have been widespread suggestions that RS issues should be taken into account in psychiatric and therapeutic practice (e.g. Crossley and Salter, 2005; Cook *et al.*, 2009; Pargament, 2011; Pargament, 2013).

Can We Distinguish Spiritual and Cultural Factors Affecting Mental Illness?

The question was highlighted for me when a psychiatrist commented that studying religion and mental health was the same as studying culture and mental health. King and Dein (1998) suggest that psychiatrists regard spirituality as 'cultural noise to be respected but not addressed directly'.

Works on cultural psychiatry normally offer much material involving spiritual issues, with RS factors subsumed under the heading of culture. Belo's story from the beginning of this chapter is one example.

To the observing ethnographer or psychiatrist, RS beliefs and practices may be seen as intrinsic to the culture. For Western psychiatrists, RS factors may seem distinct from culture only when they appear in patients from the same cultural group as the psychiatrist. But we can see from the examples that began this chapter that discussions about clinical management among the patient's own group often seem to involve strategies that are specifically RS. This helps to understand the importance for users of the RS sanctioning and origins of their behaviour – as with Belo and Jonah – and also the importance of the religious endorsement of clinical interventions. Understanding of emic perspectives is therefore important (Weiss *et al.*, 1992): Belo, Jonah and Ellen all felt their behaviour was spiritually inspired. Also, it was important for Belo to accept that the hen sacrifice would be spiritually valid, for Jonah to accept that his rabbi approved his psychiatric treatment, and for Ellen to know that her fellow church members thought she should have medicine. These behaviours and decisions were embedded in particular cultural contexts, but it is the spiritual dimensions that have special significance for understanding and clinical management.

Can We Generalize from Western, Christian Studies on RS Factors in Relation to Mental Health to Other Cultures?

There are two suggestions in particular that need airing. One is that religion has generally benign effects on health and mental health (e.g. Koenig *et al.*, 2012). This is a broad conclusion: some effects are null, and some are negative. Some aspects and styles of RS may be unhelpful. Outstanding examples have emerged from Pargament and his collaborators (e.g. Pargament *et al.*, 2011) on styles of religious coping that impact on well-being: for example, belief that G-d is supportive is helpful, belief that G-d is angry is reliably associated with poor outcomes.

Studies of religion and mental health have problems with research methods. Most studies have involved a cross-sectional design; most researchers have studied the relations between measures of RS and health/mental health at one point in time. This makes it difficult to draw conclusions about causality. Prospective studies would enable firmer conclusions, but there are (as yet) few of these. The biggest problem, in the context of our present concerns, is the narrow range of religious traditions (mainly Christian) and cultures (North American and other Western cultures). There have been only

a small number of studies of Hindus, Jews, Muslims and other groups.

So the first suggestion that needs examining in the transcultural context is that RS may be beneficial for mental health. The rich ethnographic material available suggests that findings from current research cannot always be generalized into other cultural contexts. It is possible that if and when spirituality is distinguished from religion, as in the case of those identified as spiritual but not religious (SBNR), the relationship of spirituality to mental health may differ from that of religion (King *et al.*, 2013), and effects may vary in different cultural contexts.

The second suggestion is that not only psychiatric but also spiritual support can be offered by a professional with appropriate training. This issue in culture-sensitive service provision is likely to become debatable in the future. Can, say a Christian minister, with knowledge and understanding of the beliefs and customs of other faiths, provide spiritual support acceptable and helpful to members of other religious traditions – Muslims, Jews, Hindus, others, even Christians of other denominational affiliations. This is contentious: members of some religious groups may be happy to receive some professional (i.e. psychiatric, clinical–psychological) mental health support from professionals outside their religious group, even if they have reservations about whether they are fully understood (e.g. Cinnirella and Loewenthal, 1999). However, they might feel that RS support needs to come from a qualified religious leader in their own tradition. Some chaplains may find that they can offer support to members of other faiths, which may be gratefully accepted, but this does not imply that this is going to serve all needs across the board, obviating the need for religiously specific support.

Having reviewed these preliminary issues – whether spirituality and religion need to be distinguished, the varied role played in psychiatry by RS issues, the difficulty of distinguishing spiritual and cultural factors, and generalizability of research on Western Christians to other groups – we now turn to examine the ways in which RS might affect prevalence, help-seeking and compliance, and diagnosis and decisions about clinical management.

Prevalence

Cultural and spiritual/religious factors may affect prevalence and referral rates for different conditions.

Depression

Overall, there is a reliable association between higher religiosity and lower levels of depression (e.g. Loewenthal, 2007; Koenig *et al.*, 2012). There are some aspects of religiosity that are exceptions to this general tendency, but a number of features of religion have now been identified that are likely to play a causal role in ameliorating or preventing depression. These include:

- Religiously based coping beliefs (Loewenthal *et al.*, 2000; Ano and Vasconelles, 2005; Pargament *et al.*, 2011; Koenig *et al.*, 2012) particularly the belief that G-d is benign and supportive.
- Social support – warm and confiding relationships, esteem, practical help, and companionship are all encouraged among religious groups (e.g. Nooney and Woodrum, 2002; Inaba and Loewenthal, 2009).
- Reduced stress, of the type that could cause depression (e.g. Loewenthal *et al.*, 1997).
- Positive mood states, many of which are religiously encouraged, play a role in reducing depressive mood and illness. These include purpose in life, joy, optimism and forgiveness (Seligman, 2002; Joseph *et al.*, 2006).

The main aspects of religion which may foster depression are first, beliefs that G-d is punishing, vengeful or simply indifferent (Pargament, 1997; Ano and Vasconelles, 2005; Pargament *et al.*, 2011), and second, situations in which religious forces encourage persecution, warfare and other horrific circumstances. However, it remains unclear whether these horrors are more likely to be encouraged in the name of religion than they are in the name of some non-religious ideology, such as socialist justice, liberty, equality and fraternity, or a Great Leap Forward. Prevalence and referral for depression are often greater among women than among men (Keyes and Goodman, 2006). Religion may be implicated here.

Religion may be perceived as supportive of the abuse of women, leading to depression. For example, married women in some cultures may have no property rights and may even be regarded as the property of their husband's families, leading to their entrapment and depression. Domestic violence against women is practised in many cultures, often with no protest from religious authorities and sometimes tacit support. Female genital mutilation (FGM) is practised in parts of Africa and the Middle East, and among immigrants to the West, especially in Muslim communities, although Muslim scholars deny that this practice is religiously authorized. Female genital mutilation has severe consequences for physical and psychological health (Loewenthal, 2013).

Gender may interact with religiously supported lifestyle factors, such as alcohol use, which impact on depression. Alcohol is used more frequently by men than by women, and in moderation it may have an anti-depressant effect. The alcohol–depression hypothesis suggests that societies in which men are as likely to be depressed as women are ones in which depression (particularly men's) is not masked by alcohol use and abuse (Loewenthal *et al.*, 2003, Loewenthal, 2009).

The overall effect in most studies is a reduced likelihood of depressed mood and illness among the religiously active, but further transcultural investigation is needed.

Anxiety and Obsessive–Compulsive Disorder

There seem to be two important and conflicting effects. First, spirituality and religious commitment are usually associated with feelings of obligation to perform religious duties. Earlier commentators, notably Freud (1907) commented that this relieved guilt, but it has become more apparent that spiritual satisfaction is an important factor. This might involve scrupulosity with regard to diet, religiously prescribed cleanliness, or caring for others, for example. Some work has indicated that religiosity is associated with higher levels of subclinical anxiety and obsessionality (Lewis, 1998). However, *clinical* levels of anxiety and obsessive–compulsive disorder are not more likely among the religiously active, though cultural–religious context can affect the shaping of symptoms (Greenberg and Witztum, 2001; Tek and Ulug, 2001).

The second important effect works in the opposite direction. Heightened spirituality, religious faith, awareness that (once one has done what is humanly possible) all is in the hands of heaven – these beliefs and states of awareness are associated with lower anxiety. This effect might be obscured by the tendency for individuals under stress to increase levels of religious and spiritual activity – notably prayer and meditation. In cross-sectional studies this can give a muddled picture. But with sufficient attention to research design, measurement and interpretation, there is now reasonable confidence about the relations between anxiety and religious/spiritual factors (Koenig *et al.*, 2012).

Psychosis

Schizophrenia has a lifetime prevalence of approximately 1 in 200 across different cultural groups. It is admitted that diagnostic criteria can vary, and there is still vigorous debate about the nature and classification of psychosis (Bentall and Beck, 2004). Variations in prevalence may be a result of variations in the occurrence and classification of culture-specific symptoms and syndromes. An important example is the misdiagnosis of fervent prayer and other religious coping behaviour as psychotic symptomatology. Moreover, meditation may precipitate manic or psychotic episodes in those already vulnerable to these disorders and screening may be advised before participation in meditation (Lustyk *et al.*, 2009).

Prevalence estimates may rest on diagnoses based on 'symptoms' which are in fact attempts to cope, stimulated by stress, often using spiritual and religious devices. These may be quite effective. This can make it difficult to disentangle the conflicting effects of culture, religion and spirituality on prevalence, but the existence of conflicting effects does not imply inconclusiveness. A further noteworthy point is that there are many culture-specific symptoms and syndromes, with religiously flavoured symptoms; again the causal roles of spiritual and religious factors are complex.

Help-Seeking and Compliance

Prevalence is not necessarily reflected in referral rates. Of the many RS factors that might affect help-seeking and referral, we can identify two broad groups: first factors affecting views about treatments and ways of coping, and second factors affecting social-psychological dynamics.

Views about Treatments and Ways of Coping: Religious Coping, Religiously Influenced Beliefs about the Efficacy and Acceptability of Different Treatments and Coping Methods

Particularly in exclusive religious groups, RS resources within the group may be seen as offering effective relief from mental health difficulties (Greenberg and Witztum, 2001; Leavey, 2008), and the practices and beliefs of mental health professionals are unacceptable religiously, spiritually harmful, and ineffective. 'We treat such problems in the community. We give the person with difficulties a boost, talking about belief, and trust in G-d, saying we must not despair ... everything is from Heaven' (Orthodox rabbi, quoted in Greenberg and Witztum, 2001). Most clients state that their RS concerns are important and they would wish them to be taken into account (D'Souza, 2002). Some early work suggested that mental health professionals were generally less religiously active than clients, and often uninterested in religious issues. Subsequent work (e.g. Cook *et al.*, 2009) suggests that mental health professionals are increasingly concerned to take RS issues into account.

The outrageously anti-religious statements of Freud and others may have helped to foster a view that it is spiritually dangerous to seek psychological help. There may be more specific concerns: mental health professionals might encourage or condone sexual or other behaviours that are not acceptable in some religions – homosexuality, for example, or speaking disrespectfully about parents (Loewenthal, 2005). Some professionals may misunderstand, misjudge or fail to consider their patient's RS concerns.

There is of course growing evidence of the effectiveness of much religious coping: prayer, trust, belief in a benevolent, fair G-d, perception of purpose – all these have been empirically shown as effective (e.g. Loewenthal *et al.*, 2000; Pargament *et al.*, 2011; Koenig *et al.*, 2012), and they are perceived as effective (Loewenthal *et al.*, 2001). There is also growing consensus that most users and potential users of mental health services are pragmatic in their use of different kinds of help for psychological problems; use is determined by availability, cost-effectiveness and confidentiality. Clients shop around until they find something accessible that works. These factors help explain the popularity of prayer, religious and spiritual healing (Sembhi and Dein, 1998; Loewenthal and Cinnirella, 1999; Hood *et al.*, 2009).

The effectiveness and accessibility of spiritually based help and coping methods, and religious barriers to seeking professional help, combine to give the result that substantial numbers of patients – up to 70 per cent or more in some studies – will have used one or more spiritually based treatment before seeking professional help.

It is unknown for what proportion of people who use RS support or help, that help is sufficiently effective, or there is 'spontaneous' remission, so that further help is not sought. Some professionals may be concerned that RS barriers to seeking professional help may result in further deterioration. This is an important concern, but there is no substantial evidence in place as yet.

Religious and Spiritual Factors Affecting Social–Psychological Dynamics: Trust for Clinicians, Stigma and the Own-Group Dilemma

There are social–psychological effects that rest on RS factors, and which affect help-seeking and referral. Foremost among these is *stigma* – the fear that one is or will be discredited by significant others. Stigmatization is a likely consequence of mental illness, particularly in close-knit religious groups (e.g. Muslim, black Christian, orthodox Jewish). For example:

- 'Our people do not want everyone to know they have a problem.'
- 'I would think that many people would prefer something more confidential than an open meeting.'
- 'What kind of people would use this (service)? Must be people who can't cope.'

While members of religious groups say that they would feel best understood by a professional who shares their religious background, they fear that this might lead to their condition becoming known:

- 'I would think twice before going to a counsellor from my community. I would not want everyone to know.'

(Examples from Cinnirella and Loewenthal, 1999; Loewenthal and Brooke-Rogers, 2004)

Stigmatization almost certainly occurs more strongly in tightly knit religious groups and collectivist social milieux, than it does in complex, urbanized, individualistic societies. So insofar as RS factors play a role in the formation and maintenance of close-knit, collectivist groups, stigmatization is a likely by-product. This is hypothetical, and empirical work on this topic is lacking.

Bear in mind that that the upside of living in a close-knit religious group is that social support is offered to the distressed: helping, listening and being made to feel wanted are all more likely in such groups, as well as increased likelihood of beneficial religious coping strategies. Mood is improved and psychological difficulties may be lessened (e.g. Loewenthal *et al.*, 2000; Nooney and Woodrum, 2002; Inaba and Loewenthal, 2009)

Adherence

Adherence in psychiatry and psychotherapy can be reflected in taking prescribed medication, keeping appointments or developing an acceptable working relationship, and these are all related to trust and confidence in the professional. Trust and confidence are likely to be higher for a professional who is seen to understand and respect clients' explanatory models (Bhui and Bhugra, 2002), including spirituality, and who can address any spiritual concerns (Fabrega *et al.*, 2000; Pargament and Tarakeshwar, 2005; Pargament, 2013).

However, caution is needed. Pargament *et al.* (2005) list some of the potential dangers of spiritually sensitive therapy, for example, overestimating the importance of spirituality. Individuals may feel that using a professional from their own cultural–religious group means that their spiritual concerns are understood, but there are also concerns about stigma and confidentiality. Even if these are resolved by finding a professional from another geographical area, where there is less likelihood of the consultation becoming known, problems can remain. As Loewenthal (2005) points out, the client may have magical expectations of the therapist, over-idealize them, and expect him or her to give advice which is not appropriate in the therapeutic situation. Dein (2002), Loewenthal and Brooke-Rogers (2004), Fernando (2005), Sue *et al.* (2009) and others have discussed some of the difficulties in implementing culturally and spiritually sensitive mental healthcare. Apart from the financial difficulties experienced by those providing such services, which almost always spring from the voluntary sector, there is limited research funding. Does cultural–religious matching of providers and clients really:

- result in more effective services,
- result in matching explanatory models (or maps), and
- improve adherence and outcomes?

Initial research findings on culture-sensitive services are promising (Sue *et al.*, 2009).

Diagnosis and Clinical Management

Diagnostic and treatment decisions can be based on patients' religious behaviours and feelings. There are also at least two diagnostic areas in which there may be biases based on information about religious behaviour and affiliation: psychosis and obsessive–compulsive disorder.

Many religions endorse and encourage spiritual experiences and behaviours which might be construed as psychotic symptoms: the hearing of voices, visions and religious practices such as glossolalia, ecstatic states, trances, dancing and other behaviours involving dissociative phenomena.

There is a growing amount of work to suggest that:

- visions, voices and experiences that may often be interpreted as spiritual are genuine from the experiential and phenomenological perspective;
- among psychotic patients, these experiences are significantly more unpleasant, uncontrollable and persistent than among others (Peters *et al.*, 1999; Davies *et al.*, 2001: Andrew *et al.*, 2008);
- a range of visions, voices and other hallucinatory experiences are extremely common among those not suffering from psychiatric problems. They are seldom reported for fear of being taken as signs of madness (e.g. Hinton *et al.*, 2005).

Nevertheless, these behaviours may be taken as symptoms of psychosis. This may be one cause of the so-called Afro-Caribbean schizophrenia 'problem': higher referral and possibly prevalence of schizophrenia among Afro-Caribbeans, in Western countries and not elsewhere. Loewenthal and Cinnirella (2003) and Cantor-Graae and Selden (2005) reported that schizophrenia is more commonly diagnosed among Afro-Caribbeans in Western countries than it is among other ethnic groups, but not in Africa or the Caribbean. This is associated with a family history of migration and may be an effect of adversity. However, there may be more than adversity at work here: Littlewood and Lipsedge (1981) found that a form of schizophrenia with a relatively good prognosis was more common among Afro-Caribbeans than among other groups, and this was characterized by 'religiously flavoured symptoms'. One explanation, based on Bhugra (2002) is that when individuals are under stress, they may adopt religious coping strategies, which decline when – for whatever reason – there is remission. Thus religious behaviours are not so much a symptom of distress but a form of coping. This is speculative, but

there is some evidence of a tendency to misdiagnose religious coping behaviour as symptomatic of psychopathology (Loewenthal, 1999).

If one knows that a religious tradition requires cleanliness before prayer, or purification from sin, for example, by confession, it is tempting to conclude that obsessive–compulsive disorder (OCD) may be fostered by these religious demands, by the over-zealous wish for spiritual purity. Nevertheless, it has been concluded that – while religiosity may be associated with non-clinical scrupulosity, and can influence which obsessional symptoms are developed in OCD – it does not actually cause OCD. Obsessive–compulsive disorder is no more prevalent among Jews than among other groups (Lipsitz *et al.*, 2009). But as with psychosis, there may a persistent diagnostic bias. Yossifova and Loewenthal (1999) and Lewis (2001) found that both clinicians, clinical trainees and lay people were more likely to diagnose OCD when a patient was described as religiously active.

Nevertheless, we cannot conclude that patient religiosity, spirituality and cultural background have a uniformly negative effect on clinical decision-making, although this is a persistent fear among potential patients. There is no striking evidence of diagnostic biases regarding conditions other than schizophrenia and OCD. In one study, Janes (2005) found that clinical outcomes were rated (by clinicians) as just as good for psychotic patients with religious symptoms, as for psychotic patients with other symptoms. Clinicians can become aware of the possibilities of diagnostic biases, and make efforts to overcome these biases (Littlewood and Lipsedge, 1997; Snowden, 2002; Cook *et al.*, 2009).

Conclusions

This chapter has looked at cultural–spiritual–religious factors and their impact in cultural psychiatry. In providing services, and in making clinical decisions, it is important to bear in mind that specific spiritual beliefs and practices are not uniform within any culture.

Three kinds of effects of religion and spirituality on mental health seem to be important. First, is that while there are some damaging effects of RS beliefs and practices, these may be outweighed by the beneficial effects. Work on how and whether these beneficial effects may be harnessed to bring clinical benefits is only in very preliminary stages. Second, there may be unhelpful diagnostic biases and clinical decisions based on patients' religiosity and spirituality, particularly perhaps when religious practices are culturally unfamiliar. It needs to be explored whether these exist for disorders other than schizophrenia and OCD, and whether they are pervasive and persistent. Third, religious coping behaviour is felt to be spiritually and psychologically beneficial. However, when individuals are under stress, there may be an increase in religious coping, and this can lead to an impression that the religious behaviour is a sign and symptom of illness. This effect needs to be explored carefully in longitudinal studies, and is a possibility that clinicians need to bear in mind.

References

Andrew, E. M., Gray, N. S. and Snowden, R. J. (2008). The relationship between trauma and beliefs about hearing voices: a study of psychiatric and non-psychiatric voice hearers. *Psychological Medicine*, **38**, 1409–1417.

Ano, G. G. and Vasconelles, E. B. (2005) Religious coping and psychological adjustment to stress: a meta-analysis. *Journal of Clinical Psychology*, **61**, 461–480, doi: 10.1002/jclp.20049.

Bentall, R. P. and Beck, A. (2004). *Madness Explained: Psychosis and Human Nature*. Harmondsworth: Penguin.

Bhugra, D. (2002). Self-concept: psychosis and attraction of new religious movements. *Mental Health, Religion and Culture*, **5**, 239–252.

Bhui, K. and Bhugra, D. (2002). Explanatory models for mental distress: implications for clinical practice and research. *British Journal of Psychiatry*, **181**, 6–7.

Broch, H. B. (2001). The villagers' reactions towards craziness: an Indonesian example. *Transcultural Psychiatry*, **38**, 275–305.

Cantor-Graae, E. and Selden, J.-P. (2005) Schizophrenia and migration: a meta-analysis and review. *American Journal of Psychiatry*, **162**, 12–24, doi: http://dx.doi.org/10.1176/appi.ajp.162.1.12.

Cinnirella, M. and Loewenthal, K. M. (1999). Religious and ethnic group influences on beliefs about mental illness: a qualitative interview study. *British Journal of Medical Psychology*, **72**, 505–524.

Cook, C., Powell, A. and Sims, A. (eds) (2009). *Spirituality and Psychiatry*. London, Royal College of Psychiatrists Publications.

Crossley, J. P. and Salter, D. P. (2005). A question of finding harmony: a grounded theory study of clinical psychologists' experience of addressing spiritual beliefs in therapy. *Psychology and Psychotherapy: Theory Research and Practice*, **78**, 295–314.

Davies, M. F., Griffiths, M. and Vice, S. (2001). Affective reactions to auditory hallucinations in psychotic, evangelical and control groups. *British Journal of Clinical Psychology*, **40**, 361–370.

Dein, S. (2002). Transcultural psychiatry. *British Journal of Psychiatry*, **181**, 535–536.

D'Souza, R. (2002). Do patients expect psychiatrists to be interested in spiritual issues? *Australasian Psychiatry*, **10**, 44–47, doi:10.1046/j.1440–1665.2002.00391.x

Fabrega, H., Jr, Lopez-Ibor, J. J., Jr, Wig, N. N. *et al.* (2000). Culture, spirituality and psychiatry. *Current Opinion in Psychiatry*, **13**, 525–530.

Fernando, S. (2005). Multicultural mental health services: projects for minority ethnic communities in England. *Transcultural Psychiatry*, **42**, 420–436.

Freud, S. (1907). Obsessive actions and religious practices. In *Collected Papers, 1907/1924*. London: Hogarth Press.

Freud, S. (1927). *The Future of an Illusion*. London: Hogarth Press.

Greenberg, D. and Witztum, E. (2001). *Sanity and Sanctity: Mental Health Work among the Ultra-Orthodox in Jerusalem*. New Haven and London: Yale University Press.

Hinton, D. E., Hufford, D. J. and Kirmayer, L. (2005). Culture and sleep paralysis. *Transcultural Psychiatry*, **42**, 5–10.

Hood, R. W., Hill, P. C. and Spilka, B. (2009). *The Psychology of Religion: An Empirical Approach*, 4th edn. New York: Guilford, p. 465.

Inaba, K. and Loewenthal, K. M. (2009). Religion and altruism. In *Oxford Handbook of the Sociology of Religion*, ed. P. Clarke and P. Beyer. Oxford: Oxford University Press, pp. 876–889.

Janes, K. (2005). Clinical psychologists' appraisals of referral letters describing clients with symptoms of psychosis with and without a religious component. *DClinPsych*, Royal Holloway, University of London.

Joseph, S., Linley, P. A. and Maltby, J. (eds) (2006). Special Issue: Positive Psychology and Religion. *Mental Health, Religion and Culture*, **9**(3), 209–212, doi: doi.org/10.1080/13694670600615227.

Keyes, C. L. M. and Goodman, S. H. (eds) (2006). *Women and Depression: A Handbook for the Social, Behavioral and Biomedical Sciences*. Cambridge: Cambridge University Press.

King, M. and Dein, S. (1998). The spiritual variable in psychiatric research. *Psychological Medicine*, **28**, 1259–1262.

King, M., Marston, L., McManus, S., Brugha, T. *et al.* (2013). Religion, spirituality and mental health: results from a national study of English households. *British Journal of Psychiatry*, **202**, 68–73, doi: 10.1192/bjp.bp.112.112003.

Koenig, H., King, D. and Carson, V. (eds) (2012). *Handbook of Religion and Health*. Oxford and New York: Oxford University Press.

Leavey, G. (2008). UK clergy and people in mental distress: community and patterns of pastoral care. *Transcultural Psychiatry*, **45**, 79–104.

Lewis, C. A. (1998). Cleanliness is next to godliness: religiosity and obsessiveness. *Journal of Religion and Health*, **37**, 49–61.

Lewis, C. A. (2001). Cultural stereotypes of the effects of religion on mental health. *British Journal of Medical Psychology*, **74**, 359–367.

Lipsedge, M. (1996). Religion and madness in history. In *Psychiatry and Religion: Context, Consensus, and Controversies*, ed. D. Bhugra. London: Routledge.

Lipsitz, J. D., Geulayov, G. and Gross, R. (2009). The epidemiology of anxiety disorders in Israel. In *Psychiatric and Behavioral Disorders in Israel*, ed. I. Levav. Jerusalem: Gefen, pp. 200–211.

Littlewood, R. and Lipsedge, M. (1981). Some social and phenomenological characteristics of psychotic immigrants. *Psychological Medicine*, **11**, 289–302.

Littlewood, R. and Lipsedge, M. (1997). *Aliens and Alienists: Ethnic Minorities and Psychiatry*, 3rd edn. London: Oxford University Press.

Loewenthal, K. M. (1999). Religious issues and their psychological aspects. In *Cross Cultural Mental Health Services: Contemporary Issues in Service Provision*, ed. K. Bhui and D. Olajide. London: W. B. Saunders.

Loewenthal, K. M. (2005). Strictly orthodox Jews and their relations with psychiatry and psychotherapy. *Transcultural Psychiatry Section, World Psychiatric Association Newsletter*, **23**, 20–24.

Loewenthal, K. M. (2007). *Religion, Culture and Mental Health*. Cambridge: Cambridge University Press.

Loewenthal, K. M. (2009). The alcohol–depression hypothesis: gender and the prevalence of depression among Jews. In *Comorbidity of Depression and Alcohol Use Disorders*, ed. L. Sher. New York: Nova Science Publishers, pp. 31–40.

Loewenthal, K. M. (2013). Religion, spirituality and culture. In *Handbook of Psychology, Religion and Spirituality*, ed. K. I. Pargament, J. Exline, J. Jones, A. Mahoney, E. Shafranske. Washington, DC: American Psychological Association.

Loewenthal, K. M. and Brooke Rogers, M. (2004). Culture sensitive support groups: how are they perceived and how do they work? *International Journal of Social Psychiatry*, **50**, 227–240.

Loewenthal, K. M. and Cinnirella, M. (1999). Beliefs about the efficacy of religious, medical and psychotherapeutic interventions for depression and schizophrenia among different cultural–religious groups in Great Britain. *Transcultural Psychiatry*, **36**, 491–504.

Loewenthal, K. M. and Cinnirella, M. (2003). Religious issues in ethnic minority mental health with special reference to schizophrenia in Afro-Caribbeans in Britain: a systematic review. In *Main Issues in Mental Health and Race*, ed. D. Ndegwa and D. Olajide. London: Ashgate.

Loewenthal, K. M., Goldblatt, V., Gorton, T. *et al.* (1997). The costs and benefits of boundary maintenance: stress, religion and culture among Jews in Britain. *Social Psychiatry and Psychiatric Epidemiology*, **32**, 200–207.

Loewenthal, K. M., MacLeod, A. K., Goldblatt, V., Lubitsh, G. and Valentine, J. D. (2000). Comfort and joy: religion, cognition and mood in individuals under stress. *Cognition and Emotion*, **14**, 355–374.

Loewenthal, K. M., Cinnirella, M., Evdoka, G. and Murphy, P. (2001). Faith conquers all? Beliefs about the role of religious factors in coping with depression among different cultural–religious groups in the UK. *British Journal of Medical Psychology*, **74**, 293–303.

Loewenthal, K. M., MacLeod, A. K., Cook, S., Lee, M. J. and Goldblatt, V. (2003). Beliefs about alcohol among UK Jews and protestants: do they fit the alcohol–depression hypothesis? *Social Psychiatry and Psychiatric Epidemiology*, **38**, 122–127.

Lustyk, M. K. B., Chawla, N., Roger, S. *et al.* (2009). Mindfulness meditation research: issues of participant screening, safety procedures, and researcher training. *Advances in Mind–Body Medicine*, **24**, 20–30.

Miller, A. (1984). Endorsement. In Abraham Amsel's *Rational Irrational Man*, New York: Feldheim.

Neeleman, J. and Persaud, R. (1995). Why do psychiatrists neglect religion? *British Journal of Medical Psychology*, **68**, 169–78.

Nooney, J. and Woodrum, W. (2002). Religious coping and church-based social support as predictors of mental health outcomes: testing a conceptual model. *Journal for the Scientific Study of Religion*, **41**, 359–368, doi: 10.1111/1468-5906.00122.

Pargament, K. (1997). *The Psychology of Religion and Coping*. New York: Guilford Press.

Pargament, K. (2011). *Spiritually Integrated Psychotherapy*. New York: Guilford.

Pargament, K. I. (ed.) (2013). *APA Handbook of Psychology, Religion and Spirituality*. Washington, DC: American Psychological Association.

Pargament, K. and Tarakeshwar, N. (eds) (2005). *Spiritually Integrated Psychotherapy. Special Issue: Mental Health Religion and Culture*, **8**, 155–238.

Pargament, K. I., Murray-Swank, N. A. and Tarakeshwar, N. (2005). An empirically-based rationale for a spiritually-integrated psychotherapy. *Mental Health, Religion and Culture*, **8**, 155–165, doi: dx.doi.org/10.1080/13694670500138940.

Pargament, K., Feuille, M. and Burdzy, D. (2011). The brief RCOPE: current psychometric status of a short measure of religious coping. *Religions*, **2**, 51–76, doi:10.3390/rel2010051.

Peters, E., Day, S., McKenna, J. and Orbach, G. (1999). Delusional ideas in religious and psychiatric populations. *British Journal of Clinical Psychology*, **38**, 83–96.

Pfeifer, S. (1994). Belief in demons and exorcism in psychiatric patients in Switzerland. *British Journal of Medical Psychology*, **67**, 247–58.

Seligman, M. (2002). *Authentic Happiness*. New York: Free Press.

Sembhi, S. and Dein, S. (1998). The use of traditional Asian healers by Asian psychiatric patients in the UK: a pilot study. *Mental Health, Religion and Culture*, **1**, 127–134.

Snowden, L. R. (2002). Bias in mental health assessment and intervention: theory and evidence. *American Journal of Public Health*, **93**, 239–243, doi: 10.2105/AJPH.93.2.239.

Srinivasan, T. N. and Thara, R. (2001). Beliefs about causation of schizophrenia: do Indian families believe in supernatural causes? *Social Psychiatry and Psychiatric Epidemiology*, **36**, 134–140.

Sue, S., Zane, N., Nagayama Hall, G. C. and Berger, L. K. (2009). The case for cultural competency in psychotherapeutic interventions. *Annual Review of Psychology*, **60**, 525–548, doi: 10.1146/annurev.psych.60.110707.163651.

Tek, C. and Ulug, B. (2001) Religiosity and religious obsessions in obsessive–compulsive disorder. *Psychiatry Research*, **104**, 99–108.

Weiss, M. G., Doongaji, D. R., Siddhartha, S. *et al.* (1992). The Explanatory Model Interview Catalogue (EMIC): contribution to cross-cultural research methods from a study of leprosy and mental health. *The British Journal of Psychiatry*, **160**, 819–830, doi: 10.1192/bjp.160.6.819.

Wilkens, K. (2009). Mary and the demons: Marian devotion and ritual healing in Tanzania. *Journal of Religion in Africa*, **39**, 295–318, doi: 10.1163/157006609X453310.

Yossifova, M. and Loewenthal, K. M. (1999). Religion and the judgement of obsessionality. *Mental Health, Religion and Culture*, **2**, 145–152.

Zinnbauer, B. J., Pargament, K. I., Cole, B. *et al.* (1997). Religion and spirituality: unfuzzying the fuzzy. *Journal for the Scientific Study of Religion*, **36**, 549–564.

Chapter 6

Lifestyle Medicine in Psychiatry

Jerome Sarris and Chee H. Ng

Editors' Introduction

In high-income countries and, increasingly, in low- and middle-income countries, changing lifestyle factors are recognized as leading to an increase in different types of illness and also are linked with chronicity of various diseases. These are known as contributing to the causation as well as perpetuation of the so-called 'diseases of lifestyle' such as obesity, hypertension, etc., which in turn affect individuals' mental health. There is no doubt that if people with diabetes or hypertension develop mental illness it becomes difficult to control both illnesses. Furthermore, it is well recognized that the economic burden of lifestyle-related diseases around the globe is greater than that of many physical illnesses. Lifestyle medicine is defined as a branch of evidence-based medicine in which comprehensive lifestyle changes (including nutrition, physical activity, stress management, social support and environmental exposures) are used to prevent, treat and reverse the progression of chronic diseases by addressing their underlying causes. Social inequalities can further contribute to this. Applying these principles in changing the way we live, can help promote better physical and mental health, and better outcomes in the event of existing ill health. There is no doubt that to deliver any of this a multidisciplinary involvement is required, as well as an active participation by the patient, their carers, families and the general population in learning about lifestyle choices and interventions and using these to improve health and outcomes. There is no health without mental health, and both domains need to be considered together, especially in addressing the rising epidemic of lifestyle-related diseases globally. A range of lifestyle-focused health programmes known to enhance both physical and mental health is being applied in many Western countries. However, it remains largely unknown as to whether such programmes are practical or functional across different cultural contexts. Current evidence suggests that the major components of lifestyle-focused health programmes to enhance mental and physical health include the adoption of physical activity and exercise, dietary modification, general psychoeducation, adequate relaxation/sleep and social interaction, use of mindfulness techniques, reduction of substance use, improvement of intersecting environmental factors, and the use of motivation and goal-setting techniques. Nevertheless, there are potential barriers, challenges and logistical considerations that need to be addressed in the implementation of such programmes within diverse cultures and populations.

Introduction

In contemporary times, lifestyle factors are increasingly linked with chronic diseases, both in terms of the causation and perpetuation of the so-called 'diseases of lifestyle'. Worldwide, the economic burden of lifestyle-related diseases in both developed and developing countries is enormous and can no longer be ignored. 'Lifestyle medicine' has been defined by the American College of Lifestyle Medicine and the European Lifestyle Medicine Organization (EULM) as a branch of evidence-based medicine in which comprehensive lifestyle changes (including nutrition, physical activity, stress management, social support and environmental exposures) are used to prevent, treat and reverse the progression of chronic diseases by addressing their underlying causes (see the EULM website at https://eulm.org). Importantly, the focus is on applying lifestyle principles to promote better physical and mental health, or in the event of existing ill health to integrate lifestyle practices into the modern medical treatment and rehabilitation. Implicit in this concept are several critical assumptions: the need for multidisciplinary involvement in delivering the comprehensive patient care plan; the active participation by the patient or healthcare consumer in making healthier lifestyle choices and implementing self-management strategies; and that psychological and mental health issues cannot be separated from the physical health domain but should considered as a whole.

The Link between Physical and Mental Health

There is growing recognition that physical and mental health interact with each other in a bidirectional manner. Apart from maintenance of physical health, modifiable lifestyle factors such as diet, exercise, sleep, use of substances and enhancement of social networks are also vital for general mental health (Sarris and Wardle, 2014; Stanley and Laugharne, 2014). There is a large body of research literature that has documented the close relationship between physical and mental health, especially concerning people with mental illness (Stanley and Laugharne, 2014). In addition, the strong link between serious mental illnesses and their pharmacological treatments with poor physical health and associated increased mortality has been well established (McElroy, 2009). Existing evidence points towards the need for an integrated health response that supports prevention and early diagnosis, treatment and management of both physical and mental health problems.

The current focus on screening and treating metabolic issues and weight gain in psychiatry has emphasized lifestyle modification programmes, especially dietary and exercise adjustment to address the interrelationship between poor physical and mental health. A review of the evidence was conducted on 24 lifestyle health programmes globally, aimed at reducing obesity and improving fitness for participants with serious mental illness (Bartels and Desilets, 2012). The authors found that while participants experienced an overall mean weight loss and/or decrease in body mass index, lifestyle interventions appear to be inconsistently successful in achieving clinically significant results. The programme elements found by the authors to have enhanced success were duration of three months or longer, and the inclusion of both education and activity-based approaches.

To create a comprehensive 'integrative' lifestyle-focused programme and move beyond a basic model which is limited to diet and exercise modification, other components such as general lifestyle and psychoeducation, mindfulness technique instruction, and motivation and goal setting skills should also be incorporated. While this may hold promise in theory, research underpinning the use of integrative programmes for mental health conditions is currently limited. To date only one study has examined the effects of combining multiple lifestyle interventions for the treatment of psychiatric disorders such as depression. This randomized controlled trial (Garcia-Toro et al., 2012) involved 80 outpatients with diagnosed major depressive disorder who were taking antidepressant treatment. The researchers provided to the 'active group' four specific lifestyle recommendations consisting of dietary modification, exercise, sunlight exposure and sleep patterns, while the control group was given just general daily patterns to follow. Blinded assessment conducted before and after six months revealed that the active group had a significantly greater reduction of depression than the control group, with 11 out of 40 people in the active group achieving depression remission, compared to only one person in the control group. While these results are encouraging, further well-controlled and rigorously designed studies employing a comprehensive lifestyle intervention are needed.

Cross-Cultural Aspects

As most of the lifestyle studies in psychiatry have been conducted in Western countries, there is an absence of data from lifestyle modification programmes being applied in non-Western countries. In addition, marked intrinsic differences in lifestyles between Western and Eastern societies imply that it is largely unknown how such programmes based on Western lifestyles would operate across diverse cultures. While some programmes have been studied in non-Western populations to address general health issues such as diabetes or smoking, there are few studies evaluating integrative lifestyle programmes in cross-cultural settings to address mental health issues. For example, a study assessed self-help (bibliotherapy) in improving psychological resilience of Thai people with moderate level depression (Songprakun and McCann, 2012). Employing a range of modules delivered over an 8-week period focusing on physical activity, socialization, psychoeducation, progressive muscle relaxation, and sleep hygiene, resulted in a significant difference in increased perceived resilience between the intervention and control group at follow up.

Lifestyle approaches to managing mental health issues for a variety of reasons may be more appealing in different cultural contexts. Among the Chinese population in Singapore, the use of mindfulness practice and traditional Chinese medicine for depressive and anxiety symptoms is regarded as acceptable and lacks the stigma of a psychiatric label (Kua and Tan, 2005). A study of common lifestyle programme components in Singapore, using a preventive psychiatry programme for depression and dementia in Chinese elderly was carried out in partnership with non-governmental organizations, the private sector and volunteers. The study explored whether psychosocial intervention through group activities, together with health education about lifestyle, diabetes mellitus and hypertension, can prevent the onset of depression and delay the progression of dementia (Wu *et al.*, 2014). The pilot study comprising 110 Chinese elderly with mild depressive or anxiety symptoms who attended weekly group meetings for three months and then monthly for 21 months. Each of the four modalities (art therapy, music-reminiscence therapy, t'ai chi exercise and mindfulness practice) resulted in lower depressive scores which persisted beyond a year (Rawtaer *et al.*, 2015). The group approach was acceptable and it is possible that exposure to social interaction when exercising may have additional psychological benefits. Therefore, this is a promising finding that a range of lifestyle programme components can improve the mood of elderly Chinese people.

There appears to be some evidence that both vegetables and fruits, which traditionally have been widely consumed in many parts of Asia, Africa and the Pacific, may lower the risk of depression (Tsai *et al.*, 2012). Further, it is of interest is that diet modification and traditional Chinese medicine, are also widely used in clinical prevention and therapy for both mental and physical illness in Taiwan, Japan, Korea and China (Wu *et al.*, 2008). However, due to the increasing availability of Westernized food choices in recent decades, dietary patterns in Asia and other non-Western regions are significantly changing (Baker and Friel, 2014). For instance, consecutive national surveys from the 1993–1996 and 2005–2008 Nutrition and Health Surveys in Taiwan found a significant increase in sugar intakes and sedentary lifestyle especially in the young generation (Pan *et al.*, 2011). The growing preference for highly processed diet or 'fast-foods' in Asia which is fashionably associated with the Western lifestyle may undermine any dietary benefits based on traditional or cultural values. Dietary patterns are diverse across the world, and while it is important for any dietary modifications

to be culturally appropriate, it is sensible to advocate a wholefood unprocessed diet as a general guide.

A particular challenge in lifestyle modification across culture is the implementation of regular physical activity and exercise. In some modernized Asian countries, jogging, basketball, aerobics and yoga are popular, but living in a subtropical climate, polluted atmosphere and dense urban environments may lead to a preference for indoor exercise and an increase in sports and gym facilities. This may be particularly relevant for countries with a hot climate such as in the Middle East where sports activities within indoor facilities may be more practical. Hence, different modes of exercise may or may not be appropriate depending on socio-economic factors, work patterns, cultural practice and available resources. Notwithstanding, the practice of traditional and inexpensive forms of exercise such as t'ai chi may be effective in both improving both physical and mental health (Wang *et al.*, 2014).

There is increasing recognition that workplace stress can affect an individual's physical and psychological health as well as result in unhealthy lifestyles and behaviours. The World Health Organization states that a healthy workplace is one in which workers and managers collaborate to use a continual improvement process to protect and promote the health, safety and well-being of all workers and the sustainability of the workplace. In many countries especially newly developed world economies this would be challenging to implement due to the culture of high workplace demands, long working hours and low leave usage. To address this issue adequately requires education and communication regarding ways to modify or eliminate sources of stress inherent in the workplace and work environment. Comprehensive plans are needed to prevent and to manage psychosocial risks factors within the broader economic and industrial contexts.

Many factors need to be considered for any lifestyle programme to be effective, not least the existing prescriptive guidelines in terms of work, lifestyle, environmental and social factors, including economic elements. There are also a range of specific considerations when developing and implementing lifestyle programmes across different cultures. It is important to have an understanding of the cultural uniqueness and diversity across the region with respect to variations in lifestyle preference, work patterns, family and community interactions (Sarris *et al.*, 2015). Thus, tailoring any lifestyle programme to the specific culture is crucial. It stands to reason that promotion and implementation of such programmes is best driven by local authorities, communities or workplaces.

Integrative Lifestyle Programmes

As discussed previously, general lifestyle elements addressed in integrative programmes should focus on encouraging a balance between meaningful work, adequate rest and sleep, judicious exercise (or physical activity), a balanced wholefood diet, positive social interaction and pleasurable hobbies, in addition to a minimizing of harmful environmental and biological influences. There are a range of general lifestyle elements that are highly modifiable (e.g. physical activity, alcohol and nicotine use), while other elements are usually modifiable such as diet or sleep/work/ rest balance or technological interface (depending on environmental, employment and economic factors). While psychoeducation may not demonstrate equal effectiveness to psychological or pharmacological treatments, it is a vital component of lifestyle programmes, by way of increasing an individual's knowledge and insight, and also by enhancing self-efficacy (Xia *et al.*, 2011).

One basic lifestyle element that can be addressed in many populations throughout Western and Eastern societies is the consideration that both smoking and alcohol use are a prevalent public health concern. Of note in Chapter 33 in this volume, these key exogenous substances that interact with liver metabolism and can either inhibit or induce the clearance of many psychotropic medications. Thus, health promotion programmes need to tackle these issues by focusing on managing the problem in a culturally appropriate way using a range of psychoeducational, counselling and pharmacotherapeutic strategies to minimize harm. Other drugs of abuse, such as betel nut, need also to be considered, as in places such as Taiwan high betel nut use remains prevalent (Chang *et al.*, 2014).

Dietary education is also a key pillar of lifestyle programmes. While such programmes have not yet been rigorously evaluated in conditions such as depression, cross-sectional studies by Akbaraly *et al.* (2009) and Jacka *et al.* (2010) have revealed that a healthy diet rich in complex carbohydrates, fruits and vegetables and lean meats, and low in processed foods, reduces the risk of depression. Altering dietary patterns by way of education and access to healthy foods may affect a variety of factors influencing mental health and the development of mood disorders

(Jacka and Berk, 2007; Quirk *et al.*, 2013). In addition to physical activity, dietary modification is the most prevalent behavioural strategy in most lifestyle programmes, primarily to reduce body weight (Foster *et al.*, 2005), but also to improve mood, self-esteem and quality of life. For example, numerous meta-analyses (Franz *et al.*, 2007; Wu *et al.*, 2009; Schaar *et al.*, 2010) have indicated that programmes combining diet and exercise components may produce significantly better long-term outcomes than interventions consisting of each strategy alone. Although evidence supporting specific nutritional advice is currently absent, a basic balanced wholefood diet including foods containing a spectrum of nutrients can be recommended. Foods that are rich in omega 3, L-tryptophan, B and C vitamins, zinc and magnesium have a range of health benefits, as they are necessary for many bodily and neurochemical functions (Werbach, 1996). These include whole grains (zinc, magnesium, B vitamins), lean meat (zinc, magnesium, protein, e.g. tryptophan), deep sea fish (essential fatty acids), green leafy vegetables (vitamin C, folate), coloured berries (vitamin C, antioxidant phenolic compounds), nuts (monounsaturated fats, vitamin E, zinc, magnesium) (Haas, 1992).

Introducing dietary modification as part of any lifestyle programme for diverse populations should take into account the context of cultural and religious considerations regarding cooking and eating habits and cuisine choices. While data indicates that the adherence to traditional dietary patterns could be beneficial, even some 'traditional' dietary patterns may be potentially improved (i.e. diets high in fatty fried foods). A growing concern as mentioned earlier is that in some modernized Asian countries there is an increasing issue of Western 'fast food' infiltration (Baker and Friel, 2014). Another potential point of dietary education is to avoid excessive salt/sodium consumption which may be prevalent in many non-Western countries (Batcagan-Abueg *et al.*, 2013).

Increasing physical activity is advised in persons with sedentary lifestyles, and is especially indicated in cases of obesity and metabolic syndrome. Associations between greater physical activity and improved mood and well-being have consistently been documented (Adams *et al.*, 2007; Deslandes *et al.*, 2009). Many clinical trials have revealed that exercise is effective in improving general mood, with meta-analyses of such trials showing a significant effect in favour of physical exercise compared with control conditions (routine care, wait list, meditation/

relaxation, or low-intensity exercise) (Sarris et al., 2008). Further, adjunctive physical activity interventions have also been found to significantly reduce depressive symptoms in individuals with diagnosed mental illness, in addition to improving a range of anthropometric measures (e.g. weight), aerobic capacity, and quality of life (Rimer et al., 2012). It is evident that adequate physical activity and exercise is of synergistic relevance given the increased burden of metabolic syndrome in individuals with psychiatric disorders (McIntyre et al., 2012). Current evidence supports the use of exercise of sufficient duration and intensity to maintain a healthy weight, and to improve mood. Importantly, research indicates that a dose-dependent effect occurs, thus programmes can encourage regular moderate to strong intensity exercise to elicit more positive results, provided it can be sustained safely (Dunn et al., 2005; Singh et al., 2005).

Encouraging culturally appropriate recreational activities may also provide an opportunity to experience pleasure, to direct the mind away from rumination and worry, and may provide a setting for increased social interaction. Global climate change and environmental degradation affecting many parts of the world are evolving public concerns; and while current data is weak in respect to an association with mental health issues, common sense suggests minimizing exposure to environmental toxins, chemicals pollutants (Genc et al., 2012) and noise pollution (Riediker and Koren, 2004). Specifically, environmental toxins (including particulate air pollution) are also an issue, having a potential effect on the central nervous system (Genc et al., 2012). Exposure to air pollution has been found in a longitudinal study of 537 elderly Koreans to be associated with an increase in depressive symptoms (Lim et al., 2012). To mitigate this concern, benefits may be found in spending time away from urbanized areas, which will result in increased exposure to fresh air and sunlight. This may be manifested as a 'nature-assisted therapy' approach (for example hikes in nature) (Annerstedt and Wahrborg, 2011). It can be noted though that the benefits of participation in organized physical recreation and spending time in nature are currently supported by a limited dataset that are mostly derived from Scandinavia (Annerstedt and Wahrborg, 2011). One interesting public health application in Japan (Takayama et al., 2014) is the recommendation of 'forest bathing', which involves advising people to spend time in forests. Preliminary evidence suggests that such exposure can improve both general mental health while altering physiological stress and immune biomarkers. Moderation of excessive technological interface (e.g. mobile phones, computers, television) may be potentially important in general lifestyle education (Walsh, 2011). Many Asian populations integrate technology into their lives as a primary work and social interface, and thus a delicate approach for balanced use is needed.

'Mindfulness' techniques may also beneficial in lifestyle programmes (Barnhofer et al., 2009), and their use has a rich history in Eastern meditative practices (Loizzo et al., 2009). The teaching of simple meditative techniques such as coordinated breathing and mental focus on the present (environment, bodily sensations, breath, emotions), may have an application in improving mood, and moderating negative behaviours such as over-eating. While the concept of meditation is varied, it can be taught as either 'open monitoring' or 'focused' forms. A key aspect of meditative practice involves the concept of 'mindfulness', which is commonly defined as the awareness which arises through paying attention in a particular way: on purpose, in the present moment and non-judgmentally (Kabat-Zinn, 1994). Mindfulness techniques can also be applied in the context of relaxation therapy, or applied into a pre-sleep routine, or eating routine. In patients with insomnia, anxiety and mood disorders, mindfulness techniques have demonstrated a large effect size for improving clinical symptoms (Hofmann et al., 2010) and have shown significant large effects in treating anxiety and depression, with gains maintained at follow up (Khoury et al., 2013).

As mindfulness-based techniques originated from Eastern cultures, applying these practices is generally well accepted in the Asian settings. Mindfulness techniques may be applied as a regular meditative practice, or in simple forms (such as breathing exercises, mindful walking or eating), or as applied psychological techniques such as mindfulness-based cognitive-behavioural therapy, or as movement-based approaches such as t'ai chi, qigong or yoga (some evidence does exist in these exercises for improving mood or reducing anxiety) (Sarris et al., 2012; Cramer et al., 2013; Yin and Dishman, 2014). Being based on ancient Taoist and Buddhist practices, common spiritual practices in East Asia include qigong, t'ai chi and various styles of meditation. In line with 'mindfulness' elements of some lifestyle programmes, these practices may be considered not only for prevention or therapy for illness, but also for self-growth. Therefore, people may practise these activities as part of their 'lifestyle', rather than as needing to be undertaken in strict therapeutic sessions. Another form of exercise that combines a 'mindfulness' element is the practice of yoga which, while originating in India, is widely practised in many Eastern and Western countries. A recent systematic review (Cramer *et al.*, 2013) found an effect on the severity of depression, with moderate evidence showing a beneficial short-term effect of yoga compared to usual care, and limited evidence compared to aerobic exercise or relaxation.

Conclusions

In the current age, the world's population is becoming more sedentary and is eating a poorer diet than previous generations, while living in the threat of worsening environmental degradation. In addition to other lifestyle factors such as excessive alcohol and nicotine use, irregular sleep patterns, psychosocial stress and increasing work pressures, the cost on both physical and mental health is unsustainable. Due to this there is a strong argument to enhance the application of lifestyle programmes across diverse cultures to improve mental and physical health globally. To address this effectively, a more integrative approach to delivering optimal healthcare is needed. Further, any intervention programme needs to be modified with consideration of cross-cultural perspectives on mental health problems and their treatment priorities; while also addressing motivational issues, time restrictions and financial constraints.

References

Adams, T. B., Moore, M. T. and Dye, J. (2007). The relationship between physical activity and mental health in a national sample of college females. *Women and Health*, **45**(1), 69–85.

Akbaraly, T. N., Brunner, E. J., Ferrie, J. E. *et al.* (2009). Dietary pattern and depressive symptoms in middle age. *British Journal of Psychiatry*, **195**(5), 408–413.

Annerstedt, M. and Wahrborg, P. (2011). Nature-assisted therapy: systematic review of controlled and observational studies. *Scandinavian Journal of Public Health*, **39**(4), 371–388.

Baker, P. and Friel, S. (2014). Processed foods and the nutrition transition: evidence from Asia. *Obesity Reviews*, **15**(7), 564–577.

Barnhofer, T., Crane, C., Hargus, E., Amarasinghe, M., Winder, R. and Williams, J. M. (2009). Mindfulness-based cognitive therapy as a treatment for chronic depression: a preliminary study. *Behaviour Research and Therapy*, **47**(5), 366–373.

Bartels, S. and Desilets R. (2012). Health Promotion Programs for People with Serious Mental Illness (Prepared by the Dartmouth Health Promotion Research Team). Washington, DC: SAMHSA-HRSA Center for Integrated Health Solutions. January.

Batcagan-Abueg, A. P., Lee, J. J., Chan, P., Rebello, S. A. and Amarra, M. S. (2013). Salt intakes and salt reduction initiatives in Southeast Asia: a review. *Asia Pacific Journal of Clinical Nutrition*, **22**(4), 490–504.

Chang, F. C., Sung, H. Y., Zhu, S. H. and Chiou, S. T. (2014). Impact of the 2009 Taiwan tobacco hazards prevention act on smoking cessation. *Addiction*, **109**(1), 140–146.

Cramer, H., Lauche, R., Langhorst, J. and Dobos, G. (2013). Yoga for depression: a systematic review and meta-analysis. *Depression and Anxiety*, **30**(11), 1068–1083.

Deslandes, A., Moraes, H., Ferreira, C. *et al.* (2009). Exercise and mental health: many reasons to move. *Neuropsychobiology*, **59**(4), 191–198.

Dunn, A. L., Trivedi, M. H., Kampert, J. B., Clark, C. G. and Chambliss, H. O. (2005). Exercise treatment for depression: efficacy and dose response. *American Journal of Preventive Medicine*, **28**(1), 1–8.

Foster, G. D., Makris, A. P. and Bailer, B. A. (2005). Behavioral treatment of obesity. *American Journal of Clinical Nutrition*, **82**(1 Suppl), 230S–235S.

Franz, M. J., VanWormer, J. J., Crain, A. L. *et al.* (2007). Weight-loss outcomes: a systematic review and meta-analysis of weight-loss clinical trials with a minimum 1-year follow-up. *Journal of the American Diet Association*, **107**(10), 1755–1767.

Garcia-Toro, M., Ibarra, O., Gili, M., *et al.* (2012). Four hygienic-dietary recommendations as add-on treatment in depression: a randomized-controlled trial. *Journal of Affective Disorders*, **140**(2), 200–203.

Genc, S., Zadeoglulari, Z., Fuss, S. H. and Genc, K. (2012). The adverse effects of air pollution on the nervous system. *Journal of Toxicology*, **2012**: 782462.

Haas, E. M. (1992). *Staying Healthy with Nutrition*. Berkeley: Celestial Arts.

Hofmann, S. G., Sawyer, A. T., Witt, A. A. and Oh, D. (2010). The effect of mindfulness-based therapy on anxiety and depression: a meta-analytic review. *Journal of Consulting and Clinical Psychology*, **78**(2), 169–183.

Jacka, F. N. and Berk, M. (2007). Food for thought. *Acta Neuropsychiatrica*, **19**(5), 321–323.

Jacka, F. N., Pasco, J. A., Mykletun, A. *et al.* (2010). Association of Western and traditional diets with depression and anxiety in women. *American Journal of Psychiatry*, **167**(3), 305–311.

Kabat-Zinn, J. (1994). *Wherever You Go, There You Are: Mindfulness Meditation in Everyday Life*. New York: Hyperion.

Khoury, B., Lecomte, T., Fortin, G. *et al.* (2013). Mindfulness-based therapy: a comprehensive meta-analysis. *Clinical Psychology Review*, 33(6), 763–771.

Kua, E. and Tan, C. (2005). Traditional Chinese medicine in psychiatric practice in Singapore. *International Psychiatry*, 8, 7–9.

Lim, Y. H., Kim, H., Kim, J. H., Bae, S., Park, H. Y. and Hong, Y. C. (2012). Air pollution and symptoms of depression in elderly adults. *Environmental Health Perspectives*, 120(7), 1023–1028.

Loizzo, J., Charlson, M. and Peterson, J. (2009). A program in contemplative self-healing: stress, allostasis, and learning in the Indo-Tibetan tradition. *Annals of the New York Academy of Sciences*, 1172, 123–147.

McElroy, S. L. (2009). Obesity in patients with severe mental illness: overview and management. *Journal of Clinical Psychiatry*, 70(Suppl 3), 12–21.

McIntyre, R. S., Alsuwaidan, M., Goldstein, B. I. *et al.* (2012). The Canadian Network for Mood and Anxiety Treatments (CANMAT) task force recommendations for the management of patients with mood disorders and comorbid metabolic disorders. *Annals of Clinical Psychiatry*, 24(1), 69–81.

Pan, W. H., Wu, H. J., Yeh, C. J., Chuang, S. Y. *et al.* (2011). Diet and health trends in Taiwan: comparison of two nutrition and health surveys from 1993–1996 and 2005–2008. *Asia Pacific Journal of Clinical Nutrition*, 20(2), 238–250.

Quirk, S. E., Williams, L. J., O'Neil, A., Pasco, J. A. *et al.* (2013). The association between diet quality, dietary patterns and depression in adults: a systematic review. *BMC Psychiatry* 13, 175.

Rawtaer, I., Mahendran, R., Yu, J. *et al.* (2015). Art, music, tai-chi and mindfulness: an evaluation of psychosocial interventions for subsyndromal depression and anxiety in older adults – a naturalistic study. *Asia-Pacific Psychiatry*, 7(3), 240–250.

Riediker, M. and Koren, H. S. (2004). The importance of environmental exposures to physical, mental and social well-being. *International Journal of Hygiene and Environmental Health*, 207(3), 193–201.

Rimer, J., Dwan, K., Lawlor, D. A., Greig, C. A., McMurdo, M., Morley, W. and Mead, G. E. (2012). Exercise for depression. *Cochrane Database of Systematic Reviews*, 7, CD004366.

Sarris, J. and Wardle, J. (2014). *Anxiety. Clinical Naturopathy: An Evidence-Based Guide to Practice*, 2nd edn. Sydney: Elsevier.

Sarris, J., Kavanagh, D. and Newton, R. (2008). Depression and Exercise. *Journal of Complementary Medicine* 7(3), 48–62.

Sarris, J., Moylan, S., Camfield, D. A. *et al.* (2012). Complementary medicine, exercise, meditation, diet, and lifestyle modification for anxiety disorders: a review of current evidence. *Evidence-Based Complementary and Alternative Medicine*, 2012, article ID: 809653.

Sarris, J., Nishi, D., Xiang, Y. T. *et al.* (2015). Implementation of psychiatric-focused lifestyle medicine programs in Asia. *Asia-Pacific Psychiatry*, 7(4), 345–354.

Schaar, B., Moose-Thiele, C. and Platen, P. (2010). Effects of exercise, diet, and a combination of exercise and diet in overweight and obese adults: a meta-analysis of the data. *Open Sports Medicine Journal*, 4, 17–28.

Singh, N. A., Stravinos, T. M., Scarbek, Y., Galambos, G., Liber, C. and Singh, M. A. F. (2005). A randomized controlled trial of high versus low intensity weight training versus general practitioner care for clinical depression in older adults. *Journals of Gerontology Series A: Biological Sciences and Medical Sciences*, 60A(6), 768–776.

Songprakun, W. and McCann, T. V. (2012). Effectiveness of a self-help manual on the promotion of resilience in individuals with depression in Thailand: a randomised controlled trial. *BMC Psychiatry*, 12, 12.

Stanley, S. and Laugharne, J. (2014). The impact of lifestyle factors on the physical health of people with a mental illness: a brief review. *International Journal of Behavioral Medicine*, 21(2), 275–281.

Takayama, N., Korpela, K., Lee, J. *et al.* (2014). Emotional, restorative and vitalizing effects of forest and urban environments at four sites in Japan. *International Journal of Environmental Research and Public Health*, 11(7), 7207–7230.

Tsai, A. C., Chang, T. L. and Chi, S. H. (2012). Frequent consumption of vegetables predicts lower risk of depression in older Taiwanese: results of a prospective population-based study. *Public Health Nutrition*, 15(6), 1087–1092.

Walsh, R. (2011). Lifestyle and mental health. *American Psychologist*, 66(7), 579–592.

Wang, F., Lee, E. K., Wu, T., Benson, H. *et al.* (2014). The effects of tai chi on depression, anxiety, and psychological well-being: a systematic review and meta-analysis. *International Journal of Behavioral Medicine*, 21(4), 605–617.

Werbach, M. (1996). *Nutritional Influences on Illness*. Tarzana, CA: Third Line Press.

Wu, D., Feng, L., Yao, S., Tian, X., Mahendran, R. and Kua, E. (2014). The early dementia prevention programme in Singapore. *The Lancet Psychiatry*, 1, 9–11.

Wu, T., Gao, X., Chen, M. and van Dam, R. M. (2009). Long-term effectiveness of diet-plus-exercise interventions vs. diet-only interventions for weight loss: a meta-analysis. *Obesity Reviews*, 10(3), 313–323.

Wu, T. H., Chiu, T. Y., Tsai, J. S. *et al.* (2008). Effectiveness of Taiwanese traditional herbal diet for pain management in terminal cancer patients. *Asia-Pacific Journal of Clinical Nutrition*, **17**(1), 17–22.

Xia, J., Merinder, L. B. and Belgamwar, M. R. (2011). Psychoeducation for schizophrenia. *Cochrane Database of Systematic Reviews*, **6**, CD002831.

Yin, J. and Dishman, R. (2014). The effect of tai chi and qigong practice on depression and anxiety symptoms: a systematic review and meta-regression analysis of randomized controlled trials. *Mental Health and Physical Activity*, 7, 135–146.

Globalization and Mental Health

Driss Moussaoui

Editors' Introduction

Globalization and the speed with which changes have occurred have been absolutely astonishing. The speed of change and access to social media as a result and expectations have changed the way we work and interact. Economic aspects of globalization have been positive in that people have become closer and trade has become easier but equally importantly it has led to psychological demands which are often urgent and pressured. Globalization has led to an increasing sense of belonging as a citizen of the world and rapid spread of ideas and news has contributed to urgent responses. Globalization has led to an acceleration of cognitive functioning, mood and technologies. With technological advances perception of time and space has changed. Movement of goods, people and ideas has become incredibly fast. Even the language is changing fast: instead of long sentences, young people prefer onomatopoeia or emoticons sent through social media networks. Interrelatedness and interconnectedness has become the norm which has led in many countries to increased nationalism and populism. Globalization has created a big problem of governance: no government is powerful enough to oppose the huge financial phenomena. In this chapter, Moussaoui reminds us that the mental and social cost of this for the individual and community is of course far from being negligible. This way of life looks from the psychopathological point of view as a hypomanic speedy life. Globalization can also contribute to cultural changes in response to this interconnectedness. Structures of traditional joint families can give way to nuclear families and associated stressors. Furthermore, social expectations change and as do networks as a result of industrialization and urbanization related to globalization. Moussaoui highlights in this chapter that globalization also contributes to changes in roles and gender role expectations for women. Globalization also has major political implications wherein people can either accept these changes willingly or reject them outright. Psychosocial effects of globalization also influence brain and physical functioning. Globalization is not likely to be reversed or go away altogether so we as clinicians need to understand its impact and manage within the framework.

Introduction

All living beings are prone to movement and hence to migration. Trees and plants travel through seeds with the winds, and each animal species tries to occupy maximum geographical niches, by adapting themselves to the various climatic specificities. Like other animals, and for millions of years, the *Homo* species (*Homo erectus*, Australopithecus) migrated very early in and outside of Africa, where they appeared for the first time, to the rest of the world (Meredith, 2011). Recent studies have suggested that the Bushmen (San people) of South Africa have DNA linked to the earliest *Homo sapiens*, dating back around 200,000 years. *Homo sapiens* headed very early through the rift region of the Great Lakes towards north and northwest Africa and towards the Middle East and Europe, expanding their migration to the Asia/Pacific region and the Americas. In north Africa (Balter, 2011), and especially in Morocco, a number of Aterian sites dating from about 80,000 years ago, have shown that there were similarities between the tools used in various sites in south and north Africa. This means that human beings transported as they journeyed their know-how, craftsmanship and their way of living from one part of Africa to another. It is of great interest that the first *H. sapiens* who inhabited the Middle East and Europe were dark skinned, and some studies suggest that some Neanderthals in Europe who lived at the same time may have had lighter coloured skin and fair/red hair. This is to say that the concept of globalization, as understood today, is in fact a very old story, which started right at the beginning of the human adventure.

The borders we know today between countries and continents were meaningless thousands years ago. For example, the Iberomaurusian civilization started about 20,000 years ago in the northern part of Morocco and in southern Spain. The groups living in this part of the world had the same habits of life (food, ornaments …) and even the same kind of medical pathologies. In one of the sites in the northeastern part of Morocco, the Taforalt grotto, the skull of a person was discovered who was operated on neurosurgically and who survived the operation, as the healing process around the operation hole was complete (Dastugue, 1962). This trephination dates back to 12,000 years ago, and the skull can be seen at the Archaeological Museum of Rabat, Morocco. Describing such society, part of it in Africa and the other part in Europe, the word civilization is not excessive at all and it easily crossed the Gibraltar straits.

It is also of interest to remember the qualitative and quantitative aspects of trade to better understand that the concept of globalization existed thousands of years ago. With the help of wheels on roads, and of ships on rivers and oceans, trade was one of the most important motivations to cross deserts, mountains and rivers, in order to exchange goods and know-how. For thousands of years, the Silk Road was one such trade network; the trade of ivory, gold and amber between pharaonic Egypt and the Baltic countries is another example. The trading ships built in the sixteenth century by the Chinese emperors were more than ten times bigger than the Columbus caravels that 'discovered' the Americas. In these migration/trade phenomena, cultures, beliefs, myths, manuscripts and religions travelled with human groups from one part of the world to the other. In the eleventh century, a copy of a book written by Avicenna in Central Asia (Persia) could be sold in the Koutoubia (literally the book market) of Marrakech, Morocco, less than a year later because of the vitality of exchanges through the Mecca pilgrimage of the Muslim religion. This is to say that migration of human beings, when it happened, also meant migration of goods and ideas.

Another aspect of migration is the courage small groups of human beings had to have to confront very difficult routes and situations in order to find a better place to live, or to achieve an aim. This included military campaigns, with or without commercial intentions. The Trojan war and the trip of Odysseus and his companions are good illustrations of such phenomena, as well as the multiple trips of the Vikings in the Atlantic and Mediterranean regions, and also the extraordinary trips of the Māori emerging from the Marquesas islands in the entire Pacific region. This is to say that migration also transports with it the image of heroes and this continues today. Only the most courageous, smart and able of the community dare to start a journey into the unknown. And this is part of the psychological motivations of migration today.

New Migrations

Among the big changes in the life of humankind during the last two centuries is the acceleration of migrations, including ideas and technologies. In the nineteenth century, the development of big steam boats speeded up colonization of Africa, Australia, India and the Americas. For the latter, migration concerned especially poor populations from north and central Europe. At the beginning of the twentieth century, about a third of the population of Sweden migrated elsewhere, especially towards the USA, because it was the poorest country of Europe. Western Europeans, especially British and French, created empires by colonizing other countries and continents, and imported natives from their empire and from poorer countries for their own interest (African slaves, soldiers during the two world wars of the twentieth century, Polish miners, Spanish, Portuguese and Maghrebian workers …). The extraordinary development of means of transportation served these purposes well: trains, ships and airplanes, but also cars and trucks. Those transportation machines became bigger, faster and cheaper, and travel became a much more democratic way of living, expanding the horizons of all. Currently, movements of populations have never before reached such magnitude in the history of humankind.

One of the most important migrations is from rural to urban areas. The United Nations estimate is that 200,000 persons move each day from the countryside to settle in cities. The urbanized population in the world in 2014 represented more than 54 per cent, as compared to 30 per cent in 1950. The urbanization figure is expected to reach 66 per cent in 2015 (United Nations, 2014). This increases tremendously the size of urban settings, making many of them become megacities (Tokyo, 38 million; Delhi, 25 million; Shanghai, 23 million; and Mexico City, Mumbai and

São Paulo, each with around 21 million inhabitants). Megacities have both good and bad aspects: anonymity and anomie, more services and crowdedness, beautiful neighbourhoods and slums, more cultural opportunities and a noisy polluted environment. The United Nations estimate is that, currently, at least one-third of the world population lives and works in a different place than the one the person was born in, and this figure will grow in the future.

International migration with settlement concerns relatively smaller numbers: the United Nations states in its report on international migration (UN, 2013) that there are 232 million migrants who settled in other countries, 41 per cent of them living in developing countries. Between 1990 and 2013, there was a 50 per cent increase in that population, and the pace of growth is increasing.

However, it is of interest to watch carefully the seasonal migrations, especially tourism. In 2014, there were 1.18 billion tourists worldwide (UN, 2015). Some religious pilgrimages reached the extraordinary figure of 120 million people, such as the Maha Kumbh Mela in Allahabad, India over a two-month period in 2013. Moreover, the International Civil Aviation Organization reports that 3.5 billion passengers buckled up for take-off in 2015, and the International Air Transport Association expects that number to be 3.8 billion in 2016 (Negroni, 2016). What was the exception in the middle of the last century, long and tedious trips, became usual and even the rule. The number of expected persons who would fly, if the growth continues as it is, might reach 18 billion people in 2050.

In parallel to physical shifts such as these ones, shared information grew up tremendously all over the world. In the late 1980s, to obtain a phone line was a privilege in a major city such as Casablanca, Morocco (5 million inhabitants). Currently, there are 58 million phone subscriptions for a population of 34 million inhabitants in the country, half of the devices being smart phones with access to the Internet.

The skyrocketing number of radio and TV stations in the second half of the twentieth century was another major development, as now almost everybody in the world can listen to or watch these channels through satellite dishes. Even the remotest areas in the world can catch these channels with satellites; when villages in the mountains have no electricity, they use car batteries to switch on a TV set. This is how information circulated at the speed of light from one part of the planet to the other. In 1960, a French psychiatrist Leguillant adopted the concept of 'still migration' (*transplantation immobile*) to designate this new way of life (Leguillant, 1960). This means that in one's own house, a person can visit other parts of the world without passport, without visa, and by paying very little money: the electrical consumption of a TV set.

Even more important was the creation and development of the Internet in the 1990s. This new dimension radically changed the life of billions of people, especially with the extraordinary development of smartphones and the multiple applications that can be run on these portable devices. Every owner of a mobile phone may become a social actor, almost a journalist on his/her own way when witnessing an event, shooting it and putting it live on social media networks. Those information and communication channels were a major factor in throwing out a number of dictators in north Africa and the Middle East in 2011–2012. This had an impact on governance in low- and middle-income countries at large and for the promotion of democracy, even if some steps forward led to tragic outcomes in some of these countries. Because of this power in the hands of all citizens, still today, some non-democratic countries in the Middle East and in Asia try to ban satellite dishes, and try to control the Internet and all its applications. On the same note, and because of the freedom acquired by the Internet, the most powerful countries in the world gather huge data on individuals and communities, with the pretext of fighting terrorism, but with the real aim of economical, political and military spying – on friends and foes alike.

This acceleration is best illustrated by the YouTube phenomenon (*Fortune*, 2013). YouTube was created in 2005, and by 2010 the monthly viewed videos were 62 billion and by 2013 they had reached 130 billion. In that year, more than 100 hours of videos were uploaded every single minute. This kind of exponential growth is seen in every single technological field, and it definitely has an impact on mental and social functioning of individuals and communities.

Psychosocial Impact of Globalization

The impact of globalization on the minds of people through these new technologies and still migrations is huge. It changed the way persons and communities perceive themselves, their governing bodies, their families and the world at large.

There are at least two good aspects to globalization: an increasing sense of being a citizen of the world, through swift information on what happens in the world in real time. More and more people do think, rightly, that what occurs in one part of the world, impacts on them and on the rest of the world. The other benefit of globalization is the availability of more goods for the neediest in the poorest countries, because of the steady decrease in prices.

Acceleration, Cognitive Functioning, Mood and Technologies

When electricity and cars were invented, they changed the perception of time and space. Days became longer, much longer than nights. Security became better with electric lighting in the streets. In a traditional Muslim society, an old lady stated the following: 'Since introduction of electric bulbs in houses, "jinn" [spirits] were frightened and fled away.' In this way, multiple lighting at night chased away the fear of darkness and gave more sense of security. This is how a technology may change traditional beliefs.

With the advent of cars, distances became less of a problem; we should remember that a trip for the French King Louis XIV from Versailles to Paris took a whole day at the beginning of the eighteenth century! We should also remember that, in 1920, a car driving at the speed of 17 km/hour was considered to be crazy. It goes without saying that a car cannot be driven the same way one rides a donkey or a mule. The cognitive demand for the car driver is much higher, and the more sophisticated a car is, the more attention, vigilance and concentration it necessitates. Decade after decade, the cognitive demand in an ever changing environment is increasing steadily. This is the case for transport, information, shopping (more and more on the Internet), money management, work – leading to an exponential growth of cognitive demand. And here, we are talking social and mental acceleration.

The best work done on the phenomenon of social acceleration is by the German sociologist, Hartmut Rosa from Iena University, who described the speeding up of all social processes (Rosa, 2013). Consumption increases everywhere in the world. For low socio-economic class persons, they ingest more food than ever before, and the poorest suffer more and more from obesity. For middle and high socio-economic classes, the consumption of goods is diversified to the extent that an important part of what is bought will be used rarely or not used at all. Time given to family and friends, time given to eat or to read is shrinking in a dramatic way. Everything goes faster and faster. People expect to receive the reply to an email 30 minutes later, and if it is not done, they sometimes call to know if the person is sick. The number of trips per year, including abroad, is also increasing fast. Half of the USA population took a plane in 2015.

Even the language is changing fast: instead of long sentences, young people prefer onomatopoeia or emoticons sent through social media networks. Another important aspect of globalization is the extraordinary development of international finance. In the 1980s, the prime minister of Italy visited the New York Stock Exchange on Wall Street. He was appalled to see that the equivalent of the annual budget of his country was traded in less than 10 minutes. Currently, the same amount is traded by computers in a fraction of second. The amount of money invested by hedge funds is US$750 trillion. This represents three times the GDP of the world. Moreover, the amount of money switching from one currency to another in the world exchange market is 5,000 billion dollars per day!

All this creates a big problem of governance: no government is powerful enough to oppose this huge financial strength, the function of which is mostly speculation – money producing money. One of the consequences of this is fluctuation of prices of essential products, such as food and energy, that is not necessarily good for the vast majority of human beings, especially the most vulnerable.

The aim of acceleration is to have more for less: more goods for less money, more information in less time, more trips in fewer days, more food with less exercise, more 'friends' on social media instead of fewer friends in real life.

The mental and social cost of this for the individual and community is of course far from being negligible. This way of life looks from the psychopathological point of view as a hypomanic speedy life. In manic patients, time flies, and in the opposite, the perceived flow of time is very slow in depression/melancholia. This was well documented by the German and French phenomenologists in psychiatry (Ludwig Binswanger, Eugène Minkowski, Hubertus Tellenbach), especially in the book *Le Temps vécu* by Minkowski (1933). One of my severely depressed patients told me once that for her, 1 minute lasted 40 hours.

According to the World Health Organization, the burden of depression and other mental health conditions is on the rise globally (WHO, 2017). Looking at the results of prevalence of depression in the general population in epidemiological surveys conducted in the United States of America every decade (Epidemiological Catchment Area, National Comorbidity Survey, National Comorbidity Survey-Replication), it shows clearly a steady increase of the prevalence of depression (Robins and Regier, 1991; Kessler *et al.*, 2005). Hence the questions are: what is the role of social acceleration in the increase of occurrence of depression in the general population and what is the role of decrease of duration of sleep in almost all societies? The metaphor that could better help understand what is happening is the following: if a number of persons are obliged to walk more and more quickly (look at the people going to their work in the morning on the metro/tube), then obliged to run more and more quickly, exhaustion will catch up. What happens then, after a certain time, is that an increasing number of persons will stop on the side of the road and will refuse even to walk. Acceleration is probably a risk factor for depression and even for other mental disorders.

In this respect, another question needs to be asked: there is an obvious decrease of sleep hours all over the world, due in part to the introduction of electricity in houses and the multiplication of screens, especially TV sets. In the US, a Gallup survey showed a loss of more than an hour per night sleep time from 1942 to 2013; it went down from 7.9 to 6.8 hours sleep per 24 hours (Jones, 2013). What is the relationship between this and the steady increase in prevalence of bipolar disorders in the general population as found in many countries of the world?

Cultural Changes and Technologies

Another major change in individuals and communities is the introduction of new cultural schemes through TV channels. A clash of cultures is then inevitable. It is remarkable to see how US American, Mexican, Brazilian, Indian or Turkish soap operas impact profoundly on the spectators worldwide, especially with translations into local languages. The structure of a traditional family can be shaken by the watching of an episode where a girl refuses to marry a boy chosen by the parents or when, as it happened recently in a Mexican series, two homosexuals amorously kiss each other. This kind of phenomenon accelerates the process towards modernization of families

and societies, and finally leads to the emergence of an individually marked thinking and discourse.

The evolution of the status of women, children and aged people is impacted by the flux of images broadcasted through satellites. This changes in depth the way traditional families and societies function.

Political Implications of Globalization

Globalization does not go without reactions, sometimes leading to adaptation, and sometimes to violent rejection. We already spoke about the use of social media for more democratization by toppling dictators in north Africa and the Middle East. There is another aspect in the interface between politics and globalization: the more globalized culture invades the world, with its sodas, jeans, fast food, malls and arrogant stock exchanges, the more reluctance it encounters, and not only in low- and middle-income countries. In the UK the recent 'Brexit' came as a surprise to many, despite the fact that economic loss for British people may accompany the exit of the United Kingdom from the European Union (EU). What made this vote possible is the low and middle class that considered that the EU is responsible for the economic difficulties of the British people, and which rejects the dilution of British identity in the bigger image of Europe. Another example is the recent race for the US presidency that shows how people think, in a very populist way, that the only manner to fight the globalized invasion, including migration/terrorism and loss of jobs because of deindustrialization, is to come back to the old specificities, including racism and contempt towards other nations. This is how President Trump's proposal to simply bar access to the USA to 1.5 billion Muslims of the world came about.

Another important political aspect is what is happening with the perception of terrorism, especially in its new form Daech (or ISIS). This terrorist organization uses new technologies to recruit fighters and to give its murderous actions maximum visibility all over the world. This is how people worldwide became deeply preoccupied with this menace. For example, all national authorities put heavy constraints on visa acquisition and on all travellers by plane in the world (3.5 billion people). If we think more rationally, we would see that most attacks happen in streets and public places, sometimes by attackers with limited means; moreover, the vast majority of killing targets Muslims. Let us compare two figures: 13,286 people were killed in the US by firearms in 2015, according to the Gun Violence Archive, and 26,819 people were injured (BBC, 2016). This is the equivalent of the deaths by the attack on the twin towers on 11 September 2001 every trimester of 2015! In comparison, in July 2016, CNN stated: 'Since declaring its caliphate in June 2014, the self-proclaimed Islamic State has conducted or inspired more than 140 terrorist attacks in 29 countries other than Iraq and Syria, where its carnage has taken a much deadlier toll. Those attacks have killed at least 2,043 people and injured thousands more' (Lister *et al.*, 2017). Needless to say that most of ISIS victims were Muslims. Another figure: in 2015, in countries such as France or Morocco, more than 4,000 persons died because of traffic accidents. Still, the Western perception today is that the main threat facing humankind is religious (mostly Muslim) terrorism, and this is due to the continuous highlighting of terrorist attacks on all TV networks.

It goes without saying that this list of psychosocial effects of globalization is by no means complete. The phenomenon of big data, the extraordinary developments in molecular biology, including the interface between machines and brain, the environmental challenges, the greater place of robots in the future, the growing importance of virtual reality, and not only as a game, are all important to consider.

The various consequences of globalization are interesting to study, but why would we psychiatrists and other mental health workers be in need of addressing such issues? What can we do practically to decrease the negative impact of globalization on individuals and communities?

What to Do?

The first necessity is to recognize that globalization has an impact on the mental status of all of us, especially the most vulnerable. Globalization is not only a process for lectures by economists or politicians, but it also must be addressed in the media by mental health professionals. The examples given here are enough to illustrate this fact.

A simple message is 'Slow down' whenever possible. It is very important for the mental health of all to not put oneself in danger because 'time is money'; if this is really the case, what is the real cost of lost health if all the time is spent to acquire money? And what is the value of money without health?

It is of essence not to be a slave of technologies, and to master their effect. Replying to emails until late at night, watching TV programmes the whole weekend, having numerous 'friends' on multiple social media, being a multi-task/multi-function person permanently, are all detrimental to health and mental health. It is of importance to highlight positive aspects of life, and time can be a precious ally or a terrible foe. To take time for leisure and for significant others is a protecting factor for mental health. The slow attitude should become a motto for a better life, even if it is considered by others as laziness.

Migration from rural to urban areas is huge. To strengthen family and social ties in all neighbourhoods, especially the poorest, is hence a major preventive measure for better mental health. Social workers and other mental health workers can do a lot to fight anomie that is known to be a risk factor for depression and suicide (Durkheim, 1897).

Another aspect of urban mental health is noise, which is detrimental to the health of people when it is excessive. The possibility of having more silence is good for mental health. In 1983, Herbert von Karajan stated in a speech given at UNESCO 'One day, silence will become one of the Human rights.'

Lastly, consider mental health at work: having time for oneself in the workplace is better understood by international companies, because the well-being of employees is a good factor for greater productivity. Some companies even have gyms, playing rooms or a place to nap during working hours. The possibility of working at a distance should also be considered for some employees.

The suggestions made in this section are in no way complete. Globalization is changing our lives dramatically and mental health workers need to do their best to dampen its bad effects. Each situation must be analysed and solutions found together with those concerned.

Concluding Remarks

Globalization always existed and will always exist. It is a very old reality that gains momentum year after year. Acceleration can make phenomena take a path that is exponential. This means that the speed of change is speeding up. The best metaphor of this is to drive a car that has an increasingly powerful engine without upgrading the brakes; the accident on that road is inevitable. The 'accelerated globalization' must be decelerated! In other words, acceleration needs more powerful brakes, and more power needs more responsibility and more ethics – individually and globally.

The psychosocial consequences of this acceleration are good in some aspects (in a sense of being a citizen of the world and having better governance and democracy), but it clearly has bad aspects for the most vulnerable. The question is on the table to know whether the accelerated globalization is or is not a major risk factor for mental health, especially mood disorders.

More research is needed in this field that is just at its beginning.

References

Balter, M. (2011). Was North Africa the launch pad for modern human migrations? *Science* **331**, 20–23.

BBC (2016). Guns in the US: the statistics behind the violence. Online article available at www.bbc.com/news/world-us-canada-34996604.

Dastugue, J. (1962). Paléopathologie. In *La Nécropole Épipaléolithique de Taforalt (Maroc oriental)*, ed. D. Ferembach, J. Dastugue, M. J. Targowla Poitrat. Edita-Casablanca, Rabat; Paris: Éditions du CNRS, pp. 133–158.

Durkheim, Emile (1897) *Le Suicide*, Paris: Presses universitaires de France.

Fortune (2013). European edition, 12 August.

Kessler, R. C., Chiu, W. T., Demler, O, Walters, E. E. (2005). Prevalence, severity, and comorbidity of 12-month DSM-IV disorders in the National Comorbidity Survey Replication. *Archives of General Psychiatry*, **62**, 617–627.

Leguillant, L. (1960). Psychopathologie de la transplantation. *Concours Médical*, **82**, 3429–3440.

Lister, Tim, Sanchez, Ray, Bixler, Mark *et al.* (2017). ISIS goes global: 143 attacks in 29 countries have killed 2,043. Online article available at cnn.com/192015/12/17/world/mapping-isis-attacks-around-the-world/.

Meredith M. (2011). *Born in Africa, the Quest for the Origins of Human Life.* Johannesburg: Jonathan Ball Publishing.

Minkowski, E. (1933). *Le Temps vécu. Étude phénoménologique et psychopathologique.* Paris: PUF-Quadrige.

Negroni, C. (2016). How much of the world's population has flown in an airplane? *Air and Space*, 6 January. Available online at www.airspacemag.com/daily-planet/how-much-worlds-population-has-flown-airplane.

Robins, L. N. and Regier, D. A. (1991). *Psychiatric Disorders in America: The Epidemiologic Catchment Area Study.* New York, NY: The Free Press.

Rosa, Hartmut (2013). *Social Acceleration: A New Theory of Modernity.* New York: Columbia University Press.

Jones, J. (2013). In US, 40% get less than recommended amount of sleep. Online article available at www.gallup.com/poll/166553/less-recommended-amount-sleep.aspx.

United Nations, Department of Economic and Social Affairs, Population Division (2013). International Migration Report.

United Nations, Department of Economic and Social Affairs, Population Division (2014). World Urbanization Prospects: The 2014 Revision, Highlights (ST/ESA/SER.A/352).

United Nations World Tourism Organization (2015). World Tourism Rankings.

World Health Organization (2017). Depression Fact Sheet. Available online at www.who.int/mediacentre/factsheets/fs369/en/.

Chapter 8

Social Media

Stephanie Solazzo, Pamela Hoffman and Margaret S. Chisolm

Editors' Introduction

Social media has become the prime source of inter-action especially among younger populations. The information and sharing of research and ideas has become much more relevant and instantaneous through the use of social media. Social media includes web, telephone apps, use of Twitter, Snapchat, Instagram, Facebook and other agencies. In this chapter, Solazzo *et al.* remind us that social media and other informatics tools are shaping how the public feel about medicine and how patients interact with their personal health information. These tools are influencing how clinicians communicate with one another and with patients, and how patients communicate among themselves. Healthcare informatics tools allow a patient's health information to be securely transmitted, electronic health portals provide secure venues by which patients can access their own personal health information, and mobile applications create and encourage an online community of patients around a particular illness or health-related issue. In research, interactions have also increasingly shifted online, expanding from the traditional, face-to-face interface of researcher and participant to one much less limited by time and space constraints. In medical education, with the help of the millennial generation, these tools have allowed learning to move beyond the confines of the traditional lecture hall. Social media have influenced clinical care, research and education. They are a powerful cultural force with the potential to both pull and push people towards an array of health-related behaviours. It is imperative that – as twenty-first-century mental health professionals – we understand social media and informatics tools and harness their power to relieve human suffering.

Introduction

Social media and other healthcare informatics tools – like their predecessors writing/reading, the printing press, radio and television – have made a significant impact on our culture. The world is smaller than ever before and understanding how these new communication tools are being used by researchers, educators, clinicians, patients and families around the world is increasingly essential to our work as twenty-first-century mental health professionals. These new tools are shaping how the public feel about medicine and how patients interact with their personal health information. As telemedicine expands access to care to countries with limited local mental health resources, these tools are also affecting how mental illness is viewed and treated around the world.

In cultures and areas where mental health is stigmatized or access to care is severely limited, healthcare informatics tools allow a patient's health information to be securely transmitted. Using secure videoconferencing technology, a patient can interact in real time with a psychiatrist far away. Telemedicine technology can help local primary care providers in the diagnosis and generation of treatment plans for their patients, often in consultation with families, all of whom live far from specialty mental health services. This technology can also facilitate continued locally based mental healthcare for these patients via ongoing consultation or direct provision of telemedicine mental health services, removing the additional social and economic burden of travelling for specialty treatment. Moreover, telemedicine provides a conduit for continuing mental health education to medical staff located in a remote community (Kaelber *et al.*, 2008).

Personal health records and patient-accessible electronic health portals have drastically changed the conceptualization of healthcare. In the previous century, patients passively accepted information and recommendations from their doctors. Now that medicine has shifted toward a shared partnership for healing, patients desire full and timely access to information and tools that promote better understanding and greater self-advocacy around illness and health (Martinez-Perez *et al.*, 2013). Electronic health portals provide secure venues by which patients can access their own personal health information as well as resources for additional shared knowledge. For example, a patient can view lab value results from a blood draw and link out to resources describing the implications of that result. Health portals allow patients to take ownership of their personal data and medical record, giving them access and control to help guide their treatment, in collaboration with their providers, and engage in prevention and other self-advocacy efforts.

Mobile healthcare applications go one step beyond online health portals to put a world of information quite literally into a patient's hands. There are now mobile applications focusing on everything from diagnosis to manualized therapies. Some mobile applications create and encourage an online community of users, offering an interactive environment for patients around a particular illness or health-related issue (Myers *et al.*, 2008). The location of the patient no longer offers the same cultural constraint; technology allows the patient to join global communities for information and support. Social media thus provide a unique method of engagement among a community of clinicians, patients, families and other care-givers. In academic settings, this community extends to researchers, research participants, educators and learners. Yet – as with any new technology – the arrival of social media is accompanied by an array of opportunities and challenges, both expected and unexpected. This chapter will examine some of these, organized around the three legs of the tripartite mission: research, education and clinical care.

In research, as elsewhere, interactions have increasingly shifted online, expanding from the traditional, face-to-face interface of researcher and participant to one much less limited by time and space constraints. Web-based communication tools enable researchers to interact with an entire world of individuals continuously creating their own online content, including that generated by recruited study participants as well as the public-at-large. These web-based tools bring with them the potential to exponentially increase participant recruitment for and participation in specific studies. They also provide access to online content generated by the user without the intent of being used for research purposes. In addition, these tools allow for increased collaboration among a world of researchers, as well

as real-time peer review and global dissemination of research results.

The use of social media in research has spurred a passionate and ongoing debate around various ethical issues, including what constitutes public vs private data and informed consent, demonstrating the absence of clear-cut ethical guidelines for conducting online human subject research (Markham and Buchanan, 2012). While most investigators defer to their local institutional review boards for an opinion regarding such ethical questions, little consensus exists among these boards on these matters. At present, the key ethical challenges identified for social media research include adequate informed consent, the loss of subject confidentiality due to searchable nature of content, and the use of child-, adolescent-, and young adult-created content (Henderson *et al.*, 2013). This last challenge is of particular concern, given that three-quarters of American teenagers have access to smartphones and 71 per cent report use of multiple social media sites (Lenhart *et al.*, 2015). Because young people are creating a significant amount of online content, consideration of the ethical quandaries surrounding social-media-based recruitment and data collection among children, adolescents and young adults is thus paramount.

The SharpTalk study – a research project funded by the National Institute for Health Research (UK) – provides a good illustration of this specific ethical dilemma. SharpTalk was designed as an online forum to encourage dialogue between healthcare providers and those young adults who engage in self-harm behaviours. Initially, the study did not receive local institutional review board approval due to the board's concerns that the investigators would not be able to preserve anonymity, ensure safety and provide adequate informed consent among participants. Faced with these concerns, the researchers argued for methods based in the conceptual model of 'ethics as process'. The investigators posited that ethics are a fluid entity between the researcher and the participant that is to be examined over time. Using this research model, participant contributions and their right to withdraw are maintained in balance with the study goals by a number of methods. For example, in this case, the investigators created multiple different chat rooms within the SharpTalk study website and provided study-specific usernames to maintain anonymity. The researchers found this approach to be an integral part of their overall risk-management strategy, reporting that participant concerns of anonymity and safety were in line with both the expectations of the local institutional review board and the study participants. Thus, for this study using this model, ethics became a collaborative project between researchers and participants, allegedly allowing for a more trustworthy environment and openness with participant participation (Sharkey *et al.*, 2011).

Alternatively other researchers have proposed a 'contextual based approach' to ethics. Website users who upload content assent to conditions-of-use agreements. Although these agreements vary widely among websites based upon the sites' goals and functions, many investigators hold the view that all such user-uploaded content rests in the public domain and thus represents an ethically acceptable data collection source. However, some ethicists argue that these conditions-of-use agreements do not necessarily satisfy the traditional criteria of informed consent held by the scientific community at large, criteria that are considered absolutely necessary for the conduct of ethically sound research. They argue for 'portable legal consent', which – in addition to the website user assenting to a conditions-of-use agreement – requires the user to assent to a voluntary relinquishing of personal information prior to the user's online content being available for research, in general. In other words, the user must explicitly consent to becoming a research participant, a process which would also include advising the participant of the right to revoke consent in the future. Although this approach preserves participant autonomy and control over their personal information, limitations abound including the blanket assent to participate in unspecified research, removal of choice for the participant to consent to some projects but not others, skewing of research samples towards tech-savvy individuals (in the United States, predominantly educated adults younger than 65 years of age), and reducing generalizability of study results.

Ethical concerns around the use of online content in research also extend to the rapidly expanding area of mobile social media healthcare applications. Considering the technologic leap made in communications in merely the last decade, the social media landscape is an ever fluid, ever-evolving environment. As research adapts to present technology, future technologic advances will pose these current ethical concerns as well as new challenges exposing the naiveté and lack of preparedness of the research community. DeCamp suggests social media technology and research ethics will continue to shape each other's development and require continuous vigilant examination of their evolving relationship (DeCamp, 2015).

Despite ethical challenges, social media provide researchers with the means to expand their academic reach. Online communities create arenas for collaboration, bridging researchers across continents and areas of scientific and medical specialty. Through platforms such as Symplur, social media tools can be collected and globally disseminated around both trending topics and events. These curated collections are a way of sharing information among the entire scientific community rather than only a few. Beyond dissemination of research topics and ideas, social media tools create a launch pad for researchers to attract attention to their own work, cultivate collaborations, and advance their scientific mission, an especially important benefit of social media for early career researchers and clinicians. As Lafferty notes, social media allow a sharing of curated knowledge that rivals the traditional literature search in its power for research development and planning (Lafferty and Manca, 2015). While some argue that social media-facilitated dissemination and impact (as measured by altmetrics) does not necessarily equate with scientific validity or importance, social media sharing of one's work may provide a new avenue for real-time peer review by the global research community. Such broad review may provide more accurate and honest critique of scientific work in comparison to review by a select group of peers (Lafferty and Manca, 2015).

Just as social media are being harnessed for research, these tools are also advancing education, which has now moved well beyond the confines of the traditional lecture hall. The millennial generation (individuals born between the early 1980s and the mid 1990s to early 2000s), also known as 'digital natives', have exerted tremendous pressure to move all aspects of education into the digital era. With focus on collaboration and active engagement, these young adults see education as a process and knowledge as malleable. These young people are the next generation of physicians and are changing the role of medical educators from transmitters of information to helpful guides. In this way, these medical learners are changing some aspects of the educational hierarchy, as they both consume and create knowledge. For a generation raised in an era of blogs, wikis, Facebook, and

Twitter, the inclusion of social media in medical school curricula is viewed more as an imperative than an option (Sandars and Morrison, 2007).

The use of social media in medical education has the potential to create a more active learning environment for trainees, one which promotes greater engagement with peers and faculty. However, given the emerging nature of these tools as applied to medical education, high-quality scholarship in this field is sparse. Although it is difficult to draw any definitive, evidence-based conclusions regarding the value of social media use in medical education, a review of the initial research looks promising (Cheston et al., 2013). For example, a study of the use of blog-based discussion forums in medical students found higher test scores among participants than non-participants (Geyer and Irish, 2008). Another study suggested that participation in an online course focusing on professionalism and humanism, which included blog discussions, protected medical students from a decline in empathy during third-year clerkships (Rosenthal et al., 2011). Yet social media and other online educational tools are not without their challenges. For instance, medical students who participated in online problem based learning groups spent more time on clinical skills assignments than students who participated in classroom groups, and faculty noted increased time requirements for blog facilitation (Raupach et al., 2009; Cheston et al., 2013). Nevertheless, more recent studies suggest social media tools can be valuable for medical education in a way that promotes lifelong learning. Twitter has shown some promise as an engaging educational tool for on-the-go learning for graduate-level trainees and beyond. One study described how general internal medicine programme directors and residents posted tweets containing de-identified teaching pearls from morning report, daily conference, grand rounds, as well as team cases. As measured by a pre- and post-study survey, residents found these tweets to be a convenient way to receive information and stay up to date, particularly when clinical duties prevented attendance at some of the educational activities (Galiatsatos et al., 2016).

Despite generally positive medical student and resident attitudes towards social media use in medical education, faculty and practising physician attitudes are more variable. A study of social media and continuing medical education noted that, while attitudes were relatively favourable across age groups, use was more clearly more prevalent among early career practitioners. In particular, physicians aged 50 and greater held more cautious opinions of social media and reported less frequent use. Furthermore, these physicians reported using social media more for social and personal interactions rather than professional use or dissemination of knowledge (Wang et al., 2012). Faculty engagement, or rather lack of engagement, professionally on social media highlights a crucial concern in medical education, adding support to learner critiques of the quality of online educational forums.

The openness of social media remains its asset and its weakness, including in the realm of medical education. Ease of access to social media allows for rapid dissemination and discussion of materials. However, participation and promotion of ideas can be deceptively unequal. As Carroll notes, 'Sometimes ego outweighs talent, unbeknownst to the reader or listener' (Carroll et al., 2016). Social media-created content can be measured by popularity and dissemination rather than scientific quality or concern with developing clinical practice. Additionally, studies and opinions perceived as less interesting or less popular – regardless of how critical they may be to medical education and clinical care – may receive less attention and/or be influenced by market-driven forces. For example, the dearth of older, more experienced practitioners on social media means that often less experienced providers are the ones facilitating online discussions. Or online discussion in healthcare forums may focus more on technology, procedural interventions and products. Thus, medical educators increasingly have a responsibility to actively participate in these virtual classrooms for the benefit of future healthcare providers and the public (Carroll et al., 2016). Involvement in lifelong learning directly correlates with career satisfaction (Afonso et al., 2014), and participation with social media may benefit faculty and seasoned physicians alike, both personally and professionally.

As the digital age is shaping the future of biomedical research and medical education, it is also influencing how providers communicate with patients and how patients communicate among themselves. Clinical communication among patients is transitioning to online and social media platforms at a remarkable pace. Peer support groups have historically played a role in the treatment of chronic and severe psychiatric and medical illness. Thus, it is not surprising that patients themselves have broken through barriers of time and space to create their own online support networks through a variety of platforms such as blogs, discussion boards, Facebook groups, and Twitter chats. Patients may seek online groups primarily for emotional support and information (Chung, 2014). For patients with particularly physically debilitating illnesses, such as multiple sclerosis, online support groups may promote more openness and greater ease of sharing emotions and information, without the added burden of mobility challenges (Davison *et al.*, 2000). Additionally some patients feel more comfortable discussing their feelings with strangers who share their illness than with family and friends (Jones *et al.*, 2011). A study of online forums for patients who identified as having bipolar disorder demonstrated that patients frequently discussed their symptoms, coping strategies, relationships with family members, as well as medications and their side effects; suggesting that online peer support groups are an important self-help tool for bipolar disorder patients, enabling them to discuss and manage their disease (Bauer *et al.*, 2013).

While greater anonymity may provide more ease of support and sharing, this indistinctness perhaps places the most vulnerable patients at risk. Facebook is the largest online social network, with 1.65 billion active users participating monthly (Statista, 2016), and has increasingly become the default method of contact between family and friends (Mehta and Atreja, 2015). Yet participation for patients with psychiatric illness may lead to adverse clinical outcomes, as some studies suggest that online participation may lead to jealousy of 'friends" lives and depression (Kross *et al.*, 2013). In addition, seeking online support for certain behavioural disorders carries other potential risks, as demonstrated by pro-anorexia websites that provide advice on food restriction and ways to conceal behaviours (Harshbarger *et al.*, 2009).

Another concern is the fact that social media sites are often mediated and controlled by non-clinician entities who are motivated by commercial rather than purely altruistic interests. Online posts place potentially private personal health information, which would otherwise be HIPAA-protected, into the hands of corporate programmers and executives. In 2014, Reuters reported on Facebook's intention to delve into healthcare, spurred by product teams realizing that patients with chronic ailments used the site for disease information (Farr and Oreskovic, 2014).

Yet Facebook's central interest stems from the potential to increase engagement and traffic with the site rather than patient care and advocacy. As Facebook already collects user information to tailor advertising, collection of health information certainly raises ethical concerns (Farr and Oreskovic, 2014; Wakefield, 2015). In 2014, Facebook published a study on emotional contagion, describing how they tracked changes in users' emotional responses based upon exposure to negative, positive or reduction of positive comments in user newsfeed (Kramer *et al.*, 2014). Facebook controlled exposure by altering its ranking algorithm that controls which content enters a user's newsfeed. The study's authors argued that, by agreeing to Facebook's user data policy when creating an account, users are consenting to research participation, and thus providing informed consent. However, this understanding of consent raises ethical concerns – beyond those previously discussed regarding big data use in general – as study leaders knowingly strove to affect user emotional state without user knowledge of participation in this specific study, or consideration of user mental and physical health. While HIPAA and privacy laws bind healthcare professionals to ethical practice of medicine, websites are not bound by these same rules of conduct and, as discussed previously, conditions-of-use agreements prove nebulous in their explanations for potential uses of data. Experiments conducted by anyone, including corporate entities, have the potential to cause clinical harm and, as always, the most vulnerable patients are placed at greatest risk.

While recognizing the importance of these concerns, it is clear that advances in technology bring with them certain benefits such as allowing clinicians to interface in real time with at-risk patients through mobile applications. The field of addiction treatment research perhaps best demonstrates the advantages of how the increased prevalence of mobile application usage can result in improved delivery of clinical care. For example, the Addiction-Comprehensive Health Enhancement Support System (A-CHESS), a mobile application designed to deliver treatment specifically for alcohol addiction, provides a number of tools for patients, including discussion groups, GPS locators for high-risk patients, 'ask an expert' features that allow patients to receive personalized responses to their questions within 48 hours, and 'panic buttons' that – upon activation – deliver encouraging statements to patients and alert appropriate providers to reach out either in person or via phone to the patient. Four months after being introduced to the A-CHESS application, approximately 73 per cent of the initial study population remained engaged, especially with the social features of the application (e.g. discussion groups, interaction with their addiction team) (McTavish *et al.*, 2012). A randomized control trial comparing residential treatment patients exposed and not exposed to the A-CHESS application showed that the exposed group reported statistically significantly fewer risky drinking days (defined as more than four drinks for men and three drinks for women consumed in a two-hour time period) compared to the unexposed group, at four, eight and twelve months after discharge (Gustafson *et al.*, 2014). Preliminary studies of relapse in patients participating with A-CHESS suggest the application may be able to predict relapse in high-risk patients, however, the percentage of patients who relapse despite mobile application usage and engagement with treatment remains relatively unknown. Though initial studies of this and other mobile applications show promise, their use as peer support remains in its nascent stages, and its potential for sustainable outcomes is not yet realized (Chih *et al.*, 2014; Chih, 2014).

Social media and other healthcare information tools have the potential to support medicine's mission as a public trust via their use in biomedical research, education and clinical care. It is also very clear that these tools have immense power to influence and shape human behaviour in ways that may be helpful or harmful to public health and mental hygiene. No consideration of these new communication tools in relation to cultural psychiatry would be complete without a discussion that recognizes how social media are a cultural force in themselves with the power to both pull and push people towards health-related behaviours in a variety of ways.

The initial normalization of cigarette smoking, followed by its stigmatization, is an example of how social expectations are able to pull individuals towards behaviours considered culturally normative for the era. In the case of cigarette smoking, initially this pull was towards smoking – at first normalized among men and later among women – to the clear detriment of public health. As the health risks of smoking became publicized (in particular by the 1964 US Surgeon General's report linking smoking and a variety of adverse health outcomes, including lung cancer), smoking rates among men dropped. The

sharp decline in smoking among men following the Surgeon General's report prompted aggressive tobacco company marketing of cigarettes to women – with products designed specifically for women like the 'Eve' cigarette brand and advertising campaigns aimed at women like 'You've come a long way, baby' by the makers of Virginia Slims. Women were initially pulled into smoking behaviour by these marketing efforts, but – with public health counter-efforts highlighting adverse health effects of smoking specific to women (especially those related to pregnancy) – smoking among women eventually declined as well. With increasing public awareness of the harmful health effects of cigarette smoking and its prohibition in various locations – airlines, at work, in bars – smoking has become increasingly more stigmatized. This stigmatization of cigarette smoking behaviour has pulled more and more individuals towards quitting (or not initiating) smoking.

The work of Christakis and others has demonstrated how people can be pulled towards certain behaviours at specific times in history because of the expectations of their particular social network or cluster (Apicella *et al.*, 2012; Christakis and Fowler, 2013; Kim *et al.*, 2015). Because social networks can now form through online connections, and social expectations can be amplified by social media, these new technologies provide a great opportunity to improve public health. However these technologies carry with them risks as well, especially for vulnerable individuals who are placed at increased risk of being pulled towards great harm by a non-normative social cluster. Consider, for instance, the case of disaffected youth who are pulled into a network of radicalized jihadists via social media-based communication tools. The expectations of this social cluster include a set of behaviours that culminate in death via suicide bombing.

Bandura's 'Bobo doll' experiments provide an excellent illustration of a slightly different kind of socially induced behavioural pull. In these classic studies, Bandura demonstrated how children are able to learn social behaviours – such as aggression – by watching the behaviour of another person (Bandura *et al.*, 1961). He showed how – by observation and imitation – psychologically normal people can be drawn into non-normative social behaviours. The field of social learning theory developed from these and other studies has important implications for the effects of social media on behaviour and health. In the age of social media, Tumblr sites created by users who discuss self-harm provide another example. Here, a non-normative social cluster models a different kind of self-harm (compared to the radicalized jihadists), which draw other vulnerable people to imitate these behaviours.

In addition to the pulls of social cluster and observation/imitation towards healthy and harmful behaviours, there are also pushes. Like pulls, pushes can also be shaped by social media tools. Pushes often come from the interaction of innate or acquired physiological drives and conditioned learning. In the realm of sexual drive, for example, online pornography and chat rooms illustrate how otherwise normal people can be pushed – via the interaction of innate sexual drive and conditioned learning – towards sexual behaviours considered non-normative, including paedophilia (Klein, 2014). Conditioned learning – based on a person seeking out repeated exposure to pornographic images especially arousing to that individual – increases drive towards this increasingly limited set of sexual images and narrows sexual preference, which has implications for not only the behaviour and health of the individual, but for families and communities.

There is little doubt that social media and other online communications technology has already made an enormous impact on society in general and medicine in particular. These new technologies are being used as social and political tools by a variety of movements with relevance to medicine (e.g. anti-vaccination, Black Lives Matter) and business interests (e.g. pharmaceutical, pornography, illicit drugs). These tools are also being used by healthcare professionals, trainees and patients, usually for the good of public health and mental hygiene, but – as potential social and political tools – they also risk being used to the detriment of public health and mental hygiene. It is imperative that – as twenty-first century mental health professionals – we recognize the potential of these tools and that we harness their power as a communication infrastructure resource aimed at our common good: to alleviate human suffering.

References

Afonso, P., Ramos, M. R., Saraiva, S., Moreira, C. A. and Figueira, M. L. (2014). Assessing the relation between career satisfaction in psychiatry with lifelong learning and scientific activity. *Psychiatry Research*, **217**(3), 210–214.

Apicella, C. L., Marlowe, F. W., Fowler, J. H. and Christakis, N. A. (2012). Social networks and cooperation in hunter-gatherers. *Nature*, **481**(7382), 497–501.

Bandura, A., Ross, D. and Ross, S. A. (1961). Transmission of aggression through imitation of aggressive models. *Journal of Abnormal and Social Psychology*, **63**, 575–582.

Bauer, R., Bauer, M., Spiessl, H. and Kagerbauer, T. (2013). Cyber-support: an analysis of online self-help forums (online self-help forums in bipolar disorder). *Nordic Journal of Psychiatry*, **67**(3), 185–190.

Carroll, C. L., Bruno, K. and von Tschudi, M. (2016). Social media and free open access medical education: the future of medical and nursing education? *American Journal of Critical Care: An Official Publication, American Association of Critical-Care Nurses*, **25**(1), 93–96.

Cheston, C. C., Flickinger, T. E. and Chisolm, M. S. (2013). Social media use in medical education: a systematic review. *Academic Medicine: Journal of the Association of American Medical Colleges*, **88**(6), 893–901.

Chih, M. Y. (2014). Exploring the use patterns of a mobile health application for alcohol addiction before the initial lapse after detoxification. *AMIA Annual Symposium Proceedings*, **2014**, 385–394.

Chih, M. Y., Patton, T., McTavish, F. M. *et al.* (2014). Predictive modeling of addiction lapses in a mobile health application. *Journal of Substance Abuse Treatment*, **46**(1), 29–35.

Christakis, N. A. and Fowler, J. H. (2013). Social contagion theory: examining dynamic social networks and human behavior. *Statistics in Medicine*, **32**(4), 556–577.

Chung, J. E. (2014). Social networking in online support groups for health: how online social networking benefits patients. *Journal of Health Communication*, **19**(6), 639–659.

Davison, K. P., Pennebaker, J. W. and Dickerson, S. S. (2000). Who talks? The social psychology of illness support groups. *The American Psychologist*, **55**(2), 205–217.

DeCamp, M. (2015). Ethical issues when using social media for health outside professional relationships. *International Review of Psychiatry (Abingdon, England)*, **27**(2), 97–105.

Farr, C., and Oreskovic, A. (2014). Exclusive: Facebook plots first steps into healthcare. *Reuters*, 3 October.

Galiatsatos, P., Porto-Carreiro, F., Hayashi, J., Zakaria, S. and Christmas, C. (2016). The use of social media to supplement resident medical education: the SMART-ME initiative. *Medical Education Online*, **21**, 29332.

Geyer, E. M. and Irish, D. E. (2008). Isolated to integrated: an evolving medical informatics curriculum. *Medical Reference Services Quarterly*, **27**(4), 451–461.

Gustafson, D. H., McTavish, F. M., Chih, M. Y., Atwood, A. K., Johnson, R. A., Boyle, M. G. *et al.* (2014). A smartphone application to support recovery from alcoholism: a randomized clinical trial. *JAMA Psychiatry*, **71**(5), 566–572.

Harshbarger, J. L., Ahlers-Schmidt, C. R., Mayans, L., Mayans, D. and Hawkins, J. H. (2009). Pro-anorexia websites: what a clinician should know. *The International Journal of Eating Disorders*, **42**(4), 367–370.

Henderson, M., Johnson, N. F. and Auld, G. (2013). Silences of ethical practice: dilemmas for researchers using social media. *Educational Research and Evaluation*, **19**(6), 546.

Jones, R., Sharkey, S., Ford, T., Emmens, T., Hewis, E., Smithson, J. *et al.* (2011). Online discussion forums for young people who self-harm: user views. *The Psychiatrist*, **35**, 364–368.

Kaelber, D. C., Jha, A. K., Johnston, D., Middleton, B. and Bates, D. W. (2008). A research agenda for personal health records (PHRs). *Journal of the American Medical Informatics Association*, **15**(6), 729–736.

Kim, D. A., Hwong, A. R., Stafford, D., Hughes, D. A., O'Malley, A. J., Fowler, J. H. *et al.* (2015). Social network targeting to maximise population behaviour change: a cluster randomised controlled trial. *The Lancet*, **386**(9989), 145–153.

Klein, C. A. (2014). Digital and divergent: sexual behaviors on the Internet. *The Journal of the American Academy of Psychiatry and the Law*, **42**(4), 495–503.

Kramer, A. D., Guillory, J. E. and Hancock, J. T. (2014). Experimental evidence of massive-scale emotional contagion through social networks. *Proceedings of the National Academy of Sciences of the United States of America*, **111**(24), 8788–8790.

Kross, E., Verduyn, P., Demiralp, E., Park, J., Lee, D. S., Lin, N. *et al.* (2013). Facebook use predicts declines in subjective well-being in young adults. *PloS One*, **8**(8), e69841.

Lafferty, N. T. and Manca, A. (2015). Perspectives on social media in and as research: a synthetic review. *International Review of Psychiatry*, **27**(2), 85–96.

Lenhart, A., Duggan, M., Perrin, A., Stepler, R., Rainie, L. and Parker, K. (2015). *Teens, Social Media and Technology Overview 2015. Smartphones Facilitate Shifts in Communication Landscape for Teens*. Washington, DC: Pew Research Center.

Markham, A. and Buchanan, E. (2012). Ethical decision-making and Internet research: recommendations from the AoIR ethics working committee (version 2.0). Association of Internet Researchers.

Martinez-Perez, B., de la Torre-Diez, I. and Lopez-Coronado, M. (2013). Mobile health applications for the most prevalent conditions by the world health organization: review and analysis. *Journal of Medical Internet Research*, **15**(6), e120.

McTavish, F. M., Chih, M. Y., Shah, D. and Gustafson, D. H. (2012). How patients recovering from alcoholism use a smartphone intervention. *Journal of Dual Diagnosis*, **8**(4), 294–304.

Mehta, N., and Atreja, A. (2015). Online social support networks. *International Review of Psychiatry*, **27**(2), 118–123.

Myers, K., Cain, S., Work Group on Quality Issues, and American Academy of Child and Adolescent Psychiatry Staff. (2008). Practice parameter for telepsychiatry with children and adolescents. *Journal of the American Academy of Child and Adolescent Psychiatry*, **47**(12), 1468–1483.

Raupach, T., Muenscher, C., Anders, S., Steinbach, R., Pukrop, T., Hege, I. *et al.* (2009). Web-based collaborative training of clinical reasoning: a randomized trial. *Medical Teacher*, **31**(9), e431–7.

Rosenthal, S., Howard, B., Schlussel, Y. R., Herrigel, D., Smolarz, B. G., Gable, B. *et al.* (2011). Humanism at heart: preserving empathy in third-year medical students. *Academic Medicine: Journal of the Association of American Medical Colleges*, **86**(3), 350–358.

Sandars, J., and Morrison, C. (2007). What is the net generation? The challenge for future medical education. *Medical Teacher*, **29**(2–3), 85–88.

Sharkey, S., Jones, R., Smithson, J., Hewis, E., Emmens, T., Ford, T. *et al.* (2011). Ethical practice in Internet research involving vulnerable people: lessons from a self-harm discussion forum study (SharpTalk). *Journal of Medical Ethics*, **37**(12), 752–758.

Statista (2016). Number of monthly active Facebook users 2008–2016. Available online at www.statista.com/statis tics/264810/number-of-monthly-active-facebook-users-worldwide/ (accessed 10 May 2016).

Wakefield, J. (2015). What is Facebook doing with my data? Online article posted 10 November. Available online at www.bbc.com/news/magazine-34776191 (accessed 10 May 2016).

Wang, A., Sandhu, N., Wittich, C., Mandrekar, J. and Beckmana, T. (2012). Using social media to improve continuing medical education: a survey of course participants. *Mayo Clinic Proceedings*, **87**(12), 1162.

Telepsychiatry
Cultural Considerations

Maryann Waugh and Jay H. Shore

Editors' Introduction

The use of videoconferencing in psychiatry is not new and has been in practice for a few decades. However, its use is increasing in many clinical settings for a number of reasons. Geographical inaccessibility of services is one such factor. In many countries with limited resources, using telepsychiatry can lead to immediate access to diagnosis and therapeutic interventions. In this chapter, Waugh and Shore describe how telepsychiatry, the use of videoconferencing to virtually connect psychiatric providers to patients, physicians, and other healthcare providers, is growing as a care modality that improves psychiatric care access to patients across a variety of care settings. By leveraging this technology, psychiatric providers increasingly encounter larger and more diverse populations of patients including those from unfamiliar communities and cultures. The challenges of culturally appropriate care are not new to psychiatry, but unique to telepsychiatry is the potential to aggravate culturally based misunderstanding and biased interpretation of behaviour through use of a virtual treatment modality. As such, cultural awareness and competency are particularly critical to ensuring positive patient–provider relationships and effective, high quality care. The purpose of the chapter is to highlight examples of effective cross-cultural telepsychiatry, identify some common elements and key components to culturally competent, virtual care delivery, and put forth practical recommendations for practitioners and organizations embarking on such cross-cultural work.

Introduction

Telepsychiatry, the use of videoconferencing to virtually connect psychiatric providers to patients, physicians, and other healthcare providers (American Psychiatric Association (APA), 2015) is growing as a care modality that improves psychiatric care access to patients across a variety of care settings (Deslich *et al.*, 2013). Telepsychiatry has been effectively used for assessment, diagnosis, medication management and psychoeducation (APA, 2015) to treat a variety of behavioural health diagnoses including mood disorders, schizophrenia, post-traumatic stress disorder, and eating disorders (Hilty *et al.*, 2013). The telepsychiatry research literature has documented positive treatment and cost outcomes that meet and, in some cases, exceed those of traditional in-person care delivery. Positive outcomes include improved behavioural health symptoms, shorter hospital stays, fewer hospital re-admissions, and increased medication adherence (Hilty *et al.*, 2013). Measures of patient acceptability are also positive and patients report similar levels of satisfaction following treatment delivered via videoconferencing or in person (Malhotra *et al.*, 2013).

By leveraging technology to mitigate care-access barriers, telepsychiatry is helping to transform psychiatric care delivery. Data aggregated across a variety of international studies found that over 70 per cent of the cost of patient and provider time and travel for a standard inpatient visit could be saved through the use of telemedicine in rural and remote areas (Spaulding *et al.*, 2010). Further, the real-time video and audio technology is increasing the number of patients a single provider can reach (Deslich *et al.*, 2013) and has the potential to address persistent health disparities for a variety of populations including rural residents, elderly and physically challenged patients, students, veterans, native populations, incarcerated persons, etc. (Deslich *et al.*, 2013; Shore *et al.*, 2006). Through these technological advances, psychiatric providers increasingly encounter larger and more diverse populations of patients including those from unfamiliar communities and cultures. As such, cultural awareness and competency are critical to ensuring positive patient–provider relationships and effective, high quality care.

Telepsychiatry and Cultural Competency

The Substance Abuse and Mental Health Services Administration (SAMHSA) defines cultural competency as 'the ability to interact effectively with people of different cultures' and clarifies that culture goes beyond race and ethnicity to include age, gender, sexual orientation, religion, socio-economic status, disability, geographical location and other characteristics (SAMHSA, 2015). The National Institute of Health (NIH) and the American Medical Association (AMA) endorse a more comprehensive definition, stating: 'Cultural and linguistic competence is a set of congruent behaviors, knowledge, attitudes, and policies that come together in a system, organization, or among professionals that enables effective work in cross-cultural situations.' They further define culture as referring to 'integrated patterns of human behavior that include the language, thoughts, actions, customs, beliefs, and institutions of racial, ethnic, social, or religious groups' and competence, as 'having the capacity to function effectively as an individual or an organization within the context of the cultural beliefs, practices, and needs presented by patients and their communities'. These agencies additionally include a patient/family-centred orientation and an appreciation of social and cultural influences that may affect medical services and treatment quality in their full explanation of cultural competency (Association of American Medical Colleges, 2005; NIH, 2016).

The goal of cultural competency is culturally appropriate care: 'the delivery of mental health services that are responsive to the cultural and linguistic concerns of all racial or ethnic minority and non-minority groups, including their psychosocial issues, characteristic styles of problem presentation, family, and immigration histories, traditions, beliefs and values' (US Public Health Service Office of the Surgeon General, 2001). This care relies on using generalized frameworks of understanding about typical cultural characteristics while avoiding derogatory stereotyping, and leaving ample space for unique individual orientations (Yellowlees et al., 2008). With a diverse patient population, and an increasingly diverse number of frameworks for cultural

understanding, it is important to remember that the act of rendering cultural competent care is an ongoing process rather than a singular event; a journey not a destination. The American Psychological Association (APA) notes that cultural humility is a useful construct for developing a process-oriented attitude to competency. This humility requires an attitude that respects the right of individuals to define the components most critical to their own cultural identity. Cultural humility puts forth the notion of cultural competency as an ongoing process framed by three major aspects: (1) a lifelong commitment to self-evaluation and self-critique characterized by flexibility and acknowledgement of the limitations of one's own knowledge; (2) addressing power imbalances inherent in the patient–provider relationship through collaboration; and (3) partnering with other people and groups to advocate for the needs of others in a systematic manner (APA, 2013).

The challenges of culturally appropriate care are not new to psychiatric providers and must remain a goal of care across all treatment settings and modalities (Tseng and Streltzer, 2004). What is unique to telepsychiatry is the potential to aggravate culturally based misunderstanding and biased interpretation of behaviour through use of a virtual treatment modality. While systems and individuals celebrate the ability of this technology to improve care access and reduce healthcare disparities, they must also remain aware of the heightened potential of cultural differences to negatively impact treatment quality (Nelson et al., 2002). Cultural humility is a particularly critical construct in the delivery of effective and patient-centred telepsychiatry, as psychiatric providers increasingly find themselves working with both individuals and organizations of unfamiliar culture.

Cultural Considerations: Individuals

As in any clinical encounter, providers must consider the patient's cultural background, his/her interpretation of behavioural health, illness and treatment plans, the impact of culture on the patient–provider relationship, and a variety of other individual factors that may impact both the therapeutic relationship and treatment outcomes (Shore et al., 2006). These factors may impact both behaviour and interpretations of verbal and non-verbal communication, including eye-contact (or lack thereof), body positioning and tone of voice (Shore et al., 2006). When the treatment modality is virtual, providers must also be aware of patients' comfort with videoconferencing, and technology in general. There are wide cultural variations in the affinity, access and skill-sets related to technology use. Race/ethnicity, education, rurality, and most strongly income, are associated with disparate technology use (Yellowlees *et al.*, 2008). Further, individuals with confidentiality-related concerns may limit disclosure over televideo, while individuals with post-traumatic stress or autistic-spectrum related disorders may disclose more through a televideo medium than in person (Shore *et al.*, 2006). The medium itself can serve to magnify, mute or change typical verbal and non-verbal communication patterns (i.e. speaking more loudly, maintaining a more direct gaze/body position). An attitude of openness and flexibility that seeks to interpret behaviour within a comprehensive multi-factor awareness will serve providers and patients in a telepsychiatry setting.

Cultural Considerations: Organizations

Remote care delivery also heightens the need for cultural humility towards the cultural organization of the originating site (the site/clinic where the patient receiving care is physically located). In a traditional care setting, the psychiatric provider would, through typical orientation or position on-boarding, be familiar with both the care clinic and its setting (i.e. hosting neighbourhood, town or county). When the psychiatric provider is instead present virtually, s/he may have never been on site, have had no exposure to the clinic environment (light, noise, temperature, administrative staff, etc.) or work flow processes, and may have little to no understanding of the cultural or local norms of the area. Virtually present providers may abruptly find themselves in the midst of a potentially unfamiliar culture, with no transition period to develop an awareness of how the organizational culture may impact patient care. Patients' experiences with the culture of the organization may impact his/her experiences with the virtual provider (Shore *et al.*, 2006).

Working across Cultures

A growing body of literature is showing that despite challenges to culturally competent telepsychiatry, high quality care and positive treatment outcomes are feasible across a variety of cross-cultural telepsychiatry situations. As previously noted, stereotypes are to be avoided, but having general frameworks from which to understand the culture of specific settings, populations and organizations, can support a culturally competent approach to telepsychiatric care (Beach *et al.*, 2005). While far from exhaustive, the following provides examples of feasible cross-cultural care delivery and highlights some of the key cultural considerations associated with successful implementation.

Feasibility of Cross-Cultural Work: Patient Culture

Feasibility with Rural Patients

Almost one-fifth of US citizens live in rural counties, which account for more than 85 per cent of the federally designated mental health professional shortage areas (Pyne *et al.*, 2010). Rural areas have higher rates of poverty and larger proportions of racial and ethnic minorities (Yellowlees *et al.*, 2008). Individuals in rural communities are less likely to receive mental health treatment because of challenges such as lack of mental health insurance, distance to providers, and increased stigma related to seeking behavioural health treatment (Pyne *et al.*, 2010). Rural residents who do receive treatment, are less likely to access evidence based practices, tend to attend fewer care sessions, begin care later after symptom onset, have more significant symptoms, and require more expensive treatment (Pyne *et al.*, 2010). Real-time teleconferencing technology has the demonstrated ability to mitigate challenges by increasing access to providers, reducing the time and cost spent in travel for patient and providers, and reducing stigma as telepsychiatry increases opportunities to access psychiatry care in primary care, home, and/or other locations (Fortney *et al.*, 2015). Patient and community culture, race/ethnicity, language and specialty-care access all impact health, and may be particularly relevant to rural residents. Survey data from primary care providers and staff at rural health clinics identified the following factors as most important to the provision of effective behavioural healthcare in rural areas: providers who value individual differences, providers who are personally dedicated to delivering high quality care, conditions that allow rural patients reasonable access to care, and having trained interpreters that speak patients' primary languages (Hilty *et al.*, 2013).

Feasibility in Hispanic Populations

The evidence for telepsychiatry as a feasible option for delivering culturally appropriate care to patients from diverse racial and ethnic backgrounds is substantial and growing (Hilty et al., 2013). Hispanic and Latino populations in the US have been identified as one particular cultural group who remain underserved despite clinical advances in the delivery for high quality depression care via traditional and videoconferencing methods (Moreno et al., 2012). Comparative cultural analysis finds that Hispanic and Latino patients differ from the overall US population in some significant demographic and health-related factors. On average, they are younger, have less education, and are of lower socio-economic status. In Hispanic populations, mental illness is associated with higher rates of comorbid/complicating factors (like obesity and diabetes). Hispanic populations have less access to quality mental healthcare, and tend to access mental healthcare more frequently in primary care versus specialty settings, and have lower rates of depression but more persistent expression for those afflicted. They also have lower rates of treatment/medication adherence; suspected at least in part, because of linguistic and educational barriers (Humberto et al., 2006).

Culturally appropriate care for this population includes sensitivities to geographic, socio-economic and language issues that can be barriers to appropriate behavioural health diagnosis and care (Humberto et al., 2006). The provision of behavioural health services, including psychiatry, within a more familiar primary care environment is one feasible approach to improving culturally appropriate care access for such patients. Research has shown positive improvements in both symptoms and quality of life ratings for Hispanic patients partaking in primary care-based depression treatment (Moreno et al., 2012). In a randomized trial of primary care based treatment as usual versus primary care co-located specialty behavioural healthcare, depressed Hispanic patients who participated in telepsychiatry had greater improvements in provider double-blind ratings of symptoms and self-ratings of quality of life (Moreno et al., 2012). These positive results show great promise for improving culturally appropriate care access for Hispanic populations by leveraging the primary care setting. Further, the videoconferencing technology was associated with improved care efficacy by allowing patients to access bilingual psychiatrists – who were not physically available in their home communities.

Feasibility with Children

Telepsychiatry has been well established as a way to increase care quality and access for children (Hilty et al., 2013). Telepsychiatry has documented efficacy for diagnosis, assessment and treatment across multiple settings including paediatric and primary care clinics, mental health centres, schools and day care centres (Savin et al., 2011). In a review of telepsychiatry with minority youth, Savin et al. (2011) note that parents have a particularly strong influence on the cultural orientation of the child. In all psychiatric encounters with youth, the provider must operate much like an ethnographer and become familiar with the parents' childrearing practices, what the family considers normal child behaviour, and how the family conceptualizes behavioural health illness and treatment. Without this familial cultural orientation, the psychiatric provider cannot accurately assess the child's ideations or behaviour, nor develop treatment plans likely to be followed and effective within the context of family goals and values. The inclusion of a virtual medium may further complicate this effort. The authors note that while the young patients are typically very comfortable with technology, parents and care-givers – such as grandparents – do not always trust the virtual psychiatrist. They recommend allowing adequate time to orient parents and care-givers to the technology, allow for small talk to give care-givers time to develop comfort with the virtual communication, and whenever possible, using local para-professionals and other healthcare practitioners to help build trust and rapport with the virtual psychiatrist (Savin et al., 2011).

Feasibility in Native American Communities

Native American populations, and particularly native veteran populations, are another group with high rates of poverty, and complex behavioural health needs; native veterans serve and suffer the consequences of military service at disproportionately higher rates as compared to the rest of the population (Shore et al., 2012).

A 2012 study evaluated the feasibility of a telepsychiatry programme leveraging university clinicians from an urban university to work with native veterans at two rural telemental health clinics. More than three-quarters of this native veteran population had PTSD, and many also held one or more additional behavioural health diagnoses. On average, these men also had three to four active physical health diagnoses, as well as high rates of self-reported social, familial, employment, and/or financial problems (Shore *et al.*, 2012). As such, this population presents a significant treatment challenge to behavioural health providers; even before considering cross-cultural challenges based on provider–patient cultural differences. Despite this myriad of challenges, pre-post chart review found trends towards decreased rates of hospitalization, associated with significant increases in measures of service utilization and treatment engagement. Of particular note was the significant increase in psychotropic medication use as recommended by Veterans Association (VA) and US Department of Defense guidelines (Shore *et al.*, 2012).

This native veteran project centred upon a cultural humility-based approach. The rural clinics were operating under a partnership between the VA, its Rural Health Resource Center and the University of Colorado Denver's Centers for American Indian and Alaska Native Health. Partner roles and responsibilities at each site were defined through ongoing regular communication and an iterative process that was based on the strengths and needs of each site's community. Additionally, each site employed an outreach worker, a native veteran responsible for administrative and technical functions who also serves as a cultural liaison between the tribe and partnering systems and providers (Shore *et al.*, 2012). In a discussion of cultural aspects critical to telepsychiatry, providers and researchers from the American Indian and Alaska Native Programs (AIANP) at the University of Colorado Health Sciences Center described this clinical outreach worker, called a tribal/telehealth outreach worker (TOW) as key to developing the trust and rapport needed for an effective patient–provider relationship in their telepsychiatry clinics. The TOW is a local community member of respect, and is often him or herself a native veteran. Not only does the TOW help patients feel more comfortable in accessing what may be an unfamiliar treatment modality (teleconferencing) and an unfamiliar healthcare practice (behavioural healthcare treatment), but they also guide the psychiatrists regarding cultural and other local issues relevant to individuals' treatment (Shore *et al.*, 2006). For example, the TOW helped link patients in the programme with traditional

healers in their local communities, enhancing the cultural competency and specificity of the care providing, increasing rapport between the clinics, patients and communities and providing care in better alignment with the community values (Shore *et al.*, 2012).

Evaluations of telemental health delivered to First Nation community members in Ontario, Canada also demonstrate the feasibility of using technology to increase care access in native communities. While not restricted to virtual psychiatric services, telemental health in these rural and remote communities was associated with increased care access and decreased healthcare costs. These communities have also proposed using the videoconferencing technology to increase local providers' access to psychoeducation and ongoing professional collaboration with a larger mental health workers' network (Gibson *et al.*, 2011).

The efficacy of telepsychiatry and telemental health in First Nation communities rests upon its ability to align with native culture. The Assembly of First Nations takes a holistic view of health, broadly supports the expansion of health technology and has passed resolutions to increase broadband capacity in Canada's First Nation communities. The Assembly has further articulated a major cultural consideration for partnering agencies and providers. They note that community empowerment and individual well-being are critical to aboriginal people and communities, particularly in light of increased violence, alcoholism and suicide related to a legacy of colonization. Assembly leaders call for health and social services systems that are designed and delivered by trained aboriginal people within an empowered self-government (Gibson *et al.*, 2011). The Brazilian National Telemedicine Programme in indigenous healthcare, while not specific to telepsychiatry, echoes these recommendations. A qualitative evaluation of their programme highlights the importance of maintaining a dialogue between all institutions involved in telehealth endeavours, and a democratic forum for ongoing process evaluating and decision-making. Similarly, they reiterate the importance of supporting native populations in efforts towards self-maintenance and social control; not simply implementing programmes aligned with the values of external provider groups (Taviera *et al.* 2014).

Feasibility of Cross-Cultural Work: Systems Culture

Distally located telepsychiatrists will likely work not just with new patient cultures, but also with new system cultures and unfamiliar clinical processes. Cross-agency work is often challenging as partner agencies navigate potentially disparate rules and regulations, processes and procedures, professional training and background, and expectations about new forms of collaboration (Savin *et al.*, 2011).

Juvenile Justice Settings

Juvenile justice settings range from community-based probation and group homes to locked detention and commitment facilities. As in any correctional institution, safety and security are top institutional priorities, which alone is a major cultural shift from a traditional behavioural health setting. Legal considerations related to licensure and malpractice may also be impacted by practising within a juvenile justice setting (Kaliebe *et al.*, 2011).

Perhaps of greatest clinical concern is that the institutional culture of a juvenile justice setting changes the dynamic of a traditional provider–patient alliance. There may be staff present in the room with the juvenile potentially impeding full patient disclosure because of lack of privacy and concern about confidentiality. Parents, care-givers, correctional staff, and/or even patients themselves may be unfamiliar or skeptical about behavioural health treatment and medication; presenting a level of treatment resistance not typical to traditional mental health settings. Further, even when parents, care-givers, correctional staff and patients are on board with a care plan, they may not have the freedom to adhere to all treatment components within the rigidity of a correctional setting (Kaliebe *et al.*, 2011).

There are often also added challenges in getting patient records – which can be a critical barrier to providing well-informed care given that histories often include comorbid mental health and substance abuse, trauma, foster care, poverty, academic challenges, aggression and failed treatment (Myers *et al.*, 2006). Working closely with institutional staff to understand the culture of the particular juvenile justice setting is critical, as is collaboratively identifying solutions to ensure the psychiatrist has access to critical information related to patient records, prior treatment and ongoing updates to legal and behavioural health status. Further, telepsychiatrists must find effective ways to develop rapport and engage youth in treatment despite the challenges of the intuitional culture and the virtual medium (Kaliebe *et al.*, 2011).

Child Welfare Settings

Youth in the child-welfare system have particularly high rates of behavioural health needs. In the United States, reports show that up to 75 per cent of youth in foster care have behavioural health needs that warrant professional attention (Landsverk *et al.*, 2009) but only about a quarter of those in need actually receive services (Burns *et al.*, 2004). Challenges to care access include a lack of coordination between child welfare and mental health agencies, failure to adequately identify youth mental health needs and scarcity of providers, among others. One potential consequence of inadequate behavioural healthcare is an over-reliance on medications – and data shows that Medicaid youth have higher numbers and doses of psychotropic and antipsychotic prescriptions. United States federal regulations now require careful monitoring of psychiatric medication for foster care youth to ensure that prescribed medications and doses are effective and limit the potential for long term and unnecessary side effects (Hilt *et al.*, 2013). Telepsychiatry has been used to mitigate some of these challenges, but effective models must work within the foster care culture. While a typical psychiatrist interaction may include a patient, or a patient and a parent/guardian, children, biological and/or foster parents, family advocates, child welfare case workers, telehealth consultants or coordinators, psychologists, and other therapists frequently attend psychiatric consultations in the child welfare system (Keilman, 2005).

There are examples of successful models of child welfare-based telepsychiatry in the literature. While not focused on the aspects of cultural competency needed to succeed in this system, the stress placed on the team-based and multidisciplinary culture is consistent across published descriptions. A 2005 study of the quality and acceptability of virtual versus in-person consultations found that psychiatrists at the University of New Mexico were able to deliver virtual services that were rated favourably as compared to in-person services by the large majority of rural child welfare-involved participants (Keilman, 2005).

Similarly, a published report described positive outcomes following a Wyoming state child welfare and Medicaid agencies collaborative telepsychiatry programme implemented with a team of distally based child psychiatrists at the University of Washington, Seattle (Hilt *et al.*, 2013). In this model, psychiatrists completed records reviews, phone consultations with child welfare case workers, televisits with patients, and follow up consultations with the child welfare multidisciplinary teams – and provided second opinions for previous youth prescriptions, and phone-based consultation to youth primary care providers. The implementation of this virtual consultative model was associated with improvement across three areas of previously identified concern for Wyoming's foster care youth: (1) high numbers and high dosages of psychotropic medication prescriptions for children under 5 years old; (2) long psychiatric hospitalization stays for youth without adequate child psychiatrist access; and (3) primary care providers concerned with their lack of youth mental health supports. These improvements were also associated with cost savings to the state (Hilt *et al.*, 2013).

In both instances, urban, university-based psychiatrists had to work not only with the rural culture of the individual and community, but also with the multidisciplinary culture of a foster care system. Working within the culture of diverse professionals and in a consultative instead of purely direct care role is very different from a typical mental health outpatient format. The team-based care was the cornerstone of the system culture, and the virtual psychiatrists adopted a consultative, team-based, and more diverse role to accommodate the needs of the patients and the system culture.

International Care

Behavioural health disorders account for 12 per cent of global disease burden according to the World Health Organization (WHO); however, only a quarter of those suffering in the developing world receive behavioural healthcare (WHO, 2014). Telemental health, including telepsychiatry, has a huge potential to positively impact global treatment disparities by bringing virtual care to underserved populations across the world. The positive potential of virtual care has been realized, and to some extent documented, in international response to natural and man-made disasters. A comprehensive review of telemental health in international and post-disaster settings notes that while more research is needed, there are strong and growing measures of successful telehealth implementation, with associated lessons learned and recommendations for clinicians providing cross-cultural virtual care in international settings (Augusterfer *et al.*, 2015). Literature on the effects of natural and man-made disasters (such as the Chernobyl disaster, the earthquake, tsunami and nuclear disaster in Japan; the armed conflict in Syria; the 9/11 attacks in the US; and the earthquake in Haiti; and others) make clear that in the wake of these disasters lies not just physical, but significant emotional trauma. Rates of post-traumatic stress disorder (PTSD) are very high after disasters, and research shows that the availability of mental health and psychosocial resources was critical to survivors' ability to recover and mitigate their trauma exposure (Boscarino, 2015).

To address global disparity and post-disaster need, international telemental health has been used effectively for a wide range of behavioural health services; from community and provider education to case consultations and direct clinical care (Augusterfer *et al.*, 2015). However, effective behavioural health treatment in international settings may be challenged by more than just issues of care access. For example, the authors describe an investigation of Syrian refugees in which 42 per cent of over 350 surveyed refugees reported symptoms consistent with PTSD. Despite measured need, only about a third of those surveyed perceived psychiatric need, and of those, less than half were willing to access care using virtual technology (Augusterfer *et al.*, 2015). In a review of disaster responses literature Boscarino (2015) notes that in addition to pre-existing vulnerabilities, a variety of social factors impact individuals' responses to traumatic episodes. These may include perceived self-esteem and self-efficacy, the perception of the threat of death, and other culturally driven interpretations related to traumatic events.

Authors Augusterfer, Mollica and Lavelle (2015) offer a variety of practical suggestions for psychiatrists and other mental health professionals based on decades of research in such challenging post-disaster, international care settings. In line with the model of cultural humility, the authors cite provider education, training and consultation as the most effective means for distally located providers to support other providers via videoconferencing technology. Similar to rural and other underserved areas previously described, these authors note that the largest care burden in international low-resource settings is borne by primary care providers. Providing these primary care providers with education and consultation: (1) increases the sustained capacity of the local providers to treat behavioural health immediately after and in an ongoing way following the disaster; (2) leaves direct treatment to providers who have greater familiarity with local culture and its impact upon treatment options and adherence; and (3) minimizes legal and licensing problems by leveraging provider-to-provider interactions and avoiding, but supporting, direct patient care (Augusterfer *et al.*, 2015).

In addition to the complications of cross-cultural international telepsychiatry, many post-disaster responses involve coordination across widely diverse agencies. Doarn and Merrell (2014) review decades of successful international post-disaster mitigation that include telehealth technology. Some successful operations involved the National Aeronautics and Space Administration (NASA) and military organizations from various countries, as well as humanitarian and other non-governmental groups. In many cases, successful virtual care efforts demand ongoing, collaborative and bilateral working relationships between the on-site providers and agencies to deliver culturally acceptable and sustainable care. For example, despite the culture of psychiatric avoidance in war-torn Somalia, another study found that tele-consultations with distal specialists were associated with an improved capacity of local clinicians to effectively manage complicated cases and an overall positive rating of the consultation experience by local providers (Augusterfer *et al.*, 2015).

Practical Recommendations and Conclusions

Practical Recommendations: Preparing for Cross-Cultural Telepsychiatry

These examples show that effective and culturally competent telepsychiatry has been documented across a variety of populations, systems and in domestic and international settings. As previously noted, however, providing culturally competent care is an ongoing journey. Because technology has made it possible to quickly expand psychiatry access to previously underserved and in-need populations, psychiatrists are increasingly and abruptly working in new and unfamiliar individual and systems cultures. This rapid deployment should not come at the expense of culturally competent care. The recommendations made in Table 9.1 are designed to provide practitioners and organizations with practical ways to prepare for the challenges of virtual cross-cultural work.

Practical Recommendations: Clinical Processes

The introduction of a virtual psychiatrist, whether into a behavioural health or a different type of partner agency, will require changes in workflow at the originating site. Providers and system leadership should spend time carefully articulating a set of clinical processes that allow for effective, efficient and culturally competent care. While many of the components in this successful clinical process will be site specific, the following recommendations will aid in ensuring culturally competent virtual care across a variety of settings.

- Work with the originating site to make sure the monitor image is appropriate for individual preferences. For example, with a patient who considers sustained eye contact disrespectful, make sure the monitor view has an appropriate zoom to the provider's eyes (Shore *et al.*, 2006).
- Make sure patients who have had less technology exposure have adequate time for orientation and opportunities to ask questions and try out the videoconferencing technology (Shore *et al.*, 2006).
- Consider using community-based health and cultural facilitators such as outreach health workers, local staff or other respected members of the local community to facilitate initial and ongoing sessions engagement between the provider, individual patients and their community. Such facilitators may help identify cultural barriers for the psychiatrist, help patients feel more comfortable with a distant provider, and provide valuable support to patient and provider as care plans are developed and implemented (Shore *et al.*, 2006).

Conclusions

Telepsychiatry is associated with improved care access, decreased care costs and improved care parity in its ability to reach underserved and/or

Table 9.1 Preparing for telehealth: recommendations for practitioners and organizations

Recommendations for practitioners

- Call upon the clinical skills used to build therapeutic alliances with patients and families and employ parallel processes for building institutional alliances that bridge cultures and improve culturally acceptable care (Savin *et al.*, 2011).
- Be aware of both individual and organization culture differences.
- Become a serious student of the cultures within which you are working.
- Make regular site visits if at all possible; and during site visits, participate in local traditions, customs and cultural events.
- Seek cultural information from a variety of sources. Consult websites, books and other published material, and use administrative sessions to ask questions.
- Identify and seek mentorship from someone in, or very familiar with, the culture.
- Be mindful of your relationship with the overall community in which you are providing care.
- Look for opportunities to build positive relationships with individuals and agencies beyond just the care site.
- Look beyond the field to psychiatry to find broad telehealth related recommendations for the effective delivery of virtual care. For example, the Brazilian National Telemedicine Program in indigenous healthcare exists to assist health professionals working in remote areas and strengthen healthcare provided to indigenous people. Their documents and evaluations provide recommendations for culturally acceptable care delivered via all types of telemedicine (Taviera *et al.*, 2014).

Recommendations for Organizations

- *Expect* problems to arise because of institutional culture differences.
- Allow space and time to raise and address cross-cultural challenges within the processes of designing and implementing telepsychiatry programmes.
- Build strategies for approaching unanticipated inter-institutional difficulties into programme structure.
- Time spent addressing administrative and clinical issues will help identify conflicting operational and clinical procedures, and will help build unified clinical teams (Savin *et al.*, 2011).
- Include site visits in project schedules and budgets.
- Have organization leadership set an example of increasing their cultural awareness, knowledge and competency by pursuits such as those recommended for practitioners.
- Acknowledge and openly discuss the challenges of cross-cultural work.
- Include time for discussing cross-cultural challenges at regular team meetings.
- Cultural-competence training exercises are promising strategies for improving providers' cultural knowledge, skills and attitudes, and patient ratings of care quality (Beach *et al.*, 2005). Consider including such training for all involved staff in project design/implementation.

remote populations (Hilty *et al.*, 2013). With these care improvements, however, come challenges to the provision of culturally competent care as providers are quickly deployed into more disparate cultural care settings. When providers are physically removed from the environment in which they render care, they may have limited knowledge of the environmental, organizational and community culture that impacts their patients. As such, the use of a videoconferencing medium to provide distant care increases the need for cultural humility in diagnosing and treating persons of different cultural backgrounds and working in organizations, systems and settings of unfamiliar culture (Shore *et al.*, 2012).

Despite challenges, there is a growing body of literature that documents successful and culturally competent applications of cross-cultural telepsychiatric care in diverse populations and systems, in domestic and international settings. This chapter has outlined a number of approaches that can help to improve culturally competent care delivery in virtual settings. Broad recommendations include increasing provider/organizational awareness of cross-cultural challenges, seeking ongoing cultural competency education within and external to the field of psychiatry, and using on-site mentorship and visits to gain first-hand experiences within new care cultures. The time spent addressing cross-cultural clinical and process issues before they become problems will help build unified clinical teams.

These suggestions are designed to increase the ability of providers and organizational leaders to be mindful of critical cultural considerations and thoughtfully adapt services to best meet the needs of their diverse patient populations.

References

American Psychiatric Association (APA) (2015). Telepsychiatry; relevance to the underserved issue. Available at: www.psychiatry.org/practice/professional-interests/underserved-communities/telepsychiatry (accessed 16 March 2016).

American Psychological Association (APA) (2013). Reflections on cultural humility. Available at: www.apa.org/pi/families/resources/newsletter/2013/08/cultural-humility.aspx (accessed 5 May 2016).

Association of American Medical Colleges (2005). Cultural competence education. Available at: www.aamc.org/download/54338/data/culturalcomped.pdf (accessed 15 March 2016).

Augusterfer, E. F., Mollica, R. F. and Lavelle, J. (2015). A review of telemental health in international and post-disaster settings. *International Review of Psychiatry*, 27(6), 540–546, doi:10.3109/09540261.2015.1082985.

Beach, M. C., Price, E. H., Gary, T. L. *et al.* (2005). Cultural competency: a systematic review of health care provider educational interventions. *Medical Care*, 43(4), 356–373.

Boscarino, J. A. (2015). Community disasters, psychological trauma, and crisis intervention. *International Journal of Emergency Mental Health*, 17, 369–371.

Burns, B. J., Phillips, S. D., Wagner, H. R., Barth, R. P., Kolko, D. J., Campbell, Y. and Landsverk, J. (2004). Mental health need and access to mental health services by youths involved with child welfare: a national survey. *Journal of the American Academy of Child and Adolescent Psychiatry*, 43(8), 960–970.

Deslich, S. A., Stec, B., Tomblin, S. and Coustasse, A. (2013). Telepsychiatry in the 21st century: transforming healthcare with technology. *Perspectives in Health Information Management*, 10(1f), 1–17, PMCID: PMC3709879.

Doarn, C. R. and Merrell, R. C. (2014). Telemedicine and e-Health in Disaster Response. *Telemedicine and e-Health*, 20(7), 605–606, doi:10.1089/tmj.2014.9983.

Fortney, J. C., Pyne, J. M., Turner, E. E. *et al.* (2015). Telepsychiatry: integration of mental health services into rural primary care settings. *International Review of Psychiatry*, 27(6), 525–539, doi: 10.3109/09540261.2015.1085838.

Gibson, K. L., Coulson, H., Miles, R., Kakekakekung, C., Daniels, E. and O'Donnell, S. (2011). Conversations on telemental health: listening to remote and rural First Nations communities. *Rural and Remote Health*, 11, 1–19.

Hilt, R. J., Romaire, M. A., McDonell, M. G., Sears, J. M., Krupski, A., Thompson, J. N., Trupin, E.W. (2013). The Partnership Access Line: evaluating a child psychiatry program in Washington state. *Journal of the American Medical Association Pediatrics*, 167(2), 162–168, doi:10.1001/2013.jamapediatrics.47.

Hilty, D. M., Ferrer, D. C., Parish, M. B., Johnston, B., Callahan, E. J., and Yellowlees, P. M. (2013). The effectiveness of telemental health: a 2013 review. *Journal of Telemedicine and E-Health*, 19(6), 444–454, doi: 10.1089/tmj.2013.0075.

Humberto, M., Escobar, J. I., and Vega, W. A. (2006). Mental illness in Hispanics: a review of the literature. *Focus*, 6(1), 23–37.

Kaliebe, K. E., Heneghan, J. and Kim, T. J. (2011). Telepsychiatry in juvenile justice settings. *Child and Adolescent Psychiatric Clinics of North America*, 20, 113–123, doi:10.1016/j.chc.2010.09.001.

Keilman, P. (2005). Telepsychiatry with child welfare families referred to a family service agency. *Telemedicine and e-Health*, 11(1), 98–101.

Landsverk, J. A., Burns, B. J., Stambaugh, L. F. and Reutz, J. A. (2009). Psychosocial interventions for children and adolescents in foster care: review of research literature. *Child Welfare*, 88(1), 49–69.

Malhotra, S., Chakrabarti, S. and Shah, R. (2013) Telepsychiatry: promise, potential, and challenges. *Indian Journal of Psychiatry*, 55(1), 3–11, doi: 10.4103/0019-5545.105499.

Moreno, F. A., Chong, J., Dumbauld, J., Humke, M. and Byreddy, S. (2012). Use of standard webcam and Internet equipment for telepsychiatry treatment of depression among underserved Hispanics. *Psychiatric Services*, 63(12), 1213–1217.

Myers, K., Valentine, J., Morganthaler, R. and Melzer, S. (2006). Telepsychiatry with incarcerated youth. *Journal of Adolescent Health*, 38, 643–648.

National Institute of Health (NIH), US National Library of Medicine, National Information Center on Health Services Research and Health Care Technology (NICHSR) (2016). Health literacy and cultural competence. Available at: www.nlm.nih.gov/hsrinfo/health_literacy.html# updated: March 2016 (accessed 15 March 2016).

Nelson, A. R., Smedley, B. D. and Stith, A. Y. (eds) (2002). *Unequal Treatment: Confronting Racial and Ethnic Disparities in Health Care*. Washington, DC: National Academies Press.

Pyne, J. M., Fortney, J. C., Tripathi, S. P., Maciejewski, M. L., Edlund, M. J. and Williams, D. K. (2010). Cost-effectiveness analysis of a rural telemedicine collaborative care intervention for depression. *Archives of General Psychiatry*, **67**(8), 812–21, doi: 10.1001/archgenpsychiatry.2010.82.

Savin, D., Glueck, D. A., Chardavoyne, J., Yager, J., and Novins, D. K. (2011). Bridging cultures: child psychiatry via videoconferencing. *Child and Adolescent Psychiatric Clinics of North America*, **20**, 125–134, doi: 10.1016/j.chc.2010.09.002.

Shore, J. H., Savin, D., Novins, D. and Manson, S. (2006). Cultural aspects of telepsychiatry. *Journal of Telemedicine and Telecare*, **12**, 116–121.

Shore, J. H., Brooks, E., Anderson, H., Bair, B., Dailey, N., Kaufmann, L. J. and Manson, S. (2012). Characteristics of telemental health service use by American Indian veterans. *Psychiatric Services*, **63**(2), 179–181, doi: 10.1176/appi.ps.201100098.

Spaulding, R., Belz, N., DeLurgio, S. and Williams, A. R. (2013). Cost savings of telemedicine utilization for child psychiatry in a rural Kansas community. *Journal of Telemedicine and e-Health*, **19**(6), 444–454, doi: 10.1089/tmj.2013.0075.

Substance Abuse and Mental Health Services Administration (SAMHSA) (2015). Cultural Competence. Available at: www.samhsa.gov/capt/applying-strategic-prevention/cultural-competence (accessed 15 April 2016).

Taveira, Z. Z., Scherer, M. D., and Diehl, E. E. (2014). Implementation of telemedicine in indigenous people's healthcare in Brazil. *Cadernos de Saúde Pública*, **30**(8), 1793–1797. http://dx.doi.org/10.1590/0102-311X00026214.

Tseng, W. and Streltzer, J. (eds), (2004). Introduction: Culture and psychiatry, in *Cultural Competence in Clinical Psychiatry*. Washington DC: American Psychiatric Publishing.

US Public Health Service Office of the Surgeon General (2001). Mental health: Culture, race, and ethnicity: A supplement to mental health: A report of the Surgeon General. Rockville, MD: Department of Health and Human Services, US Public Health Service.

World Health Organization (WHO) (2014). Mental disorders: Fact sheet. Geneva: World Health Organization. Available at: www.who.int/mediacentre/factsheets/fs396/en/ (accessed 15 April 2016).

Yellowlees, P., Marks, S., Hilty, D. and Shore, J. H. (2008). Using e-health to enable culturally appropriate mental healthcare in rural areas. *Telemedicine and e-Health*, **14**(5), 486–492, doi: 10.1089/tmj.2007.0070.

Chapter 10

Ethnic Inequalities and Cultural-Capability Framework in Mental Healthcare

Kamaldeep Bhui, Rubens Dantas, Antonio Ventriglio and Dinesh Bhugra

Editors' Introduction

There is considerable evidence in literature, as has been shown consistently in this volume, that rates of some types of mental illness are higher in black and ethnic minority groups when compared with other groups, especially majority groups. This has been attributed to a number of reasons, of which misdiagnosis keeps being referred to. The explanations for ethnic inequalities are multilayered, and include social inequalities, socio-economic factors, gender and age. A large number of factors including explanatory models affect where, when and how help is sought as well as clinical assessments and outcomes of therapeutic consultations. There is no doubt that values of majority cultures dramatically influence these processes especially as a result of acculturation and equally importantly acculturative stress can contribute to distress. Explanatory models held by patients and carers will dictate which pathways to professional care they follow. Help-seeking is also determined by the personal, folk and social resources an individual has.

Bhui *et al.* explore the major causes of ethnic variations in the patterns of health service usage, which are many, and include cultural variations in explanations of distress, knowledge about the local care systems, geographical and emotional accessibility of services. The culture of healthcare delivery can also influence attitudes towards patients, their carers and their problems. There is no doubt that these processes are mediated through social and cultural factors, including lifestyle. They suggest that a cultural-capability framework which assesses cultural identity, explanatory models, individual and organizational dynamics along with a clear emphasis on reflexivity in the assessment may enable the clinician to engage cultural minorities in decision-making and engagement in therapeutic alliances. This may diminish inequalities in experience of healthcare and outcomes. Inequalities in need for mental healthcare are particularly stark in some clinical settings, such as forensic

care or primary care. Some ethnic groups are over-represented in each of these settings. Community and organizational factors also play a role in help-seeking, as well as dissatisfaction with such approaches. Inequalities in healthcare emerge from consequences of the actions of individual practitioners and organizational cultures working together. Cultural capability includes sensitivity, awareness, empathy, knowledge and adjustment to consultation and treatment according to cultural factors if services are to be used effectively by patients.

Introduction

Ethnic inequalities in healthcare are universal and exist across medical specialties. To complicate matters further often gender, age, social class and educational status create a complex picture related to inequalities but of these cultural and ethnicity driven factors are probably most significant. Ethnic-minority groups often also have increased rates of certain physical illnesses thereby causing comorbidities and hence contributing to high levels of morbidity and differential help seeking.

Decades of British psychiatric research demonstrate ethnic inequalities in service use, experiences and benefit from services (Department of Health, 2003). A similar picture is described in USA studies, confirming ethnic disparities in access to services and interventions, as well as variations in clinical outcomes (Snowden, 2003; US Department of Health and Human Services, 2001; van Ryn and Fu, 2003). A number of mechanisms are proposed to explain the higher incidence of schizophrenia among some black and ethnic-minority patients and the higher rates of using inpatient care and compulsory detention. These processes are mediated, not uniquely through biological or genetic predispositions alone, but through social and cultural mediators such as lifestyle, social networks, expectations and attitudes to mental health services, coping styles and socio-cultural vulnerabilities (Sharpley, *et al.*, 2001). It is known that the culture influences help-seeking behaviour and characteristic expressions of distress (Bhui *et al.*, 2002; Gater *et al.*, 1991). It is also possible that the cultures of healthcare organizations and professional practice can reduce access to desired interventions among some ethnic groups; for example, coronary artery bypass grafts and angioplasty are less frequently performed for South Asians needing revascularization for ischemic heart disease (Feder *et al.*, 2002). At the same time, health professionals may impose undesirable interventions on some ethnic groups; for example, compulsory detentions among black Caribbean people (Bhui *et al.*, 2003). The major causes of ethnic variations in the patterns of mental health service use are many. Although much of the data upon which this chapter is based arises from the UK context, the potential explanations are of importance in other countries including the North American continent, where the data for black people in the UK are mirrored in the reported service-used data for African Americans (US Dept of Health and Human Services, 2001).

Although much attention is given to ethnic minorities and their contact with mental health services, migration alongside ethnicity must also be considered as a risk factor for mental healthcare. Recent studies show that the incidence of psychosis is higher among migrants (above all black migrants from Africa) and refugees. Increased risk of psychosis among black Caribbean migrants and their descendants has been described since the 1960s (Tortelli *et al.*, 2015). Moreover, refugees report an increased risk of schizophrenia and other non-affective psychotic disorders compared with non-refugee migrants from similar regions of origin (Hollander *et al.*, 2016). Anderson *et al.* (2015) point out that psychosocial and cultural factors associated with migration may contribute to the risk of psychotic disorders.

Ethnic variations of health status are often explained away as being secondary to social inequalities. Social inequalities are invariably evident following migration and resettlement. In particular, migrants who flee persecution have not usually prepared for their residence in a new country, may leave their own country impulsively, and, necessarily, seek employment to secure monies, accommodation and food. Entering the employment market and social integration involves overcoming obstacles such as language differences, prejudice and different work cultures. For professionals migrating to the UK to seek work, along with migration rules there are distinct national certification and regulation requirements, so their former qualifications, income levels and status may be eroded following the migration experience. Social inequalities appear to be transmitted through cultures and society; consecutive generations continue to face similar obstacles as those faced by new immigrants, but their expectations and skills in negotiating these obstacles are different. Berry (1997) has outlined how bi-culturally proficient migrants are more able to access resources, whilst sustaining their identification with their culture of origin. D'Anna-Hernandez *et al.* (2015) reported that acculturative stress among Mexican women did contribute to increased levels of depression during pregnancy. Kim *et al.* (2014) highlight that there is a geographical variation linked with ethnic variations.

Thus an integrated cultural identity reflects, and perhaps encourages, more successful adaptation. However, the relationship between migration and wealth is complex. Although migration controls are usually in place to restrict immigration, so as to limit the perceived drain on scarce resources, recent data compiled by the Home Office in the UK show that migration is actually profitable for host nations (Dobson *et al.*, 2001). Studies in Germany, the United States and the UK show that foreign-born people contribute more to the state in taxation than they consume in benefits and social security. Nonetheless, some groups fare badly. Caribbean-origin black people have very high rates of unemployment, whilst Bangladeshi and Pakistani people have the lowest incomes in the UK. Unemployment and other deprivation indicators are known to be related to, and are possibly aetiological risk factors for, mental health problems (Fryers *et al.*, 2003). Although social inequalities explain a great deal of ethnic inequalities in health, they do not fully explain these. Other factors, such as discrimination, have independent effects (Nazroo, 2003). Cultures of adversity and impoverishment shape opportunities for health gains through health promotion, and choice over service use. National policies attending to migrant well-being can inadvertently be detrimental if they encourage cultural identities that are not adaptive, for example, through an emphasis on assimilation: giving up one's culture of origin and adopting host cultural values (Berry, 1997). In this context, this chapter describes ethnic inequalities of access to mental health services in the UK, and then focuses specifically on methods to improve the cultural capability of mental health services and clinical practice.

There is no doubt that racial discrimination at many levels can contribute to ethnic inequalities which in turn affect mental health and health outcomes. A systematic review of 121 studies on discrimination against people with mental health problems, especially adolescents, children and young people, showed statistically significant associations with racial discrimination found in 76 per cent of outcomes examined (Priest *et al.*, 2013). Not surprisingly, statistically significant associations were also found between racial discrimination and positive mental health (e.g. self-esteem, resilience), behaviour problems, well-being, and pregnancy/birth outcomes.

Psychiatric and Forensic Services in the UK

There are higher rates of non-affective psychosis among black Caribbean people, with the highest rates in the second generation, so dismissing biological and genetic predisposition among black people as a plausible explanation (Harrison *et al.*, 1988; Hutchinson *et al.*, 1997; Sharpley *et al.*, 2001). Few studies have examined first-incidence data among other groups, although some studies indicate that South Asians in the UK are less likely to use inpatient care but have a similar incidence of schizophrenia (Gupta, 1991; King *et al.*, 1994). Rates of compulsory admission have increased in England in recent decades, and this trend is accelerating (Weich *et al.*, 2014). Age of the adult population and ethnic density along with higher levels of deprivation can account for the markedly higher rates of compulsory inpatient treatment in urban areas (Keown *et al.*, 2016).

A consistent finding is that African Caribbean people have higher rates of psychiatric admissions, both compulsory and voluntary, and over-representation in psychiatric forensic services (Bhui *et al.*, 1995; Coid *et al.*, 2000). Although the background to this in the UK is that the rate of detention is going up all the time for all patients, so African Caribbean populations may be particularly sensitive indicators of a general trend, but that they are so affected and over such a long period of time needs better understanding. This contrasts with similar rates of psychosis (broadly defined) across population samples of ethnic minorities (Nazroo, 1997). Over-engagement in forensic psychiatric and general psychiatric

services, when preliminary data suggest similar rates of population level psychoses, require explanations that reflect different risk factors for African Caribbean people, and/or different pathways and influences on help-seeking and treatment options across ethnic groups. Similar account needs to be given for lower representation in inpatient care, despite apparently similar risk of incident schizophrenia among South Asians in the UK.

Such effects may be articulated by less social support leading to more crises contacts (Cole *et al.*, 1995) and delayed contact with services. It is possible that early care experiences, and failures of such care, can become established patterns of interaction with all carers, including service providers. So given the higher rates of single parents and 'within-family unofficial fostering' among Caribbean people, less secure attachment (Arai and Harding, 2002) with parental figures may be replicated in more avoidant or distant relationships with services (Adshead, 1998; Mallett *et al.*, 2002).

Professional perceptions of greater risk among black people may in part be fuelled by black people not wishing to engage voluntarily. A consequence is that more coercive and compulsory legal powers are used (van Ryn and Fu, 2003). This tendency not to reach an alliance may feed professionals' perceptions of dangerousness and criminality (Lewis *et al.*, 1990), by public mistrust of mental health services (McLean *et al.*, 2003; Sainsbury Centre for Mental Health, 2003), and by patients' dissatisfaction with services (Parkman *et al.*, 1997). An additional controversy is to what extent diagnostic uncertainty can be attributed to ethnic variations in affective and non-affective symptom prevalence (Hickling *et al.*, 1999; Kirov and Murray, 1999). These studies suggest more 'manic' or 'excited' presentations among Caribbean origin people, perhaps with greater religious flavour (Littlewood and Lipsedge, 1998). If black people are presenting in crisis more often than other cultural groups, and there are ethnic variations in the symptoms being presented, then clinical assessments among black people are more often conducted in crisis, a situation that is not conducive to weighing complex decisions. Consequently, crises will generate more conservative and risk-averse approaches to clinical management.

Actual differences in levels of past violence, aggression or offending behaviour may also explain the tendency of professionals to be less tolerant of voluntary treatment or voluntary disengagement among black people (Wessely, 1998). So, if the risk factors among minorities militate against voluntary treatment, then this may explain the excess compulsory admission rate and over-representation in specialist and forensic care. Yet, recent data on Mental Health Act admissions showed that Caribbeans were no more likely to have violent presentation or substance misuse problems when admitted to prison or to secure psychiatric facilities (Bhui et al., 1998; Lelliott et al., 2001). A similar picture emerges when looking at data on forensic populations. A national cross-sectional study of over 3,000 prisoners found that fewer black and South Asian male prisoners reported childhood traumas and conduct disorder (Coid et al., 2002b). Fewer black people received previous psychiatric treatment compared to whites. Different rates of offending and lower rates of psychiatric morbidity may explain the relative excess of sentenced black prisoners in comparison with white sentenced prisoners (Coid et al., 2002a). In a study of men remanded to Brixton Prison, in comparison with white men, the courts were less likely to seek a psychiatric report among black people (black African, Caribbean and black British combined: 20–28 per cent; white 41 per cent). Black people were more likely to be identified as needing a psychiatric report at the time of reception into prison (black African and black Caribbean: 50–59%), whilst black British people, specifically, were more likely to be identified as having a mental health problem in the courts, at reception to the prison, or later during remand whilst on the prison wings (Bhui et al., 1998). This tendency to not be identified to have a mental health problem until in the prison, or at least after court appearance, was confirmed by Coid et al., 2002b. So, black subgroups may have distinct experiences that are patterned according to their identity (black British vs African Caribbean self-rated identity), and if there appear to be few risk factors for aggression, other than specific offences, what can account for the over-representation in forensic and secure services?

Are black people less likely to comply with conditions of bail, or to come back for outpatient appointments? Black people are more dissatisfied with consecutive contacts with inpatient admission environments (Parkman et al., 1997), and so may fear voluntary engagement with agencies of which they are suspicious and in which they have little confidence (McLean et al., 2003; Sainsbury Centre for Mental Health 2003). This

may explain more absconding from inpatient care (Falkowski et al., 1990) and less likelihood of voluntary engagement in community programmes of mental healthcare. An alternative explanation is that there are ethnic variations in perceptions of what constitutes mental illness. For example, Pote and Orrell (2002) report that African Caribbean people were less likely to view 'thought disorder' as pathological; Bangladeshis were less likely to conclude that hallucinations and suspiciousness were mental health problems. Therefore, some of the objections of specific ethnic groups may be explained by divergent professional–patient conceptualizations of what constitutes a mental health problem. Bhui found ethnic variations in explanatory models for common mental disorders, and ethnic variations in general practitioners' assessments of common mental disorders (Bhui et al., 2002) thus leading to uncertainty in clinical encounter. Faced with uncertainty about the patterns of symptoms presented by culturally different groups, clinicians may also be influenced by the social circumstances of patients. Lower patient incomes, more severe disorders and less experienced physicians, are all reported to be more commonly found by ethnic minorities presenting to services and explain less psychosocial talk in the consultation (Cooper-Patrick et al., 1999). Young and Rabiner (2015) observed that there were clear racial/ethnic differences in parent-reported barriers to accessing children's health services. Hispanic parents reported higher levels of socio-economic and stigma-related barriers as more inhibiting than did African American parents. Beevert et al. (2014) also reported variation in help-seeking among children indicating that severity may be an important factor in help-seeking.

As mentioned previously, gender expectations may also play a role. Casey et al. (2008) showed among Native American males that their attitudes and knowledge of diabetes affected help-seeking. Fernández de la Cruz(2015) showed that in services ethnic minority patients with obsessive–compulsive disorders were seen less frequently. The reasons for such variations are many including varying explanatory models. Saloner et al. (2014) suggest that black and Hispanic youth were significantly less likely than whites to complete treatment for both alcohol and marijuana. Completion rates were similar for whites, Native Americans, and Asian Americans.

Alegria et al. (2013) reported that in their study in the USA, Asians had lower prevalence rates of probable lifetime PTSD, compared with African

Americans who had higher rates in contrast with non-Latino whites, even after adjusting for type and number of exposures to traumatic events indicating that cultural values may play a role. Malhotra *et al.* (2015) demonstrated that race and ethnicity were significant predictors in the usage of outpatient services.

Primary Care

A systematic review of the evidence on ethnic variations in access to specialist psychiatric care concluded that African Caribbean groups are more likely to be referred to specialist care by GPs, and least likely to be recognized to have a mental disorder in primary care (Bhui *et al.*, 2003). South Asians are more likely to visit their general practitioners, are considered to present somatic manifestations of mental distress more commonly than other groups, are less likely to have a recognized mental disorder than white groups, and even if this is recognized, they are the least likely to be referred to specialist care by GPs (Bhui *et al.*, 2003). Van Ryn and Fu (2003), using data from the USA, describe a valuable schema for understanding cognitive distortion in the assessment of perceived clinical needs and risks among ethnic groups. They argue that such errors of judgement are influenced by provider beliefs about help-seeking and providers' interpretation of symptoms; these influence diagnostic practice, decision-making and the recommended choice of interventions.

Help-seeking behaviour itself can shape the response of providers, and the provider behaviour can, in turn, shape the presentation of symptoms. For example, it is known that the earlier a physical symptom is presented in the primary-care consultation, the more likely it is that the general practitioner assigns a physical diagnosis (Tylee *et al.*, 1995). A study of primary-care presenters in South London demonstrated that, for similar levels of common mental disorder (anxiety and depression combined), general practitioners more often assigned a mental-illness label to white English people than to Punjabi Asians, who, despite having similar levels of somatic symptoms, were more often assigned a somatic-illness label in accordance with the general stereotype (Bhui *et al.*, 2001). Thus, general practitioners' expectations, congruent with their gatekeeper role, and their reliance on physical idioms of distress, lead them to underestimate the severity of common mental disorders among South Asians (Bhui *et al.*, 2003; Kirmayer, 2001). From the USA, Hahm *et al.* (2015) reported that for depression screening in primary care black and ethnic minority individuals were less likely to receive this. Clear ethnic differences were observed. Among both males and females, blacks and Asians were less likely but Latinos were more likely to be screened for depression in comparison with white Americans. Interestingly, severity of depression played a role in healthcare. Among those with moderate or severe depression, black males and females, Latino males, and Asian males and females were less likely than whites to receive any mental healthcare. The disparity in screening between blacks and whites was greater among females compared with males but in mental healthcare disparity between Latinos and whites was greater among males than females.

Encountering physicians of a different race/ethnic group has been shown to be associated with distrust and a lack of satisfaction among African Americans in the USA (Corbie-Smith, Thomas and St George, 2002; Doescher *et al.*, 2000). In contrast, a British study of primary-care presenters found that GPs of South Asian background were not better at recognizing mental disorders among South Asians (Odell *et al.*, 1997, Jacob *et al.*, 1998). Indeed, South Asian GPs were poorer at recognizing mental disorders among South Asian patients than were GPs of other cultural backgrounds (Odell *et al.*, 1997). Similarly, from a pool of South Asian GPs, Punjabi and non-Punjabi GPs were equally able to recognize common mental disorder among Punjabi or non-Punjabi patients, but South Asian GPs were less effective in recognizing common mental disorders among English women (Bhui *et al.*, 2001). Thus gender–culture consultation dynamics are equally important to assess.

Despite international research showing that there are a finite number of emotions that are recognized in all societies and cultures (surprise, disgust, fear, anger, contempt, happiness and sadness; Shiori *et al.*, 1999), it is known that the accurate recognition of these emotional states varies with culture of the observer (Elfenbein and Ambady, 2002, 2003; Shiori *et al.*, 1999), and becomes more precise the greater the exposure to the cultures in which emotions are being assessed. It may be that, when assessing emotional states across cultures and socio-economic groups, the emotional content is not fully appreciated, and that such fine-grain omissions account for some of the dissatisfaction of ethnic minorities.

Community and Organizational Factors

Consultation outcomes do not rely only on patient characteristics, but also on clinician characteristics, and organizational factors. The knowledge, skills and resources of the care provider interact with those of the patient, leading to a complex negotiation of meanings and actions during and after a consultation. These negotiations are constrained by the values each participant brings to the consultation, and the expected role each participant assumes. The care provider has the additional context of their organization culture, and its policies, ethos and flexibility (or lack of it). Yet, all patients do not become patients until they elect to consult health professionals. Before this they may consult the community's social and folk sector of healthcare provision, in which family, friends and folk healers are active agents (Grewal and Lloyd, 2002; Kleinman, 1980). Different cultural groups have different explanatory models that dictate distinct recommended pathways to secure care and recovery. Help-seeking from healthcare services may therefore be triggered at quite different stages of the access chain by people from distinct cultures. Furthermore, communities and individuals from distinct ethnic groups have coping strategies and resiliency promoting behaviours/beliefs that may also mediate quite distinct pathways into care and recovery (Sproston and Bhui, 2002).

Some organizations can foster and display beneficial levels of cultural awareness and competency to manage the health and social care needs of ethnic minorities, whereas others simply function in a colour and culture blind approach and offer a fixed package of interventions and delivery systems, irrespective of culture (Cross et al., 1989). Cross et al. (1989) assert that there are six stages in the progression from cultural destructiveness, through incapacity, blindness, precompetence, competence, and then proficiency. Might such findings reflect discrimination? Discrimination can be defined on the basis of individual prejudicial intentions of healthcare providers, or by organizational policies and procedures, which compound distress, do not address existing healthcare needs and perhaps even add to healthcare needs through neglect. Not all inequalities of access are necessarily discriminatory, or undesirable. For example, the lower recognition of mental disorders among South Asian patients by general practitioners may, in fact, be the outcome of a shared decision by GP and patient not to proceed with referral to specialist care. Such a decision is not necessarily thought about in an explicit manner, but emerges through the negotiated and contested meanings and values and expectancies that arise in a consultation. For example, the different assessments among South Asians in primary care may reflect cultural idioms of distress that do not trigger the same concern in a GP as might more classic complaints of depression and suicidal thinking presented among white British patients. General practitioners generally act to exclude serious mental illness, and do not always consider anxiety and depression to be serious as confirmed by studies showing that GP assessments of depression have high specificity but low sensitivity (Bhui et al., 2000; Chew-Graham et al., 2002; Jacob et al., 1998). Such processes, even if they involve a shared decision between GP and patient, may deprive some patients of appropriate and timely interventions, although this may be explained away as patients exercising choice in accord with their culturally determined belief systems (Sproston and Bhui, 2002). Prady et al. (2016) noted that ethnic minority women with common mental disorders were given fewer non-pharmaceutical interventions. The dilemma is whether to impose a medical, psychiatric or sociological intervention, each with attendant risks and benefits. Or, go along with culturally unique explanations and prescriptions of treatment, for example, to alter diet to improve mood, risking chronicity, suicide attempts, loss of job and relationship difficulties.

An alternative cause of poorer outcome for minorities may be that the interventions, service delivery systems and access issues are irrelevant because an accepted intervention is ineffective in a specific ethnic group. This could be considered as an issue in the use of talking treatments for some ethnic groups who do not see this as a relevant part of recovery, wanting more immediate instrumental action to assist with housing, benefits, employment and prejudice (Fenton and Karlsen, 2002). Or, an intervention may not be as effective or carry with it adverse consequences that diminish its value as an intervention when applied to other cultural or ethnic groups. For example, differing profiles of drug metabolism and drug efficacy in different cultural groups mean that Asian people need lower doses of anti-psychotic, and that African Americans can benefit from smaller doses of antidepressant (Bhugra and Bhui, 2001; Lin et al., 1995). A lack of knowledge about these issues can lead to a poorer experience of service contact for some ethnic groups, and some may not be willing to tolerate future bad experiences leading to disengagement. This will not foster confidence among patients who feel that their complaints are unheard. Complaints about medication being sedative, or causing side effects may have a pharmacological basis, but may also reflect differing attitudes to medication as a way of controlling emotions. For example, among Sikh and Islamic scriptures the use of intoxicants to control suffering, as opposed to devotion to God to overcome and tolerate suffering, is condemned (Bhui, 1999). Under the influence of such teachings and spiritual practices, medication and physicians are subordinate to supernatural influences, and so medication is avoided. Therefore, evidence-based interventions may not lead to equal benefit or be equally acceptable as an intervention.

Inequalities in outcome cannot always be considered organizational failures to deliver effective services. However, if ethnic minorities do not feel that mental health services are there to serve their best interests, how can they subject themselves to this system of care of which they are suspicious? Professionals may justify this as an inevitable part of the care of the mentally ill. Nonetheless, it does leave the impression among the public that liberty is threatened, choice is removed and inappropriate or ineffective treatments might be forced upon them. Interestingly, Nieuwenhuijsen *et al.* (2015) observe that lack of recovery opportunities at work plays a major role in ethnic variations in outcomes.

Inequalities are consequences of the actions of individual practitioners and organizational cultures acting together. Social exclusion is mirrored in the economy of healthcare manifesting as alienation, non-participation and an absence of public corporate ownership which erodes any effort to provide services by consent. The service-user movement largely ensures accountability and participation, rather than any promise of improved clinical outcomes (Crawford *et al.*, 2002). Such approaches, if fully inclusive of ethnic minorities, may actually improve the inequalities of access, not due to changes in individual action by care providers, but by differing thresholds for patients to subject themselves to voluntary treatment mediated by more trust and ownership in the system of care. Such action will also ensure that the values and organizational practices that oppress are open to persistent transformation leading to more attractive and acceptable practices. Such a shift in values of organizations may also lead to a shift in professional values. The whole movement in cultural psychiatry, once a marginalized speciality, has now raised fundamental questions about the constitution of mental healthcare. Thus, it holds lessons for mental healthcare generally, and any service solution will reap benefits for all patients, and not only those from the minority groups.

Cultural Capability, Policies and Practice

Every single patient has culture as does every single mental health professional. Thus an understanding of cultural values and factors is the basic first step in understanding what the patient is going through. Clinicians may over- or under-diagnose illness behaviours if they are not aware of what is seen as normal and what is seen as deviant in that particular culture. Without knowing the norms of the patient's culture, the clinician is not always likely to assess cognition and affect. Thus, sharing ethnicity and cultural background may help somewhat but it cannot be taken for granted that this would help. Understanding the experiences, the ethnographic accounts and the impact of the patient's cultural peers can help. Knowing the patient's culture's sources of power whether these are political, economic or mythological is useful. An awareness of patient's socio-cultural milieu (within which the individual lives and functions) is essential in understanding the idioms of distress, pathways into care and psychopathology, and may also help in increasing treatment adherence. Understanding the patient's cultural framework of reference enables the clinician to empathize with the distress. The tendency is to project different social images or personality types when using different languages (these could equally be language of clinical transaction). We recognize that for the patients to speak another language (a secondary language) may have uncertain consequences for the clinical encounter. Bilingual patients may choose to withhold information if they are interviewed only in their secondary language. They may not be able to express affect easily but may express facts easily. Cultural framework of reference thus has to incorporate the individual's functioning within which language is a firm part of the identity. The choice of language combined with 'medical' or technical language will bring problems of its own. Culturally adapted psychotherapies, and ethnographic and motivational assessment are effective and favoured by patients and carers (Bhui *et al.*, 2015a).

Certain aspects of the mental-state examination cannot be translated, e.g. ambivalence, social withdrawal. A critical first step in the clinical encounter is for the mental health professional to identify and recognize the cultural dimension by becoming aware of his or her own cultural encumbrances. Patients may well have strong feelings about their culture and about the culture of the mental health professional they are facing. These feelings can be positive as well as negative.

Cultural relativism relates to the differences in beliefs, feelings, behaviours, tradition, social practices and technological arrangements that are found among diverse people of the world (Fabrega, 1989). Using biopsychosocial approaches means that the clinician must be aware of relativist values. Fabrega's argument is that both psychiatric illness and culture meaningfully implicate humans as holistic and symbolic creatures. By arguing for the importance of specific social and cultural factors in the content, experience, expression or distribution of a psychiatric or other illness, a relativist is committed to a qualitative, descriptive and ethnographic approach in understanding the patient's experiences. Understanding social factors such as inequalities in employment or housing and cultural factors such as role of family, child-rearing practices, religions and dietary taboos will enable the mental health professional to speak in a language the patient feels comfortable with. Simply ticking boxes to say that mental health professionals are culturally capable will not do.

In order to address inequalities of access to services and experiences of services, there have been calls for cultural sensitivity, awareness and more recently for cultural competency of all professionals. Park *et al.* (2005) observed that residents (trainees) often complained of not being aware and sensitive to cultural factors as a result of not being trained in the subject. In a qualitative study they reported that most residents acknowledged the importance of cross-cultural care yet reported little formal training in this area and consequently they wanted more formal training which was not pandering to stereotypes. Problematically most of the sample had developed ad hoc, informal skills to care for diverse patients. They reported receiving mixed messages about cross-cultural care. In spite of

Table 10.1 Capability framework

- Performance: what people need to possess and what they need to achieve
- Ethical: integrating knowledge, values, and social awareness into professional practice
- Reflective practice
- Implement evidence based interventions
- Lifelong learning
- Negotiate above principles with new cultural frame of reference, ethical values and absence of evidence base

being told that cultural awareness was important, lack of structured training led to coping behaviours rather than skills based on formally taught best practices. Interestingly, Holdaway *et al.* (2015) suggest that professional migrants may have a role to play in responding to discrimination and inequalities.

'Cultural competency' is often reduced to knowledge about specific cultural groups, and tends to be applied concretely as if competence were a static entity that once acquired can be taken for granted. More recently, the term 'cultural capability' has been adopted. This includes elements of ability in more general terms, referring to possession of skills, knowledge, and powers, or something being possible. Capability also refers to the possession of an aptitude, especially one that derives from a person's character. It includes (1) awareness, (2) competency around particular tasks, skills, knowledge, and attitudes to practice and (3) the ability to progress learning in new situations. Thus it mandates reflective practice, continuing professional development, the acquisition of transferable skills and self-efficacy in learning. It is relevant not only to cultural working practices, but to all mental healthcare, and indeed all professional care (see Table 10.1; Sainsbury Centre for Mental Health, 2003), but specific modifications and programme enhancement are necessary for a comprehensive culturally capable workforce to be developed. Through such a programme, the detailed competencies can be set within a framework of culturally capable practice that will adapt to new populations to make possible a truly multiculturally effective service. Within such cultural models sub-cultural values may require attention (Samu and Suaalii-Sauni, 2009).

Abel and Frohlich (2012) offer an alternative. They describe structure–agency linkages to target in order to reduce social inequalities in health. They propose life chances (structure) are related to choice-based life conduct (agency) and suggest capability as a useful means to reduce social inequalities in health at perhaps both social and individual levels which can then take into account both structural conditions and individual responsibilities. There is no doubt that people's capabilities to be active for their health form a critical and crucial concept in public health. However, a key challenge is that black and ethnic minority individuals may be so neglected by the system that they are unable to develop these capabilities. Yang *et al.* (2014) studied Chinese immigrants in New York and noted that these individuals were guided by frameworks of structural discrimination and 'what matters most' – a cultural mechanism which determined any meaningful participation in the community. Structural vulnerabilities included being in an inferior position and made access to affordable mental health services problematic. This may reflect the US healthcare system itself. However, more interestingly, such structural inferiority inevitably led to a depreciated sense of self, which further contributed to alienation, isolation and poor capacity to engage in social interactions.

These issues have been under continuing consideration for over two decades. In the UK, the Department of Health launched *Inside/Outside* (2003), a framework for the eradication of ethnic inequalities of mental healthcare that goes far beyond service provision. This document emphasizes not only cultural capability by developing the workforce, but also encourages measures to improve public mental health and community resilience by recommending significant investments in community development workers to promote well-being, community inclusion and improved communication as well as routes to influence service development. There is also a framework for research, which promises more ethical research studies with more equitable funding of projects. The impact of this policy document is yet to be assessed; however, one of the unique aspects of this policy is that it was put out to a national consultation that specifically targeted Caribbean-origin black people, South Asians, and Chinese people, including service users and carers. A policy document titled *Delivering Race Equality*, following *Inside/Outside*, placed more emphasis on organizational strategies, and the use of the Race Relations Amendment Act as a lever to ensure compliance. These policies considered in isolation demonstrate different facets of a necessary process to eradicate

ethnic inequalities, and provide more appropriate care. Bhui *et al.* (2012) propose that race, ethnicity and culture in history and their representation in unconscious and conscious thought are significant factors in developing cultural competence training. They also point out that tackling inequities requires personal development and the emergence and containment of primitive anxieties, hostilities and fears on the part of both providers and users thus both majority and minority communities need to look at this.

The American Psychiatric Association sets out how to undertake a cultural formulation to enhance existing practices when assessing mental status of patients (Griffith, 2002). This emphasizes enquiry about cultural identity and explanatory models. This should take place alongside an assessment of the impact on the therapeutic relationship of culture of the professional and/or patient. Cultural factors related to the socio-cultural environment (discrimination, unemployment, asylum laws) should also be considered as factors that impact on mental health. Finally, there should be an overall statement outlining any culturally relevant aspects of diagnosis and treatment. Professionals should take particular care to ensure that the rationale for the treatment is understood, and does not break any cultural taboos, or undermine any cherished cultural beliefs, as this may lead to potential non-compliance. Most importantly, any further investigations that are necessary should be stated explicitly, including the gathering of more information and assessment with voluntary or specialist providers. Tseng (2003) sets out different perspectives of cultural capability: sensitivity, awareness, empathy, knowledge, adjusting the relationship between a patient and the mental health professional and treatment modifications. These descriptions are essentially clinical practice-based solutions. Bhui and Bhugra (1998) extended individual practice-based solution to ones involving the community, voluntary organizations, and independent providers, including experiential, behavioural, cognitive-behavioural, motivational systems of learning that take account of subjective experiences of distress. Bhui *et al.* (1995) outlined how opportunities to address discrimination experiences within services had to be enshrined in equal-opportunities policies, alongside flexibility in the interventions and service components that were available, in accordance with the most effective model of culturally capable services as defined by Moffic and Kinzie (1996). They argue for innovation in service structures and styles of delivery to optimally manage distress in the cultural group of interest. The emphasis on removing the organizational constraints to culturally capable practice are now more evident; there is a greater focus on values and attitudes, and reviewing changes in the characteristics of organizations (Bhui, 2002; Siegel *et al.*, 2003). These approaches mandate the inclusion of organizational performance standards for training, education, employment practices and policies, values and attitudes, language differences, accessibility, appropriateness, attractiveness of services and continual feedback from communities. These are now being enshrined in performance indicators for organizations, to ensure all aspects of an organization's activities are cognizant of the need to place cultural capability at the centre of discussions about clinical effectiveness and governance. The recommendations are derived largely from clinicians and organizations that have grappled with the challenge of providing culturally appropriate services. As such, they are a natural development in a chain of proposed solutions that have been implemented, evaluated and modified to promote culturally capable mental healthcare. In the UK, individual 'cultural competence' training was announced to be necessary for all practitioners; but the same ambition to make organizations culturally capable has not been realized, albeit, the Race Relations Amendment Act in the UK requires all public bodies to ensure they are acting in a non-discriminatory manner. Apart from using culture brokers and culture mediators, Corrigan *et al.* (2014) recommend developing the role of peer navigators in mental health services as these have been used in cancer.

Delivering Race Equality (DRE) Programme and Cultural Consultation Services

Delivering Race Equality in Mental Health Care (DRE; 2005–2010) was an action plan for achieving equality and tackling discrimination in mental health services in England for all people of black and minority ethnic (BME) status, including those of Irish or Mediterranean origin and east European migrants (Moffat *et al.*, 2009a). The programme was based on three actions: more appropriate and responsive services, community engagement and better information. Improving pathways to care is an important part of UK government policy on delivering equitable

treatment for black and minority ethnic (BME) patients (Sass *et al.*, 2009). In fact, black and ethnic minorities show different pathways to care services and different routes out of care (Moffat *et al.*, 2009b). The project revealed that keys to success include a reflective use of team strengths, engagement of stakeholders from boardroom to clinical teams, transformational leadership, transmission of leadership to more appropriate leaders for different stages of the project, a reflective learning style that permits obstacles to be embraced and managed, and cycles of movement between 'ideological' and 'operational' phases of the project.

Bhui *et al.* (2015b) reported experiences and outcomes from a new type of cultural consultation service (CCS). This is a multi-component and systemic complex intervention offered over 18 months in East London to specialist mental health providers in one of the poorest regions of the UK. The CCS model is an adaptation of the McGill model, which uses ethnographic methodology and medical anthropological knowledge (Owiti *et al.*, 2014). The method and approach not only contribute both to a broader conceptual and dynamic understanding of culture, but also to learning of cultural competence skills by healthcare professionals. The service received 900 clinically related contacts and 99 in-depth consultations. Global functioning and psychopathology of patients improved and costs per patient decreased. Clinicians felt the cultural consultation service helped to improve the treatment plan (71%), engagement (50%), medication compliance (21%) and earlier discharge (7%). Understanding the cultures of care showed that clinical and managerial over-structuring of care prioritizes organizational proficiency (Ascoli *et al.*, 2012). Given the need to apprehend narratives in care practice, especially at times of disputed evidence, cultural consultation processes may be an appropriate paradigm to address intersectional inequalities (Bhui *et al.*, 2012).

Conclusions

It is clear that a range of possible explanations for these inequalities can be proposed. These include the influence of culture on the illness behaviour, the effects of cultural identity and explanatory models in the consultation process, and the lack of cultural capability of services and professional practices. Institutionalized and individual factors must be addressed to eradicate undesirable inequalities.

References

Abel, T. and Frohlich, K. (2012). Capitals and capabilities: linking structure and agency to reduce health inequalities. *Social Science and Medicine*, 74(2), 236–244.

Adshead, G. (1998). Psychiatric staff as attachment figures: understanding management problems in psychiatric services in the light of attachment theory. *British Journal of Psychiatry*, 172, 64–69.

Alegría, M., Fortuna, L. R., Lin, J. Y. *et al.* (2013). Prevalence, risk, and correlates of posttraumatic stress disorder across ethnic and racial minority groups in the United States. *Medical Care*, 51(12),1114–1123, doi: 10.1097/MLR.0000000000000007.

Anderson, K. K., Cheng, J., Susser, E. *et al.* (2015). Incidence of psychotic disorders among first-generation immigrants and refugees in Ontario. *Canadian Medical Association Journal*, 187(9), E279–286, doi: 10.1503/cmaj.141420.

Arai, L. and Harding, S. (2002). *African Caribbeans: Generational Effects of Health: A Review*. London: MRC.

Ascoli, M., Palinski, A., Owiti, J. A., de Jongh, B., Bhui, K. S. (2012). The culture of care within psychiatric services: tackling inequalities and improving clinical and organisational capabilities. *Philosophy, Ethics and Humanity in Medicine*, 7(12), 1–8, doi: 10.1186/1747–5341-7-12.

Berry, J. (1997). Immigration, acculturation, adaptation. *Applied Psychology*, 46, 5–68.

Bevaart, F., Mieloo, C. L., Wierdsma, A. *et al.* (2014). Ethnicity, socio-economic position and severity of problems as predictors of mental health care use in 5- to 8-year-old children with problem behaviour. *Social Psychiatry and Psychiatric Epidemiology*, 49(5), 733–742.

Bhugra, D. and Bhui, K.(2001). *Cross Cultural Psychiatry: A Practical Guide*. London: Arnold.

Bhui, K. (1999). Common mental disorders: prevalence, explanatory models and GP assessments among Punjabi and English primary care attenders. MD thesis. Institute of Psychiatry, University of London.

Bhui, K. (2002). *Racism and Mental Health*. London: Jessica Kingsley Publishing, p. 202.

Bhui, K. and Bhugra, D. (1998). Training and supervision in effective cross cultural mental health services. *Hospital Medicine*, 59(11), 861–865.

Bhui, K., Christie, Y. and Bhugra, D. (1995). The essential elements of culturally sensitive psychiatric services. *International Journal of Social Psychiatry*, 41, 242–256.

Bhui, K., Brown, P., Hardie, T. *et al.* (1998). African-Caribbean men remanded to Brixton Prison. Psychiatric and forensic characteristics and outcome of final court appearance. *British Journal of Psychiatry*, 172, 337–344.

Bhui, K., Bhugra, D. and Goldberg, D. (2000). Cross-cultural validity of the Amritsar Depression Inventory and the General Health Questionnaire amongst English and Punjabi primary care attenders. *Social Psychiatry and Psychiatric Epidemiology*, 35(6), 248–254.

Bhui, K., Bhugra, D., Goldberg, D. *et al.* (2001). Cultural influences on the prevalence of common mental disorder, general practitioners' assessments and help-seeking among Punjabi and English people visiting their general practitioner. *Psychological Medicine*, 31(5), 815–825.

Bhui, K., Bhugra, D. and Goldberg, D. (2002). Causal explanations of distress and general practitioners' assessments of common mental disorder among Punjabi and English attendees. *Social Psychiatry and Psychiatric Epidemiology*, 37, 38–45.

Bhui, K., Stansfeld, S., Hull, S. *et al.* (2003). Ethnic variations in pathways to and use of specialist mental health services in the UK. Systematic review. *British Journal of Psychiatry*, 182, 105–116.

Bhui, K., Ascoli, M. and Nuamh, O. (2012). The place of race and racism in cultural competence: what can we learn from the English experience about the narratives of evidence and argument? Transcultural Psychiatry, 49(2), 185–205, doi: 10.1177/1363461512437589.

Bhui, K. S., Aslam, R. W., Palinski, A. *et al.* (2015a) Interventions to improve therapeutic communications between black and minority ethnic patients and professionals in psychiatric services: systematic review. *British Journal of Psychiatry*, 207(2), 95–103, doi: 10.1192/bjp.bp.114.158899.

Bhui, K. S., Owiti, J. A., Palinski, A. *et al.* (2015b) A cultural consultation service in East London: experiences and outcomes from implementation of an innovative service. *International Review of Psychiatry*, 27(1), 11–22, doi: 10.3109/09540261.2014.992303.

Cavanaugh, Casey L., Taylor, Christopher A., Keim, Kathryn S. *et al.* (2008). Cultural perceptions of health and diabetes among Native American men. *Journal of Health Care for the Poor and Underserved*, 19(4), 1029–1043.

Chew-Graham, C. A., Mullin, S., May, C. R. *et al.* (2002). Managing depression in primary care: another example of the inverse care law? *Family Practice*, 19, 632–637.

Coid, J., Kahtan, N., Gault, S. *et al.* (2000). Ethnic differences in admissions to secure forensic psychiatry services. *British Journal of Psychiatry*, 177, 241–247.

Coid, J., Petruckevitch, A., Bebbington, P. *et al.* (2002a). Ethnic differences in prisoners. 1: criminality and psychiatric morbidity. *British Journal of Psychiatry*, 181, 473–480.

Coid, J., Petruckevitch, A., Bebbington, P. *et al.* (2002b). Ethnic differences in prisoners. 2: risk factors and psychiatric service use. *British Journal of Psychiatry*, 181, 481–487.

Cole, E., Leavey, G., King, M. *et al.* (1995). Pathways to care for patients with a first episode of psychosis: a comparison of ethnic groups. *British Journal of Psychiatry*, **167**, 770–776.

Cooper-Patrick , L., Gallo, J., Gonzales, J. *et al.* (1999). Race, gender, and partnership in the patient–physician relationship. *Journal of the American Medical Association*, **828**(6), 583–589.

Corbie-Smith, G., Thomas, S. B. and St George, D. M. (2002). Distrust, race, and research. *Archives of Internal Medicine*, **162**, 2458–2463.

Corrigan, P. W., Pickett, S., Batia, K., Michaels, P. J. (2014). Peer navigators and integrated care to address ethnic health disparities of people with serious mental illness. *Social Work in Public Health*, **29**(6), 581–593, doi: 10.1080/19371918.2014.893854.

Crawford, M. J., Rutter, D., Manley, C. *et al.* (2002). Systematic review of involving patients in the planning and development of health care. *British Medical Journal*, **325**, 1263.

Cross, T. L., Barzon, B. J., Dennis, K. W. *et al.* (1989). *Towards a Culturally Competent System of Care: A Monograph on Effective Services for Minority Children Who Are Severely Emotionally Disturbed*. Washington, DC: CASSP Technical Assistance Center, Georgetown University Child Development Center.

D'Anna-Hernandez, K. L., Aleman, B., Flores, A. M. (2015). Acculturative stress negatively impacts maternal depressive symptoms in Mexican-American women during pregnancy. *Journal of Affective Disorders*, **176**, 35–42, doi: 10.1016/j.jad.2015.01.036.

Department of Health (2003). *Inside/Outside*. London: Department of Health.

Dobson, J., Koser, K., McLaughlan, G. and Salt, J. (2001). *International Migration and the United Kingdom: Recent Patterns and Trends*. London: Home Office. RDS Occasional Paper No. 75.

Doescher, M. P., Saver, B. G., Franks, P. *et al.* (2000). Racial and ethnic disparities in perceptions of physician style and trust. *Archives of Family Medicine*, **9**(10), 1163.

Elfenbein, H. A. and Ambady, N. (2002). On the universality and cultural specificity of emotion recognition: a meta-analysis. *Psychology Bulletin*, **128**(2), 203–235.

Elfenbein, H. A. and Ambady, N. (2003). When familiarity breeds accuracy: cultural exposure and facial emotion recognition. *Journal of Personal and Social Psychology*, **85**(2), 276–290.

Fabrega, H. (1989). Cultural relativism and psychiatric illness. *Journal of Nervous and Mental Disease*, **177**, 415–425.

Falkowski, J., Watts, V., Falkowski, W. *et al.* (1990). Patients leaving hospital without the knowledge or permission of staff: absconding. *British Journal of Psychiatry*, **156**, 488–490.

Feder, G., Crook, A. M., Magee, P. *et al.* (2002) Ethnic differences in invasive management of coronary disease: prospective cohort study of patients undergoing angiography. *British Medical Journal*, **324**(7336), 511–516.

Fenton, S. and Karlsen, S. (2002). Explaining mental distress: narratives of cause. In *Ethnic Differences in the Context and Experience of Psychiatric Illness: A Qualitative Study*, ed. W. O'Connor and J. Nazroo. London: The Stationery Office, pp. 17–27.

Fernández de la Cruz, L., Llorens, M., Jassi, A. *et al.* (2015). Ethnic inequalities in the use of secondary and tertiary mental health services among patients with obsessive-compulsive disorder. *British Journal of Psychiatry*, **207**(6), 530–535, doi: 10.1192/bjp.bp.114.154062.

Fryers, T., Melzer, D. and Jenkins, R. (2003). Social inequalities and the common mental disorders: a systematic review of the evidence. *Social Psychiatry and Psychiatric Epidemiology*, **38**, 229–237.

Gater, R., de Almeida e Sousa, B., Barrientos, G. *et al.* (1991). The pathways to psychiatric care: a cross-cultural study. *Psychological Medicine*, **21**, 761–774.

Grewal, I. and Lloyd, K. (2002). Use of services. In *Ethnic Differences in the Context and Experience of Psychiatric Illness: A Qualitative Study*, ed. W. O'Connor and J. Nazroo, London: The Stationery Office, pp. 51–60.

Griffith, E. and Committee on Cultural Psychiatry of the Group for the Advancement of Psychiatry (2002). *Cultural Assessment in Clinical Psychiatry*. Washington DC: American Psychiatric Publishing, Inc.

Gupta, S. (1991). Psychosis in migrants from the Indian subcontinent and English-born controls. A preliminary study on the use of psychiatric services. *British Journal of Psychiatry*, **159**, 222–225.

Hahm, H. C., Cook, B. L., Ault-Brutus, A., Alegría, M. (2015). Intersection of race–ethnicity and gender in depression care: screening, access, and minimally adequate treatment. *Psychiatric Services*, **66**(3), 258–264, doi: 10.1176/appi.ps.201400116. Epub 1 December 2014.

Harrison, G., Owens, D., Holton, A. *et al.* (1988). A prospective study of severe mental disorder in Afro-Caribbean patients. *Psychological Medicine*, **18**, 643–657.

Hickling, F. W., McKenzie, K., Mullen, R. *et al.* (1999). A Jamaican psychiatrist evaluates diagnoses at a London psychiatric hospital. *British Journal of Psychiatry*, **175**, 283–285.

Holdaway, J., Levitt, P., Fang, J. and Rajaram, N. (2015). Mobility and health sector development in China and India. *Social Science and Medicine*, **130**, 268–276.

Hollander, A. C., Dal, H., Lewis, G., Magnusson, C., Kirkbride, J. B., Dalman, C. (2016). Refugee migration and risk of schizophrenia and other non-affective psychoses: cohort study of 1.3 million people in Sweden. *British Medical Journal*, **352**, i1030, doi: 10.1136/bmj.i1030.

Hutchinson, G., Takei, N., Bhugra, D. *et al.* (1997). Increased rate of psychosis among African Caribbeans in Britain is not due to an excess of pregnancy and birth complications. *British Journal of Psychiatry*, **171**, 145–147.

Jacob, K. S., Bhugra, D., Lloyd, K. and Mann, A. (1998). Common mental disorders, explanatory models and consultation behaviour among Indian women living in the UK. *Journal of the Royal Society of Medicine*, **91**(2), 66–71.

Keown, P., McBride, O., Twigg, L. *et al.* (2016). Rates of voluntary and compulsory psychiatric in-patient treatment in England: an ecological study investigating associations with deprivation and demographics. *British Journal of Psychiatry*, **209**(2), 157–161, doi: 10.1192/bjp. bp.115.171009.

Kim, G., Parton, J. M., Ford, K. L. *et al.* (2014). Geographic and racial–ethnic differences in satisfaction with and perceived benefits of mental health services. *Psychiatry Services*, **65**(12), 1474–1482, doi: 10.1176/appi. ps.201300440.

King, M., Coker, E., Leavey, G. *et al.* (1994). Incidence of psychotic illness in London: comparison of ethnic groups. *British Medical Journal*, **309**, 1115–1119.

Kirmayer, L. (2001). Cultural variations in the clinical presentation of anxiety and depression: implications for diagnosis and treatment. *Journal of Clinical Psychiatry*, **62**, 22–28.

Kirov, G. and Murray, R. M. (1999). Ethnic differences in the presentation of bipolar affective disorder. *European Psychiatry*, **14**, 199–204.

Kleinman, A. (1980). *Rethinking Psychiatry*. New York: Free Press.

Lelliott, P., Audini, B. and Duffett, R. (2001). Survey of patients from an inner-London health authority in medium secure psychiatric care. *British Journal of Psychiatry*, **178**, 62–66.

Lewis, G., Croft-Jeffreys, C. and David, A. (1990). Are British psychiatrists racist? *British Journal of Psychiatry*, **157**, 410–415.

Lin, K. M., Anderson, D. and Poland, R. E. (1995). Ethnicity and psychopharmacology: bridging the gap. *Psychiatric Clinics of North America*, **18**, 635–647.

Littlewood, R. and Lipsedge, M. (1998). *Aliens and Alienists: Ethnic Minorities and Psychiatry*. London: Unwin Hyman.

Malhotra, K., Shim, R., Baltrus, P. *et al.* (2015). Racial/ethnic disparities in mental health service utilization among youth participating in negative externalizing behaviors. *Ethnicity and Disease*, **25**(2), 123–129.

Mallett, R., Leff, J., Bhugra, D. *et al.* (2002). Social environment, ethnicity and schizophrenia: a case-control study. *Social Psychiatry and Psychiatric Epidemiology*, **37**, 329–335.

McLean, C., Campbell, C. and Cornish, F. (2003). African-Caribbean interactions with mental health services in the UK: experiences and expectations of exclusion as

(re)productive of health inequalities. *Social Science and Medicine*, **56**, 657–669.

Moffat, J., Sass, B., McKenzie, K., Bhui, K. (2009a). Enhancing pathways and mental healthcare for BME groups: learning between the ideological and operational. *International Review of Psychiatry*, **21**(5), 450–459, doi: 10.1080/09540260802202075.

Moffat, J., Sass, B., McKenzie, K., Bhui, K. (2009b). Improving pathways into mental health care for black and ethnic minority groups: a systematic review of the grey literature. *International Review of Psychiatry*, **21**(5), 439–449, doi: 10.1080/09540260802204105.

Moffic, H. S. and Kinzie, J. D. (1996). The history and future of cross cultural psychiatric services. *Community Mental Health Journal*, **32**(6), 581–592.

Nazroo, J. (1997). *Ethnicity and Mental Health*. London: Policy Studies Institute.

Nazroo, J. Y. (2003) The structuring of ethnic inequalities in health: economic position, racial discrimination, and racism. *American Journal of Public Health*, **93**, 277–284.

Nieuwenhuijsen, K., Schene, A. H., Stronks, K., *et al.* (2015). Do unfavourable working conditions explain mental health inequalities between ethnic groups? Cross-sectional data of the HELIUS study. *BMC Public Health*, **15**, 805, doi: 10.1186/s12889-015-2107-5.

Odell, S. M., Surtees, P. G., Wainwright, N. W. *et al.* (1997). Determinants of general practitioner recognition of psychological problems in a multi-ethnic inner-city health district. *British Journal of Psychiatry*, **171**, 537–541.

Owiti, J. A., Ajaz, A., Ascoli, M. *et al.* (2014). Cultural consultation as a model for training multidisciplinary mental healthcare professionals in cultural competence skills: preliminary results. *Journal of Psychiatric and Mental Health Nursing*, **21**(9),814–826, doi: 10.1111/jpm.12124.

Park, E., Betancourt, J., Kim, M., Maina, A., Blumenthal, D. and Weissman, J. (2005). Mixed messages: residents' experiences learning cross-cultural care. *Academic Medicine*, **80**(9), 874–880.

Parkman, S., Davies, S., Leese, M. *et al.* (1997). Ethnic differences in satisfaction with mental health services among representative people with psychosis in south London: PRiSM study 4. *British Journal of Psychiatry*, **171**, 260–264.

Pote, H. and Orrell, M. (2002). Perceptions of schizophrenia in multicultural Britain. *Ethnicity and Health*, **7**(1), 7–20.

Prady, S. L., Pickett, K. E., Gilbody, S. *et al.* (2016). Variation and ethnic inequalities in treatment of common mental disorders before, during and after pregnancy: combined analysis of routine and research data in the Born in Bradford cohort. *BMC Psychiatry*, **16**, 99, doi: 10.1186/s12888-016-0805-x.

Priest, N., Paradies, Y., Trenerry, B., Truong, M., Karlsen, S. and Kelly, Y. (2013). A systematic review of studies examining the relationship between reported racism and health and well-being for children and young people. *Social Science and Medicine*, **95**, 115–127.

Sainsbury Centre for Mental Health (2003). *Circles of Fear*. London: Sainsbury Centre for Mental Health.

Saloner, B., Carson, N., Lê Cook, B. (2014). Explaining racial/ethnic differences in adolescent substance abuse treatment completion in the United States: a decomposition analysis. *Journal of Adolescent Health*, **54**(6), 646–653, doi: 10.1016/j.jadohealth.2014.01.002.

Samu K. S., Suaalii-Sauni T. (2009). Exploring the 'cultural' in cultural competencies in Pacific mental health. *Pacific Health Dialog*, **15**(1), 120–130.

Sass, B., Moffat, J., Bhui, K., McKenzie, K. (2009). Enhancing pathways to care for black and minority ethnic populations: a systematic review. *International Review of Psychiatry*, **21**(5), 430–438, doi: 10.1080/09540260802204121.

Sharpley, M. S., Hutchinson, G., Murray, R. M. *et al.* (2001). Understanding the excess of psychosis among the African-Caribbean population in England: review of current hypotheses. *British Journal of Psychiatry*, **178**, S60–S68.

Shioiri, T., Someya, T., Helmeste, D. and Tang, S. W. (1999). Misinterpretation of facial expression: a cross-cultural study. *Psychiatry and Clinical Neuroscience*, **53**(1), 45–50.

Siegel, C., Hugland, G. and Chambers, E. D. (2003). Performance measures and their benchmarks for assessing organisational cultural competency in behavioural health and care service delivery. *Administration and Public Policy in Mental Health*, **31**(2), 141–170.

Snowden, L. R. (2003). Bias in mental health assessment and intervention: theory and evidence. *American Journal of Public Health*, **93**, 239–243.

Sproston, K. and Bhui, K. (2002). Coping mechanisms. In *Ethnic Differences in the Context and Experience of Psychiatric Illness: A Qualitative Study*, ed. W. O'Connor and J. Nazroo. London: The Stationery Office, pp. 41–50.

Tortelli, A., Errazuriz, A., Croudace, T., *et al.* (2015). Schizophrenia and other psychotic disorders in Caribbean-born migrants and their descendants in England: systematic review and meta-analysis of incidence rates, 1950–2013. *Social Psychiatry and Psychiatric Epidemiology*, **50**(7), 1039–1055, doi: 10.1007/s00127-015-1021-6.

Tseng, W. S. (2003). *Clinician's Guide to Cultural Psychiatry*. San Diego, CA: Academic Press.

Tylee, A., Freeling, P., Kerry, S. *et al.* (1995). How does the content of consultations affect the recognition by general practitioners of major depression in women? *British Journal of General Practice*, **45**, 575–578.

US Department of Health and Human Services (2001). *Mental Health, Culture, Race and Ethnicity: A Supplement to Mental Health: A Report of the Surgeon General*. Washington, DC: US Department of Health and Human Services.

van Ryn, M. and Fu, S. S. (2003). Paved with good intentions: do public health and human service providers contribute to racial/ethnic disparities in health? *American Journal of Public Health*, **93**, 248–255.

Weich, S., McBride, O., Twigg, L., *et al.* (2014). *Variation in Compulsory Psychiatric Inpatient Admission in England: A Cross-Sectional, Multilevel Analysis*. Southampton (UK): NIHR Journals Library; Health Services and Delivery Research.

Wessely, S. (1998). The Camberwell Study of crime and schizophrenia. *Social Psychiatry and Psychiatric Epidemiology*, **33** (Suppl. 1), S24–S28.

Yang, L., Chen, F., Sia, K., Lam, J., Lam, K., Ngo, H., Lee, S., Kleinman, A. and Good, B. (2014). 'What matters most': a cultural mechanism moderating structural vulnerability and moral experience of mental illness stigma. *Social Science and Medicine*, **103**, 84–93.

Young, A. S. and Rabiner, D. (2015). Racial/ethnic differences in parent-reported barriers to accessing children's health services. *Psychological Services*, **12**(3), 267–273, doi: 10.1037/a0038701.

Psychopathology and the Role of Culture
An Overview

Dinesh Bhugra, Matthew Kelly and Antonio Ventriglio

Editors' Introduction

It has been well recognized that cultures play a major role in our lives in a number of ways. Not only that cultures influence our cognitions, social interactions and the way we are brought up, in times of distress we use terms and expressions which are very strongly influenced by cultures. The cultures in which we are born start to affect us before birth, for example the way in which nurseries (if they exist) are decorated, diets of mothers, etc. After birth the way the children are dressed and the way they are brought up. In many cultures male children are dressed in female clothes to fool the spirits into not affecting male children. We absorb culture through patterns of child-rearing, from peers, folk tales, media, education in schools and universities, places of employment and many other sources. It must be recognized that the relationship between culture and development and perpetuation of psychopathology remains complex and multi-faceted. The way distress is expressed in help-seeking is very strongly affected by culture. Culture also influences healthcare systems as well as dictating funding for healthcare and how the resources are utilized. Bhugra, Kelly and Ventriglio, in this chapter, provide an overview of the relationship between culture and psychopathology in the context of social factors and social conditions which may cause mental disorders. It is well recognized that social determinants affect illnesses in varying ways. Building on Tseng's work in the previous edition of this volume, the authors recognize that culture can cause psychiatric distress and illness, cultures make people choose patterns of description and how psychopathology is modelled and how behaviours get exaggerated as well as how cultures influence responses to distress. It is inevitable that culture has a broader, more direct effect on minor as opposed to major psychiatric disorders on all these levels but it is true to say that idioms of distress whether these are to do with minor or major psychiatric disorders are likely to be affected by cultural values.

Introduction

Culture is a critical part of the environment within which we live and work and grow up and die. Culture are a set of beliefs, values, expectations and rites and rituals. The reasons cultures affect emotions are a result of many interacting factors. Cultures teach us which emotions are acceptable and how these are manifested and how emotions and their expressions can be seen as deviant or abnormal and hence pathological. For example, using metaphors to express distress is common across cultures even though metaphors may vary. Culture can influence child-rearing, accepted patterns and cognitive schema which in turn influence the individual's inner world view.

As Kirmayer highlights in this volume (see Chapter 1), culture has potentially three meanings. These include cultivation, culture as a set of beliefs and lastly anthropological studies. In addition, Kirmayer reminds us that cultural psychiatry has been an integral part of psychiatry. There have been discussions and debates within cultural psychiatry, whether cultural psychiatry should focus on relativist positions or universalist positions. There is no doubt that from a clinical perspective it is important to make sense of individual experiences in the context of the environment within which they live and function. As a result of globalization, the emergence of global health has again produced a Euro–US centric medicine and clinical practice. Migration of millions of individuals who may well require healthcare is compounded by migration of healthcare providers who may have different sets of priorities. Therefore it becomes crucial to provide an overview of how cultures affect and influence not only emotional distress but how distress is expressed and understood by healthcare providers.

As Kirmayer has noted in Chapter 1 in this volume, early commentaries on medicine by travellers around the globe reflected differences not only on skin colour but also habits, rites and rituals and differences in sickness and the role shamans played in managing illnesses. With the spread of the British empire inevitably academics and anthropologists moved with the empire and observed 'the other' and created descriptions which were often from a white superior position in which natives were seen as exotic, often stupid and under-developed. This created a basis for racism which has continued to this day. Often these observers saw odd behaviours and immediately branded oddities as pathology often without recognizing the contexts. American anthropologists focused their attention mostly on indigenous populations and their healing practices. Kirmayer, in Chapter 1, also reminds us that early observations saw universality of psychiatric disorders. Historically, comparative psychiatry gave way to cross-cultural psychiatry and subsequently to 'new' cross-cultural psychiatry followed by cultural psychiatry.

Culture and Psychopathology

It is important to understand the relationship between culture and psychopathology. As Tseng (1997) argues, it is important to note that cultures define abnormality. As Offer and Sabshin (1974) highlight, normality can be distinguished from abnormality in four ways: experts agreeing that something is not right; deviation from the norm or the mean; assessment of functioning; and lastly by social judgement. Tseng (1997) urges that clinicians need to be aware to explore which of these four approaches have been identified in defining abnormality and in addition be very clear about the limitations of each approach.

Historical Development

Between anthropologists and clinicians in colonized countries, racial differences between the rulers and the ruled were observed which led to a recognition that many communities were inferior, e.g. Germans and Irish migrant populations were seen to be ill and this susceptibility to illness and resistance to treatment reflected their status (Wittkower and Prince, 1974). As a result of colonialism, the British constructed asylums which were Victorian in design and in some countries separate asylums/wards were constructed for the white people so that the ruled individuals should not see their masters as ill (see Bhugra and Littlewood, 2001). The impact of these observations also led to recognition and description of culture-bound syndromes (see Chapter 14 in this

volume). The recognition of these syndromes confirmed in the mind of the clinicians that the natives were exotic and often more ill and difficult to manage. Unique or rare psychopathology in these groups created a sense of adventure and need for identifying mental illness. In some ways such an identification brought more light on to psychopathology and also often ignored the contribution and comorbidity of physical and mental illness. Oda *et al.* (2005) note that the early views of 'alienists' was that insanity was rare among 'primitive' people and that insanity increased with civilization. Kraeplin's interest in classification of mental illness also led to his exploring whether such classifications could be applied across countries. When he travelled to the Far East, he noted that it was indeed possible to use his classifications in other cultures though symptoms may have included some differences (Jilek, 1995). Since then it is well known that, for example in depression, feelings of guilt are perhaps more common in Judeo-Christian cultures whereas shame may be more common in many socio-centric societies.

Bogousslavsky and Moulin (2009) suggest that neurology played a major role in the development of modern psychiatry. Choudhary and Kirmayer (2009) make a similar point. However, this does not appear to be the case in development of cultural psychiatry. Earlier studies related to cultural comparisons were part of the comparative psychiatry or ethnopsychiatry. When Opler (1959) studied cultural/ethnic differences in symptoms of schizophrenia among Italian Americans and Irish Americans in New York he recognized that these groups differed on seven out of ten variables. Some of these variables may appear odd now – they included homosexuality, preoccupation with sin and guilt especially as part of depression or obsessive–compulsive disorders, physical or somatic complaints and chronic alcoholism. The findings that more Italian patients compared with Irish patients had overt homosexual tendencies during psychotic conditions, behaviour problems and attitudes of rejecting authority are not generalizable to these groups now and need to be carefully understood in the context of the period. Both groups were largely Roman Catholic which may also have had something to do with feelings of sin and guilt especially among the Irish. Irish patients also showed higher than expected rates of chronic alcoholism. It is entirely possible that these findings are related to ethnicities or national characteristics rather than actual symptoms. Murphy *et al.* (1963) studied 26 symptoms or signs of schizophrenia in different cultures and regions. This was a prelude to the subsequent studies by the World Health Organization (WHO) – the International Pilot Study of Schizophrenia and Determinants of Outcome in Severe Mental Disorders. However, whereas Murphy's study gave a list of symptoms to participating psychiatrists, the latter two studies had much stronger assessment tools even though these were criticized for having a Western bias. Not surprisingly, Murphy reported that the distribution of symptoms of schizophrenia varies according to social and cultural factors. It became clear that in many Asian countries symptoms of schizophrenia showed a relatively high prevalence of the simple and catatonic varieties and lower than expected rates of subtypes and a lower prevalence of the paranoid subtype of schizophrenia in their clinical settings.

In the 1970s, WHO launched the International Pilot Study of Schizophrenia (IPSS), with nine centres namely: Aarhus (Denmark), Agra (India), Cali (Colombia), Ibadan (Nigeria), London (UK), Moscow (USSR), Taipei (Taiwan, China), Washington (USA), and Prague (Czechoslovakia) (WHO, 1973). It was the first formal comparative study with multiple centres in different parts of the world and used standardized tools to collect clinical and social information. One of the major important findings was that there was a core set of symptoms which were almost universal whereas there were also soft symptoms which varied dramatically across cultures. The core symptoms were positive symptoms such as auditory hallucinations and experiences of control and negative symptoms such as lack of insight. The findings indicated that some core symptoms were common across cultures and settings whereas others were more strongly influenced by cultures. It was also revealed that, among all the patients studied from all the centres, there were clear differences in subtypes of schizophrenia. The findings revealed that rates of catatonic subtype varied and were reported mostly from low-income countries and confirmed variations in subtypes of schizophrenia across cultures. The subsequent study, the WHO Determinants of Outcome in Severe Psychiatric Disorders (DOSMeD; Jablensky *et al.*, 1991) confirmed these findings.

A groundbreaking study by Hollingshead and Redlich (1958) revealed that social class played a role in rates of schizophrenia and low social class showed higher rates, thereby proposing a social theory of psychopathology which included social disorganization as a possible cause (Faris and Dunham, 1939) related to poverty, breakdown of social communication and urbanicity contributing to high rates of psychopathology. This was countered by social drift (Meyerson, 1941; Clausen and Kohn, 1959). Hare (1956) proposed a social attraction hypothesis arguing that social disorganization in some inner-city areas can attract individuals with schizophrenia who may find social contact aversive.

Social cohesion has been recognized as a protective factor for patients (Chance 1964). In addition, in recent times the concept of social capital has taken hold. There is no doubt that certain social conditions may contribute to a higher prevalence of mental disorders, but it is highly unlikely that they will 'cause' disorders but may simply increase vulnerability.

Different Ways Culture Contributes to Psychopathology

The issue is not whether social and cultural factors influence psychopathology, but in what ways they do. It can be argued that culture contributes to psychopathology in different ways but psychopathology that is predominantly determined by biological factors is less likely to be influenced by cultural factors and any such influence may well be secondary or peripheral. In contrast, psychopathology that is predominantly determined by psychological factors is attributed more to cultural factors. This basic distinction is necessary in discussing different levels of cultural impact on various types of psychopathologies.

Tseng (1997) developed the model of culture and psychopathology and initially suggested three different types of cultural impact on psychopathology. These included culture contributing to phenomenology by shaping of symptoms; variations of psychopathology as a syndrome; unique psychopathology as in culture bound syndromes and frequency of psychopathology. The cultural influences on precipitating, perpetuating and presenting factors can be seen as too simplistic. Tseng (2001) went on to expand on these observations to create six different ways in which culture can contribute to psychopathology (Tseng, 2001: 178–183). These are covered in the following subsections.

Pathogenic Effects

Cultures can cause direct effects on psychopathology by forming or 'generating' it. Cultural ideas and beliefs contribute to stress leading to psychopathology. This cultural stress may be related to culturally demanded performance especially in the context of culturally prescribed roles with special duties which lead on to feelings of inadequacy and anxiety. Not being able to deal with culturally shared specific cultural beliefs will contribute to stress and anxiety. Tseng (2001) illustrates that culturally related psychopathology may lead to culturally related, specific syndrome. He gives an example of the folk belief that if the penis shrinks into the abdomen, this will cause death, leading to panic and people who believe this experience may tie weights to their penis to ensure that shrinking does not take place. Similarly semen-loss anxiety can be related to strong cultural beliefs about the importance of semen in individual well-being.

Pathoselective Effects

Members of a society or culture may select consciously or otherwise certain culturally influenced reaction patterns leading to manifestation of certain psychopathologies. Tseng (2001) illustrates this with an example from Japan where in response to a hopeless situation, the whole family commits suicide (Ohara, 1963). The response of males in the Malayan peninsula to run *amok* is very strongly culturally influenced. Such responses are related to common mental disorders most of the time.

Pathoplastic Effects

Cultures modify the way distress is expressed thus modelling or 'plastering' the manifestations of psychopathology. Culture affects the contents of symptoms and expressions used. Tseng (2001) illustrates this by giving examples that delusional content of individuals will vary according to whichever grandiose figure they identify with or which figure is more popular or important in their society. Similarly contents of delusions will depend upon social and economic as well as cultural factors. Thus culture will affect the psychopathology in such a way that the disorders could be recognized as 'atypical', 'subtypes' or 'variations' of disorders officially recognized in the current Western classification system. However, it must be recognized that sometimes there may not be any overlap with Western classificatory systems.

Pathoelaborating Effects

It is well recognized that although some patterns of behaviour are universal others may become exaggerated to the extreme in some cultures through cultural reinforcement (Simons, 1996). Tseng (2001) illustrates this with the example of *latah* which is observed in Malaysia. It is characterized by the sudden onset of a transient dissociative attack induced by startling. According to Tseng (2001) suicidal behaviour is another behaviour strongly influenced by culture. Japan is well known for acts of *hara-kiri*, or *seppuku*, which is a very formal and culturally sanctioned act performed by a warrior, or samurai, as an honourable way of ending their own life (rather than surrendering to the enemy and being humiliated). Tseng (2001) goes on to illustrate many other reasons for committing suicide: as a means of punishment, or to atone for wrongfulness. Thus there are many types of suicide in Japan such as *oyako-shinju* (parent–child double suicide), *ikka-shinjiu* (family suicide), *jio-shi* (double suicide by a couple due to an obstructed affair), or *kan-shi* (when a subordinate commits suicide to transmit loyal advice to an authority figure). Similarly, till around nineteenth century, the self-sacrifice of a Hindu widow on the death of her husband described as *sati* has been described as non-pathogenic suicide in India (Bhugra, 2005).

Pathofacilitative Effects

Pathofacilitative effects suggest that some types of psychopathology are more common in some cultures compared with others. Tseng (2001) argues that cultural factors may not actually change the manifestation of the psychopathology too much i.e. the clinical picture can still be recognized and categorized. However, cultural factors do contribute significantly to the frequent occurrence of certain mental disorders in a society at particular times. Therefore, the 'facilitating' effect of culture makes it comparatively easier for certain psychopathologies to develop. This may lead to an increase in their frequency but this variation may also depend upon other social, economic and cultural factors. Tseng (2001) illustrates the excessive concern with body weight and the perception of slimness as beauty in some cultures to be strongly influenced by cultural values and expectations. Westermeyer (1973) has argued that liberal attitudes towards gun control, leading to more weapon-related violence or homicidal behaviour, are strongly influenced by cultures. Cultural attitudes to alcohol consumption as well as availability will influence rates of alcoholism.

Pathoreactive Effects

Pathoreactive effects of culture influence not only people's beliefs about their experiences related to emotional distress what terms they use to attribute the distress. Tseng (2001) thus argues that it is inevitable that the clinical picture of the mental disorder will be coloured by the cultural reaction of the individual. However, it must also be recognized that the understanding of the carers and family members will also colour the patient's expectations. He illustrates this by descriptions of *susto* (meaning fright in Spanish) used by people in Latin America to refer to the condition of loss of soul (Rubel, 1964; Rubel *et al.*, 1985). The fear is that even though everyone has a soul, the soul may depart if the individual is frightened or startled. Consequently the person who has lost his/her soul will manifest certain morbid mental conditions and illness behaviours which may be seen as spiritual factors but the clinical manifestations are very likely to be heterogeneous (Gillin, 1948). Tseng (2001) goes on to emphasize that it is culture-related because the morbid condition is 'interpreted' according to folk and cultural concepts of causation and interventions. Tseng (2001) also uses post-traumatic stress disorder (PTSD) as another example of pathoreactive effects. In some societies soldiers with PTSD get benefits and better pensions and a sympathetic attitude is thus likely to influence the numbers of people who will seek help and also present in clinical settings.

Cultural Influences on Different Groups of Psychopathology

From a cultural perspective, it is useful to recognize not only the actual spectrum of psychopathology but also that of severity because interpretations of severity and non-response will be very strongly affected by cultural values. As far as severity is concerned, Tseng (2001) sees that as primarily biological causation. However, cultural factors also influence biological factors. As mentioned previously, contents of symptoms – be they seen as minor or major illnesses – are very likely to be strongly influenced and closely related to culture. Interestingly, Tseng also highlights the role of each of these six relationships with different

psychiatric disorders. López and Guarnaccia (2000) suggest that our understanding of culture and psycho-pathology has increased in the past few decades and this has continued in the last decade with cultural formulation now being an integral part of DSM-5 (APA, 2013).

Organic Mental Disorders

By definition, organic mental disorders are caused by organic aetiological factors. Although one could argue culture does not have a 'direct' causal effect on these disorders. However, dietary habits and taboos may play a role. For example, neurocysticercosis is not as common in many countries as the parasite can be transmitted through food, especially pork meat (although poor sanitation is also a major cause, the disease being transmitted through uncooked food and drink which has been infected by human faeces). Furthermore, the manifestation of the disorder will be almost similar irrespective of their ethnic or cultural backgrounds although the contents of symptoms and clinical presentation will be directed by culture in a pathofacilitating manner.

Similar to the example of neurocysticercosis, Tseng (2001) highlights the example of kuru seen among the Fore tribe people of New Guinea. The rate of mortality was 1 per cent, especially among women. The tribe saw kuru as being caused by witchcraft. However, kuru is one of the transmissible spongiform encephalopathies, or prion diseases, it attacks the central nervous system after a long incubation period and is transmitted through victims eating the brains of dead people. This was confirmed by Keesing (1976) who reminds us that it was the custom for Fore women to ritually eat the bodies and brains of their dead relatives, hence transmission of the disease. Therefore it can be seen that this culture-rooted behaviour and habit of eating human brains contributes significantly to the genesis of organic disorders.

Sexually transmitted diseases play a role and their treatment and attitudes vary across cultures leading to organic mental disorders. As Tseng (2001) reminds us, while culture is not a direct causative factor in these organic mental disorders, a society's attitude toward sexual behaviour, particularly outside marriage, and its tolerance of promiscuity, will certainly affect the sexual behaviour of its members. This is particularly evident in the case of HIV transmission and consequent mental illness as in some cultures it is believed that having sex with virgins can cure HIV; thus the prevalence of sexually transmitted diseases and resulting mental complications.

Major Psychiatric Disorders: Schizophrenia

Readers are directed also to look at specific chapters in this volume for further details. As mentioned earlier, the DOSMeD study (Jablensky *et al.*, 1991) was led by the WHO. This study had 12 centres: Aarhus (Denmark), Agra and Chandigarh (India), Cali (Columbia), Dublin (Ireland), Honolulu and Rochester (USA), Ibadan (Nigeria), Moscow (USSR), Nagasaki (Japan), Nottingham (UK) and Prague (Czechoslovakia). Jablensky *et al.* (1991: 45–52), found that using a stricter definition of schizophrenia the incidence rates did not differ widely among the centres similar to many other epidemiological studies.

Tseng (2001) reminds us that there seems to be some evidence that there may well be possible patho-reactive effects on schizophrenia. The 2 year follow up of the WHO's International Pilot Study of Schizophrenia (IPSS) revealed that the level of social development had a certain relation to the short-term prognosis of schizophrenia. The 2 year outcome was better in developing societies compared with developed societies (Sartorius *et al.*, 1977). It is possible that family, social and cultural factors may have pathoreactive effects on functional psychoses, such as schizophrenia, resulting in different prognoses. Sartorius *et al.* (1978) postulated that less stigma and more family support may result in better outcome.

Affective Disorder: Depression

Depression is an interesting illness to study because the word does not appear in many languages but the experiences of feeling depressed and its causation are understood (see Bhugra, 1996). For a considerable period it had been thought that depression did not exist in native populations (Bhugra and Littlewood, 1997). Individuals may use other pathways and may not see depression as an illness but as a response to life's ups and downs. As has been demonstrated by Bhugra *et al.* (1997a, b), Punjabi women seek help from religious leaders for their feelings of sadness and feeling low in mood. Thus actual presentation needs to be looked at. Understanding of feeling low and tired

may lead to physical investigations rather than receiving psychiatric help. Culturally moulded presentations will dictate pathways into care.

Another complicating factor is that people may not believe in mind–body dualism and present and seek help for somatic complaints. Simon *et al.* (1999) from the World Health Organization study of psychological problems in general practices in 15 countries found that one in ten people presenting with physical complaints had major depression. Interestingly, they observed that patients were more likely to present with physical symptoms if they did not have a personal relationship with the physicians. It is entirely possible that people may feel that as they are going to see a doctor they need to present with physical symptoms. It has been noted that not only rates of depression vary within the same country, actual symptoms too vary (Bhugra 1996; Bhugra *et al.* 1997c).

In a classic study, Pfeiffer (1968) observed that the 'core' symptoms of depression (i.e. change of mood, biological symptoms such as changes in libido, sleep and appetite, and hypochondriacal symptoms) were similar across cultures. However, other symptoms, such as feelings of guilt and shame as well as suicidal tendencies varied across cultures. Other studies have confirmed this (Binitie, 1975; Sartorius, 1975). Suicidal behaviours and wishes can be expressed in culturally appropriate ways. As Islam proscribes suicide, Waziri (1973) reported that the majority of depressed patients in Afghanistan expressed 'death wishes' instead of suicidal intentions or thoughts. In many countries around the world the act of suicide is illegal, thereby creating a degree of confusion about the act and its value to the individual. Thus culture can cause a pathoplastic effect.

The presence or absence of guilt and shame is very strongly influenced by cultures. Prince (1968) found that in Africa, mental–emotional self-castigation is rare or absent in the early stages of depressed patients. Similarly, Murphy *et al.* (1967) observed that Christianity (and Judaism) may cause feelings of guilt, though El-Islam (1969) argues that levels of education and literacy influence levels of guilt. With many cultures in transition it will be interesting to compare these rates across cultures. Bhugra *et al.* (1997c) found that the notion of shame was more prevalent in north India but anecdotal evidence suggests that this may be changing as a result of cultural transition.

Similar to the schizophrenia studies, the WHO instigated a number of studies looking at rates of depression across cultures using standardized methods especially using clusters of symptoms (Sartorius *et al.*, 1983) in five study centres in four countries: Basel (Switzerland), Montreal (Canada), Nagasaki (Japan), Tehran (Iran) and Tokyo (Japan). Using the WHO Schedule for Standardized Assessment of Depressive Disorders (SADD) and specific diagnostic criteria of the International Statistical Classification of Diseases and Related Health Problems, ninth version (ICD-9) a total of 573 patients were examined. Patients in all the sites had high frequencies of sadness, joylessness, anxiety, tension, lack of energy, loss of interest, concentration difficulties and feelings of inadequacy. However, there was a considerable degree of variation in the frequencies of presentation across centres. Not surprisingly, guilt feelings were present in two-thirds (68%) of Swiss patients, but in only one-third (32%) of the Iranian patients. On the other hand more than half (57%) of Iranian patients had somatic symptoms compared with only a quarter (27%) of patients in Canada. Patients in Nagasaki, Montreal and Basel were more anergic and showed higher levels of psychomotor retardation than those in Tokyo and Tehran.

Depression and its prevalence may not always be clearly identified as it may be mixed with anxiety and pain or somatic symptoms. Depression varies in severity and there are many recognized subtypes of depression which must be taken into account in any research activity. Like the organic mental disorders, it is likely that more severe forms of depression are caused by biological factors but as Marsella *et al.* (1985) argue, the actual symptoms may well vary as modified by cultural values (pathoplasticity) and reactions to symptoms (pathoreactive).

Perhaps, from a cultural psychiatric point of view, one of the most useful areas of study is that of the psychological causes of depression, especially reactive depression rather than endogenous may offer a better understanding of cultural–pathology interactions. It has been hypothesized that separation in childhood may well contribute to certain psychiatric disorders including depression (Bhugra *et al.* 1999). Separation from or loss of a parent in childhood and of a spouse in adulthood may contribute to depression.

It can be argued that how a culture and society views death and ritualizes mourning will also affect the occurrence of depression. In cultures where bereavement and rituals related to it are expected to last for a year, it is possible that response to loss may

well be different. In Samoa, death is seen as a natural event in life and the community provides effective support when someone dies (Ablon, 1971). Thus abnormal grief reaction must be understood in such contexts defined by cultures. Fernando (1975) studied social and family factors in depressed patients of Jewish and protestant origins and noted that increasing paternal inadequacy and weakening ethnic links and religious faith were related to depressive ills among Jews, but not among protestants.

Depression is likely to be the commonest psychiatric disorder around the globe by 2020 and deserves further detailed study looking at and ascertaining cultural factors and the impact of culture and society on development and persistence of depression as well as pathways people take in seeking help.

Substance Abuse and Dependency

Mental disorders associated with substance abuse and/or dependency are basically biophysiological in nature; however, there is room for psychological input. Culture has pathoselective and pathofacilitative effects on the prevalence of abuse. In the religious context if drinking is proscribed, associated problems are likely to be lower. Indulgence in alcohol and other substance intoxication may well be a way of dealing with stress.

It is entirely possible that with rapid sociocultural change, particularly associated with cultural uprooting, substance abuse tends to increase sharply, particularly among youngsters.

Suicidal Behaviour

As already mentioned, suicidal behaviour and acts are very strongly influenced by cultures. Suicidal behaviour may be more suitable for cross-cultural comparison than other kinds of psychopathology but when the act is illegal it is difficult to get accurate figures. Furthermore, suicide is not a homogeneous clinical phenomenon. Suicidal behaviour may be a result of severe psychiatric disorders, a secondary reaction towards stigmatized mental disorders that are chronic or untreatable. It may be associated with substance abuse or dependence. Many suicidal behaviours may be a result of reactions to stress in daily life.

As described in the chapter on suicide in this volume, there is a rather wide range of rates among the different countries. The range of difference in rates is very wide in contrast to other psychiatric disorders, such as schizophrenia, which have a difference of merely several times. Many of the very-low-rate countries are Muslim or Catholic societies that have prohibitive religious attitudes toward self-killing. Rates of suicide depend upon a number of factors including social, economic and political climate. La Vecchia *et al.* (1994) stated that, over time, the figures for suicide rates are relatively favourable in less developed areas of the world, including Latin America and several countries in Asia, however, with cultures in transition and increased urbanization this may well change dramatically.

Common Psychiatric Disorders

Among minor psychiatric disorders, conversion and dissociative disorders are good examples of the rich effects of culture. Tseng (2001) goes on to point out that the prevalence of conversion or dissociation varies greatly among different societies (due to patho-facilitating effects). He reminds us that it may be that in some societies, in contrast to other forms of psychopathology, it is preferable to deal with stress (pathoselective effects) by repressing or dissociating the painful emotion. There is no doubt that cultures and societies will respond and react in different ways to the phenomena of conversion or dissociation (pathoreactive effects). Conversion is a well-recognized phenomenon in expressing social distress. Matten (2015) has suggested that from the second century BCE, and with Hippocratic precedent, ancient medical writers described a condition they called *hysterike pnix* or 'uterine suffocation'. He argues that uterine suffocation was, in modern terms, a functional somatic syndrome characterized by chronic anxiety and panic attacks. He reminds us that there exist a number of similar panic-type syndromes in modern populations, indicating that cultures continue to pathofacilitate distress in a physical way.

Neurasthenia is another psychiatric disorder that deserves attention. Originally the syndrome included core symptoms of mental fatigue, associated with poor memory, poor concentration, irritability, headaches, tinnitus, insomnia and other vague somatic complaints. This diagnostic category was included only in the second edition of the *Diagnostic and Statistical Manual* (DSM-II) in 1968. Again interestingly the term was removed from the next edition in 1980. In many parts of the world, especially in China, the term continues to be deployed and is a culturally sanctioned diagnosis and way of expressing distress. In China the term neurasthenia, a translation of the Chinese term *shenjing suairuo* (nerve-weakened disorder), became a commonly accepted medical term. The concept of *shenjing suairuo* is compatible with the traditional Chinese medical concept of *shen-kui* (kidney-deficiency disorder). The term is widely used and easily understood and accepted by the layperson, as well. Kleinman (1982) conducted a clinical study of patients diagnosed by Chinese clinicians as having neurasthenia, and observed that 87 per cent of the patients he examined could be 're-diagnosed' as having a depressive disorder according to Western criteria. However, many prominent Chinese psychiatrists insisted that neurasthenia was a recognized psychiatric disorder distinct from depressive disorders (Yan, 1989; Young, 1989; Zhang, 1989). Thus parallel diagnoses need to be looked at closely in research and clinical criteria.

Personality Disorders

Apart from the observation whether personality disorders are true medical conditions, it can be argued that different cultures emphasize different personality traits and characteristics as ideal. Furthermore, cultures themselves define abnormal and deviancy especially in the context of behaviours which are closely related to personality which thus becomes a culture-relative exercise. Therefore, cultures define and describe boundaries which reflect specific values, ideas, world view, resources and social structure of the society (Foulks, 1996).

When attempting to define personality disorder we are best to refer to the most recent universally agreed diagnostic criteria, the DSM-5 (APA, 2013). Within personality disorder diagnoses it is cluster B personality disorders that receive the most attention within the literature. Characterized by dramatic, emotional and erratic traits, patients diagnosed with cluster B personality disorders usually present with issues regarding poor impulse control and emotional regulation. The reason for this focus on cluster B disorders, in particular borderline and antisocial, is most simply explained by the fact that these individuals are subsequently most likely to appear before emergency psychiatric services and within forensic settings (Mulder, 2012). They are therefore more likely to place services under strain with regard to cost and resources (NICE, 2009). Given the current need to better understand and treat these disorders from both an ethical and economic perspective, along with the large evidence bases surrounding them, this chapter will focus on the cultural differences between these two personality disorders specifically.

Within the DSM-5 (APA, 2013) antisocial personality disorder (ASPD) is diagnosed following impairments in the self-functioning in terms of identity which is ego-centric, driven by personal gain, self-esteem derived through perceived power and self-direction guided by personal gratification with an absence of pro-social norms and subsequent failure to comply with normal ethics and lawful behaviour. These impairments can be seen within interpersonal functions presenting as a lack of empathy for others, incapacity for intimate relationships and pathological personality traits which can be antagonistic in the forms of manipulative, deceitful, callous, hostile behaviour and disinhibited irresponsible, impulsive and risk taking.

Dependent personality disorder is defined as 'having difficulty making everyday decisions without an excessive amount of advice and reassurance from others', and 'needing others to assume responsibility for most major areas of his or her life'. This definition needs careful unpicking, depending on whether the person being identified thus is living in an individualistic or a collectivist society. In a collectivist or socio-centric society, considering, consulting with, or depending on others is a cultural expectation and norm that does not necessarily imply that the person is suffering from dependency. The concept of antisocial personality disorder is also defined by the failure to conform to 'social norms', however they are defined, and identified by the culture. Thus there is an epidemiological challenge in comparing rates across different cultures and societies, because methodologically, the surveys are one-point studies and not necessarily a longitudinal study of behaviours. It can be argued that antisocial personality disorder, due to its nature, is the easiest to identify and study as long as social norms are clearly identified.

The Epidemiological Catchment Area (ECA) study in the United States found that among the three ethnic groups surveyed, namely, Caucasian American, African American, and Hispanic American, the lifetime prevalence rates of antisocial personality disorder were found to be 2, 2.3 and 3.4 per cent, respectively. Robins *et al.* (1991) therefore claimed that, in the United States, there were no racial differences in the prevalence of antisocial personality disorder. However,

the racial distribution of the United States' prison population reflects racial disparity which continues to this date. Kosson *et al.* (1990) reported that African Americans, who comprise less than 13 per cent of the general population, represented 45 per cent of the prisoners in the United States. Thus overpathologizing bias toward African Americans may have resulted in more subjects sentenced to prison under the diagnosis of antisocial personality disorder (Lopez, 1989) but this needs further exploration. Alarcón and Foulks (1995) argue that the criteria for diagnosing antisocial personality are inappropriate for settings in which value systems and behavioural rules encourage learning to be violent as a protective strategy for survival. This observation also highlights the specific issues about majority communities' ability and power to pathologize minority communities.

Lynn (2002), after studying several facets of psychopathic personality disorder, showed that there were differences between blacks and Native Americans (high values), Hispanics (intermediate levels), lower values in whites and the lowest values in East Asians. He attributed these different to genetic factors but Zuckerman (2003) saw these differences as a consequence of social class, historical circumstance and their positions in Western society rather than of racial genetics. This debate highlights the role of social factors in behaviour patterns.

As mentioned earlier, there are comparatively fewer studies across cultures looking at personality disorders for a number of reasons. However, when the questionnaire used in the Epidemiological Catchment Area (ECA) study in the United States was translated into Chinese and applied in an epidemiological study in Taiwan (Hwu *et al.*, 1989), researchers found that the prevalence of antisocial personality disorder was only 0.14 per cent in Taiwan compared to around 3 per cent that was found in the United States (Compton *et al.*, 1991). However, there are methodological issues related to the way specific questions are framed.

Schrier *et al.* (2013) found that the association between personality factors and disorders or symptoms of anxiety and depression was very similar in three ethnic groups in the Netherlands, and surprisingly found that all show the typical profile of high neuroticism and low extraversion, agreeableness and conscientiousness.

In an interesting overview, Cooke (1997) hypothesized that individualistic societies, in contrast to collective societies, are more likely to produce glibness and superficiality, grandiosity, promiscuity and multiple marital relationships, together with a lack of responsibility within relationships. This observation confirms that antisocial behaviour is subject to the pathofacilitating effect of cultures. However, it must also be recognized that not all members of an individualistic society are likely to be individualistic. Ryder *et al.* (2014) suggest that separate dimensions in assessing personality disorder in Asians may be needed. Wallace (2015) argues that cultural norms and social interaction are synergistic with individual and group cognition and their disorders. He puts forward a model that suggests that 'atomistic models of economic interaction are increasingly characterized as divorced from reality by heterodox economists' and may play a role in creating high rates of psychopathic and antisocial personality disorder and obsessive–compulsive disorder in the West, which may well be Western culture-bound syndromes or in those societies which are undergoing social disintegration.

Cultural Communicability of Psychopathology

Although it can be argued that psychiatric symptoms differ from communicable symptoms, various epidemics of sharing of symptoms, such as in *koro*, mass hysteria, epidemic panic disorder, indicate that social and cultural factors play a significant role in the occurrence of these phenomena. Pathogenic, pathoselective, pathoplastic and pathofacilitating effects are all significant factors in the development of psychologically contagious collective mental disorders. The contagious nature of some psychiatric disorders needs further exploration (Ventriglio and Bhugra, 2017).

Studies of the *koro* epidemics from Southeast Asian countries such as China, Thailand and India, indicate that symptoms communicated through various causative factors are: commonly shared folk belief (that shrinking of the penis could potentially result in death); the existence and exaggeration of community anxiety (due to conflict or disasters, be they natural or man-made) which serves as the grounds for the occurrence of the community-based, massive anxiety attack; the transmission of anxiety, fear, and panic among people, which promotes the contagious occurrence of the epidemic disorder. *Folie à deux* and *folie à famille* and epidemic hysteria are other conditions which are shared psychopathologies.

Culture-Related Specific Psychiatric Syndromes

Culture-bound syndromes are mental conditions whose occurrence or manifestation is closely related to cultural factors. Increasingly, they are seen as culture-related specific syndromes because these are usually unique, with special clinical manifestations in that specific culture. These are not easily classifiable conditions as they do not fit neatly into classificatory systems (Tseng, 2001: 211–263). These are discussed further in this volume by Bhugra *et al.*, in Chapter 14.

Therefore, cultural factors play a significant role in development and maintenance of these syndromes. In most cases, the pathogenic, pathoselective, pathoplastic, pathoelaborating, pathofacilitating and pathoreactive effects of culture all contribute to the development of these symptoms. Although Draguns (1980) argues that culture has a moderate, but not unlimited, impact on psychopathology (depending on the cultural group involved and the nature of the cultural influence), we contend that for certain conditions this impact can be major.

Cultural input in these conditions is so significant that these culture-related specific syndromes are often unevenly distributed. However, with increased globalization and other factors such as industrialization and urbanization in many cultures, the culture-specificity of these conditions is beginning to change. As discussed elsewhere in this volume, previously it was thought that culture-related specific syndromes were 'bound' to particular ethnic groups or cultural units hence they were recognized as 'culture-bound syndromes'. Recently, this view has changed to express the thoughts that such syndromes may well be closely related to certain cultural features, but are not necessarily 'bound'. These conditions therefore, may occur across the boundaries of ethnicity, society or cultural units, as long as they have common cultural 'traits', 'elements' or 'themes' that contribute directly to the formation of such pathologies (see Sumathipala *et al.*, 2004). Cultures do affect symptoms but these are no longer confined to specific cultures only.

Conclusions

There is no doubt that culture affects psychopathology in different ways from causing the actual psychopathology (psychogenic effect) through to actual contribution to the selection of psychopathology (pathoselective effect). Cultures shape and modify the clinical manifestation of the psychopathology (pathoplastic effect). Cultural values may promote the occurrence of certain pathologies (pathofacilitating effect) or elaborate on the nature of psychopathology (pathoelaborating effect) as well as influence the way society reacts to the occurrence of psychopathology (pathoreactive effect). There is little doubt that these effects can be differential on individuals and conditions.

It is important for clinicians to note and be trained in the process of clinical assessment and the evaluation of psychopathology especially as related to the impact of culture. Of course clinical assessment is a dynamic and ongoing process. The process must include how the patient perceives distress, expresses it – what idioms are selected, how they respond to it, and communicate with others as well as the clinician. Obviously the patient's educational, socioeconomic and other factors will play a role in the expression and help-seeking. Similarly the clinician's personality, professional orientation and clinical experience, cultural identity, including value system and concept of normality and pathology, will affect their clinical skills including assessment, judgement and management of psychopathology. Cultural competence is good clinical practice and a competent clinician will have suitable culturally orientated attitudes to understand, assess and evaluate the psychopathologies of patients from diverse cultural backgrounds.

Acknowledgements

Professor Wen-Shing Tseng contributed this chapter to the first edition of this book. Sadly he passed away in 2012. We dedicate this chapter to his memory and have kept the theme and structure as he had and updated the chapter.

References

Ablon, J. (1971). Bereavement in a Samoan community. *British Journal of Psychology*, 44, 329–337.

Alarcón, R. and Foulks, E. (1995). Personality disorders and culture: contemporary clinical views, Part A. *Cultural Diversity and Mental Health*, 1, 3–17.

Bhugra, D. (1996). Depression across cultures. *Primary Care Psychiatry*, 2(3), 155–165.

Bhugra, D. (2005). Sati: a type of non-psychiatric suicide. *Crisis*, 26(2), 73–77.

Bhugra, D. and Littlewood, R. (eds) (2001). *Colonialism and Psychiatry*. New Delhi: Oxford University Press.

Bhugra, D., Baldwin, D. and Desai, M. (1997a). Focus groups: implications for primary and cross-cultural psychiatry. *Primary Care Psychiatry*, 3(1), 45–50.

Bhugra, D., Baldwin, D. and Desai, M. (1997b). A pilot study of the impact of fact sheets and guided discussion on knowledge and attitudes regarding depression in an ethnic minority sample. *Primary Care Psychiatry*, 3(3), 135–140.

Bhugra, D., Gupta, K. R. and Wright, B. (1997c). Depression in north India: comparison of symptoms and life events with other patient groups. *International Journal of Psychiatry in Clinical Practice*, 1, 83–87.

Bhugra, D., Mallett, R. and Leff, J. (1999). Schizophrenia and African Caribbeans: a conceptual model of aetiology. *International Review of Psychiatry*, 11(2), 145–152.

Binitie, A. (1975). A factor-analytical study of depression across cultures (African and European). *British Journal of Psychiatry*, 127, 559–563.

Bogousslavsky, J. and Moulin, T. (2009). From alienism to the birth of modern psychiatry: a neurological story? *European Neurology*, 62, 257–263, doi:10.1159/00235594.

Chance, N. (1964). A cross-cultural study of social cohesion and depression. *Transcultural Psychiatric Research Review*, 1, 19–24.

Choudhury, S. and Kirmayer, L. J. (2009). Cultural neuroscience and psychopathology: prospects for cultural psychiatry. *Progress in Brain Research*, 178, 263–283, doi: 10.1016/S0079-6123(09)17820-2.

Clausen, J. A. and Kohn, M. L. (1959) Relations of schizophrenia to the social structure of a small city. In *Epidemiology of Mental Disorders*, ed. B. Pasamanick. Washington, DC: American Association for the Advancement of Science.

Comton, W. M., Helzer, J. E., Hwu, H. G. *et al.* (1991). New methods in cross-cultural psychiatry: psychiatric illness in Taiwan and the US. *American Journal of Psychiatry*, 148, 1697–1704.

Cooke, D. J. (1997). Psychopaths: oversexed, overplayed but not over here? *Criminal Behaviors and Mental Health*, 7(1), 3–11.

Draguns, J. G. (1980). Psychological disorders of clinical severity. In *Handbook of Cross-Cultural Psychology: Psychopathology*, vol. 6, ed. H. C. Triandis and J. G. Draguns. Boston: Allyn and Bacon.

El-Islam, M. F. (1969). Depression and guilt: a study at an Arab psychiatric clinic. *Social Psychiatry*, 4, 56–58.

Faris, R. and Dunham, H. (1939). *Mental Disease in the Chicago Area*. Chicago: University of Chicago Press.

Fernando, S. J. M. (1975). A cross-cultural study of some familial and social factors in depressive illness. *British Journal of Psychiatry*, 127, 46–53.

Foulks, E. F. (1996). Culture and personality disorders. In *Culture and Psychiatric Diagnosis: A DSM-IV Perspective*, ed. J. E. Mezzich, A. Kleinman, H. Fabrega, Jr and L. Parron. Washington, DC: American Psychiatric Press, pp. 243–252.

Gillin, J. (1948). Magical fright. *Psychiatry*, **11**, 387–400.

Hare, R. (1956). Mental illness and social condition in Bristol. *Journal of Mental Science*, **102**, 349–357.

Hollingshead, A. B. and Redlich, F. C. (1958). *Social Class and Mental Illness: A Community Study*. New York: John Wiley.

Hwu, H. G., Yeh, E. K. and Chang, L. Y. (1989). Prevalence of psychiatric disorders in Taiwan defined by the Chinese Diagnostic Interview Schedule. *Acta Psychiatrica Scandinavica*, **79**, 136–147.

Jablensky, A., Sartorius, N., Ernberg, G., *et al.* (1991). *Schizophrenia: Manifestations, Incidence and Course in Different Cultures: A World Health Organization Ten-Country Study. Psychological Medicine, Monograph Supplement*, **20**. Cambridge: Cambridge University Press.

Jilek, W. G. (1995). Emil Kraepelin and comparative socio-cultural psychiatry. *European Achives of Psychiatry and Clinical Neuroscience*, **245**, 231–238.

Keesing, R. M. (1976). *Cultural Anthropology: A Contemporary Perspective*. New York: Holt, Rinehart and Winston, p. 219.

Kleinman, A. (1982). Neurasthenia and depression: a study of somatization and culture in China. *Culture, Medicine and Psychiatry*, **4**, 117–190.

Kosson, D. S., Smith, S. S. and Newman J. P. (1990). Evaluating the construct validity of psychopathy in black and white male inmates: three preliminary studies. *Journal of Abnormal Psychology*, **99**, 250–259.

La Vecchia, C., Lucchini, F. and Levi, F. (1994). Worldwide trends in suicide mortality, 1955–1989. *Acta Psychiatrica Scandinavica*, **90**, 53–64.

Lopez, S. R. (1989). Patient variable biases in clinical judgement: conceptual overview and methodological considerations. *Psychological Bulletin*, **106**, 184–203.

Lynn, R. (2002). Racial and ethnic differences in psychopathic personality. *Personality and Individual Differences*, **32**(2), 273–316.

Marsella, A. J., Sartorius, N., Jablensky, A. and Fenton, F. R. (1985). Cross-cultural studies of depressive disorders: an overview. In *Culture and Depression: Studies in the Anthropology and Cross-Cultural Psychiatry of Affect and Disorder*, ed. A. Kleinman and B. Good. Berkeley: University of California Press.

Mattern, S. P. (2015). Panic and culture: hysterike pnix in the Ancient Greek World. *Journal of the History of Medicine and Allied Sciences*, **70**(4), 491–515, doi: 10.1093/jhmas/jru029.

Meyerson, A. (1941). Review of mental disorders in urban areas. *American Journal of Psychiatry*, **96**, 995–997.

Murphy, H. B. M., Wittkower, E. D., Fried, J. and Ellenberger, H. F. (1963). A cross-cultural survey of schizophrenic symptomatology. *International Journal of Social Psychiatry*, **9**, 237–249.

Murphy, H. B. M., Wittkower, E. D. and Chance, N. (1967). Cross-cultural inquiry into the symptomatology of depression: a preliminary report. *International Journal of Psychiatry*, **3**(1), 6–22.

NICE (2009). Borderline personality disorder: recognition and management. *National Institute for Health and Clinical Excellence*. NICE guideline (CG78).

Oda, A. M. G. R., Banzato, C. E. M. and Dalgalarrondo, P. (2005). Some origins of cross-cultural psychiatry. *History of Psychiatry*, **16**(2), 155–169.

Ohara, K. (1963). Characteristics of suicides in Japan, especially of parent–child double suicide. *American Journal of Psychiatry*, **120**(4), 382–385.

Opler, M. K. (1959). Cultural differences in mental disorders: an Italian and Irish contrast in the schizophrenia – USA. In *Culture and Mental Health: Cross-Cultural Studies*, ed. M. K. Opler. New York: Macmillan Company.

Pfeiffer, W. (1968). The symptomatology of depression viewed transculturally. *Transcultural Psychiatric Research Review*, **5**, 121–124.

Prince, R. (1968). The changing picture of depressive syndromes in Africa: is it fact or diagnostic fashion? *Canadian Journal of African Studies*, **1**, 177–192.

Robins, L. N., Tipp, J. and Pryzbeck, T. (1991). Antisocial personality. In *Psychiatric Disorders in America: The Epidemiologic Catchment Area Study*, ed. L. N. Robins and D. A. Rogers. New York: Free Press.

Rubel, A. J. (1964). The epidemiology of a folk illness: susto in Hispanic America. *Ethnology*, **3**, 268–283.

Rubel, A. J., O'Nell, C. W. and Collado, R. (1985). The folk illness called susto. In *The Culture-Bound Syndromes*, ed. R. C. Simons and C. C. Hughes. Dordrecht: D. Reidel.

Ryder, A. G., Sun, J., Dere, J. and Fung, K. (2014). Personality disorders in Asians: summary, and a call for cultural research. *Asian Journal of Psychiatry*, **7**(1), 86–88, doi: 10.1016/j.ajp.2013.11.009.

Sartorius, N. (1975). Epidemiology of depression. *WHO Chronicle*, **29**, 423–427.

Sartorius, N., Jablensky, A. and Shapiro, R. (1977). Two-year follow-up of the patients included in the WHO International Pilot Study of Schizophrenia. *Psychological Medicine*, **7**, 529–541.

Sartorius, N., Jablensky, A. and Shapiro, R. (1978). Cross-cultural differences in the short-term prognosis of schizophrenic psychoses. *Schizophrenia Bulletin*, **4**, 102–113.

Sartorius, N., Davidian, H., Ernberg, G. *et al.* (1983). *Depressive Disorders in Different Cultures: Report on the WHO Collaborative Study on Standardized*

Assessment of Depressive Disorders. Geneva: World Health Organization.

Schrier, A. C., de Wit, M. A., Krol, A., *et al.* (2013). Similar associations between personality dimensions and anxiety or depressive disorders in a population study of Turkish-Dutch, Moroccan-Dutch, and native Dutch subjects. *Journal of Nervous and Mental Disease*, **201**(5), 421–428, doi: 10.1097/NMD.0b013e31828e110d.

Simon, G. E., VonKorff, M., Piccinelli, M., Fullerton, C. and Ormel, J. (1999). An international study of the relation between somatic symptoms and depression. *New England Journal of Medicine*, **341**(18), 1329–1335.

Simons, R. C. (1996). *Boo! Culture, Experience, and the Startle Reflex*. New York: Oxford University Press.

Sumathipala, A., Siribadanna, S. H. and Bhugra, D. (2004). Culture bound syndromes: the story of dhat syndrome. *British Journal of Psychiatry*, **184**, 200–209.

Tseng, W. S. (1997). Overview: culture and psychopathology. In *Culture and Psychopathology: A Guide to Clinical Assessment*, ed. W. S. Tseng and J. Streltzer. New York: Brunner/Mazel, pp. 1–27.

Tseng, W. S. (2001). *Handbook of Cultural Psychiatry*. San Diego: Academic Press.

Ventriglio, A. and Bhugra, D. (2017). Communicability of symptoms in psychiatry. *International Journal of Social Psychiatry*, **63**(2), 89–90.

Wallace, R. (2015). Closed-system 'economic' models for psychiatric disorders: Western atomism and its culture-bound syndromes. *Cognitive Processing*, **16**(3), 279–290, doi: 10.1007/s10339-015-0659-z.

Waziri, R. (1973). Symptomatology of depressive illness in Afghanistan. *American Journal of Psychiatry*, **130**, 213–217.

Westermeyer, J. (1973). On the epidemic of *amok* violence. *Archives of General Psychiatry*, **28**, 873–876.

WHO (1973). *The International Study of Schizophrenia*. Geneva: World Health Organization.

Wittkower, E. D. and Prince, R. (1974). A review of transcultural psychiatry. In *American Handbook of Psychiatry*, 2nd edn, vol. **2**, *Child and Adolescent Psychiatry, Sociocultural and Community Psychiatry*, ed. G. Capan. New York: Basic Books, pp. 535–550.

Yan, H. Q. (1989). The necessity of retaining the diagnostic concept of neurasthenia. *Culture, Medicine and Psychiatry*, **13**(2), 139–145.

Young, D. S. (1989). Neurasthenia and related problems. *Culture, Medicine and Psychiatry*, **13**(2), 131–138.

Zhang, M. Y. (1989). The diagnosis and phenomenology of neurasthenia: a Shanghai study. *Culture, Medicine and Psychiatry*, **13**(2), 147–161.

Zuckerman, M. (2003). Are there racial and ethnic differences in psychopathic personality? A critique of Lynn's (2000) racial and ethnic differences in psychopathic personality. *Personality and Individual Differences*, **35**(6), 1463–1469.

Developmental Aspects of Cultural Psychiatry

Joseph Westermeyer

Editors' Introduction

The development of psychiatry as a medical specialty and discipline has moved from the observational to the social and, in the last few decades, to an increased emphasis on genetic and gene–environmental interactions in the causation of psychiatric disorders. The emphasis on cultural psychiatry and impact of cultural factors on psychiatric disorders has varied between western Europe and the USA. In Europe, especially in Britain, the anthropologists often followed the colonial masters in observing the natives and their rituals in their natural habitat. These led to misconceptions about diagnosis and a management of psychiatric cases but, more importantly, it meant that the traditional ways of dealing with mentally ill individuals and mental illness were criticized, looked down upon and in some cases traditional manuals and texts even destroyed. The traditions, however, survived perhaps because of the oral tradition of history and information being passed on across generations.

In this chapter Westermeyer sets out the global context within which cultural psychiatry has emerged and started to make its presence felt. He observes that cultural psychiatry has many features in common with social psychiatry in that both relate to social institutions such as family, community and psychiatric institutions. There are distinctions between two types of psychiatry as well in that their focus is somewhat different. Illustrating the historical context by using migration as an example and the notions of racial and ethnic superiority/inferiority become more apparent. Current status of cultural psychiatry follows on from two different traditions – European and American. Westermeyer notes that differences between social psychiatry and cultural psychiatry persist in spite of attempts to use terms such as socio-cultural psychiatry. The use of different social units across the two specialties and the relative importance of nation state provide clear pointers in different directions in which the two specialties lead.

In the last few decades or so, cultural psychiatrists have become involved in providing services and directing service planning for migrant or minority ethnocultural groups. Cultural consultation and acting as cultural brokers have been important steps forward in making psychiatric services accessible. Westermeyer makes a strong case for psychiatry to move into international psychiatry away from national psychiatries. This has also to be seen in the context of globalization.

Introduction

Cultural psychiatry includes numerous subfields, some more theoretical in nature and others more practical in orientation. These areas range from early tomes on culture and psychoanalysis, such as *Totem and Taboo* (Freud, 1918), to latter-day research on the psychiatric genome (Bartels *et al.*, 2004) and ethnopsychopharmacology (Lin *et al.*, 1993). The following four précis exemplify valuable contributions to our understanding of psychiatric disorder and treatment achieved through cultural research.

Psychopathology across Cultures

Early investigators in cultural psychiatry described symptoms, signs, and course of disorder, noting similarities and differences across cultures. Emil Kraeplin began observing differences among hospitalized psychiatric patients in eastern and central Europe, later replicating these studies in Asian countries (Boroffka, 1990). Delusions, for example, show highly overlapping themes (e.g. persecutory, grandiose, nihilistic) and content (e.g. religious-spiritual, political, preternatural), but in distributions that vary greatly over time among differing cultures and in single cultures undergoing change (Westermeyer, 1988b). Later investigators, such as Tsung Y. Lin (Lin, 1989) and Alexander Leighton (Leighton, 1981), expanded this stratagem in the mid 1900s with their epidemiological studies of various disorders within and across populations. These studies revealed small differences in the prevalence of certain psychotic disorders, e.g. schizophrenia, bipolar I disorder, and extreme ranges from 0 to 10 per cent crude prevalence rates for some behavioural disorders, e.g. substance-use disorder, eating disorder (Westermeyer, 1988a). These descriptive and epidemiological approaches to the understanding of psychiatric disorder vis-à-vis culture continue to the present time, girded by use of psychiatric rating scales, scheduled psychiatric interviews, genomic and neuroimaging studies (Tseng, 2003). Concurrently, social scientists had shown interest in socio-cultural aspects of psychiatric topics, as exemplified by Emile Durkheim's study of social factors affecting suicide rates in France during the later 1800s (Durkheim, 1951).

Cultural Factors Preventing or Precipitating Psychiatric Disorder

Cultural psychiatrists assessed specific cultural features as pathogens. Examples included political extrusion of sub-groups as refugees (Fazel et al., 2005) and the influence of inflexible social roles or sex-related mores in generating psychopathology (Al-Issa, 1982). Studies of culture as resource emphasized the 'intimate social network' in fostering resilience (Speck and Attneave, 1974) and culturally prescribed family strategies for adaptive grieving and other coping (Knafl and Gilliss, 2002).

Cross-Cultural Psychiatric Care

After 1950, increased travel resulted in psychiatrists from one culture rendering care to patients from other cultures. International travellers included refugees, foreign students, tourists, foreign 'guest workers', and others (Westermeyer, 1989b). Over recent years, more ethnic minorities and remote rural dwellers have relocated to urban areas. The clinical imperatives stemming from these novel migrations have greatly stimulated practical aspects of cross-cultural psychiatry. Areas of enhanced knowledge and skill have included the role of the translator in psychiatric evaluation (Westermeyer, 1990), the psychiatrist's cultural norms and their potential influence on diagnosis (Comas-Diaz and Jacobsen, 1991), clinical presentations or syndromes influenced by culture (Abbey and Garfinkel, 1991), reliability of cross-cultural diagnoses (Westermeyer

and Sines, 1979), and applicability of psychometrics across languages and cultures (Wittchen et al., 1991). Since many patients in cross-cultural contexts are fleeing war and/or political oppression, assessment and care of trauma-related disorders has become a prominent feature in much cross-cultural care (Jaranson et al., 2004; Hollifield et al., 2006).

Ethnopsychiatry: Care in Cultural Context

Ethnopsychiatry studies have examined systems of care, ranging from efficacy to inequalities of care (Gaines, 1992). Analyses have addressed outcomes in the professional mainstream, e.g. hospitals and clinics (Collins et al., 1992), and in other assorted settings, e.g. over-the-counter sales, indigenous or folk healing and acculturation therapy (Szapocznik et al., 1986). Patient-centred surveys have encompassed access to care and patient satisfaction. On the micro-level, the role of ritual and ceremony in treatment and healing has been assessed (Johnson et al., 1995). One clinician evaluated Native American perspectives towards their own recovery during treatment (Thompson, 1996).

Historical Origins of Social and Cultural Psychiatry

Social psychiatry and cultural psychiatry differ in the monocultural emphasis of the former and the bi- or multicultural emphasis of the latter. Contrasts in these two psychiatric fields suggest differing developmental trajectories, from their original founding, to current functions, and their future potentials. Nonetheless, social psychiatry possesses many features in common with cultural psychiatry (Gruenberg, 1983). For example, social psychiatry considers psychiatry as related to social institutions: the family, community, licensing bodies, economics, education, politics, law, and public health. Social psychiatrists may explore the socio-dynamics of psychiatric institutions, such as clinics, hospitals, research institutes, academic centres and professional guilds, as they can impact patient care beneficially or adversely. Social research goals may encompass deeper understanding of special groups of patients (e.g. students, military units, factory workers), social circumstances affecting patients (e.g. disasters, racism), social therapies (e.g. family, group, milieu, industrial, recreational), and social consequences of psychiatric disorder (Blendon et al., 1995; Mollica et al., 2002).

Social and cultural psychiatry may seem nearly indistinguishable at first glance, since both fields concern groups of people vis-à-vis psychiatric disorder and treatment. However, they have been separate fields with relatively limited overlap or interaction – a paradox made comprehensible by realizing their differing historical origins and evolutions. Social psychiatry first appears in the efforts of Pare, Rush and others to deliver humanistic care to institutionalized psychiatric patients during the late 1700s and early 1800s (Farr, 1994). European renaissance-era psychiatric institutions had grown from ancient Greco-Roman spas and later medieval Arab–Islamic psychiatric asylums (in Bagdad, Cairo and elsewhere), which utilized rest, quiet, baths and massage to restore mental well-being (Okasha, 2001). As urban populations grew and responsibility for the mentally ill became unclear, psychiatric institutions came to resemble prisons more than hospitals. These efforts in western Europe and North America to restore humanistic asylum arose in a particular socio-philosophical setting. Individual rights and the dignity of the individual, in the vanguard of social thinking, were extended to the care of those with psychiatric disorder, including alcohol and drug disorders. At this early stage of social psychiatry development, a cultural psychiatry cannot yet be discerned.

Later in the 1800s, research by the first social scientists presaged work by social psychiatrists in the early 1900s. Social concerns with child raising, working conditions, social equity, and social influences in ameliorating or exacerbating psychiatric disorder began in this era. During this period, Kraeplin, Freud, Roheim and other psychiatrists first began considering the effects of cultural influences on psychiatric disorder (Freud, 1918; Roheim, 1926). By mid-century, innovators in cultural psychiatry were working around the globe, e.g. Morris Carstairs (Britain), Frantz Fanon (Caribbean–France–Algeria), T. Y. Lin (Taiwan), H. B. M. Murphy (Canada), T. A. Lambo (Nigeria), C. A. Sequin (Peru), Eric Wittkower (Canada) and P. M. Yap (Hong Kong). Their early contributions addressed topics still current in the field: i.e. substance use across ethnic groups, folk healers vis-a-vis university-trained physicians, epidemiology, culture-bound or culture-related syndromes, colonial-racist impacts on clinical phenomena, and migration as stressor/pathogen.

Early on, cultural psychiatrists began to employ novel research methods. For example, psychiatric epidemiologists Odegaard and Malzberg compared the prevalence of various psychiatric disorders across ethnic and migrating groups during the 1930s and 1940s (Odegaard, 1932; Malzberg, 1940). Unlike the wholly qualitative descriptions of the earlier generation, they employed methods that were inductive and quantitative, as well as qualitative. Their studies, replicable and liable to statistical analysis, marked a shift from descriptive or philosophical treatises to scientific enterprises.

By the mid twentieth century another genera of cultural psychiatrists emerged. This group had training in both psychiatry and one of the social sciences (e.g. anthropology, sociology, epidemiology, economics, public health). Alexander Leighton, an early exemplar of a psychiatrist–anthropologist, worked in a US-established relocation camp for Japanese Americans during World War II (Leighton, 1981). He and colleagues Dorothea Leighton (Leighton and Leighton, 1941) and J. A. Lambo (Lambo, 1955), played seminal roles in the establishment of cultural psychiatry as an international field within psychiatry, as well as an academic field in universities.

During the 1970s the numbers of psychiatrists writing on cultural psychiatry topics increased geometrically. African psychiatrists, influenced by Lambo and other mentors, published work related to cultural changes occurring in Africa (Ifabumuyi and Rwegellera, 1979). Australian, British and Canadian psychiatrists studied groups at home and abroad, contributing important new methodologies while doing so (Krupinski et al., 1973; Wintrob, 1973; Leff, 1974). Many Americans from minority ethnic or immigrant groups undertook work rooted in their extensive cross-cultural clinical experiences (Wintrob and Diamen, 1974; Gaviria and Wintrob, 1975; Spiegel, 1976; Favazza and Oman, 1978). A few Europeans examined psychiatric changes occurring over time within their own cultures (Steinbrunner and Scharfetter, 1976). Importantly, the Mental Health Division of the World Health Organization led large, definitive studies with both practical and theoretical implications (Sartorius et al., 1978). By 1980 an international cultural psychiatry was well established. Several journals supported this progress, some of them devoted only to cultural psychiatry (i.e. *Transcultural Psychiatric Research Reviews*; *Culture, Medicine, and Psychiatry*) and others covering the field more broadly but publishing cultural articles of general interest (i.e. *British Journal of Psychiatry*,

Indian Medical Journal, Journal of Nervous and Mental Disease) symbolized the coming-of-age for the field.

Early Social Psychiatry Developments and their Effects on Cultural Psychiatry

Child Psychiatry

An early clinical endeavour in social psychiatry was the development of child-study/child-care centres in the 1920s, based on the notion that early care might prevent subsequent psychiatric disorder. Several decades later cultural psychiatrists undertook studies of children from a cultural perspective. Many of these studies focused on refugee children and adolescents (Williams and Westermeyer, 1984; Ahearn and Athey 1991; Sack *et al.*, 1996; Savin *et al.*, 1996), thus paralleling the studies being undertaken among refugee adults. Additional work consisted of cross-cultural differences in the clinical assessment of children and their families (Tseng *et al.*, 1982), culture and the abuse of children (Berry-Caban and Brue, 1999), and possible cross-generational effects of war and genocide (Leon *et al.*, 1981).

Refugees and Other Traumatized Populations

During the post-World War II era, many African, Asian, Latin American and European countries assigned social psychiatry a principal role in developing health services (Mohan, 1973; Bhugra and Till, 2013), at a time when individual-focused, psychoanalytic thinking dominated North American mental health services (Romano, 1995). Many psychiatrists who developed social psychiatry were suckled on the social chaos of World War II. They learned first-hand the power of social disorganization to undermine human communities with their fragile veneer of civilization. They also learned the value of social institutions to protect, organize and give meaning to human existence. The brightest and ablest of them turned these war-wrought lessons to the care of the psychiatric casualties – those whose lives, families and communities were being undermined by the wartime trauma and psychosocial epidemics following World War II (Pedersen, 1949; Cameron, 1968; Wyman, 1989).

Social psychiatry in Europe began in a context of want and reconstruction, but reached fruition in a milieu of relative wealth. This broad-based effort grew from new modes of psychiatric care and rehabilitation springing from numerous sources. One survivor–innovator, psychiatrist Vladimir Houdolin, identified the growing problem of alcoholism and developed detoxification facilities and employee-assistance programmes (Savelli and Marks, 2015). Ambrose Uchtenhagen, discerning the drug abuse epidemic among the 'lost youth' of modern Europe, established creative therapeutic communes, industrial rehabilitation, heroin maintenance and methadone maintenance in rural settings (Angst, 1999). Norman Sartorius led World Health Organization efforts in developing an international psychiatry founded on rational planning and scientific understanding (Sartorius and Janca, 1996). These and other social psychiatry leaders developed new psychiatric theories and institutions to meet modern demands. As evidence for this new field, the *International Journal of Social Psychiatry* appeared. Several chairs of social psychiatry were appointed in Europe, Asia and Latin America. National societies for the advancement of social psychiatry appeared, subsequently leading to the International Society of Social Psychiatry.

Early Lessons in Cultural Psychiatry

The Experiences with Immigration

In the mid 1800s, during a period of heavy immigration, American psychiatrists observed that immigrants had higher-than-expected prevalence of disabling mental conditions (Malzberg, 1930). Originally focused on immigrants themselves, further investigations revealed that several European countries (England and Germany in particular) were sending criminals, debtors, unemployed persons and institutional inmates to the United States at public expense. As an outgrowth of these studies, immigration procedures to screen immigrants disabled by mental disorder were established. International agreements were negotiated, so that disabled persons might be returned to their communities of origin at the expense of shipping companies and the countries of emigration. These early treaties did much to solve the social–financial crisis presented by disabled immigrants – an expense greater than public education in several American states. Regrettably, these experiences also begat theories purporting to 'prove' the inherent superiority – or inferiority – of specific national or ethnic groups. The political corollaries of these theories were writ large in the subsequent European Holocaust of the 1940s (Nadler and Ben-Slushan, 1989).

To test notions of migration, culture and psychopathology scientifically, the Norwegian psychiatrist Odegaard conducted a milestone hospital-based epidemiological study of emigrant Norwegians to Minnesota in the United States, comparing them to Norwegians who remained at home and to native-born Norwegian Americans (Odegaard, 1932). Tsung Y. Lin later extended Odegaard's findings in the first field-based epidemiology of psychiatric disorder, comparing Han Chinese immigrants with the aboriginal peoples of Taiwan. Alexander Leighton's efforts to embed cultural psychiatry in academia further advanced the field (Leighton 1981). These and similar endeavors from 1930 to 1950 provided a solid foundation for the work of cultural psychiatrists in the latter half of the twentieth century.

Confluence of Need and Expertise

Following World War II, cultural psychiatry studies began pouring out of nations with significant immigrant populations. These included especially Australia (Krupinski, 1967), Canada (Tyhurst, 1977), and the United Kingdom (Cox, 1976). In Norway, Eitinger (himself a refugee from Nazi prison camps) led an effort to study the most traumatized of refugees accepted by that country (Eitinger, 1961). H. B. M. Murphy and his European colleagues – working in Switzerland, France and other European countries under the auspices of the United Nations – were early contributors to the cross-cultural care and resettlement of refugees (Murphy, 1955). The principles of European social psychiatry current at the time demanded that all persons have access to psychiatric services, regardless of wealth or ethnicity. This strategy required that each clinician work efficiently and effectively with scores, if not hundreds of ethnic peoples whose life ways flowed outside the societal mainstream. In order to treat psychiatric disorders among minorities and refugees (not previously done in any concerted fashion), clinicians had to acquire additional knowledge, skill, attitudes and experience.

Later waves of refugees from the anti-Communist uprisings in 1950s eastern Europe produced additional important findings from Canada emphasizing the pathways from pre-migration to acute presentation (Mezey, 1969; Tyhurst, 1977). The flood of Southeast Asian refugees throughout the world

likewise contributed new concepts, understanding, and methods to cultural psychiatry (Kinzie *et al.*, 1982; Beiser and Fleming, 1986; Westermeyer, 1989a; Mollica *et al.*, 1990; Hauff and Vaglum, 1994). The diaspora from African nations in recent years has further challenged the field (Jaranson *et al.*, 2004).

In the 1960s and 1970s a new generation of cultural psychiatrists became interested in treatment – a departure from earlier psychiatrists interested more in epidemiology, diagnostic categories and clinical assessment methods. Scores of psychiatrists joined in this effort. Among the earliest was John Spiegel, who underscored the relevance of cultural transference and counter-transference for cross-cultural psychiatric assessment, mutual trust and clinical care (Spiegel, 1976).

Seminal studies on cultural psychiatry topics were accepted in such psychiatric journals as *Acta Psychiatrica Scandinavica, British Journal of Psychiatry, Journal of Nervous and Mental Disease, Medical Anthropology, Culture, Medicine and Psychiatry, Psychological Anthropology, Transcultural Psychiatry* and *World Psychiatry*. The Society for the Study of Psychiatry and Culture (SSPC), organized in the 1970s, has an annual meeting and newsletter. Currently, several hundred African, Asian, Australian, European and American psychiatrists identify themselves as cultural psychiatrists, with a like number of anthropologists, epidemiologists, sociologists and social psychologists working on topics relevant to cultural psychiatry.

Social and Cultural Psychiatry: An Analysis of Similarities and Differences

As noted earlier, cultural and social psychiatry come from different origins, both in terms of original purposes, differing social and cultural contexts, and founding leaders. Further, they have remained largely separate entities. In view of historical differences, the failure of the integrative term *socio-cultural psychiatry* to gain wide acceptance can be understood – despite its occurrence in published articles (Coombs and Globetti, 1986; Westermeyer, 1992). Each subfield tends to emphasize a different social unit. Social psychiatry has focused on social institutions and psychiatric patients. In contrast, cultural psychiatry has focused on the psychology of the patient and the clinician as culturally derived or influenced, and the assessment and care of patients from cultural backgrounds notably different from those of their clinicians. Another difference is the relative importance of the nation state. From the standpoint of social psychiatry, the nation state is the 'universe' of interest. Viewed from cultural psychiatry, any one nation state is simply a single case study among many case studies. Given this difference in orientation, cultural psychiatrists might perceive social psychiatrists as ethnocentric. On the contrary, social psychiatrists might view cultural psychiatrists as overly relativistic. This separation of social and cultural psychiatrists contrasts with the tight union of biological psychiatrists, who share journals and annual meetings despite their roots in highly diverse anatomical, biochemical, embryological, genetic, histological, physiological, neuro-imaging, neuro-psychological, psychopharmacological and other biological sciences. Despite their differences, social and cultural psychiatry have benefitted each other in numerous ways. In the opening sections, we have considered ways in which social psychiatry has fostered cultural psychiatry. In the next section, we will review contributions of cultural psychiatry to social psychiatry.

Contributions of Cultural Psychiatry to Social Psychiatry

Cultural psychiatry has made its greatest contribution to social psychiatry in those settings in which a large number of culturally or ethnically diverse patients seek psychiatric services. One contribution has been the development of methods to assess psychopathology across cultures and languages. This contribution has been relevant for those social psychiatric programmes and clinics serving foreign students, immigrants, refugees and guest workers. These methods, useful both clinically and for research purposes, have included the following:

- translation of rating scales and psychometric instruments from one language/culture to another language/culture;
- selection, training and collaboration with psychiatric interpreters;
- pathoplasticity (and lack thereof) in various psychiatric conditions;
- rates of psychopathology among different migrating groups;

- syndromes common to certain cultures;
- use of the anthropological literature or cultural consultants in assessing a patient's world view, cognition and behaviour.

Cultural psychiatry has also contributed to the cross-cultural treatment of psychiatric patients from cultures not familiar to the clinician. These contributions have consisted of the following:

- the role of cultural transference and countertransference in facilitating and/or impeding the clinician–patient relationship;
- common features of psychotherapy apt to be beneficial across cultural and ethnic boundaries;
- bio-ethnic similarities and differences in pharmacodynamics and pharmacokinetics of psychotropic agents.

Increased understanding of migration and psychopathology has revealed increased rates of virtually all psychiatric disorders, including pathogenic social problems such as divorce and juvenile delinquency. An excess of certain conditions among migrants has been well known, such as depressive symptoms, paranoid symptoms, *folie à deux/famille/milieu* syndromes and psychosomatic symptoms. Back-migration into labour-exporting populations (e.g. Ireland, Bavaria, Mexico and the Caribbean) has been associated with concentration of psychopathology into those groups who contribute guest workers or migratory workers to other countries and regions. Onset of psychopathology in relation to duration since relocation has shown tendencies for depression to occur early, alcoholism and drug addictions to occur later, and schizophrenia to occur independent of time since migration (Westermeyer, 1989b).

Cultural psychiatry has revealed rates of psychiatric disorder that can be extraordinarily high. For example, lifetime prevalence rates of schizophrenia or bipolar disorder have not exceeded a percentage or two of most populations, unless one lives in a society that exports workers to other areas, as have Martha's Vineyard, Bavaria, the Caribbean, Ireland and Mexico (Westermeyer, 1989b). Depressive disorders and anxiety disorders often soar following natural disasters or prolonged civil disturbance. Social phobia has been prevalent among ethnic minorities who are economically disadvantaged relative to those living around them (Regier *et al.*, 1984). Alcohol and drug use disorders can increase to levels that seriously undermine the social fabric binding an entire people.

For example, lifetime adults-only alcohol use disorder prevalence among some Native Americans has reached 20–25 per cent (Boehnlein *et al.*, 1993). Lifetime adults-only prevalence of opium addiction among certain Asian poppy farmers has ranged from 16 to 24 per cent (Westermeyer, 1982). These lifetime prevalence rates are consistent with estimated lifetime risk among males of 40 to 60 per cent and among females of 20 to 25 per cent due to premature mortality lowering the lifetime prevalence rate observed in survivors. Such findings can guide social psychiatrists in planning for preventive and clinical services.

For several decades, national and international agencies have charged cultural psychiatrists with delivering services. Such circumstances have occurred during development of psychiatric services for minority groups and relief of fleeing or resettled refugees. Cultural psychiatrists have served in the following capacities:

- consulting to local professionals, clinics, hospitals and programmes not familiar with assessment and treatment of foreign-born or minority ethnic groups;
- training foreign-born or minority persons to serve as psychiatric interpreters;
- staffing outpatient clinics, day programmes or inpatient units;
- establishing services for torture victims, post-traumatic disorders, solo parents, delayed or missed grief, and 'acculturation therapy' for those failing to acculturate.

An International Psychiatry

The separate existence of an entire national psychiatric classification system in one country (e.g., the *Diagnostic and Statistical Manual*, or DSM, in the United States) and a number of national psychiatric categories in the International Classification of Disease or ICD verifies that psychiatry still operates in the era of 'national psychiatries'. For more than a century, surgery, medicine and paediatrics have functioned as international clinical and scientific fields. Unless we can have one international diagnostic schema, we remain a less-than-equal partner within medicine. Progress in the field will be stymied by conceptual differences, communication gaps and the inability to apply research findings universally.

Despite problems, cross-cultural diagnostic understanding is growing. Agreement between the ICD and DSM systems has occurred at times, and diagnostic rapprochement has limited the national syndromes listed in recent ICDs. In collaboration with social, biological and other psychiatric experts, cultural psychiatrists are contributing to improved understanding of disorders across cultures.

Controlled Studies across Nation States

Collaboration among nation states may potentially aid our knowledge of psychiatric policy and programmes – areas in which tradition, local laws and management idiosyncrasies can impede scientific progress. As countries or provinces/states utilize similar and diverse interventions, the consequences of their decisions can be assessed and compared. The expansion of methadone maintenance of opioid dependence in several countries over the last few decades comprises an example. Such studies require comparable sampling and data collection – tasks for which the World Health Organization is well suited. Although difficult, it might even be feasible to conduct crossover studies among countries. For example, countries 1 to 5 might apply intervention X, while countries 6 to 10 might use intervention Y. After assessing the effects of these interventions, the countries might then switch interventions, with countries 1 to 5 using intervention Y and countries 6 to 10 using intervention X. Although complex international efforts seem beyond achievement, in fact such collaboration has already occurred in the study of nosocomial infection on 1417 intensive care units in 14 European countries (Vincent *et al.*, 1995). If such international collaboration is feasible for nosocomial infections, collaboration should also be feasible for more common problems with greater mortality, morbidity and economic cost such as depression, schizophrenia and substance use disorders.

Statecraft Regarding Psychiatric Disorders

Statecraft – the art and science of conducting state affairs – in relation to substance use disorders, pathological gambling, eating disorder, and other behavioural and psychiatric conditions remains at a rudimentary level in most countries (Westermeyer, 1999). On the contrary, statecraft is fairly sophisticated in areas related to road building, international commerce, and maternal–child healthcare. In the absence of an international statecraft vis-à-vis these disorders, each society must learn largely through its own mistakes and occasional blind luck. Attention to history and cross-national comparisons can reduce repetition of the same costly mistakes.

In the alcoholism field, principles of statecraft have been evolving over centuries for alcohol disorder control (Popham *et al.*, 1976; Pardes, 1975) continuing down to the present time. One of the earliest efforts was the containment of the Gin Epidemic in England during the 1600s and 1700s (Rodin, 1981). Effective interventions have included legislation on alcohol production, importation, taxation, hours and locations of off/on premises sale, age limitations and drinking under certain conditions, such as driving and working. Legislation requiring establishment and funding of prevention, early intervention and treatment–rehabilitation have shown positive results. Several countries have decreased alcohol-related problems (especially in middle-aged men) after several decades of trial and error, learning hard-won lessons that could be replicated in other countries. Even in countries having notable success in reducing alcohol problems overall, alcohol problems among women and young males have either not improved or become worse, indicating the need for further international cooperation with age- and gender-specific efforts.

Statecraft in the drug addiction field began with the efforts of several oriental nations trying to contain tobacco and opium dependence in the 1600s. Despite its centuries-old history in Asia (Terry and Pellens, 1928; Tamura, 1989), drug addiction statecraft remains at an early developmental stage in most of the world, as evidenced by dramatic shifts in drug-control policies and preventive approaches (Westermeyer, 1976). For example, the pharmacology and epidemiology of various drug use problems showed little or no relationship to drug policies in 12 countries of Europe (Reubank, 1995); instead, findings suggested that informal social controls and socio-cultural attitudes were more important in determining drug addiction prevalence than was official government policy. The need for international cooperation in this area grows ever more critical as many countries open their national boundaries, possess greater disposable income and permit easier access to addictive substances – factors that favour drug addiction epidemics (Gerevic and Bacskai, 1995).

References

Abbey, S. E. and Garfinkel, P. E. (1991). Neurasthenia and chronic fatigue syndromes: the role of culture in making a diagnosis. *American Journal Psychiatry*, **148**(12), 1628–1646.

Ahearn, F. L. and Athey, J. L. (eds) (1991). *Refugee Children: Theory, Research, and Services*. Baltimore, MD: Johns Hopkins University Press.

Al-Issa, I. (1982). Does culture make a difference in psychopathology? In *Culture and Psychopathology*, ed. I. Al-Issa. Baltimore: University Park Press, pp. 3–29.

Angst, J. (1999). Laudatio Ambros Uchtenhagen. *European Addiction Research*, **5**(2), 97–101.

Bartels, M., Boomsma, D. I., Hudziak, J. J. *et al.* (2004). Disentangling genetic, environmental, and rater effects on internalizing and externalizing problem behavior in 10-year-old twins. *Twin Research*, **7**(2), 162–175.

Beiser, M. and Fleming, J. A. E. (1986). Measuring psychiatric disorder among Southeast Asian refugees. *Psychological Medicine*, **16**, 627–639.

Berry-Caban, C. S. and Brue, K. C. (1999). Child abuse and neglect among Central Americans: the role of social violence. *Psychline*, **3**(1), 26–31.

Bhugra, D. and Till, A. (2013). Public mental health is about social psychiatry. *International Journal of Social Psychiatry*, **59**(2), 105–106.

Blendon, R. J., Scheck, A. C., Donelan, K. *et al.* (1995). How white and African Americans view their health and social problems: different experiences, different expectations. *Journal of the American Medical Association*, **273**(4), 341–346.

Boehnlein, J. K., Kinzie, J. D., Leung, P. K. *et al.* (1993). The natural history of medical and psychiatric disorder in an American Indian community. *Culture, Medicine and Psychiatry*, **16**, 543–554.

Boroffka, A. (1990). Emil Kraeplin (1856–1926). *Transcultural Psychiatric Research Review*, **27**, 228–237.

Cameron, D. C. (1968). Youth and drugs: a world view. *Journal of the American Medical Association*, **206**, 1267–1271.

Collins, D., Dimsdale, J. and Wilkins, D. (1992). Consultation/liaison psychiatry utilization patterns in different cultural groups. *Psychosomatic Medicine*, **54**, 240–245.

Comas-Diaz, L. and Jacobsen, F. M. (1991). Ethno-cultural transference and countertransference in the therapeutic dyad. *Journal Orthopsychiatry*, **61**(3), 392–402.

Coombs, D. W. and Globetti, G. (1986). Alcohol use and alcoholism in Latin America: changing patterns and sociocultural explanations. *International Journal of Addictions*, **21**, 59–81.

Cox, J. L. (1976). Psychiatric assessment of the immigrant patient. *British Journal Hospital Medicine*, **16**, 38–40.

Durkheim, E. (1951). *Le Suicide (1897) [Suicide: A Study in Sociology]*. New York, The Free Press.

Eitinger, L. (1961). Pathology of the concentration camp syndrome. *Archives General Psychiatry*, **5**, 79–87.

Farr, C. B. (1994). Benjamin Rush and American psychiatry. *American Journal of Psychiatry*, **151**(Suppl. 6), 65–73.

Favazza, A. and Oman, N. (1978). Foundations of cultural psychiatry. *American Journal of Psychiatry*, **135**, 293–303.

Fazel, M., Wheeler, J. and Danesh, J. (2005). Prevalence of serious mental disorder in 7000 refugees resettled in Western countries: a systematic review. *The Lancet*, **365**, 1309–1314.

Freud, S. (1918). *Totem and Taboo*. New York, Dodd Mean.

Gaines, A. D. (1992). *Ethnopsychiatry: The Cultural Construction of Professional and Folk Psychiatries*. New York, State University of New York Press.

Gaviria, M. and Wintrob, R. M. (1975). The foreign medical graduate who returns home after postgraduate training in the USA: a Peruvian case study. *Journal of Medical Education*, **50**, 167–175.

Gerevic, J. and Bacskai, E. (1995). Drug problems and drug policy: a Hungarian point of view. *European Addiction Research*, **1**, 50–60.

Gruenberg, E. (1983). The origins and directions of social psychiatry: commentary. *Integrative Psychiatry*, **1**, 93–94.

Hauff, E. and Vaglum, P. (1994). Chronic posttraumatic stress disorder in Vietnamese refugees: a prospective community study of prevalence, course, psychopathology, and stressors. *Journal of Nervous and Mental Disease*, **182**(2), 85–90.

Hollifield, M., Jenkins, J., Lian, N. *et al.* (2006). Assessing war trauma in refugees: properties of the Comprehensive Trauma Inventory – 104 (CTI-104). *Journal Traumatic Stress*, **19**(4), 527–540.

Ifabumuyi, O. I. and Rwegellera, G. G. (1979). Koro in Nigerian male patients: a case report. *African Journal of Psychiatry*, **5**, 103–105.

Jaranson, J. M., Butcher, J. N, Halcon, L. *et al.* (2004). Somali and Oromo refugees: correlates of torture and trauma. *American Journal of Public Health*, **94**(4), 591–598.

Johnson, D. R., Feldman, S. C., Lubin, H. and Southwick, S. M. (1995). The therapeutic use of ritual and ceremony in the treatment of post-traumatic stress disorder. *Journal of Traumatic Stress*, **8**(2), 283–298.

Kinzie, J. D., Manson, S. M., Vinh, D. T. *et al.* (1982). Development and validation of a Vietnamese language depression rating scale. *American Journal of Psychiatry*, **139**(10), 1276–1281.

Knafl, K. and Gilliss, C. (2002). How families managed chronic conditions: an analysis of the concept of normalization. *Research in Nursing and Health*, **9**, 215–222.

Krupinski, J. (1967). Sociological aspects of mental ill-health in migrants. *Social Science and Medicine* **1**, 267–281.

Krupinski, J., Stoller, A. and Wallace, L. (1973). Psychiatric disorder in East European refugees now in Australia. *Social Science and Medicine*, **7**, 31–49.

Lambo, T. A. (1955). Role of cultural factors in paranoid psychosis among the Yoruba tribe. *The Journal of Mental Science*, **101**, 239–266.

Leff, J. P. (1974). Transcultural influences on psychiatrists' rating of verbally expressed emotion. *British Journal of Psychiatry*, **125**, 336–340.

Leighton, A. (1981). Culture and psychiatry. *Canadian Journal of Psychiatry*, **26**, 522–529.

Leighton, A. H. and Leighton, D. C. (1941). Elements of psychotherapy in Navaho religion. *Psychiatry*, **4**, 515–523.

Leon, G. R., Butcher, J. N., Kleinman, M., Goldberg, A. and Almagor, M. (1981). Survivors of the Holocaust and their children: current status and adjustment. *Journal of Personality and Social Psychology*, **41**(3), 503–516.

Lin, K. M., Poland, R. E. and Nakasaki, G. (eds)(1993). *Psychopharmacology and Psychobiology of Ethnicity*. Washington, DC: American Psychiatric Press, Inc.

Lin, T. Y. (1989). Neurasthenia in Asian cultures. *Culture, Medicine and Psychiatry*, **13**, 105–241.

Malzberg, B. (1930). Mental disease and the 'melting pot'. *Journal of Nervous and Mental Disease*, **72**, 379–395.

Malzberg, B. (1940). *Social and Biological Aspects of Mental Disease*. Utica, NY: New York State Hospital Press.

Mezey, A. G. (1969). Personal background, emigration and mental disorder in Hungarian refugees. *Journal of Mental Science*, **106**, 618–627.

Mohan, B. (1973). *Social Psychiatry in India*. Calcutta: Minerva.

Mollica, R. E., Cui, X., McInnes, K. and Massagli, M. P. (2002). Science-based policy for psychosocial interventions in refugee camps: a Cambodian example. *Journal of Nervous and Mental Disease*, **190**, 158–166.

Mollica, R. F., Wyshak, G., Lavelle, J., Truong, T., Tor, S. and Yang, T. (1990). Assessing symptom change in Southeast Asian refugee survivors of mass violence and torture. *American Journal of Psychiatry*, **147**(1), 83–88.

Murphy, H. B. M. (ed.) (1955). *Flight and Resettlement*. Paris: UNESCO.

Nadler, A. and Ben-Slushan, D. (1989). Forty years later: long-term consequences of massive traumatization as manifested by holocaust survivors from the city and the kibbutz. *Journal of Consulting and Clinical Psychology*, **57**, 287–293.

Odegaard, O. (1932). Emigration and insanity: a study of mental disease among the Norwegian born population of Minnesota. *Acta Psychiatrica et Neurologica Scandinavica*, **4**(Supplement), 1–206.

Okasha, A. (2001). Mental health and psychiatry in the Middle East: historical development. *Eastern Mediterranean Health Journal*, **7**, 336–347.

Pardes, A. (1975). Social control of drinking among the Aztec Indians of Mexoamerica. *Journal of Studies on Alcohol and Drugs*, **36**, 1139–1153.

Pedersen, S. (1949). Psychopathological reactions to extreme social displacements (refugee neurosis). *Psychoanalysis Review*, **36**, 344–354.

Popham, R. E., Schmidt, W. and de Lint, J. (1976). The effects of legal restraint on drinking. *The Biology of Alcoholism*, vol. 4: *Social Aspects of Alcoholism*, ed. B. Kissin and H. Begleiter. New York, Plenum Press, pp. 579–625.

Regier, D. A., Myers, J. K., Kramer, M. *et al.* (1984). The NIMH Epidemiological Catchment Area program. *Archives of General Psychiatry*, **411**, 934–941.

Reubank, K. H. (1995). Drug use and drug policy in western Europe. *European Addiction Research*, **1**, 32–34.

Rodin, A. E. (1981). Infants and gin mania in 18th century London. *Journal of the American Medical Association*, **245**, 1237–1239.

Roheim, G. (1926). The scapegoat. *Psychoanalytic Review* **13**, 235–236.

Romano, J. (1995). Reminiscences: 1938 and since. *American Journal of Psychiatry*, **151**(Suppl. 6), 83–89.

Sack, W. H., Clarke, G. N. and Seeley, J. (1996). Multiple forms of stress in Cambodian adolescent refugees. *Child Development*, **67**, 107–116.

Sartorius, N. and Janca, A. (1996). Psychiatric assessment instruments developed by the World Health Organization. *Social Psychiatry and Psychiatric Epidemiology*, **31**, 55–69.

Sartorius, N., Jablensky, A. and Schapiro, R. (1978). Cross cultural differences in the short-term prognosis of schizophrenic psychosis. *Schizophrenia Bulletin*, **4**, 102–113.

Savelli, M. and Marks, S. (eds) (2015). *Psychiatry in Communist Europe: Mental Health in Historical Perspective*. Basingstoke, England: Palgrave Macmillan.

Savin, D., Sack, W. H., Clarke, G. N., Meas, N. and Richart, J. (1996). The Khmer adolescent project: III. A study of trauma from Thailand's site II refugee camp. *Journal of the American Academy of Child and Adolescent Psychiatry*, **35**, 384–391.

Speck, R. W. and Attneave, C. (1974). *Family Networks*. New York: Vintage Books.

Spiegel, J. P. (1976). Cultural aspects of transference and countertransference revisited. *Journal of the American Academy of Psychoanalysis*, **4**, 447–467.

Steinbrunner, S. and Scharfetter, C. (1976). Changes in delusional psychoses: a historical transcultural comparison. *Archiv Psychiatrie Nervenkrankeheitan*, **222**, 47–60.

Szapocznik, J., Santisteban, D., Rio, A., Perez-Vidal, A., Kurtines, W. and Hervis, O. (1986). Bicultural Effectivenss Training (BET): an intervention modality for families experiencing intergenerational/intercultural conflict. *Hispanic Journal of Behaviour Sciences*, **8**, 303–330.

Tamura, J. (1989). Japan: stimulant epidemics past and present. *UN Bulletin on Narcotics*, **41**, 81–93.

Terry, C. E. and Pellens, M. (1928). *The Opium Problem*. Montclair, NJ: Patterson Smith.

Thompson, J. W. (1996). Native American perspectives. In *Culture and Psychiatric Diagnosis: A DSM-IV Perspective* ed. J. E. Mezzich, A. Kleinman, H. Fabrega and D. Parron. Washington, DC: American Psychiatric Press, Inc., pp. 31–33.

Tseng, W., McDermott, J. and Ogino, K. (1982). Cross cultural differences in parent–child assessment: USA and Japan. *International Journal of Social Psychiatry*, **28**, 305–317.

Tseng, W. S. (2003). *Clinician's Guide to Cultural Psychiatry*. San Diego: Elsevier.

Tyhurst, L. (1977). Psychosocial first aid for refugees. *Mental Health and Society*, **4**, 319–343.

Vincent, J. L., Bihari, D. H., Suter, P. M., Bruining, H. A. and White, J. (1995). The prevalence of nosocomial infection in intensive care units in Europe. *Journal of the American Medical Association*, **274**(8), 639–644.

Westermeyer, J. (1976). The pro-heroin effects of anti-opium laws in Asia. *Archives of General Psychiatry*, **33**(9), 1135–1139.

Westermeyer, J. (1982). *Poppies, Pipes and People*. Los Angeles: University of California Press.

Westermeyer, J. (1988a). National differences in psychiatric morbidity: methodological issues, scientific interpretations and social implications. *Acta Psychiatrica Scandinavica*, **78**(Supplement 344), 23–31.

Westermeyer, J. (1988b). Some cross cultural aspects of delusions. In *Delusional Beliefs*, ed. T. F. Oltmanns and B. A. Maher. New York: Wiley Interscience, pp. 212–229.

Westermeyer, J. (1989a). *Mental Health for Refugees and Other Migrants: Social and Preventative Approaches*. Springfield, IL: Chas. Thomas.

Westermeyer, J. (1989b). *The Psychiatric Care of Migrants: A Clinical Guide*. Washington, DC: American Psychiatry Press, Inc.

Westermeyer, J. (1990). Working with an interpreter in psychiatric assessment and treatment. *Journal of Nervous and Mental Disease*, **178**, 745–749.

Westermeyer, J. (1992). The sociocultural environment in the genesis and amelioration of opium dependence. In *Anthropological Research: Process and Application*, ed. J. Poggie, B. DeWalt, W. Dressler. New York, State University of New York Press, pp. 115–132.

Westermeyer, J. (1999). Addiction, community and the state: a review. *American Journal of Addictions*, **8**, 279–287.

Westermeyer, J. and Sines, L. (1979). Reliability of cross-cultural psychiatric diagnosis with an assessment of two rating contexts. *Journal of Psychiatric Research*, **15**(3), 199–213.

Williams, C. and Westermeyer, J. (1984). Psychiatric problems among adolescent Southeast Asian refugees: a descriptive study. *Journal of Nervous and Mental Disease*, **171**, 79–85.

Wintrob, R. M. (1973). Toward a model for effective mental health care in developing countries. *Psychopathologie Africaine*, **9**, 285–294.

Wintrob, R. M. and Diamen, S. (1974). The impact of cultural change on Mistassini Cree youth. *Canadian Psychiatric Association Journal*, **19**, 331–342.

Wittchen, H., Robins, L., Cottler, L., Sartorius, N., Burke, J. and Regier, D. (1991). Cross cultural feasibility, reliability and sources of variance of the Composite International Diagnostic Interview (CIDI). *British Journal of Psychiatry*, **159**, 645–653.

Wyman, M. (1989). *DPs: Europe's Displaced Persons, 1945–1951*. New York: Cornell University Press.

Explanatory Models in Psychiatry

Mitchell G. Weiss

Editors' Introduction

When a person falls ill or develops symptoms, they have an idea of what is wrong with them, what may have caused it and what is needed in order to get better and get functional. These models are strongly influenced by cultural values, educational and economic status, past experiences, age and many other factors. Weiss reminds us that over nearly four decades the illness explanatory model framework has been a valued resource for clinically applied medical anthropology, motivating consideration of culture in mainstream clinical practice and research in cultural psychiatry and other areas of medicine. This chapter examines the concept and its interdisciplinary underpinnings. The explanatory model framework developed from distinction between illness and disease. The former was what affected patients and what they saw as the problem, and the latter was the medical model. There is no doubt that in order to engage with and work jointly a common understanding about the explanatory model is indicated. This way, patients' needs and concerns can be met in a more holistic way. Furthermore the concept of emic and etic derived from linguistics allows researchers and clinicians alike to explore the patients' distress using emic (from within) instruments and understanding. Weiss reminds us that like the dichotomy of disease and illness, etic and emic orientations provide a fundamental technical distinction between professional (etic) explanatory models in psychiatry and mental health and personal (emic) ways of explaining experience and life in cultural worlds. The framework has been useful in community studies of mental health and other areas of public health. Research strategies attentive to emic explanatory models have a role to play for planning psychiatric services, reducing the treatment gap and advancing other interests on the agenda of global mental health. Questions about how emic explanatory models relate to complementary features of cultural identity, gender, stigma, risk, self-help, help-seeking and health services utilization remain

relevant. Kleinman's succinct guide to assessment continues to enable research, and various research instruments have also been developed based on mixed methods, qualitative and quantitative approaches (e.g. EMIC, SEMI, MINI, BEMI-C). As a fundamental principle guiding development of the Cultural Formulation Interview for DSM-5, the impact of the emic explanatory model framework on clinical training and practice is increasing. It has been firmly established in the lexicon of culture, health and illness.

Introduction

Over nearly four decades the illness explanatory model framework has been a valued resource for clinically applied medical anthropology, motivating consideration of culture in mainstream clinical practice and research in cultural psychiatry and other areas of medicine and public health. Working with explanatory models enables health professionals to evaluate clinical problems based on not only what they know about medical problems from their professional disciplinary training but also informed from the vantage points of patients and family caretakers who are directly affected. Applying anthropological principles to the process of clinical assessment also enhances empathy and contributes to a more effective therapeutic alliance.

This chapter examines the framework and its underpinnings, explaining how Kleinman's conceptualization of illness explanatory models relates to other kinds of *explanatory models* – same term but different meaning – that are also commonly used in psychiatry, medicine and in many other scientific disciplines that endeavour to explain topical interests of their field. An overview of the literature indicates the appeal of illness explanatory models for health professionals and social scientists. It also acknowledges limitations. We consider the various approaches and instruments that have been developed and used to study explanatory models of illness for research and in clinical practice.

Kleinman's Explanatory Models

The illness explanatory model framework was developed by Arthur Kleinman in the mid 1970s as a product of interdisciplinary activity in the fields of psychiatry, medicine and medical anthropology. In his extensive writing, Kleinman created a technical term that has been elaborated by him and others with reference to his original definition: 'Notions about an episode of sickness and its treatment that are employed by all those engaged in the clinical process' (Kleinman, 1980: 105). The scope of these notions was broad, encompassing illness experience, its meaning and treatment preferences. The definition made a point of distinguishing personal views of people who were directly concerned, not just professionals, and he distinguished a focus on specific episodes of illness both from general beliefs about illness and from scientific theories based on research and/or professional training. 'Such general beliefs belong to the health ideology of the different health care sectors' (Kleinman, 1980: 104).

Notwithstanding rootedness in broad ethnographic conceptual underpinnings, restricted interpretations have focused solely on perceived causes of illness (also termed causal attributions), thereby ignoring other aspects of illness experience, preferred treatment and relevant context. In that regard, both for better and for worse, the conceptualization in practice has been somewhat malleable and sometimes reshaped according to the interests and priorities of clinicians and researchers who work with it. Although a sharper focus may have operational advantages for pursuing some particular research aims, overly simplifying explanatory models and promoting expectations of a 'technical fix' may detract from, instead of enhance, culturally sensitive and empathic clinical interactions (Kleinman, 1981: 375).

Kleinman's formulation of illness explanatory models regarded them as neither singular nor static. Inasmuch as they were representations of personal experience, meaning, ideas and expectations, they were not expected to be fully coherent, logical or fixed. He contrasted essential characteristics of 'vagueness, multiplicity of meanings, frequent changes and lack of sharp boundaries between ideas and experience' with professional theories characterized by 'single

causal trains of scientific logic' (Kleinman, 1980). The field of psychiatry itself, however, is also notable for its multiplicity of theories (Eisenberg, 1977; Littlewood, 1990). Unlike professional theories, however, which are expected to be at least relatively coherent and stable for those who accept that theory, Kleinman's illness explanatory models of patients and their families permitted juxtaposition of logically challenged elements, and they were subject to change over time and in response to interventions, clinical course and life events. These points are well-recognized by researchers and clinicians who work with the framework. As Mathew and colleagues (2010) explain, 'Explanatory models of illness are often multiple, dynamic and change over time.'

At the outset, motivating interests in illness explanatory models were based on their value for culturally sensitive clinical practice in psychiatry (Kleinman, 1978a) and medicine (Kleinman *et al.*, 1978). It was also expected that the explanatory model framework would be applied to cultural studies of health systems (Kleinman, 1978b). As a framework for ethnomedical study, explanatory models were well-suited to explain the significance of different 'clinical realities' of practitioners and patients. Kleinman (1977b) asserted: 'There simply is no escaping the conceptions of sickness held by patients, communities, practitioners and researchers.' The approach appeared relevant at the time for developing ethnomedical models (Fabrega, 1975), distinguishing illness and disease (Eisenberg, 1977) and for elaborating semantics of illness (Good, 1977).

Conceptually, some adjustment of the clinical formulation is required to work with the framework in community studies. The focus on illness episodes that motivate help-seeking do not necessarily fit the priorities of community respondents, because they are not necessarily troubled by a current illness. Appropriate adjustments to the approach are required to make the community assessment relevant and manageable. Kleinman's earlier enthusiasm turned to scepticism. He felt that various efforts to simplify clinical assessment for clinicians had rendered the idea of explanatory models too simplistic for anthropological research. In his rethinking of the 'discourse between anthropology and medicine', Kleinman gave up on explanatory models as a relevant tool for ethnographic study, notwithstanding enduring confidence in their clinical value: 'Clinically, the explanatory model approach may continue to be useful, but ethnography has fortunately moved well beyond this early formulation' (Kleinman, 1995: 9). The literature reviewed later in this chapter, however, shows that with appropriate adjustment, tools and study designs, the explanatory model framework has remained useful in community studies of mental health and public health, if not ethnography.

Conceptual Underpinnings

The explanatory model framework took shape during a period notable for complementary interdisciplinary developments. Eisenberg (1977) elaborated the technical distinction of disease and illness, which has become a fundamental principle of clinically applied medical anthropology and cultural psychiatry. He argued that more attention was required for a new understanding of illness that better represented and enabled response to patients' priorities and needs. The emergence of George Engel's enhanced *biopsychosocial* medical model addressed similar concerns about an overly biomedical approach (Engel, 1977).

The emic and etic framework advanced by Kenneth Pike applied principles of linguistic anthropology to broader interests of cultural anthropology (Pike, 1967). Loosely referred to as insider and outsider perspectives for social analysis, the approach was controversial at the time (Headland *et al.*, 1990). Like the dichotomy of disease and illness, however, etic and emic orientations provide a fundamental technical distinction between professional (etic) explanatory models in psychiatry and mental health and personal (emic) ways of explaining experience and life in cultural worlds. Subsequently, the controversy faded, and the relevance of the emic designation has been widely acknowledged as an essential feature of the illness explanatory model framework (Weiss, 1997; Patel and Mann, 1997; Lloyd *et al.*, 1998).

One may also impute underpinnings of explanatory models deeply rooted in the field of psychiatry and traceable to essential features of the phenomenology proposed by Karl Jaspers in 1912. Broome (2002) implied that a complementary tension required consideration of 'the patients' symptoms in light of their world view'. Rudell and colleagues (2009) suggest comparable features of Kleinman's explanatory models and Leventhal's formulation of *illness representations* with reference to psychological self-regulatory theory accounting for the behavioural response to physical threats.

Emic Illness Explanatory Models and Etic Professional Models for Psychiatry and Mental Health

Although defined with reference to illness episodes for clinical utility, Kleinman's illness explanatory models are also commonly invoked for widely held theoretical orientations of communities, cultural groups and professionals. Anthropologists had previously referred to *explanatory models* before Kleinman appropriated these words as a technical term referring to illness episodes. For example, in a study of the Ashanti traditional medicine in Ghana and its relationship to psychiatry, Twumasi noted that 'the educated and the young tend to look down upon traditional explanatory models of illness' (Twumasi, 1972: 60). This anthropological interest in acknowledging various orientations, perspectives and ways of interpreting experience as a feature of cultural groups differs from the ways that other health professionals and scientists think about explanatory models. For them, an explanatory model is a statement of theory developed as a product of the work of science that endeavours to explain topical interests of a discipline.

In the field of psychiatry, interest in models of illness pre-dated both Kleinman's formulation of explanatory models and Eisenberg's distinction of disease and illness (Siegler and Osmond, 1966). When Kendler (2008) analysed 'explanatory models of psychiatric illness', he was not referring to emic views of non-professionals; he was considering professional psychiatric theories and how well they served the interests of psychiatric practice. Professional scientific explanatory models may be relatively more descriptive or predictive. Another common specialized denotation of the term refers to statistical explanatory models, which enable corrections for confounding and provide valid approaches to analyse data sets for both descriptive and predictive models (Katz, 2003). When scientists and health professionals refer to explanatory models resulting from their work, validity is based on scientific research findings, professional experience and academic study. These explanatory models are essentially etic, and their value derives from their coherence, comprehensiveness and/or usefulness.

Although etic professional explanatory models may include or be based on consideration of emic explanatory models, the latter are fundamentally different. Bhui and colleagues (2006) gloss the term as 'personal explanations for mental distress'. Considering interest of the outline for cultural formulation of DSM-IV in explanatory models, Alarcon (2009) refers to ethnography as enabling assessment of a 'patient-owned perspective', considered with reference to interests. The validity of an emic explanatory model of illness, however, whether it refers to ideas about an illness episode or general illness beliefs, derives from accuracy in representing the experience, meaning, ideas about treatment and other aspects of illness according to a patient or other informant, regardless of scientific support for their ideas.

Such explanatory models provide a complementary contribution to management of divergent emic and etic considerations in expectations and the approach to treatment (Mavundla *et al.*, 2009). The coherence, comprehensiveness, rational construction and predictive capacity may be immaterial, because eliciting and working with this kind of explanatory model fosters an empathic understanding of potentially diverse orientations, perspectives, priorities and values of patient, family and clinician participants in the clinical process. Research suggests that concordant illness explanatory models of patients and clinicians predicts patients' satisfaction (James *et al.*, 2014), better even than shared ethnicity (Callan and Littlewood, 1998).

Apart from clinical interests resulting in large measure from a process that facilitates empathy and a therapeutic alliance, research interests are often concerned with patterns of explanatory models characteristic of particular mental health problems, cultural groups and how features of explanatory models may relate to risk, clinical management, course, outcome and other practical considerations. In that regard, data from a number of emic illness explanatory models may be analysed to generate etic professional explanatory models. This has been an early and enduring interest of the field (Blumhagen, 1980; Bhui *et al.*, 2006), although different terms are typically used for professional explanatory models to avoid the confusion of the same term referring to two distinct concepts in one report. To make sense of the diverse literature of *explanatory models*, however, the confusion is unavoidable, and it must be acknowledged and resolved.

Literature of Explanatory Models

To provide a rough estimate of health research interest in emic explanatory models of illness, a literature search of PubMed through to 30 June 2016 retrieved 1710

entries for search criteria of explanatory model(s) (singular or plural) as a text word in titles or abstracts. The earliest PubMed citation was an article in 1962, a 'critical review and explanatory models' of sensory deprivation (Kenna, 1962), and all of the citations until 1980 referred to etic professional explanatory models. The first PubMed reference to a study of emic illness explanatory models was an article in 1980 published in *Culture, Medicine and Psychiatry* (CMP) on 'hyper-tension' as a folk illness (Blumhagen, 1980).

To sharpen the focus on cultural psychiatry, our interest here, a search for articles on explanatory model(s) and either psychiatry or mental health identified 461 articles cited in PubMed over the same period. The abstract or full article for each of these citations was evaluated to distinguish those addressing emic illness explanatory models ($n = 275$, 60.0%) or etic professional explanatory models ($n = 183$, 40.0%). Three citations were excluded because they were only marginally related to psychiatry or mental health. Figure 13.1 indicates the number of these emic and etic citations annually. Kleinman was the founding editor of CMP, and this journal accounted for the largest portion of articles dealing with emic explanatory models ($n = 29$, 10.6%); other journals with three or more publications are listed in Table 13.1.

This metric of PubMed citations indicates a pattern of increasing interest over the years, and the relative frequency of emic and etic explanatory models publications in the medical literature. Intended as indicative rather than comprehensive, the approach does not provide a precise account. Some important articles are missed because they do not use the term in the title or abstract (e.g. Littlewood, 1990; Pattanayak and Sagar, 2012) – and relevant books (Kleinman, 1980), grey literature and journal articles (especially those in social science journals) may not be indexed in PubMed. On the other hand, articles on explanatory models but not psychiatry or mental health are intentionally excluded.

Topical Interests

Prominent topical interests of this literature include a focus on common mental disorders (Patel *et al.*, 1997; Jacob *et al.*, 1998; Bhui *et al.*, 2006) – especially depression, somatization and persisting related questions about neurasthenia (Weiss *et al.*, 1995; Henningsen *et al.*, 2005; Paralikar *et al.*, 2011). Other priority topics include psychoses (Scheper-Hughes, 1987; Larsen, 2004; Bhikha *et al.*, 2015), suicide (Zadravec *et al.*, 2006; Parkar *et al.*, 2009;

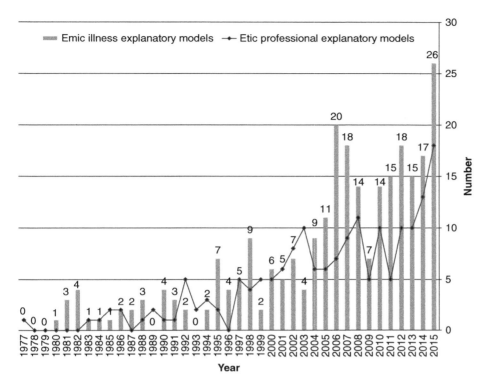

Figure 13.1 PubMed citations for 'explanatory model(s)' in title or abstract, and 'psychiatry' or 'mental health' in any field, annually through 2015

Chowdhury *et al.*, 2013; Hagaman *et al.*, 2013), substance-related addictive disorders (Costain, 2008; Penka *et al.*, 2008; Taieb *et al.*, 2012; Nadkarni *et al.*, 2013), dementia (Hinton *et al.*, 2005; Faure-Delage *et al.*, 2012; Giebel *et al.*, 2016a), personality disorders (Alarcon and Leetz, 1998) and psychosocial issues arising from primary medical problems (Loewe and Freeman, 2000; Chipimo *et al.*, 2011; Shackelton-Piccolo *et al.*, 2011; Owiti *et al.*, 2015).

In short, the literature covers cultural aspects of a full range of well-recognized mental health problems and various cross-cutting challenges for adult, child and geriatric psychiatry. Treatment preferences and help-seeking are among the major interests of this literature (Ying, 1990; Sheikh and Furnham, 2000; Bhugra and Flick, 2005; Okello and Neema, 2007), and the research agenda has included studies of clinicians and traditional healers (Stein, 1986; Joel *et al.*, 2003). The experience and social impact of stigma have also been important cross-cutting interests (Raguram *et al.*, 1996; Chowdhury *et al.*, 2001; Charles *et al.*, 2007; Lin, 2013). Specialized interests also include challenging end-of-life issues and palliative care (Downs *et al.*, 2006).

The explanatory model literature has been particularly concerned with questions of clinical care in multicultural societies, especially the problems and efforts to provide culturally sensitive care of ethnic minorities and migrants (McCabe and Priebe, 2004; Guzder *et al.*, 2013; Leavey *et al.*, 2016); questions of trust pose a challenge for research to guide culturally sensitive care of such groups. Analysis of the social impact of cultural representations of mental illness has also been considered with reference to explanatory models, including the impact of films (Atilola and Olayiwola, 2013). Following in the wake of the 'new cross-cultural psychiatry', explanatory models have provided a useful framework in the transition of the field from prior interests in identifying exotic culture-bound disorders to acknowledgement and response to pervasive aspects of culture (Kleinman, 1977a; Kirmayer and Jarvis, 1998). Strategies for current priorities of global mental health recognize the relevance of explanatory models for research, planning to reduce the treatment gap and provision of culturally sensitive and acceptable mental health services (Patel *et al.*, 2016).

147

Table 13.1 Number of PubMed citations through 2015 for journals that published at least three articles on emic illness 'explanatory model(s)' and either 'psychiatry' or 'mental health'

Journal	Citations	Percentage
Culture, Medicine and Psychiatry	29	10.55
International Journal of Social Psychiatry	19	6.91
Transcultural Psychiatry	18	6.55
Social Science and Medicine	17	6.18
British Journal of Psychiatry	13	4.73
Social Psychiatry and Psychiatric Epidemiology	7	2.55
Asian Journal of Psychiatry	6	2.18
Psychological Medicine	5	1.82
Qualitative Health Research	4	1.45
Journal of Affective Disorders	4	1.45
International Journal of Mental Health Nursing	3	1.09
BMC Psychiatry	3	1.09
National Medical Journal of India	3	1.09
Journal of Nervous and Mental Disease	3	1.09
BMC Health Services Research	3	1.09
Current Opinion in Psychiatry	3	1.09
International Review of Psychiatry	3	1.09
European Psychiatry	3	1.09
Canadian Journal of Psychiatry	3	1.09
Psychiatric Services	3	1.09
Total citations	275	100.00

Criticism and Defence

In addition to this literature acknowledging the appeal of explanatory models for research in cultural psychiatry, questions at the outset challenged the value of a clinically oriented explanatory model framework for social analysis and critical study of health systems. In his comments on Kleinman's presentation at a conference of the National Science Foundation in 1976 on theory in medical anthropology (Kleinman, 1978b), Ronald Frankenburg asserted 'that it is necessary to situate the analysis of a cultural system within a system of political economy, not just to give lip service to the presence of both social and cultural systems' and 'that to change a medical system, critical analyses of it must be located outside the conventional framework of medical practice' (reported by Thomas, 1978).

A later critique by Alan Young argued that clinical paradigms were inherently inferior to political economic and social models of health and illness. Young presented his critique in two papers, one in a provocative editorial published in CMP (Young, 1981), which sparked eight rejoinders published in a subsequent issue by clinicians and social scientists, and Young's second article on the anthropologies of illness and sickness in the *Annual Review of Anthropology* (Young, 1982). Like Frankenburg, Young also asserted that because Kleinman's interest in medical beliefs and practices is essentially clinical, it is inadequate to deal with priorities that are essentially social. He asserted that two critical problems with the explanatory model approach made it inappropriate for analysis of social relations of sickness: it confuses the class basis of power relationships with an interpersonal feature of relationships, and it fails to define sickness as a process for socializing disease and illness. As indicated earlier in this chapter, Kleinman later came to accept this argument criticizing explanatory models for social analysis.

Nevertheless, Young's and other critiques of the clinical relevance of explanatory models have been less influential. William and Healy (2001) argued that explanatory models were essentially 'reified and implicitly static', suggesting that the term *models* should be replaced with *maps*. Young and others proposed other operational adjustments to reformulate or replace the explanatory model framework with an account of *prototypes, chain links* and *explanatory accounts* (Stern and Kirmayer, 2004; see also the section on exclusively qualitative assessment on page 150). Although presented as alternative *knowledge structures*, prototypes and chain links may be regarded as alternatives only if one accepts Young's critique that explanatory models are necessarily fixed and coherent. Otherwise the new terms are not alternatives but rather operational elaborations refining and elaborating the sources and underlying associations and linkages of experience and ideas that constitute explanatory models – i.e. more complementary than contradictory. Similar points about the contexts and interrelationships of concepts had already been elaborated with reference to semantic analysis, causal webs and the role of social networks: 'Patient and family EMs often do not possess single referents but represent semantic networks that loosely link a variety of concepts and experiences' (Kleinman, 1980: 106–107; see also p. 108, figure 4).

Among the eight rejoinders to Young's critique in CMP, Blumhagen (1981) explained the value and clinical utility of the explanatory model framework based on experience working with it. Over the years, as indicated in the literature noted in the previous section, others have also affirmed positive experience and the value of the framework in clinical settings for cultural psychiatry (e.g. see Bhui and Bhugra, 2002). Consistent with experience in India, showing that patients may 'simultaneously hold multiple and possibly contradictory beliefs' (Jacob, 2010), experience in other settings with diverse ethnic groups is similarly notable for multiple, simultaneously contradictory explanatory models (Lloyd *et al.*, 1998; McCabe and Priebe, 2004), indicating the value of a pluralistic account for coping with different aspects of a health problem (Johnson *et al.*, 2012).

Research Instruments

The format for assessing explanatory models in the field of cultural psychiatry primarily involves clinical interviews with patients, family caretakers and clinicians. Community studies or research in the absence of an index patient as a focus of the interview typically make use of illness vignettes, enabling comparative analysis of various views about the mental health problem portrayed in the vignette. Although several explanatory model interviews and frameworks have been developed as instruments for wider use beyond a single study, many investigators have also designed study-specific interviews or guides to meet the needs of their particular research aims. That was in fact the norm before semi-structured interviews became available in the late 1990s, but even after, many investigators continue to use their own study-specific interview agenda, consistent with Kleinman's early advice.

Kleinman sketched his recommended approach for eliciting explanatory models using 'ethnoscientific elicitation procedures' in home-based studies and in

> **BOX 13.1** Questions suggested by Kleinman for eliciting details of patients' explanatory models
>
> 1. What do you call your problem? What name does it have?
> 2. What do you think has caused your problem?
> 3. Why do you think it started when it did?
> 4. What does your sickness do to you? How does it work?
> 5. How severe is it? Will it have a short or long course?
> 6. What do you fear most about your sickness?
> 7. What are the chief problems your sickness has caused for you?
> 8. What kind of treatment do you think you should receive? What are the most important results you hope to receive from the treatment?
>
> Source: Kleinman (1980: 106)

clinical interviews by indicating 'a genuine, nonjudgmental interest in patients' beliefs'. The in-depth ethnographic approach he suggested begins with 'general, open-ended questions', and it may proceed with eight suggested questions to elicit further detail about the features of patients' explanatory models (Kleinman, 1980: 106). Adjustment is required, though not explicit, to reframe these questions for family caretakers or other potential respondents among participants in the clinical process. Although the approach is presented in a footnote (rather than a chapter or designated section of the book), these questions and suggestions for using them have been highly influential and widely quoted in the literature of explanatory model studies (see Box 13.1). They have provided a framework both for study-specific interviews and for the development of several approaches to explanatory model interviewing intended for use beyond a single study.

Integrated Quantitative and Qualitative Explanatory Model Interviews

Two approaches intended for mixed quantitative and qualitative study rooted in these eight questions have been developed and adapted for use in various settings: EMIC interviews (explanatory model interview catalogue; Weiss, 1997) and the SEMI (short explanatory model interview; Lloyd *et al.*, 1998). Developments in psychiatric epidemiological survey research motivated both of these approaches. Acknowledging a desire to complement etic with emic accounts of mental health problems, use of these instruments is often paired with psychiatric diagnostic and psychopathology assessments (e.g. GHQ-12, SCID and other instruments). Both EMIC and SEMI were also explicit in their priority of integrating quantitative and qualitative interests of explanatory model research. The scope and the range of interests covered by the two approaches are similar, and each involves local adaptation for the needs of a particular study. Consideration of the name of the illness, presenting problems and priority symptoms, seriousness, perceived causes, treatment preferences and help-seeking history are addressed. Both also focus on a current illness episode but may optionally include illness vignettes to elicit general illness beliefs. Interviews based on both strategies have been verified for interrater reliability.

The EMIC Framework

The EMIC approach involves an elicitation strategy that combines open-ended questions followed by category-specific follow-up, a data form and an analytic strategy that weights categorical responses reported spontaneously, in response to the category-specific probes and/or identified as superlative (i.e. most troubling aspect of illness experience, most important perceived cause, first source of outside help and so forth). This enables a computation of the prominence of a reported category. Item-specific qualitative narratives are noted or preferably recorded for transcription. The principles and strategy have been elaborated as a methodology for cultural epidemiology that includes integration of quantitative analysis and thematic analysis of qualitative narratives (Weiss, 2001; Weiss, 2017). Current research with EMIC interviews makes use of Android-based tablet computing to administer, enter, record and upload interview data. This approach to tablet-based integrated qualitative and quantitative interviewing has been validated with reference to paper-based interviews (Giduthuri et al., 2014). Audio recordings are time stamped by screen swipes for automated coding of interview notes and access to item-specific audio-recorded narratives even before transcription. The scope and length of EMIC interviews vary according to study aims.

The SEMI Framework

Development of the SEMI was explicitly intended to provide a shorter and less complex interview based solely on open-ended questions, and it has been suggested that it is easier to use than EMIC interviews. An approach to post-coding of qualitative SEMI interview responses is recommended as an alternative to the coding strategy used in EMIC interviews. Emic categories in the analysis of qualitative notes or transcripts of responses to questions of the SEMI are coded as either reported or not reported to derive variables that enable quantitative analysis (Savarimuthu et al., 2010). Results are typically reported as frequencies of analysis categories and analysed for associations based on study aims.

Exclusively Qualitative Assessment

As an alternative to integrated qualitative and quantitative assessments, a purely qualitative approach has been developed to overcome concerns about the limitations of quantitative methods for ethnographic study. The McGill Illness Narrative Interview (MINI) is a product of these efforts (Groleau et al., 2006). It was motivated by concerns that EMIC and SEMI interviews 'may not produce narratives of sufficient spontaneity and depth to allow more intensive methods of narrative and discourse analysis'. The structure of the MINI is shaped by 'the nature of knowledge structures underlying illness narratives'. It is also an effort to demonstrate the salience of essential elements of Young's critique of explanatory models described earlier in this chapter (Young, 1981; Young, 1982).

Narratives elicited by administration of the MINI are intended for analysis and coding with reference to three types of reasoning about representations: (1) explanatory models (identified as causal thinking or causal attributions); (2) prototypes (reasoning based on analogy and prior personal or shared experience); and (3) chain complexes (linkages between past experience and current symptoms in the absence of explicit causal connections or prototypes). The interview itself is structured in five parts: (1) initial illness narrative, (2) prototype narrative, (3) explanatory model narrative, (4) services and response to treatment, and (5) impact on life.

A high degree of sophistication and intensive training is required for interviewers, both in technical aspects and disciplinary contexts of the interview. Interviewers are expected to be able to engage effectively with interviewees and to respond to questions about their own family and professional identities. It is also recommended that if 'an interviewee is found to be withholding too much information as a result of social identity, power and position, the only solution may be to replace the interviewer by one whose social status is deemed more appropriate in terms of gender, ethnocultural background or other salient aspects of identity' (Groleau *et al.*, 2006: 680).

One of the five sections of the interview refers explicitly to explanatory models, elaborating various aspects of causal reasoning. All 46 questions of the MINI, however, are fully consistent with the broader scope and interests of explanatory model interviewing. But the exclusively qualitative theory-driven structure and analytic coding strategy, and the level of training required to administer and analyse MINI interview data are distinctive.

Exclusively Quantitative Assessment

Several instruments have been developed with the aim of simplifying assessment and avoiding comprehensive qualitative assessment, mindful of limitations of time and training in order to enhance the feasibility and acceptability of the tool for wider use. The three approaches noted here make use of a checklist for their respective interests of (1) assessing comprehensive features of illness explanatory models, (2) using a set of screening questions and (3) making an indirect assessment.

BARTS Explanatory Model Inventory: Checklist (BEMI-C)

The BEMI-C was developed as the checklist version of a more extended explanatory model interview (Rudell *et al.*, 2009). It was abridged as a checklist and the analytic approach was developed as acknowledgement that 'clinicians do not usually have the time and resources to undertake a detailed and unstructured exploration of EMs or qualitative data analysis' (Bhui *et al.*, 2006). The initial report of its development aimed to assess the feasibility of a relatively simple self-report checklist for comprehensive assessment of explanatory models of common mental disorders, and to determine whether perceived causes of mental health problems (distress) are related to treatment preferences and whether explanatory models are influenced more by ethnicity than mental disorders.

The original instrument, which has been adapted in subsequent studies, was based on a comprehensive formulation of illness explanatory models, and it addressed five domains: identity (41 items; i.e.

identification of the illness, not personal cultural identity), causes (40 items), timeline (cyclical or duration), consequences (26 items) and preferred interventions (18 items). Assessed items for each of these domains are analysed with reference to thematic groups using appropriate statistics for comparing groups and analysing associations pertinent to research questions.

Based on concerns about feasibility and acceptability, the approach omits a qualitative assessment. It was initially used on a sample of people reporting 'any problem or difficulty in the past month' but not necessarily seeking treatment for that problem. The BEMI-C is intended for use in surveys and research studies in settings where constraints limit the feasibility and acceptability of a qualitative assessment. Recent research has produced a dementia-specific tool for study of South Asian minorities in the UK, considering its value and broader use (Giebel *et al.*, 2016b).

Mental Distress Explanatory Model Questionnaire (MDEMQ)

Among the earliest assessments of explanatory models, the MDEMQ was developed to study beliefs about illness causation (Eisenbruch, 1990). Although intended to meet the needs of clinicians with limited time and training, it was pilot tested on a sample of college students. Respondents were asked to consider 'any sort of mental distress' and how anybody, including the respondent, might explain the cause with reference to 46 potential categories. Each category is coded on a five-point Likert scale ranging from not at all likely to highly likely. Multidimensional scaling was used in the original study to analyse the questionnaires, and results are presented with reference to classification of the categories as indicating non-Western or Western physiology, and mystical or stress-related causes.

The MDEMQ has been used to compare beliefs about mental illness causation among groups of Christian, Buddhist and no-religious-affiliation students in Singapore (Mathews, 2011) and to relate ideas about cause to help-seeking among Asian and Western adults (Sheikh and Furnham, 2000).

Explanatory Model Association Task (EMAT)

An indirect approach to assessment has been developed to adapt measures of task latency self-attribution to assess causal attributions of health problems. Concern that patients, especially ethnic minority patients, may distort their real views to present more socially desirable responses was the motivation for this alternative to direct-assessment interviews (Ghane *et al.*, 2012). The EMAT was constructed to make this assessment and to validate results by comparison with a direct assessment using the perceived cause section of an explanatory model interview. A pilot study was done with Dutch college students with 'a relatively serious physical or mental problem' in the previous 5 years, which served as the reference condition for the assessment.

Clinical Interests and Tools

Notwithstanding extensive use for research, it has been practical clinical interest and the relevance for training in cultural psychiatry that motivates much of the appeal of the explanatory model framework for cultural psychiatry. The framework has long been a focal interest in the development of clinically applied medical anthropology in psychiatry and general practice. Littlewood (1991) described the relevance of medical anthropology and the disease–illness framework for consultation-liaison services, psychotherapy, cognitive therapy, and for group and milieu work on inpatient units. Nearly two decades ago, all patients on his psychosomatic ward at University College Hospital, London, were asked to complete an explanatory model questionnaire. Others have also been concerned that despite evidence that shared concepts of illness are associated with more satisfied patients (Callan and Littlewood, 1998), clinicians too often lack the clinically relevant social science skills to assess and work with illness explanatory models (Bhui and Bhugra, 2002). The need for appropriate frameworks and instruments for supervision and training curricula has long been clear (Alarcon *et al.*, 1999).

The interests of research and clinical practice are complementary, but each must proceed with methods based on their own distinct priorities. Although training in the use of research tools may contribute to clinical competence, instruments and agendas cannot be assumed to be interchangeable. Clinical methods that are useful in practice may be inadequate for research if they lack a strategy for translating clinical information into research data; research instruments that work well and provide suitable data for analysis to achieve study aims may be unwieldy in routine practice and unsuitable if they lack feasibility and acceptability for clinical use.

Psychiatric assessment is appropriately concerned with diagnostic evaluation and biopsychosocial contexts. Cultural psychiatry highlights the importance of dual core specialty interests, namely, cultural features of illness and the context of cultural identity – defined by group identities, ways of life, race, ethnicity, interpersonal networks, social interactions, economic resources and political status. For the cultural assessment of illness, eliciting explanatory models may be regarded as a core competency.

Outline for Cultural Formulation and the Cultural Formulation Interview

In the DSM-IV, a framework for cultural assessment was included to address cultural issues in clinical assessment (DSM-IV, Appendix I). The five sections of this outline for cultural formulation (OCF) consider cultural features of (1) personal identity, (2) explanations of the illness (i.e. explanatory models), (3) psychosocial environment and level of functioning, (4) the relationship with the clinician and (5) an overall cultural assessment. Development of the OCF was a product of an advisory group on culture and diagnosis, which aimed to provide a framework for clinical training and practice and thereby enhance the cultural sensitivity of mainstream psychiatry. The OCF has also been used as a guideline for case reports published in the psychiatric literature (Lewis-Fernandez, 1996).

Although the OCF provided a framework for clinicians to consider cultural priorities relevant for clinical care, questions remained about how to work with that framework. To clarify and respond to this ambiguity, a cultural formulation interview (CFI) was developed, tested and included in the DSM-5 (APA, 2013: 749–759; Lewis-Fernandez *et al.*, 2014). In addition to the core CFI for an individual with an identified problem, typically a patient, the DSM-5 also includes a similarly structured informant version for a family care-giver or someone else who knows the clinical problem and social context. In addition, 12 supplementary modules to elaborate particular interests of the CFI are readily available online, and a module on explanatory models is first among them.

Although the four major sections of the CFI address all the issues identified in the OCF, the structure is different. The first two sections of the CFI on (1) cultural definition of the problem and (2) perceptions of cause, context and support refer explicitly to explanatory models. A subsection on cultural identity is embedded in the latter. The remaining two sections deal with cultural aspects of treatment preferences, which are also relevant interests of explanatory models, though not explicitly designated as such in the CFI: (3) self-coping and past help–seeking and (4) current help-seeking. The supplementary module on explanatory models includes questions elaborating each of these standard issues: general understanding of the problem, perceived causes, anticipated course and expectations of help-seeking and treatment. Three questions on illness prototypes, incorporating questions about the source of ideas about the explanatory model, are also included in this module.

Although the scope and questions of the CFI are similar to questions of various research instruments, the CFI was developed as a clinical tool rather than as a research instrument. Research skills, study designs and data management plans would need to be developed if a version of the CFI were to be adapted for use as a research instrument. Operational research questions, however, about its clinical usefulness, feasibility, acceptance and overall value have been studied to validate the CFI (Paralikar *et al.*, 2015; Lewis-Fernandez *et al.*, 2017), and barriers to implementation have been examined qualitatively (Aggarwal *et al.*, 2013).

Conclusion

As a product of interdisciplinary development, the illness explanatory model framework provides a lens for examining emic understandings of illness in various settings. An expanding literature on the topic indicates the framework remains as much a priority as ever. Although enthusiasm for use in ethnographic studies has waned, it continues to be relevant and useful in community studies of mental health and other areas of public health. Research strategies attentive to emic explanatory models have a role to play for planning psychiatric services, reducing the treatment gap and advancing other interests on the agenda of global mental health. Questions about how emic explanatory models help to explain the significance of complementary features of cultural identity, gender, stigma, risk, self-help, help-seeking and use of available health services remain priorities of cultural psychiatry. Kleinman's succinct guide continues to guide assessment of explanatory models, and various research instruments have

also been developed for mixed-methods, qualitative and quantitative approaches to research. As a key feature of the CFI and the OCF, the illness explanatory model framework plays an increasingly important role in culturally sensitive clinical training and practice. It has been firmly established in the lexicon of culture, health and illness.

References

Aggarwal, N. K., Nicasio, A. V., Desilva, R., Boiler, M. and Lewis-Fernandez, R. (2013). Barriers to implementing the DSM-5 cultural formulation interview: a qualitative study. *Culture, Medicine and Psychiatry*, **37**, 505–533.

Alarcon, R. D. (2009). Culture, cultural factors and psychiatric diagnosis: review and projections. *World Psychiatry*, **8**, 131–139.

Alarcon, R. D. and Leetz, K. L. (1998). Cultural intersections in the psychotherapy of borderline personality disorder. *American Journal of Psychotherapy*, **52**, 176–190.

Alarcon, R. D., Westermeyer, J., Foulks, E. F. and Ruiz, P. (1999). Clinical relevance of contemporary cultural psychiatry. *Journal of Nervous and Mental Disease*, **187**, 465–471.

American Psychiatric Association (APA) (2013). *Diagnostic and Statistical Manual of Mental Disorders, 5th edn (DSM-5)*. Washington, DC: APA.

Atilola, O. and Olayiwola, F. (2013). Frames of mental illness in the Yoruba genre of Nigerian movies: implications for orthodox mental health care. *Transcultural Psychiatry*, **50**, 442–454.

Bhikha, A., Farooq, S., Chaudhry, N., Naeem, F. and Husain, N. (2015). Explanatory models of psychosis amongst British South Asians. *Asian Journal of Psychiatry*, **16**, 48–54.

Bhugra, D. and Flick, G. R. (2005). Pathways to care for patients with bipolar disorder. *Bipolar Disorders*, **7**, 236–245.

Bhui, K. and Bhugra, D. (2002). Explanatory models for mental distress: implications for clinical practice and research. *British Journal of Psychiatry*, **181**, 6–7.

Bhui, K., Rudell, K., and Priebe, S. (2006). Assessing explanatory models for common mental disorders. *Journal of Clinical Psychiatry*, **67**, 964–971.

Blumhagen, D. (1980). Hyper-tension: a folk illness with a medical name. *Culture, Medicine and Psychiatry*, **4**, 197–224.

Blumhagen, D. W. (1981). On the nature of explanatory models. *Culture, Medicine and Psychiatry*, **5**, 337–340.

Broome, M. (2002). Explanatory models in psychiatry. *British Journal of Psychiatry*, **181**, 351–352.

Callan, A. and Littlewood, R. (1998). Patient satisfaction: ethnic origin or explanatory model? *International Journal of Social Psychiatry*, **44**, 1–11.

Charles, H., Manoranjitham, S. D., and Jacob, K. S. (2007). Stigma and explanatory models among people with schizophrenia and their relatives in Vellore, south India. *International Journal of Social Psychiatry*, **53**, 325–332.

Chipimo, P. J., Tuba, M. and Fylkesnes, K. (2011). Conceptual models for mental distress among HIV-infected and uninfected individuals: a contribution to clinical practice and research in primary-health-care centers in Zambia. *BMC Health Services Research*, **11**, 7.

Chowdhury, A. N., Sanyal, D., Bhattacharya, A., Dutta, S. K., De, R., Banerjee, S. *et al.* (2001). Prominence of symptoms and level of stigma among depressed patients in Calcutta. *Journal of the Indian Medical Association*, **99**, 20–23.

Chowdhury, A. N., Banerjee, S., Brahma, A., Hazra, A. and Weiss, M. G. (2013). Sociocultural context of suicidal behaviour in the Sundarban region of India. *Psychiatry Journal*, **2013**, 486081.

Costain, W. F. (2008). The effects of cannabis abuse on the symptoms of schizophrenia: patient perspectives. *International Journal of Mental Health Nursing*, **17**, 227–235.

Downs, M., Small, N. and Froggatt, K. (2006). Explanatory models of dementia: links to end-of-life care. *International Journal of Palliative Nursing*, **12**, 209–213.

Eisenberg, L. (1977). Disease and illness. Distinctions between professional and popular ideas of sickness. *Culture, Medicine and Psychiatry*, **1**, 9–23.

Eisenbruch, M. (1990). Classification of natural and supernatural causes of mental distress. Development of a Mental Distress Explanatory Model Questionnaire. *Journal of Nervous and Mental Disease*, **178**, 712–719.

Engel, G. L. (1977). The need for a new medical model: a challenge for biomedicine. *Science*, **196**, 129–136.

Fabrega, H., Jr (1975). The need for an ethnomedical science. *Science*, **189**, 969–975.

Faure-Delage, A., Mouanga, A. M., M'belesso, P., Tabo, A., Bandzouzi, B., Dubreuil, C. M. *et al.* (2012). Socio-cultural perceptions and representations of dementia in Brazzaville, Republic of Congo: the EDAC Survey. *Dementia and Geriatric Cognitive Disorders Extra*, **2**, 84–96.

Ghane, S., Kolk, A. M. and Emmelkamp, P. M. (2012). Direct and indirect assessment of explanatory models of illness. *Transcultural Psychiatry*, **49**, 3–25.

Giduthuri, J. G., Maire, N., Joseph, S., Kudale, A., Schaetti, C., Sundaram, N. *et al.* (2014). Developing and validating a tablet version of an illness explanatory model interview for a public health survey in Pune, India. *PLoS One*, **9**, e107374.

Giebel, C., Challis, D., Worden, A., Jolley, D., Bhui, K. S., Lambat, A. *et al.* (2016a). Perceptions of self-defined memory problems vary in South Asian minority older people who consult a GP and those who do not: a mixed-method pilot study. *International Journal of Geriatric Psychiatry*, **31**, 375–383.

Giebel, C. M., Jolley, D., Zubair, M., Bhui, K. S., Challis, D., Purandare, N. *et al.* (2016b). Adaptation of the Barts Explanatory Model Inventory to dementia understanding in South Asian ethnic minorities. *Aging and Mental Health*, **20**, 594–602.

Good, B. J. (1977). The heart of what's the matter: the semantics of illness in Iran. *Culture, Medicine and Psychiatry*, **1**, 25–58.

Groleau, D., Young, A. and Kirmayer, L. J. (2006). The McGill Illness Narrative Interview (MINI): an interview schedule to elicit meanings and modes of reasoning related to illness experience. *Transcultural Psychiatry*, **43**, 671–691.

Guzder, J., Yohannes, S. and Zelkowitz, P. (2013). Helpseeking of immigrant and native born parents: a qualitative study from a Montreal child day hospital. *Journal of the Canadian Academy of Child and Adolescent Psychiatry*, **22**, 275–281.

Hagaman, A. K., Wagenaar, B. H., McLean, K. E., Kaiser, B. N., Winskell, K. and Kohrt, B. A. (2013). Suicide in rural Haiti: clinical and community perceptions of prevalence, etiology, and prevention. *Social Science and Medicine*, **83**, 61–69.

Headland, T. N., Pike, K. L. and Harris, M. (1990). *Emics and Etics: The Insider/Outsider Debate*. Newbury Park, CA: Sage.

Henningsen, P., Jakobsen, T., Schiltenwolf, M. and Weiss, M. G. (2005). Somatization revisited: diagnosis and perceived causes of common mental disorders. *Journal of Nervous and Mental Disease*, **193**, 85–92.

Hinton, L., Franz, C. E., Yeo, G., and Levkoff, S. E. (2005). Conceptions of dementia in a multiethnic sample of family caregivers. *Journal of the American Geriatrics Society*, **53**, 1405–1410.

Jacob, K. S. (2010). The assessment of insight across cultures. *Indian Journal of Psychiatry*, **52**, 373–377.

Jacob, K. S., Bhugra, D., Lloyd, K. R. and Mann, A. H. (1998). Common mental disorders, explanatory models and consultation behaviour among Indian women living in the UK. *Journal of the Royal Society of Medicine*, **91**, 66–71.

James, C. C., Carpenter, K. A., Peltzer, K. and Weaver, S. (2014). Valuing psychiatric patients' stories: belief in and use of the supernatural in the Jamaican psychiatric setting. *Transcultural Psychiatry*, **51**, 247–263.

Joel, D., Sathyaseelan, M., Jayakaran, R., Vijayakumar, C., Muthurathnam, S. and Jacob, K. S. (2003). Explanatory models of psychosis among community health workers in South India. *Acta Psychiatrica Scandinavica*, **108**, 66–69.

Johnson, S., Sathyaseelan, M., Charles, H., Jeyaseelan, V. and Jacob, K. S. (2012). Insight, psychopathology, explanatory models and outcome of schizophrenia in India: a prospective 5-year cohort study. *BMC Psychiatry*, **12**, 159.

Katz, M. H. (2003). Multivariable analysis: a primer for readers of medical research. *Annals of Internal Medicine*, **138**, 644–650.

Kendler, K. S. (2008). Explanatory models for psychiatric illness. *American Journal of Psychiatry*, **165**, 695–702.

Kenna, J. C. (1962). Sensory deprivation phenomena: critical review and explanatory models. *Proceedings of the Royal Society of Medicine*, **55**, 1005–1010.

Kirmayer, L. J. and Jarvis, E. (1998). Cultural psychiatry: from museums of exotica to the global agora. *Current Opinion in Psychiatry*, **11**, 183–189.

Kleinman, A. M. (1977a). Depression, somatization and the 'new cross-cultural psychiatry'. *Social Science and Medicine*, **11**, 3–10.

Kleinman, A. (1977b). Culture, and illness: a question of models. *Culture, Medicine and Psychiatry*, **1**, 229–231.

Kleinman, A. (1978a). Clinical relevance of anthropological and cross-cultural research: concepts and strategies. *American Journal of Psychiatry*, **135**, 427–431.

Kleinman, A. (1978b). Concepts and a model for the comparison of medical systems as cultural systems. *Social Science and Medicine*, **12**, 85–95.

Kleinman, A. (1980). *Patients and Healers in the Context of Culture: An Exploration of the Borderland between Anthropology, Medicine, and Psychiatry*. Berkeley: University of California Press.

Kleinman, A. (1981). On illness meanings and clinical interpretation: not 'rational man', but a rational approach to man the sufferer/man the healer. *Culture, Medicine and Psychiatry*, **5**, 373–377.

Kleinman, A. (1995). *Writing at the Margin: Discourse between Anthropology and Medicine*. Berkeley: University of California Press.

Kleinman, A., Eisenberg, L. and Good, B. (1978). Culture, illness, and care: clinical lessons from anthropologic and cross-cultural research. *Annals of Internal Medicine*, **88**, 251–258.

Larsen, J. A. (2004). Finding meaning in first episode psychosis: experience, agency, and the cultural repertoire. *Medical Anthropology Quarterly*, **18**, 447–471.

Leavey, G., Loewenthal, K. and King, M. (2016). Locating the social origins of mental illness: the explanatory models of mental illness among clergy from different ethnic and faith backgrounds. *Journal of Religion and Health*, **55**(5), 1607–1622.

Lewis-Fernandez, R. (1996). Cultural formulation of psychiatric diagnosis. *Culture, Medicine and Psychiatry*, **20**, 133–144.

Lewis-Fernandez, R., Aggarwal, N. K., Bäärnhielm, S., Rohlof, H., Kirmayer, L. J., Weiss, M. G. *et al.* (2014). Culture and psychiatric evaluation: operationalizing cultural formulation for DSM-5. *Psychiatry*, **77**, 130–154.

Lewis-Fernandez, R., Aggarwal, N. K., Lam, P. C., Galfalvy, H., Weiss, M. G., Kirmayer, L. J. *et al.* (2017). Feasibility, acceptability and clinical utility of the Cultural Formulation Interview: mixed-methods results from the DSM-5 international field trial. *British Journal of Psychiatry*, **210**, 290–297.

Lin, S. Y. (2013). Beliefs about causes, symptoms, and stigma associated with severe mental illness among 'highly acculturated' Chinese-American patients. *International Journal of Social Psychiatry*, **59**, 745–751.

Littlewood, R. (1990). From categories to contexts: a decade of the 'new cross-cultural psychiatry'. *British Journal of Psychiatry*, **156**, 308–327.

Littlewood, R. (1991). From disease to illness and back again. *The Lancet*, **337**, 1013–1016.

Lloyd, K. R., Jacob, K. S., Patel, V., St Louis, L. L., Bhugra, D. and Mann, A. H. (1998). The development of the Short Explanatory Model Interview (SEMI) and its use among primary-care attenders with common mental disorders. *Psychological Medicine*, **28**, 1231–1237.

Loewe, R. and Freeman, J. (2000). Interpreting diabetes mellitus: differences between patient and provider models of disease and their implications for clinical practice. *Culture, Medicine and Psychiatry*, **24**, 379–401.

Mathew, A. J., Samuel, B. and Jacob, K. S. (2010). Perceptions of illness in self and in others among patients with bipolar disorder. *International Journal of Social Psychiatry*, **56**, 462–470.

Mathews, M. (2011). Assessment and comparison of culturally based explanations for mental disorder among Singaporean Chinese youth. *International Journal of Social Psychiatry*, **57**, 3–17.

Mavundla, T. R., Toth, F., and Mphelane, M. L. (2009). Caregiver experience in mental illness: a perspective from a rural community in South Africa. *International Journal of Mental Health Nursing*, **18**, 357–367.

McCabe, R. and Priebe, S. (2004). Explanatory models of illness in schizophrenia: comparison of four ethnic groups. *British Journal of Psychiatry*, **185**, 25–30.

Nadkarni, A., Dabholkar, H., McCambridge, J., Bhat, B., Kumar, S., Mohanraj, R. *et al.* (2013). The explanatory models and coping strategies for alcohol use disorders: an exploratory qualitative study from India. *Asian Journal of Psychiatry*, **6**, 521–527.

Okello, E. S. and Neema, S. (2007). Explanatory models and help-seeking behavior: pathways to psychiatric care among patients admitted for depression in Mulago hospital, Kampala, Uganda. *Qualitative Health Research*, 17, 14–25.

Owiti, J. A., Greenhalgh, T., Sweeney, L., Foster, G. R. and Bhui, K. S. (2015). Illness perceptions and explanatory models of viral hepatitis B and C among immigrants and refugees: a narrative systematic review. *BMC Public Health*, 15, 151.

Paralikar, V., Agashe, M., Sarmukaddam, S., Deshpande, S., Goyal, V. and Weiss, M. G. (2011). Cultural epidemiology of neurasthenia spectrum disorders in four general hospital outpatient clinics of urban Pune, India. *Transcultural Psychiatry*, 48, 257–283.

Paralikar, V. P., Sarmukaddam, S. B., Patil, K. V., Nulkar, A. D. and Weiss, M. G. (2015). Clinical value of the cultural formulation interview in Pune, India. *Indian Journal of Psychiatry*, 57, 59–67.

Parkar, S. R., Nagarsekar, B. and Weiss, M. G. (2009). Explaining suicide in an urban slum of Mumbai, India: a sociocultural autopsy. *Crisis*, 30, 192–201.

Patel, V. and Mann, A. (1997). Etic and emic criteria for non-psychotic mental disorder: a study of the CISR and care provider assessment in Harare. *Social Psychiatry and Psychiatric Epidemiology*, 32, 84–89.

Patel, V., Todd, C., Winston, M., Gwanzura, F., Simunyu, E., Acuda, W. et al. (1997). Common mental disorders in primary care in Harare, Zimbabwe: associations and risk factors. *British Journal of Psychiatry*, 171, 60–64.

Patel, V., Xiao, S., Chen, H., Hanna, F., Jotheeswaran, A. T., Luo, D. et al. (2016). The magnitude of and health system responses to the mental health treatment gap in adults in India and China. *The Lancet*, 388(10063), 3074–3084.

Pattanayak, R. D. and Sagar, R. (2012). A qualitative study of perceptions related to family risk of bipolar disorder among patients and family members from India. *International Journal of Social Psychiatry*, 58, 463–469.

Penka, S., Heimann, H., Heinz, A. and Schouler-Ocak, M. (2008). Explanatory models of addictive behaviour among native German, Russian-German, and Turkish youth. *European Psychiatry*, 23(Suppl 1), 36–42.

Pike, K. L. (1967). Etic and emic standpoints for the description of behavior. In *Language in Relation to a Unified Theory of the Structure of Human Behavior*, 2nd rev. edn. The Hague, the Netherlands: Mouton and Co., pp. 37–72.

Raguram, R., Weiss, M. G., Channabasavanna, S. M. and Devins, G. M. (1996). Stigma, depression, and somatization in South India. *American Journal of Psychiatry*, 153, 1043–1049.

Rudell, K., Bhui, K. and Priebe, S. (2009). Concept, development and application of a new mixed method assessment of cultural variations in illness perceptions:

Barts Explanatory Model Inventory. *Journal of Health Psychology*, 14, 336–347.

Savarimuthu, R. J., Ezhilarasu, P., Charles, H., Antonisamy, B., Kurian, S. and Jacob, K. S. (2010). Post-partum depression in the community: a qualitative study from rural south India. *International Journal of Social Psychiatry*, 56, 94–102.

Scheper-Hughes, N. (1987). 'Mental' in 'Southie': individual, family, and community responses to psychosis in South Boston. *Culture, Medicine and Psychiatry*, 11, 53–78.

Shackelton-Piccolo, R., McKinlay, J. B., Marceau, L. D., Goroll, A. H. and Link, C. L. (2011). Differences between internists and family practitioners in the diagnosis and management of the same patient with coronary heart disease. *Medical Care Research and Review*, 68, 650–666.

Sheikh, S. and Furnham, A. (2000). A cross-cultural study of mental health beliefs and attitudes towards seeking professional help. *Social Psychiatry and Psychiatric Epidemiology*, 35, 326–334.

Siegler, M. and Osmond, H. (1966). Models of madness. *British Journal of Psychiatry*, 112, 1193–1203.

Stein, H. F. (1986). 'Sick people' and 'trolls': a contribution to the understanding of the dynamics of physician explanatory models. *Culture, Medicine and Psychiatry*, 10, 221–229.

Stern, L. and Kirmayer, L. J. (2004). Knowledge structures in illness narratives: development and reliability of a coding scheme. *Transcultural Psychiatry*, 41, 130–142.

Taieb, O., Chevret, S., Moro, M. R., Weiss, M. G., Biadi-Imhof, A., Reyre, A. et al. (2012). Impact of migration on explanatory models of illness and addiction severity in patients with drug dependence in a Paris suburb. *Substance Use and Misuse*, 47, 347–355.

Thomas, A. (1978). Discussion on Arthur Kleinman's paper. *Social Science and Medicine*, 12B, 95.

Twumasi, P. A. (1972). Ashanti traditional medicine and its relation to present-day psychiatry. *Transition*, 50–63.

Weiss, M. G. (1997). Explanatory Model Interview Catalogue (EMIC): framework for comparative study of illness. *Transcultural Psychiatry*, 34, 235–263.

Weiss, M. G. (2001). Cultural epidemiology: an introduction and overview. *Anthropology and Medicine*, 8, 5–29.

Weiss, M. G. (2017). The promise of cultural epidemiology. *Taiwanese Journal of Psychiatry* (Taipei). 31, 8–24.

Weiss, M. G., Raguram, R. and Channabasavanna, S. M. (1995). Cultural dimensions of psychiatric diagnosis: a comparison of DSM-III-R and illness explanatory models in south India. *British Journal of Psychiatry*, 166, 353–359.

William, B. and Healy, D. (2001). Perceptions of illness causation among new referrals to a community mental health team: 'explanatory model' or 'exploratory map'? *Social Science and Medicine*, 53, 465–476.

Ying, Y. W. (1990). Explanatory models of major depression and implications for help-seeking among immigrant Chinese-American women. *Culture, Medicine and Psychiatry*, **14**, 393–408.

Young, A. (1981). When rational men fall sick: an inquiry into some assumptions made by medical anthropologists. *Culture, Medicine and Psychiatry*, **5**, 317–335.

Young, A. (1982). The anthropologies of illness and sickness. *Annual Review of Anthropology*, **11**, 257–285.

Zadravec, T., Grad, O. and Socan, G. (2006). Expert and lay explanations of suicidal behaviour: comparison of the general population's, suicide attempters', general practitioners' and psychiatrists' views. *International Journal of Social Psychiatry*, **52**, 535–551.

Culture-Bound Syndromes
Past, Current Status and Future

Dinesh Bhugra, Rubens Dantas and Antonio Ventriglio

Editors' Introduction

Cultures in traditional or less developed societies were seen as containing clinical conditions which were seen as exotic and esoteric which were not 'seen' in other cultures. The history of clinical anthropology followed two different routes in western Europe and North America. By and large in the colonial times the anthropologists studied the ruled (colonized people) populations. On the other hand, in North America, the focus was on studying native and aboriginal groups. As a result, the clinicians who went to work in the colonies decided that certain conditions occurred only as a result of civilization and that the colonized people could possibly not suffer from these. On the other hand, some clinical conditions were seen 'exclusively' in certain ethnic groups and were a result of under-development of the brain leading to behaviours which were uncivilized. *Amok*, seen in the Malay archipelago, was criminalized by the British. Consequently, a previously acceptable social behaviour expressing distress became criminal behaviour. Thus those who suffered from it were sent to prison. There is clear evidence that a similar condition has been reported from other cultures but not seen as criminal.

Using *amok* as an example, among other so-called culture-bound syndromes, Bhugra *et al.* set the scene on the development of the concept of culture-bound syndromes. They argue that all psychiatric syndromes are affected by culture and are within this boundedness. Running *amok* in the Far East is no different from individuals taking guns and shooting randomly and indiscriminately at school children in the USA. *Latah* has similar hyperstartle response in other cultures. *Dhat* or semen-loss anxiety as seen in a culture-bound manner in the Indian subcontinent has been historically reported in many developed countries. Using historical accounts, the authors argue that, in North America, cornflakes and

crackers were invented and marketed as a treatment for masturbation in the nineteenth century. These anxieties are related to prevalent social and economic factors and should be seen as studies in that particular context. They welcome the DSM-5 proposals to abandon the term 'culture-bound syndromes' as it stands.

Introduction

The role of culture in affecting the idioms of distress and how these are expressed where help is sought and who provides the help and how resources are allocated is well known. Over the past two to three decades there has been an increasing attention paid to the role culture plays in developing and expressing idioms of distress, explaining the distress and modulating when, where from and how help is sought. In this chapter we do not propose to discuss the historical development of cultural psychiatry which is described elsewhere in this volume (see Chapter 1). However, it must be noted that the historical aspects were also very strongly influenced by the research interests, movement and narratives of anthropologists from the west (Europe and, to a lesser extent, America) to the rest of the world. The British anthropologists followed the path of the imperial and colonial rulers. This paved the way for the 'coming of age' of not only anthropology but also psychiatry, initially of social psychiatry which subsequently and gradually gave way to cultural psychiatry. As a consequence of imperialism and colonialism, indigenous methods and practice of medicine were suppressed in large parts of the world, leading to folk-healing practices being seen as second grade interventions. In addition, 'new' clinical diagnoses and categories were created and imposed on the ruled population. Thus, distress which may have been expressed in social idioms became medicalized and new syndromes were created.

In this chapter we aim to evaluate the status of culture-bound syndrome in modern-day clinical practice by studying the historical development of three well-known culture-bound syndromes in detail. These are *dhat* (semen-loss anxiety), *latah* and *amok*. Although we aim to touch upon other culture-bound syndromes (*susto* and *koro*), our contention in the first edition of this text that time had come to abandon these concepts and the reasons we put forward has come to pass in DSM-5, which describes only nine conditions which are strongly influenced by cultures which report them but even these have multiple other psychiatric conditions with these experiences.

Definitions

The so-called culture-bound syndromes (CBS) were described under a broad rubric which focused on the exotic and unusual nature of the symptoms. Whereas Littlewood and Lipsedge (1985) refer to these as episodic and dramatic reactions specific to a particular community and as locally defined discrete patterns of behaviour, Hughes (1996) also saw these as unique and distinctive but in those who are seen as 'the others' (i.e. those individuals who form a group which is outside the main group, immaterial of how it is defined). The inclusion of these syndromes in cultural psychiatry was seen as a reflection of their Eurocentric heritage where these syndromes had been institutionalized in the classificatory systems (Murphy, 1977; Haldipur, 1980). Hughes (1996) recommends that phenomenologists need to go beyond the semantic difficulties of using what is called 'label-grip', i.e. the paralysis of analytic acumen created by (perceived) powerful labels of culture-bound syndrome. Historical and contextual analysis of such symptoms therefore becomes of great interest so that one begins to understand and identify the stages and time when these symptoms became pathologized and medicalized.

Ayonrinde and Bhugra (2015) noted that over the last five to six decades there has been a clear evolution of the concept from culture-bound psychogenic psychoses to culture-bound syndromes which became culture-specific disorders and then giving way to cultural concepts of distress. The DSM-5 has adapted the term cultural concepts of distress. Ayonrinde and Bhugra (2015) assert that globalization and urbanization are likely to influence changes in prevalence of culture-bound syndromes.

Traditionally, culture-bound syndromes were defined as rare, exotic with unpredictable and chaotic behaviours at their core with individuals experiencing these being seen as uncivilized (Bhugra and Jacob, 1997). These authors suggested that such behaviours were placed in the context of Western diagnostic systems without any cultural links between environmental stressors and social environment and consequently symptoms which in the past had been often tolerated and accepted in the social-cultural context became medicalized. In some conditions legal proscriptions were the first step before medicalization.

Two decades ago, Hughes and Wintrob (1995) called for a contextual (and by implication sociocultural) frame of reference for understanding clinical significance of these conditions. Yap (1962) suggested that the variety of terms used to describe these conditions be replaced by atypical culture-bound psychogenic pychoses, which he subsequently shortened to culture-bound syndromes (Yap, 1969). This cultural context relies on the type of culture an individual comes from. It is critical that the treating clinician is familiar with the context which may allow better therapeutic engagement. Hofstede (1980, 1984) based on his work in large companies offers five dimensions of cultures which include the individualistic (ego-centric)/ collectivist (socio-centric) dimension; distance from the centre of power; long-term orientation; masculine/feminine dimension; and uncertainty avoidance. Within each culture, individuals can be ego-centric (idiocentric) or socio-centric (allocentric). The individualist cultures focus on I-ness, where kinship links are weaker and the individual may or may not focus on the immediate (nuclear) family. Studies have demonstrated that, with increasing gross national product (GNP), rates of divorce and crime go up. In collectivist cultures, kinship forms the basis of identity and relationships with group solidarity and sharing of material and non-material resources. Individuals in certain settings may behave in a collective fashion even if they are in individualistic societies, but the important fact remains that more often than not, they will behave like the society they were brought up in (Bhugra, 2005). However, as a result of rapid urbanization and globalization traditional attitudes and behaviours are changing leading to cultures-in-transition where some of the old order but not all is being replaced by differing expectations.

Society and Illness

The importance of this distinction into socio-centric and ego-centric (or collectivist and individualistic) societies and individuals is embedded in differential rates of common mental disorders in these populations and crime figures as well (Maercker, 2001). Maercker (2001) demonstrates that societies with different economic, social and political structures will have differential rates of crime, disorder and pathways into care. Thus with changes in cultures, values may change and traditional descriptions and views of culture-bound syndromes have given way to the notions of more diffuse presentations.

As noted previously, and often equated with ethnic psychoses (Devereux, 1956) and hysterical psychoses (Yap, 1969), culture-bound syndromes were seen as unclassifiable and exotic (Arieti and Meth, 1959) which meant that research into these conditions remained very limited. The range of names and characteristics indicate that the nosology of these syndromes has been problematic from their very genesis. The usage of the suffix 'bound' to illustrate the boundedness of these symptoms to individual cultures is both its problem and the perceived solution. As has been noted in DSM-5, it is fairly clear that the underlying pathology of most of these syndromes is not confined to one culture, and by stating that these are culture-bound to indicate their boundaries are defined by cultures leads to a possible confusion in understanding the conditions.

Hughes (1985) pointed out that the labels of atypical psychoses and exotic syndromes implied a degree of deviance from a standard diagnostic base. This tension between this abnormality (in the eyes of the observing group) and normality (in the eyes of culture within which it is generated) indicates the underlying conflict. Exotic becomes foreign, exciting, deviant and different, thereby confirming the diagnosis in 'the other'. The patient who is already 'the other' in relationship to the clinician and the diagnostician thus has another layer of otherness conferred upon them, making it difficult to place the diagnosis in the true cultural context and creating double jeopardy for them. It is useful to reiterate that diagnosis of psychiatric condition is not only Eurocentric but often also androcentric and anthropocentric.

Both the major diagnostic classificatory systems of ICD-10 (WHO, 1992) and DSM-5 (APA, 2013) have been amended to incorporate culture as a factor in the diagnosis, and these diagnostic formulations are explicitly committed to taking a theoretically neutral position including aetiological, perpetuating and precipitating factors.

Varieties of Culture-Bound Syndromes

A large number of culture-bound syndromes were identified and interested readers are referred to the volume by Simons and Hughes (1985). Historically, hundreds of conditions were described, DSM-5 has reduced these to nine conditions.

First, in this chapter, we use three main syndromes to illustrate that most of the symptoms also appear in other cultures and are not confined to a single culture. Second, we report that the prevalence of similar symptoms varies according to economic factors and perhaps social evolution of cultures.

Dhat

Dhat, or semen-loss anxiety syndrome, is derived from the Sanskrit word *dhatu* (metal) and refers to constituent parts of the body. *Dhat* is colloquially expressed as a synonym for semen. Wig (1960) described the *dhat* syndrome (semen loss) as consisting of vague somatic symptoms of fatigue, weakness, anxiety, loss of appetite, guilt and symptoms of sexual dysfunction attributable to loss of semen following nocturnal emissions or masturbation, or loss through urine.

Indian historical texts describe the symptoms of semen-loss anxiety. In Ayurvedic texts dating from between 5000 BCE and the seventh century, the process of semen production was described as 'food converts to blood which converts to flesh which converts to marrow and the marrow is ultimately converted to semen. It is said that it takes 40 days for 40 drops of food to be converted to one drop of blood and 40 drops of blood to one drop of flesh and so on' (Bhugra and Buchanan, 1989). Thus historical concepts as part of cultural memory influence the individual psyche and knowledge, and semen starts to take on a precious existential importance. These ideas then not only explain but also actively compound the degree of weakness experienced by the individual and the physical symptoms of anxiety and depression then give rise to somatic symptoms. These notions of semen loss and resulting weakness associated with anxiety and depression are seen across the Indian subcontinent. This perceived weakness is so dominating that the traditional healers – vaids and hakims, following Ayurvedic or Unani systems respectively – advertise their fares and clinic timings widely.

In an intriguing study from Chandigarh in North India, Malhotra and Wig (1975) studied 175 individuals aged 30–50 in the community and, using a case vignette, explored the public perceptions of semen loss, its aetiology and potential management. The variety of responses giving reasons and management strategies were clearly associated with social class of the respondents. Whereas one-third of respondents did not favour any interventions at all, those respondents from social class IV were more likely than any other group to see nocturnal emission and semen loss as abnormal and least likely to see psychological persuasion as a mode of treatment. This group saw diet and marriage as potential management strategies, along with avoiding bad company, masturbation and access to erotic literature. The authors called the *dhat* syndrome a sex neurosis of the Orient and concluded that susceptible individuals react to the belief system of semen loss. This seeking of medical interventions and doctors or others providing intervention thus confirms the underlying or resulting real or perceived physical complaints.

A majority of the rest of the studies from the Indian subcontinent relate to clinical populations. In these studies with patients as particpants, the syndrome is described and diagnosed as a separate entity and many studies do not give the associated psychiatric diagnosis. Thus, sometimes the syndrome is seen and recognized as a culture-bound syndrome. Our contention is that this approach reflects a historical anomaly and looking at some of the detailed data it would appear that:

- the syndrome is accompanied by easily and clinically recognizable common mental disorders; and
- its descriptions abound in other cultures (European and Western) as well.

Chadda and Ahuja (1990) studied 52 patients who had volunteered passage of *dhat* in the urine as their presenting complaint in the clinic and 80 per cent were said to have accompanying hypochondriacal symptoms, although these clinical descriptions do not make clear whether the diagnosis of hypochondriasis was made by patients or clinicians or what specific criteria were used to define such hypochondriasis (see Table 14.1). Interestingly, they report that seven patients (who did not have hypochondriasis) had 'pure' *dhat* syndrome. Our contention is that it is possible that this preoccupation with *dhat* itself is a hypochondriacal preoccupation. Bhatia and Malik (1991), in another study from the same centre in north India, reported that of 144 consecutive patients attending a sexual dysfunction clinic, 93 presented with passing *dhat*. On assessing these 93 cases using Hamilton rating scales and ICD-9 diagnostic categories, a significant number had one or more somatic symptoms of which physical weakness was the commonest. One-third reported sexual problems and half scored above seven on the Hamilton scale for depression. Nearly one-third received no psychiatric diagnosis. These authors report 'pure' *dhat* syndrome in a much larger proportion in 60 (41.7%) patients.

Using a case control design study, Chadda (1995) compared those presenting with *dhat* with controls who had neurotic disorders. He defined *dhat* in the urine as *dhat* syndrome although not all sufferers of *dhat* syndrome acknowledge this. Nearly half were reported to have depressive disorder, 18% had anxiety disorder and 32% had somatoform disorders – the figures for controls were 54, 30 and 16%, respectively, which reflect the source of data collection for the controls. However, the validity of diagnosis and associated psychiatric diagnosis can be questioned. Similar findings of depression in 52 per cent and 16 per cent having anxiety disorders had been previously reported in 1985 by Singh from another part of north India (Singh, 1985). Grover *et al.* (2015a) reported on 106 subjects presenting with *dhat* and compared them with those presenting with depression and a group presenting with somatoform disorders. Interestingly, the age of onset of *dhat* was around 22 years. In another study Grover *et al.* (2015b) suggest that *dhat* may be a precursor to depression rather than the other way around. Other authors (Dhikav *et al.*, 2008) have also reported high levels of depression (as high as 66%) in individuals presenting with *dhat*. Thus it is entirely possible that somatization may present as bodily concerns related to semen loss which may also occur in other settings. Similar findings have been reported among South Asians in other countries too (Menéndez *et al.*, 2012) among rural attendees with high levels of psychological distress (Gautham *et al.*, 2008). Prakash *et al.* (2016) observed that it may be possible to subdivide the syndromes. Udina *et al.* (2013) emphasize the heterogeneity of the syndrome, thus reflecting differential emphasis on presentation and help-seeking.

Table 14.1 Findings of studies conducted in clinical settings

Study	Setting	No.	Inclusion criteria	Presenting symptom	Attributes to semen loss	Duration of semen loss	Mode of loss (one or more)					
							in sleep	with urine	masturbation	sex heter.	sex homo.	other
Behete and Natraj (1984)	Psychiatric outpatient clinic at Psychiatry Dept Institute of Med. Sci. India	50	Consecutive referrals. Main complaint of *dhat* discharge	Associated symptoms: impotence, marital problems, premature ejaculation, weakness, others??	No, this was the presenting symptom itself	Less than 3 months to more than 1 year	? Yes unclear	? Yes unclear	? Unclear as given if a cause	? Unclear		
Singh, 1985	Psychiatric outpatient clinic, Ptia, India	50	Consecutive patients of male potency disorder and complaint of *dhat* (N-30)	Primary complaint of loss of semen but accompanied by mental and physical symptoms	Unclear. No reference attribution	Not reported	No? NR?	Yes	No? NR?	No? NR?	No? NR?	No NR?
De Silva and Dissanayeke (1989) Descriptive Study	Referrals to a university psychiatric clinic in Sri Lanka	38	Clear – see the next column. They belonged to four different clinical presentations	Four different groups: (1) Excessive loss of semen (2) Specific sexual dysfunction (3) Anxiety about present or future sexual function (4) Multiple phys/psych symptoms	The presenting complaint. Yes Yes Yes	6 months – 20 years	Yes*	Yes	Yes*	Yes	Yes*	Yes
Chadda and Ahuja (1990) Descriptive Study	University psychiatric clinic in India/ Delhi	52	Passage of *dhat* in urine was presenting feature but has elicited somatic symptoms		Yes (all)	1–12 months			Yes*	Yes*	Yes	Yes

* indicated seen in majority/common NR – not reported.

In a study from Sri Lanka, de Silva and Dissanayake (1989) reported that in their cohort of 38 cases recruited from a sexual dysfunction clinic, various explanations of semen loss were offered. These included excessive loss of semen or associated sexual or physical dysfunction and the accompanying belief that loss of semen was harmful. A majority of individuals reported continuing loss of semen and the duration varied from 6 months to 20 years. More than 50 per cent were found to have somatic symptoms. More than half (53%) received a diagnosis of anxiety, 40% of hypochondriasis and 5% stress reaction. The sample size is small but it indicates the presence of psychological and somatic symptoms to be significant. From the same clinic, Deveraja and Sasaki (1991) collected data from 35 patients who had been attributing their symptoms to loss of semen. Although the numbers are small, 50 per cent reported somatic symptoms and one-third (35%) reported sexual deficiencies. Using an 18-item questionnaire, they found that Sri Lankan students were more likely to believe in semen loss.

Ventriglio *et al.* (2015) propose that *dhat* may be seen as an idiom of distress. Menon *et al.* (2013) indicate that conflicting explanations may be present. The heterogeneity and difficulties in measuring comorbidities may further lead to diagnostic confusion in certain cultures and clinical settings.

In China

Similar observations related to semen loss causing weakness have also been reported from China. However, texts in China suggest that women have the ability to steal vital fluid from men and this loss of semen can lead to disease (Bottero, 1991). Weakness in Chinese people is seen as due to loss of vital energy (*qu*). Excessive loss of semen through sexual intercourse or masturbation creates anxiety because semen is said to contain *jing* (the essence of *qu*) which, when lost, produces weakness (Kleinman, 1988). Yap (1965) posits that a healthy exchange of *yin* and *yang* in sexual intercourse maintains a balance. Following masturbation, nocturnal emission or homosexual intercourse, *yang* may be lost but without corresponding gain of *yin*, and the resulting imbalance therefore leads to disease. This has been associated with epidemics of *koro* (another so-called culture-bound syndrome where the individual holds the belief that the penis is shrinking into the body and disappearing; Yap, 1965; Rin, 1966; Tseng *et al.*, 1988; see later).

Taoist teaching in ancient China believed that seminal essence was held in the lower part of the male abdomen, and the purpose is to increase the amount of life-giving seminal essence (*ching*) through sexual stimulus while at the same time avoiding possible loss (Bullough, 1976). It was essential that the woman reach orgasm in intercourse so that the man would receive her *yin* essence; the more *yin* essence he himself received without giving out his precious male substance, the greater his strength will grow and this could be achieved through *coitus reservatus* – keeping the penis in the vagina but avoiding orgasm. Another technique was to practise *huan ching pu nao* (making the *ching* return to nourish the brain), suggesting that this method and positive thinking would lead to the essence of semen to ascend and rejuvenate parts of the body. Masturbation for men was seen as leading to a loss of vital essence. Manipulation of genitals without orgasm was encouraged, but involuntary emissions were viewed with concern as these led to weakness in men caused by fox spirits.

Views on Semen Loss in the West

The West has not been immune from anxieties related to semen loss. From the times of Hippocrates and Aristotle, semen has been considered extremely important for the healthy functioning of the individual. Although Greeks in ancient times saw masturbation as a natural substitute for those men lacking the opportunity for sexual intercourse, they also believed that the semen supplied the form and the female supplied the matter fit for shaping. Galen, following the example of Aristotle, stated:

> Certain people have an abundant warm sperm which incessantly arouses the need of excretion: however, after its expulsion, people who are in this state experience a languor at the stomach orifice, exhaustion, weakness, and dryness of the whole body. They become thin, their eyes grow shallow . . .
>
> (Galen, 1963)

Thus this clear description is not too dissimilar from that of the modern *dhat* syndrome (see Table 14.2).

Pre-dating the Christian era, Jewish writers also acknowledged that deposit of semen anywhere else other than in the vagina was unacceptable. The male then had to become ritually pure after such emission and a short period of continence was normally required. Masturbation was regarded as a crime deserving the death penalty according to one Talmudic writer. Bullough (1976) points out that

Table 14.2 Timeline of the historical perspective and development of beliefs related to 'semen loss'

Person	Period	Comments
Agnivasa	*c.* 1500 BCE	Charaka Samhita – *An Indian Treatise on Medicine*
Susruta	*c.* sixth century BCE	Susruta Samhita – An *Indian Treatise on Surgery* (the traditional Ayurvedic knowledge of the above two named teachers was systematized and edited in these two texts between 600 BCE and AD 1000 – *samhita* means 'collection'). Semen is the most concentrated, perfect and powerful bodily substance. Its preservation guarantees health and longevity
Hippocrates	*c.* 460–377 BCE	*Diseases II*: Semen supplies the form to the human body
Aristotle	384–322 BCE	'Sperms are the excretion of our food, or to put it more clearly, as the most perfect component of our food'
Celsus	AD 50	'It results in death due to consumption'
Galen	AD 130–201	Involuntary loss was termed as 'gonorrhoea' – it robs the body of its vital breath; 'losing sperm amounts to losing the vital spirits'; exhaustion, weakness, dryness of the whole body, thinness, eyes growing hollow, are the resulting symptoms
Giovanni Sirubaldi	1642	Added gout as caused by semen loss (in *Geneanthropeia*, Europe's first textbook on sexuality)
Jean-Etienne Dominique Esquirol	1772–1840	'One of the most common cases of melancholia and dementia and also commonly suicide'
Andrew Tissot	1728–1797	'Losing one ounce of sperm is more debilitating than losing forty ounces of blood' in *Treatise on the Diseases Produced by Onanism*. His basic tenet was that debility, disease and death are the outcome of semen loss
Henry Maudsley	1835–1918	Semen loss, especially if it occurs through masturbation, results in serious mental illness
George Beard	1839–1883	'One of the commonest explanations of neurasthenia is wastage of sexual energy, often in the form of nocturnal emissions (involuntary emissions)'
Sigmund Freud	1856–1939	'Neurasthenia in males is acquired at puberty and becomes manifest in the patient's twenties. Its source is masturbation, the frequency of which runs completely parallel to that of male neurasthenia'. Freud opposes Steckel's view that semen loss has no pernicious effect on brain functioning
The Lancet (articles and editorials by George Dangerfield and W. H. Ranking)	1840–1843	'On physical disability, mental impairment and moral degeneration caused by seminal loss'; 'The symptoms, pathology, causes and treatment of spermatorrhoea'

fear of loss of semen was well known, but why this loss of semen was so feared is not entirely clear. However, Bullough hypothesizes that the loss of semen may imply the failure on the male's part to procreate and replenish the Earth which was seen as their basic duty. It is, of course entirely possible that unexpected or inappropriate loss of semen may lead to reduction of the tribe, thereby making the tribe vulnerable to other factors perhaps leading to eventual elimination. In Western European cultures, masturbation was often prohibited using religious grounds and rationale. Even nocturnal emissions were seen as a sin and it required three nights of an hour-long standing vigil, provided the sinner had been given an adequate diet of beer and meat. If he had been on a rigid diet, the sinner was required to sing 28 or 30 psalms or to undertake extra work. Apparently, it was assumed that a person who has been fasting would have less control over his bodily processes, hence involuntary nocturnal emissions in these individuals were less serious.

The attitudes to non-heterosexual behaviour and loss of semen varied in the Middle Ages (see Bullough, 1976 for a further discussion). However, for our purposes, Tissot's writings in the eighteenth century provide an interesting overview (Tissot, 1974). He believed that, even with an adequate diet, the body could waste away through diarrhoea, blood loss and seminal emission. Semen caused the beard to grow and muscles to thicken, hence involuntary semen loss weakened the male. Frequent intercourse was dangerous in itself but the most dangerous loss of semen was when the individual lost it through unnatural means and the most debilitating loss was through masturbation. Such loss of semen led to cloudiness of ideas and madness, decay of bodily powers, acute pains in the head, pimples on the face, eventual weakness of the power of generation (as indicated by impotence, premature ejaculation, gonorrhoea, priapism and tumours of the bladder) and disordering of the intestines. This is again not dissimilar to the symptoms and concerns of the patients who present with *dhat*. Tissot gave scientific credibility to the Western hostility to sex. The similarities between the then prevalent hostility to sex in the West and current hostility to sex in the Orient are uncanny. From being a sex-positive society, Hindu culture has become obsessed with procreation, and the main purpose of sex is procreation rather than pleasure. The historical impact of colonialism and before that centuries of Mughal rule may have contributed to this shift of attitudes. The emerging middle classes of the eighteenth century in the West embraced Tissot's ideas with great enthusiasm, and sexual purity became a way of distinguishing themselves from the sexual promiscuity of the noble and the lower classes, which is again very similar to attitudes among burgeoning middle classes in many low- and middle-income countries. Tissot (1764/1974) led the Western world into an age of masturbatory, or shall we say *dhat* insanity. Though Tissot's work did not reach the USA until 1832, his influence was apparent in the writings of Benjamin Rush – father of American psychiatry. Rush believed that all diseases could be caused by debility of the nervous system and propounded that careless indulgence in sex would lead to seminal weakness, impotence, dysuria, tabes dorsalis, pulmonary consumption, dyspepsia, dimness of sight,

vertigo, epilepsy, hypochondriasis, loss of memory, myalgia, fatuity and eventual death (Rush, 1812).

Sylvester Graham advocated graham flour (unbolted wheat) and graham cracker as a cure for debility, skin and lung disease, headaches, nervousness and weakness of the brain – much of which he believed resulted from sexual excess. Graham (1834) blamed orgasm on the abuse or misuse of sexual organs. Over-indulgence in sex caused languor, lassitude, muscular relaxation, general debility and heaviness, depression of spirits, loss of appetite, indigestion, faintness and a sinking feeling in the pit of the stomach, increased susceptibility of skin and lungs, feebleness of circulation, chilliness, headache, melancholy, hypochondria, hysterics, feebleness of senses, impaired vision, loss of memory, epilepsy, insanity, apoplexy, etc. Like the Ayurvedic perceptions, Graham believed that the loss of an ounce of semen was equivalent to the loss of several ounces of blood, with the result that every time a man ejaculated he lowered his life force and exposed his system to diseases. These attitudes are not dissimilar to attitudes held by patients presenting with *dhat* syndrome.

In nineteenth century France, Lallemand (1839) also was concerned with involuntary loss of semen, which would possibly lead to insanity. Acton (1871), an English physician, also encouraged men to engage in sex infrequently so that they would not lose their energy through prolonged sexual activity. He maintained that the worst kind of seminal emission was masturbation.

Kellogg (of the breakfast cereal fame) (1882) believed that the nervous shock accompanying the exercise of the sexual organs was the most profound to which the nervous system was subject, and described a long list of symptoms including physical and psychological – 'the dangers were terrible to behold, senile genital excitement produced intense congestion and led to irritation, priapism, piles and prolapsus of rectum, atrophy of the testes, varicocoele, nocturnal emissions and general exhaustion'. His cereals were developed as a panacea for treating masturbation. It has been argued that this may have also been a result of overproduction of corn! Every loss of semen was regarded as equivalent to the loss of four ounces of blood and, although the body could eventually replace the loss, it took time for it to recuperate (Hunter, 1900).

In the 1840s, articles on the involuntary discharge of seminal fluid dominated *The Lancet*. Dangerfield

(1843) suggested that, as a result of involuntary discharge:

> the patient complains of weakness, restlessness and listlessness, his manners are shy and nervous with a remarkable timidity and indisposition to answer questions, his complexion is generally pale, slightly emaciated, gradually loses memory, has dull pain, and feeling of weakness especially in the lower extremities, along with fatigue. On further investigations, the physician will find that he has been afflicted for some time with seminal emissions during sleep accompanied by libidinous dreams.

In a comprehensive review, Darby (2001) suggests that male circumcision was advocated as a cure for spermatorrhoea (as well as masturbation) and this was the testing ground on which regular medical practitioners sought to establish their credentials and to demarcate themselves from quacks(!). He argues that William Acton in Britain and George Beaney in Australia were representatives of the battle for professional turf and the medical right to manage all the functions of the body. Unfortunately for the regular doctors, until circumcision became an option, the treatments they offered differed little from those of their rivals. Walker (1985, 1987, 1994) points out that nineteenth-century medical orthodoxy held that any seminal loss weakened the system.

In Australia they followed the line of the colonialists, who in turn were pushing for various treatments for semen loss. Darby (2001) points out that it was not always possible to draw a hard and fast line between regular doctors and quacks – the former exhibited plenty of evidence of ignorant faddism and eccentricity, while the latter frequently offered more humane and less damaging treatments. Beaney graduated from Edinburgh and settled in Melbourne in 1857; he published extensively on the damaging effects of spermatorrhoea, suggesting that semen was more precious than blood and that treatments for spermatorrhoea were effective if victims avoided the quacks. Spermatorrhoea was defined as an abnormal emission of the seminal fluid, and 'that of all the diseases to which man is liable, there are few others which induce so much mental anxiety as this; it embitters all the victim's [sic] social relations and subjects him to the harrowing reflection that he is the object of the taunts and jeers of those about him' (Beaney, 1870).

Masturbation was both a specific form of spermatorrhoea and its cause, which then ruined the nervous equilibrium of the sexual system. The consequences of masturbation and spermatorrhoea included inflammation of the urethra, bladder irritation, disturbed sleep, erotic dreams, confusion of mind, vertigo, wakefulness, depression, tuberculosis, epilepsy and impotence. Darby (2001) suggests that Beaney's views are religious tub-thumping and not scientific. However, it is entirely possible that Beaney is merely reflecting the prevalent view of spermatorrhoea and the semen-loss anxiety. In making his views more culturally specific to Australian manhood, Beaney makes the point that the relatively free and easy life of the Antipodes, the more relaxed social structure and the more intimate mingling of the sexes may indeed lead to increasing sexual precocity among children, thus magnifying the threat to Australian manhood. The treatments recommended included Sitz baths, alcohol and chemical compounds like potassium bromide and phosphorus and application of electricity to the nervous system. Gradually, circumcision came to be seen as a treatment for these sexual urges. Thus it would appear that, in the nineteenth-century colonies too, the anxieties related to semen loss persisted. Whether the clinicians were reflecting their own anxieties or those of their patients remains a moot point. What is clear is that semen-loss anxiety is neither a new condition nor confined to the Orient and neither is its presentation or explanations of the consequences.

The scientific backing to morality and making sexual activity prohibitive continued unabated in the nineteenth and early twentieth centuries. The impact of these on the 'patients' is uncertain but there is little doubt that a lot of the writings of Graham, Kellogg and others were directed at the general population as part of the public education. Therefore, there must have been a need for such advice because most of these monographs went into several editions and were translated into several languages. Needless to say, similarities between their writings and the present-day descriptions of *dhat* are striking.

We have presented historical data from among the studies from the West (Australia is included in the west in this context), and our contention is that with industrialization and colonization, the anxiety about semen loss in the West may have diminished and the same may well happen in South Asia as well, as cultures evolve and change. If we understand *dhat* as a culture-bound syndrome, the historical evidence indicates that it was prevalent in Europe, the USA and Australia in the nineteenth century but never seen as culture-bound. It may have disappeared in response to changing social and economic factors, whereas it carries on as is, in South Asia. We believe that the universality of symptoms of anxiety (in this case secondary to fear or actual loss of semen) has to be acknowledged. Although there are discrepancies in the data from modern-day India and only descriptions exist in the eighteenth and nineteenth century, it proves that *dhat* syndrome is not culture-bound and it is not an exotic neurosis of the Orient. Furthermore, it is our contention that the *dhat* syndrome as described in the literature from the Indian subcontinent is not always a homogeneous entity; and although syndromes by definition are heterogeneous, the symptoms described are more likely to be psychological or psychosomatic, even though their attribution to *dhat* may be culture influenced. Our contention is that collectivist societies allow anxiety to be expressed in a way that is secretive, and semen loss in the context of procreation becomes significant. It is thus also possible that semen-loss anxiety disappeared in the West as family and kinship structures changed. Whether industrialization and urbanization contributed to this change needs further exploration. In cultures-in-transition it is entirely possible that the same changes will occur a few decades from now. The idioms of distress will also change according to educational status so it is entirely likely that presentations and explanations will also change.

There is no doubt that, as Tseng (2001) has asserted, cultures do influence psychopathology through pathogenetic, pathoselective, pathoplastic, pathoelaborating, pathofacilitating and pathoreactive effects (also see Chapter 11). However, we believe that the interaction between the individual and the culture remains extremely complex. Even if culture is being pathofacilitatory or pathoreactive, the individual pathology can be, and will be, influenced by other factors, such as personality traits, educational and economic status, peer and family support available to the individual, alternative explanations of the experience, etc. The society and cultures do dictate pathways into help-seeking and care and resources – economic, political and human-allocated. Tseng (2001) proposes that these syndromes be sub-grouped according to the six impacts of cultures, but we believe that DSM-5 has done the right thing by abandoning this category altogether and focusing on multi-axial systems which include cultural factors in aetiology and management. *Dhat* provides an illustration that,

when looked at carefully, these conditions transcend cultural boundaries and any variations should be seen in the cultural/individual context.

We believe that attribution patterns on explanatory models regarding semen-loss anxiety need to be studied in different cultures in order to confirm what we have hypothesized. We accept that loss of semen is a shared belief reported from certain societies. It may be that this is reported because the clinicians and the researchers are aware of it and therefore are willing to ask questions regarding such an attribution. Certainly in the clinical practice in the West, the topic hardly ever comes up and clinicians do not explore the topic.

Latah

Latah is often described as a classical example of a culture-bound syndrome (Bhugra and Jacob 1997). Provoked usually by a short, loud noise or a prod in the ribs, it constitutes a dissociative state with altered consciousness, coprolalia, echolalia, echopraxia and, in extremely severe cases, 'command automation'. Yap (1952) described the condition as occurring in middle-aged women of the Malay or other indigenous races of Southeast Asia. The clinical features include sudden onset after an acute fidget, episodic echolalia, echopraxia and coprolalia and is induced by sudden touching in poor vulnerable individuals. Local culture sees this as a state rather than a 'disease' (Friedman, 1982). In a study, 50 cases of *latah* were diagnosed in 12,000 Malaysians. Of the 50 cases, 7 had a clinical diagnosis of schizophrenia, neurosis or adjustment reaction; another 14 had mixed diagnoses and were all women. The cases had sexual conflict as an associated factor (Chiu *et al.*, 1972). Simons (1985) described three types of *latah* – immediate response, attention captive and the role *latah*. The role *latah* is strongly influenced by social factors and the individuals are mostly female and have marginal social status. Yap (1952) saw coprolalia as a publicly sanctioned expression of sexual undertones, as did Murphy (1976).

Winzeler in an ethnographic study summarized *latah* paradox as the proposition that while *latah* can only be understood in highly specific culture terms unique to the Javanese (or to the Javanese and other Malay peoples), it occurs also among various distant peoples as well (Winzeler, 1995: 3). Writing about *latah* and *amok* has been in conjunction with other favourite colonialist topics, which created and perpetuated images of Malays as mentally deficient, thereby justifying and indeed encouraging the European domination (Alatas, 1977: 48). Dreissen and Tijssen (2012) point out that startle syndromes are paroxysmal and show stimulus sensitivity which may make them respond to benzodiazepines.

Winzeler (1995) concurs with this observation but is generous in his interpretation that these orientalist observers did not mean to do so. Included in the accounts are the general observations about the Malayan character, which might indicate inferiority and a possible improvement under European rule. In the context of *latah*, this observation becomes further complicated because the focus of study is sexual and among women. The perceived nervous, sensitive and volatile nature of the colonized was not confined only to the Malay but also to other ruled populations who had to be saved from themselves. Although initially written about by Western psychiatrists and observers, subsequently local psychiatrists such as Yap contributed to these observations.

The earliest record of *latah* is said to be in 1849 (Winzeler, 1995). Exotic startle patterns were also reported from places as far apart as Maine and Siberia in the last quarter of the nineteenth century and similar patterns also emerged from descriptions in Norway, Iceland and Madagascar (Winzeler, 1995: 33). Yap (1952: 515) too noted that the French, Italian, Dutch and English observers had used the term *latah* in non-Malaysian instances. Thai, Indonesian, Philippine, French Canadian, Lapp and African descriptions of conditions similar to latah have been offered. In Indonesia sometimes a term *gigiren* is used (Winzeler, 1995: 40) which is roughly similar to *mali mali* used in the Philippines and *bahtschi* in Thailand. In cases of *bahtschi* the people affected were women, factory workers and migrants to urban areas. 'Jumping' was described among the French Canadians in rural Maine where responses were provoked by startle or commands given in a quick lowered voice and the affected individuals will then imitate voices and actions (Beard, 1886). These observations indicate a universality of this process. Winzeler (1995: 41) points out that these actions were seen as exotic and therefore to be explained away by reference to arctic or tropical climates, non-Caucasian racial constitutions and outlandish customs and beliefs. Nearly a century later, Chapel (1970) and Kunkle (1967) found and reported on such cases. Among the Lapps similar behaviour was found (Collinder, 1949: 152). Although women were seen to

be affected more commonly, the African–Arabian type of *latah* and the French Canadian variety affects men more commonly. Automatic obedience is less likely in the Arab–African variety, as is coprolalia. These differences may reflect the type of society and cultural norms and values as well as cultural status of the individuals, which may influence the symptom content.

Winzeler (1995), in his ethnographic study from the centre of the coastal plain in Malaysia, suggests that the term *latah* has been used in different ways. It can be used as talking nonsense, or a particular pattern of behaviour or a tendency/vulnerability to such behaviours. Two forms of *latah* were observed – these were startlers or followers. He found that although children may play at *latah*, the condition is largely limited to adults (Winzeler, 1995: 62). More common among women (attributed to women having less soul or blood than men) and the poor, *latah* has become a stylized, more or less common, pattern of behaviour.

Winzeler (1995: 75) emphasizes that, although *latah* has been analysed both as a startle reaction (Simons, 1980, 1983) and as a fear reaction (Yap, 1952), these are closely related. Startle has been associated with both magical transformations and magical power. The relationships between *latah*, shamans and midwives and trance states are well known. Bhidayasiri and Truong (2011) in describing three types of startle include *latah* as one of the varieties. They note that it can be seen as a protective function against injury. Bakker *et al.* (2013) indicate that following their startle response, *latah* patients showed stereotyped responses including vocalizations and echo phenomena thereby supporting the classification of *latah* as a 'neuropsychiatric startle syndrome'. This indicates that individuals who tend to show hyperstartle reflexes are seen across countries.

There is no doubt that, whatever form *latah* takes, it has symbolic meaning and by providing an opportunity for tomfoolery and aggressive teasing along with sexual humour, it allows an expression which is otherwise inhibited. *Latah* allows an inversion of dominant cultural standards of polite and proper behaviour (Winzeler, 1995: 99). Winzeler (1995: 129) argues forcefully that *latah*, whether true or imitative, must be seen as a form of trance and understood in that light. Thus this would avoid what would appear to be serious danger of turning this into a medicalized experience.

Susto

Susto refers to fright or some loss and represents a disorder among Latinos in the US, Central and South America and Mexico, and the main worry is related to experience of fear. It is seen as an event which by its fearful nature leads the soul to leave the body, and results in unhappiness, sickness and social withdrawal. Such feelings may persist for years after the initial fright. The core symptoms of poor or increased appetite, too little or excess sleep, feeling low, poor motivation, low self-worth, somatic symptoms of aches and pains may be seen. At a clinical level all these symptoms can be seen as reflecting depression; whether that is mild or moderate or severe remains to be ascertained. Rubel *et al.* (1984) studied three communities in Central America. *Susto* patients were identified using a number of clear criteria, along with levels of social stress and levels of psychiatric impairments as well as those of organic disease. Patients with *susto* had significantly higher levels of psychiatric pathology, and an average of 5.15 diseases per patient were diagnosed. The prevalence of mental disorders was different across the three communities studied. Digestive disorders were more common among the patients of *susto* when compared with controls. On objective laboratory tests, levels of haemoglobin indicated that patients were more likely to be anaemic compared with controls. Rubel *et al.* (1984: 112) point out that they utilized an open system model emphasizing interactions among the social, emotional and biological dimensions of individuals. These authors found that *susto* was associated with the person's perceptions of their inadequacy in the performance of their social roles. The aggregation of symptoms indicated an organic causation. It can be argued that the 'stress' of the fright may push the individual towards a depression-like condition.

Amok

Amok describes a syndrome with an element of dissociation where an individual commits furious or violent assault of homicidal intensity often associated with the indigenous population of the Malaysian archipelago (Carr and Tan, 1976). The predominant and most dramatic aspect of the syndrome is mass assault which would warrant placing it in the impulse control category (Bhugra and Jacob, 1997). Of the ten cases of true *amok* reported by Carr and Tan (1976), seven had delusions and/or hallucinations at the time of admission. Alcohol (Westermeyer, 1982) and cerebral malaria (van Loon, 1927) have been reported as contributory factors. Folk explanations include *amok* as a step towards preparing for war and a response to strict hierarchical society. *Amok* is often seen as a culture-bound syndrome, but similar attacks as exemplified by many episodes in the USA such as the Columbine School massacre are no different than attacks of *amok* but are never seen or discussed as such.

Koro

Koro is often reported from China and countries of Southeast Asia (probably originating from the Japanese word signifying tortoise) and usually the male sufferer has a primary feeling that his penis is shrinking into the body with a fear of impending death. Females who experience this may feel that their nipples or vulva are shrinking leading to panic (Crozier, 2011). It is not uncommon to have associated feelings of depersonalization. Folk explanations include worry and guilt about sex (Yap, 1965) and changes in socio-economic status. Perceptions of size are also changed. It has been reported from other parts of the world, including an epidemic in Nigeria. *Koro* is a syndrome in which it is felt that the penis (or sometimes the nipples or vulva) is retracting, with deleterious effects for the sufferer. In modern psychiatry, it is considered a culture-bound syndrome (CBS). Crozier (2011) offers an explanation of *koro* as a good example of culture-bound syndrome against the backdrop of emerging ideas about culture and psychiatry dating from the late colonial period, especially in Africa, which are central to modern ideas about transcultural psychiatry. It has been reported in cases with a diagnosis of schizophrenia (Afonso *et al.*, 2013), psychosis (Ramamourty *et al.*, 2014), Cotard's syndrome in a Spanish male (Alvarez *et al.*, 2012), in Greece (Ntouras *et al.*, 2010, in Bengal (Chakraborty and Sanyal, 2012; Kumar *et al.*, 2014), Oman (Al-Sinawi *et al.*, 2008), thus indicating that far from being confined to certain specific cultures, it occurs widely as a syndrome as well as a comorbid condition.

The Relationship between Psychiatric Disorders and Culture-Bound Syndromes

Figure 14.1 describes the relationship between psychiatric and culture-bound disorders. Many conditions such as eating disorders, shoplifting,

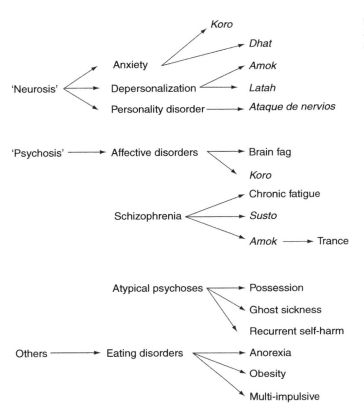

Figure 14.1 Interaction between psychiatric disorders and culture-bound syndromes. (Modified from Bhugra and Jacob, 1997.)

parasuicide, agoraphobia and flashing have been described as Western culture-bound syndromes (Littlewood and Lipsedge, 1985; Rittenbaugh, 1982; Winzeler, 1995). Increasingly, with changes in socio-economic conditions and power structures there, these too are beginning to appear in low- and middle-income countries.

The DSM-5 (APA, 2013) recognizes that there is seldom a one-to-one correspondence of any cultural concept with a DSM diagnosis. There is an explicit acknowledgement that such correspondence is likely to be one-to-many in either direction. There is an implicit recognition that symptoms which may be seen in many DSM disorders may well be included in a single folk concept. The DSM-5 notes that three concepts of syndromes, idioms and explanations are more relevant to clinical practice than the old concepts of culture-bound syndromes

Whereas DSM-IV (APA, 1994a) and DSM-IV TR (APA, 1994b) offered an outline for cultural formulation (where multi-axial diagnostic assessments were supplemented by a systematic review of the individual's cultural background and the role of the cultural context in the expression and evaluation of symptoms and dysfunction), DSM-5 has absorbed this to create the cultural formulation interview. There is now a clear recognition that cultural differences between the individual seeking help and clinician offering such help will influence the therapeutic relationship and interventions between them. There is no doubt that cultural identity of the individual is crucial in a number of ways in influencing idioms of distress and where the individuals seek help from. Therefore, cultural explanations of the distress acknowledged and understood by the individual along with psychological, social and cultural environment, their levels of functioning under these circumstances and the therapeutic relationship between the individual and clinician, are important. If all these factors are taken into account and used seriously in diagnoses, then the scope for culture-bound syndromes becomes even more limited. The DSM-5 does retain the category of cultural concepts of distress which highlight nine conditions which were previously considered as culture-bound syndromes (APA, 2013). The nine conditions are:

1. *ataque de nervios*
2. *dhat* syndrome
3. *khyal cap*
4. *kufungisisa*
5. *maladi moun*
6. *nervios*
7. *shenjing shuairuo*
8. *susto*
9. *taijin kyofusho*.

Several of these syndromes reflect patients' levels of anxiety, related to perceived weakness of the nervous system and may not be seen as clinical or medical conditions. Clinicians therefore must be cautious in exploring these and not turn these into medical or psychiatric conditions. Each of these conditions is linked with multiple other conditions within DSM-5. A balanced understanding between illness and disease experiences is critical.

Conclusions

There are significant problems in the use of terms such as culture-bound syndromes because all psychiatric conditions are arguably culture bound. It is important to recognize that cultures influence how distress is expressed; how it is understood and analysed and how help is sought as well as sources for help. Culture-bound syndromes reflect the colonial past of the country and state. It is important to recognize that cultures play a key role in all types of distress and explanatory models that people use.

Acknowledgments

Athula Sumathipala and Sisira Siribaddana contributed to the chapter in the first edition.

References

Acton, W. (1871). *The Functions and Disorders of the Reproductive Organs in Childhood, Youth, Adult Age, and Advanced Life Considered in their Physiological, Social and Moral Relations*. London: J. and A. Churchill.

Afonso, P., Saraiva, S. and Gameiro, Z. (2013). Schizophrenia presenting with koro-like symptoms. *Journal of Neuropsychiatry and Clinical Neurosciences*, 25(1), E32–E32.

Alatas, S. H. (1977). *The Myth of the Lazy Native*. London: Frank Cass.

Al-Sinawi, H., Al-Adawi, S. and Al-Guenedi, A. (2008). Ramadan fasting triggering koro-like symptoms during acute alcohol withdrawal: a case report from Oman. *Transcultural Psychiatry*, 45(4), 695–704.

Alvarez, P., Puente, V., Blasco, M., Salgado, P., Merino, A. and Bulbena, A. (2012). Concurrent koro and Cotard syndromes in a Spanish male patient with a psychotic depression and cerebrovascular disease. *Psychopathology*, 45(2), 126–129.

American Psychiatric Association (APA) (1994a). *Diagnostic and Statistical Manual of Mental Disorders*, 4th edn (DSM-IV). Washington, DC: APA.

American Psychiatric Association (APA) (1994b). *Diagnostic and Statistical Manual of Mental Disorders-TR, (DSM-IV-TR)*. Washington, DC: APA.

American Psychiatric Association (APA)(2013). *Diagnostic and Statistical Manual of Mental Disorders, 5th edn. (DSM-5)*. Washington, DC: APA.

Arieti, S. and Meth, J. (1959). Rare, unclassifiable, collective and exotic syndromes. In *American Handbook of Psychiatry*, ed. S. Arieti. New York: Basic Books.

Ayonrinde, O. and Bhugra, D. (2015). Culture-bound syndromes. In *Troublesome Disguises*, ed. D. Bhugra and G. Malhi. Chichester: Wiley Blackwell, pp. 231–251.

Bakker, M., van Dijk, J., Pramono, A., Sutarni, S. and Tijssen, M. (2013). Latah: an Indonesian startle syndrome. *Movement Disorders*, 28(3), 370–379.

Beaney, G. J. (1870). *Spermatorrhoea in its Physiological, Medical and Legal Aspects*. Melbourne: Walker Publishers.

Beard, G. M. (1886). Experiments with the 'Jumpers' or 'Jumping Frenchmen' of Maine. *The Journal of Nervous and Mental Disorders*, 7, 487–491.

Behere, P. B. and Nataraj, G. S. (1984). Dhat syndrome: the phenomenology of a culture-bound sex neurosis of the Orient. *Indian Journal of Psychiatry*, 26(1), 76–78.

Bhatia, M. S. and Malik, S. C. (1991). Dhat syndrome: a useful diagnostic entity in Indian culture. *British Journal of Psychiatry*, 159, 691–695.

Bhidayasiri, R. and Truong, D. (2011). Startle syndromes. *Handbook of Clinical Neurology*, 100(32), 421–430.

Bhugra, D. (2005). Cultural identities and cultural congruency: a new model for evaluating mental distress in immigrants. *Acta Psychiatrica Scandinavica*, 111(2), 84–93.

Bhugra, D. and Buchanan, A. (1989). Impotence in ancient Indian texts. *Sexual and Marital Therapy*, 4, 87–92.

Bhugra, D. and Jacob, K. S. (1997). Culture-bound syndromes. In *Troublesome Disguises: Underdiagnosed Psychiatric Syndromes*, ed. D. Bhugra and A. Munro. Oxford: Blackwell Science, pp. 296–334.

Bottero, A. (1991). Consumption by semen loss in India and elsewhere. *Culture, Medicine and Psychiatry*, 15, 303–320.

Bullough, V. L. (1976). *Sexual Variance in Society and History*. Chicago: University of Chicago Press.

Carr, J. and Tan, E. (1976). In search of the true *amok: amok* as viewed within the Malay culture. *American Journal of Psychology*, 133, 1295–1299.

Chadda, R. K. (1995). Dhat syndrome: is it a distinct clinical entity? *Acta Psychiatrica Scandinavia*, 91, 136–139.

Chadda, R. K. and Ahuja, N. (1990). Dhat syndrome: a sex neurosis in Indian subcontinent. *British Journal of Psychiatry*, 156, 577–579.

Chakraborty, S. and Sanyal, D. (2012). An outbreak of koro among 19 workers in a jute mill in south Bengal. *Industrial Psychiatry Journal*, 20(1), 58.

Chapel, J. L. (1970). Gilles de la Tourette's Syndrome: latah, myriachit and jumpers revisited. *New York State Journal of Medicine*, 1, 2201–2204.

Chiu, T. L., Tong, J. E. and Schmidt, K. E. (1972). A clinical and survey study of latah in Sarawak. *Psychological Medicine*, 2, 155–165.

Collinder, B. (1949). *The Lapps*. Princeton, NJ: Princeton University Press.

Crozier, I. (2011). Making up koro: multiplicity, psychiatry, culture, and penis-shrinking anxieties. *Journal of the History of Medicine and Allied Sciences*, 67(1), 36–70.

Dangerfield, G. N. (1843). The symptoms, pathology, causes, and treatment of spermatorrhoea. *The Lancet*, I, 211–216.

Darby, R. (2001). A source of serious mischief. In *Understanding Circumcision*, ed. G. C. Denniston, F. M. Hodges and M. F. Milos. New York: Kluwer Academic Press, pp. 153–197.

De Silva, P. and Dissanayeke, S. A. W. (1989). The loss of semen syndrome in Sri Lanka: a clinical study. *Sex and Marital Therapy*, 4(2), 195–204.

Deveraja, R. and Sasaki, Y. (1991). Semen loss syndrome: a comparison between Sri Lanka and Japan. *American Journal of Psychotherapy*, xlv, 1, 14–20.

Devereux, G. (1956). Normal and abnormal. In *Some Uses of Anthropology, Theoretical and Applied*, ed. J. B. Casagrande and T. Gladwin. Washington, DC: Anthropological Society of Washington.

Dhikav, V., Aggarwal, N., Gupta, S., Jadhavi, R. and Singh, K. (2008). Depression in dhat syndrome. *The Journal of Sexual Medicine*, 5(4), 841–844.

Dreissen, Y. and Tijssen, M. (2012). The startle syndromes: physiology and treatment. *Epilepsia*, 53, 3–11.

Friedman, C. T. H. (1982). The so called hysteropsychoses: latah, windigo and pibloktoq. In *Extraordinary Disorders of Human Behaviour*, ed. C. T. H. Friedman, and R. Faguet. New York: Plenum, pp. 215–228.

Galen (1963 reprint). *On the Passion and Error of the Soul* (trans. P. W. Hawkins). Columbus, OH: Ohio State University Press.

Gautham, M., Singh, R., Weiss, H., Brugha, R., Patel, V., Desai, N., Nandan, D., Kielmann, K. and Grosskurth, H.

(2008). Socio-cultural, psychosexual and biomedical factors associated with genital symptoms experienced by men in rural India. *Tropical Medicine and International Health*, 13(3), 384–395.

Graham, S. (1834). *A Lecture to Young Men on Chastity*. Boston: C. H. Pierce.

Grover, S., Gupta, S. and Avasthi, A. (2015a). Psychological correlates and psychiatric morbidity in patients with dhat syndrome. *Indian Journal of Psychiatry*, 57(3), 255.

Grover, S., Gupta, S., Mehra, A. and Avasthi, A. (2015b). Comorbidity, knowledge and attitude towards sex among patients with dhat syndrome: a retrospective study. *Asian Journal of Psychiatry*, 17, 50–55.

Haldipur, C. V. (1980). The idea of cultural psychiatry: a comment on the foundations of cultural psychiatry. *Comprehensive Psychology*, 21, 206–211.

Hofstede, G. (1980). *Culture's Consequences*. Beverly Hills, CA: Sage.

Hofstede, G. (1984). *Culture's Consequences (abridged)*. Beverly Hills, CA: Sage.

Hughes, C. C. (1985). Glossary. In *Culture-Bound Syndromes: Folk Illnesses of Psychiatric and Anthropological Interest*, ed. R. C. Simons and C. C. Hughes. Dordrecht: Reidel, pp. 469–505.

Hughes, C. C. and Wintrob, R. M. (1995). Culture-bound syndromes and the cultural context of clinical psychiatry. In *Review of Psychiatry*, ed. J. M. Oldham and M. Riba. Washington DC: APA Press.

Hunter, W. J. (1900). *Manhood: Wrecked and Rescued*. New York: Health Culture Company.

Kellogg, J. H. (1882). *Plain Facts for Old and Young*. Burlington, IA: I. F. Senger.

Kleinman, A. (1988). *The Illness Narratives: Suffering, Healing and the Human Condition*. New York: Basic Books.

Kumar, R., Phookun, H. and Datta, A. (2014). Epidemic of Koro in north east India: an observational cross-sectional study. *Asian Journal of Psychiatry*, 12, 113–117.

Kunkle, E. C. (1967). The 'Jumpers' of Maine: a reappraisal. *Archives of Internal Medicine*, 119, 355–358.

Lallemand, M. (1839). *On Involuntary Seminal Discharges* (trans. W. Wood). Philadelphia: A. Waldier.

Littlewood, R. and Lipsedge, M. (1985). Culture-bound syndromes. In *Recent Advances in Psychiatry*, ed. K. Granville-Grossman. Edinburgh: Churchill Livingstone.

Maercker, A. (2001). Association of cross-cultural differences in psychiatric morbidity with cultural values: a secondary data analysis. *German Journal of Psychiatry*, 4, 17–23.

Malhotra, H. K. and Wig, N. N. (1975). Dhat syndrome: a culture-bound sex neurosis of the Orient. *Archives of Sexual Behaviour*, 4(5), 519–528.

Menéndez, V., Fernández-Suárez, A., Placer, J., García-Linares, M., Tarragon, S. and Liso, E. (2012). Dhat syndrome, an emergent condition within urology in Spain. *World Journal of Urology*, **31**(4), 941–945.

Menon, V., Shrivastava, M. and Kattimani, S. (2013). Is semen loss syndrome a psychological or physical illness? A case for conflict of interest. *Indian Journal of Psychological Medicine*, **35**(4), 420.

Murphy, H. B. M. (1976). Notes for a theory on latah. In *Culture-Bound Syndromes: Ethno-psychiatry and Alternate Therapies*, ed. W. P. Lebra. Honolulu: University of Hawaii Press, pp. 3–21.

Murphy, H. B. M. (1977). Transcultural psychiatry should begin at home. *Psychological Medicine*, 7, 369–371.

Ntouros, E., Ntoumanis, A., Bozikas, V., Donias, S., Giouzepas, I. and Garyfalos, G. (2010). Koro-like symptoms in two Greek men. *BMJ Case Reports*, 15 March, doi: 10.1136/bcr.08.2008.067.

Prakash, S., Sharan, P. and Sood, M. (2016). A study on phenomenology of dhat syndrome in men in a general medical setting. *Indian Journal of Psychiatry*, **58**(2), 129.

Ramamourty, P., Menon, V. and Aparna, M. (2014). Koro presenting as acute and transient psychosis: implications for classification. *Asian Journal of Psychiatry*, **10**, 116–117.

Rin, H. (1966). Koro: a consideration on Chinese concepts of illness and case illustrations. *Transcultural Psychiatry*, **15**, 23–30.

Rittenbaugh, C. (1982). Obesity as a culture-bound syndrome. *Cultural Medicine and Psychiatry*, **6**, 347–361.

Rubel, A. J., O'Neill, C. W. and Collado-Ardón, R. (1984). *Susto: A Folk Illness*. Berkeley, CA: University of California Press.

Rush, B. (1812). *Medical Inquiries and Observations upon the Diseases of the Mind*. Philadelphia: Kimber and Richardson.

Simons, R. C. (1980). The resolution of the latah paradox. *Journal of Nervous and Mental Disorders*, **168**, 195–206.

Simons, R. C. (1983). Latah II: problems with a purely symbolic interpretation. *Journal of Nervous and Mental Disease*, **171**, 168–175.

Simons, R. C. (1985). The resolution of the latah paradox. In *Culture-Bound Syndromes: Folk Illnesses of Psychiatric and Anthropological Interest*, ed. R. Simons and C. C. Hughes. Dordrecht: Reidel, pp. 43–62.

Simons, R. C. and Hughes, C. C. (eds) (1985). *Culture Bound Syndromes*. Dordrecht: Rendel.

Singh, G. (1985). Dhat syndrome revisited. *Indian Journal of Psychiatry*, **27**(2), 119–122.

Tissot, S. A. (1764/1974). A treatise on the diseases produced by onanism. In *The Secret Vice Exposed: Some Arguments against Masturbation*, ed. C. Rosenberg and C. Smith-Rosenberg. New York: Arno Press. First published 1764, London: J. Pridden.

Tseng, W.-S. (2001). *Handbook of Cultural Psychiatry*. San Diego, CA: Academic Press.

Tseng, W.-S., Mo, K. M., Hsu, J. *et al.* (1988). A sociocultural study of koro epidemics in Guangdong. *American Journal of Psychiatry*, **145**, 1538–1543.

Udina, M., Foulon, H., Valdés, M., Bhattacharyya, S. and Martín-Santos, R. (2013). Dhat syndrome: a systematic review. *Psychosomatics*, **54**(3), 212–218.

Van Loon, F. H. G. (1927). Amok and latah. *Journal of the Abnormal and Social Psychology*, **21**, 434–444.

Ventriglio, A., Ayonrinde, O. and Bhugra, D. (2015). Relevance of culture-bound syndromes in the 21st century. *Psychiatry Clin Neurosci*, **70**(1), 3–6.

Walker, D. (1985). Continence for a nation: seminal loss and national vigour. *Labour History*, **48**, 1–14.

Walker, D. (1987). Modern nerves, nervous moderns: notes on male neurasthenia. *Australian Cultural History*, **6**, 49–63.

Walker, D. (1994). Energy and fatigue. *Australian Cultural History*, **13**, 164–178.

Westermeyer, J. (1982). Amok. In *Extraordinary Disorders of Human Behaviour*, ed. C. T. Friedmann and R. A. Faguet. New York: Plenum, pp. 173–190.

Wig, N. N. (1960). Problems of the mental health in India. *Journal of Clinical and Social Psychiatry (India)*, **17**, 48–53.

Winzeler, R. (1995). *Latah in Southeast Asia: The History and Ethnography of a Culture Bound Syndrome*. Cambridge: Cambridge University Press.

World Health Organization (WHO) (1992). *ICD-10 Classification of Mental and Behavioural Disorders*. Geneva: World Health Organization.

Yap, P. M. (1952). The latah reaction: its pathodynamics and nosological position. *Journal of Nervous and Mental Disease*, **98**, 515–564.

Yap, P. M. (1962). Words and things in comparative psychiatry with special reference to exotic psychosis. *Acta Psychiatrica Scandinavica*, **38**, 157–182.

Yap, P. M. (1965). Koro: a culture-bound depersonalised syndrome. *British Journal of Psychiatry*, **111**, 43–50.

Yap, P. M. (1969). The culture-bound reactive syndromes. In *Mental Health Research in Asia and the Pacific*, ed. W. Caudill and T. Y. Lin. Honolulu: East–West Center Press.

Chapter 15

Psychiatric Epidemiology and its Contributions to Cultural Psychiatry

Robert Kohn and Kamaldeep Bhui

Editors' Introduction

Cultures affect rates of mental illness and epidemiology provides us with the tools to understand how rates of various psychiatric disorders vary and what the potential causes and explanatory factors can be. The relationship between cultural psychiatry and psychiatric epidemiology remains in a constructive tension. Although in certain fields of cultural psychiatry studies are problematic because of small numbers, the basic premise of epidemiology, usually requiring large data sets, can be employed provided the interpretation of the findings is clearly contextualized. The measurement of psychopathology across cultures using the same set of tools especially if they have been developed and validated in one population but used in another is fraught with major difficulties. The category fallacy under these circumstances raises critical questions. It is also of interest that often these assessment tools move from Euro–US centric settings to the rest of the world, rather than the other way around. It is important to recognize conceptual equivalence and validity as well. In this chapter Kohn and Bhui examine the contribution of psychiatric epidemiology to cultural psychiatry, and some controversial questions. They argue that over the last several decades psychiatric epidemiology has undergone at least three generations of evolution, followed most recently by a fourth generation from which cultural epidemiology has emerged as a new branch of epidemiology, taking in perspectives from medical anthropology, epidemiology and public health. The implications of these changes are significant, both for research and clinical practice. There is no doubt that there are common clinical features in many psychiatric conditions which are seen and recognized in different cultural settings. Kohn and Bhui urge that psychiatric epidemiology must take cultural factors into account.

Introduction

The methodological advances of psychiatric epidemiology revealed the limitations of earlier psychiatric research. These critiques had implications for the use of diagnostic instruments, and for the methodological advances needed to study cultures and compare mental health problems in diverse cultural groups. Psychiatric epidemiologists have undertaken cross-national comparisons, but have not always paid attention to the critiques of cultural psychiatry and anthropology. From a public health point of view, these advances have highlighted the significant burden of mental illness in many societies in the world, and the need for greater emphasis on providing mental healthcare. Availability of care may vary from indigenous practices within the lay and folk sectors of healing, to the use of statutory services.

Three critical questions arise in the role of psychiatric epidemiology in cultural psychiatry:

- Have these methodological advances preserved the meaning of culture (the emic) in the research of heterogeneous populations?
- Is it valid and appropriate that research instruments used for case ascertainment and establishment of disability in one culture and society, be translated and adapted for use across differing groups of people; or should instruments always be constructed ground-up for every single cultural group?
- Perhaps, a more challenging question is whether DSM-IV/DSM-5 or ICD-10/ICD-11 can be applied universally.

If the answer to some or all of those questions were in the negative, research findings from conventional psychiatric epidemiology might legitimately be challenged. Much effort on cultural issues is seen in the development of DSM-5, with the introduction of the cultural formulation interview, sections on cultural issues throughout, and the cultural formulation no longer in an appendix. Field trials contributed to this effort, although the methods and processes for ICD-11 are yet (at the time of writing) to be made public.

If epidemiological methods do not address these three critical quesions, clues from epidemiological studies about aetiology and treatment would then be open to suspicion. Indeed, some have argued that comparative epidemiology and psychiatric research does not have a place in researching culturally diverse populations, that each population perhaps requires a special ethnography to epidemiology practice that is internally coherent and meaningful and only then to be compared with imported concepts and methods. The socio-cultural influences in mental healthcare and measuring mental disorders perhaps make studies of psychiatric disorders especially vulnerable, but similar arguments might be made about cardiovascular disease or cancer around psychosocial and lifestyle related risk factors and interventions. Such statements might be interpreted to imply that the study of culture should be restricted to anthropologists or sociologists using qualitative methods; alternatively, research of cultural groups has also been proposed to only be possible if people from the culture of interest undertake the research either as service users or sufferers of mental health problems, or even as professional researchers. The latter proposition requires a substantial commitment to build capacity for research among diverse groups, by recruiting researchers from diverse cultural backgrounds. The implications are that there are whole new methodologies and concepts to discover, before we can make use of existing evidence; clearly such a tenet is theoretically pure but practically inefficient and unlikely to be resourced.

Psychiatric Epidemiology: A Brief History

Epidemiology is the study of the distribution of diseases, disorders or conditions in populations, and the factors that contribute to that distribution. The goals of psychiatric epidemiology are to describe the occurrence of mental or behavioural disorders; determine the risk factors associated with their onset, course and outcome; provide data for programmed planning and evaluation in the domains of prevention, care and rehabilitation; and assist in the determination of clinical syndromes.

One of the first major attempts to examine the true prevalence of mental disorders in the community was conducted by Jarvis in 1855 in Massachusetts, USA (Jarvis, 1971). His study included both treated and untreated cases in the community. Jarvis found that the Irish immigrants to the state were at increased risk for psychopathology, a result due to individuals in the pauper class having 64 times higher risk of 'insanity'. Since this seminal study, psychiatric epidemiology has undergone at least three discernible generations of methodological advancement (Dohrenwend and Dohrenwend, 1982), and now a fourth. Each generation has improved its methods of data collection and the classification of disorders and the criteria used for measurement of disorders.

The First Generation

From the turn of the last century to World War II, studies consisted of interviews with informants and agency records in order to ascertain persons with mental disorders in the community (Dohrenwend and Dohrenwend, 1974). The two main problems with studies of that period were, incomplete case ascertainment and lack of reliability or validity in clinical diagnoses, as the latter were taken at face value. This period highlights the problems associated with making determinations of prevalence or risk factors from treated cases; persons in treatment are not a random sample of all people with mental disorders (Cohen and Cohen, 1984; Kohn *et al.*, 1997). In addition, due to the uncertainty about the validity of clinical diagnoses, as opposed to more precisely measured diagnosis obtained from diagnostic interview schedules, the potential for biased and inaccurate prevalence estimates and risk factor profiles becomes self-evident.

The Second Generation

Following World War II, studies used an expanded definition of psychiatric disorders with the introduction of the *Diagnostic and Statistical Manual* (American Psychiatric Association, 1952). In this group of studies, community residents were directly interviewed usually by a single psychiatrist or by a team headed by a mental health professional. Except for a few North American studies such as the Stirling County (Leighton *et al.*, 1963a), in Canada, and the Midtown Manhattan Study, in the USA (Srole *et al.*, 1962), these interviews typically did not employ standardized data collection procedures (Lin, 1953). Studies in developing countries were frequently conducted by researchers from other societies, for example, Leighton *et al.* (1963b), a North American psychiatrist, investigated the Yoruba in Nigeria. This practice may introduce bias, and may actually retain ethnocentric and culturally invalid methods.

Case identification in the second generation studies were made by psychiatrists following evaluation of protocols collected by interviewers. The second generation of psychiatric epidemiology also used screening scales comprised of symptom items. These scales, such as the general health questionnaire (Goldberg *et al.*, 1976), attempted to screen and distinguish cases from non-cases using empirically determined cutoff scores (Shrout *et al.*, 1986). This second generation resulted in a number of advances in psychiatric epidemiology including: the use of survey methods and probability samples of community respondents; the development of reliable impairment scales used in psychiatric research today; the recognition that there was no single cause of mental illness; and the focus on social and cultural influences on mental health (Dohrenwend and Dohrenwend, 1982). This second generation, however, had a number of limitations. Impairment scales assumed a unitary dimension to mental illness and did not examine specific diagnostic categories limiting the usefulness for cultural psychiatry research. This generation of studies emphasized the role that stress had on psychiatric disorder, and with few exceptions, they ignored other causes such as genetics, infections, early childhood experience and biological factors that may vary across cultures, and indeed applied similar thresholds for case ascertainment across cultural, national and ethnic groups. These studies also overlooked the difficulties of classifying race, culture and ethnic group, and did not address the problems of recruitment of hard to reach groups into research.

The Third Generation

This era of research evolved the explicit diagnostic criteria and produced structured clinical interview schedules, both of which contributed to improved diagnostic reliability, of syndromes as defined by conventional psychiatric field studies mainly among Euro-American populations. Among the earliest instruments used was the Present State Examination (PSE; Wing *et al.*, 1977) which was geared to generate diagnoses consistent with the International Classification of Disease (ICD) criteria (World Health Organization, 1978). In addition, there were instruments such as the Schedule for Affective Disorders and Schizophrenia

(SADS; Endicott and Spitzer, 1978) which generated diagnoses according to Research Diagnostic Criteria (RDC; Spitzer *et al.*, 1978); and the Diagnostic Interview Schedule (DIS; Robins *et al.* 1981) that generated *Diagnostic and Statistical Manual III* (DSM-III) diagnoses (American Psychiatric Association, 1980). More recently, new third-generation instruments have been developed, such as the Standardized Psychiatric Examination (SPE; Romanoski and Chahal, 1981), the Revised Clinical Interview Schedule (CIS-R; Lewis and Pelosi, 1990), and the Schedules for Clinical Assessment in Neuropsychiatry (SCAN; Wing *et al.*, 1990), which use ICD criteria, largely based on the PSE. These instruments also enabled a symptom-based analysis of mental distress, and could therefore explore symptom clusters within any one diagnostic group. The Composite International Diagnostic Interview (CIDI; Robins *et al.*, 1988) generates diagnoses according to both ICD-10 (World Health Organization, 1992) and DSM-IV (American Psychiatric Association, 1994) criteria.

There remain two major issues facing this third generation of psychiatric epidemiological studies: the cross-cultural validity of the diagnostic criteria used and the cross-cultural reliability of interview schedules, which are administered by lay interviewers. The difficulties around recruitment to studies, and engagement of socially excluded groups in the research process became more openly acknowledged as researchers engaged with the observations of anthropologists, sociologists and cultural psychiatrists. However, cultural factors aside, each of the advances did help to better test the association between sociodemographic variables and specific mental disorders, with greater validity and precision. Have these three stages of development in psychiatric epidemiology translated into a better understanding of cultural psychiatry issues?

The Alliance between Culture and Psychiatric Epidemiology

There are good reasons to conclude that psychiatric epidemiology has provided insights into the understanding of mental illness within and across cultural groups. Psychiatric prevalence surveys have been conducted already in nearly all regions of the world, including in some developing countries (Bromet *et al.*, 2011; Puac-Polanco *et al.*, 2015). These studies have provided results which are compelling as universally valid findings.

First, no society is immune from mental illnesses; these are common and are among the most disabling medical conditions in both the developed and developing world (WHO, 2001). These studies have shown that gender differences across specific psychiatric disorders are nearly universal, such as the 2:1 female to male ratio found for major depression, with rare exceptions (Egeland and Hostetter, 1983; Levav et al., 1997). Schizophrenia has been shown to consistently be more prevalent among individuals in the lower social classes (Goldberg and Morrison, 1963; Dohrenwend et al., 1992; Kohn et al., 1998). The elderly, contrary to earlier beliefs, are now thought to have lower rates of mental illness than younger cohorts, except for dementia (Gum et al., 2009). Traumatic events that occur to both individuals and groups, and man-made or natural catastrophes, have been shown to have short-term as well as long-lasting effects on mental health (North et al., 1999; Mollica et al., 2001; Sharon et al., 2009). In addition, new insights have been gained with regard to immigration and mental health; for example, non-traumatized immigrants may have better mental health outcomes than the second generation in open societies (Breslau et al., 2006), and the country one immigrates to may result in differential psychological distress (Flaherty et al., 1988a).

Cross-National Comparisons and Cultural Psychiatry

Cross-national comparisons have been used in psychiatric epidemiology to provide insights into cultural differences in the risk and outcome of specific psychiatric disorders. The determinants of the outcomes study from the World Health Organization (Jablensky et al., 1992) raised substantive issues relevant to cultural psychiatry, namely, that schizophrenia is a universal disease, that the rates vary little across countries, and the possibility that individuals with schizophrenia in developing countries may have better outcomes. However, at variance with this popular textbook view is the finding that if the raw data with confidence intervals are inspected the incidence rates are consistent for narrowly defined schizophrenia, but not for broadly defined schizophrenia. Indeed, even for narrowly defined schizophrenia the investigation probably

did not have the power to detect smaller differences. Furthermore, the prognosis of schizophrenia is thought to be better in developing countries, and this does require explanation (Hooper et al., 2007). Although some assert this axiom requires more nuanced research around the realities of living with severe mental illness in a resource poor country (Cohen et al., 2008).

A number of studies using the DIS (Weissman et al., 1997) and the CIDI (Bijl et al., 2003) worldwide have made cross-national comparisons and showed communalities across countries. The similarities across studies may be more meaningful than their differences, since the latter can be attributed to methodological variability between studies. Psychiatric epidemiology is now attempting to address these methodological shortcomings; for example, the World Mental Health Survey, a multi-country epidemiological effort, is designed to reduce the issue of problems related to methodological variability (World Mental Health Survey Consortium, 2004).

Do these cross-national comparisons contribute to cultural psychiatry? Indeed, one might question whether cultural psychiatry as a body of research and practice claims to own cross-national comparisons, or do these simply fall into international psychiatry as a form of universalism, minimizing cultural issues. Tseng (2001) proposed that:

> In a strict sense, psychiatric epidemiology does not relate closely to cultural psychiatry, even when cross-ethnic, racial, societal, or national comparative epidemiological studies are carried out, unless the epidemiological investigations are conducted in conjunction with an examination of core cultural variables, namely the beliefs, values, and attitudes of subjects, their families, or others in the community surveyed.

One might argue that culture is found at several levels (Figure 15.1). At the individual and group levels there is scope to learn about shared cultural beliefs and attitudes, that are multilayered and ambiguous and contradictory but shape a shared attitude or intentionality of cultural groups; and then there are cognitive representations and more accepted beliefs, and then unconscious experience and attitudes, of groups and individuals, that influence the way people perceive their world and relate to suffering, illness and recovery.

Where does culture exist: in society, in a local region, in a town, among sub-groups such as families

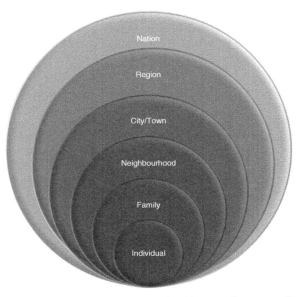

Figure 15.1 Where is culture located and how is to be measured?

or congregations, or does it exist within the mind of one person? Where should research on culture be focused? Tseng's proposition suggests that cultural psychiatry research should focus on families, and take account of the emic perspective, adhering to the traditional social–anthropological endeavours proposed by Kleinman (1977). However, we propose that other bodies of evidence and research can contribute to cultural psychiatry, especially if they are interrogated in order to complement more emic studies, and by ensuring that methods do reflect more scientific measures of, for example, race, ethnic group, etc.

For example, the finding that children of immigrants are at increased risk for schizophrenia (Cantor-Graee *et al.*, 2003) for some ethnic groups, such as African Caribbean to England (Sharpley *et al.*, 2001), but not others, such as those that immigrated to the Netherlands (Selten *et al.*, 2001), constitute a bona fide cultural psychiatric-related finding that generates intriguing hypotheses for investigation. Indeed, most biological or physiological hypotheses have been unfruitful, and so environmental factors are favoured and cultural factors beyond social conditions appear to play a significant role. However, the attitudes, beliefs and values of the subjects were not explicitly investigated. Also, the study of variables such as religious affiliation, gender, socio-economic status, immigration, trauma, war, race or ethnic origin within a country or across countries constitutes a valid

contribution to cultural psychiatry. Variations of risk factors or rates across these groups require explanation, and further in-depth research.

Cross-Cultural Applicability of Psychiatric Epidemiological Instruments

Experience shows that adapting an instrument for cross-cultural use is often more cost-effective and facilitates cross-cultural comparisons better than developing new instruments to measure similar constructs. The complexity of translating an instrument varies depending on how much the construct being measured differs between the two cultures. Procedures for translating instruments across cultural groups have been well outlined (Sartorius and Kuyken, 1994; Bhui *et al.*, 2003). Admittedly, the often used back-translation technique is not beyond criticisms. Bilingual translators may be able to achieve equal back-translations yet fail to achieve optimal interpretations of the meaning of the item. Also, after an instrument is translated, it is still necessary to evaluate the adapted version in the target population. Aside from translation issues, several questions regarding validity and reliability need to be answered before such an instrument can be applied (Flaherty *et al.*, 1988b). Content equivalence: are the items that make up the concept in the original culture relevant to the host culture? Semantic equivalence: do the translated items have the same meaning in the target culture? Technical equivalence: do the methods of data collection yield different results in the target culture? Criterion equivalence: how do the results of the adapted version of the instrument compare to independent criteria measuring the same construct? Conceptual equivalence: are the same variables being measured? However, most psychiatric epidemiological studies do not adapt these approaches in full, often adhering to an ethnocentric approach, one in which the researcher mistakenly assumes that the concepts completely overlap in the two cultures.

Frequently, as noted above, instruments are used with individuals that differ from the population in which the instruments were originally developed and normed, a methodological danger that has a substantive impact. This results in the risks of making skewed interpretations of results if the populations differ on some latent variable. Examples of such methodological shortcomings are readily available in the psychiatric epidemiology literature; rarely are these standards met beyond good-faith efforts at accurate translations and small reliability studies in the now widely used large-scale psychiatric epidemiological surveys across countries (Wittchen, 1994). For example, are the extremely low rates of psychopathology in China (Wang *et al.*, 1992; Shen *et al.*, 2006), Nigeria (Gureje *et al.*, 2006), and Taiwan (Hwu *et al.*, 1989) based on studies using the DIS and CIDI, reality or artefact? Advances have been made; researchers in dementia have been partially successful in developing culturally fair instruments (Hendrie *et al.*, 1995). Ongoing epidemiological research on schizophrenia and other mental disorders in Ethiopia appears to demonstrate that culturally valid studies in distinct cultural settings are possible (Alem *et al.*, 1999). There are limits, however, to the incorporation of local cultural constructs into an instrument in use, lest it loses the capacity to measure the intended original construct and still be able to serve in cross-cultural studies (Canino *et al.*, 1997).

What are reasonable methodological expectations for valid research taking into account cost constraints? To conduct validity and reliability studies for each instrument and on every cultural group, although ideal, is economically not feasible, and may raise insurmountable obstacles for any meaningful epidemiological research.

Early on in the third generation of psychiatric epidemiological research data were collected using mental health professionals (Levav *et al.*, 1993). The norm now is the use of lay interviewers employing a fully structured diagnostic instrument, in part due to the high costs of psychiatrically trained personnel. In addition, the current size of the large-scale prevalence studies resulted in lay interviewers becoming a financial and logistical necessity. What has been lost with these instruments and interviewers is the ability to carefully probe and interpret behaviour in a clinically and culturally meaningful manner, as responses to fully structured interview schedules are to be accepted at face value regardless of the presenting behaviour. For example, someone who is actively hallucinating but denies it in the initial probing would be recorded as not having a psychotic symptom. Reliability studies examining inter-rater reliability against semi-structured instruments administered by mental health professionals have shown good agreement for many (Ustun *et al.*, 1997), but not all disorders, in particular schizophrenia and somatization disorder, and frequently panic disorder, generalized anxiety

disorder, and dysthymia (Wittchen, 1994). Psychiatric epidemiology unfortunately has had to compromise the ability to obtain data that are richer in their ability to derive cultural interpretation and meaning for the economics and constraints of the research environment.

Application of Universal Diagnostic Systems

Perhaps the most important contribution to come out of psychiatric epidemiology, and yet the most controversial, is the application of a universal diagnostic system and criteria such as the ICD and DSM. If one takes the position that psychiatric nosological systems cannot be applied cross-culturally as they are imposed constructs devoid of a meaningful cultural context (Mezzich *et al.*, 1992), then most of psychiatric epidemiology has made little to no contribution to cultural psychiatry. Alternatively, it may be argued that cultural-bound syndromes, as represented in diagnostic manuals as cogent and absolute entities, do not exist, and may even be classifiable elsewhere within the current nosological system (Lopez-Ibor, 2003). Fabrega (1994) has placed psychiatric diagnostic systems in their proper perspective alluding to the tension created by its use internationally: 'Although in theory applicable to all people regardless of population/genetic, national, or cultural background, it is used by clinicians of highly specific cultural origin, and in settings characterized by distinctive cultural traditions about sickness, healing, non-sickness or health, and social behaviour.'

Psychiatric epidemiology does offer the possibility to examine whether symptom criteria differ across different populations, and if symptom criteria can be applied similarly across groups. Only once we have a better understanding of the genetic basis of mental illness, can this controversy be resolved regarding whether the phenotypic presentation of mental illness is indeed highly variable across cultures. Until the genetic basis of mental illness becomes reality, culturally based studies in psychiatric epidemiology are faced with what Kleinman (1977, 1988) terms a category fallacy in diagnosis. However, this straw man is easy to attack, and destroy, if diagnostics are misunderstood to simply be an operationalized and value-free enterprise. Rather, diagnosis should be a process in which the emic is understood alongside the etic, and in which the clinician explores relevance, cultural appropriateness of behaviours and beliefs, and reflects on the transference and counter-transference including attention to race and ethnic factors, differences, similarities in the consulting room. The ICD and DSM are not intended for use as representations of hard scientific facts, but are the best we have in an evolving nosology of benefit to the majority of patients, and worth considering in clinical practice which may actually diverge from the ostensibly valid and universal systems in order to truly reflect the distress experiences as felt and lived by people, service users and patients. The Outline for Cultural Formulation as described in DSM-5 does set out a humanistic process and not a technology. Genetic epidemiological and dimensional classifications of psychopathology are likely to enable more complex and less static categorical classifications; these will be more difficult for clinicians to use, and for patients to understand, but they will retain greater potential for authentic representations of psychopathology, and may be more able to embrace cultural dimensions/factors as variables that should be considered for their central importance in resilience, recovery and illness behaviour.

The Fourth Generation of Psychiatric Epidemiology and Global Mental Health

The fourth and current generation of psychiatric epidemiology has been focused on a strong emphasis on the search for specific risk factors, both biological and psychosocial. Current psychiatric epidemiological studies have coincided with the emergence of global mental health (Kohn, 2014). The finding that mental disorders contribute a disproportionate amount to the global burden of disease is a result of a better understanding of the prevalence of mental illness and its risk factors. The high treatment gap combined with the excess disability due to mental illness, in particular in low- and middle-income countries, has led psychiatric epidemiology also to start to focus on primary and secondary prevention, scaling-up mental health (Kohn et al., 2004; Eaton et al., 2011).

However, the global mental health movement is not without controversy. Cultural psychiatry and global mental health, although sharing domains of interest, grew from distinct lineages (de Jong, 2014). Critics of the global mental health movement suggest that mental disorders are viewed as universal without

taking into account that mental distress is culturally and socially mediated. However, a synergy is needed between cultural psychiatry and global mental health (de Jong, 2014). Developing programmes that scale up mental health in low- and middle-income countries is not feasible without cultural psychiatry. Epidemiological studies that include concepts of distress can improve identification of risk groups and assessment of culturally salient intervention outcomes (Kohrt et al., 2014). Global mental health and the evolution of the fourth generation of psychiatric epidemiology has increased the opportunity for further synergy with cultural psychiatry with the development of cultural epidemiology.

The linkage with big data and policy influence is welcomed, yet such major transnational movements carry with them risks of oversight of the more nuanced local realities and belief systems that drive poor mental health and need to be captured to lead to recovery. In the global burden of disease studies mental illnesses are seen as discrete single dimension diagnostic categories, rather than as more complex and intersectional elements of illness experience that are determinants of premature mortality for many chronic diseases. The cultural constructions of illness and influences on programmes of prevention and treatment are also overlooked at a global level, but relegated to local action plans creating some disparity in terms of resources and potential impacts for patients and public mental health.

Cultural Epidemiology: A Brief Introduction

There are several foci that must be addressed within psychiatric epidemiology. First, studies using methodological advances that combine cultural variables and qualitative data into epidemiological surveys need to be more commonplace (de Jong and van Ommeren, 2002). This type of epidemiological research Weiss (2001) has termed cultural epidemiology, when studies apply locally valid categories of experience, meaning and behaviour into them. Second, psychiatric epidemiological studies that test cultural psychiatric hypotheses need to be further fostered in developing countries and special populations in developed countries using local investigators. Third, psychiatric epidemiology should incorporate assessments of risk factors that are primarily cultural: attitudes and behaviours that are culturally based in

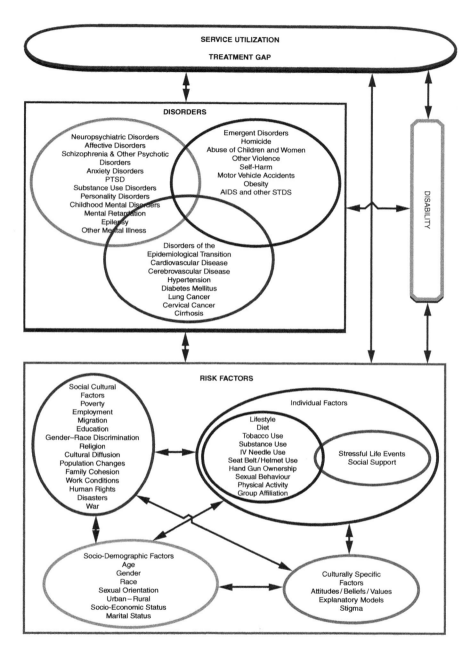

Figure 15.2 Disorders and conditions of concern for psychiatric epidemiology

the research design; this may provide opportunities to test epidemiological theories, albeit instruments and analytic techniques will need re-examination. For example, adjusting for ethnic group cannot be undertaken uncritically; stratifying by ethnic group will lead to smaller sample sizes but must be recommended in the first instance, and ethnic/cultural groups should reflect the requirements of hypotheses and not just the convenient ethnic/cultural group classifications used

in census and politically motivated data sources. Fourth, psychiatric epidemiology focused on cultural psychiatry should also address public health issues that allow for service planning, and addressing local and global population needs.

To make psychiatric epidemiology more relevant to the cultural context of changes that are currently occurring in societies and the increased focus on behavioural and lifestyle issues, psychiatric epidemiology must include, in addition to the traditional neuropsychiatric disorders, an increased emphasis on emergent disorders and disorders of the epidemiological transition, that examine individual risk factors, socio-demographic, socio-cultural factors, and culturally specific factors across the lifespan, for a range of conditions (Figure 15.2).

Conclusions

To sum up, psychiatric epidemiology across its three generations has made important contributions to cultural psychiatry, including the demonstration that there are universalities in the presentation of psychopathology. It has also shown that diagnostic criteria and instruments can be applied across different populations and cultures. These accomplishments have not been without controversy, leaving open the argument that psychiatric epidemiological studies all too frequently ignore the cultural context of the populations being studied thus adding little to the study of cultural psychiatry. However legitimate this debate is, psychiatric epidemiology remains an integral component of cultural psychiatry research. At a minimum, it provides the latter both tools and methodologies, thus further contributing to secure the scientific evidence required to be a credible evidence-based field of study. Cultural epidemiology is now gathering momentum, but is likely to be challenging, given it requires greater stringency as far as research methods go, a stringency that will be perceived as a nuisance by the culturally blind and naive clinician and researcher.

References

Alem, A., Kebede, D., Woldesemiat, G., Jacobsson, L. and Kullgren, G. (1999). The prevalence and socio-demographic correlates of mental distress in Butajira, Ethiopia. *Acta Psychiatrica Scandinavica Supplementum*, 397, 48–55.

American Psychiatric Association (1952). *Mental Disorders: Diagnostic and Statistical Manual*. Washington DC: American Psychiatric Association.

American Psychiatric Association (1980). *Diagnostic and Statistical Manual of Mental Disorders*, 3rd edn. Washington DC: American Psychiatric Association.

American Psychiatric Association (1994). *Diagnostic and Statistical Manual of Mental Disorders*, 4th edn. Washington DC: American Psychiatric Association.

Bhui, K., Mohamud, S., Warfa, N., Craig, T. J. and Stansfeld, S. A. (2003). Cultural adaptation of mental health measures: improving the quality of clinical practice and research. *British Journal of Psychiatry*, 183, 184–186.

Bjil, R. V., de Graff, R., Hiripi, E. *et al.* (2003). The prevalence of treated and untreated mental disorders in five countries. *Health Affairs*, 22, 122–133.

Breslau, J., Aguilar-Gaxiola, S., Kendler, K. S. *et al.* (2006). Specifying race–ethnic differences in risk for psychiatric disorder in a USA national sample. *Psychological Medicine*, 36, 57–68.

Bromet, E., Andrade, L. H., Hwang, I., *et al.* (2011). Cross-national epidemiology of DSM-IV major depressive episode. *BMC Medicine*, 26, 90.

Canino, G., Lewis-Fernandez, R. and Bravo, M. (1997). Methodological challenges in cross-cultural mental health research. *Transcultural Psychiatry*, 34, 163–184.

Cantor-Graae, E., Pedersen, C. B., McNeil, T. F. and Mortensen, P. B. (2003). Migration as a risk factor for schizophrenia: a Danish population-based cohort study. *British Journal of Psychiatry*, 182, 117–122.

Cohen, A., Patel, V., Thara, R. and Gureje, O. (2008). Questioning an axiom: better prognosis for schizophrenia in the developing world? *Schizophrenia Bulletin*, 34, 229–244

Cohen, P. and Cohen, J. (1984). The clinician's illusion. *Archives of General Psychiatry*, 41, 1178–1182.

De Jong, J. T. (2014). Challenges of creating synergy between global mental health and cultural psychiatry. *Transcultural Psychiatry*, 51, 806–828.

De Jong, J. T. and van Ommeren, M. (2002). Toward a culture-informed epidemiology: combing qualitative and quantitative research in transcultural contexts. *Transcultural Psychiatry*, 39, 422–433.

Dohrenwend, B. P. and Dohrenwend, B. S. (1974). Social and cultural influences on psychopathology. *Annual Review of Psychology*, 25, 417–452.

Dohrenwend, B. P. and Dohrenwend, B. S. (1982). Perspective on the past and future of psychiatric epidemiology. The Rema Lapouse Lecture. *American Journal of Public Health*, 72, 1271–1279.

Dohrenwend, B. P., Levav, I., Shrout, P. E. *et al.* (1992). Socio-economic status and psychiatric disorders: the causation–selection issue. *Science*, 255, 946–952.

Eaton, J., McCay, L., Semrau, M., *et al.* (2011). Scale up of services for mental health in low-income and middle-income countries. *The Lancet*, 378, 1592–603.

Egeland, J. A. and Hostetter, A. M. (1983). Amish Study, I: affective disorders among the Amish, 1976–1980. *American Journal of Psychiatry*, 140, 56–61.

Endicott, J. and Spitzer, R. L. (1978). A diagnostic interview: the Schedule for Affective Disorders and Schizophrenia. *Archives of General Psychiatry*, 35, 837–844.

Fabrega, H., Jr (1994). International systems of diagnosis in psychiatry. *Journal of Nervous and Mental Disease*, 182, 256–263.

Flaherty, J. A., Kohn, R., Levav, I. and Birz, S. (1988a). Demoralization in Soviet-Jewish immigrants to the

United States and Israel. *Comprehensive Psychiatry*, **29**, 588–597.

Flaherty, J. A., Gaviria, F. M., Pathak, D. *et al.* (1988b). Developing instruments for cross-cultural psychiatric research. *Journal of Nervous and Mental Disease*, **176**, 257–263.

Goldberg, D. P., Rickels, K., Downing, R. and Hesbacher, P. (1976). A comparison of two psychiatric screening tests. *British Journal of Psychiatry*, **129**, 61–67.

Goldberg, E. M. and Morrison, S. L. (1963). Schizophrenia and social class. *British Journal of Psychiatry*, **109**, 785–802.

Gum, A. M., King-Kallimanis, B. and Kohn, R. (2009). Prevalence of mood, anxiety, and substance abuse disorders for older Americans in the National Comorbidity Survey-Replication. *American Journal of Geriatric Psychiatry*, **17**, 769–781.

Gureje, O., Lasebikan, V. O., Kola, L. and Makanjuola, V. A. (2006). Lifetime and 12-month prevalence of mental disorders in the Nigerian Survey of Mental Health and Well-Being. *British Journal of Psychiatry*, **188**, 465–471.

Hendrie, H. C., Osuntokun, B. O., Hall, K. S. *et al.* (1995). Prevalence of Alzheimer's disease and dementia in two communities: Nigerian Africans and African Americans. *American Journal of Psychiatry*, **152**, 1485–1492.

Hooper, K., Harrison, G., Janca, A. and Sartorius, N. (eds) (2007). *Recovery from Schizophrenia: An International Perspective*. Oxford: Oxford University Press.

Hwu, H. G., Yeh, E. K. and Chang, L. Y. (1989). Prevalence of psychiatric disorders in Taiwan defined by the Chinese Diagnostic Interview Schedule. *Acta Psychiatrica Scandinavica*, **79**, 136–147.

Jablensky, A., Sartorius, N., Ernberg, G. *et al.* (1992). Schizophrenia: manifestations, incidence and course in different cultures. A World Health Organization Ten-Country Study. *Psychological Medicine*, monograph supplement, 20.

Jarvis, E. (1971). *Insanity and Idiocy in Massachusetts: Report of the Commission of Lunacy (1855)*. Cambridge, MA: Harvard University Press.

Kleinman, A. (1977). Depression, somatization and the new cross-cultural psychiatry. *Social Science and Medicine*, **11**, 3–10.

Kleinman, A. (1988). *Rethinking Psychiatry: From Cultural Category to Personal Experience*. New York: Free Press.

Kohn, R. (2014). Trends and gaps in mental health disparities. In *Global Mental Health: Essential Concepts*, ed. S. O. Okpaku. New York: Cambridge University Press, pp. 27–38.

Kohn, R., Levav, I., Dohrenwend, B. P., Shrout, P. E. and Skodol, A. E. (1997). Jews and their intraethnic vulnerability to affective disorders, fact or artifact? II: evidence from a cohort study. *Israel Journal of Psychiatry and Related Sciences*, **34**, 149–156.

Kohn, R., Dohrenwend, B. P. and Mirotznik, J. (1998). Epidemiologic findings on selected psychiatric disorders in the general population. In *Adversity, Stress, and Psychopathology*, ed. B. P. Dohrenwend. New York: Oxford University Press, pp. 235–284.

Kohn, R., Saxena, S., Levav, I. and Saraceno, B. (2004). The treatment gap in mental health care. *Bulletin of the World Health Organization*, **82**, 858–866.

Kohrt, B. A., Rasmussen, A., Kaiser, B. N. *et al.* (2014). Cultural concepts of distress and psychiatric disorders: literature review and research recommendations for global mental health epidemiology. *International Journal of Epidemiology*, **43**, 365–406.

Leighton, A. H., Lambo, T., Hughes, J. M., Leighton, D. C., Murphy, J. and Maclin, D. (1963b). *Psychiatric Disorders among the Yoruba*. Ithaca, New York: Cornell University Press.

Leighton, D. C., Harding, J. S., Macklin, D. B., Hughes, C. C. and Leighton, A. H. (1963a). Psychiatric findings of the Stirling County Study. *American Journal of Psychiatry*, **119**, 1021–1026.

Levav, I., Kohn, R., Dohrenwend, B. P. *et al.* (1993). An epidemiologic study of mental disorders in a 10-year cohort of young adults in Israel. *Psychological Medicine*, **23**, 691–707.

Levav, I., Kohn, R., Golding, J. and Weissman, M. M. (1997). Vulnerability of Jews to affective disorders. *American Journal of Psychiatry*, **154**, 941–947.

Lewis, G. and Pelosi, A. J. (1990). *Manual of the Revised Clinical Interview Schedule (CIS-R)*. London: MRC Institute of Psychiatry.

Lin, T. (1953). A study of the incidence of mental disorder in Chinese and other cultures. *Psychiatry*, **16**, 313–336.

Lopez-Ibor, J. J., Jr (2003). Cultural adaptations of current psychiatric classifications: are they the solution? *Psychopathology*, **36**, 114–119.

Mezzich, J. E., Fabrega, H., Jr and Kleinman, A. (1992). Cultural validity and DSM-IV. *Journal of Nervous and Mental Disease*, **180**, 4.

Mollica, R. F., Sarajlic, N., Chernoff, M., Lavelle, J., Vukovic, I. S. and Massagli, M. P. (2001). Longitudinal study of psychiatric symptoms, disability, mortality, and emigration among Bosnian refugees. *Journal of the American Medical Association*, **286**, 546–554.

North, C. S., Nixon, S. J., Shariat, S. *et al.* (1999). Psychiatric disorders among survivors of the Oklahoma City bombing. *Journal of the American Medical Association*, **282**, 755–762.

Puac-Polanco, V. D., Lopez-Soto, V. A., Kohn, R., Xie, D., Richmond, T. S. and Branas, C. C. (2015). Previous violent events and mental health outcomes in Guatemala. *American Journal of Public Health*, **105**, 764–771.

Robins, L. N., Helzer, J. E., Croughan, J. and Ratcliff, K. S. (1981). National Institute of Mental Health Diagnostic Interview Schedule: its history, characteristics, and validity. *Archives of General Psychiatry*, **38**, 381–389.

Robins, L. N., Wing, J., Wittchen, H. U. *et al.* (1988). The Composite International Diagnostic Interview: an epidemiologic instrument suitable for use in conjunction with different diagnostic systems and in different cultures. *Archives of General Psychiatry*, **45**, 1069–1077.

Romanoski, A. J. and Chahal, R. (1981). *The Standardized Psychiatric Examination.* Baltimore, MD: Johns Hopkins University School of Medicine, Department of Psychiatry and Behavioural Sciences.

Sartorius, N. and Kuyken, W. (1994). Translation of health status instruments. In *Quality of Life Assessment: International Perspectives*, ed. J. Orley and W. Kuyken. New York: Springer-Verlag, pp. 3–18.

Selten, J. P., Veen, N., Feller, W. *et al.* (2001). Incidence of psychotic disorders in immigrant groups to the Netherlands. *British Journal of Psychiatry*, **178**, 367–372.

Sharon, A., Levav, I., Brodsky, J., Shemesh, A. A., and Kohn, R. (2009). Psychiatric disorders and other health dimensions among Holocaust survivors six decades later. *British Journal of Psychiatry*, **195**, 331–335.

Sharpley, M. S., Hutchinson, G., Murray, R. M. and McKenzie, K. (2001). Understanding the excess of psychosis among the African-Caribbean population in England: review of current hypotheses. *British Journal of Psychiatry*, **178**(Suppl. 40), 60–68.

Shen, Y. C., Zhang, M. Y., Huang, Y., Q. *et al.* (2006). Twelve-month prevalence, severity, and unmet need for treatment of mental disorders in metropolitan China. *Psychological Medicine*, **36**, 257–267.

Shrout, P. E., Dohrenwend, B. P. and Levav, I. (1986). A discriminant rule for screening cases of diverse diagnostic types: preliminary results. *Journal of Consulting and Clinical Psychology*, **54**, 314–319.

Spitzer, R. L., Endicott, J. and Robins, E. (1978). Research diagnostic criteria: rationale and reliability. *Archives of General Psychiatry*, **35**, 773–782.

Srole, L., Langer, T. S., Michael, S. T., Opler, M. K. and Rennie, T. A. (1962). *Mental Health in the Metropolis: The Midtown Manhattan Study.* New York: McGraw Hill.

Tseng, W. S. (2001). *Handbook of Cultural Psychiatry.* San Diego, CA: Academic Press, pp. 195–209.

Ustun, B., Compton, W., Mager, D. *et al.* (1997). WHO study on the reliability and validity of the alcohol and drug use disorder instruments: overview of methods and results. *Drug Alcohol Dependence*, **47**, 161–169.

Wang, C. H., Liu, W. T., Zhang, M. Y. *et al.* (1992). Alcohol use, abuse, and dependency in Shanghai. In *Alcoholism in North America, Europe, and Asia*, ed. J. E. Helzer and C. J. Canino. New York: Oxford University Press, pp. 264–286.

Weiss, M. G. (2001). Cultural epidemiology: an introduction and overview. *Anthropology and Medicine*, **8**, 1–29.

Weissman, M. M., Bland, R. C., Canino, G. J. *et al.* (1997). The cross-national epidemiology of panic disorder. *Archives of General Psychiatry*, **54**, 305–309.

Wing, J. H., Nixon, J., Mann, S. A. and Leff, J. P. (1977). Reliability of the PSE (ninth edition) used in a population survey. *Psychological Medicine*, **7**, 505–516.

Wing, J. K., Babor, T., Brugha, T. *et al.* (1990). SCAN: schedules for clinical assessment in neuropsychiatry. *Archives of General Psychiatry*, **47**, 589–593.

Wittchen, H. U. (1994). Reliability and validity studies of the WHO: Composite International Diagnostic Interview (CIDI): a critical review. *Journal of Psychiatric Research*, **28**, 57–84.

World Health Organization (1978). *Mental Disorders: Glossary and Guide to their Classification in Accordance with the Ninth Revision of the International Classification of Diseases.* Geneva: World Health Organization.

World Health Organization (1992). *The ICD-10 Classification of Mental and Behavioural Disorders: Clinical Descriptions and Diagnostic Guidelines.* Geneva: World Health Organization.

World Health Organization (2001). *The World Health Report 2001 Mental Health: New Understanding New Hope.* Geneva: World Health Organization. Available online at www.who.int/whr/2001/en/ (accessed 24 July 2017).

World Mental Health Survey Consortium (2004). Prevalence, severity, and unmet need for treatment of mental disorders in the World Health Organization World Mental Health surveys. *Journal of the American Medical Association*, **291**, 2581–2590.

Chapter 16

Acculturation and Identity

John W. Berry

Editors' Introduction

Cultures are never static. Cultures change and evolve in response to a number of factors and in a bi-directional way they also change individuals. The individuals influence cultures as a consequence of globalization, rapid urbanization and industrialization in many countries and settings. Some of the cultural characteristics and inherent traits in individuals are more prone to changes than others. The impact of one culture on another depends upon a number of factors, such as the purpose of such contact, the degree and the duration of this contact. If one culture invades another for political and economic reasons, the outcome is more likely to be different and may lead to deculturation than if the contact is through media at a distance where changes may be slow rather than sudden. Berry, in this chapter, defines acculturation as a process of cultural and psychological change in cultural groups, families and individuals following intercultural contact. Cultural identity refers to the ways in which individuals establish and maintain connections with, and a sense of belonging to, various groups. Embedded within cultural identity are micro-identities of the individual such as gender, religion, sexual orientation, etc. some of which can be hidden and others are obvious. The processes and outcomes of these processes are highly variable, with large group and individual differences. This chapter focuses on describing some of these processes, the strategies people use to deal with them, and the adaptations that result. Three questions are raised: how do individuals and groups seek to acculturate? How well do they succeed? Are there any relationships between how they go about acculturation and their psychological and socio-cultural success? Berry notes that the commonest strategy is integration (defined as preferring to maintain one's cultural heritage while seeking to participate in the life of the larger society), rather than assimilation, separation or marginalization which is likely to be most adaptive.

Acculturation: Cultural and Individual

Acculturation is the process of cultural and psychological change that takes place as a result of contact between cultural groups and their individual members (Redfield, Linton and Herskovits, 1936). Such contact and change occurs during colonization, military invasion, migration and sojourning (such as tourism, international study and overseas posting); it continues after initial contact in culturally plural societies, where ethnocultural communities maintain features of their heritage cultures. Adaptation to living in culture-contact settings takes place over time; occasionally it is stressful, but often it results in some form of mutual accommodation. Acculturation and adaptation are now reasonably well understood, permitting the development of policies and programmes to promote successful outcomes for all parties.

The initial research interest in acculturation grew out of a concern for the effects of European domination of colonial and indigenous peoples. Later, it focused on how immigrants (both voluntary and involuntary) changed following their entry and settlement into receiving societies. More recently, much of the work has been involved with how ethnocultural groups and individuals relate to each other, and change, as a result of their attempts to live together in culturally plural societies. Nowadays, all three foci are important, as globalization results in ever-larger trading and political relations: indigenous national populations experience neo-colonization, new waves of immigrants, sojourners and refugees flow from these economic and political changes, and large ethnocultural populations become established in most countries.

Graves (1967), introduced the concept of psychological acculturation, which refers to changes in an individual who is a participant in a culture contact situation, being influenced both directly by the external (usually dominant) culture, and by the changing culture (usually non-dominant) of which the individual is a member.

There are two reasons for keeping the cultural and psychological levels distinct. The first is that, in cross-cultural psychology, we view individual human behaviour as interacting with the cultural context within which it occurs; hence separate conceptions and measurements are required at the two levels (Berry et al., 2011). The second is that not every individual enters into the new culture, and participates in it, or changes in the same way; there are vast individual differences in psychological acculturation, even among individuals who live in the same acculturative arena (Sam and Berry, 2016).

A framework that outlines and links cultural and psychological acculturation, and identifies the two (or more) groups in contact (Berry and Sam, 2016) provides a map of those phenomena which I believe need to be conceptualized and measured during acculturation research. At the cultural level we need to understand key features of the two original cultural groups prior to their major contact, the nature of their contact relationships, and the resulting dynamic cultural changes in both groups and in the emergent ethnocultural groups, during the process of acculturation. The gathering of this information requires extensive ethnographic, community-level work. These changes can be minor or substantial, and range from being easily accomplished through to being a source of major cultural disruption. At the individual level, we need to consider the psychological changes that individuals in all groups undergo, and their eventual adaptation to their new situations. Identifying these changes requires sampling a population and studying individuals who are variably involved in the process of acculturation. These changes can be a set of rather easily accomplished behavioural shifts (e.g. in ways of speaking, dressing, eating and in one's cultural identity) or they can be more problematic, producing acculturative stress as manifested by uncertainty, anxiety and depression (Berry, 2006). Adaptations can be primarily internal or psychological (e.g. sense of well-being, or self-esteem) or socio-cultural (Ward, 1996), linking the individual to others in the new society as manifested, for example, in competence in the activities of daily intercultural living.

Cultural Identity

During acculturation, individuals have to deal with the question: 'Who am I?' Although this question has many dimensions (such as age, gender, social class, religion), we are concerned here with the cultural dimension of the question. Considerable research (e.g. Berry, 1999; Birman et al., 2010; Liebkind et al., 2016; Phinney, 1990) has revealed evidence for a complex pattern of thoughts, feelings and social relationships that make up a person's cultural identity. This complexity is particularly evident during the course of development (Beiser et al., 2015; Motti-Stefanidi et al., 2012; Umaña-Taylor et al., 2014).

As for acculturation, the issue of one's cultural identity comes to the fore during intercultural contact: individuals engage with two systems of cultural norms, beliefs and practices, and attempt to sort out who they are in relation to these two ways of living. Cultural identity involves, at its core, a sense of attachment or commitment to a cultural group, and is thus a cultural as well as a psychological phenomenon. In this sense it requires the existence of a cultural group, which can be actual and viable at present, remembered from one's past, or imagined in one's future. And, as for acculturation, cultural identity involves the possibility of change, both over time, and from situation to situation. This malleability renders it difficult to pin down as a relatively stable feature of an individual's psychological make-up.

Intercultural Strategies

Not all groups and individuals undergo acculturation in the same way; there are large variations in how people seek to engage the process. These variations have been termed acculturation strategies (Berry, 1980). A parallel concept of identity strategies (Camilleri and Malewska-Peyre, 1997) has been proposed to specify the variations in the ways that individuals may identify themselves during intercultural contact and the ensuing process of acculturation. Which strategies are used depends on a variety of antecedent factors (both cultural and psychological); and there are variable consequences (again both cultural and psychological) of these different strategies. These strategies consist of a number of (usually related) components, including attitudes and behaviours. Preferences about how to live interculturally, and the actual behaviours that are exhibited in day-to-day intercultural encounters reveal marked variations from group to group and from person to person. These variations in ways of acculturating are sometimes referred to as the 'how?' question in acculturation research (Berry et al., 2006).

Acculturation Strategies

The centrality of the concept of acculturation strategies can be illustrated by reference to each of the components included in the acculturation framework mentioned earlier (Berry and Sam, 2016). At the cultural level, the two groups in contact (whether dominant or non-dominant) usually have some notion about what they are attempting to do (e.g. colonial policies, or motivations for migration), or what is being done to them, during the contact. Similarly, the kinds of changes that are likely to occur will be influenced by their strategies. At the individual level, both the behaviour changes and acculturative stress phenomena are now known to be a function, at least to some extent, of what people try to do during their acculturation; and the longer term outcomes (both psychological and socio-cultural adaptations) often correspond to the strategic goals set by the groups of which they are members.

Four acculturation strategies have been derived from two basic issues facing all acculturating peoples. These issues are based on the distinction between orientations towards one's own group, and those towards other groups (Berry, 1980). This distinction is rendered as (1) a relative preference for maintaining one's heritage culture and identity and (2) a relative preference for having contact with and participating in the larger society along with other ethnocultural groups. It has now been well demonstrated that these two dimensions are empirically, as well as conceptually, independent from each other (Ryder et al., 2000). This two dimensional formulation is presented in Figure 16.1.

These two issues can be responded to on attitudinal dimensions, represented by bipolar arrows. For purposes of presentation, generally positive or negative orientations to these issues intersect to define four acculturation strategies. These strategies carry different names, depending on which ethnocultural group (the dominant or non-dominant) is being considered. From the point of view of non-dominant groups (on the left of Figure 16.1), when individuals do not wish to maintain their cultural identity and seek daily interaction with other cultures, the assimilation strategy is defined. In contrast, when individuals place a value on holding on to their original culture, and at the same time wish to avoid interaction with others, then the separation alternative is defined. When there is an interest in both maintaining one's original culture, while in daily interactions with other groups, integration is the option. In this case, there is some degree of cultural integrity maintained, while at the same time seeking, as a member of an ethnocultural group, to participate as an integral part of the larger social network. Finally, when there is little possibility or interest in cultural maintenance (often for reasons of enforced cultural loss), and little interest in having relations with others (often for reasons of exclusion or discrimination) then marginalization is defined. This presentation was based on the assumption that non-dominant groups and their individual members have the freedom to choose how they want to acculturate. This, of course, is not always the case. When the dominant group enforces certain forms of acculturation, or constrains the choices of

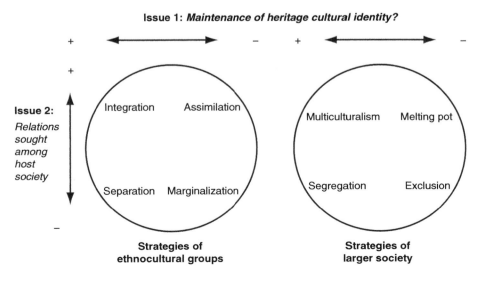

Issue 1: *Maintenance of heritage cultural identity?*

Figure 16.1 Acculturation strategies in ethnocultural groups and in the larger society. (Also see Figure 4.4.)

Issue 2:
Relations sought among host society

Integration   Assimilation

Separation   Marginalization

Multiculturalism   Melting pot

Segregation   Exclusion

Strategies of ethnocultural groups

Strategies of larger society

non-dominant groups or individuals, then other terms need to be used (see below).

Integration can only be 'freely' chosen and successfully pursued by non-dominant groups when the dominant society is open and inclusive in its orientation towards cultural diversity. Thus a mutual accommodation is required for integration to be attained, involving the acceptance by both groups of the right of all groups to live as culturally different peoples. This strategy requires non-dominant groups to adopt the basic values of the larger society, while at the same time the dominant group must be prepared to adapt national institutions (e.g. education, health, labour) to better meet the needs of all groups now living together in the plural society.

These two basic issues were initially approached from the point of view of the non-dominant ethnocultural groups. However, the original anthropological definition clearly established that both groups in contact would change and become acculturated to each other. Hence, a third dimension was included: that of the powerful role played by the dominant group in influencing the way in which mutual acculturation would take place (Berry, 1974). The inclusion of this third dimension produces the right side of Figure 16.1. Assimilation when sought by the dominant group is termed the 'melting pot'. When separation is forced by the dominant group it is 'segregation'. Marginalization, when imposed by the dominant group, is 'exclusion'. Finally, integration, when diversity is a widely accepted feature of the society as a whole, including by all the various ethnocultural groups, is called 'multiculturalism'.

With the use of this framework, comparisons can be made between individuals and their groups, and between non-dominant peoples and the larger society within which they are acculturating. The ideologies and policies of the dominant group constitute an important element of intercultural research (see Berry *et al.*, 1977; Bourhis *et al.*, 1997), while the preferences of non-dominant peoples (their acculturation strategies) are a core feature in acculturation research (Berry *et al.*, 1989). Inconsistencies and conflicts between these various acculturation preferences are commonly sources of difficulty for acculturating individuals. Generally, when acculturation experiences cause problems for acculturating individuals, we observe the phenomenon of acculturative stress, with variations in levels of adaptation. These phenomena are sometimes referred to as the 'how well?' question in acculturation research.

Identity Strategies

A parallel approach to understanding variations in how individuals engage their intercultural worlds uses the concept of identity strategies. This approach has been developed by Camilleri and colleagues (Camilleri and Malewska-Peyre, 1997). These *stratégies identitaires* have clear similarities to the various acculturation strategies discussed earlier.

Just as the notion of acculturation strategies is based on two underlying dimensions (own cultural maintenance, and involvement with other cultures), there is now a consensus that how one thinks of oneself (i.e. one's cultural identity) is also constructed along two dimensions (Phinney, 1990; Phinney and Baldelomar, 2011). The first is identification with one's heritage or ethnocultural group, and the second is identification with the larger or dominant society. These two aspects of cultural identity have been referred to in various ways: ethnic identity and civic identity (Kalin and Berry, 1995) and ethnic identity and national identity (Berry *et al.*, 2006). Moreover (as for the acculturation dimensions) these dimensions are independent of each other (in the sense that they are not negatively correlated, or that more of one does not imply less of the other).

These two identity dimensions have both theoretical and empirical similarities with the four acculturation strategies: when both identities are asserted, this resembles the integration strategy; when one feels neither, then there is a sense of marginalization; and when one is strongly emphasized over the other, then the cultural identities resemble either the assimilation or separation strategies. Evidence for this link is found in numerous empirical studies where acculturation strategies and cultural identities have both been assessed. For example, these two strategies have been examined together by Georgas and Papastylianou (1998) among samples of ethnic Greeks remigrating to Greece. They found that those with a 'Greek' identity were high on the assimilation strategy, those with a 'mixed' (e.g. Greek–Albanian) were highest on integration, and those with an 'indigenous' (e.g. 'Albanian') identity were highest on separation. These findings are consistent with expectations about how acculturation and identity strategies should relate to each other. In a large international study of immigrant youth (Berry *et al.*, 2006), this consistent pattern was also found: those who preferred integration had strong ethnic and national identities; those who preferred either assimilation or separation had a strong identity with one, but weak identity with the other group; and those who preferred marginalization, had weak identities with both groups.

In their work on identity strategies, Camilleri and Malewska-Peyre (1997) draw a distinction between a 'value identity' (what an individual would like to be ideally; cf. acculturation attitudes) and their 'real identity' (what an individual is like at the present time; cf. acculturation behaviours). These two aspects of identity can be very similar or very different (cf. the discrepancy between acculturation attitudes and behaviours). In the case of discrepancy, individuals will usually strive to reduce the difference between the two. During intercultural encounters, non-dominant individuals (e.g. Muslim migrants in France, where most of Camilleri and Malewska-Peyre's work has been done) may begin to perceive a greater difference between their real self (as rooted in their own culture), and a new ideal self that is communicated, perhaps imposed, by the dominant French society. For Camilleri and Malewska-Peyre (1997), such discrepancies are particularly large among immigrant adolescents, who often share the values of their peers in the dominant society, in opposition to those of their parents' heritage culture group. This frequently leads to conflict that needs to be resolved using various strategies to preserve an individual's 'coherence of identity'.

One of these identity strategies is to maintain 'simple tolerance', avoiding identity conflict by clinging to one's heritage cultural values, and ignoring or rejecting challenges to these from the dominant culture; this identity strategy resembles the acculturation strategy of separation. A second identity strategy is that of 'pragmatism' in the face of pressure to adapt to the dominant culture. In this case, young immigrants maintain 'traditionalist' identity and behaviour in their relationships with their parents (and their heritage cultural community), and a 'modernist' orientation with their peers; this may also be seen as a 'chameleon identity'. When such a combination is possible, it resembles one form of the integration acculturation strategy. Another strategy that resembles integration is that of 'conflict avoidance by complex coherence'. In this case, individuals use a 'strategy of maximization of advantages' in which the most advantageous aspects of each culture are selected and interwoven into one's identity. Of course, when one's heritage culture no longer contributes to one's sense of self, then exclusive identification with the dominant society may take place, resembling the assimilation acculturation strategy. Alternatively, when both the heritage and dominant cultures are not part of one's identity (which is the case frequently of young immigrants in Europe), the situation of marginalization is present.

Acculturative Stress

Three ways to conceptualize outcomes of acculturation have been proposed by Berry (1992; see Figure 16.2). In the first conception (behavioural shifts) we observe those changes in an individual's behavioural repertoire that take place rather easily, and are usually non-problematic. This process encompasses three sub-processes: culture shedding, culture learning

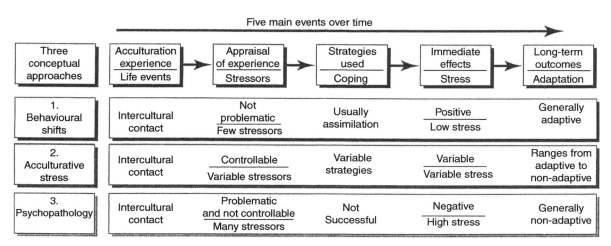

Figure 16.2 The process of acculturation and adaptation, with three conceptual approaches

and culture conflict. The first two involve the selective, accidental or deliberate loss of behaviours, and their replacement by behaviours that allow the individual a better 'fit' in with the larger society. Most often, this process has been termed 'adjustment' (Ward, 1996), since virtually all the adaptive changes take place in the non-dominant acculturating individual, with few changes occurring among members of the larger society. These adjustments are typically made with minimal difficulty, in keeping with the appraisal of the acculturation experiences as non-problematic. However, some degree of conflict may occur, which is usually resolved by the acculturating person yielding to the behavioural norms of the dominant group. In this latter case, assimilation is the most likely outcome.

When greater levels of conflict are experienced, and the experiences are judged to be problematic but controllable and surmountable, then the second approach (acculturative stress) is the appropriate conceptualization (Berry, 2006; Berry et al., 1987). In this case, individuals experience change events in their lives that challenge their cultural understandings about how to live. These change events reside in their acculturation experiences, hence the term 'acculturative' stress. In these situations, they come to understand that they are facing problems resulting from intercultural contact that cannot be dealt with easily or quickly by simply adjusting or assimilating to them. Drawing on the broader stress and adaptation paradigms (e.g. Lazarus and Folkman, 1984), this approach advocates the study of the process of how individuals deal with acculturative problems on first encountering them, and over time. In this sense, acculturative stress is a stress reaction in response to life events that are rooted in the experience of acculturation.

A third approach (psychopathology) has had long use in clinical psychology and psychiatry. In this view, acculturation is usually seen as problematic; individuals usually require assistance to deal with virtually insurmountable stressors in their lives. However, contemporary evidence (e.g. Beiser, 2000; Berry and Kim, 1988; Berry et al., 2006; Sam et al., 2016) shows that most people deal with stressors and re-establish their lives rather well, with health, psychological and social outcomes that approximate those of individuals in the larger society.

Instead of using the term culture shock (see Ward et al., 2001) to encompass these three approaches, we prefer to use the term acculturative stress for two reasons. First, the notion of shock carries only negative connotations, while stress can vary from positive (eustress) to negative (dis-stress) in valence. Since acculturation has both positive (e.g. new opportunities) and negative (e.g. discrimination) aspects, the stress conceptualization better matches the range of affect experienced during acculturation. Moreover, shock has no cultural or psychological theory, or research context associated with it, while stress (as noted above) has a place in a well-developed theoretical matrix (i.e. stress–coping–adaptation). Second, the phenomena of interest have their life in the intersection of two cultures; they are intercultural, rather than cultural in their origin. The term culture implies that only one culture is involved, while the term acculturative draws our attention to the fact that two cultures are interacting, and producing the problematic phenomena. Hence, for both reasons, I prefer the notion of acculturative stress to that of culture shock.

Relating these three approaches to acculturation strategies, some consistent empirical findings allow the following generalizations (Berry, 1997). For behavioural shifts, fewest behavioural changes result from the separation strategy, while most result from the assimilation strategy; integration involves the selective adoption of new behaviours from the larger society, and retention of valued features of one's heritage culture; and marginalization is often associated with major heritage culture loss, and the appearance of a number of dysfunctional and deviant behaviours (such as delinquency, and substance and familial abuse). For acculturative stress, there is a clear picture that the pursuit of integration is least stressful (at least where it is accommodated by the larger society), while marginalization is the most stressful; in between are the assimilation and separation strategies, sometimes one, sometimes the other being the less stressful. This pattern of findings holds for various indicators of mental health (Berry and Kim, 1988; Schmitz, 1992), and for self-esteem (Phinney et al., 1992).

Individuals engage in the appraisal of these experiences and behavioural changes. When they are appraised as challenging, some basic coping mechanisms are activated. Lazarus and Folkman (1984) have identified two major coping functions: problem-focused coping (attempting to change or solve the problem) and emotion-focused coping (attempting to regulate the emotions associated with the problem). Endler and Parker (1990) have identified a third: avoidance-orientated coping. It is not yet clear how the first two coping strategies relate to acculturation strategies since both forms of coping are likely to be involved in assimilation and integration. However, the third (avoidance) closely resembles the separation and possibly the marginalization strategies.

Adaptation: Psychological and Socio-Cultural

As a result of attempts to cope with these acculturation changes, some long-term adaptations may be achieved. As mentioned earlier, adaptation refers to the relatively stable changes that take place in an individual or group in response to external demands. This was referred to earlier as the 'how well?' question. Moreover, adaptation may or may not improve the 'fit' between individuals and their environments. It is thus not a term that necessarily implies that individuals or groups change to become more like their environments (i.e. adjustment by way of assimilation), but may involve resistance and attempts to change their environments, or to move away from them altogether (i.e. by separation). In this usage, adaptation is an outcome that may or may not be positive in valence (i.e. meaning only well-adapted). This bipolar sense of the concept of adaptation is used in the framework in Figure 16.2, where long-term adaptation to acculturation is highly variable ranging from well to poorly adapted, varying from a situation where individuals can manage their new lives very well, to one where they are unable to carry on in the new society.

Adaptation is also multifaceted. The initial distinction between psychological and socio-cultural adaptation was proposed and validated by Ward (1996). Psychological adaptation largely involves one's psychological and physical well-being, while socio-cultural adaptation refers to how well an acculturating individual is able to manage daily life in the new cultural context. While conceptually distinct, they are empirically related to some extent (correlations between the two measures are in the +0.4 to +0.5 range). However, they are also empirically distinct in the sense that they usually have different time courses and different experiential predictors. Psychological problems often increase soon after contact, followed by a general (but variable) decrease over

time; socio-cultural adaptation, however, typically has a linear improvement with time. Analyses of the factors affecting adaptation reveal a generally consistent pattern. Good psychological adaptation is predicted by personality variables, life-change events, and social support while good socio-cultural adaptation is predicted by cultural knowledge, degree of contact, and positive inter-group attitudes.

Research relating adaptation to acculturation strategies allows for some further generalizations (Berry, 1997; Ward, 1996). For all three forms of adaptation, those who pursue and accomplish integration appear to be better adapted, while those who are marginalized are least well adapted. And again, the assimilation and separation strategies are associated with intermediate adaptation outcomes. While there are occasional variations on this pattern, it is remarkably consistent, and parallels the generalization regarding acculturative stress.

The most comprehensive evidence for the relationship between how people acculturate and how well they adapt comes from the study of immigrant youth mentioned earlier (Berry et al., 2006). Individuals who carry out their intercultural lives in an 'integrative' way of acculturating (i.e. those who preferred integration, had positive identities with and had social contacts with peers from both groups, and were able to speak both languages) had positive psychological and socio-cultural adaptation. In sharp contrast, poor adaptation was the outcome for those youth who were 'diffuse' in their way of acculturating (with a pattern made up of unclear acculturation attitudes and weak identities with both groups). In second place, with respect to how well they were adapting, were youth with an 'ethnic' orientation to acculturation (a preference for separation, a strong ethnic but a weak national identity, and close ties with peers from their own group but weak ties with members in the national society). And third, somewhat surprisingly, were adolescents with a 'national' orientation to acculturation (a preference for assimilation, a strong national but a weak ethnic identity, and close ties with peers from the national society, but weak ones with peers from their own ethnic group). This pattern of relationships between how and how well people manage their acculturation has clear implications for their well-being, and some further implications for professionals in clinical practice and schools, and for policy makers in various levels of government.

Implications

For policy makers, it is now evident that policies that promote assimilation do not lead to well-adapted individuals who are in the process of acculturation. This long-standing preference of many countries to try to absorb immigrants and members of ethnocultural groups into some homogeneous single national culture has no research support. Even worse is any public policy that leads to their marginalization, combining the exclusion of immigrants or refugees from participation in the larger society, and the denial of their own cultural rights. Segregation as a policy also lacks research support, although there is some evidence (Berry *et al.*, 2006) that when sought by acculturating individuals and groups (i.e. separation), moderately good psychological adaptation results. The large body of evidence in support of integration (and of multiculturalism as a public policy) provides ample evidence for pursuing this way of organizing intercultural living in culturally plural societies.

At the individual level, including clinical practice in counselling, psychology, psychiatry, and social work, the same evidence supports the encouragement of individuals to maintain or regain their links with both cultures. Of course, the vast individual differences in acculturation and identity strategies outlined in this chapter make it essential to first discover *how* each individual is trying to live. Tools are available to make this determination (Van de Vijver *et al.*, 2016), and should be employed to find out both how they are currently, and how they would prefer to, live interculturally. On this basis, and with the knowledge that an integrative way is usually preferable, efforts can be made to guide acculturating individuals towards more positive adaptations.

Acknowledgement

This book chapter was prepared within the framework of the Basic Research Program at the National Research University Higher School of Economics (HSE) and supported within the framework of a subsidy by the Russian Academic Excellence Project '5-100'.

References

Beiser, M., (2000). *Strangers at the Gate*. Toronto: University of Toronto.

Beiser, M. Puente-Duran, S. and Hou, F. (2015). Cultural distance and emotional problems among immigrant and refugee youth in Canada: findings from the New Canadian Child and Youth Survey. *International Journal of Intercultural Relations*, 49, 33-45.

Berry, J. W. (1970). Marginality, stress and ethnic identification in an acculturated Aboriginal community. *Journal of Cross-Cultural Psychology*, 1, 239–252.

Berry, J. W. (1974). Psychological aspects of cultural pluralism: unity and identity reconsidered. *Topics in Culture Learning*, 2, 17–22.

Berry, J. W. (1980). Acculturation as varieties of adaptation. In *Acculturation: Theory, Models and Findings*, ed. A. Padilla. Boulder: Westview, pp. 9–25.

Berry, J. W. (1992). Acculturation and adaptation in a new society. *International Migration*, 30, 69–85.

Berry, J. W. (1997). Immigration, acculturation and adaptation. *Applied Psychology: An International Review*. 46, 5–68.

Berry, J. W. (1999). Aboriginal cultural identity. *Canadian Journal of Native Studies*, 19, 1–36.

Berry, J. W. (2006). Stress perspectives on acculturation. In *Cambridge Handbook of Acculturation Psychology*, ed. D. Sam and J. W. Berry, Cambridge: Cambridge University Press, pp. 43–57.

Berry, J. W. (in press). Theories and models of acculturation. In *Oxford Handbook of Acculturation and Health*, ed. S. Schwartz. New York: Oxford University Press.

Berry, J. W. and Kim, U. (1988). Acculturation and mental health. In *Health and Cross-Cultural Psychology*, ed. P. Dasen, J. W. Berry and N. Sartorius. Newbury Park: Sage, pp. 207–236.

Berry, J. W. and Sam, D. L. (2016). Conceptual issues. In *Cambridge Handbook of Acculturation Psychology*, 2nd edn, ed. D. L. Sam and J. W. Berry. Cambridge: Cambridge University Press, pp. 11–29.

Berry, J. W., Kalin, R. and Taylor, D. (1977). *Multiculturalism and Ethnic Attitudes in Canada*. Ottawa: Supply and Services.

Berry, J. W., Kim, U., Minde, T. and Mok. D. (1987). Comparative studies of acculturative stress. *International Migration Review*, 21, 491–511.

Berry, J. W., Kim, U., Power, S., Young, M. and Bujaki, M. (1989). Acculturation attitudes in plural societies. *Applied Psychology: An International Review*, 38, 185–206.

Berry, J. W., Phinney, J. S., Sam, D. L. and Vedder, P. (eds) (2006). *Immigrant Youth in Cultural Transition: Acculturation, Identity and Adaptation across National Contexts*. Mahwah: Erlbaum

Berry, J. W., Poortinga, Y. H., Breugelsman, S., Chasiotis, A. and Sam, D.L. (2011). *Cross-Cultural Psychology: Research and Applications*, 3rd edn. New York: Cambridge University Press.

Birman, D., Persky, I., & Chan, W. Y. (2010). Multiple identities of Jewish immigrant adolescents from the former Soviet Union: an exploration of salience and impact of ethnic identity. *International Journal of Behavioral Development*, **34**, 193–205, doi:10.1177/0165025409350948.

Bourhis, R., Moise, C., Perreault, S. and Senecal, S. (1997). Towards an interactive acculturation model: a social psychological approach. *International Journal of Psychology*, **32**, 369–386.

Camilleri, C. and Malewska-Peyre, H. (1997). Socialisation and identity strategies. In *Handbook of Cross-Cultural Psychology,* vol. 2, *Basic Processes and Human Development*, ed. J. W. Berry, P. R. Dasen and T. S. Saraswathi. Boston: Allyn and Bacon, pp. 41–68.

Endler, N. and Parker, J. (1990). Multidimensional assessment of coping. *Journal of Personality and Social Psychology*, **58**, 844–854.

Georgas, J. and Papastylianou, D. (1998). Acculturation and ethnic identity: the remigration of ethnic Greeks to Greece. In *Key Issues in Cross-Cultural Psychology*, ed. H. Grad, A. Blanco and J. Georgas. Lisse: Swets and Zeitlinger, pp. 114–127.

Graves, T. (1967). Psychological acculturation in a tri-ethnic community. *South-Western Journal of Anthropology*, **23**, 337–350.

Kalin, R. and Berry, J. W. (1995). Ethnic and civic self-identity in Canada: analyses of the 1974 and 1991 national surveys. *Canadian Ethnic Studies*, **27**, 1–15.

Lazarus, R. S. and Folkman, S. (1984). *Stress, Appraisal and Coping*. New York: Springer.

Liebkind, K., Mähönen, T. A., Varjonen, S. and Jasinskaja-Lahti, I. (2016). Acculturation and identity. In *Cambridge Handbook of Acculturation Psychology*, 2nd edn, ed. D. L. Sam and J. W. Berry. Cambridge: Cambridge University Press, pp. 30–49.

Motti-Stefanidi, F., Berry, J. W., Chryssochoou, X., Sam, D. L. and Phinney, J. (2012). Positive immigrant youth adaptation in context: developmental, acculturation, and social psychological perspectives. In *Capitalizing on Migration: The Potential of Immigrant Youth*, ed. A. Masten, K. Liebkind and D. Hernandez. Cambridge: Cambridge University Press, pp. 117–158.

Phinney, J. (1990). Ethnic identity in adolescents and adults. *Psychological Bulletin*, **108**, 499–514.

Phinney, J. S. and Baldelomar, O. A. (2011). Identity development in multiple cultural contexts. In *Bridging Cultural and Developmental Approaches to Psychology: New Syntheses in Theory, Research and Policy*, ed. L. Arnett Jensen. New York: Oxford University Press, pp. 161–186.

Phinney, J., Chavira, V. and Williamson, L. (1992). Acculturation attitudes and self-esteem among school and college students. *Youth and Society*, **23**, 299–312.

Redfield, R., Linton, R. and Herskovits, M. (1936). Memorandum on the study of acculturation. *American Anthropologist*, **38**, 149–152.

Ryder, A., Alden, L. and Paulhus, D. (2000). Is acculturation unidimensional or bidimensional? *Journal of Personality and Social Psychology*, **79**, 49–65.

Sam, D. L. and Berry, J. W. (eds) (2016). *Cambridge Handbook of Acculturation Psychology*, 2nd edn. Cambridge: Cambridge University Press.

Sam, D. L., Jasinskaj-Lahti, I., Ryder, A. and Hassan, G. (2016). Acculturation and health. In *Cambridge Handbook of Acculturation Psychology*, 2nd edn, ed. D. L. Sam and J. W. Berry. Cambridge: Cambridge University Press, pp. 504–524.

Schmitz, P. (1992). Acculturation styles and health. In *Innovations in Cross-Cultural Psychology*, ed. S. Iwawaki, V. Kashima and K. Leung. Amsterdam: Swets and Zeitlinger, pp. 360–370.

Umaña-Taylor, A. J., Quintana, S. M., Lee, R. M., Cross, W. E., Rivas-Drake, D., Schwartz, S. J., Syed, M., Yip, T., Seaton, E. and Ethnic and Racial Identity in the 21st Century Study Group (2014). Ethnic and racial identity during adolescence and into young adulthood: an integrated conceptualization. *Child Development*, **85**, 21–39.

Van de Vijver, F., Berry, J.W. and Celenk, O. (2016). Assessment of acculturation. In *Cambridge Handbook of Acculturation Psychology*, 2nd edn, ed. D. L. Sam and J. W. Berry. Cambridge: Cambridge University Press, pp. 93–114.

Ward, C. (1996). Acculturation. In *Handbook of Intercultural Training*, ed. D. Landis and R. Bhagat, 2nd edn. Newbury Park: Sage, pp. 124–147.

Ward, C., Bochner, S. and Funham, A. (2001). *The Psychology of Culture Shock*. London: Routledge.

Cultural Consonance

William W. Dressler

Editors' Introduction

The relationship between the individuals and their culture is often taken for granted but not understood very clearly. The relationship between the culture and people's mental health, needs to be explored. Cultural consonance allows an inspection and understanding of how individual beliefs and behaviours pan out on the broader cultural values. This can be further complicated by beliefs and behaviours of clinicians in relation to the patients too. 'Cultural consonance' is the degree to which individuals approximate shared cultural models in their own beliefs and behaviours. Research indicates it is a potent predictor of health outcomes. Dressler and his colleagues have developed the idea further and they suggest that: (1) cultural consonance can be successfully measured in a variety of settings and a variety of cultural domains; (2) cultural consonance is associated with several outcomes, including depressive symptoms, blood pressure, immune-system function, body habitus and nutrient intake; (3) cultural consonance mediates the effects of social class and race/ethnicity on outcomes; (4) cultural consonance can be measured in cultural models that have a very wide social distribution as well as in cultural models that have a more narrow social distribution; and (5) cultural consonance in different cultural domains intersects in complex ways, relative to the social distribution of cultural models. Cultural consonance can also affect the outcomes, and therefore it becomes critical to understand this concept clearly. This body of work suggests that this is a useful theoretical orientation and measurement model for continuing research on culture and mental health, as well as other health outcomes.

Introduction

The relationship between culture, understood as a property of social aggregates (especially whole societies, but sometimes smaller aggregates such as organizations), and the individuals who make up those social aggregates, has been a conundrum in the social sciences. Often it seems that social scientists write about culture as though it was either completely reproduced in the minds and behaviours of individuals, hence making an individual level of analysis unnecessary; or, alternatively, that culture in the aggregate is a mere averaging of individual thoughts and behaviours, rendering that aggregate quality of culture epiphenomenal. Neither of these perspectives is particularly useful.

A satisfactory resolution of this problem is particularly important in the study of cultural influences on human health. Without a useful account of how culture in the aggregate gets translated into individual understanding and social practice, the way in which culture affects health will remain something of a mystery.

My aim in this chapter is to present a theory of culture that resolves the difficult conceptual issues involved, and that has a related set of research methods with which dimensions of culture can be measured at the individual level. This is a theory of 'cultural consonance', or the degree to which individuals, in their own beliefs and behaviours, approximate the prototypes for belief and behaviour that are encoded in shared cultural models (Dressler, 2005). As I will argue, this general idea of a match (or, sometimes more importantly, a mismatch) between shared understandings and expectations for behaviour, and the way in which that behaviour is realized in individual lives, is not new. Indeed, in many respects this is precisely what Freud (1930) addressed in *Civilization and its Discontents*, or Durkheim (1951) in *Suicide*. What separates the concept of cultural consonance from earlier attempts to resolve this issue are the simultaneous developments of new concepts and research methods in the cognitive sciences (D'Andrade, 1995).

The approach I will present evolved from earlier anthropological studies of culture, stress and disease (Dressler, 2010). These studies examined the broad cross-cultural differences in rates of disease, especially cardiovascular disease and mental illness, observed throughout the twentieth century, particularly in the years following World War II. These differences in disease rates accompanying processes of modernization and globalization were not easily explained by conventional risk factors. The stresses associated with cultural change were posited to underlie these epidemiologic patterns, and models of psychological stress and disease were adapted to cross-cultural research in an attempt to specify the process. As results accumulated, however, it became more apparent that a core feature of the process involved the fundamental question of culture and the individual. In contexts of changing understanding and expectation, to what extent could the individual successfully incorporate those new expectations into his or her own behaviour? In any social context, whether it be one of social change or not, what are the implications of a lack of fit between the individual and their environment? These questions have been raised before (e.g. Cassel *et al.*, 1960), but a satisfactory account of this process awaited new concepts and methods.

Background to a Theory of Cultural Consonance

A theory of cultural consonance begins with the assumption that culture is both learned and shared, and that the locus of culture is both within individual human beings and in the aggregate social groups made up of human beings. This seeming contradiction is resolved when the concept of sharing is elaborated to mean, in part, 'distributed' (Sperber, 1985). Following Goodenough (1996), culture is defined as the learned, shared knowledge that one must possess to function adequately in a social group. It is important not to confuse the meaning of the term knowledge with closely related concepts like belief. Here, knowledge is used in Searle's (1995) sense of the understandings that constitute human institutions. For example, to 'know' something about marriage in American society is to know that social expectations are such that one individual will marry one other individual; they will live independently of their families; they will pool economic resources; they will raise common children; they will anticipate sexual exclusivity; and they will enter the union with the expectation of a lifelong commitment. To 'believe' something about marriage in American society is to

adopt an evaluative stance relative to all or parts of that definition of marriage. But the definition constitutes (or creates, or constructs) that social institution.

Of course, employing the example of marriage as cultural knowledge at this point in American history immediately alerts us to the fact that such knowledge can be contested. And this is useful for realizing that there can be a divergence of understanding within an overall sharing of culture. Neither opponents nor proponents of same-sex marriage regard the basic underlying cultural institution as including any form of polygyny, for example. Rather, the contested part of the understanding of the institution involves the gender of the participants. So, basic cultural knowledge can be widely shared, even when the disputed features of culture seem so prominent.

The pattern of the distribution knowledge within a social group is an empirical issue. That is, this knowledge could be widely shared; it could be weakly shared and highly contested; it could be concentrated within one or more social sub-groups; or it might be widely shared but with specific points of contention. This distribution of knowledge means, at the least, that individuals command differing degrees of cultural knowledge; at the same time, even if any given individual does not him- or herself have very elaborate knowledge of a particular cultural domain, there is a sense of the collective, that 'we' think or do certain kinds of things (Searle, 1995). It is this distributive quality of culture that makes it an aggregate property of a social group while, at the same time, locating it squarely within the cognitive structures of individuals (Gatewood, 2012).

The form that cultural knowledge takes is described well by current culture theory in cognitive anthropology (D'Andrade, 1995; Kronenfeld, 2011). Cultural knowledge exists in varying degrees of schematicity or modularity, so that the term 'cultural model' can be used as a shorthand way of denoting this knowledge that is skeletal, in outline form, and shared. The cultural model of a domain includes the elements of that domain and the semantic, functional, and causal relationships that are understood to exist among those elements, as well as how that domain links with other domains. The modular form of cultural knowledge makes it highly generalizable. For example, in the oft-cited example of a model for going to eat in a restaurant, understanding how this process works generally applies to French, German, Latin American and Chinese restaurants in the United

States (D'Andrade, 1995). The cultural schema can be tailored and applied to many specific instances.

Cultural models will vary considerably in abstraction and their links to other models. For example, a model of small-scale commercial transactions (i.e. how to buy something) can be incorporated into many more comprehensive models (e.g. going on holiday).

Again, however, to be truly a cultural model, this modular knowledge must be shared. It is a shared understanding of what are, in many cases, arbitrary models of the world that gives those models causal potential (D'Andrade, 1995). Assessing sharing has been a major problem in culture theory and research. With the advent of the cultural consensus model, however, a systematic way for evaluating the degree of sharing, or consensus, in a cultural domain became available (Romney et al., 1986; Weller, 2007). In cultural consensus analysis, agreement among a set of respondents (and in many applications a small set, e.g. around 30, is sufficient) is evaluated by first collecting their responses to a set of questions that sample knowledge of a domain. Then, a kind of statistical thought experiment is conducted in which an aggregate model of the 'culturally best' responses is proposed, and the degree to which each informant's responses match that aggregate model is evaluated. If, overall, there is a relatively high degree of correspondence between each informant's set of responses and the hypothesized culturally best model, then it can be said that there is consensus regarding that knowledge, and it is further reasonable to infer that each individual is using the same or a very similar model. Note that the responses to the questions by each informant, and the aggregate responses, are generated by each informant's knowledge of the cultural model, but these are not the model per se. The cultural model remains a hypothetical construct of which we have evidence, but which we do not observe directly. We can observe each individual putting their knowledge of the cultural model to use.

Cultural Consensus and Cultural Consonance

There are several important theoretical and methodological advances provided by the cultural consensus model. First, sharing can be unambiguously evaluated. Second, consensus can be quantified, and low consensus versus high consensus cultural domains

(and everything in between) can be identified. Third, intracultural diversity can be examined in several ways. The degree to which some individuals match the aggregate model better than others in their own knowledge can be quantified in terms of the cultural competence coefficient (which is literally the correlation of the individual's profile of responses and the hypothesized aggregate model). The higher this coefficient, the more effectively an individual's responses replicate the responses of the group as a whole. These cultural competence coefficients can then be compared by social category, to determine what the mean level of competence is of individuals in different social categories. At the same time, it is also possible to identify 'residual agreement', or sub-group agreement that exists within the context of overall consensus. And there may be more than one consensus model for a domain, which can be detected using cultural consensus analysis. Fourth, the culturally best set of responses is estimated in the analysis; these represent the most likely answers to those questions offered by any generally culturally competent member of that society, and, given the level of cultural consensus, it is possible to define the confidence in the reliability and generalizability of the responses (Dressler et al., 2015a; Gatewood, 2012).

In summary, a theory of cultural models and the cultural consensus model provide a means for resolving the apparent paradox of culture as a term the referent of which is both an aggregate and the individual. Cultural models are located in the heads of individuals, to be sure, but cultural models have certain aggregate properties in that such models (not mental models in general, but *cultural* models specifically) are distributed across minds. The size and shape of the cultural model can only be extracted from responses of a sample of individuals, and the resulting model is not some simple averaging of individual thoughts and ideas, but rather takes into account the fact that some individuals are more competent in that model than others. The culturally best set of responses estimated from cultural consensus analysis gives higher weight to individuals who are more culturally competent.

This approach enables us to describe what is prototypical and appropriate in a given cultural domain, as that is understood within a social group. One critique that has been traditionally levelled against cognitive approaches in culture theory is that they deal with how things are thought to be and not with actual practice or behaviour. Bourdieu (1990) in particular has argued that the study of cognitive orientations as constructive of understanding must be linked both to the position of an individual in the social structure and to the ways in which culturally constructed knowledge is realized in practice. The link of cultural model and behaviour is likely to be imperfect for two reasons. First, in many domains, the cultural model will provide only general guidelines for behaviour that must be sorted out in the context of specific influences and constraints within a given context. (It is worth noting, too, that a theory of cultural models leaves ample room for individual agency, within certain limits.) Second, some individuals, while they know the model, will be unable to act on it. In many instances this inability to act on a model will be a function not of the individual's motivation, but of limits placed on the individual action, principally as a function of social and economic constraints (Dressler et al., 2015b). What this means is that for some people, under some circumstances, there will be a gap between their knowledge of what is culturally prototypical and what they themselves are doing. The link of individual practice to shared cultural models is a measurable phenomenon. I have proposed the term 'cultural consonance' for this link, defined specifically as the degree to which individuals, in their own beliefs and behaviours, approximate the shared expectations encoded in cultural models.

A number of authors anticipated the theoretical construct of cultural consonance. Sapir (1927) suggested that it would be worthwhile to examine what he called 'social behaviour,' defined as individual behaviour patterns related to cultural patterns, as distinct from purely idiosyncratic behaviour. Much later, Cassel et al. (1960) employed a similar idea specifically in the context of the study of migration, arguing that, among migrants to a novel cultural setting, there may be a mismatch between the values, expectations and social practices of the migrant and the corresponding social and cultural patterns of the host society, the result being a stressful inconsistency (see also Bhugra, 2004). French et al. (1974) proposed a concept of 'person–environment fit' to describe the consistency between an individual's attitudes and the values of a particular social setting. This basic idea of a mismatch between the individual and his or her social and cultural environment is thus not a new one.

The construct of cultural consonance can be regarded as distinct from earlier approaches in two senses. First, as argued thus far, a theory of cultural consonance is embedded in a cognitive theory of culture, and so is more explicit in describing the larger environment of shared meaning in which individuals act. Second, there is a clear set of research procedures associated with the theory of cultural consonance for determining the degree of sharing within a particular cultural domain, and then in turn connecting shared meaning to individual belief and behaviour (Borgatti, 1999). There is thus a direct, measured link from collective representation to individual practice. Because of this clear measurement model, we have argued that measures of cultural consonance can be regarded as having high 'emic validity' (Dressler and Oths, 2014). In anthropology, an emic approach refers to a description of culture in the terms that members of a society themselves use to categorize the world around them, rather than using categories derived from the experience of the observer (D'Andrade, 1995). These categories are, in short, meaningful to participants in a social setting, and may or may not be meaningful to the observer. In conventional approaches, the validity and reliability of a measurement usually hinges on whether or not that measurement is acceptable to a community of researchers. The measurement of cultural consonance, on the other hand, starts by first examining how participants construct the world around them, and from that creates systematic measures that order individuals along a continuum defined by the terms they themselves use (Dressler et al., 2005a).

The question is: what are the psychological and biological costs of low cultural consonance?

Cultural Consonance and Health Outcomes

Cultural consonance and its associations with health outcomes have been examined by our research group in four major studies, three conducted in urban Brazil and one in the African American community of a small city in the southeastern United States (Dressler, 2005; Dressler and Bindon, 2000; Dressler et al., 2016a). The Brazilian studies examined a variety of outcomes, including blood pressure, depressive symptoms, body composition, C-reactive protein, and food intake; the US study focused exclusively on blood pressure. Cultural consonance is an extremely flexible concept in the sense that a person's consonance could be measured within virtually any cultural domain. The initial studies of cultural consonance focused on the cultural domains of lifestyle and social support. These domains describe the emic, lived experience of individuals with respect to two major dimensions of social life: social status and social integration. Lifestyle refers to the accumulation of material goods and related leisure time practices. As Veblen (1899) pointed out in the nineteenth century, lifestyle is a way of projecting into mundane social interaction a claim to a particular social status. Although Veblen is usually associated with the notion of 'conspicuous consumption' with respect to lifestyles, he also argued that the majority of people aspire to what he called 'a common standard of decency'; that is, individuals seek not to exceed local standards of lifestyle, but rather to attain what is collectively regarded as a 'good life', often more a kind of modest domestic comfort than a high level of consumption. In examining cultural models of lifestyle in Brazil and in the African American community, this is precisely what we found (although the specific content of models differs between societies).

Social support refers to the help and assistance that individuals can anticipate and receive in times of felt need. There are several facets to social support, and one that has received relatively little attention is the cultural model of social support. In our work, we have found that there are shared models of appropriate sources of social support in relation to specific kinds of problems. These tend to be quite variable across societies. For example, in Brazil, the cultural model of social support is somewhat like a series of concentric circles around the individual, with family and friends forming the inner circles, and less intimate relationships forming the outer circle. At the same time, there are distinct kinds of problems for which certain kinds of supporters can be approached, even if they are regarded as less intimate. In the African American community, there is a distinction between kin and non-kin supporters, with one or the other set of supporters being preferred within different social contexts (Dressler and Bindon 2000; Dressler et al., 2005a).

In both studies we confirmed, using cultural consensus analysis, that there were broadly shared cultural models of lifestyle and social support. Then, in survey research, we asked individuals specifically about their own lifestyles and patterns of social support. Cultural consonance is measured by how closely an individual's reported behaviour corresponds to the

culturally prototypical patterns described by the cultural models. In Brazil, we found higher cultural consonance in both dimensions to be associated with lower blood pressure, fewer reported symptoms of depression, lower alcohol intake, and lower body fat and body mass index (Dressler et al., 1997, 1998, 2002; Dressler et al., 2004). In the African American community, we found an interaction between cultural consonance in lifestyle and cultural consonance in social support, such that for all respondents higher cultural consonance in lifestyle was associated with lower blood pressure, but the association was stronger for individuals who also had high cultural consonance in social support (Dressler and Bindon, 2000).

More recent work in Brazil has enabled us to extend the cultural consonance model in several ways. First, using more precise methods of data collection and analysis from cognitive anthropology (Borgatti, 1999), we have confirmed the outlines of the cultural models of lifestyle and social support from previous studies. Furthermore, we have found that cultural consensus models in these cultural domains and others (see later) are stable over a 10-year period (Dressler et al., 2015a). Not only are these cultural consensus models stable, they do not vary significantly by age, gender or social class.

Second, we have expanded the cultural domains examined, by including national identity, family life, occupational and educational aspirations, and food. These cultural domains were selected for study both on the basis of their theoretical interest and on the basis of ethnographic observation. For example, with respect to the cultural domain of family life, there is ample theoretical justification for its inclusion in any study of health outcomes, and the family as a cultural domain is the focus of much interest and discussion in everyday discourse in Brazil. Food is also a focus of much interest in Brazil (DaMatta, 1985). From a theoretical standpoint, it is useful to separate the cultural meaning of food from nutrient intake, examining food as a cultural domain (Oths et al., 2003). Finally, there has been considerable historical interest in national identity in the social sciences (Gorer, 1948), and cultural domain analyses and the measurement of cultural consonance afforded a novel approach to its examination.

The research we have carried out in Brazil has enabled us to examine cultural consonance and health from a number of angles. One question guiding this work has involved the specificity of the effects of cultural consonance. There are some domain-specific effects of cultural consonance. For example, the associations of cultural consonance in lifestyle and cultural consonance in social support in relation to arterial blood pressure have been replicated (Dressler *et al.*, 2005b), but cultural consonance in other domains appears not to be related to blood pressure. Similarly, cultural consonance in social support is associated with C-reactive protein (an indicator of immune system stimulation and a risk factor for coronary artery disease), but no other measure of cultural consonance is (Dressler *et al.*, 2016b).

On the other hand, we found that measures of cultural consonance tend to converge in a kind of generalized cultural consonance. Specifically, in a factor analysis, cultural consonance in the domains of lifestyle, social support, family life and national identity all loaded on a single factor, while cultural consonance in several dimensions of food loaded an independent factor; then, using factor scores, we found that higher cultural consonance on each of these was independently associated with lower depressive symptoms, although the factor describing consonance in social factors (i.e. lifestyle, family life) had an association with depressive symptoms twice as large as that of cultural consonance in food (Dressler *et al.*, 2007a). These measures of generalized cultural consonance were also associated with lower body mass and body fat (Dressler *et al.*, 2012).

These results and ethnographic work led us to hypothesize that cultural consonance in the domains of lifestyle, social support, family life, national identity and occupational/educational aspirations were all meaningfully organized as lifespan developmental goals. A cultural consensus study demonstrated that all of these domains described specific goals in life in Brazil, and they revolved around the central goal of achieving the respect and recognition of others. Then, in a cultural consonance study, we found that cultural consonance in these five domains all loaded a single principal component, and this measure of cultural consonance in life goals was the strongest predictor of depressive symptoms, controlling for demographic variables as well as for stressful life events, locus of control and frustration tolerance (Dressler *et al.*, 2016c).

With respect to the independent association of cultural consonance and health outcomes, we found that cultural consonance completely mediates the association of socio-economic status and health (Dressler *et al.*, 2015b).

We also carried out a 2-year follow-up study of cultural consonance and depressive symptoms in Brazil (Dressler *et al.*, 2007b). Controlling for baseline values of depressive symptoms and cultural consonance, change in cultural consonance over a 2-year period was associated with change in depressive symptoms, controlling for standard demographic variables and stressful life events occurring over that 2-year period.

Finally, we have incorporated a gene–environment interaction component into the research on depressive symptoms. In a non-random subsample drawn from the longitudinal study just described, respondents were genotyped for a single nucleotide polymorphism (SNP) in the 2A receptor for serotonin (–1486 G/A; rs6311). There was a significant interaction between this SNP and cultural consonance (specifically in the cultural domain of family life) such that for persons with the AA genotype the inverse association of cultural consonance with depressive symptoms was stronger than for persons with the GG or GA genotypes. Because this was a non-random subsample, however, sampling error could have confounded the results; therefore, we undertook a replication study with a much larger and more representative sample. In that larger sample, the cultural consonance–gene interaction was not replicated (Dressler *et al.*, 2016d).

In additional analyses of those data, however, we found a gene–environment interaction involving the 2A serotonin receptor SNP and childhood adversity. Persons who reported experiencing childhood adversity (such as death of a parent or severe socialization) also reported more depressive symptoms as an adult if they were an AA genotype, while there was little association of childhood adversity and depressive symptoms for persons with GG or GA genotypes. This replicates a widely documented gene–environment interaction (Caspi *et al.*, 2010). We hypothesized that this childhood adversity–gene interaction might be mediated by cultural consonance in family life, suggesting that learning the cultural model as a child and then incorporating the cultural model of the family into one's own life – cultural consonance – could be compromised. Results showed that cultural consonance in family life did indeed completely mediate the association of the childhood adversity–gene interaction with depressive symptoms. Individuals with the AA genotype and high childhood adversity reported significantly lower cultural consonance in family life than persons with the GG or GA genotypes, and in turn reported higher depressive symptoms (Dressler *et al.*, 2016a).

Work by Other Investigators

A number of other investigators have incorporated the theory and method of cultural consonance into their work, independently corroborating the results from our research group. Sweet (2010) examined cultural consonance in lifestyle and blood pressure within a sample of African American adolescents in a major city in the United States. In keeping with the role of material culture as a marker of social status, she hypothesized that there would be a well-defined cultural consensus model of lifestyle items that symbolized being a successful teen, and that lower cultural consonance with that model would result in higher blood pressure. She found a strongly shared and quite detailed model of a valued lifestyle, emphasizing particular material goods such as specific cell phones and brands of shoes. The association of cultural consonance and blood pressure, however, depended on parental socio-economic status. Where parental socio-economic status was low, increasing cultural consonance was associated with increasing blood pressure; where parental socio-economic status was high, increasing cultural consonance was associated with lower blood pressure.

Reyes-Garcia and her colleagues (2010) employed cultural consonance in lifestyle to examine psychological well-being among the Tsimane' of lowland Bolivia. The Tsimane' are an ethnic group with systematic variation in the degree to which they have become involved in market economies, with some villages having a virtual subsistence economy (based on horticulture, hunting and fishing) while other villages, closer to market centres, depend more on sales of produce and some wage labour. These investigators developed a cultural consensus model of lifestyle items necessary to be a successful Tsimane'. Then, in survey research, they found that higher cultural consonance was associated with reports of higher subjective well-being.

Dengah (2013, 2014) carried out research among Brazilian Pentecostals. While Brazil remains the world's largest Catholic country, adherents to various Pentecostal Protestant denominations grew dramatically throughout the twentieth and into the twenty-first century. He developed a cultural consensus model of what it means to be a 'good' *evangélico* (as Pentecostals are referred to in Brazil), which was ordered around living 'the complete life' (*a vida completa* in Portuguese). Elements of this model included private devotional acts (belief, prayer), receiving material benefits of faith, and engaging in public demonstrations of faith (especially speaking in tongues). Adherents with high cultural consonance in the model of the complete life reported fewer depressive symptoms. Dengah (2015) also included measures of cultural consonance in family life and lifestyle. Interestingly, he found a synergistic effect among these measures of cultural consonance. The inverse association of cultural consonance in family life and lifestyle with depressive symptoms was enhanced by cultural consonance in the complete life.

In a quite different social context, Snodgrass *et al.* (2013) examined cultural models of success in both the real world and the world of Azeroth, a virtual reality for players of the multi-player Internet video game 'World of Warcraft' (or 'WoW'). In WoW, players assume identities represented by their avatars and join with other players to wage war, pursue heroic quests and accumulate virtual goods and status. In their research, involving ethnographic research with players in local groups and online survey research, these researchers first developed cultural consensus models of what participants regarded as being successful in both the real world and in WoW. There was some overlap in elements of the models, but they turned out to be quite distinct. Then, in survey research, they measured cultural consonance with each model and related that to a modified scale of Internet addiction. They found that measures of cultural consonance of success in the real world and success in WoW were statistically independent, and that each was associated with Internet addiction, but in opposite directions. Persons high in cultural consonance in the real world had lower Internet addiction scores, while persons high in cultural consonance in WoW had higher Internet addiction scores.

Issues in the Study of Cultural Consonance

This theory of cultural consonance, and its associated measurement model, deals with a number of difficult issues. Perhaps most importantly, it takes seriously the two sides of culture: as an environment of shared meaning that refers to an aggregate, and as a set of understandings that individuals learn within that environment of shared meaning. It then takes the additional step of examining how individuals are differentially able to put those understandings into practice in their own behaviour. Results thus far suggest that there are psychological and physiological costs to low cultural consonance.

What mediates the effects of cultural consonance? We examined this question in one study, hypothesizing that perceived stress would mediate the influence of cultural consonance on depressive symptoms. Interestingly, while there was a partial mediation of the influence of cultural consonance, the mediating effect of perceived stress was actually quite small, indicating that a more subtle and nuanced process must be at work (Balieiro *et al.*, 2011).

At one level, cultural consonance shapes an individual's sense of how the world works, in the terms discussed by Aaron Antonovsky (1979) many years ago. Antonovsky argued that a person who maintained good health in its broadest sense would have a world view that he described as a 'sense of coherence', defined as:

> ... a global orientation that expresses the extent to which one has a pervasive, enduring though dynamic feeling of confidence that one's internal and external environments are predictable and that there is a high probability that things will work out as well as can reasonably be expected. (Antonovsky 1979: 123)

Individuals with a higher level of cultural consonance share an understanding with their peers of how the world is supposed to work, and their world, in fact, conforms to that expectation. On the other hand, the individual with a lower level of cultural consonance is faced with a world in which things simply do not work out in accordance with expectation.

At another level, cultural consonance helps to mediate mundane social interaction. A fundamental motive in social interaction is to receive confirmation from others of a basic social status, even in relatively anonymous interactions in mass society. Our cultural consonance, as we embody that status and as we strategically reveal our position in the symbolic space of culture, helps to define our presentation of self. Where that cultural consonance does not support a claim to a basic social status, recognition, respect and confirmation can be withheld. Over time, these 'micro-stressors' in everyday social interaction can take their toll both psychologically and physiologically (Scheepers *et al.*, 2009).

These linked processes are especially acute in the cultural domains we have studied because cultural competence in the domains is so widely and uniformly distributed. That is, 'everyone' (within the limits of individual competences) knows the models, but not everyone is able to enact those models in their lives. It is this sense of 'incoherence' that is likely to be stressful and contribute to the risk of disease.

One of the more interesting questions emerging in research on cultural consonance concerns the convergent, competing and synergistic effects of cultural consonance in different domains. Our research suggests that cultural consonance in the different domains we have studied converges around the cultural theme of life goals, and that a measure combining cultural consonance in all the specific domains is a potent correlate of mental health (Dressler *et al.*, 2016c). Dengah (2015) on the other hand found interactive effects among cultural consonance in different cultural domains, while Snodgrass and colleagues (2013) found cultural consonance in different domains to have opposite effects. Clearly, culture is a complex phenomenon. There is as yet little well-developed theory about how cultural models in different domains link and under what circumstances. Similarly, there are only the barest outlines of how cultural consonance in different domains might converge, or not. Clearly, however, the ways in which cultural consonance in different domains may or may not converge has implications for individual mental health, and future research to help clarify these basic socio-cultural processes would be helpful.

In the final analysis, the theory of cultural consonance and the results from the empirical analysis of this theory suggest that, in health, culture matters. Individuals live out their lives in a space of meaning constructed out of shared cultural models. Where their personal beliefs and behaviours situate them in this space can have profound implications for their well-being.

Acknowledgements

Research on which this chapter is based was funded by the National Institutes of Health, USA (HL45663), and the National Science Foundation, USA (BNS9020786, BCS0091903 and BCS1026429). These studies were conducted with my long-time collaborators James R. Bindon, Mauro C. Balieiro, Kathryn S. Oths, Rosane P. Ribeiro and José Ernesto dos Santos.

References

Antonovsky, A. (1979). *Health, Stress, and Coping*. San Francisco, CA: Jossey-Bass.

Balieiro, M. C., dos Santos, M. A., dos Santos, J. E. and Dressler, W. W. (2011). Does perceived stress mediate the effect of cultural consonance on depression? *Transcultural Psychiatry*, **48**(5), 519–538.

Bhugra, D. (2004). Cultural identities and cultural congruency: a new model for evaluating mental distress in immigrants. *Acta Psychiatrica Scandinavia*, **111**, 84–93.

Borgatti, S. P. (1999). Elicitation techniques for cultural domain analysis. In *Ethnographer's Toolkit: Enhanced Ethnographic Methods*, vol. 3, ed. J. J. Schensul, *et al.* Walnut Creek, CA: Altamira Press, pp. 115–151.

Bourdieu, P. (1990). *In Other Words: Essays Toward a Reflexive Sociology*, ed. M. Adamson (trans.). Stanford, CA: Stanford University Press.

Caspi, A., Hariri, A. R., Holmes, A., Uher, R. and Moffitt, T. E. (2010). Genetic sensitivity to the environment: the case of the serotonin transporter gene and its implications for studying complex diseases and traits. *American Journal of Psychiatry*, **167**, 509–527.

Cassel J. C., Patrick, R. and Jenkins, C. D. (1960). Epidemiological analysis of the health implications of culture change. *Annals of the New York Academy of Sciences*, **84**, 938–949.

D'Andrade, R. G. (1995). *The Development of Cognitive Anthropology*. Cambridge: Cambridge University Press.

DaMatta, R. (1985). *A Casa e a Rua*. São Paulo, Brasil: Editora Brasiliense.

Dengah, H. J. F. (2013). The contract with God: patterns of cultural consensus across two Brazilian religious communities. *Journal of Anthropological Research*, **69**, 347–372.

Dengah, H. J. F. (2014). How religious status shapes psychological well-being: cultural consonance as a measure of subcultural status among Brazilian Pentecostals. *Social Science and Medicine*, **114**, 18–25.

Dressler, W. W. (2005). What's *cultural* about bio*cultural* research? *Ethos*, **33**, 20–45.

Dressler, W. W. (2010). Culture and the stress process. In *A Companion to Medical Anthropology*, ed. M. Singer and P. Erickson. New York: Wiley-Blackwell, pp. 119–134.

Dressler, W. W. and Bindon, J. R. (2000). The health consequences of cultural consonance: cultural dimensions of lifestyle, social support and arterial blood pressure in an African American community. *American Anthropologist*, **102**, 244–260.

Dressler, W. W. and Oths, K. S. (2014). Social survey methods. In *Handbook of Methods in Cultural Anthropology*, 2nd edn, ed. H. R. Bernard and C. C. Gravlee. Lanham, MD: AltaMira Press, pp. 497–515.

Dressler, W. W., Balieiro, M. C. and dos Santos, J. E. (1997). The cultural construction of social support in Brazil: associations with health outcomes. *Culture, Medicine and Psychiatry*, **21**, 303–335.

Dressler, W. W., Balieiro, M. C. and dos Santos, J. E. (1998). Culture, socio-economic status and physical and mental health in Brazil. *Medical Anthropology Quarterly*, **12**, 424–446.

Dressler, W. W., Balieiro, M. C. and dos Santos, J. E. (2002). Cultural consonance and psychological distress. *Paidéia: Cadernos de Psicologia e Educação*, **12**, 5–18.

Dressler, W. W., Ribeiro, R. P., Balieiro, M. C., Oths, K. S. and dos Santos, J. E. (2004). Eating, drinking and being depressed: the social, cultural and psychological context of alcohol consumption and nutrition in a Brazilian community. *Social Science and Medicine*, **59**, 709–720.

Dressler, W. W., Borges, C. D., Balieiro, M. C. and dos Santos, J. E. (2005a). Measuring cultural consonance: examples with special reference to measurement theory in anthropology. *Field Methods*, **17**, 531–555.

Dressler, W. W., Balieiro, M. C., Ribeiro, R. P. and dos Santos, J. E. (2005b). Cultural consonance and arterial blood pressure in urban Brazil. *Social Science and Medicine*, **61**, 527–540.

Dressler, W., Balieiro, M., Ribeiro, R., and dos Santos, J. (2007a). Cultural consonance and psychological distress: examining the associations in multiple cultural domains. *Culture, Medicine and Psychiatry*, **31**, 195–224.

Dressler, W., Balleiro, M., Ribeiro, R. and dos Santos, J. (2007b). A prospective study of cultural consonance and depressive symptoms in urban Brazil. *Social Science and Medicine*, **65**, 2058–2069.

Dressler, W. W., Oths, K. S., Balieiro, M. C., Ribeiro, R. P. and dos Santos, J. E. (2012). How culture shapes the body: cultural consonance and body mass in urban brazil. *American Journal of Human Biology*, **24**, 325–331.

Dressler, W. W., Balieiro, M. C. and dos Santos, J. E. (2015a). Finding culture change in the second factor: stability and change in cultural consensus and residual agreement. *Field Methods*, **27**, 22–38.

Dressler, W. W., Balieiro, M. C., Ribeiro, R. P. and dos Santos, J. E. (2015b). Culture as a mediator of health disparities: cultural consonance, social class, and health. *Annals of Anthropological Practice*, **39**, 214–231.

Dressler, W. W., Balieiro, M. C., Ferreira de Araújo, L., Silva, W. A., Jr and dos Santos, J. E. (2016a). Culture as a mediator of gene-environment interaction: cultural consonance, childhood adversity, a 2A serotonin receptor polymorphism, and depression in urban Brazil. *Social Science and Medicine*, **160**, 109–117.

Dressler, W. W., Balieiro, M. C., Ribeiro, R. P. and dos Santos, J. E. (2016b). Culture and the immune system: cultural consonance in social support and C-reactive protein in urban Brazil. *Medical Anthropology Quarterly*, **30**, 259–277.

Dressler, W. W., Balieiro, M. C. and dos Santos, J. E. (2016c). Cultural consonance in life goals and depressive symptoms in urban Brazil. *Journal of Anthropological Research*, 73(1), 43–65.

Dressler, W. W., Balieiro, M. C., de Araújo, L. F., Silva, W. A., Jr and dos Santos, J. E. (2016d). The interaction of cultural consonance and a polymorphism in the 2A serotonin receptor in relation to depression in Brazil: failure to replicate previous findings. *American Journal of Human Biology*, 28, 936–940.

Durkheim, E. (1951). *Suicide: A Study in Sociology*. G. Simpson (ed.), J. A. Spaulding (trans.) Glencoe, IL: Free Press.

French, J. R. P., Rogers, W. and Cobb, S. (1974). Adjustment as person–environment fit. In *Coping and Adaptation*, ed. G. V. Coelho, D. A. Hamburg and J. E. Adams. New York: Basic Books, pp. 316–333.

Freud, S. (1930). *Civilization and its Discontents*. J. Riviere (trans.) London: Hogarth Press.

Gatewood, J. B. (2012). Cultural models, consensus analysis, and the social organization of knowledge. *Topics in Cognitive Science*, 4, 362–371.

Goodenough, W. H. (1996). Culture. In *Encyclopedia of Cultural Anthropology*, ed. D. Levinson and M. Ember, New York: Henry Holt, pp. 291–299.

Gorer, G. (1948). *The American People: A Study in National Character*. New York: Norton.

Kronenfeld, D. B. (2011). Afterword: one cognitive view of culture. In *A Companion to Cognitive Anthropology*, ed. D. B. Kronenfeld, G. Bennardo, V. C. de Munck and M. D. Fischer. Malden, MA: Wiley-Blackwell, pp. 569–583.

Oths, K. S., Carolo, A. and dos Santos, J. E. (2003). Social status and food preference in southern Brazil. *Ecology of Food and Nutrition*, 42, 303–324.

Reyes-García, V., Gravlee, C., McDade, T., Huanca, T., Leonard, W. and Tanner, S. (2010). Cultural consonance and psychological well-being. *Culture, Medicine and Psychiatry*, 34, 186–203.

Romney, A. K., Weller, S. C. and Batchelder, W. H. (1986). Culture as consensus: a theory of culture and informant accuracy. *American Anthropologist*, 88, 313–338.

Sapir, E. (1927). The unconscious patterning of behaviour in society. In *The Unconscious: A Symposium*. New York: Alfred A. Knopf, pp. 114–142.

Scheepers, D., Ellemers, N. and Sintemaartensdijk, N. (2009). Suffering from the possibility of status loss: physiological responses to social identity threat in high status groups. *European Journal of Social Psychology*, 39, 1075–1092.

Searle, J. (1995). *The Construction of Social Reality*. New York: Free Press.

Snodgrass, J. G., Dengah, H. J. F., Lacy, M. G. and Fagan, J. (2013). A formal anthropological view of motivation models of problematic MMO play: achievement, social, and immersion factors in the context of culture. *Transcultural Psychiatry*, 50, 235–262.

Sperber, D. (1985). Anthropology and psychology: towards an epidemiology of representations. *Man*, 20, 73–89.

Sweet, E. (2010). 'If your shoes are raggedy you get talked about': symbolic and material dimensions of adolescent social status and health. *Social Science and Medicine*, 70, 2029–2035.

Veblen, T. (1899). *The Theory of the Leisure Class*. New York: Macmillan.

Weller, S. C. (2007). Cultural consensus theory: applications and frequently asked questions. *Field Methods*, 19, 339–368.

Chapter 18

Neurotic Disorders

Anxiety and Fear Related, Dissociative and Bodily Distress Disorders

Geetha Desai and Santosh K. Chaturvedi

Editors' Introduction

Neurotic disorders are perhaps the commonest mental disorders. These consist of many mental disorders, like depressive disorders, anxiety and fear related, dissociative, and bodily distress disorders. This category has undergone vast changes in terms of nomenclature, nosology and clinical practice. In this chapter, Chaturvedi and Desai provide an overview of the concept of neurosis, and the transformations it has gone through over the decades. Not only the nomenclature has changed but the research evidence and treatment modalities have become clearer in many settings along with the role of culture. Neurosis, considered a maladaptive pattern of behaviour following a stressful situation which leads to an avoidance of responsibility and the stressful situation itself, presents with anxiety symptoms. The anxiety provoking situations in the past should have resulted in excessive nervousness, depression or bodily symptoms. The diagnosis of common mental disorders is influenced by culture and the importance given to symptoms and the meaning assigned by the clinician will also depend upon culture at large but importantly their own culture. These symptoms may reflect a failure to cope but may also be a cry for help, requiring support and understanding from the friends, families and professionals. The diagnosis of neurosis is influenced (to a considerable degree) by the subject's perception of illness. The cultural factors may influence the symptom presentation, help-seeking and the explanations for the illnesses. The presentations of many of the so called erstwhile neurotic disorders show varying patterns of abnormal illness behaviours.

Introduction

The term 'neurosis' has been ascribed various meanings and definitions, including being named as the 'worried well'! There has been an effort to abandon this term; however, it is still used by physicians and many psychiatrists in their clinical practice. In ICD-10 all neurotic disorders have been clubbed under the rubric 'neurotic, stress related and somatoform disorders'. In DSM-5, the term 'neurotic disorders' has not been used at all. In the ICD-11, neurotic disorders are proposed to be included as anxiety and fear related disorders, dissociative disorders and bodily distress disorders. Depressive neurosis and neurotic depression are included in the category for dysthymic disorders, anxiety neurosis is included in generalized anxiety disorder. Anankastic neurosis and obsessive–compulsive neurosis are included in obsessive–compulsive disorders, and hypochondriacal neurosis is included under hypochondriasis.

Neuroticism is a dimension of personality that captures trait individual differences in the tendency to experience negative thoughts and feelings. Barlow *et al.* (2014) provide a fresh perspective on the developmental origins of neuroticism – a dimension of temperament marked by elevated stress reactivity resulting in the frequent experience of negative emotions. This negative affectivity is accompanied by a pervasive perception that the world is a dangerous and threatening place, along with beliefs about one's inability to manage or cope with challenging events.

Neurosis, as a disorder, is considered a maladaptive pattern of behaviour (or reaction), following a stressful situation, which tends to avoid responsibility (instead of facing up to the stress) and the stressful situation itself. Three factors, which have to be taken into consideration while making a diagnosis of a neurotic disorder, are as follows:

1. There should be an evidence of stress (or a stressful situation) of recent origin which should have some temporal relationship with the development of symptoms. Many times a presumed or perceived stress rather than an actual stress may be present.

2. The reaction to this stress (actual or presumed) should appear to be maladaptive, i.e. instead of

coping and facing the stress, there is a tendency to avoid the stress and its consequences.

3. There should be an evidence of anxiety proneness. The anxiety provoking situations in the past should have resulted in excessive nervousness, depression or somatic symptoms.

Incidentally, in most cases routinely diagnosed as a neurotic disorder, the above factors are not taken into consideration or there is a lack of clear-cut evidence for the stress, anxiety proneness, or tendency to avoid stress or responsibilities. Interestingly, stress and coping have a close association with cultural factors.

Cultural aspects of mental disorders including neurosis have been studied extensively. The phenomenological experience and expression of that experience differs across cultures and these affect the diagnosis and labelling of disorders. Not only do the diagnoses differ across cultures, but the importance given to symptoms and the meaning assigned by the psychiatrist depending on their cultural background also differ. The diagnosis of neurosis is influenced to a considerable degree by the subject's perception of illness. The cultural factors may influence the symptom presentation; help-seeking and the explanations for the illnesses. Epidemiological studies of neurotic disorders have proved to be challenging, mainly due to differences in the concepts of neurosis. The various manifestations of neurotic disorders in different cultural settings contribute to this difficulty. Various neurotic disorders are discussed here in terms of epidemiology, symptoms and treatment with some reference to the role of cultural factors.

Dysthymia (Neurotic Depression)

Dysthymia includes neurotic depression and depressive neurosis in the proposed ICD-11. It is one of the commonest psychiatric diagnoses in patients attending psychiatric clinics, psychiatric outpatient departments or mental health facilities. Though it is commonly encountered, its concept, nosological status, aetiology, course and management are poorly understood. Patients with somatic symptoms, anxiety, depression, dysphoria or any other unclear psychopathology are labelled as having neurotic depression. This category is also used for cases that develop depression secondary to or as a reaction to any emotional precipitating factor (reactive depression or depressive reaction).

In the West, a new approach to the understanding of depressive disorders has emerged over the last five decades or so, and the studies have focused more on dysthymic disorders, atypical depression, characterological depression, minor depression, etc. But for many clinicians, it is a habit to diagnose these cases as neurotic depression. Various factors have been taken into consideration while making a diagnosis of neurotic depression. As mentioned previously, there should be evidence of stress (presumed or perceived) of recent origin, which should have some temporal relationship with the development of symptoms. The reaction to the previously mentioned stress should appear to be maladaptive and there should be some evidence of anxiety proneness. The anxiety provoking situations in the past should have resulted in excessive nervousness, depression or somatic symptoms.

Epidemiology

Patients with neurotic depression usually remain in outpatient treatment. They may form nearly 25–30 per cent of all psychiatric patients in a general hospital psychiatric set-up, and nearly 10–15 per cent of the psychiatric hospital population. In the general population, neurotic depression was reported to be nearly 10–20 per 1,000 population. It is more common in women and the commonest age groups are between 20 and 35 years. Since the label of neurotic depression is no longer being used in classificatory systems, estimates of its prevalence in the recent past are lacking.

Clinical Features

The commonest signs and symptoms are feelings of sadness, weeping spells, lack of interest in surroundings and activities of daily life. Sadness is non-pervasive and becomes less on removing the person from the stressful situation. The symptoms are generally worse in the evening. Depressive cognitions may occur at the same time as the feelings of sadness. The patient usually tends to blame others or the environment, and do not hold themselves responsible for their symptoms. The feelings of anxiety, tension and nervousness, along with autonomic symptoms are invariably present. The feelings of guilt, self-depreciation and self-blame may be absent. The reactivity of mood is preserved. Somatic symptoms or bodily complaints are present in many of the cases. The common bodily complaints are headache, body ache, and pain in the back, feelings of weakness, fatigue and palpitations. Lack of appetite is mild and there may be periods of overeating. The lack of appetite usually does not lead to loss of weight. Sleep is disturbed in many cases, the commonest disturbances being either difficulty in falling asleep or intermittent awakenings. Alternatively, hypersomnia may be present. Suicide itself is generally not a feature of neurotic depression but suicidal gestures or attempts may occur frequently. Depressive personality traits may be evident in some cases.

The core features of depression have attracted a great deal of attention in the cross-cultural studies. The most salient feature of depression is a distinction between psyche and soma or the mind–body dualism. This distinction is evident in the formulation of depressive disorders which revolve around particular affects and associated somatic symptoms. The latter are relatively easy to ascertain across cultures. The difficulty lies in determining the presence of depressed mood as defined in the West, because of assumptions about emotion and its phenomenology. In many cultures there are essentially no terms to describe depression and internal emotional states. The absence of such terms does not in itself preclude the existence of related affect, or even analogous categories of illness. Certain cultures discourage displays of extreme sadness and sorrow. In many cultures, an illness with features of depression is called by other local names (nervous problem) in order to shift the emphasis to the physical nature of the illness (which is acceptable), from the emotional one (which may not be acceptable).

Shenjing shuairuo, known as neurasthenia in the West, is a condition highly prevalent among the Chinese. It is characterized by feelings of physical and mental exhaustion, difficulty concentrating, memory loss, fatigue and dizziness. A number of associated physical complaints similar to those seen in depression include difficulty in sleeping, appetite disturbance, sexual dysfunction, headaches and irritability. There is an ongoing debate regarding whether or not this is a Chinese label for depressive disorders. *Shenjing shuairuo* is associated with lesser stigma than the term depression. In Central and South America, many people attribute illness to an acute fright (*susto, espanto, pasmo*). Similar ideas are found in Asia and Africa. An intense fright leads to a sudden flight of the soul from the body. This 'soul loss' is the underlying cause of the illness. Despite its explicit links to fright, *susto* may be associated more closely with depression than with anxiety disorders.

Anxiety Disorders

The experience of fear in response to threat of injury that accompanies fight-or-flight response is a universal phenomenon. Even though anxiety is a universal phenomenon, the context in which it is experienced, the interpretations of its meaning, and the responses to it, are strongly influenced by cultural beliefs or practices. Earlier studies examined cultural differences on self-report measures of anxiety symptoms, and established significant differences in prevalence. In epidemiological studies significant differences in rates of anxiety disorders have been noted among ethnocultural groups. Mexican Americans have higher rates of simple phobias. A cross-national study involving surveys in the United States, Canada, Puerto Rico, Germany, Taiwan, Korea and New Zealand found comparable rates. Although many anxiety disorders show comparable prevalence among major ethnocultural groups in the general population, substantial differences in rates are found in clinical epidemiologic studies, probably due to differential patterns of help-seeking.

Cross-cultural studies have found substantial differences in the symptomatology of anxiety. These include differences in the prominence and type of specific fears as well as associated somatic, dissociative and affective symptoms and syndromes. A variety of culture-related forms of anxiety disorders have also been identified including *koro* in south and east Asia, semen-loss anxiety syndrome (*dhat, jiryan* in India, *sukra praneha* in Srilanka, *shen-k'uei* in China), *tai-jinkyofusho* in Japan, as well as various 'nervous fatigue' syndromes, including ordinary *shinkeishitsu* in Japan, brain fag in Nigeria and neurasthenia in China. Cultural influences are apparent in the content and focus of anxiety disorders. (see Chapter 14.)

Generalized Anxiety Disorders (GAD)

Epidemiology

Prevalence rate of GAD ranges from 2.5 to 6.4 per cent. The 1-year prevalence rate for men is around 2 per cent and 4.3 per cent for women.

Clinical Features

The main symptoms of GAD are: worry and apprehension, free floating anxiety, motor tension like restlessness, inability to relax, headache, aching of the back and shoulders and stiffness of the muscles, autonomic hyperactivity, experienced as sweating, palpitation, dry mouth, epigastric discomfort and giddiness. However, the intensity and frequency of these symptoms are less as compared to those of other anxiety disorders such as panic disorder, social phobia and simple phobia. These patients often complain of difficulty in concentrating, poor memory and heightened sensitivity to noise. The appearance of these patients is characteristic, and includes a strained face, horizontal folds in the forehead, restless and fidgety with pale skin and sweating. Sleep disturbance may present as a difficulty in falling sleep and intermittent awakening. Other less prominent symptoms of GAD are tiredness, depressive symptoms, obsessional symptoms and depersonalization.

Differential Diagnosis

Generalized anxiety disorders need to be differentiated from some common psychiatric and physical disorders. In depressive disorders, anxiety is often a symptom of depression and depressive symptoms can also occur in an anxiety disorder. It is therefore useful to make the diagnosis on the basis of the severity of two kinds of symptoms and by the order in which they appear. Thus, whichever type of symptom appears first and is more severe is considered the primary condition. Patients with schizophrenia sometimes complain of only anxiety, especially in the initial part of the assessment interview. In order to avoid misdiagnosis, the patient may be asked what their explanation is about the origin or cause of his anxiety symptoms. Alcohol or drug use can mask the underlying GAD. It is helpful to determine whether the GAD is primary or secondary. If the patient reports more anxiety symptoms in the morning, it would suggest the possibility of alcohol dependence. Some people consume alcohol or drugs in order to reduce their anxiety.

Panic Disorder (PD)

Epidemiology

The lifetime prevalence of panic attacks is 10 per cent. The lifetime prevalence of panic disorders is 1.5 to 3.5 per cent. Morbidity and impairment of quality of life in panic disorder are comparable to those of depression.

Clinical Features

The first panic attack is often totally spontaneous. The major symptoms are extreme fear and a sense of impending doom. Physical signs include palpitation,

tachycardia, dyspnoea and sweating. The attack is brief, and usually lasts for 10 to 30 minutes, rarely longer. Some patients may experience depersonalization and syncopal attacks during these episodes. In between attacks patients may have anticipatory anxiety about having another attack. Hyperventilation may produce respiratory alkalosis and other symptoms. Comorbidity is very common in PD; around 30 to 90 per cent of patients with PD have comorbid anxiety disorders, and around 50 per cent have major depression. A study of patients referred to the psychiatric outpatient clinic in Qatar found that panic disorders typically involved fear of after death than of dying per se. Cultural beliefs may make unusual symptoms salient and clinicians unfamiliar with the local idioms of distress may be misled, at times to the extent of considering such patients psychotic. This is particularly likely when cultural differences make dissociative symptoms more prevalent.

The Nigerian culture-related syndrome of *ode-ori* is characterized by prominent somatic symptoms including culture-specific symptoms such as feelings of heat in the head, or sensations of parasites crawling in the head. Sensations of worms crawling in the head are common non-specific somatic symptoms in equatorial Africa that may be prominent symptoms of panic disorders or generalized anxiety disorder as well as other psychiatric disorder. *Ode-ori* may also be associated with paranoid fears of malevolent attack by witchcraft. Such fears are common in societies where witchcraft is practised or is a part of local belief.

Differential Diagnosis

The presence of thyroid, parathyroid, adrenal and substance-related disorders can cause symptoms of panic attacks. Symptoms like chest pain, especially in predisposed patients with cardiac risk factors, may warrant further cardiac tests. Situational-bound panic attacks may indicate conditions like phobia, OCD and depressive disorder.

Phobic Anxiety Disorders

This group of disorders is characterized by anxiety and phobic symptoms which occur only in particular circumstances, avoidance of the situations which provoke anxiety and also the experience of anticipatory anxiety. Common phobias are simple phobia, social phobia and agoraphobia.

Simple phobia

Epidemiology

Lifetime prevalence of simple phobia is 4 per cent in men and 13 per cent in women.

Clinical Features

There are phobias confined to highly specific situations such as certain animals, heights, thunder, darkness, flying, closed spaces, dentistry, sight of blood and fear of exposure to specific diseases, and many others. Diagnosis is made when a person exposed to the above mentioned situations, experiences psychophysiological manifestations of anxiety and subsequently avoids such fear-provoking situations.

Differential Diagnosis

Phobic disorders need to be differentiated from other disorders that have fear as a symptom. Hypochondriasis is characterized by fear of having a disease, contrary to the reassurance given by the doctors. Specific disease phobia is the fear of contracting the disease, and hence avoiding situations which may produce the disease. Obsessive–compulsive disorder patients may avoid knives because they have an obsessive fear of killing someone, whereas patients with a specific phobia involving knives may avoid the same for fear of cutting themselves.

Social Phobia

Epidemiology

Social phobias are almost equally prevalent in men and women. The 1-year prevalence of social phobia has been estimated as 7 per cent for men and 9 per cent for women.

Clinical Features

In social phobia inappropriate anxiety is experienced in situations in which the person is observed and could be criticized. They tend to avoid such situations. The situations include restaurants, canteens, dinner parties, seminars, board meetings, etc. The Japanese form of social phobia, *taijinkyofusho*, provides an example of the interaction of cultural beliefs and practices with anxiety. The core symptom is the fear that one will offend or make others uncomfortable through inappropriate social behaviour and self-presentation including staring, blushing, emitting an offensive odour or having a physical blemish or mis-shapen features. This fits with Japanese preoccupation with the proper public presentation of self in society. A study of Japanese–American students and a community sample of adults in Hawaii found that symptoms of *taijinkyofusho* were substantially correlated with those of social phobia. Although there were no differences between Asian and Western students in mean levels of *taijinkyofusho* symptoms, higher levels of *taijinkyofusho* symptoms (but not other social phobia symptoms) were found among less acculturated individuals, lending some support to the notion that the distinctive feature of *taijinkyofusho* is associated with Japanese culture. There is also a difference in the value psychiatrists in Japan and the United States assign to feelings of victimization, the Japanese viewing them as more or less normal while their Western counterparts, when confronted with Japanese cases, tend to view such feeling as persecutory or delusional. This leads Western psychiatrists to diagnose Japanese cases of *taijinkyofusho* as paranoia and paranoid schizophrenia. Furthermore, while the *taijinkyofusho* sufferer feels victimized by their symptoms, the feeling of victimization is primarily expressed in terms of embarrassment or unpleasantness the symptoms are thought to arouse in others.

Differential Diagnosis

Patients with social phobia experience anxiety only when confronted with the phobic stimulus unlike in panic disorder. Patients with agoraphobia are often comforted by the presence of another person in an anxiety provoking situation, whereas a patient with social phobia may become more anxious in the presence of other people. Differentiation from anxious avoidant personality disorder may be difficult and the assessment needs to be supplemented with a detailed case personal history and extensive interviews. Avoidance may be a symptom of depression, but it would be accompanied by other characteristic depressive symptoms. Subjects with schizoid personality disorder have a lack of interest in interaction rather than the fear of socializing like in social phobia.

Agoraphobia

Epidemiology

One-year prevalence of agoraphobia without panic disorder varies between 1.7 and 3.8 per cent and the lifetime prevalence is about 6 to 10 per cent.

Clinical Features

Patients with agoraphobia avoid situations where help is not easily available. The term agoraphobia includes fears not only of open spaces but also situations like crowded stores, closed spaces, busy streets and wherever there is a difficulty of immediate or easy escape to a safe place. It is one of the most incapacitating phobic disorders. Two groups of symptoms are described in agoraphobics, panic attacks and anxious cognitions about fainting and going crazy. Severely affected individuals often become completely housebound, especially women. Most patients are less anxious when accompanied by a trusted person or a family member. Depressive symptoms, depersonalization and obsessional thoughts may also be present.

Differential Diagnosis

Differential diagnosis includes all the medical disorders which cause symptoms of anxiety or depression. Psychiatric differential diagnosis includes major depressive disorder, social phobia, generalized anxiety disorder, panic disorder, paranoid personality disorder, avoidant personality disorder and dependent personality disorder.

Separation Anxiety Disorder

Separation anxiety disorder is characterized by marked and excessive fear or anxiety about separation from specific attachment figures. In children, separation anxiety typically focuses on parents or other family members; in adults it is typically a partner or children. Separation anxiety presents with thoughts of harm, reluctance to go to school or work, recurrent excessive distress upon separation, reluctance or refusal to sleep away from the person attached to, and recurrent nightmares about separation.

Dissociative or Conversion Disorder

Conversion and dissociative disorders were previously considered as subtypes of hysteria. The common theme shared by the hysterical disorders was a partial or complete loss of function of body parts or loss of normal integration between memories of the past, awareness of identity and immediate sensations, and control over bodily movements. Hysterical neurosis is believed to be gradually becoming infrequent in the West though it is a common diagnosis in the developing countries. The decline in hysteria in the West has been accompanied by a compensatory rise in the incidence of anxiety and depression. Conversion may be a means of expressing forbidden feelings or ideas, as a kind of communication when direct verbal communication is blocked.

Some culture-bound syndromes like *latah* and *amok* represent means of expressing anger and rage when it is not culturally permissible. These are regarded as variants of hysteria. There is a tendency to avoid the use of the term hysteria in view of its many and varied meanings. In DSM-IV, this group of disorders is characterized by symptoms or deficits involving voluntary motor or sensory functions. Dissociative amnesia, fugue and identity disorder are classed together in a separate category of dissociative disorders. In ICD-10 these conditions are classified as dissociative disorders.

Epidemiology

Lifetime prevalence of having conversion symptoms is reported to be around 33 per cent; however, conversion disorders are much less prevalent, and in many Western and developed countries, conversion disorders have disappeared. Some studies from general hospital psychiatry units report that 5 to 16 per cent of psychiatric consultations are diagnosed as conversion disorders. The female to male ratio varies from 2:1 to 5:1.

Clinical Features

Clinical features are mainly motor symptoms like abnormal gait, manifesting as staggering, ataxia with gross jerks and inability to stand without support (astasia-abasia). Pseudoseizures, hysterical blindness and sensory symptoms like anaesthesia, hyperesthesia and paraesthesia are common conversion symptoms. Psychogenic vomiting, urinary retention, pseudocyesis (pseudo-pregnancy), globus hystericus (feeling of lump in the throat), and some visual disturbances are described under conversion disorder.

Clinical Presentations

Dissociative Amnesia

The main feature is loss of memory of important recent, usually traumatic events. Invariably the onset is sudden, and very often the events are physically or emotionally traumatic, like accidents or unexpected bereavements. Amnesia may be localized and rarely complete or generalized. Personal identity usually remains unchanged and an apparent unconcern about the memory loss is observed frequently.

Dissociative amnesia is generally short-lasting and self-limited.

Dissociative Fugue

Dissociative fugue has all the features of dissociative amnesia, along with an apparently purposeful journey away from home or place of work during which self-care is maintained. After establishing a new residence, occupation and identity, the person has no memory of the past and is not aware that the memories are missing. Fugue often remits spontaneously and recurs rarely. The memories of events during the fugue state may be recalled under hypnosis. Those patients with conflict may require prolonged psychotherapeutic interventions.

Dissociative Identity Disorder

This is also known as multiple personality disorder and has been reported predominantly in the West and is rare in the developing countries. The important characteristic feature of multiple personality disorder is the presence of two or more distinct personalities within a single individual with only one of them being manifest at a time. The cause of this disorder is largely unknown; however, traumatic events in childhood either of physical or sexual abuse are commonly reported. The change from one personality to another is often sudden and dramatic. Each personality is complete, with its own memories, characteristic personal preferences and behavioural patterns. The personalities may be of either sex and may be disparate and extremely opposite. Nothing unusual is found in the mental status of these patients except for amnesia for the events which occurred during the previous personality. Often prolonged interviews and multiple contact with the patient may lead the clinician to arrive at a diagnosis of multiple personality disorder.

Trance and Possession Disorder

The central feature of dissociative trance disorder is the temporary alteration in the state of consciousness or loss of customary sense of personal identity without replacement by an alternate identity. An associated narrowing of the awareness of surroundings and also some stereotyped behaviours maybe present. Episodes occur in discrete attacks and there is amnesia for the trance state. In possession attacks, an episodic alteration in the state of consciousness is characterized by the replacement of the customary sense of personal identity by a new identity. These could be stereotyped and culturally determined behaviours or movements that are experienced as being controlled by the possessing agent. Trance and possession states can occur in various religious and cultural contexts. It becomes a disorder only when it occurs involuntarily or is unwanted and also when it intrudes into ordinary activities by occurring outside religious or other culturally accepted situations. Possession states and trance are common in the Indian subcontinent.

Other dissociative phenomena of interest are *latah* and *amok*. *Latah* is well described among Malaysians. It is characterized by hypersensitivity to fright or startle, often with echopraxia, echolalia, command obedience, and dissociative or trance like behaviour. *Amok* is characterized by homicidal frenzy, preceded by brooding and followed by amnesia. (See Chapter 14.)

Bodily Distress Disorder

Somatoform disorders have been described as bodily distress disorders in the ICD-11. These are characterized by physical complaints for which no obvious, serious and demonstrable organic findings can be discerned. There is some evidence or presumption that psychological factors, stresses or conflicts seem to be initiating, exacerbating and maintaining the somatic symptoms.

The terms and description have been revamped in DSM-5. This is done to modify the arbitrary use of the number of symptoms to diagnose somatoform disorders. Also the subcategories were not very useful and had no clear validity. Hence in DSM-5 they have been renamed as somatic symptoms and related disorders which include somatic symptoms disorder, illness anxiety disorders, conversion disorders, factitious disorders, psychological factors affecting medical conditions.

Clinical Picture

The main clinical features are multiple, recurrent and frequently changing physical symptoms, which have usually been present for several years. Most patients have a long and complicated history of consulting several doctors. Symptoms include gastrointestinal sensations, multiple skin symptoms, sexual complaints and menstrual irregularities. The presentation of bodily symptoms in most cultures, regardless of source, constitutes an idiom of distress. In many cultures, the presentation of personal or social distress in the form of somatic complaints is the norm. In the past, somatization was believed to be a phenomenon in non-Western countries, now it is established that it is a worldwide phenomenon, though it appears commonly in developing countries. In an effort to explain such cultural differences, models that incorporate mind/body schemas prevalent in various cultures have been studied. In the West, mental and physical health is seen as arising out of mind and body respectively. In non-Western countries the body is understood as a whole rather than a dualistic model seen in the West.

The types of symptoms presented in different cultural settings are diverse. In Latin America, certain somatoform disorders are described. *Ataque de nervios* is commonly reported in Puerto Rican and Caribbean subjects. It commonly follows stressful events and manifests as somatization and dissociative symptoms, with dramatic behavioural correlates. *Ataques* are common in women, particularly those who are older, unmarried and with low levels of education. The common somatic manifestations of *ataque de nervios* are headache, trembling, palpitations, stomach disturbances, a sensation of heat rising to the head, numbness of extremities and at times pseudo-seizures, fainting or unusual spells. Hot and cold syndromes are the cultural dimensions reported by Puerto Ricans that may affect their health-use patterns is the 'hot–cold' theory of disease and therapies.

Hwa byung is a Korean folk illness label commonly used by patients suffering from a multitude of somatic and psychological symptoms, including constricted, oppressed, or pushing-up sensations in the chest, palpitations, heat sensations, flushing, headache, epigastric mass, dysphoria, anxiety, irritability and difficulty in concentration. It is said to be a common condition that afflicts less-educated, middle-aged married women in times of stress.

Somatic neurosis is a chronic neurotic syndrome among Muslim women in India who report multiple somatic symptoms. This somatic neurosis is different from anxiety neurosis and depressive neurosis. Socio-cultural factors may be contributing to these differences.

Understanding about aetiology of somatoform disorders is intriguing. Emotional deficits, cognitive biases and abnormal perception of body signals have been considered to form somatic cognitions.

Hypochondriasis or Illness Anxiety Disorders

Epidemiology

Six-month prevalence rates of 4 to 6 per cent among the general medical patient population have been reported. There are no significant differences in social status, education and marital status. The age of onset is most commonly between 20 and 30 years of age. Illness anxiety disorders are being used currently in DSM-5 in place of hypochondriasis and have specific care seeking and care avoiding.

Clinical Features

There are mainly physical complaints without any demonstrable underlying organic pathology, which are described with minute specific details. The symptoms reflect no recognizable disease pattern. There is also a persistent refusal to accept the advice and reassurance of several different doctors that there is no physical illness or abnormality underlying the symptom. In hypochondriacal disorder, the patient tends to ask for investigations to determine or confirm the nature of the underlying disease.

The culture-related syndrome *koro* involves an intense acute fear that the penis is shrinking into the body and when involution is complete, the sufferer will die. *Koro* affects individuals who are vulnerable due to pre-existing anxiety, sexual, reproductive and relationship concerns, recent stressful life events, and, perhaps, suggestibility. This is a cultural variant of hypochondriacal disorder.

Neurasthenia

Neurasthenia, also known as chronic fatigue syndrome (CFS), is a condition of uncertain cause commonly ascribed to the effect of stresses of modern life on the human nervous system. Many physicians have observed that the symptoms of chronic fatigue are not readily explained by organic disease or psychiatric conditions. Consequently, it became regarded as a 'medically unexplained' condition. In ICD-10 the syndrome is included under 'other neurotic disorders'. Neurasthenia is the commonest neurotic disorder in China (see earlier). In a survey conducted in China neurasthenia was nearly twice as commonly diagnosed as depressive neurosis. This term is readily accepted by the medical practitioners there and has less stigma attached to it.

Clinical Features

Primary complaints in neurasthenia are tiredness and fatigue. This fatigue lasts for months to years, and typically begins soon after a viral fever or exposure. In addition to fatigue, the syndrome is characterized by myalgias and cognitive changes such as forgetfulness and poor concentration. Patients may complain of sexual weakness also, which needs to be addressed in the light of cultural background, and needs to differentiate from *dhat* syndromes in men or women. In young males in the Indian subcontinent, *dhat* syndrome manifests as bodily, mental or sexual weakness attributed to loss of semen, by masturbation, sexual activity or loss of 'semen' in the urine. In women, tiredness, fatigue and exhaustion is attributed to passage of normal vaginal discharge, this is considered as loss of vital elements, akin to semen in men.

In Japan, other types of neurasthenia are recognized, namely neurasthenia, neurasthenic reaction or reactive neurasthenia and pseudo-neurasthenia. In China, neurasthenia or *shenjing shuairou* meaning weakness of nerves is reported by intellectual individuals with probable socio-political factors underlying the cause. In Taiwan neurasthenia is regarded as a clinical entity and called as *shinkei-shitsu*, which is characterized by obsessive and introverted personality traits and sociophobic symptoms. The role of cultural factors in the development, presentation, and management of neurotic disorders needs to be appreciated. The explanatory models employ the cultural formulation to get an understanding of the disorder. The neurotic symptoms reflect a cry for help, an indication of the failing coping methods and need for support and understanding from their family, friends and professionals. These need to be understood and addressed under the unique cultural framework of the individual.

Illness Behaviours and Neurosis

Illness behaviours are the ways the person responds and reacts to their bodily symptoms. The behaviours are considered as abnormal in individuals who have maladaptive ways of perceiving and reacting to their health status. Culture has a significant role in illness behaviours. Cultural factors impact the way they perceive their health based on the norms in the culture and utilization of health systems. The presentations of many of the so called erstwhile neurotic disorders show varying patterns of abnormal illness behaviours.

References

American Psychiatric Association (2013). *Diagnostic and Statistical Manual of Mental Disorders*, 5th edn, Washington DC: American Psychiatric Association.

Barlow, D. H. (2003). *Anxiety and its Disorders*. New York: Guilford Press.

Barlow, D. H., Ellard, K. K., Sauer-Zavala, S., Bullis, J. R., Carl, J. R. (2014). The origins of neuroticism. *Perspectives in Psychololgy and Sciences*, **9**, 481–496.

Barsky, A. J. and Klerman, G. L. (1983). Overview: hypochondriasis, bodily complaints and somatic styles. *American Journal of Psychiatry*, **140**, 273–283.

Bass, C. and Potts, S. (1993). Somatoform disorders. In *Recent Advances in Clinical Psychiatry*, ed. K. G. Grossman. Edinburgh: Churchill Livingstone, pp. 143–163.

Brown, T. A. (1997). The nature of generalized anxiety disorder and pathological worry. Current evidence and conceptual model. *Canadian Journal of Psychiatry*, **42**, 817–825.

Carota, A. and Calabrese, P. (2014). Hysteria around the world. *Frontiers of Neurological Neurosciences*, **35**, 169–180.

Chaturvedi, S. K. (1993). Neurosis across culture. *International Review of Psychiatry*, **5**, 181–194.

Chaturvedi, S. K. and Bhugra, D. (2007) The concept of neurosis in a cross-cultural perspective. *Current Opinion in Psychiatry*, **20**, 37–45.

Chaturvedi, S. K. and Joseph, S. (2005). Neurotic, stress-related and somatoform disorders. In *Handbook of Psychiatry: A South Asian Perspective*, ed. D. Bhugra, G. Ranjith and V. Patel. New Delhi: Viva Publishers, pp. 247–270.

Chaturvedi, S. K. and Parameswaran, S. (2015). Hysteria: history and critiques. *International Encyclopedia of Social and Behavioural Sciences*, vol. **11**, 2nd edn, ed. James Wright. Amsterdam: Elsevier, 506–511.

Clark, D. A., Beck, A. T. and Beck, J. S. (1994). Symptom differences in major depression, dysthymia, panic disorder and generalized anxiety disorder. *American Journal of Psychiatry*, **151**, 205–209.

Escobar, J. I. (1995) Transcultural aspects of dissociative and somatoform disorders. *Psychiatric Clinics of North America*, **18**, 555–569.

Gelder, M., Gath, D. and Mayou, R. (eds) (1996). Anxiety, obsessive compulsive and dissociative disorders. In *Oxford Textbook of Psychiatry*, 3rd edn. New York: Oxford University Press.

Halligan, P. W., Bass, C. and Marshall, J. C. (2001). *Contemporary Approaches to the Study of Hysteria.* Oxford: Oxford University Press.

Kaplan, H. I. and Sadock B. J. (eds) (1995). Anxiety disorders. In *Comprehensive Textbook of Psychiatry*, 6th edn. Baltimore: Williams and Wilkins.

Kirmayer, L. J., Allan Young, A. and Hayton, B. C. (1995). The cultural context of anxiety disorders. *Psychiatric Clinics of North America*, **18**, 503–521.

Lipowski, Z. J. (1998). Somatization. The concept and its clinical application. *American Journal of Psychiatry*, **145**, 1358–1368.

Marks, I. M. (1969). *Fears and Phobias*. London: Heinemann.

Marshall, J. R. (1997). Panic disorder: a treatment update. *Journal of Clinical Psychiatry*, **58**(1), 36–42.

Noyce, R. and Hoehn-Saric, R. (1998). *The Anxiety Disorders*. Cambridge: Cambridge University Press.

Pearce, S. and Miler, A. (1993). Chronic pain. In *Recent Advances in Clinical Psychiatry*, ed. K. G. Grossman. Edinburgh: Churchill Livingstone, pp. 123–142.

Perkins A. M., Arnone D., Smallwood J., Mobbs D. (2015). Thinking too much: self-generated thought as the engine of neuroticism. *Trends in Cognitive Science* **19**(9), 492–498.

Pierre, J. M. (2012). Mental illness and mental health: is the glass half empty or half full? *Canadian Journal of Psychiatry*, **57**, 651–658.

Ross, G. A., Miller, S. D., Reagon, P. *et al.* (1990). Structured interview data on 102 cases of multiple personality disorder for four centers. *American Journal of Psychiatry*, **147**, 596–601.

Sharma, P. and Chaturvedi, S. K. (1995). Conversion disorder revisited. *Acta Psychiatrica Scandinavica*, **92**, 301–304.

Stein, D. J. and Hollander, E. (2002). Generalized anxiety, panic and obsessive compulsive disorders. In *Textbook of Anxiety Disorders*, ed. Dan J. Stein, Eric Hollander and Barbara O. Rothbaum. Washington DC: American Psychiatric Publishing Inc.

Uhde, T. W., Trancer, M. E., Black, B. *et al.* (1991). Phenomenology and neurobiology of social phobia. Comparison with panic disorder. *Journal of Clinical Psychiatry*, **52**, 31.

Wessely, S., Hotopf, M. and Sharpe, M. (1998). *Chronic Fatigue and its Syndromes*. Oxford: Oxford University Press.

WHO (2016). Website for ICD-11 Beta Draft (Mortality and Morbidity Statistics) available at http://apps.who.int/cla ssifications/icd11/browse/l-m/en. (accessed 30 May 2016).

Chapter 19

Schizophrenia and Related Psychoses

Assen Jablensky

Editors' Introduction

Schizophrenia occurs across cultures though actual presentation and help-seeking as well as outcome will depend upon a number of factors. Jablensky in this chapter reminds us that the comparative study of schizophrenia and other psychoses across different populations and cultures gained in scope and momentum with the research programme of the World Health Organization from the 1960s onwards. These studies set the scene and actual standards for cross-cultural epidemiology. He suggests that schizophrenia essentially represents a spectrum of clinical syndromes with some internal cohesion and likely shared genomic underpinnings. The existence of a specific brain disease (or diseases) underlying these conditions points to a schizophrenia syndrome. This remains a hypothesis, notwithstanding the variety of neurobiological and cognitive features or tentative susceptibility genes associated with the disorder. He argues that the question whether cases diagnosed as schizophrenia in different cultures are phenotypically homologous is of critical importance, considering that the biological basis of the disorder still eludes us and no objective diagnostic test is available. He concludes that at present, no single, or major, environmental risk factor influencing the incidence of schizophrenia or other psychoses has been conclusively demonstrated. It is therefore, inevitable that studies using large samples may well give us further clues and direction to evaluate potential risk factors, antecedents and predictors, for which the present evidence is inconclusive.

Introduction

Interest in the manifestations and frequency of mental disorders in non-Western cultures, primarily the psychoses, dates back to the colonial era. In the nineteenth century, British, Dutch and French colonial administrators imported into their overseas dependencies the 'enlightened' asylum model of care for the mentally ill and built mental hospitals for custodial care of patients with intractable chronic illness and 'dangerous' psychotics. In 1903, Kraepelin travelled to Java and, after several weeks spent at the Buitenzorg (now Bogor) hospital, came to the conclusion that the basic forms of dementia praecox and manic-depressive insanity in the Javanese were generically the same as those in Europe, though 'racial characteristics, religion and customs' might modify their clinical manifestations. Although Kraepelin saw in this primarily a confirmation of his nosological system, he anticipated 'rich rewards' for the potential of comparative research to 'throw light on the causes of mental disorder' and proposed 'comparative psychiatry' as the systematic study of mental disorders and personality traits across different cultures (Kraepelin, 1904).

However, during the decades to follow, the sources on the epidemiology of schizophrenia and other psychotic disorders in non-European cultures remained restricted to mental hospital statistics or rudimentary field surveys undertaken by psychiatrists or colonial public health administrators. Typically, the conclusion was that 'true' schizophrenia and depression were rare among indigenous peoples, but that chronic psychotics were well tolerated in the community. The ideological framework in which such early observations were embedded varied between benign paternalism and overt racism. In a monograph published by the World Health Organization, Carothers (1953) claimed that the paucity of structured delusional contents and the lack of systematization of delusions in 'the African' could be explained by a congenital underdevelopment of the frontal lobes of the brain. Similar assumptions led other authors to conclude that depression was rare in sub-Saharan Africa or in Asia because of the lack of Judaeo-Christian cultural values which made the experience of guilt possible.

The sketchy and often distorted picture of the epidemiology of psychoses in the developing countries started to change in the post-colonial era when locally born psychiatrists, educated in the West, entered practice and teaching in their countries. Though trained in the colonial metropolis, they were keen to understand the nature of mental disorders in their own cultures and to introduce culturally appropriate alternatives to the colonial mental hospital, such as the 'psychiatric village' (German, 1972). In a series of studies on schizophrenia among the Yoruba in Nigeria, Lambo (1965) pointed to the limitations of the Western diagnostic concepts when applied to African cultures. In Asia, Yap (1974) charted systematically the so-called 'culture-bound syndromes' and highlighted their differentiation from schizophrenia. The first epidemiological surveys which generated incidence and prevalence data on psychoses, including schizophrenia, were carried out by Rin and Lin (1962) in Taiwan; Leighton *et al.* (1963) in Nigeria; and Raman and Murphy (1972) in Mauritius. In addition to indigenous investigators, European and North American psychiatrists and anthropologists laid the foundations of cross-cultural psychiatry in which psychosis research featured prominently. Since the late 1950s, a number of epidemiological surveys were carried out in India and China. Although the methods and diagnostic criteria used were rarely described, these surveys provided data of considerable historical interest on general trends and patterns, reviewed by Murphy (1982).

The comparative study of schizophrenia and other psychoses across different populations and cultures gained in scope and momentum with the research programme of the World Health Organization initiated in the 1960s. Two multi-centre studies, the International Pilot Study of Schizophrenia (IPSS; WHO, 1973, 1979; Leff *et al.*, 1992) and Determinants of Outcome of Severe Mental Disorders (Sartorius *et al.*, 1986; Jablensky *et al.*, 1992) generated a wealth of cross-sectional and follow-up data on over 2,000 cases of schizophrenia and related disorders in 16 geographically defined areas in 12 countries in Africa, the Americas, Asia and Europe. These studies utilized for the first time standardized diagnostic criteria and assessment methods in community and hospital-based data collection by teams of local psychiatrists and other mental health workers who not only had been trained to use such research tools but participated in their development. Although the areas covered by the WHO studies were not exhaustive of all the variation that may exist in the incidence of schizophrenia and related conditions, this research provided a unique database enabling direct comparisons of the population rates, psychopathology and outcomes of the major psychoses across various cultures.

Schizophrenia: Phenotypic Comparability across Populations

Despite the availability of ICD-10 and DSM-IV/DSM-5 criteria that aim to facilitate its reliable diagnostic identification, schizophrenia essentially represents a spectrum of clinical syndromes with some internal cohesion and likely shared genomic underpinnings. The existence of a specific brain disease (or diseases) underlying these syndromes is still a hypothesis, notwithstanding the variety of neurobiological and cognitive features or tentative susceptibility genes, associated with the disorders. Thus, the question whether cases diagnosed as schizophrenia in different cultures are phenotypically homologous is of critical importance, considering that the biological basis of the disorder still eludes us and no objective diagnostic test is available. To claim that schizophrenia and its spectrum disorders are universal implies that their features can be reliably identified in different populations; consistent associations with age and gender are present; and course, outcome, and response to treatment show common patterns. Importantly, no population has yet been found to be free of schizophrenia and its related disorders. Although no single symptom is pathognomonic, the overall clinical presentation of schizophrenia is remarkably similar across cultures. Acutely ill patients in different cultural settings describe the same characteristic symptoms, such as hallucinatory voices commenting in third person on their thoughts and actions, thoughts being taken away or broadcast, or their surroundings being imbued with special meaning. Negative symptoms, such as psychomotor poverty, social withdrawal, and amotivation, commonly occur irrespective of the cultural setting. The conclusion that patients diagnosed with schizophrenia in different cultures suffer from the same disorder is further supported by the similar age- and sex-specific distribution of the onset of symptoms, which peak in late adolescence or early adulthood and, in females, have a second, lower peak after age 35. Considering the variety of social norms and beliefs about illness across cultures, the similar ways in which the core symptoms of schizophrenia are experienced and described by people in various cultures is striking, suggesting that the pathophysiological basis of the disorder may be similar in different populations.

Notwithstanding such similarities, variations seem to exist that may affect its recognition and treatment. Lambo (1965) described a characteristic symptom-complex in Nigeria consisting of anxiety, depression, vague hypochondriacal concerns, bizarre magico-mystical ideas, episodic twilight or confusional states, atypical depersonalization, emotional liability, and retrospective falsification of memory based on hallucinations or delusions. Variants of the syndrome, such as an acute onset form and a catatonic subtype appear to be more common in traditional rural communities. In the WHO ten-country study (Jablensky *et al.*, 1992) acute onset characterized 40.3% and catatonic schizophrenia 10.3% of all the cases in the low-income countries, compared to 10.9% and 1.2% in the high-income countries respectively. A common clinical problem in some low-income countries is the differentiation of schizophrenia from psychoses due to infectious or parasitic diseases. In particular, African trypanosomiasis often results in a symptomatic psychosis which has a slow, insidious onset and may mimic schizophrenia. Since a variety of infectious, parasitic, and nutritional diseases are endemic in the developing world, it has been suggested that a high proportion of the cases of schizophrenia in those populations may in fact be symptomatic psychoses accompanying physical diseases. However, among some 500 individuals with psychotic illnesses, screened in India and Nigeria for the WHO ten-country study, only 11.7 per cent were excluded on grounds of having a physical disease that might explain their psychotic symptoms. Problems of differential diagnosis may arise in respect of organic brain disorders, but it is unlikely that the majority of schizophrenic illnesses in the Third World can be attributed to underlying organic aetiology.

All this being said, schizophrenic disorders in non-Western populations can be reliably distinguished from the acute transient psychoses, the so-called culture-bound syndromes, and probably the affective disorders, although the boundary with the latter has not been sufficiently explored and some symptomatic overlap may exist. Family morbidity data are still scarce but where such information is available, it suggests that genetic factors contribute to the transmission of schizophrenia in the same way as in the developed countries.

Prevalence

Table 19.1 presents an overview of prevalence studies conducted in different populations at different times, selected on broad criteria of sample representativeness and of diagnostic assessment likely to be compatible with present-day criteria. The studies differ widely in many respects of methodology but have in common a high intensity of case finding. The term 'census' refers to surveys aiming at ascertaining every member of an entire community or a population sample. Several were repeat surveys, in which the original sample was traced and re-examined after an interval of ten or more years (the findings on follow-up are quoted in brackets).

These studies have produced point prevalence estimates in the range of 1.4 to 7.1 per 1,000 population at risk. However, in most instances these are raw (non-standardized) figures which may not be directly comparable due to demographic confounders such as age structure of the population, mortality and migration, and thus may not reflect the true variation across different populations. Thus, the question whether any major differences exist in the prevalence of schizophrenia in different populations and cultures has no simple answer. The majority of studies have found similar prevalence rates, though a small number of populations (referred to later) clearly deviate from the central tendency. The magnitude of such deviations in schizophrenia is typically modest when compared to other multifactorial diseases, such as diabetes, ischaemic heart disease or multiple sclerosis, in which 30-fold (or greater) differences in prevalence across populations are not uncommon.

Incidence

Incidence rates provide a better estimate of the 'force of morbidity' (the probability of disease occurrence at a given point in time). The estimation of incidence depends on how reliably the point of onset can be identified. Since it is not possible at present to determine with any accuracy the beginnings of the putative cerebral dysfunction underlying schizophrenia, the onset of the disorder is usually defined as the point in time when its symptoms reach the threshold of recognition. The first hospitalization is not a good

Table 19.1 Selected prevalence studies of schizophrenia

Author	Country	Population	Method	Prevalence per 1,000
Studies in developed countries				
Brugger (1931)	Germany	Area in Thuringia (n = 37,561)	Census	2.4
Strömgren (1938); Bøjholm and Strömgren (1989)	Denmark	Island population (n = 50,000)	Repeat census	3.9 (3.3)
Lemkau et al. (1943)	USA	Household sample	Census	2.9
Essen-Möller et al. (1956); Hagnell (1966)	Sweden	Community in southern Sweden	Repeat census	6.7 (4.5)
Crocetti et al. (1971)	Croatia	Household sample	Census	5.9
Rotstein (1977)	Russia	Population sample (n = 35,590)	Census	3.8
Robins and Regier (1991)	USA	Aggregated data across 5 ECA sites	DIS interviews	7.0
Jeffreys et al. (1997)	UK	London health district (n = 112,127)	Census, sample interviewed (n = 172)	5.1
Jablensky et al. (2000)	Australia	Four urban areas (n = 1,084,978)	Census, sample interviewed (n = 980)	5.9
Studies in developing countries				
Rin and Lin (1962); Lin et al. (1989)	Taiwan	Population sample	Repeat census	2.1 (1.4)
Dube and Kumar (1972)	India	Four areas in Agra (n = 29,468)	Census	2.6
Padmavathi et al. (1987)	India	Urban (n = 101,229)	Census	2.5
Salan (1992)	Indonesia	Area in Jakarta (n = 100,107)	Key informants, sample interviewed	1.4
Waldo (1999)	Kosrae (Micronesia)	Island population (n = 5,500)	Key informants, sample interviewed	6.8
Kebede and Alem (1999)	Ethiopia	District south of Addis Ababa (n = 227,135)	Key informants, sample interviewed	7.1
Zhang et al. (1998); Phillips et al. (2004)	China (mainland)	Population sample (n = 19,223)	Census	5.3

index, since the interval between the 'true' onset of overt symptoms and the point at which diagnosis is made and treatment initiated (the 'duration of untreated psychosis', or DUP) is likely to vary across different settings and cultures. A better approximation is provided by the time of the first contact with any psychiatric or general medical service at which an incipient or ongoing psychotic illness is recognized and diagnosed for the first time.

Table 19.2 presents findings from 13 incidence studies of schizophrenia. Studies that have used a 'broad' definition of schizophrenia (ICD-8 or ICD-9)

Table 19.2 Selected incidence studies of schizophrenia

Author	Country	Population	Method	Rate per 1,000
Europe and North America				
Ødegaard (1946)	Norway	Total population	First admissions, 1926–1935 ($n = 14,231$)	0.24
Häfner and Reimann (1970)	Germany	City of Mannheim ($n = 330,000$)	Case register	0.54
Liebermann (1974)	Russia	Moscow district ($n = 248,000$)	Follow-back of prevalent cases	0.20 (male); 0.19 (female)
Helgason (1964)	Iceland	Total population	First admissions, 1966–1967 ($n = 2,388$)	0.27
Castle et al. (1991)	UK	London (Camberwell)	Case register	0.25 (ICD); 0.17 (RDC); 0.08 (DSM-III)
Nicole et al. (1992)	Canada	Area in Quebec ($n = 338,300$)	First admissions	0.31 (ICD); 0.09 (DSM-III)
McNaught et al. (1997)	UK	London health district ($n = 112,127$)	Two censuses 5 years apart	0.21 (DSM-IIIR)
Brewin et al. (1997)	UK	Nottingham	Two cohorts of first contacts (1978–1980 and 1992–1994)	0.14 (0.09) (ICD-10)
Haukka et al. (2001)	Finland	Finnish birth cohorts 1950–1969	National hospital discharges register	0.62 (male) 0.49 (female)
Scully et al. (2002)	Ireland	Two rural counties ($n = 104,089$)	First contacts 1995–2000	0.14 (male) (DSM-IV) 0.05 (female)
Asia, Caribbean and South America				
Raman and Murphy (1972)	Mauritius	Total population ($n = 257,000$)	First admissions	0.24 (Africans); 0.14 (Indian Hindus); 0.09 (Indian Moslems)
Lin et al. (1989)	Taiwan	Three communities ($n = 39,024$)	Household survey	0.17
Rajkumar et al. (1993)	India	Area in Chennai ($n = 43,097$)	Household survey	0.41
Hickling and Rodgers-Johnson (1995)	Jamaica	Total population ($n = 2.46$ m)	First contacts	0.24 (broad); 0.21 (restrictive)
Mahy et al. (1999)	Barbados	Total population ($n = 262,000$)	First contacts	0.32 (broad); 0.28 (restrictive)
Selten et al. (2005)	Surinam	Total population ($n = 481,000$)	First contacts	0.18

suggest that rates based on first admissions or first contacts vary about threefold, between 0.17 and 0.54 per 1,000 population per year. Studies using more restrictive criteria, such as the Research Diagnostic Criteria (Spitzer et al., 1978), DSM-III and its successors, or ICD-10, report incidence rates that are two to three times lower than those based on 'broad' criteria.

Comparative Incidence Data: The WHO Ten-Country Study

To date, the only study which has generated directly comparable incidence data for different populations is the WHO ten-country investigation (Sartorius *et al.*, 1986; Jablensky *et al.*, 1992). Incidence rates were estimated from first-in-lifetime contacts with any 'helping agency' (which included traditional healers in the developing countries), monitored prospectively over a 2-year period of case finding. Potential cases and key informants were interviewed by clinicians using standardized instruments, and the timing of onset was ascertained for the majority of patients. For 86 per cent of the 1,022 patients the first manifestation of diagnostic symptoms of schizophrenia was within the year preceding their first contact and, therefore the first-contact rate was accepted as a reasonable proxy for the onset of psychosis. Two definitions of 'caseness' were used: a 'broad' clinical classification comprising ICD-9 schizophrenia and paranoid psychoses, and a restrictive definition, which included core or 'nuclear' schizophrenia with Schneiderian first-rank symptoms (Wing *et al.*, 1974). The rates for the 12 study areas are shown in Table 19.3.

The differences between the rates of 'broad' schizophrenia (0.16–0.42 per 1,000) across the study areas were statistically significant ($p < 0.001$, two-tailed test); however, those for nuclear schizophrenia were not. Since nuclear schizophrenia represented a subset of the cases of broad schizophrenia, greater scatter and wider confidence intervals could be expected for the nuclear rates. However, this was not the case, suggesting that nuclear schizophrenia is phenotypically more homogeneous and occurs at a similar frequency in different populations. Subsequently, replications of the design of the WHO ten-country study using the same instruments and procedures have been carried out with very similar results by investigators in India (Rajkumar *et al.*, 1993), the Caribbean (Hickling and Rodgers-Johnson, 1995; Mahy *et al.*, 1999), and the UK (McNaught *et al.*, 1997; Brewin *et al.*, 1997).

Variation in the Incidence and Prevalence of Schizophrenia across Populations: How Much Similarity and How Much Difference?

Two systematic reviews of the literature (Goldner *et al.*, 2002; McGrath *et al.*, 2004) highlight the

Table 19.3 WHO ten-country study: annual incidence rates per 1,000 population at risk, age 15–54

Country	Area	Broad definition*			Restrictive definition**		
		Male	Female	Both sexes	Male	Female	Both sexes
Colombia	Cali	0.14	0.06	0.10	0.09	0.04	0.07
Czech Republic	Prague	0.06	0.12	0.09	0.04	0.08	0.06
Denmark	Aarhus	0.18	0.13	0.18	0.09	0.05	0.07
India	Chandigarh (rural)	0.37	0.48	0.42	0.13	0.09	0.11
India	Chandigarh (urban)	0.34	0.35	0.35	0.08	0.11	0.09
Ireland	Dublin	0.23	0.21	0.22	0.10	0.08	0.09
Japan	Nagasaki	0.23	0.18	0.21	0.11	0.09	0.10
Nigeria	Ibadan	0.11	0.11	0.11	0.09	0.10	0.10
Russia	Moscow	0.25	0.31	0.28	0.03	0.03	0.02
UK	Nottingham	0.28	0.15	0.24	0.17	0.12	0.14
USA	Honolulu, HA	0.18	0.14	0.15	0.10	0.08	0.09
USA	Rochester, WA	0.15	0.14	0.15	0.09	0.08	0.09

Notes
  * ICD-9

** Diagnosis of 'nuclear' schizophrenia (S+) assigned by the computer algorithm CATEGO (Wing *et al.*, 1974) on the basis of symptoms subsequently incorporated into the ICD-10 diagnostic criteria for schizophrenia existence of variation in schizophrenia rates across geographical regions. A good deal of this variation may be attributed to methodological differences between the studies, including study design and coverage of case finding (hospital-based, field surveys, case registers, birth cohorts), sample size, diagnostic practices, and methods of data analysis. For example, birth cohort studies and case registers tend to produce higher rates than field surveys and hospital admission studies (Bresnahan *et al.*, 2000). Notwithstanding such bias and limitations, real variation is undoubtedly present (as in any human disease) and the interesting research questions concern its extent and sources as clues to a better understanding of aetiology. Since schizophrenia is a low incidence disorder (though its chronicity and associated burden of disability place it high on the public health agenda), variation would be much more visible to the naked eye in the comparison of rates obtained from relatively small geographical areas and communities. In a study of an ethnically and socio-economically homogeneous rural region in Ireland with a total population of 29,542 (Youssef *et al.*, 1991; Scully *et al.*, 2004) the overall prevalence of 3.9 per 1,000 was well within the 'modal' range, but analysis by small district electoral divisions revealed highly significant variation in rates, ranging from 0.0 to 29.4 per 1,000. Similar variation has been reported in the Roscommon study, a genetic epidemiological investigation in another region of Ireland (Kendler *et al.*, 1996). Such local variation stands in stark contrast to the more uniform rates usually found in studies of large urban areas or at national level and is attributable to a number of factors, including spatial clustering of cases due to shared genetic vulnerability within extended pedigrees; differential mobility and mortality; and differential exposure to risk factors influencing intrauterine growth and early neurodevelopment. Such (and other, still to be discovered) effects may give rise to 'outlier' pockets of high or low incidence and prevalence which tend to cancel each other out in larger population agglomerations. Their systematic study, though involving considerable methodological difficulties, has been unduly neglected in favour of the 'macro' epidemiology of psychoses.

Populations and Groups with Unusually High and Low Rates: Genetic Isolates

Isolate populations are characterized by origins in a small number of ancestors, a high degree of inbreeding, and a restricted admixture of immigrants, due to geographical or cultural seclusion over multiple generations, sometimes ranging over thousands of years. Such populations may vary considerably in size, but are likely to be less heterogeneous with regard to genetic make-up and environmental exposures, than the panmictic (outbred) populations constituting the world's majority, in which theoretically all individuals are potentially mating partners. The so-called young isolates comprise up to 20–30 generations, and typically have arisen following drastic population size reductions (bottlenecks) due to wars, famine, religious persecution or other cataclysms. Subsequent population expansion results in a more uniform genetic background, including wider intervals of linkage disequilibrium, a more uniform environment and lifestyle, and significantly higher or lower prevalence of certain diseases, including psychiatric disorders. If coupled with availability of genealogical memory or records, such isolates present unique opportunities for genetic linkage and association studies of Mendelian (monogenic) diseases, and, possibly, complex traits, including schizophrenia, bipolar disorder and other psychiatric syndromes (Varilo and Peltonen, 2004).

A number of isolated populations in different parts of the world – including Finland, Iceland and northern Sweden, the Pima Indians, the Bedouins, the inhabitants of the Central Valley of Costa Rica, several areas in Quebec, as well as religious communities, such as the Old Order Amish, the Hutterites and the Mennonites – have been studied by epidemiologists and geneticists with a view to identifying large pedigrees, informative for complex diseases ranging from asthma and diabetes to schizophrenia and bipolar disorder. Not all of these studies have produced incidence and prevalence rates, but several examples where this has been accomplished highlight the extent of variation in the frequency of psychoses that exists in such unusual groups.

High rates of psychoses (two to three times the national or regional rate) have been reported for population isolates in northern Sweden (Böök *et al.*, 1978) and several areas in Finland (Hovatta *et al.*, 1997). Though the whole population of Finland shares some features of an ancient isolate (approximately 2,000 years), the northern and eastern regions of Finland have been settled relatively recently (in the sixteenth to seventeenth centuries) and one particular sub-region with a current population of 18,000 was founded by 40 families at the end of the seventeenth century, i.e. 12 generations back (Arjärvi *et al.*, 2004).

Genetic-epidemiological studies in this isolate estimate the lifetime risk of schizophrenia at 2.2 per cent, compared to 1.2 per cent for the whole of Finland (Hovatta et al., 1997). A recent case-register based study of a birth cohort (14,817 individuals) from this region established a lifetime prevalence of 1.5 per cent for schizophrenia spectrum psychotic disorders (Arajärvi et al., 2005).

Daghestan in the northern Caucasus (Russian Federation) is a region that has been inhabited for over 3,000 years by small ethnic groups constituting together at least five genetically distinct populations, varying considerably in their morbidity patterns. The highest lifetime risk for schizophrenia (4.95%) has been reported from one such highland subisolate of approximately 3,000 members (Bulayeva et al., 2005). The population of the whole region consists of 26 ethnic subisolates in which the lifetime risk of schizophrenia was found to vary from 1.46 per cent to 4.95 per cent, i.e. the highest risk estimate ever reported for an isolate population.

The population of the Palau islands (Micronesia), currently 20,470 people, has been geographically and ethnically isolated from other Pacific populations for nearly 2,000 years. A genetic epidemiological study of treated cases estimated the lifetime risk of schizophrenia at 2.77% in males and 1.99% in females, i.e. high in excess of the 'modal' risk of about 1% reported for large outbred populations. All of the 160 Palau cases were concentrated in 59 families, each traceable to a single common founder, with 11 of them having 5 to 11 affected members each (Myles-Worsley et al., 1999).

At the other extreme, the lowest known prevalence rate of schizophrenia in any population (and a very low rate of bipolar disorder) has been found among the Hutterites in South Dakota, a Protestant sect of European descent whose members have lived since the 1870s in closely knit, endogamous rural communities in Manitoba (Canada) and South Dakota (US). According to preserved pedigree records, all of the present 35,000 Hutterites are descendants of fewer than 90 ancestors who lived in the eighteenth and early nineteenth century. Reduced genetic heterogeneity and communal lifestyle with minimum variation in environmental exposures make this population an ideal laboratory for a variety of disease studies (Ober et al., 2001; Newman et al., 2004), including psychiatric disorders. An early epidemiological study, in which the entire population of several Hutterite communities was screened, resulted in a schizophrenia lifetime prevalence of 1.1 per 1,000 (Eaton and Weil, 1955). Subsequent reanalysis of the data using DSM-IIIR criteria (Torrey, 1995), and a repeat survey (Nimgaonkar et al., 2000) replicated the original finding. Both genetic (low frequency of psychosis-predisposing alleles) and lifestyle factors (protective community support) have been proposed as an explanation for the unusually low rate of psychosis. Negative selection for individuals with schizoid traits who fail to adjust to the communal lifestyle and eventually migrate without leaving progeny has also been suggested, but not definitively proven. Low rates have also been reported for certain Pacific island populations. Two surveys in Taiwan (Rin and Lin, 1962; Lin et al., 1989), separated by 15 years during which major social changes took place, found that the prevalence of schizophrenia decreased from 2.1 to 1.4 per 1,000. In both surveys, the aboriginal Taiwanese had significantly lower rates than the mainland Chinese who had migrated to the island after World War II.

High Rates of Psychosis in Ethnic Minorities, Migrants and Refugees

The effects of migration on the incidence of psychosis have been studied extensively since the 1930s (Ødegaard, 1932). The publication of the first report of an increased prevalence of psychoses among African Caribbean minority groups in the UK (Hemsi, 1967), was followed by an increasing number of studies showing very high incidence rates of schizophrenia (about 0.6 per 1000) in the African Caribbean population in the UK (Bhugra et al., 1997; Harrison et al., 1997). A recent systematic review of the incidence of psychotic disorders in Caribbean-born migrants and their descendants in the UK (Tortelli et al., 2015) established that higher incidence rates among black Caribbean groups have been in existence for more than 60 years (incidence rate ratio, IRR = 4.7 relative to the reference 'white British' population). Moreover, the authors found that ethnic minorities, including the black Caribbeans, having been exposed to cumulative social disadvantage since childhood, had 'more complex pathways to care ... and may receive worse mental health care'. Similar conclusions were drawn from a large school-based study of ethnic minority youth in the Netherlands (Adriaanse et al., 2015), comparing the prevalence of psychotic experiences in Moroccan-Dutch (9.5%) and Turkish-Dutch (7.1%) minority children and adolescents relative to their native Dutch counterparts (3.1%). Perceived discrimination was found to be the main psychosocial factor associated with the findings. Such elevated rates of psychotic experiences, particularly in the Moroccan-Dutch children seemed to parallel the very high incidence rates of adult psychotic disorders in this minority ethnic group and might be predictive of adult psychopathology. Interestingly, minority status is not necessarily associated with an elevated risk for psychotic disorders, as shown by Suvisaari *et al.* (2014) in a study comparing the Swedish-speaking minority and the Finnish-speaking majority in Finland. While Swedish speakers made up approximately 5% of the population, their prevalence of schizophrenia spectrum disorders amounted to 0.7%, compared to 1.5% in the Finnish-speaking majority. However, as a group Swedish speakers tended to have a higher socio-economic position and longer life expectancy, leading the authors to conclude that 'social capital may be protective against schizophrenia'.

Refugees and asylum seekers represent a population group which is ethnically heterogeneous but nearly homogeneous in their exposure to severe stress related to war, natural disasters and political, racial or religious persecution. According to United Nations data on forced displacement and migration, in 2015 some 244 million people (3.3 per cent of the world's population) have been living outside their country of origin (Katona, 2016), and their number is rapidly increasing. With some exceptions (e.g. Logue *et al.*, 2015) psychiatric research on the whole is not catching up with these massive population shifts. However, one recent well-designed epidemiological study (Hollander *et al.*, 2016) has addressed the issue of refugee migration and risk of schizophrenia in a large cohort study of 1.3 million people in Sweden. The cohort was comprised of 88.4% people born in Sweden of two Swedish parents; 9.8% non-refugee migrants from the Middle East, north and sub-Saharan Africa, Asia and eastern Europe; and 1.8% refugees from the same regions. The linked data were extracted from the Swedish national registers which include all people resident in Sweden since 1932 who have been assigned a personal identity number, anonymized for the purposes of research. The database amounted to 8.9 million person years of follow-up. The incidence rate of non-affective psychotic disorders was 38.5 per 100,000 person years in the Swedish-born; 80.4 per 100,000 in the migrants; and 126.4 per 100,000 in the refugees. This corresponded to hazard ratios of 1.75 in migrants and 2.90 in refugees, compared to the Swedish born.

Thus, refugees were 1.66 times more likely than migrants to develop non-affective psychotic disorders. The authors conclude that refugees face 'substantially elevated rates of schizophrenia and other non-affective psychoses, in addition to ... other mental, physical and social inequalities ... our findings support the possibility that exposure to psychosocial adversity increases the risk of psychosis'.

Similar findings of nearly fourfold excess over the general population rate have been reported for the Dutch Antillean and Surinamese immigrants (Selten *et al.*, 1997), and for Moroccans and other non-Western immigrants in the Netherlands (Veling *et al.*, 2006). Research to date has not identified definitively any specific cause explaining this phenomenon. Little evidence has been presented to support earlier suggestions that these psychotic illnesses might be explained as substance-induced episodes or acute transient psychoses. Neither the cross-sectional symptom picture, nor the course and outcome of these disorders present any atypical features that would set them apart from ICD-10 or DSM-IIIR/DSM-IV schizophrenia (Harrison *et al.*, 1999; Hutchinson *et al.*, 1999). Incidence studies in the Caribbean (Hickling and Rodgers-Johnson, 1995; Bhugra *et al.*, 1999; Selten *et al.*, 2005) do not indicate any excess schizophrenia morbidity in the countries of origin from which migrants are recruited. Explanations in terms of biological risk factors, such as increased incidence of obstetric complications or maternal influenza, have been put to the test but found no support (Hutchinson *et al.*, 1997; Selten *et al.*, 1998).

A potentially important finding is the increased incidence of schizophrenia among the siblings of second-generation African Caribbean index cases, as compared to the incidence of schizophrenia in the siblings of white index cases with schizophrenia (Hutchinson *et al.*, 1996). Such increases in the morbid risk within sibships (in the absence of a similar increase in the risk among parents) suggest a lowered threshold for the expression of the disorder in carriers of susceptibility alleles that might be induced by environmental stress. Hypotheses involving psychosocial risk factors, such as lack of a supportive community structure, acculturation stress, demoralization resulting from racial discrimination, and blocked opportunity for upward social mobility have been proposed (Bhugra *et al.*, 1999) but not yet definitively tested. Although psychosocial adversity is most likely to affect the majority of immigrants, a plausible pathogenetic mechanism involving specific gene–environment interactions and linking such stress to the incidence of psychosis remains to be demonstrated.

Course and Outcome

Systematic investigations into the course and outcome of schizophrenia were initiated by Kraepelin (1919) who believed that the natural history of the disorder could provide a provisional validation of the disease concept until final verification could be achieved by establishing the brain pathology and aetiology. Arguably, the greatest extent of variation in schizophrenia across populations and cultures is manifest in the course and outcome of the disorder. Early reports, based on small clinical samples, pointed to a less disabling course and a high rate of recovery from schizophrenic psychoses in developing countries such as Mauritius (Raman and Murphy, 1972) and Sri Lanka (Waxler, 1979) in cases that, according to 'Western' prognostic criteria, should have a poor outcome. Selection bias could not be ruled out in such studies based on hospital admissions; standard assessment procedures and explicit diagnostic criteria were not used; and clinical improvement could have been confounded with the social adjustment many patients achieve in a comparatively undemanding environment. Thus, room was left for doubts about the validity of findings of a better prognosis of schizophrenia in non-Western environments.

Many of these methodological issues were addressed in the WHO multi-centre studies by employing standardized assessment and more refined measures of course and outcome than in previous research. In the International Pilot Study of Schizophrenia (IPSS; WHO 1973, 1979), the 2- and 5-year follow-up assessments of patients indicated significantly higher proportions of patients in India, Colombia and Nigeria having better outcomes on all dimensions than patients in the high-income countries. The initial psychotic episode had remitted during the 5-year follow-up in as many as 42 per cent of the patients in India and 33 per cent of the patients in Nigeria, whereas the majority of patients in the developed high-income countries had experienced persisting psychotic symptoms and disablement. In either setting, patients with good and poor outcomes could not be clearly distinguished on the basis of their initial symptoms, though they all met the ICD-9 criteria for a diagnosis of schizophrenia.

Nevertheless, the IPSS was not free of bias, since patients were recruited from hospitals. Bed availability and admission policies could have led to over-inclusion of chronic cases in the developed countries and of recent-onset, acute cases in the developing countries. Such confounding factors were largely eliminated in the subsequent WHO ten-country study (Jablensky et al., 1992), in which uniformly assessed first-episode cases were assessed upon their first contact with community or hospital services. The 2-year follow-up (and longer-term follow-up in several of the centres) provided ample confirmation of the finding that the outcome of schizophrenia was generally better in developing than in developed countries (Table 19.4).

Table 19.4 Two-year course and outcome in the WHO ten-country study: developed and developing countries

Course and outcome measures	% patients in developing countries	% patients in developed countries
Remitting, complete remissions	62.7	36.8
Continuous or episodic, no complete remission	35.7	60.9
Psychotic < 5% of follow-up	18.4	18.7
Psychotic > 75% of follow-up	15.1	20.2
No complete remission during follow-up	24.1	57.2
Complete remission for > 75% of follow-up	38.3	22.3
On antipsychotic medication > 75% of follow-up	15.9	60.8
No antipsychotic medication during follow-up	5.9	2.5
Hospitalized for > 75% of follow-up	0.3	2.3
Never hospitalized	55.5	8.1
Impaired social functioning throughout follow-up	15.7	41.6
Unimpaired social functioning > 75% of follow-up	42.9	31.6

Analysis of the data led to the conclusion that the better overall pattern of course and less disabling outcome in the developing countries was primarily due to a significantly greater percentage of patients remaining in a stable remission of symptoms over longer periods after recovery from an acute psychotic episode, rather than to milder or shorter psychotic episodes. This pattern was significantly predicted by setting (developing/developed country), acute onset, being married or cohabiting with a partner, and having access to a supportive social network. Being female was generally associated with a more favourable outcome. The length of remissions was unrelated to antipsychotic treatment, which generally was administered for much shorter periods of time to patients in the low-income countries. Independently of the WHO studies, a high proportion of better outcomes of schizophrenia in developing countries has been reported by numerous investigators (Kulhara and Chandiramani, 1988; Ohaeri, 1993; Thara et al., 2004).

The factors underlying the better outcome of schizophrenia in developing countries remain insufficiently understood but, in a very general sense, are likely to involve interactions between genetic variation and specific aspects of the environment. Differences in the course and outcome of a disease across and within populations may be related to varying frequencies of predisposing or protective alleles coding for proteins involved in neurodevelopment, neurotransmitter and receptor regulation, or intracerebral signalling between brain subsystems. In a large study conducted by the International Schizophrenia Consortium (de Candia et al., 2013) additive genetic variation in schizophrenia risk was compared in samples of African descent ($N = 2,142$) and European descent ($N = 4,990$). The genetic correlation between the two samples was 0.66 (highly significant), suggesting that 'many schizophrenia risk alleles are shared across ethnic groups and pre-date the African-European divergence'. While such genetic similarities undoubtedly exist, nothing specific can at present be said as to their role in the course and outcome of schizophrenia. However, a strong effect of the psychosocial environment is entirely plausible, considering the contrasts between developing and developed countries with regard to social support systems, kinship networks and beliefs about mental disease (Warner, 1983). It is, therefore, unlikely that the differences in the course and outcome of schizophrenia across populations and cultures could be explained by the operation of a single factor. The observed differences may result from the additive or interactive effects of: (a) genetic and pathophysiological differences between acute and insiduously arising schizophrenic syndromes which may have differential propensities towards recovery and stabilization; (b) lower incidence in traditional societies of the type of chronic stress to which people with schizophrenia are particularly vulnerable; (c) higher probability in traditional societies of an individual–environment fit that minimizes social isolation and withdrawal and prevents the development of secondary disabilities.

As regards (b), the WHO ten-country study found that the index of expressed emotion (EE), a short-range predictor of psychotic relapse, was as effective in Indian families (Wig et al., 1987) as in European and North American families, but that high-EE families were significantly rarer in India than in Denmark or the UK. This established a potentially important and specific cultural difference. If this finding could be replicated in other settings in developing countries, the relative rarity of at least one type of pathogenic stress in the daily environment of schizophrenic individuals would be demonstrated. However, it is unlikely that EE is the only type of stress to which schizophrenic individuals respond with psychotic exacerbation. Murphy (1982) proposed four criteria for schizophrenia-evoking stress: (1) a situation demanding action or decision; (2) complexity or ambiguity of the information supplied to deal with the task; (3) unless resolved, the situation demanding action or decision persists; (4) the person has no 'escape route' available. Each one of the components of the putative model may occur at different frequencies in traditional and industrialized societies, a proposition that should be testable epidemiologically or experimentally. As regards (c), the most important differences between traditional cultures and the industrial Western societies concern the sick role and beliefs and practices related to mental illness. The suggestive power of magical-mystic explanations of mental illness and of traditional healing practices may not cure schizophrenia but is likely to lower the barriers to spontaneous recovery and reintegration in the community. Generally, the findings of a better outcome for schizophrenia in traditional societies are compelling and set a research agenda that may lead to discoveries with fundamental implications for the management and treatment of schizophrenia in both developing and developed countries.

Acute and Transient Psychotic Disorders

Acute psychoses, different from schizophrenia or manic-depressive illness, were first described in French psychiatry as *bouffées délirantes* (Magnan and Legrain, 1895), and as *cycloid psychoses* (Kleist, 1921; Leonhard, 1995) in German psychiatry. The clinical picture overlaps with the *psychogenic psychoses* described by Danish psychiatrists (Wimmer, 1916; Strömgren, 1986) and the *schizophreniform psychoses* described by Langfeldt (1939) in Norway. These disorders represent a modest fraction of psychiatric morbidity in Western countries but are considered common in many parts of the developing world. Their correct and timely recognition is important because of their benign prognosis which is quite different from the outcome of schizophrenia or major mood disorders. ICD-10 includes a separate rubric (F23) with five subdivisions and diagnostic guidelines which aim at differentiating such acute psychoses from schizophrenia. Since little is known about their pathophysiology and genetics, this group of disorders provides a rewarding field of inquiry for clinical and epidemiological research. Common features of these states include rapid onset ('out of the blue'), few prodromal signs, dramatic and variable symptom presentation, short duration and equally rapid recovery with few residual signs. Often, but by no means always, they arise in response to psychosocial or physiological stress, but there is no characteristic family history, and the premorbid personality is inconspicuous. Recurrence of such episodes is the rule but the relapse rate is lower than in schizophrenia or affective disorder.

The French concept of *bouffées délirantes* is probably the earliest description of an acute transient psychosis. The term refers to a brief non-organic psychosis which typically presents with a sudden onset of fully formed, thematically variable delusions and hallucinations against a background of mild clouding of consciousness and fluctuating affect, and typically results in spontaneous recovery with some probability of relapse. Mental trauma is either absent or plays a minor role in the causation of *bouffées délirantes*, whose aetiology was primarily attributed to a vulnerable mental constitution. The description of the *cycloid psychoses* includes sudden onset, pervasive delusional mood, variable delusions, hallucinations in any modality, labile affect and psychomotor disturbances (excitement or inhibition). Stressful life events may precipitate a psychotic episode but the content of the psychotic experiences does not reflect the traumatic event. Leonhard emphasized the polarity of the dominant disturbance in cycloid psychoses and distinguished three subtypes: (1) 'anxiety-happiness psychosis' (extreme shifts of affect between intense fear and ecstatic elation); (2) 'motility psychosis' (impulsive hypermotility and psychomotor inhibition); (3) 'confusion psychosis' (incoherent pressure of speech and mutism). The duration varies from days to a few weeks but recovery is always complete, though there is a risk of further episodes in which much the same symptoms tend to recur.

The concept of *psychogenic psychosis*, introduced by Sommer (1894) and later elaborated by Jaspers (1963) and Scandinavian psychiatrists, defined a psychotic reaction, originating in traumatic experiences, which is psychologically understandable in terms of several criteria: (1) its content reflects the nature and significance of the psychic trauma; (2) there is a temporal relationship between the trauma and the onset; (3) removal of the traumatizing factor results in recovery; (4) the overall prognosis is good. However, the extent to which transient psychotic illnesses actually meet the criteria set by Jaspers and Wimmer is uncertain as few studies have attempted to explore its validity.

Conclusion: Prospects for Epidemiology in the Search for the Causes of Psychoses

Important insights into the nature and causes of psychotic disorders, primarily schizophrenia and its spectrum, have been gained from population-based studies, although essential questions still remain unanswered. With regard to schizophrenia, the clinical syndrome appears to be robust and identifiable reliably in diverse populations and cultures, suggesting that a common pathophysiology and likely common genetic predisposition underlie its manifestations. At the level of large population aggregates, no major differences in incidence and morbid risk have to date been detected, though small geographical area variations exist and appear to be related to a mix of risk factors whose effects may be attenuated in large, heterogeneous populations.

The study of 'atypical' populations, such as genetic isolates or minority groups, may be capable of detecting unusual variations in the incidence of schizophrenia and other psychoses that could provide novel clues to the aetiology and pathogenesis of these disorders. Notwithstanding the difficulties in the genetic dissection of complex disorders, emerging powerful methods of genomic analysis will eventually identify polymorphisms and haplotypes associated with schizophrenia risk. The majority are likely to be in genes of small effect, although one cannot rule out the possibility that rare polymorphisms of moderate or major effect will also be found, especially in isolate populations or at the level of neurocognitive and neurophysiological abnormalities underlying the disorder. Establishing their population frequency and associations with a variety of phenotypes, including personality traits, will be a major task for comparative epidemiology.

At present, no single, or major, environmental risk factor influencing the incidence of schizophrenia or other psychoses has been conclusively demonstrated. Further studies using large samples are required to evaluate potential risk factors, antecedents and predictors, for which the present evidence is inconclusive. The relationship between genotype and phenotype in schizophrenia is likely to be mediated by complex causal pathways involving gene–gene and gene–environment interactions, 'programmable' neural substrate, and stochastic events. Three models of the joint effects of genotype and environment have been proposed (Kendler and Eaves, 1986): (1) the effects of predisposing genes and environmental factors are additive and increase the risk of disease in a linear fashion; (2) genes control the sensitivity of the brain to environmental insults; and (3) genes influence the likelihood of an individual's exposure to environmental pathogens, e.g. by fostering certain personality traits.

A complementary research strategy proceeds from evidence that the ICD-10 or DSM-IV clinical diagnoses of schizophrenia and other non-affective psychoses may not represent relevant phenotypes for genetic research (Jablensky, 2006). This leads to an exploration of alternative, intermediate phenotypes (or 'endophenotypes'), such as neurocognitive abnormalities, or temperament and character traits associated with schizophrenia that may be expressed in both affected individuals and their asymptomatic biological relatives. A prerequisite for the application of this approach is the establishment of population prevalences for such endophenotypes in epidemiological samples.

Current epidemiological research is increasingly making use of existing large databases, such as cumulative case registers or birth cohorts to test hypotheses about risk factors in case-control designs. Methods of genetic epidemiology are increasingly being integrated within population-based studies. These trends predict a bright future for epidemiology in the unravelling of gene–environment interactions that are likely to be the key to the understanding of the aetiology of psychoses. In this context, research into psychotic disorders in non-Western populations can provide valuable information on the genetic heterogeneity, the impact of the environment, and the course and outcome of psychotic disorders. Both traditional communities and societies undergoing transition in their social organization can contribute critically to the better understanding of the relationships between culture and mental disorder and the variety of human experience in coping with mental illness.

References

Adriaanse, M., van Domburgh, L., Hoek, H. W., Susser, E., Doreleijers, T. A. H. and Veling, W. (2015). Prevalence, impact and cultural context of psychotic experiences among ethnic minority groups. *Psychological Medicine*, **45**, 637–646.

Arajärvi, R., Haukka, J., Varilo, T. *et al.* (2004). Clinical phenotype of schizophrenia in a Finnish isolate. *Schizophrenia Research*, **67**, 195–205.

Arajärvi, R., Suvisaari, J., Suokas, J. *et al.* (2005). Prevalence and diagnosis of schizophrenia based on register, case record and interview data in an isolated Finnish birth cohort born 1940–1969. *Social Psychiatry and Psychiatric Epidemiology*, **40**, 808–816.

Bhugra, D., Leff, J., Mallett, R., Der, G., Corridan, B. and Rudge, S. (1997). Incidence and outcome of schizophrenia in Whites, African-Caribbeans and Asians in London. *Psychological Medicine*, **27**, 791–798.

Bhugra, D., Mallett, R. and Leff, J. (1999). Schizophrenia and African-Caribbeans: a conceptual model of aetiology. *International Review of Psychiatry*, **11**, 145–152.

Bøjholm, S. and Strömgren, E. (1989). Prevalence of schizophrenia on the island of Bornholm in 1935 and in 1983. *Acta Psychiatrica Scandinavica*, **79**, suppl. 348, 157–166.

Böök, J. A., Wetterberg, L. and Modrzewska, K. (1978). Schizophrenia in a North Swedish geographical isolate, 1900–1977. Epidemiology, genetics and biochemistry. *Clinical Genetics*, **14**, 373–394.

Bresnahan, M. A., Brown, A. S., Schaefer, C. A., Begg, M. D., Wyatt, R. J. and Susser E. S. (2000). Incidence and cumulative risk of treated schizophrenia in the Prenatal Determinants of Schizophrenia Study. *Schizophrenia Bulletin*, **26**, 297–308.

Brewin, J., Cantwell, R., Dalkin, T., Fox R. *et al.* (1997). Incidence of schizophrenia in Nottingham. *British Journal of Psychiatry*, **171**, 140–144.

Brugger, C., (1931). Versuch einer Geisteskrankenzählung in Thüringen. *Zeitschrift für gesamte Neurologie und Psychiatrie*, **133**, 252–390.

Bulayeva, K. B., Leal, S. M., Pavlova, T. A. *et al.* (2005). Mapping genes of complex psychiatric diseases in Daghestan genetic isolates. *American Journal of Medical Genetics (Neuropsychiatric Genetics)*, **132B**, 76–84.

Carothers, J. C. (1953). *The African Mind in Health and Disease. A Study of Ethnopsychiatry.* Geneva: World Health Organization.

Castle, D., Wessely, S., Der, G., Murray, R. M. (1991). The incidence of operationally defined schizophrenia in Camberwell, 1965–84. *British Journal of Psychiatry*, **159**, 790–794.

Crocetti, G. J., Lemkau, P. V., Kulcar, Z., Kesic, B. (1971). Selected aspects of the epidemiology of psychoses in Croatia, Yugoslavia. II. The cluster sample and the results of the pilot survey. *American Journal of Epidemiology*, **94**, 126–134.

De Candia, T. R., Lee, S. H., Yang, J., Gejman, P. V. *et al.* (2013). Additive genetic variation in schizophrenia risk is shared by populations of African and European descent. *American Journal of Human Genetics*, **93**, 463–470.

Dube, K. C. and Kumar, N. (1972). An epidemiological study of schizophrenia. *Journal of Biosocial Science*, **4**, 187–195.

Eaton, J. W. and Weil, R. J. (1955) *Culture and Mental Disorders.* Glencoe, IL: The Free Press.

Essen-Möller, E., Larsson, H., Uddenberg, C. E., and White, G. (1956). Individual traits and morbidity in a Swedish rural population. *Acta Psychiatrica Neurologica Scandinavica*, Suppl. 100.

German, G. A. (1972). Aspects of clinical psychiatry in sub-Saharan Africa. *British Journal of Psychiatry*, **121**, 461–479.

Goldner, E. M., Hsu, L., Waraich, P., Somers, J. M. (2002). Prevalence and incidence studies of schizophrenic disorders: a systematic review of the literature. *Canadian Journal of Psychiatry*, **47**, 833–843.

Häfner, H. and Reimann, H. (1970). Spatial distribution of mental disorders in Mannheim, 1965. In *Psychiatric Epidemiology*, ed. E. H. Hare, and J. K. Wing. Oxford: Oxford University Press.

Hagnell, O. (1966). *A Prospective Study of the Incidence of Mental Disorder.* Lund: Svenska Bokforlaget.

Harrison, G., Glazebrook, C., Brewin, J., Cantwell, R., Dalkin, T., Fox, R., Jones, P., Medley, I. (1997). Increased incidence of psychotic disorders in migrants from the Caribbean to the United Kingdom. *Psychological Medicine*, **27**, 799–806.

Harrison, G., Amin, S., Singh, S., Croudace, T. and Jones, P. (1999). Outcome of psychosis in people of African-Caribbean family origin. *British Journal of Psychiatry*, **175**, 43–49.

Haukka, J., Suvisaari, J., Varilo, T. and Lönnqvist, J. (2001). Regional variation in the incidence of schizophrenia in Finland: a study of birth cohorts born from 1950 to 1969. *Psychological Medicine*, **31**, 1045–1053.

Helgason, T. (1964). Epidemiology of mental disorders in Iceland. *Acta Psychiatrica Scandinavica*, Suppl. 173.

Hemsi, L. K. (1967). Psychiatric morbidity of West Indian immigrants. *Social Psychiatry*, **2**, 95–100.

Hickling, F. W. and Rodgers-Johnson, P. (1995). The incidence of first-contact schizophrenia in Jamaica. *British Journal of Psychiatry*, **167**, 193–196.

Hollander, A. C., Dal, H., Lewis, G., Magnusson, C., Kirkbride, J. B. and Dalman, V. (2016). Refugee migration and risk of schizophrenia and other non-affective psychoses: cohort study of 1.3 million people in Sweden. *British Medical Journal*, **352**, i1030.

Hovatta, I., Terwilliger, J. D., Lichtermann, D., Mäkikyrö, T., Suvisaari, J., Peltonen, L., Lönnqvist, J. (1997). Schizophrenia in the genetic isolate of Finland. *American Journal of Medical Genetics (Neuropsychiatric Genetics)*, **74**, 353–360.

Hutchinson, G., Takei, N., Bhugra, D. *et al.* (1996). Morbid risk of schizophrenia in first-degree relatives of White and African-Caribbean patients with psychosis. *British Journal of Psychiatry*, **169**, 776–780.

Hutchinson, G., Takei, N., Bhugra, D. *et al.* (1997). Increased rate of psychosis among African-Caribbeans in Britain is not due to an excess of pregnancy and birth complications. *British Journal of Psychiatry*, **171**, 145–147.

Hutchinson, G., Takei, N., Sham P., Harvey, I. and Murray, R. M. (1999). Factor analysis of symptoms in schizophrenia: differences between White and Caribbean patients in Camberwell. *Psychological Medicine*, **29**, 607–612.

Jablensky, A. (2000). Epidemiology of schizophrenia: the global burden of disease and disability. *European Archive of Psychiatry and Clinical Neuroscience*, **250**, 274–285.

Jablensky, A. (2006). Subtyping schizophrenia: implications for genetic research. *Molecular Psychiatry*, **11**, 815–836.

Jablensky, A., Sartorius, N., Ernberg, G., Anker, M., Korten, A., Cooper, J. E., Day, R. and Bertelsen, A. (1992). Schizophrenia: manifestations, incidence and course in different cultures. A World Health Organization ten-country study. *Psychological Medicine*, Monograph Suppl. 20, 1–97.

Jablensky, A., McGrath, J., Herrman, H., Castle, D., Gureje, O., Evans, M., Carr, V., Morgan, V., Korten, A., Harvey, C. (2000). Psychotic disorders in urban areas: an overview of the Study on Low Prevalence Disorders. *Australian and New Zealand Journal of Psychiatry*, **34**, 221–236.

Jaspers, K. (1963). *General Psychopathology*. Manchester: Manchester University Press.

Jeffreys, S. E., Harvey, C. A., McNaught, A. S., Quayle, A. S., King, M. B. and Bird, A. S. (1997). The Hampstead Schizophrenia Survey 1991. I: Prevalence and service use comparisons in an inner London health authority, 1986–1991. *British Journal of Psychiatry*, **170**, 301–306.

Katona, C. (2016). Non-affective psychosis in refugees. *British Medical Journal*, **352**, i1279.

Kebede, D. and Alem, A. (1999). Major mental disorders in Addis Ababa, Ethiopia. I. Schizophrenia, schizoaffective and cognitive disorders. *Acta Psychiatrica Scandinavica* **100**, 11–17.

Kendler, K. S. and Eaves, L. J. (1986). Models for the joint effects of genotype and environment on liability to psychiatric illness. *American Journal of Psychiatry*, **143**, 279–289.

Kendler, K. S., Karkowski-Shuman, L. and Walsh, D. (1996). Age at onset in schizophrenia and risk of illness in relatives. Results from the Roscommon study. *British Journal of Psychiatry*, **169**, 213–218.

Kleist, K. (1921). Autochtone Degenerationspsychosen. *Zeitschrift für die gesamte Neurologie und Psychiatrie*, **69**, 1–11.

Kraepelin, E. (1904). Vergleichende Psychiatrie. *Zentralblatt für Nervenheilkunde und Psychiatrie*, **27**, 433–437. (English translation in *Themes and Variations in European Psychiatry*, ed. S. R. Hirsch and M. Shepherd, Bristol: John Wright and Sons, 1974, pp. 3–6.)

Kraepelin, E. (1919). *Dementia Praecox and Paraphrenia*. Edinburgh: Livingstone.

Kulhara, P. and Chandiramani, K. (1988). Outcome of schizophrenia in India using various diagnostic systems. *Schizophrenia Research*, **1**, 339–349.

Lambo, T. A. (1965). Schizophrenia and borderline states. In *Transcultural Psychiatry*. CIBA Foundation Symposium, ed. A. V. De Reuck and S. R. Porter. London: Churchill.

Langfeldt, G. (1939). *The Schizophreniform States: A Katamnestic Study Based in Individual Re-Examinations*. London: Oxford University Press.

Leff, J., Sartorius, N., Jablensky, A., Korten, A. and Ernberg, G. (1992). The International Pilot Study of schizophrenia: five-year follow-up findings. *Psychological Medicine*, **22**, 131–145.

Leighton, A. H., Lambo, T. A., Hughes, H. H., Leighton, D. C., Murphy, J. M. and Macklin, D. B. (1963). *Psychiatric Disorder among the Yoruba*. Ithaca: Cornell University Press.

Lemkau, P. V., Tietze, C. and Cooper, M. (1943). A survey of statistical studies on the prevalence and incidence of mental disorder in sample populations. *Public Health Reports*, **58**, 1909–1927.

Leonhard, K. (1995). *Classification of Endogenous Psychoses and their Differentiated Etiology*,

second, revised and enlarged edition. Vienna; New York: Springer.

Liebermann, Y. I. (1974). The problem of incidence of schizophrenia: material from a clinical and epidemiological study (in Russian). *Zhurnal nevropatologii i psikhiatrii Korsakov* **74**, 1224–1232.

Lin, T. Y., Chu, H. M., Rin, H. *et al.* (1989). Effects of social change on mental disorders in Taiwan: observations based on a 15-year follow-up survey of general populations in three communities. *Acta Psychiatrica Scandinavica*, **79**, Suppl. 348, 11–34.

Logue, M. W., Amstadter, A. B., Baker, D. G. *et al.* (2015). The Psychiatric Genomics Consortium Posttraumatic Stress Disorder Workgroup: posttraumatic stress disorder enters the age of large-scale genomic collaboration. *Neuropsychopharmacology*, **40**, 2287–2297.

Magnan, V. and Legrain, M. (1895). *Les Dégénérés. État mental et syndromes épisodiques*. Paris: Rueff et Cie.

Mahy, G. E., Mallett, R., Leff, J., Bhugra, D. (1999). First-contact incidence rate of schizophrenia on Barbados. *British Journal of Psychiatry*, **175**, 28–33.

McGrath, J., Saha, S., Welham, J. *et al.* (2004). A systematic review of the incidence of schizophrenia: the distribution of rates and the influence of sex, urbanicity, migrant status and methodology. *BMC Medicine*, **2**, 13.

McNaught, A., Jeffreys, S. E., Harvey, C. A. *et al.* (1997). The Hampstead Schizophrenia Survey 1991. II. Incidence and migration in inner London. *British Journal of Psychiatry*, **170**, 307–311.

Murphy, H. B. M. (1982). *Comparative Psychiatry*. Berlin: Springer.

Myles-Worsley, M., Coon, H., Tiobech, J. *et al.* (1999). Genetic epidemiological study of schizophrenia in Palau, Micronesia: prevalence and familiality. *American Journal of Medical Genetics (Neuropsychiatric Genetics)*, **88**, 4–10.

Newman, D. L., Hoffjan, S., Bourgain, C. *et al.* (2004). Are common disease susceptibility alleles the same in outbred and founder populations? *European Journal of Human Genetics*, **12**, 584–590.

Nicole, L., Lesage, A. and Lalonde, P. (1992). Lower incidence and increased male : female ratio in schizophrenia. *British Journal of Psychiatry*, **161**, 556–557.

Nimgaonkar, V. L., Fujiwara, T. M., Dutta, M. *et al.* (2000). Low prevalence of psychoses among the Hutterites, an isolated religious community. *American Journal of Psychiatry*, **157**, 1065–1070.

Ober, C., Abney, M. and McPeek, M. S. (2001). The genetic dissection of complex traits in a founder population. *American Journal of Human Genetics*, **69**, 1068–1079.

Ødegaard, Ø. (1932). Emigration and insanity: a study of mental disease among Norwegian born population in Minnesota. *Acta Psychiatrica Neurologica Scandinavica*, **7** (suppl 4), 1–206.

Ødegaard, Ø. (1946). A statistical investigation of the incidence of mental disorders in Norway. *Psychiatric Quarterly*, **20**, 381–401.

Oheari, J. U. (1993). Long-term outcome of treated schizophrenia in a Nigerian cohort. Retrospective analysis of 7-year follow-ups. *Journal of Nervous and Mental Diseases*, **181**, 514–516.

Padmavathi, R., Rajkumar, S., Kumar, N. and Manoharan, A. (1987). Prevalence of schizophrenia in an urban community in Madras. *Indian Journal of Psychiatry*, **31**, 233–239.

Phillips, M. R., Yang, G., Li, S., Li, Y. (2004). Suicide and the unique prevalence pattern of schizophrenia in mainland China: a retrospective observational study. *The Lancet*, **364**, 1062–1068.

Rajkumar, S., Padmavathi, R., Thara, R. (1993). Incidence of schizophrenia in an urban community in Madras. *Indian Journal of Psychiatry*, **35**, 18–21.

Raman, A. C. and Murphy, H. B. M. (1972). Failure of traditional prognostic indicators in Afro-Asian psychotics: results from a long-term follow-up study. *Journal of Nervous and Mental Diseases*, **154**, 238–247.

Rin, H. and Lin, T. Y. (1962). Mental illness among Formosan aborigines as compared with the Chinese in Taiwan. *Journal of Mental Science*, **198**, 134–146.

Robins, L. N. and Regier, D. A. (eds) (1991) *Psychiatric Disorders in America. The Epidemiologic Catchment Area Study*. New York: The Free Press.

Rotstein, V. G. (1977). Material from a psychiatric survey of sample groups from the adult population in several areas of the USSR (in Russian). *Zhurnal Nevropatologii i Psikhiatrii Korsakov*, **77**, 569–574.

Salan, R. (1992). Epidemiology of schizophrenia in Indonesia (the Tambora I study). *ASEAN Journal of Psychiatry*, **2**, 52–57.

Sartorius, N., Jablensky, A., Korten, A., Ernberg, G., Anker, M., Cooper, J. E., Day, R. (1986). Early manifestations and first-contact incidence of schizophrenia in different cultures. *Psychological Medicine*, **16**, 909–928.

Scully, P. J., Quinn, J. F., Morgan, M. G. *et al.* (2002). First-episode schizophrenia, bipolar disorder and other psychoses in a rural Irish catchment area: incidence and gender in the Cavan-Monaghan study at 5 years. *British Journal of Psychiatry*, **181**, Suppl. 43, s3–s9.

Scully, P. J., Owens, J. M., Kinsella, A. and Waddington, J. L. (2004). Schizophrenia, schizoaffective and bipolar disorder within an epidemiologically complete, homogeneous population in rural Ireland: small area variation in rate. *Schizophrenia Research*, **67**, 143–155.

Selten, J. P., Slaets, J. and Kahn, R. S. (1997). Schizophrenia in Surinamese and Dutch Antillean immigrants to the Netherlands: evidence of an increased incidence. *Psychological Medicine*, **27**, 807–811.

Selten, J. P., Slaets, J. and Kahn, R. (1998). Prenatal exposure to influenza and schizophrenia in Surinamese and Dutch Antillean immigrants to the Netherlands. *Schizophrenia Research*, **30**, 101–103.

Selten, J. P., Zeyl, C., Dwarkasing, R., Lumsden, V., Kahn, R. S. and van Harten, P. N. (2005). First-contact incidence of schizophrenia in Surinam. *British Journal of Psychiatry*, **186**, 74–75.

Sommer, R. (1894). *Diagnostik der Geisteskrankheiten*. Vienna: Urban and Schwarzenberg.

Spitzer, R. L., Endicott, J. and Robins, E. (1978). Research Diagnostic Criteria: rationale and reliability. *Archives of General Psychiatry*, **35**, 773–782.

Strömgren, E. (1938). Beiträge zur psychiatrischen Erblehre, auf Grund der Untersuchungen an einer Inselbevölkerung. *Acta Psychiatrica Neurologica Scandinavica*, Suppl. 19.

Strömgren, E. (1986). The development of the concept of reactive psychoses. *Psychopathology*, **20**, 62–67.

Suvisaari, J., Opler, M., Lindbohm, M. L. and Sallmen, M. (2014). Risk of schizophrenia and minority status: a comparison of the Swedish-speaking minority and the Finnish-speaking majority in Finland. *Schizophrenia Research*, **159**, 303–308.

Thara, R. (2004). Twenty-year course of schizophrenia: the Madras Longitudinal Study. *Canadian Journal of Psychiatry*, **49**, 564–569.

Torrey, E. F. (1995). Prevalence of psychosis among the Hutterites: a reanalysis of the 1950–53 study. *Schizophrenia Research*, **16**, 167–170.

Tortelli, A., Errazuriz, A., Croudace, T. *et al.* (2015). Schizophrenia and other psychotic disorders in Caribbean-born migrants and their descendants in England: systematic review and meta-analysis of incidence rates, 1950–2013. *Social Psychiatry and Psychiatric Epidemiology*, **50**, 1039–1055.

Varilo, T. and Peltonen, L. (2004). Isolates and their potential use in complex gene mapping efforts. *Current Opinion in Genetics and Development*, **14**, 316–323.

Veling, W., Selten, J. P., Veen, N. *et al.* (2006). Incidence of schizophrenia among ethnic minorities in the Netherlands: a four-year first-contact study. *Schizophrenia Research*, **86**, 189–193.

Waldo, M. C. (1999). Schizophrenia in Kosrae, Micronesia: prevalence, gender ratios, and clinical symptomatology. *Schizophrenia Research*, **35**, 175–181.

Warner, R. (1983). Recovery from schizophrenia in the Third World. *Psychiatry*, **46**, 197–212.

Waxler, N. E. (1979). Is outcome for schizophrenia better in non-industrial societies? The case of Sri Lanka. *Journal of Nervous and Mental Diseases*, **176**, 144–158.

WHO (1973). *Report of the International Pilot Study of Schizophrenia*, vol. **1**. Geneva: World Health Organization.

WHO (1979). *Schizophrenia. An International Follow-Up Study*. Chichester: Wiley.

Wig, N. N., Menon, D. K., Bedi, H., *et al.* (1987). Expressed emotion and schizophrenia in north India. I. Cross-cultural transfer of ratings of relatives' expressed emotion. *British Journal of Psychiatry*, **151**, 156–160.

Wimmer, A. (1916). Psykogene Sindssygdomsformer. In *St Hans Hospital 1816–1915, Jubilee Publication*. Copenhagen: Gad, pp. 85–216.

Wing, J. K., Cooper, J. E. and Sartorius N. (1974). *The Measurement and Classification of Psychiatric Symptoms*. London: Cambridge University Press.

Yap, P. M. (1974). *Comparative Psychiatry. A Theoretical Framework*. Toronto: University of Toronto Press.

Youssef, H. A., Kinsella, A. and Waddington, J. L. (1991). Evidence for geographical variation in the prevalence of schizophrenia in rural Ireland. *Archives of General Psychiatry*, **48**, 254–258.

Zhang, W. X., Shen, Y. C., Li, S. R. (1998). Epidemiological surveys on mental disorders in 7 areas in China. *Chinese Journal of Psychiatry*, **31**, 69–71.

Chapter 20

Affective Disorders Coloured by Culture: Why the Pigment of Depression is More Than Skin Deep

Gin S. Malhi and Yulisha Byrow

Editors' Introduction

It is estimated that in a few years' time the global burden of disease related to depression and its prevalence will overtake most other physical illnesses and depression will become the most common illness. Depression is a highly prevalent disease and is also a leading cause of disability. In this chapter Malhi and Byrow discuss the discrepancy in the reported prevalence of depression across cultures; with higher rates reported in high-income countries (Western) than in low–middle income countries (non-Western). Thus it is entirely possible that either the recognition of normal human experiences is turning into medicalization or that there is a genuine increase due to a number of social and cultural factors. These authors propose that the differences in the definition of depression across cultures as well as the interpretation of depression within the context of collectivist and individualist cultures may contribute to the observed differences in prevalence rates. They also explore whether there are differences in the expression of depressive symptoms across different cultures as well as the influence that differing social factors can have on both the experience of depression and its reporting. Malhi and Byrow propose that a particularly important facet to consider is that of treatment, in particular, how factors associated with culture, such as stigma, can affect treatment engagement, adherence, and outcome.

Introduction

Depression is recognized globally as a major mental health problem and major depressive disorder is ranked between the first and fourth leading causes of years lived with disability (YLD) in over 21 regions worldwide. Its prevalence rates vary from about 3% (Japan) to 16.9% (United States), with most countries falling within the range of 8 to 12% (Andrade et al., 2003). Counterintuitively, the lifetime prevalence of depression is on average lower in low- to middle-income countries (e.g. less than 10% prevalence was observed in Pondicherry, Mexico, Shenzen, South Africa) (11.1%) as compared to high-income countries (14.6%) – reaching up to 18% in France, the Netherlands, New Zealand and USA (Kessler and Bromet, 2013). Nevertheless, it is ranked as the number one leading cause of YLD in Central Latin America, Southeast Asia, Central Asia, Andean Latin America and Oceania impacting 4.33 per cent of the global population (Vos et al., 2012). Therefore it appears that although prevalence rates are lower than those observed in Western societies, depression remains a leading cause of disability and source of economic burden in non-Western societies.

Epidemiological evidence indicates that there is a discrepancy between reported prevalence rates of depression with higher rates observed in Western than non-Western cultures. There are likely to be many reasons for this discrepancy, which likely encompass numerous biological, psychological, social and lifestyle factors (see Malhi et al., 2015) that may either predispose individuals to, or protect them from, developing depression. Culture infiltrates all of these domains (biological, psychological and social), subsequently influencing reported prevalence rates.

In this chapter we first adopt a broad approach to understanding disparate prevalence rates in depression by examining differences in Eastern and Western definitions of depression, and depression in the context of collectivist and individualist cultures. Second, a more specific and granular examination of depression across cultures is presented where the potential explanations for this discrepancy are discussed. Generally speaking the reasons for differences are attributed to: (1) the expression of depressive symptoms, which is predictably subject to variation across cultures, and necessarily introduces significant biases in measurement when implementing Western definitions of depression; and

(2) social factors also vary across cultures, which undoubtedly affect the rate at which symptoms of depression are reported and perhaps even experienced. Last, we discuss the current status of treatment availability across different cultures and the factors that may influence treatment engagement, adherence and outcome.

Defining Depression

Customarily psychiatrists and psychologists use the biomedical approach to define depression which draws upon Western concepts. Central to this methodology is the idea that the diagnosis of a specific mental illness requires the presence of particular criteria – usually a combination of symptoms – that occur irrespective of culture. In contrast, the ethnographic approach, commonly used by anthropologists, suggests that although the symptoms as defined by the biomedical approach are likely to occur in diverse cultural settings, the significance of these symptoms for individuals necessarily varies depending on cultural context (Tsai and Chentsova-Dutton, 2002).

Major depressive episodes (MDEs) as defined by DSM are fundamentally a Western construct (see Table 20.1). However, DSM-5 also recognizes a series of culture specific concepts of distress, such as *shenjing shuairuo* (Mandarin), which translates to 'weakness of the nervous system', and notably

conceptualization along these lines blurs the boundaries that attempt to separate disorders. Consequently, non-Western concepts can usually be mapped onto a range of mental disorders including mood (major depressive disorder, persistent depressive disorder), anxiety (generalized anxiety disorder, social anxiety disorder, specific phobia), post-traumatic stress disorder, and somatic symptom disorders. Similar constructs exist in other cultures, for example, India (*ashaktapanna*) and Japan (*shinkei-suijaku*), and interestingly, many of these disorders bear similarities to the Western concept of neurasthenia, propagated in 1868 by the American neurologist, George Beard. This is not altogether surprising given that he suggested that the 'illness' (neurasthenia) was associated with an increased pressure created by modern civilization; he maintained that it was very much an 'American disease'. Conversely, Gilbert Ballet (1908) proposed that this 'disease' was not specific to America and considered neurasthenia to be synonymous with 'nervous exhaustion' because it was thought to be caused by emotions associated with depression (e.g. 'vexation, anxiety, disappointment, remorse'). Central to these historical depictions is the manifestation of depressive symptoms as physical symptoms. Over time, however, the concept of neurasthenia lost relevance for Western cultures and was therefore excluded from the third edition of the DSM (DSM-III). Kleinman in the 1980s suggested that the diagnosis of neurasthenia was highly prevalent in

Table 20.1 Brief overview of DSM-5 defined depressive episodes

Major depressive episode/disorder (MDE/MDD)	Persistent depressive disorder (PDD/dysthymia)

• Five or more of the following symptoms present during the same 2-week period:
 	
  • depressed mood
  • loss of interest or pleasure in almost all activities
  • weight loss or changes in appetite
  • sleep disturbances
  • psychomotor retardation or activation
  • fatigue
  • feelings of worthlessness or guilt
  • difficulty concentrating
  • suicidal ideation.
 	
• At least one of the symptoms present must be depressed mood or loss of interest.
• These symptoms must cause clinically significant distress or impairment.
	• Depressed mood occurring for most of the day, more days than not, for a minimum period of 2 years.
	• At least two of the following symptoms present during depression:
	
	  • changes in appetite
	  • sleep disturbances
	  • fatigue
	  • low self-esteem
	  • difficulty concentrating
	  • feelings of hopelessness.
	
	• There has never been a period of 2 months or more where the individual has not experienced these symptoms.
	• These symptoms must cause clinically significant distress or impairment.

China (*shenjing shuairuo*) and manifested there by way of bodily symptoms including weakness, fatigue, tiredness, headaches, dizziness and gastrointestinal afflictions (Kleinman, 1982). His seminal work emphasizes that depression can manifest differently depending on the cultural context in which it occurs.

Collectivist vs Individualist Cultures: 'We' vs 'Me'

Predominantly considered a Western value or ideal, individualism prioritizes autonomy above goals associated with the broader group, and places greater emphasis on self-esteem and the pursuit of personal happiness (Steptoe *et al.*, 2007). In contrast, collectivist cultures attach greater importance to valuing the needs of the family unit, or group, above the needs of the individual. Furthermore, collectivist cultures place importance on respecting social codes and values that are central to their culture, and accommodating the needs and expectations of others in order to maintain tradition through balanced and cooperative interactions within society (Dwairy, 2002; Nasir and Al-Qutob, 2005). For example, *Moysara* in Arabic cultures refers to a positive value whereby one may conceal one's own point of view in order to get along with others and save them from embarrassment (Dwairy, 2002; Nasir and Al-Qutob, 2005). However, this 'quality' could potentially hinder the detection of depression and potentially reinforce stigma surrounding mental illness.

Studies of individualism suggest that it is related to lower levels of depression, an effect which occurs independently of economic status and perception of control over one's life (Steptoe *et al.*, 2007). Therefore given that Western societies are more individualistic than collectivistic it follows that one would expect higher prevalence rates of depression in non-Western cultures where collectivism is more prevalent. However, according to current world health estimates the reciprocal appears to be true. Hence, the concept of individualism and collectivism provides an ideal framework to contextualize and understand the aetiology of depression and differences in the experience of depression across cultures.

Cultural Fit

Initially, there was a widely held view that the personality dimension of extraversion was central to adaptation across cultures (Ward and Chang, 1997). However

research findings were inconsistent, for example, extraversion was a significant predictor of psychological adjustment for Malaysian and Singaporean students residing in New Zealand but not for Malaysian students in Singapore (Ward and Kennedy, 1993). Consequently, theories have been modified and now consider the link between individualism and collectivism and mental health to be a function of 'cultural fit' (Caldwell-Harris and Aycicegi, 2006; Triandis, 2001; Ward and Chang, 1997). Broadly, cultural fit refers to the synergy of an individual's personality profile within the cultural norms of a society; with research findings highlighting that larger differences in extraversion scores between American students (residing in Singapore) and local students were related to greater severity of depressive symptoms (Ward and Chang, 1997). By extension the discrepancy between an individual's level of collectivist values (allocentrism) and individualist values (idiocentrism) and the prevailing cultural norms is likely to influence psychological well-being. Caldwell-Harris and Aycicegi (2006) investigated the relationship between allocentrism and idiocentrism and mental health in a collectivist (Istanbul, Turkey) and individualist (Boston, USA) society. Their findings have shown that for those in Boston, collectivism was positively associated with depression (as well as social anxiety disorder, obsessive–compulsive disorder, and dependent personality disorder), conversely for those in Istanbul individualism was positively associated with personality disorders (e.g. borderline, paranoid, narcissistic personality disorders). Taken together these findings highlight the complexity of the relationship between an individual's values and beliefs, those of the broader culture/society in which they reside, and their psychological well-being. Furthermore, it highlights the importance of considering inherent variability amongst individuals within the broader context of culture.

Biological Differences between Individualistic and Collectivistic Cultures

In terms of neurobiology, studies have shown differences in the activation of neural regions implicated in social cognition between collectivist and individualist oriented individuals (Chiao *et al.*, 2009). Specifically, for those with collectivistic values, activity within the anterior rostral region of the medial prefrontal cortex was greater when viewing contextual descriptions of the self (e.g. 'When talking to my mother + I am casual'), while those with individualistic values showed greater activation in this region when viewing general descriptions of the self (e.g. 'In general + I am assertive'). Furthermore, differences in neural regions engaged during perception, attention and processing have also been observed between collectivist and individualist groups (Liddell *et al.*, 2015). This emerging area of research highlights that there is likely a neurobiological basis associated with differences in cultural values. Furthermore, these findings provide insight into the influence of culture and social context on neural processing and development.

Genetics research has shown that individuals with the short allele of the serotonin transporter gene (5-HTT) are more likely to experience depression when exposed to a number of stressful life experiences, compared to those carrying the long allele (Caspi *et al.*, 2003). Interestingly, findings from studies examining population genetics suggest that in East Asian populations individuals with the short allele (approximately 80%) are over-represented compared to European populations (approximately 40%). Once again this pattern does not fit with the observed distribution of depression worldwide and further underscores the importance of addressing the central and intriguing question: why is the prevalence of depression seemingly greater in Western countries? To answer this question Chiao and Blizinsky (2010) compared the frequency of the short allele of the 5-HTT gene and the prevalence of depressive symptoms across 29 countries. Their findings indicate that across the regions studied collectivism and the frequency of the short allele were negatively associated with both mood and anxiety symptoms. More broadly, these findings highlight that collectivism can serve as a protective factor. Potentially the inherent desire to preserve social harmony and consider the needs of others before those of the individual creates a degree of social support that may protect against the development of depressive symptoms. For example, a study by Taylor and colleagues (2006) showed that individuals with 5-HTT short alleles (short/short) and who reported increased positive life events compared to negative ones, had the lowest levels of depressive symptoms in the sample. Other findings have shown that social life events are particularly salient for those with the short/short 5-HTT genotype and in contrast non-social events are not associated with affect (Way and Taylor, 2010). These findings support the reciprocal

nature of the gene–environment interaction and highlight that particular genotypes can influence the relationship between social events and the expression of depressive symptoms. Regarding negative or stressful life events Kilpatrick and colleagues (2007) examined long/long and short/short 5-HTT genotypes exposed to a natural disaster. Their findings indicate that those with the short/short 5-HTT genotype were at no greater risk for developing depressive symptoms than those with the long/long 5-HTT genotype, if they perceived that they were well supported socially. Those individuals with the short/short 5-HTT allele that did not have adequate social support had approximately a 4.5 times greater risk of developing depressive symptoms (Kilpatrick *et al.*, 2007). Again, these significant findings suggest that collectivism can protect against the development of psychopathology.

Factors Introducing Cultural Bias

There are several factors which can introduce a cultural bias and influence the observed prevalence rates of depression, as well as cross-cultural comparisons more generally, despite using the same method of measurement across regions. These can include a *construct bias* whereby the construct being evaluated (depression) is not universally defined or indeed understood and may also be associated with different symptom profiles across countries. This is different from *item bias*, which refers to specific items present in structured or semi-structured measures of depression that may not be familiar terms in other cultures, or are negatively stigmatized within particular cultures (Juhasz *et al.*, 2012; Van de Velde *et al.*, 2010).

Cross-Cultural Differences in Symptom Profiles

These differences in prevalence rates may be a result of cultural differences in terms of the specific symptoms associated with a diagnosis of depression. The very definition of depression is culture bound – specifically to Western cultures even though the symptoms associated with depression are known to vary depending upon the cultural context in which they occur. In a key study, Weissman and colleagues (1996) reviewed studies examining depressive symptoms as experienced by those in the United States, New Zealand, Canada, France, Germany, Italy, Lebanon, Taiwan and Korea. Their findings indicate that insomnia and loss of energy were the only symptoms that occurred in the majority of depressed participants across all countries examined. In contrast, symptoms of poor appetite were common in the majority of patients only in Lebanon, Taiwan and Korea; feelings of worthlessness/guilt in the United States, Canada, France, Korea and New Zealand and slowed thinking commonly occurred in Canada, Lebanon, Taiwan and Korea. Furthermore, symptoms of weight loss, increased appetite, hypersomnia, retardation, agitation and decreased sexual interest were not common in any of the regions examined. Therefore, this study showed similar depressed symptom profiles for respondents in most Western countries (US, France and New Zealand) and Asian countries (Korea and Taiwan), with the most distinctive symptom profile originating from Lebanon (common symptoms included: poor appetite, insomnia, loss of energy and slowed thinking).

Iwata and Buka (2002) examined the depressive symptom profiles of undergraduate students in East Asia, North America and South America. Approximately half of the items on the Center for Epidemiologic Studies Depression Scale, specifically two items associated with affect, three with somatic symptoms, and one with interpersonal problems, were differentially associated with culture (Iwata and Buka, 2002). These findings offer support for the hypothesis that there are indeed diverse symptom profiles of depression across different cultures.

Regarding somatization, an interesting trend emerging from the literature suggests that certain parts of the world, namely, China, Japan, India, Latin America and Africa report a higher degree of somatization symptoms related to depression than Western countries (Draguns and Tanaka-Matsumi, 2003). Similarly, Halbreich and colleagues (2007) report that somatic symptoms such as fatigue, sleep disturbance and pain were prominent and perceived as depression in India, Brazil, Peru, Venezuela, Morocco and Tunisia. A study examining the symptom profiles of depressed Iranian patients showed that the most frequently reported symptoms were headache (15.2%), irritability (10.6%) and pain (10.4%). In contrast, the classic depressive symptoms associated with Western countries, such as low mood, loss of interest, and hopelessness were reported by 8, 2.8 and 0.2 per cent of patients respectively (Seifsafari et al., 2013). Furthermore, these findings also showed that somatic symptoms were more common in patients from rural areas, who were female, married and with lower levels of education.

Similarly, in Eastern cultures it is often thought that depression manifests chiefly with physical symptoms and less so in terms of emotional symptoms (e.g. sadness, anhedonia) (Kleinman, 2004). However, evidence from recent research highlights that this may not necessarily be the case. For example, one study found that Asian Americans did not over-report somatic symptoms, however, European Americans endorsed affective symptoms to a greater extent than Asian Americans (Kalibatseva et al., 2014). Investigating symptoms associated with a diagnosis of mood disorders (including bipolar depression, depressive episode, recurrent major depressive disorder, persistent mood disorder or other mood disorder) in ten Asian countries (China, Hong Kong, India, Indonesia, Japan, Korea, Malaysia, Singapore, Taiwan and Thailand) a recent study has shown that the three most common symptoms experienced by individuals with depression are sadness, loss of interest and insomnia. Notably, these findings were consistently reported across different countries, income levels, and regions. They also report that vegetative symptoms were more commonly reported than mood or cognitive symptoms (Chee et al., 2015). Using the same sample another study examined symptom profiles of participants diagnosed with a depressive episode or recurrent depressive disorder and similarly found that persistent sadness (73.1%), loss of interest (52.9%), and insomnia (63.8%) were the three most commonly reported symptoms across regions (Park et al., 2015). Other somatic symptoms including psychomotor agitation/retardation and poor appetite were present in 22.7 per cent and 32.7 per cent of the sample, respectively. A study by Yen and colleagues (2000) examined depressive symptoms reported by Chinese, Chinese American, and Caucasian American students. Interestingly this study found that Chinese students reported significantly lower levels of somatic symptoms than their Caucasian American counterparts and that there were no differences in somatic symptoms reported by Chinese American and Caucasian American students. Taken together these findings suggest that there is mixed evidence supporting that somatic symptoms encompass the central features of depressive symptoms in Asian populations and cast doubt on suggestions that somatization could account for differences in prevalence rates observed across cultures.

Conversely, other studies have adopted an ethnographic approach to examine depression symptom profiles in different cultures. The qualitative analysis of interviews with 40 depressed patients revealed a theme called 'centrality of sleeplessness' whereby some patients alleged that their symptoms related to affect or mood occurred as a result of insomnia (Lee *et al.*, 2007). This theme seems to mirror the quantitative (biomedical approach) study by Park and colleagues (2015), which identified that insomnia was among the three most commonly reported symptoms across various countries in Asia. Interestingly, Lee and colleagues (2007) found that depressive symptoms as defined by Western classification systems (i.e. DSM) were generally relevant to contemporary Chinese individuals with depression and that sadness and depressed mood, although implicitly relayed during the interview, were commonly reported. However, differences in the experience of depression compared to Western cultures also emerged with individuals expressing symptoms in relation to both psychological and physical sensations e.g. *xintong* meaning 'heart pain'. The authors argue that this is inherently different to the Western idea of somatization, which asserts that psychological pain can be converted into bodily symptoms and that psychological and physical symptoms are separate constructs. Rather they suggest that the mind and body are not considered separate constructs in Chinese culture and thus psychological symptoms of distress are commonly expressed in terms of physical symptoms or a combination of both.

Taken together these findings reveal that the 'classic' features of depression e.g. anhedonia, sadness, etc. as framed by a Western definition of depression are in fact experienced by non-Western individuals, but because less emphasis is placed on these symptoms in non-Western societies these 'traditional' symptoms of depression are under-reported.

The Perception of Depression

A core feature of depression, and affective disorders, is the inability to experience positive emotions described clinically as anhedonia. However the converse, negative affect, features even more prominently in depressed individuals, and has been the primary target for first line treatments such as cognitive-behavioural therapy and antidepressants (Malhi

et al., 2015). Research shows that a complex relationship exists between factors such as positive affect, negative affect, stress and depression. Findings suggest that individuals with a history of depression experience lower levels of positive affect and greater levels of negative affect when exposed to stress and this nexus between stress and depression is moderated by positive affect (O'Hara *et al.*, 2014). Therefore the ability to experience positive affect is likely an important protective factor against depressed mood.

Cultural factors can also influence the experience and expression of emotion, with many researchers suggesting that the experience of emotion is largely dependent on cultural context (e.g. Kleinman and Good, 1985). It is widely recognized that those with East Asian cultures and values tend to experience lower levels of positive affect than individuals with western cultural values. Stemming from the Western ideal of autonomy and the pursuit of self-happiness, positive emotions are seen as essential to adaptive psychological functioning. In contrast, East Asian cultures place less emphasis on the experience of positive emotions. For example, they are less inclined to maximize positive and minimize negative emotions, are more likely to experience negative affect during positive situations, and thus embody a more balanced view of positive and negative emotions (Sims *et al.*, 2015). Instead they tend to value positive emotions associated with feeling calm, peaceful and relaxed while their Western counterparts tend to value positive feelings that are associated more with being excited, enthusiastic and energetic (Tsai *et al.*, 2006). These differential ideals lead to discrepancies regarding the expression of emotions in these cultures. For example, studies conducted on Japanese populations have shown that these individuals tend to inhibit the expression of positive affect compared to Western populations (USA) while there were no differences between groups observed when responding to negatively valenced items (Iwata and Buka, 2002; Iwata *et al.*, 1995). Similarly, inhibited expression of positive emotions has been observed in Korean and Chinese cultures (Cho and Kim, 1998; Yen *et al.* 2000). Interestingly, experiencing a lack of high arousal positive emotions (e.g. excitement and enthusiasm) is not key to the development of depression in these Asian cultures. Instead it appears that the discrepancy between the desire to feel low arousal positive emotions (e.g. calm and peaceful) and their actual experience of these emotions is linked to depression.

Conversely, in Western cultures discrepancies in the desire to feel high arousal positive emotions and their actual experience of these emotions *is* linked to depression (Tsai *et al.*, 2006). Clearly, the findings of this line of inquiry have important implications for both understanding depressive symptoms across cultures and their effective treatment.

Social Factors that Can Influence Depression across Cultures

Gender Roles

Gender is an important determinant of mental health, and one which is inextricably linked to human rights issues such as gender discrimination and gender-related violence. Globally, higher rates of depression have been reported in females than males; specifically unipolar depression is twice as common in females than males (World Health Organization, n.d.). However, beyond statistical differences in prevalence rates, gender has the potential to influence the risk, onset and course of illness, and treatment outcome associated with depression. For example, in terms of suicide, the majority of people, sampled across nine countries, that die from suicide are male, but in fact, suicide attempts are more common among females than men (Weissman *et al.*, 1999). Furthermore, in some countries, for example China, the suicide rate is higher among females than males in rural areas. Indeed, gender inequality is a worldwide phenomenon, but this discrepancy is particularly prevalent amongst more traditional societies.

The presence of certain social factors may predispose women to higher rates of depression including a greater chance of abuse (both physical and sexual), gender discrimination, poorer living and working conditions, less access to resources, and lower social position. Results from WHO surveys indicate that the frequency and severity of these factors is positively associated with the prevalence of mental health problems in women (World Health Organization, n.d.). A study examining mental health literacy amongst the Qatar general population showed a general deficiency in mental health knowledge. Furthermore, in this sample, females held more negative beliefs concerning mental illness than males (Bener and Ghuloum, 2010). Other findings point to factors related to socio-economic and family status, and explain about 20 per cent of the variance associated with the

discrepancy in depressive symptoms between males and females, across 23 European regions. Interestingly and importantly the study was unable to establish a connection between these factors and depression in countries that had a large gender related disparity in depressive symptoms (Van de Velde *et al.*, 2010), highlighting the innate complexity of the relationship between gender, culture, and depression. Overall these findings suggest that the disparity in depression prevalence rates between men and women is likely to stem from the subordinate position of women in many cultures and influence not only suicide rates but also their beliefs and attitudes about mental health problems.

Religion

Religion is another social factor that is inextricably linked with culture. It is relatively well documented that religious involvement is associated with lower levels of depression (Bonelli and Koenig, 2013). For example, after controlling for various sociodemographic factors a longitudinal study conducted over 14 years showed that there was a 22 per cent lower risk of depression for individuals who regularly attend (at a minimum monthly) religious services (Balbuena *et al.*, 2013). While the majority of findings to date have been overwhelmingly positive, there are some studies, which highlight the complexity of the relationship between religion and mental health. For instance, a meta-analysis showed that positive religious coping was associated with lower levels of depression, anxiety and distress but in those with negative religious coping the levels of these experiences were in fact higher (Ano and Vasconcelles, 2005). To explain this the authors point to a possible bidirectional relationship between religion and depression, such that feelings of rejection or punishment by God could lead to feelings associated with depression (i.e. guilt), and on the other hand those with primary depressive symptoms may experience feelings of punishment or abandonment as a result of their own negative self-beliefs (Ano and Vasconcelles, 2005). Other studies have examined this relationship between religion and depression, and also investigated the role of stressful situations. Findings from a meta-analysis examining these factors indicate that religiousness associated with a lower severity of depressive symptoms across all levels of stress, but that this relationship is particularly pronounced only in those experiencing psychosocial distress (Smith *et al.*, 2003). Therefore research findings suggest a relatively robust association between religion and depressive symptoms, but remarkably, there is a notable lack of research investigating this association across different cultures. Thus it would be interesting to further investigate the role of religion as a potential protective factor, particularly in developing regions where the population may be exposed to greater levels of traumatic or stressful life events.

Cross-Cultural Factors Affecting Treatment for Depression

Differing levels of treatment seeking across cultures has direct implications for the observed prevalence rates of depression. Findings from WHO surveys (World Health Organization, 2014) reflect a staggering disparity between high-income (189 treated cases per 100,000 population) and low-income (10 treated cases per 100,000 population) countries in terms of the treatment of moderate–severe depression. Furthermore, in terms of healthcare expenditure a WHO survey of 194 countries conducted in 2014 indicates that 32 per cent do not have a standalone policy for mental health and 49 per cent do not have a standalone mental health law. Furthermore, low- to middle-income countries spend less than US\$2 per capita per year with a significant amount of funds going to inpatient care i.e. mental hospitals. In contrast, high-income countries spend more than US\$50 per capita. Therefore, there are large discrepancies in terms of the number of mental health beds available, mental health workers, outpatient services, and welfare support between low–middle income and high-income countries (World Health Organization, 2014).

Examining the rate of treatment for depression in 63 countries, Smits and Huijts (2015) demonstrate that the chance of receiving treatment is high in European countries and low in African countries. Their findings suggest that this discrepancy is likely due to differences in treatment seeking between countries rather than differences in the prevalence of depressive symptoms. To further examine potential reasons for these differences the authors investigated the influence of a number of factors on treatment rates in general and specifically treatment rates for those with depressive symptoms. Factors such as urbanization, unemployment, no live in partner, completing primary school, female and elderly people have a higher chance of being treated. In terms of

broad country characteristics, those living in wealthier countries have a greater chance of receiving treatment for depression, while other factors such as accessibility of medical personnel, income inequality and enrolment in high school, did not have a significant relationship with treatment for depression. Other studies have shown that factors such as employment status and financial strain are related to symptoms of depression rather than income per se (Zimmerman and Katon, 2005).

Therefore, the low levels of care in these countries are likely due to several factors including access to services. However, other broader cultural values are also thought to influence low levels of mental health treatment in developing countries such as social structure, the lack of awareness of mental health problems and the widespread stigma associated with mental illness and its treatment.

Stigma

Mental health related stigma is a universal phenomenon that can occur on multiple levels. Social stigma refers to broader social groups perceiving and acting against other individuals who do not conform to a stereotypical ideal. Structural stigma occurs when institutions endorse policies and procedures that work against/marginalize those with mental illness. Lastly, internalized stigma refers to beliefs and attitudes directed toward the self that are associated with negative stereotypes of mental illness (Corrigan *et al.*, 2005). Findings from population surveys conducted in 16 countries suggest that individuals with mood or anxiety disorders report higher rates of stigma than those with chronic physical illnesses. Despite being a worldwide phenomenon, individuals with depression perceived greater levels of associated stigma in developing countries (31.2%) than those in developed countries (20%) (Alonso *et al.*, 2008).

Research indicates that differing cultural values are particularly relevant for understanding stigma associated with mental illness (Abdullah and Brown, 2011). As has been discussed, Asian cultures generally value collectivism, conforming to societal norms, achievement, and the impact of an individual's actions on the family unit and therefore in terms of stigma associated with depression, Fogel and Ford (2005) reported that depressed Asian Americans perceived greater levels of stigma when considering friends, employers and family than depressed Caucasian Americans. Furthermore, individuals with mental illness are often stigmatized and can often be viewed as the source of embarrassment and shame on their parents and the family unit. For example in Bangalore, India, marriage to an individual with a mental illness, or into a family unit associated with mental illness, is often regarded extremely unfavourably, however, concerns about marriage were less consistently encountered in London, UK samples (Weiss *et al.*, 2001). Predictably research shows that stigma associated with mental illness is related to lower treatment adherence (Livingston and Boyd, 2010) and negatively impacts treatment seeking and engagement with treatment (Corrigan *et al.*, 2014). These values are also reflected in Arabic society's attitude toward depression with findings from a qualitative study suggesting that patient and family opposition to a diagnosis of depression represents a prominent and sometimes unassailable barrier to treatment (Nasir and Al-Qutob, 2005). A recent study conducted in Iraq demonstrated that only one in seven Iraqi patients with major depressive episodes received any form of treatment (Al-Hamzawi *et al.*, 2015). Similarly, low rates of treatment for depression have been reported in other countries in the Middle East, such as Lebanon (Karam *et al.*, 2006).

Thus the stigmatization of depression and indeed all mental health problems in general remains a worldwide predicament. Not only does it deter individuals from seeking treatment, it also affects the reporting of depressive symptoms.

Conclusion

In this chapter we have shown that depression occurs worldwide but that its prevalence varies enormously across cultures. Many individual and societal cultural factors contribute to the development of depression, however, these do not readily explain the differences observed at population levels. It is likely that many other cultural factors hitherto unidentified play a significant role in the evolution and expression of depression that may help explain the observed variance of depression across cultures and also point to a potential model that provides a better framework for understanding the cultural pathogenesis of depression. A key factor that no doubt confounds and contributes to the detection and causation of depression respectively, is that of stigma, which is very much culture-bound and influenced by societal values. Hence, alongside mental health initiatives that suitably train professionals, it is imperative that world health campaigns and programmes that

raise awareness amongst communities also aim to educate, and directly address cultural factors that contribute to the stigma associated with mental illness. Until this is achieved the prevalence of depression worldwide will remain obscured by culture – even though its biological pigments are clearly more than skin deep.

References

Abdullah, T. and Brown, T. L. (2011). Mental illness stigma and ethnocultural beliefs, values, and norms: an integrative review. *Clinical Psychology Review*, 31(6), 934–948, doi: http://doi.org/10.1016/j.cpr.2011.05.003.

Al-Hamzawi, A. O., Bruffaerts, R., Bromet, E. J., Alkhafaji, A. M. and Kessler, R. C. (2015). The epidemiology of major depressive episode in the Iraqi general population. *PLoS ONE*, 10(7), 1–14, doi: http://doi.org/10.1371/journal.pone.0131937.

Alonso, J., Buron, A., Bruffaerts, R., He, Y., Posada-Villa, J., Lepine, J. P. *et al.* (2008). Association of perceived stigma and mood and anxiety disorders: results from the World Mental Health Surveys. *Acta Psychiatrica Scandinavica*, 118(4), 305–314, doi: http://doi.org/10.1111/j.1600–0447.2008.01241.x.

Andrade, L., Caraveo-Anduaga, J., Berglund, P., Bijl, R., De Graaf, R., Vollebergh, W. *et al.* (2003). Epidemiology of major depressive episodes. Results from the International Consortium of Psychiatric Epidemiology. *International Journal of Methods in Psychiatric Research*, 12 (1), 3–21.

Ano, G. G. and Vasconcelles, E. B. (2005). Religious coping and psychological adjustment to stress: a meta-analysis. *Journal of Clinical Psychology*, 61(4), 461–480, doi: http://doi.org/10.1002/jclp.20049.

Balbuena, L., Baetz, M. and Bowen, R. (2013). Religious attendance, spirituality, and major depression in Canada: a 14-year follow-up study. *Canadian Journal of Psychiatry*, 58(4), 225–232.

Bener, A. and Ghuloum, S. (2010). Gender differences in the knowledge, attitude and practice towards mental health illness in a rapidly developing Arab society. *The International Journal of Social Psychiatry*, 57(5), 480–486, doi: http://doi.org/10.1177/0020764010374415.

Bonelli, R. M. and Koenig, H. G. (2013). Mental disorders, religion and spirituality 1990 to 2010: a systematic evidence-based review. *Journal of Religion and Health*, 52(2), 657–673, doi: http://doi.org/10.1007/s10943-013-9691-4.

Caldwell-Harris, C. L. and Aycicegi, A. (2006). When personality and culture clash: the psychological distress of allocentrics in an individualist culture and idiocentrics in a collectivist culture. *Transcultural Psychiatry*, 43(3), 331–361, doi: http://doi.org/10.1177/1363461506066982.

Caspi, A., Sugden, K., Moffitt, T. E. *et al.* (2003). Influence of life stress on depression: moderation by a polymorphism in the 5-HTT gene. *Science*, **301**(5631), 386–389, doi: http://doi.org/10.1126/science.1083968.

Chee, K. Y., Tripathi, A., Avasthi, A. *et al.* (2015). Country variations in depressive symptoms profile in Asian countries: findings of the Research on Asia Psychotropic Prescription (REAP) studies. *Asia-Pacific Psychiatry*, **7**(3), 276–285, doi: http://doi.org/10.1111/appy.12170.

Chiao, J. Y. and Blizinsky, K. D. (2010). Culture-gene coevolution of individualism-collectivism and the serotonin transporter gene. *Proceedings of the Royal Society of Biological Sciences*, **277**(1681), 529–537, doi: http://doi.org/10.1098/rspb.2009.1650.

Chiao, J. Y., Harada, T., Komeda, H. *et al.* (2009). Neural basis of individualistic and collectivistic views of self. *Human Brain Mapping*, **30**(9), 2813–2820, doi: http://doi.org/10.1002/hbm.20707.

Cho, M. J. and Kim, K. H. (1998). Use of the Center for Epidemiologic Studies Depression (CES-D) Scale in Korea. *Journal of Nervous and Mental Disease*, **186**, 304–310.

Corrigan, P. W., Kerr, A. and Knudsen, L. (2005). The stigma of mental illness: explanatory models and methods for change. *Applied and Preventive Psychology*, **11**(3), 179–190, doi: http://doi.org/10.1016/j.appsy.2005.07.001.

Corrigan, P. W., Druss, B. G. and Perlick, D. (2014). The impact of mental illness stigma on seeking and participating in mental health care. *Psychological Science in the Public Interest: A Journal of the American Psychological Society*, **15**(2), 37–70, doi: http://doi.org/10.1177/1529100614531398.

Draguns, J. G. and Tanaka-Matsumi, J. (2003). Assessment of psychopathology across and within cultures: issues and findings. *Behaviour Research and Therapy*, **41**(7), 755–776, doi: http://doi.org/10.1016/S0005-7967(02)00190-0.

Dwairy, M. (2002). Foundations of psychosocial dynamic personality theory of collective people. *Clinical Psychology Review*, **22**(3), 343–360, doi: http://doi.org/10.1016/S0272-7358(01)00100-3.

Fogel, J. and Ford, D. E. (2005). Stigma beliefs of Asian Americans with depression in an Internet sample. *Canadian Journal of Psychiatry*, **50**(8), 470–478.

Halbreich, U., Alarcon, R., Calil, H. *et al.* (2007). Culturally-sensitive complaints of depressions and anxieties in women. *Journal of Affective Disorders*, **102**, 159–176.

Iwata, N. and Buka, S. (2002). Race/ethnicity and depressive symptoms: a cross-cultural/ethnic comparison among university students in East Asia, North and South America. *Social Sciences and Medicine*, **55**(12), 2243–2252, doi: http://doi.org/10.1016/S0277-9536(02)00003-5.

Iwata, N., Roberts, C. R. and Kawakami, N. (1995). Japan–U.S. comparison of responses to depression scale items among adult workers. *Psychiatry Research*, **58**(3),

237–245, doi: http://doi.org/10.1016/0165-1781(95)02734-E.

Juhasz, G., Eszlari, N., Pap, D. and Gonda, X. (2012). Cultural differences in the development and characteristics of depression. *Neuropsychopharmacologia Hungarica*, **14**(4), 259–265, doi: http://doi.org/10.5706/nph201212007.

Kalibatseva, Z., Leong, F. T. L. and Ham, E. H. (2014). A symptom profile of depression among Asian Americans: is there evidence for differential item functioning of depressive symptoms? *Psychological Medicine*, **44**(12), 2567–78, doi: http://doi.org/10.1017/S0033291714000130.

Karam, E. G., Mneimneh, Z. N., Karam, A. N., Fayyad, J., Nasser, S. C., Chatterji, S. and Kessler, R. C. (2006). Prevalence and treatment of mental disorders in Lebanon: a national epidemiological survey. *The Lancet*, **367**(9515), 1000–1006, doi: http://doi.org/10.1016/S0140-6736(06)68427-4.

Kessler, R. C. and Bromet, E. J. (2013). The epidemiology of depression across cultures. *Annual Review of Public Health*, **34**, 119–138, doi: http://doi.org/10.1146/annurev-publhealth-031912-114409.

Kilpatrick, D. G., Koenen, K. C., Ruggiero, K. J. *et al.* (2007). The serotonin transporter genotype and social support and moderation of posttraumatic stress disorder and depression in hurricane-exposed adults. *American Journal of Psychiatry*, **164**(11), 1693–1699, doi: http://doi.org/10.1176/appi.ajp.2007.06122007.

Kleinman, A. (1982). Neurasthenia and depression: a study of somatization and culture in China. *Culture, Medicine and Psychiatry*, **6**(2), 117–190, doi: http://doi.org/10.1007/BF00051427.

Kleinman, A. (2004). Culture and depression. *New England Journal of Medicine*, **351**(10), 951–953, doi: http://doi.org/10.1097/00005053-198801000-00010.

Kleinman, A. and Good, B. (1985). *Culture and Depression: Studies in the Anthropology and Cross-Cultural Psychiatry of Affect and Disorder*. Berkeley: University of California Press.

Lee, D. T. S., Kleinman, J. and Kleinman, A. (2007). Rethinking depression: an ethnographic study of the experiences of depression among Chinese. *Harvard Review of Psychiatry*, **15**(1), 1–8, doi: http://doi.org/10.1080/10673220601183915.

Liddell, B. J., Das, P., Battaglini, E., Malhi, G. S., Felmingham, K. L., Whitford, T. J. and Bryant, R. (2015). Self-orientation modulates the neural correlates of global and local processing. *PLoS ONE*, **10**(8), 1–17, doi: http://doi.org/10.1371/journal.pone.0135453.

Livingston, J. D. and Boyd, J. E. (2010). Correlates and consequences of internalized stigma for people living with mental illness: a systematic review and meta-analysis. *Social Science and Medicine*, **71**(12), 2150–2161, doi: http://doi.org/10.1016/j.socscimed.2010.09.030.

Malhi, G. S., Bassett, D., Boyce, P. *et al.* (2015). Royal Australian and New Zealand College of Psychiatrists clinical practice guidelines for mood disorders RANZCP Guidelines. *Australian and New Zealand Journal of Psychiatry*, **49**(12), 1087–1206, doi: http://doi.org/10.1177/0004867415617657.

Nasir, L. S. and Al-Qutob, R. (2005). Barriers to the diagnosis and treatment of depression in Jordan. A nationwide qualitative study. *The Journal of the American Board of Family Medicine*, **18**(2), 125–131, doi: http://doi.org/10.3122/jabfm.18.2.125.

O'Hara, R. E., Armeli, S., Boynton, M. H. and Tennen, H. (2014). Emotional stress-reactivity and positive affect among college students: the role of depression history. *Emotion (Washingtons DC)*, **14**(1), 193–202, doi: http://doi.org/10.1037/a0034217.

Park, S.-C., Lee, M.-S., Shinfuku, N., Sartorius, N. and Park, Y. C. (2015). Gender differences in depressive symptom profiles and patterns of psychotropic drug usage in Asian patients with depression: findings from the Research on Asian Psychotropic Prescription Patterns for Antidepressants study. *Australian and New Zealand Journal of Psychiatry*, **49**(9), 833–841, doi: http://doi.org/10.1177/0004867415579464.

Seifsafari, S., Firoozabadi, A., Ghanizadeh, A. and Salehi, A. (2013). A symptom profile analysis of depression in a sample of Iranian patients. *Iranian Journal of Medical Sciences*, **38**(1), 22–29.

Sims, T., Tsai, J. L., Jiang, D., Wang, Y., Fung, H. H. and Zhang, X. (2015). Wanting to maximize the positive and minimize the negative: implications for mixed affective experience in American and Chinese contexts. *Journal of Personality and Social Psychology*, **109**(2), 292–315, doi: http://doi.org/10.1037/a0039276.

Smith, T. B., McCullough, M. E. and Poll, J. (2003). Religiousness and depression: evidence for a main effect and the moderating influence of stressful life events. *Psychological Bulletin*, **129**(4), 614–636, doi: http://doi.org/10.1037/0033-2909.129.4.614.

Smits, F. and Huijts, T. (2015). Treatment for depression in 63 countries worldwide: describing and explaining cross-national differences. *Health and Place*, **31**(2015), 1–9, doi: http://doi.org/10.1016/j.healthplace.2014.10.002.

Steptoe, A., Tsuda, A., Tanaka, Y. and Wardle, J. (2007). Depressive symptoms, socio-economic background, sense of control, and cultural factors in university students from 23 countries. *International Journal of Behavioral Medicine*, **14**(2), 97–107, doi: http://doi.org/10.1007/BF03004175.

Taylor, S. E., Way, B. M., Welch, W. T., Hilmert, C. J., Lehman, B. J. and Eisenberger, N. I. (2006). Early family environment, current adversity, the serotonin transporter promoter polymorphism, and depressive symptomatology. *Biological Psychiatry*, **60**(7), 671–676, doi: http://doi.org/10.1016/j.biopsych.2006.04.019.

Triandis, H. (2001). Individualism, collectivism and personality. *Journal of Personality*, **69**(6), 907–924, doi: http://doi.org/10.1111/1467-6494.696169.

Tsai, J. L. and Chentsova-Dutton, Y. (2002). Understanding Depression across Cultures. In *Handbook of Depression*, 2nd edn, ed. I. Gotlib and C. Hammen, New York: Guilford Press, pp. 467–491, doi: http://doi.org/10.1017/CBO9781107415324.004.

Tsai, J. L., Knutson, B. and Fung, H. H. (2006). Cultural variation in affect valuation. *Journal of Personality and Social Psychology*, **90**(2), 288–307, doi:http://doi.org/10.1037/0022-3514.90.2.288.

Van de Velde, S., Bracke, P. and Levecque, K. (2010). Gender differences in depression in 23 European countries. Cross-national variation in the gender gap in depression. *Social Science and Medicine*, **71**(2), 305–313, doi: http://doi.org/10.1016/j.socscimed.2010.03.035.

Vos, T., Flaxman, A. D., Naghavi, M. *et al.* (2012). Years lived with disability (YLDs) for 1160 sequelae of 289 diseases and injuries 1990–2010: a systematic analysis for the Global Burden of Disease Study 2010. *The Lancet*, **380**(9859), 2163–2196, doi: http://doi.org/10.1016/S0140-6736(12)61729-2.

Ward, C. and Chang, W. C. (1997). 'Cultural fit': a new perspective on personality and sojourner adjustment. *International Journal of Intercultural Relations*, **21**(4), 525–533, doi: http://doi.org/10.1016/S0147-1767(97)00023-0.

Ward, C. and Kennedy, A. (1993). Where's the 'culture' in cross-cultural transition? Comparative studies of sojourner adjustment. *Journal of Cross-Cultural Psychology*, **24**(2), 221–249.

Way, B. M. and Taylor, S. E. (2010). Social influences on health: is serotonin a critical mediator? *Psychosomatic Medicine*, **72**(2), 107–12, doi: http://doi.org/10.1097/PSY.0b013e3181ce6a7d.

Weiss, M. G., Jadhav, S., Raguram, R., Vounatsou, P. and Littlewood, R. (2001). Psychiatric stigma across cultures: local validation in Bangalore and London. *Anthropology and Medicine*, **8**(1), 71–87, doi: http://doi.org/10.1080/13648470120063906.

Weissman, M. M., Bland, R. C., Canino, G. J. *et al.* (1996). Cross-national epidemiology of major depression and bipolar disorder. *Journal of the American Medical Association*, **276**(4), 293–9, doi: http://doi.org/10.1001/jama.1996.03540040037030.

Weissman, M. M., Bland, R. C., Canino, G. J. *et al.* (1999). Prevalence of suicide ideation and suicide attempts in nine countries. *Psychological Medicine*, **29**, 9–17, doi: http://doi.org/10.1017/S0033291798007867.

World Health Organization (n.d.). *Department of Mental Health and Substance Dependence: Gender Disparities in Mental Health World.* Geneva.

World Health Organization (2014). *Mental Health Atlas.* Geneva.

Yen, S., Robins, C. J. and Lin, N. (2000). A cross-cultural comparison of depressive symptom manifestation: China and the United States. *Journal of Consulting and Clinical Psychology,* **68**(6), 993–999, doi: http://doi.org/10.1037//0022-006X.68.6.993.

Zimmerman, F. J. and Katon, W. (2005). Socio-economic status, depression disparities, and financial strain: what lies behind the income–depression relationship? *Health Economics,* **14**(12), 1197–1215, doi: http://doi.org/10.1002/hec.1011.

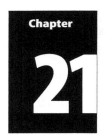

Substance Misuse

Shamil Wanigaratne and John Strang

Editors' Introduction

Addictions of different types have been around for a long time in the history of humankind. The reasons for using legal and illegal substances are many, and often complex. In many cultures such a use is well known and well described in scriptures across many faiths. Human beings use these substances to make themselves feel happier, to 'drown their sorrows' and for a variety of reasons. The use of alcohol and other substances of addiction varies dramatically across cultures and is dictated by cultural norms and societal expectations as well as availability. The global prevalence of associated disorders and patterns of use and abuse indicates the nature of influence that cultures have. In this chapter, Wanigaratne and Strang highlight that an understanding of the continuum of the use and abuse of substances is fundamental to developing interventions which will be culturally acceptable. They argue that comorbidity in psychiatric disorders with substance misuse is worth examining from a cultural perspective. Within migrant groups, patterns of use of specific substances such as *khat* may mirror those from the country of origin. The legal and illegal nature of certain substances adds another dimension to management as well as diagnosis. Using *khat* as an example, the authors point out the relationship between socialization and *khat* use in different nations. The possibility of medicalizing some of the problems must be kept in mind. The use of interventions also has to be culture sensitive and culturally appropriate.

Introduction

Ah, my Belove'd, fill the Cup that clears To-DAY of past Regrets and future Fears: To-morrow! – Why, To-morrow I may be Myself with Yesterday's Sev'n thousand Years.
  Omar Khayya'm (1048–1122; FitzGerald, 1859)

The use of mind altering or intoxicating substances has been part of human lifestyle from the beginning of time. As food and eating are often defining features of a culture, so are the intoxicants. Just as eating is essential for survival but can give rise to disorders culture bound or otherwise, intoxicants too similarly become problematic in many societies, although the type of intoxicant and society's tolerance vary. The cultural history of substance use points to three distinct patterns of substance use; religious use, medicinal use and recreational use (Crocq, 2007). All three patterns of use may have led to the pursuit of more potent compounds throughout the ages (Vetulani, 2001). Unfortunately, ethnicity and culture are lacking in many of the current dominant conceptualizations and formulations. By considering the contribution of culture, we can not only further our understanding of the nature and aetiology of substance use disorders and the pattern of presentation of these disorders, but can also inform the design of effective interventions both to treat and prevent these problems (Oyefoso, 1994). This chapter examines the continuum of substance use, misuse and dependence and how culture interacts with perceptions, attitudes and formulations when substance use is seen as problematic. It also summarizes what is known about global prevalence data for different substances of use/misuse, and the different responses to tackle what is seen as a growing worldwide substance misuse problem. We also explore what is considered to be a 'problem' and the extent to which culture influences what is seen as pathological. The example of *khat* will be presented in relation to what happens to a substance when it moves outside its original cultural context.

The smoking of the waterpipe will also be considered in relation to the increasing concerns about the associated health effects. Beyond definitions, this chapter also looks at how cultural perspectives/formulations could be used to help interventions at an individual, societal and global level.

Global Prevalence Picture

The United Nations Office for Drugs and Crime (UNODC) and the World Health Organization (WHO) monitor the prevalence of drugs, alcohol and tobacco use through published studies and country reports and produce regular reports on the changing picture globally. Examining the variations in the picture, culture undoubtedly plays a role in prevalence together with factors such as availability, economics, law enforcement and geopolitics. The most recently published (the World Drug Report) estimates suggest that over 246 million people used an illicit drug in 2013, an increase of 3 million over the past year (UNODC, 2015). An estimated 27 million people are suffering from a drug use disorder or dependence with 12.19 million people injecting drugs (UNODC, 2015). Although, from all accounts, there is an increase in drug use, with the increase in world population the prevalence rates remain stable. In relation to alcohol use, the WHO Global Information System on Alcohol and Health (GISAH) indicates that per capita consumption of alcohol has increased steadily in most countries and most regions in the world (WHO, 2014). Whilst the most recent headline estimated figures of global prevalence of alcohol use disorder are not available, a significant increase from the 2005 estimate of 76 million is to be expected with the increasing trends. It is estimated that there are over a billion tobacco smokers (WHO, 2016), although the rates are beginning to fall in some countries.

The World Drug Report (UNODC, 2015) estimates the annual rate of drug related deaths to be 187,100 in 2013. Examining the use of substances such as alcohol and tobacco, which are legal in most countries, the pictures of health burden and socio-economic consequences are amplified. For example, the estimated annual alcohol related deaths were 3.3 million in 2012 (WHO, 2014) and tobacco related deaths were estimated to be 6 million (WHO, 2016).

The above headlines point to the enormous health and social burden of substance use disorders today. Alcohol use alone is attributed to 4 per cent of the global disease burden (Room et al., 2005; Rehm et al.,

2009). The findings of the Global Burden of Disease study 2010 indicate the contribution of substance use to mental health disease burden is also considerable (Whiteford et al., 2013).

On the other hand, from an economic perspective, the legal substance industry is also a major source of revenue for most governments globally. It is not difficult to argue that the revenue factor dampens the enthusiasm of any government to intervene to reduce the consumption of these substances. On the other hand, a great deal of effort and resources in Western industrialized nations and international bodies (who are in turn influenced by them) go into combating illegal drugs such as cannabis, cocaine, heroin and amphetamines. International conventions and agreements that are driven by Western industrialized countries, especially when they decide on legality or illegality of substances, can therefore be accused of ignoring cultural perspectives of substance use, making some cultural practices that had gone on for centuries illegal overnight (Charles and Britto, 2001). It can be argued that cultural psychiatry could play a major role in enhancing our understanding of the cultural and social practices involved, which in turn may influence and result in changing some internationally held views and local legislation. An excursion into this area must also look at substances such as *khat* and betel nut, whose use is specific to certain cultures or regions in the world. Examining the use and misuse of these substances enables us to see the factors upon which our current concepts of substance misuse and dependence are developed. The current situation with these substances, particularly *khat*, gives us insight into the process of how the legality or illegality of some substances is determined. Instead of attempting to deconstruct our current conceptualizations and definitions, examining the very live debate about the status of *khat* more than illustrates how our existing concepts were formed.

From a psychiatric point of view, the picture of comorbidity or the co-occurrence of mental health problems with substance misuse becomes hugely important, as it is a significant challenge in the clinical area. The interaction between substance use and mental health problems and various causal models is also worth examining from a cultural perspective. For example, the use of cannabis in early teens and its suggested link with the development of psychosis (McGhee et al., 2000; Patton et al., 2002;

Clough *et al.*, 2005) is worth examining, as cannabis use is very much part of a number of cultures. Substance use and misuse among immigrant communities is a major consideration within this context. In Western countries there are often myths about substance misuse among immigrant communities. Taking the United Kingdom as an example, there is a perception among the public and many professionals that substance misuse among ethnic minorities is greater than in the indigenous population; however, there is no evidence to support this belief, and indeed there is some evidence to support the opposite (McCambridge and Strang, 2005). Nevertheless, there is evidence to show that substance use among immigrants is greater than compared with those living in their countries of origin (Wanigaratne *et al.*, 2001). There is also evidence for ethnic differences for consumption of different substances in countries such as the United Kingdom (Best *et al.*, 2001). This is undoubtedly mediated by culture.

The Continuum of Substance Use, Misuse/Dependence

The issue of substance use vs problematic use is fundamental to an examination of this area from a cultural perspective. It can be argued that this is the most crucial issue in the field of addictions. The philosophical question of what is normal, and what is abnormal, is at the heart of psychiatry and abnormal psychology and is decided by society and cultures. In most instances, the line to define normal is drawn on a pragmatic basis on an assumption of common and societal values, which are strongly influenced by dominant religious or political forces. For example, in Islamic countries use of psychoactive substances is forbidden by religion and not culturally acceptable. In this context 'substance use' and 'substance misuse' are understood to be and treated the same. In other words, the use of all forms of psychoactive substances is seen as 'misuse'. The Q'uran states in several verses that intoxicants are forbidden, hence within Muslim communities no distinction may be made between alcohol and psychoactive substance 'use' and 'misuse', as drinking alcohol and the consumption of any substance which clouds the mind are forbidden (Baasher, 1981). On the other hand if we look at a historical perspective, Hamarneh (1972), in his paper 'Pharmacy in medieval Islam and history of drug addiction', describes the use of poppy (opium),

hashish and *khat* in some countries in the Middle East for pharmaceutical and non-pharmaceutical purposes and some practices associated with Islam, for a considerable period.

The reader is referred to anthropological explorations of alcohol use by Douglas (1987) and the work of Heath (1976, 1978) for a more in-depth exploration of this issue. For the purpose of this chapter, it is important to delineate the basic concepts and issues. In our modern thinking, legality of a substance appears to be one of the key factors influencing where the line is drawn between the 'normal' and 'problematic'. Society is a key factor in determining whether a substance is harmful. At present, Eurocentric or northern hemispheric values may be most influential in the definitions.

The degree of 'control' an individual has over their substance use is key in the conceptualizations of 'addiction', which has become synonymous with what is seen as problematic substance use. Biological changes within the individual's brain or 'neuroadaptation' as a result of substance use is another factor. Problematic substance use, which is essentially the concern of psychiatry, psychology and other mental health professions, is seen as falling into two categories. These are 'dependence' (implying both physical and psychological dependence) and 'abuse or harmful use'. There has, for a long time, been remarkable agreement between the two dominant international diagnostic classification systems, the DSM classification system of the USA and the WHO ICD classification system. The concordance between the definitions of both diagnostic systems is probably due to the fact that they are both based on the seminal work of Griffith Edwards in the UK (Edwards and Gross, 1976) in trying to establish a working definition of alcohol dependence. The validity of the dependence syndrome described in the previous DSM-IV system and ICD-10 for different substances and in different cultures has been investigated by the WHO in 12 different countries (Nelson *et al.*, 1999). The findings largely support the content validity of the two systems for alcohol, opioids and cannabis, but not for other substances. The DSM-5 system combines the substance abuse and dependence categories into single disorder of substance use disorders (SUD) with a continuum of severity and it also adds craving and compulsion to use, as a diagnostic criteria (DSM-5, 2013). The ICD-11, the new revision of the WHO classification system is due to be published in 2018 and is currently undergoing field trials placing particular emphasis on culture. Greater convergence between the two systems is expected.

Neither DSM nor ICD systems are without their critics from a cultural perspective.

Emphasizing the power of norms (culture) in terms of motivating addictive behaviours in his excessive appetite theory of addictions, Orford (2001) strongly criticizes the DSM and ICD systems:

> ... at the very core of addiction, according to this view, is not so much attachment *per se* but rather conflict about attachment. The restraints, controls and disincentives that create conflict out of attachment are personally, socially and culturally relative. No definition of addiction or dependence, however arbitrary, will serve all people, in all places, at all times. From this perspective, systems such as DSM and ICD which claim universality may in fact be standing in the way of scientific progress by leading us to believe that such absolutes might exist.
>
> (Orford, 2001: 29)

The merits and consequences of ignoring the cultural context when defining substance misuse problems will be further explored in this chapter.

Cultural Context and Substance Use

The DSM-5 definition of substance use disorder takes into consideration negative social consequences of substance use such as legal problems resulting from substance use in its criteria. An individual being arrested for being in possession or using an illegal substance would meet one of the criteria laid down in the diagnostic system. The question of legality of a substance and its relationship with concepts of substance misuse is paramount in examining the dominant diagnostic systems from a cultural perspective. As stated earlier, use of different mind-altering substances has been part of many cultures for hundreds if not thousands of years. References to opium in Sumerian ideograms in about 4000 BCE and Assyrian medical tablets of 700 BCE and cannabis in China and the east several thousand years BCE can be cited as examples (Berridge and Edwards, 1987). The use of opium, cannabis and cocaine for medical and recreational purposes in nineteenth-century England and the changes in attitude, social context and legal status from common use to 'dangerous drugs' are charted in the classic text *Opium and the People* (Berridge and Edwards, 1987). Outside the Western world, exploring 'substance use in India', Charles and Britto (2001) outline the implications of international covenants and agreements and state that 'countries such as India had to criminalise traditions that were centuries old and accept the homogeneous definition of drug addiction and its management'. The decision to adhere to demands, made under the pressure of the World Bank and the IMF, is reported to have transformed the drug scene in many parts of India, which had a tradition of controlled use of cannabis and opium products for well over a thousand years (Charles and Britto, 2001: 467). India is a country that can boast of being a melting pot of many cultures. Most of the world religions are practised by citizens of India and many of its cultures encourage the use of mind-altering substances for medical, religious and social use. The traditional systems of medicine in India (e.g. Ayurveda, Siddha, Unani and Tibbi), as well as home remedies, tribal medicine and folk medical practices, use cannabis and opium as components of treatment (Chopra and Chopra, 1990; Britto and Charles, 2000). Even when legislation in countries allows for medicinal use of banned substances (e.g. Narcotic Drugs and Psychotropic Substance Act, 1985), these actions can backfire: thus in India implementation in terms of providing a licensing and distribution structure has been unsatisfactory, forcing individuals to act outside the law. In Sri Lanka, a systematic method of distributing opium to traditional practitioners was devised but in the year 2000 the 'international donor community' forced it to stop this. There are also many examples in India where cannabis is associated with social and religious ceremonies particularly among the Hindu festivals (e.g. Shivaratri and Holi) and aid practices such as meditation by yogis and sadhus (Fisher, 1975; Charles and Britto, 2001). Similarly, there are many examples from traditional Indian social and cultural practices where cannabis, opium and other mind-altering substances are used (e.g. during marriage ceremonies) (Chopra and Chopra, 1990; Masihi and Desai, 1998).

This section briefly outlines the implication of one aspect of a diagnostic system, namely legality and its ramifications from a cultural perspective. It must be emphasized that legality or legal problems are not the only issues that need to be taken into consideration when assessing and intervening with substance misusers from a cultural perspective.

The Culture of Poverty and Substance Misuse

The link between poverty and substance misuse has been established in many countries. Recent studies in Sri Lanka have shown how poverty itself gives rise to a culture that promotes and maintains substance use, particularly drinking (Baklien and Samarasinghe, 2003). The 'culture of poverty' or 'poor culture' makes drinking an integral part of it and traps the individual by giving him/her an identity within it and by subtle and direct means preventing the individual from escaping poverty. It is as if poverty not only makes the channels into substance misuse easier to slide down, but also makes the channels of exit more difficult to negotiate. Customs and traditions promote the use of alcohol and at the same time, ensuring that the individual gets deeper into financial difficulties, thus making it impossible to overcome poverty. The individual finds that acceptance of current circumstances is more adaptive than trying to overcome them (Baklien and Samarasinghe, 2003). In such cultures alcohol use and related behaviours such as domestic violence become accepted public norms. Mental health problems and associated manifestations such as 'learnt helplessness' become intertwined in this tapestry. Interventions to reduce alcohol consumption have to go hand in hand with poverty alleviation work taking into consideration the subtleties and mechanisms of their interdependence.

What Happens When a Substance Moves from One Cultural Context to Another? The Case of *Khat*

Khat is also known as *qat, chat* and *miraa*. The botanical name for *khat* is *Catha edulis*. It is an evergreen plant which grows in high altitudes in the eastern African and Arabian Peninsula. The chewing of *khat* is a pastime that was recommended by mystics and commenced around the tenth century (Kandela, 2000). *Khat* is structurally similar to amphetamine. It has two major psychoactive ingredients, cathinone and cathine (which have similarities to the amphetamines). Cathinone is chemically unstable, and is only present in the first couple of days after harvesting of the plant. The leaves of the *khat* plant are chewed by the user. *Khat* must be chewed a short time after picking for maximum effect. Sometimes, *khat* is also drunk in tea with honey.

Several million people are frequent users of *khat* (Kalix and Breaden, 1985). *Khat* is often linked to the Islamic faith because many users are Muslim. A prevalence study conducted in Ethiopia found that 80 per cent of users were Muslim, who reported using *khat* in order to gain a good level of concentration for prayer (Alem *et al.*, 1999). However, Islam prohibits the consumption of alcohol or of any substance that veils the mind. The use of intoxicants and alcohol are prohibited in various verses in the Q'uran:

> O you who believe! Intoxicants and gambling are abomi-nations of Shatans handiwork. So strictly avoid all that in order that you may be successful.
> (Al-Ma'idah 5:90)

There is a whole social process that occurs in relation to *khat* use. The principal effects of *khat* are increased alertness, increased ability to concentrate, confidence, friendliness, contentment and flow of ideas. Many use *khat* to study (Kennedy, 1987). *Khat* is also used for medicinal purposes. In women, it is used to relieve headaches and to assist in childbirth (Stevenson *et al.*, 1996). It is also used as an aphrodisiac (Kirkorian, 1984).

People go to the market to buy fresh *khat* around midday. It is usually sold in bundles wrapped in banana leaves. The quality varies according to price. After buying *khat* in the market, people go and have a steam bath or eat a hot curry (Kennedy, 1987). This makes them thirsty, so they drink water or soft drinks. This enhances the effect of chewing *khat*. *Khat* is usually chewed in company after around 3 pm. In Yemen, men group together at a '*khat* party'. Wealthy homes have a room set aside for this purpose, known as *mafraj* (Weir, 1985). Whilst chewing *khat*, the men also smoke the water pipe/*shisa*/*narghile*. During the *khat* session, men talk about business and personal affairs. The *khat* is stored in the men's cheeks in a ball. It is never swallowed.

Health Implications of Using *Khat*

There is some debate about whether *khat* can cause dependence (Cox and Rampes, 2003). Some state that there is no evidence of physical dependence (Ghodse, 2002) and most users report no physical withdrawal symptoms with cessation of *khat* (Cox and Rampes, 2003). There are a number of negative health consequences which have been reported with the use of *khat*. Oral consumption of *khat* in the Arabian Peninsula has been associated with oesophageal cancer (Gunaid *et al.*, 1995). The first case of *khat*-induced psychosis was reported over 40 years ago (Carothers, 1965), although very few cases of psychosis due to *khat* use have been reported, despite its heavy use in East Africa and Arab countries (Pantellis *et al.*, 1989). In an annual report of the eastern Mediterranean region, the World Health Organization expressed concern about the continued use of *khat*, especially in Yemen (WHO, 2000).

In addition to the physical and psychological side effects of chewing *khat*, its impact on the family has also been reported. Inevitably, there are social and economic implications as the family income is diverted to fund the habit (Kalix, 1984). Men who chew *khat* can also spend many hours outside the home, leaving their wives to care for the children.

The Impact of Migration on *Khat* Use

Reports of *khat* use in the UK began to circulate in newspapers from the mid 1980s (Hogg and Rogers, 1985; Pantellis *et al.*, 1989). Cathinone became controlled under the Misuse of Drugs Act (1971). In 2014 the UK joined the USA and some European countries, such as France to prohibit *khat*. The impact of this is still being assessed. Cultivation and trade in *khat* was banned in Saudi Arabia over 50 years ago (Zaghoul *et al.*, 2003). Kuwait, Morocco and Egypt have a preventative ban on *khat*. Yemen has tried on many occasions to dissuade people from chewing *khat*.

Somalian users were studied in Italy (Nencini *et al.*, 1989). They found that, whilst *khat* was easily available, it cost more than cocaine and alcohol. The general pattern of use they found was that users met at the weekends to chew *khat* in order to participate in community social life and not for the effects of the drug alone. Somalians' use of *khat* in the UK has also been studied (Griffiths *et al.*, 1997). In this study, 207 Somalians were interviewed; 76 per cent had increased their use since coming to the UK. Some reported moderate depression and a minority reported severe depression. Adverse effects of chewing *khat* were sleeplessness, anxiety and depression. Another study of Somalians in the UK (Nabuzoka and Badhadhe, 2000) found that chewing *khat* had a social dimension, occupied a significant proportion of users' time and was associated with other drug use. Most users reported negative health effects, but said that they used *khat* to cope with feelings of dislocation from their country of origin and as a form of recreation.

More recently, there has been an emerging pattern of *khat*-induced psychosis in London (Cox and Rampes, 2003) and in Australia (Stefan and Mathew, 2005). *Khat*-induced psychosis is often associated with increased consumption (Cox and Rampes, 2003). It is thought that 25 per cent of cases improve with the cessation of use of *khat*. The remainder respond swiftly to anti-psychotic medication (Stefan and Mathew, 2005).

Should We Be Concerned about *Khat*?

Should we be medicalizing *khat* or should we view it as a harmless indigenous substance with strongly associated cultural and social roots? It would be relatively easy to medicalize and prohibit *khat* use. However, this would then deny users the opportunity to exercise their own right to decide whether to chew it or not. In contrast, alcohol is tolerated in many societies, at least to some extent, despite the evidence of major problems for some who drink. Could a similar approach be taken with *khat*? Anthropologists hold a very different view of alcohol in comparison to their medical colleagues (Douglas, 1987). They have contributed to the study of alcohol by considering the social aspect of its usage. Perhaps they have a role to play in the case of *khat* outside its normal context. Medicalizing *khat* reduces the importance of, and role of, the social aspects. *Khat* parties may have a positive effect on users' psychological well-being by connecting them to members of their community. However, it would seem that use of *khat* does, at times, result in psychosis. Further studies need to be conducted from an anthropological and social perspective, in order to enhance our understanding of the use of *khat* outside its original cultural context.

Smoking the Waterpipe

The waterpipe is also known as the *shisha*, 'hubble bubble pipe', 'hookah', arghile, narghile. It has been smoked for around 400 years (Knishkowy and Amitai, 2005). There are differing opinions about where the practice first started. Some believe it started in India, others believe it started in Turkey (Onder *et al.*, 2002).

The waterpipe consists of a glass vase/bottle with a metal body and a hose pipe with a mouthpiece. The glass vase/bottle part of the waterpipe is partially filled with water. The small bowl at the top of the pipe is then heated using charcoal and the tobacco, called *maasel*, is placed in a small bowl on top of the pipe. The smoke travels through the water before it is inhaled by the user via a hose pipe. The *maasel* comes in many flavours, such as cherry, mint, strawberry and apple. The smell of the smoke can be very pleasant. Smoking the waterpipe is a social activity and people usually pass the hose part of the pipe to each other. To refuse to share a pipe is seen as insulting. The smoking session lasts from 30 to 45 minutes. It should be noted that sometimes users mix tobacco with cannabis (Knishkowy and Amitai, 2005).

Prevalence data on smoking the waterpipe are scarce and probably inaccurate, as they do not capture those who smoke at home. Use of the waterpipe is increasing in all Arab societies (Maziak *et al.*, 2004; Maziak *et al.*, 2006). In Middle Eastern countries it seems to be particularly popular with women and has opened up a permitted social world for women in many countries. With globalization and the increase in migration, we are likely to see an increase in its use elsewhere (Knishkowy and Amitai, 2005). The extent of waterpipe smoking in the West by migrants is unknown.

Given that the waterpipe is smoked in many Arab societies, it is worth considering the Islamic perspective on smoking the waterpipe. In Islam, actions which are permissible are known by the Arabic word *halal*. Actions which are forbidden are known by the Arabic word *haram*. In our experience of working with Islamic scholars, most view smoking the waterpipe as neither *halal* nor *haram*. It is viewed as *makrooh*. *Makrooh* is an Arabic word which means disliked or not recommended.

Since little was known about the health effects of smoking the waterpipe, New York University convened the first International Conference on Waterpipe Tobacco Smoking in Abu Dhabi in 2013, bringing together experts and authorities on the subject from around the world. This meeting has stimulated research and reviews and new information contradicting previously held beliefs has emerged. In a subsequent review, El-Zaatari *et al.* (2015) have outlined adverse short-term and long-term health effects including, cardiovascular, respiratory, periodontal, cancer, osteoporosis, perinatal problems and increased vulnerability to infections. This review reinforces the view that waterpipe smoking is associated with some of the health problems seen with cigarette smoking (WHO, 2005). Based on their review they call for stronger regulation of waterpipe smoking in view

of its growing popularity among young people and women (El-Zaatari *et al.*, 2015).

Interventions for Substance Misuse Problems

We have illustrated here how culture plays a part in substance use and misuse and how this aspect is often ignored in definitions and conceptualizations in the field. It is also a fact that, in every community and in every country, there are individuals whose substance use becomes problematic to themselves and/or to others. This would be the case whether one operates within the dominant diagnostic systems (DSM and ICD) or not, although what may be considered a 'case' may differ. Whether or not an intervention is required will be influenced by the extent to which the substance is deemed, at that time in that particular society, to be problematic, as well as on the basis of other considerations such as co-occurring mental health problems. Treatment in general would involve a medical intervention such as detoxification or substitute medication and a range of psychosocial interventions. These interventions are described in numerous texts (e.g. Institute of Medicine, 1990; Seivewright, 2000; Ghodse, 2002; Edwards *et al.*, 2003) and will not be explored here. Instead, some examples from the limited literature of non-western traditional interventions in the treatment of alcohol- and drug-misuse problems will be outlined. Reviews of traditional interventions in this area are rare. Jilek (1994), in a scholarly review, outlines a number of non-Western treatment approaches in a number of countries and societies including Asia (Buddhist, Hmong shamanic rituals based on Islamic traditions, Taoist traditions, Hindu and Arab Islamic traditions), North America (Eskimo Spirit Movement, Native American ceremonials, Indian Shaker Church), Central and South America (Mexican, Ecuadorian and Peruvian folk healing) and Southern Africa (Afro-Christian cults). Whilst there are significant variations in the philosophies, rituals, interventions and rehabilitation approaches in these non-Western treatments, some common themes and patterns also emerge (Jilek, 1994). The interventions or programmes are generally group based, although individual counselling may also take place. The programmes are invariably abstinence based and may be aimed at a single substance such as opiates and alcohol or poly-substance use. Whilst these interventions are grounded in a particular country, culture or community, hence widely different, there are strong themes or factors that emerge as critical. The following factors can be distilled from a variety of programmes:

- strong belief or religious component
- aversive component/experience
- cathartic abreaction
- herbal medication component (reversing withdrawal effects and reducing craving, e.g. Spencer *et al.*, 1980; Yang and Kwok, 1986; Shanmugasundaram *et al.*, 1986)
- use of sedatives and prolonged periods of sleep
- physiotherapies (e.g. steam baths, massage, hydrotherapies)
- traditional treatments such as acupuncture
- symbolic rituals (e.g. old self in a coffin, burning opium pipes, etc.)
- repetitive rituals (Naikan therapy Japan)
- transcendental meditation and yogic practices (relaxation)
- rituals that involve altered states of consciousness
- ceremonial/community aspect
- active involvement of family and community.

In traditional treatments, in spite of considerable variety in procedure, most of them follow the general principle of initial internal purgation and external cleansing from chemical and spiritual pollution combined with sedative alleviation of withdrawal symptoms, followed by spiritual didactic counselling (Jilek, 1994). The main features held in common in these traditional approaches are the ritual use of culturally valid symbolism, words and acts and may have an overt and covert commonality with Western therapeutic community approaches. It can be argued that these approaches may have directly and indirectly influenced each other, hence the commonality. There are also examples where a Western therapeutic community model has been adapted and modified incorporating local religious and cultural traditions. The Mithuru Mithuro movement in Sri Lanka is such an example, where the therapeutic community model has been adapted to incorporate Buddhist practices and Sri Lankan traditions in the rehabilitation of drug- and alcohol-dependent individuals.

Evaluating these programmes from a Western positivist methodology that would meet the criteria for evidence of effectiveness is problematic for a number of reasons, which are outlined in the next section.

Nevertheless, some of these programmes have been evaluated and these reports paint a very positive picture. Most programmes report a very low drop-out rate (80–90%) and six-month abstinence rates of up to 70 per cent. A programme in Egypt integrating an Islamic spiritual approach found that the compliance rate was higher than other non-religious programmes and was more cost-effective (Baasher and Abu El Azayem, 1980). In Thailand the outcomes of traditional treatment centres have been found to be comparable with government treatment centres (Poshyachinda, 1980; Westermeyer, 1980). In Malaysia a study looking at outcomes of traditional treatment methods taking non-traceable patients as failures found 1-year abstinence rates ranging from 8 per cent to 35 per cent (Spencer *et al.*, 1980). In Japan, Naikan therapy showed outcomes of 53 per cent abstinence in 6 months, 49 per cent in 1 year (Takemoto *et al.*, 1979). In Malawi a study showed an average 2.8 years of abstinence after joining a healing church (Peltzer, 1987). On the other hand, folk treatment in Central and South America, where abstinence was the expressed goal, only reduced consumption and improved personal and family function was achieved (Singer and Borrero, 1984).

Cultural Competence

If those receiving treatment and those providing treatment are from the same culture it is reasonable to expect that the carers share the same beliefs and values and are sensitive to the nuances of their culture. In such cases it can be argued that negative attitudes towards substance users and rigid religious beliefs are the only factors that could get in the way of good practice, with a word of caution that cultures are rarely homogeneous. Often those who provide treatment come from a different culture to those receiving treatment. This is particularly the case in countries and societies that could be called multicultural. This is where in psychiatry and the field of mental health there is a need for cultural competence in those who provide services (Davis, 1998). There are reviews that suggest positive outcomes in user satisfaction as a result of cultural training of staff (Beach *et al.*, 2005; Smedley *et al.*, 2003). Cultural competence interventions in substance misuse treatment settings in the form of training that focuses knowledge, awareness and skills have been shown to have positive results and are recommended (Delphin-Rittmon *et al.*, 2016).

Research Perspective

One of the nine biggest questions facing the field of addictions today is 'why are some individuals, strata in society, ethnic groups and cultures more susceptible to addictions than others?' (West, 2006). We put forward five guiding principles to be borne in mind in such work:

1. It is valuable to incorporate the diverse perspectives of different disciplines – medical anthropology, sociology, psychiatry and psychology – when researching culture in isolation within different paradigms.

2. There is a need for good epidemiological data that also looks at history, traditions and cultural contexts of substance use.

3. Assessments and study of mental health and substance use must be undertaken with an awareness of specific influence of culture, and how culture could mediate (i.e. beliefs).

4. Avoid importing potentially inappropriate treatments developed in other contexts and for other communities, and do not seek to impose preconceptions of the effectiveness of traditional treatment programmes and approaches.

5. Consider the potential worth of separate culturally sensitive integration of efforts to integrate traditional approaches to Western countries that have large immigrant and ethnically diverse populations.

To illustrate the challenges facing research in this area, the scientific evaluation of traditional treatment programmes can be taken as an example. Jilek (1994) outlines six possible constraints to the process. These include:

1. The sacred or arcane character of the ceremonies.

2. The healer's practices and prescriptions are often considered private or clan property.

3. The healer's reluctance to divulge information because of negative experience of enquiring authorities interested in illicit drug use.

4. The interfering effects of experimental research with the conduct of traditional ceremonies.

5. The difficulty of evaluating the merits of a single therapeutic method when several are often combined (this is a problem in evaluating most substance-misuse treatments).

6. The practical difficulties in conducting outcome studies by case follow up, due to the lack of reliable records. These difficulties can only be overcome if varying methodologies used by different disciplines are combined in evaluation work. Such an approach would enable the same rigour to be applied to evaluation of a traditional programme that is acceptable to Western evidence databases.

The effect of globalization and social media on culture and substance misuse is an area that needs urgent research attention. Globalization and liberalization of markets have made drugs more available and cheaper but the effectiveness of supply containment policies and drug demand reduction policies working together is yet to be demonstrated (e.g. Costa Sorti and De Grauwe, 2009). Social media can inform the world of a new synthetic drug and how to obtain it in a matter of seconds. The impact of this on substance misuse in young people and on existing cultures is an area of research that is wide open.

Conclusions

Substance use is as old as humanity itself. At present, there is a body of evidence that points to a trend in the increase of mind-altering substances which may be due to a number of factors such as globalization, increased travel, stresses in modern living as well as an increase in leisure time. 'Culture' very much plays a part in determining which mind-altering substance is used and the patterns of substance use in many societies. In every society there is a cost involved in the use of mind-altering substances. This cost could be in the form of a health burden to the individual and ultimately to the society; economic burden; disruption to family life and fabric of society; an increase in crime.

It can be argued that, in any society, despite the overall cost or burden to that society, compared to the overall number of people who might be using mind-altering substances it is a relatively small proportion of individuals whose substance use becomes problematic. For some of these individuals, there may be a predisposition to problems with substances or other mental health problems. But this must be considered against our background understanding of the considerable elasticity of the levels of problems with alcohol and tobacco – which vary greatly between societies and communities and over time – and for which factors such as price and availability are major influences on the extent of use and on associated harm. Some of these individuals may develop mental health problems as a result of their substance use and some individuals may develop a dependence on a mind-altering substance. Psychiatry and psychology are disciplines that are called upon to explain and define problems in this area and intervene to help individuals. Cultural considerations have not always been evident in the work of psychiatrists, clinical psychologists and researchers in this area. In Western countries where there are immigrant groups from different cultures, it is difficult to conceive how effective prevention and treatment for substance misuse problems for these individuals can be found without exploration of the cultural context. Incorporating relevant traditional practices into Western treatment programmes could only enhance the effectiveness of these treatments for individuals from different cultural backgrounds. Globally, where there is great pressure to tackle the rising substance misuse problems and governments seek Western-style interventions to deal with it, perhaps an approach where both Western and traditional treatment options are made available to individuals and where appropriate combining these methods should be attempted. Scientific evaluation of these efforts should also go hand in hand if we are to overcome what is seen as a global pandemic.

References

Alem, A., Kebede, D. and Kullgreen, G. (1999). The prevalence and socio demographic correlates of khat chewing in Butajira, Ethiopia. *Acta Psychiatrica Scandinavica Suppl.*, **387**, 84–91.

Baasher, T. A. (1981). The use of drugs in the Islamic world. *British Journal of Addiction*, **76**, 233–243.

Baasher, T. A. and Abu El Azyem, G. M. (1980). Egypt (2): the role of the mosque in treatment. In *Drug Problems in the Sociocultural Context: A Basis for Policies and Programme Planning*, ed. G. Edwards and A. Arif. Public Health Papers, WHO, No. 73, pp. 131–134.

Baklien, B. and Samarasinghe, D. (2003). *Alcohol and Poverty*. Colombo: Forut.

Beach, M. C., Price, E. G., Gary, T. L. *et al.* (2005). Cultural competency: a systematic review of health care provider educational interventions. *Medical Care*, **43**(4), 356–373.

Berridge, V. and Edwards, G. (1987). *Opium and the People: Opiate Use in Nineteenth-Century England*. New Haven: Yale University Press.

Best, D., Rawaf, S., Rowley, J., Floyd, K., Manning V. and Strang, J. (2001). Ethnic and gender difference in drinking and smoking among London adolescents. *Ethnicity and Health*, **6**, 51–57.

Britto, G. and Charles, M. (2000). *Use of Opium and Cannabis Products by Traditional Medical Practitioners*. Mumbai: NARC.

Carothers, J. C. (1965). Miraa as a case of insanity. *The East African Medical Journal*, **22**, 4–6.

Charles, M. and Britto, G. (2001). *The Socio-cultural Context of Drug Use and Implications for Drug Policy*. UNESCO, Oxford: Blackwell Publishers, pp. 467–474.

Chopra, R. N. and Chopra, I. C. (1990). *Drug Addiction with Special Reference to India*. New Delhi: Council of Scientific and Industrial Research.

Clough, A. R., d'Abbs, P., Cairney, S. *et al.* (2005). Adverse mental health effects of cannabis use in two indigenous communities in Arnhem Land, North Territory, Australia: exploratory study. *Australian and New Zealand Journal of Psychiatry*, **39** (7), 612–620.

Costa Storti, C. and De Grauwe, P. (2009). The cocaine and heroin markets in the era of globalisation and drug reduction policies. *International Journal of Drug Policy* **20**, 488–496, doi: 10.1016/j.drugpo.2009.02.004

Cox, G. and Rampes, H. (2003). Adverse effects of khat: a review. *Advances in Psychiatric Treatment*, **19**, 456–463.

Crocq, M. A. (2007). Historical and cultural aspects of man's relationship with addictive drugs. *Dialogues in Clinical Neuroscience*, **9**(4), 355–361.

Davis, K. (1998). Race, health status and managed health care. In *Cultural Competence for Healthcare Professionals Working with African American Communities: Theory and Practice*, ed. F. L. Brisbane. Rockville, MD: US Department of Health and Human Services.

Delphin-Rittmon, M. E., Flanagan, E. H., Bellamy, C. D. *et al.* (2016). Learning from those we serve: piloting a culture competence intervention co-developed by university faculty and persons in recovery. *Psychiatric Rehabilitation Journal*, **39**(1), 14–19, doi: 10.1037/prj0000155.

Douglas, M. (1987). *Constructive Drinking. Perspectives on Drink from Anthropology*. Cambridge: Cambridge University Press.

Edwards, G. and Gross, M. M. (1976). Alcohol dependence: provisional description of a clinical syndrome. *British Medical Journal*, **1**(6017), 1058–1061.

Edwards, G., Marshall, E. J. and Cook, C. (2003). *The Treatment of Drinking Problems: A Guide for the Helping Professions*. Cambridge: Cambridge University Press.

El-Zaatari, Z. M., Chami, H. A. and Zaatari, G. S. (2015). Health effects associated with waterpipe smoking. *Tobacco Control*, **24**, i31–i43, doi: 10.1136/tobaccocontrol-2014-051908.

Fisher, J. (1975). Cannabis in Nepal: an overview. In *Cannabis and Culture*, ed. V. Rubin. The Hague: Mouton Publishers.

FitzGerald, E. (1859). *The Ruba'ya't of Omar Khayya'm*. London: Bernard Quaritch.

Ghodse, H. (2002). *Drug and Addictive Behaviour. A Guide to Treatment*, 3rd edn. Cambridge: Cambridge University Press.

Griffiths, P., Gossop, M., Wickenden, S., Dunworth, J., Harris, K. and Lloyd, C. (1997). A transcultural pattern of drug use: Qat in the UK. *British Journal of Psychiatry*, **170**, 281–284.

Gunaid, A., Sumairi, A. Shidrawi, A. A. *et al.* (1995). Oesophageal and gastric carcinoma in the Republic of Yemen. *British Journal of Cancer*, **71**, 409–410.

Hamarneh, S. (1972). Pharmacy in medieval Islam and the history of drug addiction. *Medical History*, **16**(3), 226–237.

Heath, D. B. (1976). Anthropological perspectives on alcohol: an historical review. In *Cross-Cultural Approaches to the Study of Alcohol: An Interdisciplinary Perspective*, ed. M. Everett, J. Waddell and D. Heath. The Hague: Mouton.

Heath, D. B. (1978). The sociocultural model of alcohol use: problems and prospects. *Journal of Operational Psychiatry*, **9**, 55–66.

Hogg, A. and Rogers, H. (1985). Arab danger drug on sale legally in Britain. *The Sunday Times*, 20 January, 1–2.

Institute of Medicine (1990). *Broadening the Base of Treatment for Alcohol Problems*. Washington DC: National Academy Press.

Jilek, W. G. (1994). Traditional healing in the prevention and treatment of alcohol and drug abuse. *Transcultural Psychiatric Research Review*, **31**, 219–258.

Kalix, P. (1984). The pharmacology of khat. *General Pharmacology*, **15**, 179–187.

Kalix, P. and Braeden, O. (1985). Pharmacological aspects of the chewing of khat leaves. *Pharmacology Review*, **37**, 149–164.

Kandela, P. (2000). Sana'a women's rights, a tourist boom and the power of khat in the Yemen. *The Lancet*, **355**, 1437–1440.

Kennedy, J. G. (1987). *The Flower of Paradise: The Institutionalised Use of the Drug Khat in North Yemen*. Dordrecht: Kluwer Academic Publishers.

Kirkorian, A. D. (1984). Kat and its use: a historical perspective. *Journal of Ethnopharmacology*, **12**, 115–178.

Knishkowy, B. and Amitai, Y. (2005). Water pipe (Narghile) smoking. An emerging health risk behaviour. *Paediatrics*, **116**, 113–119.

Masihi, E. J. and Desai, D. B. (1998). *Culture and Drug Use in Saurashtra*. Mumbai: NARC.

Maziak, W., Fouad, F. M., Asfar, T. *et al.* (2004). Prevalence and characteristics of narghile smoking among university students in Syria. *International Journal of Tubercular Disease*, **8**, 882–809.

Maziak, W., Ward, K. D., Afifi Soweid, R. A. and Eissenberg, T. (2006). Tobacco smoking using the waterpipe: a re-emerging strain in global epidemic. *Tobacco Control*, **12**, 327–333.

McCambridge, J. and Strang, J. (2005). Can it really be this black and white? An analysis of the relative importance of ethnic group and other sociodemographic factors to patterns of drug use and related risk among young Londoners. *Drugs: Education Prevention and Policy*, **12**, 149–159.

McGee, R., Williams, S., Poulton, R. and Moffitt, T. (2000). A longitudinal study of cannabis use and mental health from adolescence to early adulthood. *Addiction*, **95**(4), 491–503.

Nabuzoka, D. and Badhadhe, F. A. (2000). Use and perception of khat among Somalis in a UK city. *Addiction Research*, **8**(1), 5–26.

Nelson, C. B., Rehm, J., Bedirhan, U. T. *et al.* (1999). Factor structures of DSM-IV substance disorder criteria endorsed by alcohol, cannabis, cocaine and opiate users: results from the WHO reliability and validity criteria. *Addiction*, **94**, 843–855.

Nencini, P., Grassi, M. C., Botan, A. A., Asseyr, A. F. and Paroli, E. (1989). Khat chewing spread to the Somali community in Rome. *Drug and Alcohol Dependence*, **23**, 255–258.

Onder, M., Oztas, M. and Arnavutt, O. (2002). Narghile (hubble bubble) smoking induced hand eczema. *International Journal of Dermatology*, **41**, 771–772.

Orford, J. (2001). Addiction as excessive appetite. *Addiction*, **96**(1), 15–31.

Oyefoso, A. (1994). Sociocultural aspects of substance use and misuse. *Current Opinion in Psychiatry*, 7, 273–277.

Pantellis, C., Hindler, C. G., and Taylor, J. C. (1989). Use and abuse of khat: a review of the distribution, pharmacology, side effects and a description psychosis attributed to khat chewing. *Psychological Medicine*, **19**, 657–668.

Patton, C., Coffey, C., Carlin, J. B., Degenhardt, L., Lynssky, M. and Hall, W. (2002). Cannabis use and mental health in young people: a cohort study. *British Medical Journal*, **325**, 1195–1198.

Peltzer, K. (1987). *Some Contributions of Traditional Healing Practices towards Psychosocial Health Care in Malawi*. Frankfurt: Fachbuch-handlung fuer Psychologie Verlag.

Poshyachinda, V. (1980). Thailand: treatment at the Tam Kraborg Temple. In *Drug Problems in the Sociocultural Context: A Basis for Policies and Programme Planning*, ed. G. Edwards and A. Arif. Public Health Papers, WHO, No. 73, pp. 121–125.

Rehm, J., Mathers, C., Popova, S., Thavorncharoensap, M., Teerawattananon, Y. and Patra, J. (2009). Global burden of disease and injury and economic cost attributable to alcohol use and alcohol-use disorders. *The Lancet*, **373**(9682), 2223–2233.

Room, R., Babor, T. and Rhem, J. (2005). Alcohol and public health. *The Lancet*, **365** (9458), 519–530, doi: http://dx.doi.org/10.1016/S0140-6736(05)17870-2.

Seivewright, N. (2000). *Community Treatment of Drug Misuse: More than Methadone*. Cambridge: Cambridge University Press.

Shanmugasundaram, E. R. B., Umarani, S. S. and Shanmugasundaram, K. R. (1986). Studies on brain structure and neurological function in alcoholic rats controlled by an Indian medicinal formula (SKV). *Journal of Ethnopharmacology*, **17**, 225–245.

Singer, M. and Borrero, M. (1984). Indigenous treatment of alcoholism: the case of Puerto Rican spiritism. *Medical Anthropology*, **8**, 246–273.

Smedley, B. D., Stith, A. Y. and Nelson, A. R. (eds) (2003). *Unequal Treatment: Confronting Racial and Ethnic Disparities in Health Care* (Committee on Understanding and Eliminating Racial and Ethnic Disparities in Health Care, Institute of Medicine). Washington DC: Academic Press.

Spencer, C. P., Heggenhougen, H. K. and Navaratnam, V. (1980). Traditional therapies and the treatment of drug dependence in Southeast Asia. *American Journal of Chinese Medicine*, **8**, 230–238.

Stefan, J. and Mathew, B. (2005). Khat chewing: an emerging drug concern in Australia? *Australian and New Zealand Journal of Psychiatry*, **39**(9), 842.

Stevenson, M., Fitzgerald, J. and Banwell, C. (1996). Chewing as a social act: cultural displacement and khat consumption in the East African communities of Melbourne. *Drug and Alcohol Review*, **15**, 73–82.

Takemoto, T., Usukine, K. and Otsu, M. (1979). A follow-up study of alcoholic patients treated by Naikan therapy. Communication to 2nd Annual Meeting on Kaikan, Kyoto.

United Nations Office on Drugs and Crime (2015). *World Drug Report*. Geneva: United Nations.

Vetulani, J. (2001). Psychoactive substances in the past and present: Part I. *Polish Journal of Pharmacology and Pharmacy*, **53**, 201–214.

Wanigaratne, S., Unninthan, S. and Strang, J. (2001). Substance misuse and ethnic minorities: issues for the UK. In *Psychiatry in Multicultural Britain*, ed. D. Bhugra and R. Cochrane. London: Gaskell.

Weir, S. (1985). *Qat in Yemen. Consumption and Social Change*. British Museum: British Museums Publications Limited.

West, R. (2006). *Theory of Addiction*. Oxford: Blackwell Publishing.

Westermeyer, J. (1980). Treatment for narcotic addiction in a Buddhist monastery. *Journal of Drug Issues*, **10**(2), 221–288.

Whiteford, H. A., Degenhardt, L., Rehm, J. Baxter, A., *et al.* (2013). Global burden of disease attributable to mental and substance use disorders: findings from the Global Burden of Disease Study 2010. *The Lancet*, **382**(9904), 1575–1586.

World Health Organization (2000). *Annual Report for Eastern Mediterranean Region*. Geneva: WHO.

World Health Organization WHO Study Group on Tobacco Product Regulation (2005). *Waterpipe Tobacco Smoking: Health Effects, Research Needs, Recommended Actions by Regulators*. Geneva: WHO.

WHO (2014). Global Status Report on Alcohol and Health available at www.who.int/substance_abuse/publications/global_alcohol_report/en/.

WHO (2016). Global Information System on Alcohol and Health (GISAH) available at www.who.int/gho/alcohol/en/.

Yang, M. M. P. and Kwok, J. S. L. (1986). Evaluation on the treatment of morphine addiction by acupuncture, Chinese herbs and opioid peptides. *American Journal of Chinese Medicine*, **14**(1–2), 46–50.

Zaghoul, A., Abdalla, A., Gammal, H. and Moselhy, H. (2003). The consequences of khat use: a review of the literature. *European Journal of Psychiatry*, **17** (2), 77–86.

Chapter 22

Culture and Mental Disorders: Suicidal Behaviour

Sarah A. Fortune and Keith Hawton

Editors' Introduction

Suicidal behaviours are seen across all cultures although the actual rates may vary according to a number of reasons, from genetic to social and cultural. In many cultures and societies the act of suicide is illegal and therefore it may be difficult to gather correct data. In other cultures due to religious reasons, the act of suicide may be proscribed which means that the actual suicidal behaviour may well be difficult to assess and manage. There are also differences in rates of suicidal ideation, suicidal acts and acts of deliberate self-harm. Fortune and Hawton in this chapter define these terms and also highlight the role acculturation may play in the actual physical act of suicide. These authors draw our attention to the fact that rates of suicide and self-harm are increasing among black females in the UK. They also emphasize the role of religion which may well be protective in some cases. Rates of self-harm can be higher than expected in displaced people due to higher levels of stress and alienation. Yet healthcare utilization can be very variable. It has been recognized that in many populations such as indigenous people, rates of suicide are raised and may well be related to urbanization and cultural transition but also related to higher levels of substance use thereby confirming a mixed complex picture. The young people may feel alienated and marginalized. Fortune and Hawton propose that many avenues of research in the field of suicidology need further investigation including social and cultural factors which may well determine national suicide prevention strategies. With increasing levels of migration it is crucial that policy makers take their individual and group vulnerabilities into account.

Introduction

Many people consider self-harm or suicide at some point in their lives. Some will engage in an act of self-harm (SH); this includes those who intend to die, but the act does not result in death (attempted suicide), and those who die by their own hand (suicide). These phenomena can be considered as successive parts of a continuum of suicidality from none to severe. Although a continuum exists, there are two main points of discontinuity. First, of those who have suicidal ideas, only a small proportion engages in some form of SH. The boundary between thoughts and an actual act of self-harm is therefore an important behavioural threshold. Second, some people engage in self-harm once, and never repeat, while others engage in self-harm several or many times during their lifetime.

In this chapter *suicide ideation* is defined as thoughts about an act of self-harm or suicide, including wishing to kill oneself, making plans of when, where and how to carry out the act, and thoughts about the impact of one's death on others. Self-harm (SH) is defined as any form of intentional self-poisoning or self-injury (such as cutting, taking an overdose, hanging, self-strangulation and running into traffic), regardless of motivation or the degree of intention to die.

In the United Kingdom, as in many other countries, suicides are classified using the International Classification of Diseases (World Health Organization, 1996). A coroner determines whether or not an unexpected death is suicide. The apparent suicide rate may partly reflect the way in which verdicts are designated by coroners, especially in relation to the number of deaths designated as suicides, due to underdetermined cause ('open' verdicts) and accidental deaths. There is significant variation around the world (Bertolote and Fleischmann, 2009); for example, a rise in youth suicide in Ireland observed in the mid 1990s was, in part, explained by a reduction in the number of 'open' or 'accidental' verdicts and a corresponding increase in 'suicide' as a verdict in addition to a real rise in the number of suicides (Cantor *et al.*, 1997).

Also, the likelihood of a death being recorded as a suicide or receiving an open verdict rather than an accidental one will be partly related to the method involved. For example, poisoning and drowning are more likely to receive accidental verdicts from coroners than other deaths involving other methods when experts in suicide research consider these to be likely suicides (Palmer *et al.*, 2015).

A key concept in the field of culture and mental health is that of acculturation. Briefly, acculturation relates to changes in cultural attitudes, values and behaviours that result from contact between two distinct cultures. Acculturative stress refers to a situation where the acculturation process causes significant problems for the individual. This has been associated with poor mental health including anxiety, depression and psychosomatic symptoms (Berry *et al.*, 2002) and also suicidality (Wyatt *et al.*, 2015). The concept of acculturative stress has been expanded into a cultural model of suicide targeted at clinicians undertaking culturally responsive assessments of suicide risk (Chu *et al.*, 2010). This model suggests that (1) culture is important in defining which stressors contribute to suicide, (2) cultural meanings of suicide have an impact on the personal suicidal process and (3) culture affects the expression of suicidal thoughts and behaviours.

Suicide and Self-Harm around the World

Rates of non-fatal suicidal behaviours and suicide vary internationally, although the available data are of inconsistent quality, making robust comparisons problematic (Phillips and Cheng, 2012). Culture and cultural influences appear to mediate the effects of international socio-political and economic trends on suicide (Bertolote and Fleischmann, 2002) and even the impact of natural disasters on suicide (Kõlves *et al.*, 2013a). It has become increasingly apparent that suicide is a major problem in low- and middle-income countries; the WHO recently estimated that nearly half of all suicides occur in China and India. Low- and middle-income countries (LMIC) combined accounted for 75 per cent of global suicides in 2012 (World Health Organization, 2016). Young adults and older women in LMIC have much higher rates of suicide than their peers living in high-income countries. In contrast, middle-aged men in wealthy countries are much more likely to die by suicide compared with men in LMIC. The male to female ratio of suicide deaths in high-income countries is 3.5:1 in contrast

with 1.6:1 in LMIC in 2012 (World Health Organization, 2016).

The prevention of premature death by suicide is identified within the Millennium Development Goals and international prevention work will continue with the new 2016–2030 Sustainable Development Goals (Norheim *et al.*, 2015).

Self-harm among Ethnic Minority Groups in the United Kingdom

Ethnicity is not currently recorded on death certificates in England and Wales. Place of birth is available and is often used as a proxy for ethnicity. However, up to half of the ethnic minority population is born in the United Kingdom (UK) leading to significant misclassification (McKenzie *et al.*, 2008). In addition, coroners appear less likely to return a verdict of suicide for ethnic minority groups (Neeleman *et al.*, 1997).

A systematic review of self-harm among minority ethnic groups in the UK was published (Bhui *et al.*, 2007) as part of NIMH UK and Department of Health strategy to 'deliver race equality'. A meta-analysis indicated higher rates of self-harm among women of South Asian descent compared with white women (RR =1.4, 95% CI 1.1 – 1.8) and lower rates among South Asian men compared with white men (RR = 0.5, 95% CI 0.4 – 0.7) (Bhui *et al.*, 2007). The authors reported lower repetition rates among South Asian and Caribbean populations and lower rates of previous self-harm among West Indians and South Asians presenting with an episode of self-harm. Interpersonal disputes and contextual stressors were more characteristic of immigrant compared with white patient populations. The data on the prevalence of psychiatric disorder were mixed with both lower and higher rates reported in various studies included in the review. Cross-cultural tension or cultural conflict in culturally specific practices and beliefs were cited in a number of included studies (Bhui *et al.*, 2007).

A more recent investigation from the Multicentre Study of Self-Harm in England, conducted in Oxford, Manchester and Derby of 20,574 individuals aged 16–64 years presenting to hospital following self-harm, showed that rates of self-harm were highest among young black females (RR = 1.90, 95% CI 1.46 – 1.98) but the relative risks for self-harm among South Asian females were similar to white females (RR = 0.99, 95% CI 0.87 – 1.11)

(Cooper *et al.*, 2010). Thus it appears that earlier patterns of high rates among South Asian females may have diminished over time. However, in a recent study of hospital presentations for self-poisoning in South London, black women presented 1.5 times as often as white women. In individuals under 24 years black women were seven times more likely to present than black men (Cross *et al.*, 2014).

In the Multicentre Study, South Asian and black women were more likely to present with poisoning using non-ingestible substances, whereas white women were more likely to present with self-injury (mainly cutting). South Asian women were significantly more likely to report partner/husband and family relationship problems compared with other women. Similar differences were observed among males, with black men more likely to use more violent methods of self-harm, including hanging and self-asphyxiation or non-ingestible substances (Cooper *et al.*, 2010).

Data from the Multicentre Study of Self-Harm in England was used to examine risk factors associated with repetition of self-harm among BME adults groups between 2000 and 2007. Data on ethnicity were known for 68.4 per cent of individuals presenting to ED, including South Asian ($n = 751$), black ($n = 468$) and white ($n = 15,705$). The risk ratio for subsequent repetition of self-harm was significantly lower among individuals from BME groups compared with white (South Asian RR = 0.69, 95% CI 0.5–0.7) and black (RR = 0.7, 95% CI 0.5 – 0.8). South Asians with a history of self-harm who presented with self-injury involving cutting, misused alcohol, did not have a partner and were under the care of psychiatric services, were at increased risk of further self-harm compared with whites. Blacks who had experienced mental health difficulties as a contributing factor to their presentation for self-harm were at increased risk of repetition compared with whites (Cooper *et al.*, 2013). In a further investigation from the Multicentre Study, South Asian and black people were less likely to die prematurely from any cause following self-harm compared with whites in a cohort of 28,512 people presenting to emergency departments following self-harm between 2000 and 2010. Black people who self-harmed were also less likely to die by suicide compared with white people (HR 0.43, 95% CI 0.19 – 0.97) (Turnbull *et al.*, 2015).

Religion is thought to offer protection against suicidal behaviour, and was examined in a study of university students in greater London ($n = 617$ total, $n = 142$ males, $n = 475$ females), just over a quarter (27%) of students had a lifetime history of self-harm. Students without a religious affiliation were more likely to report five or more episodes of self-harm (15.4%) compared with Christian (10%), Muslim (6.6%) or Hindu/Sikh (0%) students. However, as in previous research, coping and emotional styles emerged as important predictors of self-harm (Borrill *et al.*, 2011).

There have been relatively few studies of self-harm among ethnic minority children and adolescents in the UK, with mixed findings probably due to small numbers and other difficulties with study design (Goodman *et al.*, 2008). In a large community-based study in schools, Hawton *et al.* (2002) found that SH was less common among Asian (6.7%) and black (6.7%) girls compared with white girls (11.6%). Rates of SH were similar among Asian (2.7%) and white males (3.3%). Data from a randomized controlled trial of therapeutic assessment compared with treatment as usual in London ($n = 70$, 12–18 years) found no difference in the proportion of white and non-white adolescents described as being suicidal (white = 9/23) compared with those engaging in non-suicidal self-injury (white = 28/47) (Ougrin *et al.*, 2012). A recent meta-analysis of intervention studies for children and adolescents who had engaged in suicidal behaviour (Ougrin *et al.*, 2015) includes data on ethnicity, but there has been little specific analysis of the impact of ethnicity on engagement and treatment responsiveness in the UK.

In the first edition of this book we reviewed several small studies that suggested differences in clinical pathways for members of ethnic minority groups. The larger, more robust epidemiological studies outlined above indicate there is still variance in the proportion of BME service users who are offered a psychiatric assessment and follow-up treatment if they present to hospital following self-harm. Thus in the Multicentre Study of Self-Harm in England, fewer ethnic minority females received a specialist psychiatric assessment and fewer black women were offered psychiatric after-care (Cooper *et al.*, 2010). Culturally responsive interventions have been demonstrated to have a positive effect on symptoms and experiences of, and adherence to, treatment (Bhui *et al.*, 2015).

Suicide among Ethnic Groups in the UK

The overall suicide rate in the UK in 2014 was 10.8 deaths per 100,000 (males 16.8 per 100,000, females 5.2 per 100,000). Since 2013, hanging has become the most common method of suicide in both genders, accounting for more than half of male deaths (55%) and two in five female deaths (42%) (Office for National Statistics, 2016). Historically, suicide mortality among migrant groups in England and Wales has showed a mixed picture, with elevated rates among women from India, those born in Scotland and Ireland and lower rates among South Asian-born males (Maynard et al., 2012).

Older studies which suggested an elevated rate of death among young South Asian women have been superseded by more recent data which indicate a fall in the suicide rate among younger South Asian women but a marked increase among South Asian women over the age of 65 years (McKenzie et al., 2008). The death rate for females born in India was 6.7 per 100,000 in 1999–2003, significantly lower than the figure of 10.9 per 100,000 in 1989–1993. Males born in Pakistan continue to have significantly lower rates of suicide compared with men born in the UK (10.3 per 100,000 vs 21.0 per 100,000) (Maynard et al., 2012).

The risk of dying by suicide among males born in Jamaica has risen dramatically since 1979 and has moved from being comparable to rates observed in English-born men to being much higher by 1999–2003 (51.9 per 100,000) (Maynard et al., 2012).

Irish-born migrants have historically had relatively high rates of self-harm and suicide and experienced racism and discrimination. Recent fluctuations in prosperity in Ireland have been associated with changing patterns of migration, although the suicide rate in Ireland among young men has tripled between 1980 and 2010, from 8.9 to 29.7 per 100,000 (Murphy et al., 2015). Data from three time periods spanning 1979–2003 continue to show elevated and slightly increasing rates of suicide in the UK among Irish-born males (39.2 per 100,000 in 1999–2003) and females (12.2 per 100,000) although there has been a moderate decrease in deaths among males born in Northern Ireland across the same time period (Maynard et al., 2012).

Data from the National Confidential Inquiry into Suicides of People in Psychiatric Care allow for more nuanced analysis. These suggest that, between 1996 and 2011, people of ethnic minority groups who were in contact with mental health services at the time of their death, or had been within the 12 months prior to their death, accounted for 6–7 per cent of all patient suicides, or approximately 70 per year (Windfuhr and Kapur, 2011). Patients from ethnic minorities more often used violent methods of death such as jumping, drowning or self-immolation. Schizophrenia was more prominent among black Caribbean and black African patients who died by suicide, with affective disorders more prominent among South Asians (Windfuhr and Kapur, 2011).

Stratified analysis from data from 1996–2001 highlighted the importance of gender and age; a high standardized mortality ratio (SMR) was found for black Caribbean and black African men aged 13–24 years in contrast with a low SMR for South Asian and black African women under 25 years and older South Asian women (40+ years). South Asian, black Caribbean and black African women in their middle years (25–39 years) all had elevated SMRs (Bhui and McKenzie, 2008). Black African males were significantly more likely to die by suicide during inpatient psychiatric admission compared with men from any other ethnic group (SMR 2.05, 95% CI 1.12 – 3.43). White British women were more likely to die by suicide while in inpatient psychiatric care, in comparison with South Asian (SMR 0.04, 95% CI 0.17 – 0.78) or black Caribbean women (SMR 0.26, 95% CI 0.09 – 0.62) (Bhui et al., 2012).

In studies of suicide deaths among migrant groups often, but not always, there is a significant correlation between the rates of suicide for these groups in the UK and the rates in their country of origin. These mixed findings suggest that immigration alone does not account for elevated risk of suicide observed (Maynard et al., 2012).

In summary, young Indian women used to have a higher risk of suicide compared with other women in the UK. However, recent data have shown a fall in suicide rates in this group, but with a marked increase among South Asian women over the age of 65 years. Lower suicide rates continue among men of Indian origin but a dramatic rise in deaths among Jamaican-born men has been seen in recent decades. Members of ethnic minority groups are more likely to use violent methods of suicide.

We now turn to considering suicidal behaviours in other countries, specifically continental Europe and Russia, the USA and Asian countries. We then examine this phenomenon in specific at-risk groups, particularly indigenous peoples.

Eastern Europe and Russia

The fall of the Berlin Wall in 1989 and the break-up of the former Soviet Union in 1991 were significant socio-political and economic events, which changed the everyday lives of the 400 million people in this region. The quality of data available to researchers about mortality in Russia has been relatively poor, in part due to interpretation of suicide as a failure of communism and a revolutionary act (Pridemore *et al.*, 2013). However, for at least four decades, Russia has had one of the highest suicide rates in the world, particularly among young men (Pitman *et al.*, 2012).

A recent cross-sectional time series study of age adjusted suicide rates between 1990 and 2008 in 13 countries from the former Soviet Union and Soviet Bloc in eastern Europe (Belarus, Estonia, Latvia, Lithuania, Moldova, Ukraine, Bulgaria, Croatia, Czech Republic, Hungary, Romania, Slovak Republic and Slovenia) showed relatively stable rates below 30 per 100,000 in Bulgaria, Czech Republic and Slovakia. The mean age standardized rates for males decreased in Hungary and Slovenia across the time period, with a rising/falling pattern observed in most other countries included in the study, with the peak in the mid 1990s (Kõlves *et al.*, 2013b). It is likely that the true rate of suicide in many of these countries is significantly underestimated given the relatively high rate of undetermined deaths in the Baltic and Slavic republics, particularly for males. Surprisingly, alcohol consumption was not associated with male suicide rates, with a negative association for female suicide rates. Increasing prevalence of general practitioners in the population appears to offer protection for males (Kõlves *et al.*, 2013b).

Alcohol consumption has been implicated as a risk factor for suicidal behaviour at both an individual and population level, with a stronger association evident in countries with more hazardous drinking patterns typified by social acceptance of heavy drinking, use of spirits and binge drinking (for a review see Norström and Rossow, 2016). A number of studies, over many decades, have demonstrated a relationship between alcohol consumption and suicide mortality in Soviet Russia (Norström and Rossow, 2016). A recent study of per capita alcohol sales and suicide rates in Russia and Belarus between 1970 and 2014 demonstrated a strong relationship between the two variables until 2002, when the pattern diverges and alcohol sales continued to rise while the suicide rate dropped (Razvodovsky, 2015). One study indicated that Russian alcohol control policies introduced in 2006 led to a 9 per cent reduction in male (but not female) suicide mortality (Pridemore *et al.*, 2013). However, more research is required given that the suicide rate had begun to decline prior to the introduction of these measures in Russia, the absence of such measures in Belarus and the large black market for alcohol in this region not captured in official consumption statistics.

There is increasing concern about the suicide rate in Poland, with it rising from 11.2 per 100,000 in 1970 to 17.0 per 100,000 in 2009 reflecting a 51.3 per cent increase. The female rate has remained relatively low and stable (4.0 per 100,000 in 1970 to 4.8 per 100,000 in 2009) while the male rate has risen from 23.1 to 35.1 per 100,000 over the same time period resulting in a male:female ratio of 7.3:1, which is unusually high. Men aged 40–54 years have the highest rates of suicide. The year on year increases observed in Poland have differed from the pattern observed in many eastern European countries of a peak in the early 1990s followed by a decline, and is more similar to two other predominantly Catholic countries of Spain and Ireland. The prevalence of hanging in Poland has increased significantly in recent years (Höfer *et al.*, 2012).

There are relatively scant data on rates of non-fatal suicidal behaviours in eastern European nations. However, a large multinational study of childhood adversity and adjustment was conducted with young adults aged 18–24 years between 2010 and 2013 in Albania, Latvia, Lithuania, Montenegro, Romania, the Russian Federation, Macedonia and Turkey (*n* = 10 696, 59.7% female). In this study 4.1% of respondents had attempted suicide, the figure being highest in Latvia (6.3%) and lowest in Montenegro (2.7%) and Macedonia (3.0%). Of interest is that 10% of participants reported a family member with experience of depression or suicidal behaviour, which was also highest in Latvia (18.8%) (Bellis *et al.*, 2014).

A recent review of suicide rates among children aged 10–14 years suggests that a number of central Asian countries, all former republics of the USSR, have experienced a significant increase in suicide among the very young. Kazakhstan and Azerbaijan recorded the greatest increases with Kazakhstan having the highest rate in the world (8.53 per 100,000 in

2000–2009), reflecting high rates of violence, abuse and exploitation (Kõlves and De Leo, 2014)

United States of America

One person dies by suicide every 13 minutes in the USA and it was the leading cause of death for all ages in 2013, accounting for 41,149 deaths (CDC, 2015b). Suicide was the second leading cause of death among young people aged 10–24 years between 1994 and 2012, with young males having consistently higher age-adjusted rates (11.9 per 100,000 in 2012) compared with their female (3.2 per 100,000) counterparts (CDC, 2015a). Firearms, suffocation/hanging[1] and poisoning are the mostly commonly used methods by young people in the USA, with a significant rise in the rates of suffocation which is particularly noticeable among females, but observed across ethnic groups and regions of the USA (CDC, 2015a). Firearms deaths have decreased since 1994 (particularly among those aged 15–19 years, Asian/Pacific youth and in the west), but remain the leading mechanism of death for young males, whereas hanging was the common method of death for females in 2001 (CDC, 2015a).

There is increasing concern about a rise in suicides among adults in their middle years (35–64 years) in the USA, with age-adjusted rates rising from 13.7 per 100,000 in 1999 to 17.6 per 100,000 in 2010. Native American/Alaskan Native (11.2 to 18.5 per 100,000) and white males (15.9 to 22.3 per 100,000) have been particularly affected (CDC, 2013). A significant increase in deaths by suffocation has also been noted in this age group, particularly amongst males. Men over 50 years and women over 60 years have the highest age-adjusted rates. Suicide rates among Native American/Alaskan native men (59.5%) and women (81%) have increased dramatically since 1999 (CDC, 2013).

Evidence from European countries of an excess of deaths during the recent economic recession appears to translate to the USA; Reeves et al. (2012) suggested that following the recent recession (beginning in 2007/8) there were 4,750 excess deaths (95% CI 2570 to 6920) and that a 1% increase in unemployment was associated with a nearly 1% increase in

suicide rate (0.79%, 95% CI 0.16 – 1.42) and could account for nearly one-quarter of excess suicides in the USA after the onset of the recession (Reeves et al., 2012).

Community-based estimates of non-fatal suicidal behaviour in the USA suggest that around 1 in 25 adults (18 years and over) have experienced suicidal ideation in the previous year, with highest prevalence among young adults 18–25 years (7.4%), those aged 26–49 (4%) and those over 50 years (2.7%). Around 1 in 100 reported making a suicide plan and 0.6 per cent had made an attempt in the previous year (Substance Abuse and Mental Health Service Administration, 2014). In comparison, estimates among students in grade 9–12 surveyed in 2015 showed (unsurprisingly) higher rates among adolescents, 17.7% making a serious plan in the previous year and 8.6% reporting an attempt (11.6% female, 5.5% male) (Kann et al., 2016). Another large NIMH-funded Collaborative Psychiatric Epidemiology Survey of 15,180 community-based respondents suggested a lifetime prevalence of suicidal ideation highest among whites (16.10%), lowest among Asians (9.02%) with intermediate levels observed among Hispanics (11.35%) and blacks (11.82%). However the observed differences were attenuated after controlling for psychiatric disorders. Then ethnic differences were no longer significant after controlling for psychiatric disorder. But second generation immigrant Hispanics had an elevated risk of suicide attempt (Borges et al., 2012).

Good quality national data are available for adolescents via the Youth Risk Behavior Survey (YRBS). Data from 2015 indicated that Hispanic females were most likely to report serious suicidal ideation in the previous 12 months (25.6%), followed by white females (22.8%) and black females (18.7%). The previous declines in self-reported suicidal ideation noted between 1991 and 2009 have been followed by a subsequent upward trend since 2009 (Kann et al., 2016). The proportion of young people reporting a suicide attempt in the YRBS study has continued to decline since 1991. In 2015, 8.6% (11.5% female, 5.5% male) of participants reported one or more suicide attempts in the previous year, with Hispanic youth most likely to report an attempt (11.3%), followed by black (8.9%) and white youths (6.8%). Both black males and females were more likely to report a suicide attempt compared with their white peers (Kann et al., 2016).

---

[1] ICD-10 code X70 is defined as 'intentional self-harm by hanging, strangulation, and suffocation'. Many commentators refer to these deaths as hanging or hanging/suffocation because a common mechanism of suffocation is hanging.

Visits to a hospital emergency department following an episode of self-harm have doubled in the USA between 1993 and 2008, to an estimated total of at least 420,000 visits per year (Ting *et al.*, 2012). Blacks (1.9 per 1,000) were somewhat more likely to attend hospital compared with whites (1.5 per 1,000), but both groups experienced similar rates of increase across the period of the study (blacks 1.14 to 2.10 per 1,000; whites 0.94 to 1.82 per 1,000). Poisoning was the most common method of self-harm (around two-thirds of visits), followed by self-injury by cutting or piercing (21%). Females made up a greater proportion of self-poisoning visits (73% vs 59%), while self-cutting was more common among males (24% vs 18%) (Ting *et al.*, 2012).

Historically, the rate of suicide among blacks in the USA was considerably lower than whites. However, suicide deaths among black youth have continued to increase (CDC, 2015a). Factors leading to suicide among the black community are not clearly understood, in part due to the low base rate of suicide in this group, although experiences of racism, discrimination, poverty and the role of religion are likely to be important (Joe *et al.*, 2008).

Gun control measures appear to have the potential to influence suicides rates in the USA, given the dominance of firearms suicides in this jurisdiction. However, such measures have had mixed success (Pitman *et al.*, 2012). In a review Swanson and colleagues (2015) examined the relationships between mental illness, gun violence and suicide in the USA and concluded that household gun ownership makes a strong contribution to suicide risk even after controlling for other factors associated with suicide. In addition, gun control measures such as background checks and stand-down periods (known as the Brady Law) have reduced suicide deaths among older males. Further restrictions on gun purchase in the District of Columbia led to a reduction in deaths by firearms without any corresponding increase by other violent methods. These differences were not observed in neighbouring states (Swanson *et al.*, 2015). It should be noted that gun control measures appear to have had little effect in Canada, but in Australia were associated with a decrease in deaths by firearms, although there was evidence of some substitution of method (Pitman *et al.*, 2012).

In summary, in the USA there is increasing concern about the rising prevalence of death by suffocation, mainly hanging, particularly among young women, and also the rising number of deaths among Native American populations. Hispanic youth are the fastest growing demographic in the US population, which has significant implications given the excess of suicidal ideation and attempts in this group. The historically low suicide rates among blacks in the USA have risen in recent years due to a significant increase in the number of deaths among young black men. Availability of firearms contributes to suicide rates and, while evidence is mixed, greater gun control probably results in decreased rates.

Asian Countries: India, Japan, Taiwan, Hong Kong, Korea, Sri Lanka and China

The prevalence of suicide in developing countries is difficult to establish. For example, in India suicide is a crime and use of previous data based on police reporting are likely to have resulted in a significant underestimate by a quarter to a third of deaths (Patel *et al.*, 2012). A recent large, nationally representative study of suicide in India suggests relatively high rates in people aged 15 years and over for both males (26.3 per 100,000, 95% CI 22.5, 28.4 per 100,000) and females (17.5 per 100,000, 95% CI 15.2, 18.4 per 100,000). This rate for women is around twice that observed in many developed countries, although similar to China. Young women aged 15–29 accounted for 56 per cent of all female suicides, with young men accounting for 40 per cent of male deaths (Patel *et al.*, 2012). Most suicides occurred in rural areas and rates were observed to be higher in southern states. Pesticide poisoning was particularly prevalent, reflecting high availability of these compounds in rural areas complicated by variable access to prompt medical care. Hanging was the second most prevalent method amongst both males and females. Self-immolation accounted for 15 per cent of female suicides. Risk factors for male suicide were drinking alcohol and working in the agricultural sector. In contrast with developed countries, being widowed, separated or divorced decreased the risk of suicide for women. In contrast to high-income countries, the male to female ratio of deaths was 1.5:1 across all ages, with near parity among those aged 15–29 years (Patel *et al.*, 2012).

In several Asian countries, including China, the rates of suicide are relatively high in older adults, despite the traditional respect for older people in Asian cultures (Phillips *et al.*, 2012). For example, in

Japan, which has had a traditionally had a high rate of suicide, the suicide rate in 2011 was 19.7 per 100,000 (OECD, 2011). Rates of suicide in Japanese men were highest among those aged 45–64 years and among those over 65 years, although rates in the latter group are decreasing. Female suicide rates were highest among elderly women (Yoshioka *et al.*, 2016a). Suicide in the elderly in Japan has been associated with physical illness, as in many other countries (Japanese Cabinet Office, 2013). Among middle-aged Japanese men, various factors, including economic pressures (Liu *et al.*, 2013) and *inseki-jisatu*, or responsibility-driven suicides to demonstrate remorse for an untoward event (Takei and Nakamura, 2004), are thought to contribute to suicides. Hanging accounted for nearly two-thirds of deaths among Japanese males 20–39 years in 1999, with jumping also relatively common (Pitman *et al.*, 2012). Increases in deaths among males and females under 45 years are in part explained by the rise of gas, overdose and hanging as methods of suicide (Yoshioka *et al.*, 2016a).

A recent meta-analysis of presentations to Japanese emergency departments (ED) following suicidal behaviour indicated they accounted for 4.7 per cent of all ED presentations, with overdose and cutting the main methods of self-harm observed. The prevalence of jumping, hanging and burning was higher than observed in a number of Western countries, although the prevalence of common psychiatric disorders was broadly comparable (Kawashima *et al.*, 2014).

A significant amount of work was done during the 1990s to create valid and reliable epidemiological estimates of suicide in China (for example Phillips *et al.*, 2002). These studies suggested that more women than men died by suicide in China and that the elderly and rural populations were particularly at risk. Since that time China has experienced significant economic growth, with consequent socio-cultural changes. Based on deaths reported by the Chinese Ministry of Health Vital Registration, Wang and colleagues (2014) found that there was a significant decrease in suicide rates in those aged 15 years and over between 2002 and 2011, with the mean national rate being 9.8 per 100,000. Since 2006, male suicide rates have been higher than female suicide rates in both urban and rural settings. Despite a general decline in suicide rates in China, rates among older people in rural China have not decreased in the same way. Rural

suicides account for 79 per cent of all suicide deaths. The male to female ratio was 1.2 in 2009 compared with the previously noted excess of female deaths. These data are a likely undercount given the lack of a comprehensive national data collection system (Chen *et al.*, 2012).

In Hong Kong a dramatic increase from 1998 onwards in suicide by charcoal burning in an airtight space, especially in young males, was linked to individuals being overwhelmed by debts who learnt of this lethal method through newspaper coverage. It resulted in a net increase in the overall suicide rate. However, the popularity of this method appears to have peaked and decreased by one-third between 2005 and 2013, in part influenced by public health measures (Chang *et al.*, 2016). This method spread to many areas in Southeast Asia in the early part of the new century, including Taiwan, Singapore, the Republic of Korea, but with significant epidemiological variation (Chang *et al.*, 2014). In Japan, for example, charcoal burning deaths contributed to a 10–20 per cent increase in overall suicide rates among those under 45 years, particularly amongst males in rural areas (Yoshioka *et al.*, 2016b), whereas in Taiwan and Hong Kong it was much more of an urban phenomenon (Chang *et al.*, 2014). Deaths due to helium inhalation, previously unknown in Hong Kong, have shown an upward trend since 2011, with people dying using this method having similar characteristics to those associated with charcoal burning deaths (Chang *et al.*, 2016).

Rates of suicide among young men in Sri Lanka are amongst the highest in the world (Pitman *et al.*, 2012) although there have been significant changes in the epidemiology of suicide, particularly since WHO Class I pesticides were banned in 1995 and paraquat, dimethoate and fenthion were banned in 2011 (Knipe *et al.*, 2014). The rates of suicide are now highest among men over 55 years, although younger women (< 35 years) have had high rates of suicide since 1976. While the bans on certain pesticides have contributed to a reduction in the overall suicide rate, age-specific rates and case-fatality rates following self-poisoning, there has been some evidence of method substitution to hanging, particularly among females and young males (Knipe *et al.*, 2014). Non-fatal self-poisoning continues to be dominated by pesticides in Sri Lanka, with a preponderance in males, with apparently low rates of psychiatric disorder and rates of repetition, in line with data from other South Asian countries. Of note, two recent studies suggest that among more urban populations the patterns often observed in developed countries, including a female preponderance and the use of paracetamol compounds for self-poisoning, may be emerging in Sri Lanka (Knipe et al., 2014).

There is increasing concern about the rapid and significant increase of suicide deaths in Korea; rates amongst males doubled from 17 per 100,000 to 39 per 100,000 between 1995 and 2009 (OECD, 2011), and have increased 280 per cent since 1985 (Jeon et al., 2016). Female rates (20 per 100,000) are the highest in the OECD (OECD, 2011).

More males than females die by suicide in all countries for which data are published, with the exception of China where the ratio is approaching 1:1. Perhaps half of all female suicides in the world occur in China (Phillips et al., 2012). Both young and elderly women are at higher risk, and rural women at greater risk than urban women (Phillips et al., 2012). Women in China have relatively low status and suicide has been associated with negative life events rather than mental health disorders. It appears that being widowed, separated or divorced are protective against suicide for women in China and India, in contrast with findings from most developed countries (Phillips et al., 2012). Globally, self-poisoning with highly toxic pesticides is possibly the most common method of suicide (World Health Organization, 2014). In rural China and India these are readily available.

Aboriginal and Indigenous Populations

An over-representation of indigenous or aboriginal populations in suicide deaths is reported from several countries. For example, First Nations people in the USA, Metis and Inuit in Canada, Sami in Arctic Norway, Australian Aborigines and New Zealand Māori (Pitman et al., 2012).

Suicide is a leading cause of death among indigenous Native Americans and Alaskan Natives at every point across the lifespan in 2015, ranking second for those aged 10–34 years (CDC, 2015b). Young adult Native American/Alaskan Natives are 1.5 times more likely than the general population to die by suicide (15–34 years, 19.5 per 100,000 vs 12.9 per 100,000). Native American/Alaskan Native adults (4.8%) and those of multi-race backgrounds (7.9%) were more

likely to report suicidal ideation in the previous year compared with white adults (4.1%) (CDC, 2015b). The Navajo tribe has much lower rates of suicide than other ethnic minority groups, which may be associated with traditional life-affirming beliefs and protection from acculturative pressures due to their large and isolated tribal area (Middlebrook et al., 2001).

In Australia there is ongoing concern about the high rates of suicidal behaviour among Australian Aboriginal and Torres Strait Islander people, particularly among the young and those in custody (Tatz, 2001). During the period 1999–2013 age-standardized rates of hospital-treated non-fatal self-harm were more than twice that of non-indigenous people (295.8 per 100,000 vs 114.0 per 100,000), and three times higher among indigenous males (247.0 per 100,000) compared with their non-indigenous peers (79.9 per 100,000) (Pointer, 2015). Female rates were highest amongst those aged 30–34 years (715 per 100,000) and 45–49 years for males (467 per 100,000). Rates of self-harm were higher among indigenous compared with non-indigenous population, and rising for the time period 2004–2013, particularly for females, against a backdrop of relatively static rates amongst the non-indigenous population (Pointer, 2015).

Aboriginal and Torres Strait Islanders have all age-standardized rates of suicide twice those of the general population, with around 100 suicide deaths per year between 2001 and 2010. In addition to the overall elevated rate there are even greater discrepancies evident among both males aged 25–29 years (90.8 deaths per 100,000), with a rate four times higher compared with non-indigenous males, and females aged 20–24 years (21.8 deaths per 100,000), with a rate five times higher than non-indigenous women of the same age (Australian Department of Health, 2013). De Leo et al. (2011) drew attention to the fact that the rate of suicide deaths among indigenous youth under 15 years (4.61 per 100,000) in Queensland was 10 times greater than non-indigenous youth (0.48 per 100,000, RR = 9.6) between 1994 and 2007.

In Australia, hanging continues to be the most common method of suicide in indigenous people, accounting for 90 per cent of suicide deaths (De Leo et al., 2011). There are significant regional differences in rates of suicide. Higher rates have been reported from Northern Territory, South Australia, Western Australia and Queensland in comparison with New South Wales

(Australian Department of Health, 2013). It has been argued that mainstream risk factors provide an incomplete understanding of Aboriginal suicide and that issues such as marginalization, lack of purpose, disintegration of social support networks, persistent grief, illiteracy and alcohol abuse contribute to suicides in this community (Tatz, 2001). A shift towards tailoring intervention programmes and evaluating their effectiveness is evident, with a recent review of suicide prevention initiatives for Australian Aboriginal communities supporting further development of programmes utilizing a whole community approach, with a focus on enhancing connectedness, belonging and understanding of cultural heritage (Ridani et al., 2015).

New Zealand continues to have the highest rate of suicide among young people aged 15–24 years in the OECD (New Zealand Ministry of Health, 2015a). Until the mid 1980s, suicide rates among Māori (indigenous peoples) were lower than non-Māori. However, there was a sharp rise in suicides among young Māori men from this time, reflecting a significant increase in overall rates of youth suicide and some changes in the collection of census data (Skegg et al., 1995), which may have increased the number of people identifying as Māori. Currently, more Māori (15.8 per 100,000) than non-Māori (9.7 per 100,000) die by suicide, with Māori females being more than twice as likely to die by suicide compared with non-Māori females. Since 2011 there appears to be a downward trend in the death rate for Māori males, but conversely a rising trend among Māori females (New Zealand Ministry of Health, 2015b). In a recent feasibility study a National Suicide Mortality Review Committee focused on young Māori as one of three groups at particularly high risk of death by suicide. Using a combination of national data regarding service use for health, police, education, statutory child protection, public housing and public accident insurance, in addition to qualitative family interviews, leverage points for future suicide prevention initiatives were identified. These included the prominence of multiple agency involvement with young Māori for concerns about child protection, high levels of contact with police, prison/probation services and mental health services. Hanging accounted for nearly all (93%) of deaths in this group, compared with 58% of men in their middle years and 57% of deaths among mental health service users (Suicide Mortality Review Committee, 2015).

In New Zealand the annual hospitalization rate following self-harm is reported as 71 per 100,000 (New Zealand Ministry of Health, 2015a), although this is likely an underestimate of the overall extent of self-harm as it does not include presentations to GPs, or patients treated in emergency departments and discharged. Māori accounted for one in five presentations, with a rate of 85 per 100,000 compared with 68 per 100,000 for non-Māori, with a rising trend in presentations evident for Māori since 2011 (New Zealand Ministry of Health, 2015a).

Indigenous youth in Arctic areas spanning Alaska, northern Canada, Iceland, Russia and several Nordic countries are part of communities subjected to significant socio-cultural transitions including urbanization and climate change. Despite the diversity of these populations, high rates of suicidal ideation (12–43%), attempts (9.5–34%) and deaths by suicide are apparent. In addition, elevated rates of substance abuse were identified in many, but not all Arctic indigenous groups (Lehti et al., 2009).

The last 10 years have seen a significant expansion of the literature on ethnic density driven by observations that some ethnic minority groups experience a protective effect when living in areas with high ethnic density (Neeleman et al., 2001). However, a recent review of UK-based studies show mixed evidence (Shaw et al., 2012), and the importance of social differentiation, income and education are becoming better understood as predictors of mental health morbidity (Mangalore and Knapp, 2012). The EMPIRIC study in the UK suggested that the poor in African Caribbean, Pakistani and Bangladeshi communities experience a greater burden of mental health morbidity compared with poor white, Irish or Indian (Mangalore et al., 2012).

In summary, there are relatively high rates of suicidal phenomena among indigenous peoples in several countries, including in America, the Arctic region, Australia and New Zealand. Young indigenous people appear particularly vulnerable to engaging in suicidal behaviours. The prevalence of hanging is striking in these populations and represents an ongoing challenge for public health prevention measures.

Asylum Seekers and Refugees

Asylum seekers and refugees face particular migration difficulties. Their migration is often forced by adverse circumstances, which themselves are associated with poor mental health. Post-migration experiences of unemployment/under-employment, social isolation, racism, and fear for the safety of loved ones may exacerbate these problems. However, there is mounting concern that the policies of deterrence adopted by a number of Western nations, which include marginal access to health services, education, employment and detention, contribute directly to elevated rates of depression, PTSD, anxiety and suicidal behaviours in this population. Duration of detention was positively correlated with the severity of psychological distress in a review of studies of detention in the UK, USA and Australia. Release from detention initially brought some improvement in distress; however, there was evidence of persisting long-term impact of detention on mental health (Robjant et al., 2009).

High rates of depression, anxiety and post-traumatic stress disorder have been found in this population (for a review see Bogic et al., 2015; Robjant et al., 2009), conditions that are associated with elevated rates of suicidal behaviour. There are relatively few large studies focusing on suicidal behaviour among asylum seekers and refugees. However, there is concern that detention centres create a 'culture of self-harm' among both children and adults (Robjant et al., 2009: 309). There has been significant media coverage of fatal and non-fatal self-harm in Australian centres on Manus Island and Naru.

Some asylum seekers may perceive suicide as preferable to forced repatriation, with the period immediately following the rejection of refugee applications being a time of particularly high risk. A case control study of 88 asylum seekers (n = 47 male, mean age = 29 years) and 88 citizens in Sweden presenting to a mental health service following an episode of suicidal behaviour found that 39 per cent of attempts were proximal to the rejection of an asylum claim, although 24 per cent of attempts occurred earlier in the asylum-seeking process. Asylum seekers were significantly more likely to describe their attempt as having lethal intent (93% vs 73.8%) and to use hanging, strangulation or suffocation. Asylum seekers were more likely to be admitted to inpatient psychiatric care, but less likely to be referred to specialist mental health services for follow-up (Sundvall et al., 2015).

Children who experience displacement or become refugees are a particularly vulnerable group, particularly those who are unaccompanied or become separated from their family group. Two recent reviews highlight the mental health difficulties of these children, particularly those who resettle in low- to middle-income countries which often lack the legal and infrastructure resources to respond to their needs (Reed et al., 2012). These authors suggest that exposure to pre-migration violence, settlement in a refugee camp and internal displacement are associated with increased risk of poor mental health (Reed et al., 2012). The second review focuses on the larger body of literature regarding mental health outcomes of children and adolescents who resettle in high-income countries. It showed that, in addition to the factors outlined earlier, female gender, perceived discrimination, exposure to post-migration violence, changes of residence, single parenthood and psychiatric difficulties experienced by parents all elevate the risk of poor mental health. Importantly, protective factors including high levels of support from parents and friends, positive educational experience and same-ethnicity foster care were protective (Fazel et al., 2012).

Overview of Aetiological Factors

Models of Migration, Mental Illness and Suicide

Aetiological factors have been addressed earlier in this chapter, but will be reconsidered in more detail in the following section. It is now generally agreed that there is a relationship between migration and mental health problems. The explanatory models for this include high morbidity in the home countries of migrants that they bring with them, biopsychosocial vulnerability among migrants, acculturative stress, misdiagnosis (particularly the use of Western nosology for non-Western groups) and racial discrimination (Bhugra and Arya, 2005). There appears to be a protective effect on mental health for adults from ethnic minorities who live in communities with high density of people from those minorities (the ethnic density effect), although some ethnic minority adolescents experience increased depression with increasing ethnic density (Shaw et al., 2012). Bhugra and Arya (2005) also hypothesize that migration from a socio-centric society to an ego-centric society leads to the greatest levels of distress and psychiatric morbidity.

The research on risk factors associated with suicidal behaviour has largely been conducted in developed countries. A review of risk factors in developing countries indicates that while some risk factors, such as gender, living in rural communities, alcohol abuse, stressful life events and a history of self-harm, appear to be generalizable to developing countries, other factors do not. For example, being single, divorced or widowed is associated with elevated risk in Western countries but may be protective in developing countries. Also, socio-cultural factors appear as least as important as mental illness in developing countries (Vijayakumar *et al.*, 2005).

Psychiatric Morbidity among Ethnic Minority Groups in the UK

Schizophrenia is associated with elevated risk of suicide (Hor and Taylor, 2010) and the rates of schizophrenia and other psychoses are higher among migrants and their descendants of black Caribbean (pooled RR 5.6, 95% CI 3.4 – 9.2), black African (pooled RR 4.7, 95% CI 3.3 – 6.8) and South Asian (particularly females) (pooled RR 2.4, 95% CI 1.3 – 4.5) groups in England. There is also emerging evidence of elevated rates among people of mixed ethnicity and non-British white migrant groups (Kirkbride *et al.*, 2012) and a sustained elevation of risk among second generation migrant groups (Bourque *et al.*, 2011). A systematic review of the course and outcome of psychosis among black Caribbean groups in the UK reports very mixed findings, although it appears this group may be more likely to experience compulsory psychiatric admission, no significant differences in the course of the illness, but are less likely to self-harm or die by suicide (Chorlton *et al.*, 2012). A study of patients in contact with mental health services within a year of their death by suicide suggested delusions and hallucinations were more common among ethnic minority groups with lower levels of suicidal ideation, emotional distress and hostility (Bhui and McKenzie, 2008).

Depression is a risk factor for both self-harm and suicide. The rates of depression and anxiety in South Asians were previously thought to be the same, or lower than, those in the general UK population. However, in a large representative sample of adults in the community age-standardized rates of common mental disorders were consistently higher among women from all ethnic groups compared with males, with this difference most notable among South Asian women (34.3%) compared with South Asian males (10.3%). South Asian women also reported higher rates of general anxiety disorder (16.3%) compared

with black (8.4%) and white (5.0%) women, and also depressive episodes in the past week (11.8% vs 1.4% and 2.7% respectively) (NHS Health and Social Care Information Centre, 2009). In a 20-year follow-up study of older adults in London rates of depression were significantly higher among South Asian (OR = 1.79, 95% CI 1.24 – 2.58) and black Caribbean (OR = 1.80, 95% CI 1.11 – 2.92) participants. Physical health difficulties in part explained elevated rates among South Asian participants, whereas socio-economic status contributed to elevated rates in black Caribbeans (Williams *et al.*, 2015).

In contrast to adults, black African and Indian children in the UK appear to have similar or better mental health compared with their white British peers. Black Caribbean, Pakistani and Bangladeshi children are not discernible from their white peers (Goodman *et al.*, 2008).

The aetiology of mental illness in migrants is complex, involving biopsychosocial factors which interact with life events during different phases of the migration process, and may be affected by factors such as culture shock, cultural identity and local ethnic density (Morgan *et al.*, 2010). Premorbid vulnerability may make some migrants more likely to develop mental illness after migration, or mental illness may contribute to reasons why others migrate. There is also increasing concern that some statutory processes, including detention, may directly contribute to poor mental health and suicidal behaviour.

The Role of Religion

The importance of religious beliefs in relation to suicidal behaviour has been debated for some time. Generally, strong religious affiliation is associated with lower rates of suicidal behaviour. Thus, for example, in a longitudinal study of a large cohort of women in the USA VanderWeele and colleagues (2016) found that attendance at religious services once per week was associated with a fivefold lower rate of suicide compared with never attending religious services. Recent reviews suggest the relationship between religion and suicide can be understood through several theoretical mechanisms, including religion forming a moral community where certain (generally positive) attitudes and behaviours are fostered, that religious integration and greater adherence to religious beliefs are associated with lower levels of acceptability of suicide and that religious networks generally increase social support available to individuals (Koenig, 2009; Stack and Kposowa, 2011).

Countries with strong religious or spiritual elements to their culture appear to have lower suicide rates (Bertolote and Fleischmann, 2002). There is some debate as to whether religion plays a role in whether or not an individual develops suicidal thoughts or behaviours, or alternatively it influences their willingness to admit to them; for example, suicide is a criminal act in a number of Islamic countries. This literature is separate to consideration of so called 'suicide-terrorists' or people who engage in acts of violence, which end in their own death and are thought to be associated with certain beliefs (for a review see Townsend, 2014).

Self-immolation is a highly lethal method of suicide. It is particularly associated with Indian culture, both in India (Patel *et al.*, 2012) and among Indian immigrants to other countries such as England (Kapur *et al.*, 2013). Women more frequently use self-immolation than men. *Sati* is an act with historical cultural and religious importance in India, and not usually associated with mental illness (Bhugra, 2005).

The Importance of Intent and Method across Cultures

The cultural meaning of suicide and method of death vary to some extent across cultures. The importance of establishing the intent or motives underlying episodes of self-harm has attracted much recent debate. Acts of self-harm may have a variety of motives or intentions. However, it also appears that across cultures there are some universal experiences that are associated with SH. In a large study of 1646 people who harmed themselves in 13 European countries, the intentions or motives for the act of SH were investigated by providing patients with a list of possible intentions and asking them to score the relevance of each to their act. Examples of possible intentions included finding one's thoughts unbearable, wanting to get away from an unbearable situation, wanting to die and wanting to get help. The pattern of intentions was extremely consistent across countries, gender and age (Hjelmeland *et al.*, 2002).

As discussed previously, there is significant variation between cultures in the methods most commonly used for suicide. The preferred methods of suicide in any given country have an impact on suicide rates, given that some methods are more lethal than others. In addition, deaths involving a certain method may increase or decrease, depending on the availability of that method. In the USA, firearms are a common method of suicide but account for a relatively small number of deaths in the UK, New Zealand and Australia. Hanging has become increasingly popular in many countries throughout the world. The substitution of method relies on both the acceptability and availability of alternative methods; the increasing rates of hanging suggest it has become an increasingly acceptable method of suicide, perhaps because of decreased access to other methods. It is also extremely accessible with a high case fatality rate. Social contagion and media coverage may also have contributed to the spread of this method.

The use of pesticides in agrarian communities such as in China, India and Sri Lanka means that a similar method (self-poisoning) is associated with much higher mortality in these countries compared with countries where analgesics are the most frequently used substances for self-poisoning (Wu *et al.*, 2012). Also, individuals in developed countries have a second level of protection due to the greater density and proximity of adequate medical services compared with people living in developing countries.

Help-Seeking and Health Service Utilization

Studies of health service utilization have identified complex interactions between cultural beliefs and help-seeking. In addition, cultural meanings of illness and treatment and explanatory models of illness are culture bound, in a way that may not fit with the health services that are available. For example, several studies have identified that somatization can be a pathway into health services for migrants experiencing depression (Bhugra, 2003). Also, as noted earlier females from ethnic minority groups presenting to hospital following self-harm in England were less likely to receive a specialist psychiatric assessment and black females were less likely to be offered psychiatric after care compared with their white counterparts. Similarly, black males were less likely to be referred to GPs for follow-up and South Asian males less likely to be referred to any follow-up services (Cooper *et al.*, 2010).

Acculturative Stress in Migrating Groups and Subsequent Generations

Acculturative stress is a dynamic construct and appears to alter over time and across generations. The findings of studies in this area are mixed. Some have found differences in acculturative stress between first- and second-generation immigrants while other studies indicate that later generations may experience greater degrees of acculturative stress, with associated increases in risk of suicidal behaviour. Discrepancies between parent and child acculturation can be a source of family stress (e.g. Wyatt *et al.*, 2015). A large community-based epidemiological study of 6,359 adults in the USA (50.9% male), showed a significant linear relationship between increased acculturation (measured by younger age at migration, lower involvement and identification with ethnic community and language) and increased risk of suicidal ideation and suicide attempts (Perez-Rodriguez *et al.*, 2014). Also in the USA, a longitudinal study of 332 students (mean age = 16.2 years, 44% male) in New York found that increased acculturative stress was associated higher rates of internalizing mental health disorders (Sirin *et al.*, 2013).

Conclusions

The findings we have reviewed in this chapter suggest that there is significant variation in rates of suicide, self-harm and suicidal ideation around the world. Developing countries such as China and India appear to have relatively high rates of suicide, particularly among women and those in rural areas. Given the populous nature of these nations, they contribute very heavily to the global burden of suicide. However, there have been recent major changes in the epidemiology of suicide in several such countries. To date, most epidemiological research has focused on developed countries. The generalizability of risk factors identified through this process to developing countries and the role of culture requires further exploration.

Despite the fact that culture influences the manifestation of mental illness, the acceptability of suicide and the preferred methods of suicide, it appears that globally there are increasing rates of suicidal behaviour among the young, particularly when measured by

potential years of life lost (PYLL), and an increasing burden in men in their middle years.

The globalization of information has resulted in rapid and wide transmission of previously unknown and very lethal methods of suicide, for example the spread of the use of charcoal burning throughout Asia. Hanging appears to be increasingly used by people, both male and female, as a method of suicide in several countries. The mechanisms underlying the apparent increased acceptability, cultural meaning and preference for this method require further research, with a focus on leverage points for prevention.

As noted previously, the ratio of female to male suicides in China and India differs from the pattern in other countries, with relatively high rates in women (although this pattern appears to be changing in China). Although it is not yet certain how Chinese women fare if they move away from their home country, South Asian women appear to experience elevated rates of psychological distress and older women in this group appear to carry an increased risk of suicide.

Indigenous peoples in many countries experience high rates of social marginalization, unemployment and substance abuse and are often over-represented in prison and welfare populations. Young people, particularly young men in indigenous populations such as Australian Aborigines, New Zealand Māori and American First Nations peoples, have high and rising rates of both fatal and non-fatal suicidal behaviours.

The relationship between migration, mental health and suicide is important. The protective influence of ethnic density needs to be investigated further due to mixed findings. There has been a great deal of public interest in the large numbers of migrants entering Europe. There is increasing evidence that government policies aimed to deter migrants may result in mental distress and suicidality, particularly the use of detention. Refugee children are a particularly vulnerable group.

National suicide prevention strategies are now in place in many developed countries around the world. They share common elements such as intervention at a public health level and a focus on high-risk groups and high-risk individuals (Zalsman *et al.*, 2016). The establishment of suicide prevention strategies in developing countries is also important. The findings presented in this chapter suggest that addressing suicide prevention in ethnic minority groups in national suicide prevention strategies involves a range of complex factors, including, for example, the awareness of commonly used methods for suicide in an ethnic group's country of origin, cultural attitudes towards suicide and help-seeking, and willingness to use locally accepted sources of help or methods of preventing distress. Therefore, suicide prevention strategies need to be strengthened by inclusion of elements that account for the differences experienced by ethnic minority groups. For example, the detection and efficacious treatment of psychiatric disorder is an important element of suicide prevention. Members of ethnic minority groups may carry the burden of increased risk for mental illness, however, there is significant work to be done in enhancing the goodness of fit between mainstream mental health services and their cultural models of health and well-being. The development of culturally responsive mental health services continues to be a challenge.

As highlighted in this chapter the data available on the rates of self-harm and suicide in many countries are poor. This makes understanding of the phenomena more challenging and presents problems for the evaluation of suicide prevention initiatives. In addition, the countries in which poor data are kept regarding suicidal behaviour are often struggling to provide basic healthcare services to their people and suicide is one of a number of serious health issues they face.

Directions for future research include establishing a clearer understanding of the magnitude of self-harm and suicide in different ethnic and cultural groups in the community including improved understanding of the meaning of suicide for women compared with men in different cultural contexts. It appears that global shifts in rates and methods of suicide are occurring. However, the role of culture continues to be poorly understood.

References

Australian Department of Health (2013). Aboriginal and Torres Strait Islander suicide: origins, trends and incidence. National Aboriginal and Torres Strait Islander Suicide Prevention Strategy. Available online at www.health.gov.au/internet/publications/publishing.ns f/Content/mental-natsisps-strat-toc~mental-natsisps-st rat-1~mental-natsisps-strat-1-ab (accessed 1 July, 2016).

Bellis, M. A., Hughes, K., Leckenby, N., *et al.* (2014). Adverse childhood experiences and associations with health-harming behaviours in young adults: surveys in eight eastern European countries. *Bulletin of the World Health Organization*, 92, 641–55.

Berry, J. W., Poortinga, Y. H., Segall, M. H., and Dasen, P. R. (2002). *Cross-Cultural Psychology: Research and Applications*, 2nd edn. New York, NY: Cambridge University Press.

Bertolote, J. M. and Fleischmann, A. (2002). A global perspective in the epidemiology of suicide. *Suicidologi*, 7, 6–8.

Bertolote, J. M. and Fleischmann, A. (2009). A global perspective on the magnitude of suicide mortality. In *Oxford Textbook of Suicidology and Suicide Prevention*, ed. D. Wasserman and C. Wasserman. Oxford: Oxford University Press, pp. 91–98.

Bhugra, D. (2003). Migration and depression. *Acta Psychiatrica Scandinavica Supplement*, **418**, 67–72.

Bhugra, D. (2005). Sati: a type of nonpsychiatric suicide. *Crisis*, **26**, 73–77.

Bhugra, D. and Arya, P. (2005). Ethnic density, cultural congruity and mental illness in migrants. *International Review of Psychiatry*, 17, 133–37.

Bhui, K. and McKenzie, K. (2008). Rates and risk factors by ethnic group for suicides within a year of contact with mental health services in England and Wales. *Psychiatric Services*, 59, 414–20.

Bhui, K., McKenzie, K. and Rasul, F. (2007). Rates, risk factors and methods of self-harm among minority ethnic groups in the UK: a systematic review. *BMC Public Health*, 7, 336.

Bhui, K. S., Dinos, S. and McKenzie, K. (2012). Ethnicity and its influence on suicide rates and risk. *Ethnicity and Health*, 17, 141–48.

Bhui, K. S., Aslam, R. H. W., Palinski, A., *et al.* (2015). Interventions to improve therapeutic communications between black and minority ethnic patients and professionals in psychiatric services: systematic review. *The British Journal of Psychiatry*, **207**, 95–103.

Bogic, M., Njoku, A. and Priebe, S. (2015). Long-term mental health of war-refugees: a systematic literature review. *BMC International Health and Human Rights*, **15**, 29.

Borges, G., Orozco, R., Rafful, C., Miller, E. and Breslau, J. (2012). Suicidality, ethnicity and immigration in the USA. *Psychological Medicine*, **42**, 1175–84.

Borrill, J., Fox, P. and Roger, D. (2011). Religion, ethnicity, coping style, and self-reported self-harm in a diverse non-clinical UK population, *Mental Health, Religion and Culture*, 14(3), 259–269.

Bourque, F., van der Ven, E. and Malla, A. (2011). A meta-analysis of the risk for psychotic disorders among first- and second-generation immigrants. *Psychological Medicine*, **41**, 897–910.

Cantor, C. H., Leenaars, A. A. and Lester, D. (1997). Under-reporting of suicide in Ireland 1960–1989. *Archives of Suicide Research*, **3**, 5–12.

CDC (2013). MMWR: Suicide among adults aged 35–64 years – United States, 1999–2010: Centres for Disease Control and Prevention.

CDC (2015a). MMWR: suicide trends among persons aged 10–24 years – United States, 1994–2012: Centres for Disease Control and Prevention.

CDC (2015b). Suicide facts at a glance, 2015. Available online at www.cdc.gov/ViolencePrevention/pdf/Suicide-DataSheet-a.pdf (accessed 1 July, 2016).

Chang, S.-S., Chen, Y.-Y., Yip, P. S. F., Lee, W. J., Hagihara, A. and Gunnell, D. (2014). Regional changes in charcoal-burning suicide rates in East/Southeast Asia from 1995 to 2011: a time trend analysis. *PLoS Medicine*, **11**, e1001622.

Chang, S.-S., Cheng, Q., Lee, E. S. T. and Yip, P. S. F. (2016). Suicide by gassing in Hong Kong 2005–2013: emerging trends and characteristics of suicide by helium inhalation. *Journal of Affective Disorders*, **192**, 162–166.

Chen, Y.-Y., Chien-Chang Wu, K., Yousuf, S. and Yip, P. S. F. (2012). Suicide in Asia: opportunities and challenges. *Epidemiologic Reviews*. **34**(1), 129–144.

Chorlton, E., McKenzie, K., Morgan, C. and Doody, G. (2012). Course and outcome of psychosis in black Caribbean populations and other ethnic groups living in the UK: a systematic review. *International Journal of Social Psychiatry*, **58**, 400–408.

Chu, J. P., Golblum, P., Floyd, R. and Bongar, B. (2010). The cultural theory and model of suicide. *Applied and Preventive Psychology*, **14**, 25–40.

Cooper, J., Murphy, E., Webb, R., Hawton, K., Bergen, H., Waters, K. and Kapur, N. (2010). Ethnic differences in self-harm, rates, characteristics and service provision: three-city cohort study. *British Journal of Psychiatry*, **197**, 212–218.

Cooper, J., Steeg, S., Webb, R., Stewart, S. L. K., Applegate, E., Hawton, K., Bergen, H., Waters, K. and Kapur, N. (2013). Risk factors associated with repetition of self-harm in black and minority ethnic (BME) groups: a multi-centre cohort study. *Journal of Affective Disorders*, **148**, 435–439.

Cross, S., Bhugra, D., Dargan, P. I., Wood, D. M., Greene, S. L. and Craig, T. K. J. (2014). Ethnic differences in self-poisoning across south London. *Crisis*, **35**, 268–272.

De Leo, D., Sveticic, J. and Milner, A. (2011). Suicide in indigenous people in Queensland, Australia: trends and methods, 1994–2007. *Australian and New Zealand Journal of Psychiatry*, **45**, 532.

Fazel, M., Reed, R. V., Panter-Brick, C. and Stein, A. (2012). Mental health of displaced and refugee children resettled in high-income countries: risk and protective factors. *The Lancet*, **379**, 266–282.

Goodman, A., Patel, V. and Leon, D. A. (2008). Child mental health differences amongst ethnic groups in Britain: a systematic review. *BMC Public Health*, **8**, 258.

Hawton, K., Rodham, K., Evans, E. and Weatherall, R. (2002). Deliberate self harm in adolescents: self report survey in schools in England. *British Medical Journal*, **325**, 1207–1211.

Hjelmeland, H., Hawton, K., Nordvik, H., *et al.* (2002). Why people engage in parasuicide: a cross-cultural study of intentions. *Suicide and Life Threatening Behaviour*, **32**, 380–393.

Höfer, P., Rockett, I. R. H., Värnik, P., Etzersdorfer, E. and Kapusta, N. D. (2012). Forty years of increasing suicide mortality in Poland: undercounting amidst a hanging epidemic? *BMC Public Health*, **12**, 1–9.

Hor, K. and Taylor, M. (2010). Suicide and schizophrenia: a systematic review of rates and risk factors. *Journal of Psychopharmacology*, **24**, 81–90.

Japanese Cabinet Office (2013). White Paper on Suicide Prevention in Japan. Tokyo: Japanese Cabinet Office.

Jeon, S. Y., Reither, E. N. and Masters, R. K. (2016). A population-based analysis of increasing rates of suicide mortality in Japan and South Korea, 1985–2010. *BMC Public Health*, **16**, 1–9.

Joe, S., Canetto, S. S. and Romer, D. (2008). Advancing prevention research on the role of culture in suicide prevention. *Suicide and Life Threatening Behavior*, **38**, 354–62.

Kann, L., McManus, T., Harris, W. A. *et al.* (2016). *Youth Risk Behavior Surveillance: United States, 2015 Morbidity and Mortality Weekly Report (MMWR)*. Rockville, MD: Centres for Disease Control and Prevention.

Kapur, N., Hunt, I. M., Windfuhr, K., Rodway, C., Webb, R., Rahman, M. S., Shaw, J. and Appleby, L. (2013). Psychiatric in-patient care and suicide in England, 1997 to 2008: a longitudinal study. *Psychological Medicine*, **43**, 61–71.

Kawashima, Y., Yonemoto, N., Inagaki, M. and Yamada, M. (2014). Prevalence of suicide attempters in emergency departments in Japan: a systematic review and meta-analysis. *Journal of Affective Disorders*, **163**, 33–39.

Kirkbride, J. B., Errazuriz, A., Croudace, T. J., Morgan, C., Jackson, D., Boydell, J., Murray, R. M. and Jones, P. B. (2012). Incidence of schizophrenia and other psychoses in England, 1950–2009: a systematic review and meta-analyses. *PLoS ONE*, **7**, e31660.

Knipe, D. W., Metcalfe, C., Fernando, R., Pearson, M., Konradsen, F., Eddleston, M. and Gunnell, D. (2014). Suicide in Sri Lanka 1975–2012: age, period and cohort analysis of police and hospital data. *BMC Public Health*, **14**, 1–13.

Koenig, H. G. (2009). Research on religion, spirituality, and mental health: a review. *Canadian Journal of Psychiatry*, **54**, 283–91.

Kõlves, K., and De Leo, D. (2014). Suicide rates in children aged 10–14 years worldwide: changes in the past two decades. *The British Journal of Psychiatry*, **205**, 283–285.

Kõlves, K., Kõlves, K. E. and De Leo, D. (2013a). Natural disasters and suicidal behaviours: a systematic literature review. *Journal of Affective Disorders*, **146**, 1–14.

Kõlves, K., Milner, A. and Värnik, P. (2013b). Suicide rates and socio-economic factors in Eastern European countries after the collapse of the Soviet Union: trends between 1990 and 2008. *Sociology of Health and Illness*, **35**(6), 956–970.

Lehti, V., Niemela, S., Hoven, C., Mandell, D. and Sourander, A. (2009). Mental health, substance use and suicidal behaviour among young indigenous people in the Arctic: a systematic review. *Social Science and Medicine*, **69**, 1194–1203.

Liu, Y., Zhang, Y., Cho, Y. T., Obayashi, Y., Arai, A. and Tamashiro, H. (2013). Gender differences of suicide in Japan, 1947–2010. *Journal of Affective Disorders*, **151**, 325–330.

Mangalore, R. and Knapp, M. (2012). Income related inequalities in common mental disorders among ethnic minorities in England. *Social Psychiatry and Psychiatric Epidemiology*, **47**, 351–359.

Maynard, M. J., Rosato, M., Teyhan, A. and Harding, S. (2012). Trends in suicide among migrants in England and Wales 1979–2003. *Ethnicity and Health*, **17**, 135–140.

McKenzie, K., Bhui, K., Nanchahal, K. and Blizard, B. (2008). Suicide rates in people of South Asian origin in England and Wales: 1993–2003. *The British Journal of Psychiatry*, **193**, 406–409.

Middlebrook, D. L., Le Master, P. L., Beals, J., Novins, D. K. and Manson, S. M. (2001). Suicide prevention in American Indian and Alaskan Native communities: a critical review of programmes. *Suicide and Life Threatening Behavior*, **31**, 132–149.

Morgan, C., Charalambides, M., Hutchinson, G. and Murray, R. M. (2010). Migration, ethnicity, and psychosis: toward a socio-developmental model. *Schizophrenia Bulletin*, **36**, 655–664.

Murphy, O. C., Kelleher, C. and Malone, K. M. (2015). Demographic trends in suicide in the UK and Ireland 1980–2010. *Irish Journal of Medical Science*, **184**, 227–235.

NHS Information Centre for Health and Social Care (2009). Adult psychiatric morbidity in England, 2007. Results of a household survey: Social Care Statistics.

Neeleman, J., Mak, V. and Wessely, S. (1997). Suicide by age, ethnic group, coroners' verdicts and country of birth. *British Journal of Psychiatry*, **171**, 463–467.

Neeleman, J., Wilson Jones, C. and Wessely, S. (2001). Ethnic density and deliberate self-harm: a small area study in south east London. *Journal of Epidemiology and Community Health*, **55**, 85–90.

New Zealand Ministry of Health (2015a). Suicide Facts: Deaths and intentional self-harm hospitalisations 2012. Wellington, New Zealand: Ministry of Health.

New Zealand Ministry of Health (2015b, 26 November). Suicide facts: 2013 data. Ministry of Health Mortality Collection. Available online at www.health.govt.nz/publication/suicide-facts-2013-data (accessed 1 July 2016).

Norheim, O. F., Jha, P., Admasu, K, *et al.* (2015). Avoiding 40 per cent of the premature deaths in each country, 2010–30: review of national mortality trends to help quantify the UN Sustainable Development Goal for health. *The Lancet*, **385**, 239–252.

Norström, T., and Rossow, I. (2016). Alcohol consumption as a risk factor for suicidal behavior: a systematic review of associations at the individual and at the population level. *Archives of Suicide Research*, 1–18.

OECD (2011). 'Suicide', in Health at a Glance 2011: OECD Indicators: OECD Publishing.

Office for National Statistics, UK. (2016). Statistical bulletin: Suicides in the United Kingdom: 2014 registrations. Registered deaths from suicide analysed by sex, age, area of usual residence of the deceased and suicide method. Available from www.ons.gov.uk/peoplepopulationand community/birthsdeathsandmarriages/deaths/bulletins/ suicidesintheunitedkingdom/2014registrations (accessed 1 August 2016).

Ougrin, D., Zundel, T., Kyriakopoulos, M., Banarsee, R., Stahl, D. and Taylor, E. (2012). Adolescents with suicidal and nonsuicidal self-harm: clinical characteristics and response to therapeutic assessment. *Psychological Assessment*, **24**, 11–20.

Ougrin, D., Tranah, T., Stahl, D., Moran, P. and Asarnow, J. R. (2015). Therapeutic interventions for suicide attempts and self-harm in adolescents: systematic review and meta-analysis. *Journal of the American Academy of Child and Adolescent Psychiatry*, **54**, 97–107.e2.

Palmer, B. S., Bennewith, O., Simkin, S., Cooper, J., Hawton, K., Kapur, N., and Gunnell, D. (2015). Factors influencing coroners' verdicts: an analysis of verdicts given in 12 coroners' districts to researcher-defined suicides in England in 2005. *Journal of Public Health*, **37**(1), 157–165.

Patel, V., Ramasundarahettige, C., Vijayakumar, L., Thakur, J. S., Gajalakshmi, V., Gururaj, G., Suraweera, W. and Jha, P. (2012). Suicide mortality in India: a nationally representative survey. *The Lancet*, **379**, 2343–2351.

Perez-Rodriguez, M., Baca-Garcia, E., Oquendo, M. A., Wang, S., Wall, M. M., Liu, S. M. and Blanco, C. (2014). Relationship between acculturation, discrimination, and suicidal ideation and attempts among US Hispanics in the National Epidemiologic Survey of Alcohol and Related Conditions. *Journal of Clinical Psychiatry*, **75**, 399–407.

Phillips, M. R. and Cheng, H. G. (2012). The changing global face of suicide. *The Lancet*, **379**, 2318–2319.

Phillips, M. R., Yang, G., Zhang, Y., Wang, L., Ji, H. and Zhou, M. (2002). Risk factors for suicide in China: a national case-control psychological autopsy study. *Lancet*, **360**, 1728–1736.

Pitman, A., Krysinska, K., Osborn, D. and King, M. (2012). Suicide in young men. *The Lancet*, **379**, 2383–2392.

Pointer, S. (2015). *Trends in Hospitalised Injury, Australia: 1999–00 to 2012–13. Injury Research and Statistics Series No. 95*. Canberra: AIHW.

Pridemore, W. A., Chamlin, M. B. and Andreev, E. (2013). Reduction in male suicide mortality following the 2006 Russian alcohol policy: an interrupted time series analysis. *American Journal of Public Health*, **103**, 2021–2026.

Razvodovsky, Y. E. (2015). Suicides in Russia and Belarus: a comparative analysis of trends. *Acta Psychopathologica*, **1**, 22.

Reed, R. V., Fazel, M., Jones, L., Panter-Brick, C. and Stein, A. (2012). Mental health of displaced and refugee children resettled in low-income and middle-income countries: risk and protective factors. *The Lancet*, **379**, 250–265.

Reeves, A., Stuckler, D., McKee, M., Gunnell, D., Chang, S.-S. and Basu, S. (2012). Increase in state suicide rates in the USA during economic recession. *The Lancet*, **380**, 1813–1814.

Ridani, R., Shand, F. L., Christensen, H., McKay, K., Tighe, J., Burns, J. and Hunter, E. (2015). Suicide prevetion in Australian Aboriginal communities: a review of past and present programs. *Suicide and Life Threatening Behavior*, **45**, 111–139.

Robjant, K., Hassan, R. and Katona, C. (2009). Mental health implications of detaining asylum seekers: systematic review. *The British Journal of Psychiatry*, **194**, 306–312.

Shaw, R. J., Atkin, K., Bécares, L., Albor, C. B., Stafford, M., Kiernan, K. E., Nazroo, J. Y., Wilkinson, R. G. and Pickett, K. E. (2012). Impact of ethnic density on adult mental disorders: narrative review. *The British Journal of Psychiatry*, **201**, 11–19.

Sirin, S. R., Ryce, P., Gupta, T. and Rogers-Sirin, L. (2013). The role of acculturative stress on mental health symptoms for immigrant adolescents: a longitudinal investigation. *Developmental Psychology*, **49**, 736–748.

Skegg, K., Cox, B. and Broughton, J. (1995). Suicide among New Zealand Māori: is history repeating itself? *Acta Psychiatrica Scandanvica*, **92**, 453–459.

Stack, S. and Kposowa, A. J. (2011). Religion and suicide acceptability: a cross-national analysis. *Journal for the Scientific Study of Religion*, **50**, 289–306.

Substance Abuse and Mental Health Service Administration (US) (2014). *Results from the 2013 National Survey on Drug Use and Health: Mental Health Findings NSDUH Series H-49*. Rockville, MD.

Suicide Mortality Review Committee (NZ) (2015). Ngā Rāhui Hau Kura. Suicide mortality review committee. Feasibility study 2014–2015. Wellington, New Zealand: Health, Safety and Quality Commission New Zealand.

Sundvall, M., Tidemalm, D. H., Titelman, D. E., Runeson, B. and Bäärnhielm, S. (2015). Assessment and treatment of asylum seekers after a suicide attempt: a comparative study of people registered at mental health services in a Swedish location. *BMC Psychiatry*, **15**, 1–11.

Swanson, J. W., McGinty, E. E., Fazel, S. and Mays, V. M. (2015). Mental illness and reduction of gun violence and suicide: bringing epidemiologic research to policy. *Annals of Epidemiology*, **25**, 366–376.

Takei, N. and Nakamura, K. (2004). Is inseki-jisatsu, responsibility-driven suicide, culture-bound? *The Lancet*, **363**, 1400.

Tatz, C. (2001). *Aboriginal Suicide Is Different. A Portrait of Life and Self Destruction*. Canberra: Australian Institute of Aboriginal and Torres Strait Islander Studies, p. 249.

Ting, S. A., Sullivan, A. F., Boudreaux, E. D., Miller, I. and Camargo, C. A., Jr (2012). Trends in US emergency department visits for attempted suicide and self-inflicted injury, 1993–2008. *General Hospital Psychiatry*, **34**, 557–565.

Townsend, E. (2014). Suicide terrorism. In *The Oxford Handbook of Suicide and Self-Injury*, ed. M. K. Nock. Oxford: Oxford University Press, p. 544.

Turnbull, P., Webb, R., Kapur, N., Clements, C., Bergen, H., Hawton, K., Ness, J., Waters, K., Townsend, E. and Cooper, J. (2015). Variation by ethnic group in premature mortality risk following self-harm: a multicentre cohort study in England. *BMC Psychiatry*, **15**, 1–8.

VanderWeele, T. J., Li, S., Tsai, A. C., and Kawachi, I. (2016). Association between religious service attendance and lower suicide rates among US women. *JAMA Psychiatry*, **73**, 845–851.

Vijayakumar, L., John, S., Pirkis, J. and Whiteford, H. (2005). Suicide in developing countries (2). *Crisis*, **26**, 112–119.

Wang, C.-W., Chan, C. L. W. and Yip, P. S. F. (2014). Suicide rates in China from 2002 to 2011: an update. *Social Psychiatry and Psychiatric Epidemiology*, **49**, 929–941.

Williams, E. D., Tillin, T., Richards, M., Tuson, C., Chaturvedi, N., Hughes, A. D. and Stewart, R. (2015). Depressive symptoms are doubled in older British South Asian and Black Caribbean people compared with Europeans: associations with excess comorbidity and socio-economic disadvantage. *Psychological Medicine*, **45**, 1861–1871.

Windfuhr, K. and Kapur, N. (2011). Suicide and mental illness: a clinical review of 15 years' findings from the UK National Confidential Inquiry into Suicide. *British Medical Bulletin*, **100**, 101–121.

World Health Organization (1996). *Multiaxial Classification of Child and Adolescent Psychiatric Disorders: ICD-10 Classification of Mental and Behavioural Disorders in Children and Adolescents*. New York: Cambridge University Press.

World Health Organization (2014). *Preventing Suicide: A Global Imperative*. Geneva, Switzerland: WHO.

World Health Organization (2016, April). WHO Suicide fact sheet. Available online at www.who.int/entity/med iacentre/factsheets/fs398/en/ (accessed 1 June 2016).

Wu, K. C.-C., Chen, Y.-Y. and Yip, P. S. F. (2012). Suicide methods in Asia: implications in suicide prevention. *International Journal of Environment Research and Public Health*, **9**, 1135–1158.

Wyatt, L. C., Ung, T., Park, R., Kwon, S. C. and Trinh-Shevrin, C. (2015). Risk factors of suicide and depression among Asian American, Native Hawaiian, and Pacific Islander youth: a systematic literature review. *Journal of Health Care for the Poor and Underserved*, **26**, 191–237.

Yoshioka, E., Hanley, S. J., Kawanishi, Y. and Saijo, Y. (2016a). Time trends in method-specific suicide rates in Japan, 1990–2011. *Epidemiology and Psychiatric Sciences*, **25**, 58–68.

Yoshioka, E., Saijo, Y. and Kawachi, I. (2016b). Spatial and temporal evolution of the epidemic of charcoal-burning suicide in Japan. *Social Psychiatry and Psychiatric Epidemiology*, **51**, 857–868.

Zalsman, G., Hawton, K., Wasserman, D., *et al.* (2016). Suicide prevention strategies revisited: 10-year systematic review. *The Lancet Psychiatry*, **3**, 646–659.

Chapter 23

Personality Disorders and Culture

Antonio Ventriglio, Matthew Kelly and Dinesh Bhugra

Editors' Introduction

Personality disorders raise a number of critical and clinical dilemmas. There is no doubt that cultures influence personality development and the way the individual's world view is formed. The notion of the self is at the core of individual personality. The existing concepts of ego-centric or individualistic self are comparable with socio-centric or collective self. It is likely that patterns of child rearing will also influence the way the personality of the individual develops. This is further complicated by various dimensions of the culture within which the individual lives and functions. The dimensions of personality add another complex angle to the diagnosis and functioning of personality disorders. In this chapter, Ventriglio *et al.* start with anthropological perspectives and then use DSM-5 and its clusters for personality disorder and explore cultural differences and consequent intervention and management strategies. The two major classification systems have problems in agreeing on some peripheral issues. The clinical distinction between personality trait and character and between personality exaggerations and disorders raises some interesting points in reaching diagnoses, and then planning and managing personality disorders. Personality traits need to be identified so that a clear distinction is made between temporary traits and habits and permanent characteristics. Cultural differences in prevalence of many personality disorders need further detailed exploration and clinicians need to see these disorders in the cultural context within which they work and within which their patients live and function. Cultural variations in the concept of selfhood also need to be taken into account while reaching diagnosis and planning any interventions and management. The authors propose that further longitudinal studies are indicated. As cultures determine pathways into help-seeking, it is important that clinicians are aware of the normative data.

Introduction

Individual personality characteristics are influenced by several factors in their development. Some of these characteristics are biologically determined, whereas others are influenced by cultural factors, parenting and peer groups. It is inevitable that all individuals carry with them certain personality traits and characteristics which, when exaggerated, become disorders. However, it is essential to recognize that as cultures define and determine what is normal, or what is abnormal behaviour, clinicians take care in ascertaining the depth and seriousness of certain characteristics.

Psychiatric diagnoses can be agreed on a number of parameters with various assessment tools and following one of the major classification systems. Personality disorders can be difficult to diagnose, and there is some debate about whether these are or should be considered to be psychiatric disorders. However, personality disorders are also linked with comorbidity with physical illness and other psychiatric disorders which may make the diagnosis even more complex. It is imperative that clinicians see personality disorder in the longitudinal context of cultural influences – from parenting, childhood to development into adulthood and indeed beyond. The core personality traits, their recognition and their exaggeration (within the ambit of personality disorder) can provide a way forward in understanding the impact of personality disorders.

Personality and Culture

Culture and personality research look at the comparative study of the connection between individuals (their behaviour patterns and mental functioning) and the environment (within which individuals are born, live and work (Le Vine, 1973). The relationship between culture and personality is complex in many ways. Culture has been defined several times in this volume, and we do not propose to repeat that here.

However, to remind ourselves, Child (1968) described personality as the complex psychological processes occurring in a human being as they function in their daily life, and motivated and directed by a number of external and internal factors. Child (1968) goes on to state that the other and narrower meaning of personality refers to a more restricted subject matter with internally determined consistencies underlying a person's behaviour or to enduring differences among people attributed to internal characteristics rather than external life factors.

Le Vine (1973) suggests that personality is the organization in the individual of those processes that intervene between environmental conditions and behavioural responses. There is no doubt that child rearing as well as processes of socialization contribute to the development of the personality. Socialization of the individual is the process by which they are transformed into functional human beings as a result of learning from other social contacts. Le Vine (1973) argues that the actual process of socialization should be seen as the process of enculturation. There is no doubt that socialization is also about impulse control. The desires which may be disruptive or destructive can be controlled by learning what is acceptable or unacceptable socially through the processes related to socialization. Socialization is also about roles and learning about roles. Thus the child is trained to participate in society, the rules of which are set by the society, thus proffering a social participation. There are also, of course, psychoanalytic explanations which argue that social organization requires that the sexual drive be sublimated into aim-inhibited forms, allowing formation of groups and networks and fellow feeling. Socialization in the psychoanalytic context can therefore be learnt through identification with the father in the resolution of the Oedipal complex. The acquisition of impulse control is also a key aspect of the actual process of socialization. One of the goals of socialization is to get the child to control negative impulses. Psychological determinism and psychological reductionism illustrate the impact of psychological factors on the individual, and are seen as independent causes of social and cultural behaviours. To make matters more complex, personality itself can be seen as its own culture. This means that the role of the culture becomes even more fundamental in our attempts to understand the relationship. These processes of underlying the achievement embedded within socialization are not necessarily divergent.

The preservation and continuity of distinctive patterns of culture, and their transmission across generations, are key aspects of cultural continuity. Le Vine (1973) argues that some authors and researchers prefer the term enculturation to socialization because enculturation explicitly means acquiring, incorporating or internalizing culture. This process may also reflect ways of communicating information, which in turn are influenced by parenting and child rearing.

Various institutions such as schools, universities, places of employment, all contribute to the processes of socialization and also with the learning of roles and behaviours. Le Vine (1973) reminds us that social institutions can be soft (such as religion, folk tales, art, etc.) or hard (group's ecology, economy, settlement patterns, social stratifications). He argues that soft institutions may place constraints on the individual rather than expressions of their needs. With the 'concretization' of religious institutions with increased bureaucracy and rigidity, it is inevitable that they become more 'traditional', thereby creating further coercion. It is worth noting that when collective activities become institutionalized, the individual's motives may become subsumed. Thus a tension between collectivist expectations and individual motives emerges which can create problems in adjustment as well as creating functioning individuals.

Le Vine (1973) argues that the divisions of institutions into two classes – primary and secondary, maintenance systems and projective systems – one of which constrains an individual's behaviour, whereas the other expresses it, although superficially attractive is also excessively simple and empirically misleading.

It is worth noting that behaviours in any culture are proscribed and punished; proscribed but not punished; permitted but not expected; expected without conscious recognition; consciously expected but not prescribed; prescribed by norms but with informal enforcement procedures; and prescribed by norms but with formal enforcement procedures. Thus it becomes clear that behaviours in personality disorders will be strongly culturally influenced. Face-to-face interactions, looking at each other, looking into one's eyes and other verbal as well as non-verbal cues, are very strongly influenced by cultures. The interaction between culture and individuals is influenced by proximal factors such as norms and expectations and distal factors such as institutions in which the individual participate and accompanying prescriptions and proscriptions.

Le Vine (1973) reminds us that deviance itself is not a unitary phenomenon and that the line between deviance and conformity is less sharp than it may appear at times. Deviance can be exaggeration or norms or as opposition to norms. It can also reflect the breakdown of norms. These three models may represent different ways of looking at types of mental illness. It is also worth recognizing that socio-cultural changes will affect personality.

Changes in personality related to culture may be related to persistence (i.e. no change occurs); breakdown (in social disintegration); progress (i.e. acquiring new forms of competence); and revitalization (which may be accompanied by cultural contraction and cultural expansion). These models can work independently but there may well be some overlap between various outcomes.

Bandura and Walters (1963) provide an early description of social learning and personality development. They argue that in social interactions, reinforcements of the behaviours play a role in changing the personality and behaviour. Some of the behavioural responses include self-control through direct reinforcement. Le Vine (1973) uses a Darwinian approach and argues that the whole development of personality includes processes of determination of character on the grounds of temperament, constitution of a life organization as well as adaptation of character to social demands put upon the personality. Embedded within cultural values and norms is the role of religious symbols, rituals and religious experiences.

Using either of the psychosocial or cultural models, it is self-evident that cultures impact upon personality in a number of ways. Some of this is related to direct influences whereas others may result from indirect factors. The perceived and real centre of power within the community and the culture will also influence the way individual personality develops.

Definitions

There are two current operational definitions of personality disorder. The International Classification of Mental and Behavioural Disorders (ICD-10) (WHO, 1992) defines a personality disorder as: 'a severe disturbance in the characterological condition and behavioural tendencies of the individual, usually involving several areas of the personality, and nearly always associated with considerable personal and social disruption'. The ICD-10 recognizes eight categories, whilst DSM-5 recognizes more categories.

Personality disorders: Within DSM-5 (APA, 2013) more than 12 types of personality disorders have been defined. These include unspecified personality disorders in the whole canon. The DSM-5 divides personality disorders into three clusters based on descriptive similarities. They include cluster A, which has paranoid, schizoid and schizotypal personality disorders, and these individuals appear odd. Cluster B includes antisocial, borderline, histrionic and narcissistic personality disorders, and these individuals often appear anxious, emotional or erratic. The third cluster, or cluster C, includes avoidant, dependent and obsessive–compulsive personality, where individuals appear fearful and anxious. Although these clusters are not validated, they do provide an overview. It must also be recognized that not all personality disorders are confined to specific clusters nor do they have clear boundaries.

General personality disorder, according to DSM-5, shows an enduring pattern of inner experience and behaviour that deviates markedly from the expectations of the individual's culture. The pattern is manifested in two (or more) of the following areas: cognition (ways of perceiving and interpreting the self, others and events); affectivity (i.e. the range, intensity, lability and appropriateness of emotional response); interpersonal functioning and impulse control. The enduring pattern is inflexible and pervasive and leads to clinically significant distress or impairment in social or occupational or other important areas of functioning. The pattern is stable and of long duration and with onset in adolescence or early adulthood. The enduring pattern is not better explained as a manifestation or consequence of another mental disorder and is not attributable to the physiological effects of a substance or another medical condition.

Personality traits are enduring patterns of perceiving, relating to and thinking about the environment and onset that are exhibited in a wide range of social and personality contexts (APA, 2013). Cultural factors must be taken into account and accurate information obtained through reliable sources in order to make sense of an individual's experiences. We do not propose to go through all the categories of personality disorder (interested readers are directed to APA, 2013). It must be emphasized that theoretically at least cultures may well play a bigger role in some types of personality disorder than others (e.g. borderline personality disorder, BPD). Similarly, gender may well play an important role in prevalence of different types of personality disorder. Paris and Lis (2013) and Jani *et al.* (2016), for example, emphasize differences in symptoms of borderline personality disorder in different cultures and note that these differences may be related to environmental factors. Miller *et al.* (2015) showed that Americans are perceived to be narcissistic, disagreeable and antisocial. They identify environmental factors as playing a role in this. Similarly, from China, Zhou *et al.* (2015) reported that Chinese somatization should be seen as distress that traditional values affect the way communication takes place. Barron *et al.* (2015) found that symptoms of schizotypal personality varied between Trinidadian and British males, and Fonseca-Pederero *et al.* (2014) among the Spanish.

Silberschmidt *et al.* (2015) found gender and cultural differences among a clinical trial sample of individuals with borderline personality disorder. Using a self-report psychopathy scale, Horan *et al.* (2014) reported that adolescents from black and Hispanic groups may not show differences from the white population. This intriguing and somewhat unexpected finding needs to be replicated. Raza *et al.* (2014) found that paranoid personality in the USA is also affected by race and illicit drug use. They showed that black individuals are more likely to have paranoid disorders.

Ryder *et al.* (2014) suggest that personality and culture are strongly intertwined. Rossier *et al.* (2013), from their study in Burkina Faso, suggested that cultural differences affect abnormal personality traits. For dependent personality disorder too, Chen *et al.* (2009) caution that there are additional cultural factors which deserve to be taken into account. To develop these observations and further cross-cultural research, Cheung *et al.* (2011) suggest that a combined etic–emic approach to the study of personality is required.

A Brief History of the Term 'Personality Disorder'

Formal personality characterization can be traced back to early Greek society (Tyrer *et al.*, 1991). Aristotle and his student, Theophrastus, developed a literary style known as 'character writing', whereby the essential features of certain common personality types were distilled into pithy verbal portraits. Examples included 'the slanderer' with his 'malevolent disposition of the soul' and the 'flatterer' who degraded himself with 'self-profiting intercourse'. In the fourth century BCE, Hippocrates described a classification of temperament (which was later modified by Galen), based on the four bodily humours: choleric (irascible), melancholic (sad), sanguine (optimistic) and phlegmatic (apathetic). Later, over the centuries, in addition to body fluids, a person's shape, size and even the contour variations in their skull were used to make predictions about the nature of their underlying personality. Tyrer *et al.* (1991) point out that, for many years, the term personality disorder has been imbued with negative qualities of degeneracy (Koch, 1891), untreatability (Maudsley, 1868) and conflict (Henderson, 1939), and a quarter of a century after their observation there appears to be little change. They illustrate eloquently some of the problems associated with the concept of personality and personality disorder. Using Schneider's (1923) definition, which sees personality disorder defined as abnormal personalities who suffer through their abnormality and through whose abnormalities society suffers, they note that this would mean that Himmler and Goering had normal personalities between 1933 and 1939; and Sakharov and Mandela were personality disordered, as they had caused suffering to themselves and to others. As they argue that definitions of personality disorder often intertwine persistent behaviour, attitudes, subjective distress and impact on relationships, a balanced weight should be given to all of these. They caution that, although personality disorder may have the characteristics of enduring traits, this should not be seen as permanent.

The first clinical separation of abnormal personality from mental illness has been attributed to Philippe Pinel, who described a series of patients who had committed impulsive aggressive acts whilst they were in possession of clear intact reasoning (Pinel, 1801). He referred to these cases as *'mania sans delire'* ('insanity without delusion'). The description of behavioural disturbance in the absence of mental illness was later pursued by an American, Benjamin Rush, who believed that there existed certain individuals who suffered from a defect of 'the moral faculties of the mind' (Rush, 1812). In a similar vein, in Britain, Pritchard used the term 'moral insanity' to describe a wide range of diverse emotional conditions which could lead to behaviour deserving social condemnation (Pritchard, 1835). The modern classification of personality disorder came about largely from the clinical observations of Kurt Schneider, who described ten types of pathological personality, which closely resemble the subtypes in the current classification schemes (Schneider, 1958).

Cross-Cultural Perspectives on Personality

Anthropologists have long been aware of cross-cultural differences in the concept of 'person'. Shweder and Bourne (1984) highlight other people's conceptions of the person and ideas about the self. There is no doubt that the concepts of the self vary across cultures (see Morris, 1994). From a psychiatric perspective, however, an alternative concept of the person described by Shweder and Bourne (1984) is that of the phenomenon which looks at the apparently alien concept, belief or value. They suggest that the concept of the *context-dependent* person (italics added) is one expression of a broader socio-centric organic view of the relationship of the individual to society, which in turn is an aspect of the holistic world view adopted by many cultures. The notion of the primacy of the self and how that is developed is an important one, especially if this varies around the socio-centric or ego-centric concepts of the individual and the society.

Morris (1994) argues that the cultural conceptions of the person and the human being as a generic social agent and as a psychological self are important. The Western conceptions of the self, according to Morris (1994), are individualistic with a relatively inflated concern with the self, which in extreme gives rise to anxiety and a sense of narcissism, but it is also materialistic and rationalistic, thereby reflecting the thought of Western culture. The self structure in the West is therefore individuated, detached, separate and self-sufficient, and Morris proposes that the concept of the Western self is to be placed in the context of cultural hegemony of capitalism and of bourgeois mode of thought. We do not propose to dwell on this argument, but raise the possibility that with changes in mode of production in traditional societies it is likely that concepts of the person would shift.

Geertz (1975), for example asserts that the Western conception of the person as a bounded, unique, more or less integrated motivational and cognitive universe. This, however incorrigible it may seem to us, is a rather peculiar idea within the context of the world's cultures.

A characteristic feature of 'Western thinking', noted by many ethnographers, is the tendency to abstract the notion of the 'individual' from the social role. In earlier human communities, a more socio-centric conception of the person has been noted. Within these cultures, the notion of the person is inextricably linked to the performance of social roles. To members of such cultures, the Western concept of the autonomous individual who is free to make choices is alien or even bizarre.

In a seminal paper entitled 'Does the concept of the person vary cross-culturally?', Shweder and Bourne compared the personality descriptions given by 17 American adults, living in Chicago, with those provided by 70 Oriya residents of Bhubaneswar, in the state of Orissa, India (Shweder and Bourne, 1984). In their free descriptions of personality, Oriyas were more concrete than Americans. They described their intimates by reference to behavioural instances and qualified their descriptions by reference to contexts. These differences were shown to be independent of the effects of education, socio-economic status and language and the authors concluded that the difference was a cultural phenomenon – so-called 'creations of the collective imagination'.

The work of Edward Sapir, Margaret Mead and Ruth Benedict has highlighted the existence of important differences in the 'personalities' of cultures (for example, Benedict's classic account of four Plains Indian cultures). It has also been recognized that shared norms of behaviour are essential to the survival of any society (Aberle et al., 1960). However, within any culture, it is acknowledged that some individuals will inevitably fail to conform and will deviate from social norms: 'These abnormals are those individuals who are not supported by the institutions of their civilisation. They are the exceptions who have not easily taken the traditional forms of their culture' (Benedict, 1934). For Benedict, normality was not an absolute quality of personality, but was 'relative to the dominant configuration of one's society'.

The work of the World Health Organization Alcohol, Drug Abuse and Mental Health Administration programme has demonstrated that, in theory, it is possible to assess personality disorder in different nations, languages and cultures using a semi-structured interview (Loranger et al., 1994).

Loranger *et al.* (1994) reported on the use of International Personality Disorder Examination (IPDE) on 716 patients from 14 centres in 11 countries. The IPDE was modified from the Personality Disorder Examination and used nearly 150 criteria over the previous 5 years to reach a diagnosis of personality disorder. Even within the sample, using ICD-10 criteria, 2.4 per cent were diagnosed as having paranoid personality disorder and with DSM-III-R the prevalence was 5.9 per cent. Antisocial personality was diagnosed in 3.2 per cent with ICD-10, but in 6.4 per cent using DSM-III-R. The prevalence of any personality disorder was 39.5 per cent using ICD-10 criteria and 51.1 per cent using DSM-III-R. They do not give findings from each centre, but the two-fold variation within two different classificatory systems presents a significant problem. In their conclusions, the authors argue that these distinctions are of such a degree because in DSM-III-R antisocial personality disorder (ASPD) includes unlawful behaviours and criminal acts, whereas ICD-10 focuses more on generic concepts such as lack of empathy. These authors also point out that the two most frequently diagnosed types in the sample as a whole are disorders that were not included in ICD-9 and DSM-II. These are borderline disorder and avoidant or anxious types. This shift indicates the impact culture and society can have on development and recognition of new diagnoses.

The only personality disorder to have been systematically studied in community surveys of psychiatric morbidity is antisocial personality disorder. Such surveys reveal important cross-cultural differences in the prevalence of this disorder. Rates vary from 0.14 per cent in Taiwan to 3.7 per cent in Canada (de Girolamo and Reich, 1993). Currently, it remains unclear as to whether such differences reflect variations in the 'true' prevalence of the disorder, or differences in the respective 'personalities' of Taiwan and Canada (i.e. reflective of differences in the willingness of Taiwanese and Canadian people to report antisocial behaviour). From the perspectives of anthropology and epidemiology, there is clearly a need for cross-cultural validation of the other personality disorder categories.

Ryder *et al.* (2015) point out that recent large-sample studies suggest that US ethnoracial groups differ in personality disorder diagnostic rates, but also that minority groups are less likely to receive treatment for personality disorder. These authors suggest that studies demonstrate that socio-economic status partly explains group differences between African Americans and European Americans. Balaratnasingam and Janca (2017) looking at Australian Aboriginal groups highlight that making a diagnosis of personality disorder in these groups is complicated by historical trauma from colonization, disruption of kinship networks, and ongoing effects of poverty and social marginalization.

Are Personality Disorders Really Diseases?

A major contribution of medical anthropology has been the distinction between 'disease' and 'illness'. Eisenberg (1977), defines illnesses as 'experiences of discontinuities in states of being and perceived role performances'. Diseases, on the other hand, are 'abnormalities in the function and/or structure of body organs and systems'. Psychiatrists have long disagreed in their concept of disease and consequently the boundaries of psychiatry are inevitably somewhat arbitrary (Kendell, 1975). It has been argued that the absence of consistent physical markers in those regarded as mentally ill means that there is no justification for labelling these people as having a disease – the term 'psychiatric disease' is merely a metaphor for alarming or socially undesirable behaviour (Szasz, 1972). Personality disorders exemplify this problem par excellence as, since the time of Schneider, the definition has stressed socially deviant behaviour. This is particularly unsatisfactory when the society from which normative behaviour is derived, may itself be 'abnormal', for example, Nazi Germany.

The highest rates of personality disorders are found among prisoners. The Office for National Statistics survey of psychiatric morbidity among prisoners in England and Wales found that the prevalence rate of personality disorders was almost 80 per cent in the remand population, with antisocial personality disorder having the highest prevalence rate (Singleton *et al.*, 1998). Defining a large proportion of the population (for example, prisoners) as sick on the basis of social deviance creates major logistical problems for mental health teams, who are then left to deal with the considerable responsibility of caring for and treating these 'sick' individuals. Indeed, over 40 years ago, Schwartz and Schwartz (1976) warned of the damaging effects of forcing psychiatrists 'into a role which is completely out of character with the traditional healing role of physician and has more in common with that of gaoler'.

In addition to concerns relating to the 'disease status' of the personality disorders are problems surrounding the reliability, validity and utility of the diagnosis. Studies of the reliability of the clinical assessment of personality disorder have shown that the agreement between clinicians' diagnoses of personality disorder is often no better than chance (Mellsop *et al.*, 1982), although the use of a standardized instrument does improve the situation. There is a paucity of longitudinal data on these disorders and therefore, the predictive validity of the diagnosis remains uncertain. Perhaps the most alarming indictment of the diagnosis is evidence suggesting that it is a label applied to patients whom health professionals dislike. In a study in which 240 psychiatrists were asked to read case vignettes, patients with an identical history, but given a previous diagnosis of personality disorder in the vignette, were rated as more difficult, annoying, attention-seeking, and less deserving of care compared to control subjects (Lewis and Appleby, 1988).

Morice (1979) argued that there was a general agreement among psychiatrists over some subtypes of personality disorders, but not in differentiating between trait and disorder. Obviously, a high degree of agreement will be seen on the basis of behaviours and lifestyles. He points out that, in the context of transcultural perspective, it is even more difficult to differentiate between trait and disorder. Reporting on rates of personality disorder, he noted a tenfold variation across studies. His ethnocentric interpretation of these findings focuses on emphasis placed on behaviour across different cultural and socioeconomic groups. He illustrates this by giving an example of aborigines using 'sorry cuts' on themselves following bereavement and aggression to others may be interpreted as culturally legitimate behaviour. The high rates of personality disorder are seen as a response by perhaps misinterpreting hostility and aggression. Using a Pintripi–English dictionary, Morice points out that there are many words that denote anger, which can be general state, state of legitimate anger and state of unsanctioned aggressive behaviour.

It is important to note that the definition of personality disorders includes 'social disruption' and it is therefore entirely possible for an individual who has no subjective distress, but who causes societal disturbance, to be labelled as unhealthy or 'diseased' (see the examples cited earlier by Tyrer *et al.* (1991)). The potentially damaging effects of being given a psychiatric label are well documented and may include a negative impact on self-esteem, marginalization and discrimination within society. Such phenomena almost certainly occur in 'personality-disordered' patients, although remain unexplored from an anthropological perspective.

Gender and Personality Disorder

The medical establishment has often been criticized for its patriarchal nature. Psychiatry has not escaped such criticism. It has been argued that a 'male view' of disease continues to dominate psychiatric thinking. Indeed, Kaplan (1983) suggests that masculine-biased assumptions about what behaviours are healthy and what behaviours are crazy are codified in diagnostic criteria; these criteria then influence diagnosis and treatment rates and patterns.

With respect to the personality disorders, women significantly outnumber men in the diagnoses of dependent, histrionic and borderline personality disorders (Russell, 1995). This finding has led to the suggestion that these disorders represent no more than exaggerated sex role stereotypes. For example, the DSM-5 criteria for histrionic personality disorder emphasize 'excessive emotionality', whilst the criteria for dependent personality disorder emphasize 'submissive behaviour' and needing 'others to assume responsibility for most major areas of his/her life'. From a research perspective, there is evidence to suggest that in a clinical setting, although application of the criteria may not be sex-biased, the application of the diagnosis may indeed be (Ford and Widiger, 1989). Similarly, there is evidence showing that although the phenomenology, risk factors, and long-term outcome of borderline and antisocial personality disorders are very similar, borderline personality disorder is more frequently diagnosed among women, whilst antisocial personality disorder occurs more frequently in men. A contemporary epidemiological view is that the difference in prevalence of these conditions reflects biological shaping of a common base of impulsive personality traits (Paris, 1997). However, some anthropologists have suggested that these disorders might be 'spurious' medical labels with cultural histories, representing values strongly congruent with familiar cultural stereotypes: the 'independent' male and the 'dependent' female (Nuckolls, 1992).

Trait-Based Classification

The idea of classifying personality disorder based on dimensional personality traits is a concept that dominates the most recent literature. The big five personality characteristics also known as the five factor model (FFM) include five distinct personality traits: openness, agreeableness, conscientiousness, neuroticism and extroversion. The model when first proposed highlighted a dynamic model of personality where genetic predisposition results in differing temperamental levels of the five basic personality traits. These traits guide goals, attributions, beliefs and the self-concept, which are expressed as a result of external influences including both cultural norms and past live events (McCrae and Costa, 1999).

The model has obtained repeated findings of cross-cultural generalizability beginning from data from originally Filipino and French translations showing clear and detailed replication of the American normative factor structure which is believed to evidence the traits as cross-cultural and abiologically based (McCrae et al., 1998). The reliability of the FFM has been found within further Eastern cultures using an Asian lexicon including Chinese (Church, 2000) and continually evidenced and validated from studies of behaviour genetics, parent–child relations, and the longitudinal stability of individual differences in cross-cultural validity within German, British, Spanish, Czech and Turkish samples ($n = 5,085$) (McCrae et al., 2000). Whilst Rolland (2002) found cross-cultural generalizability in 16 different cultures clearly showing the cross-cultural validity of neuroticism, openness and conscientiousness and more culturally sensitive extraversion and agreeableness traits.

Building upon this cross-cultural validity, research has since begun to link the clinical use of FFM traits within the diagnosis of personality disorder, first proposed by Costa and Widiger (1994). Saulsman and Page (2004) have investigated this possibility using 15 independent samples analysing how personality disorders are different and similar with regard to underlying FFM personality traits. Results showed that each disorder displays a five-factor model profile that is meaningful and predictable given its unique diagnostic criteria. Findings revealed that the most predominantly consistent personality dimensions underlying a large number of the personality disorders are positive associations with neuroticism and negative associations with agreeableness. The results evidence how the use of FFM could potentially help with regard to obtaining a cross-cultural clarification system for personality disorder assessment and treatment.

Presentation of Early Symptoms

When typically considering epidemiology within medicine we are referring to the analysis of patterns, causes and effects of health and disease conditions in defined populations. However, to apply normal epidemiological principles in the study of personality disorder we would have to assume a heterogeneity of presentation in the symptoms. When considering BPD and ASPD across cultures we see two very distinct differences in terms of presentation. Antisocial personality disorder is a global and cultural phenomenon often referred to colloquially as 'psychopathy' and 'sociopathy'. The classifications of ASPD appear pan cultural, with prevalence and diagnosis levels appearing to have increased overtime (Kessler et al., 1994). Borderline personality disorder, however, appears to vary both in terms of cross-cultural prevalence and clinical presentation (Jani et al., 2016).

One of the potential issues affecting the presentation of symptoms is the cultural boundaries by which we define them. Such a question fractures the field of study into two distinct philosophical ideas to the exact reason for the presenting symptomatic behaviours: a deviation from scientifically agreed cognitive-behavioural norms or simply socio-cultural differences? When exploring cultural variations the obvious differences fall between ego-centric and socio-centric societies as has already been discussed in Chapter 12 on Psychopathology. As previous research has noted these values are reflected within the Chinese psychiatric diagnostic system, which rarely considers a diagnosis of personality disorder due to the high individualistic nature of symptomology (Tang and Huang, 1995). China specifically doesn't even categorize the symptoms of BPD (Yang et al., 2000) therefore resulting in low to non-existent levels of BPD diagnosis.

More recent research has observed this difference in Western and Eastern cultural values and its effect on the presentation and development of psychopathology. Caldwell-Harris and Ayçiçegi (2006) administered clinical and personality scales to a non-clinical sample of students studying in either an individualist culture (Boston, USA) or a collectivist culture (Istanbul, Turkey). For students residing in Boston, collectivism scores were positively correlated with depression, anxiety and dependent personality. Individualism scores negatively correlated with these traits. The opposite was obtained for students residing in Istanbul where individualism positively correlated with scales for borderline and antisocial personality disorder. Collectivism was associated with low report of symptoms on these scales. The results not only show the differences in values between Eastern and Western society but also indicate having a personality style which conflicts with the values of society is associated with psychiatric symptoms, in particular, personality disorder. Investigating personality disorder prevalence within the United States, Grant *et al.* (2008) used face-to-face interviews with 34,653 adults participating in the Wave 2 National Epidemiologic Survey on Alcohol and Related Conditions to find the lifetime prevalence of BPD to be 5.9% (99% CI: 5.4–6.4). There were no significant differences in the rates of BPD between men (5.6%, 99% CI: 5.0–6.2) and women (6.2%, 99% CI: 5.6–6.9). Borderline personality disorder was, however, more prevalent among Native American men, younger and separated/divorced adults, and those with lower incomes and education. It was less prevalent among Hispanic men and women and Asian women. What the results of this research demonstrate is as expected those living chaotic lives or within lower socio-economic environments have a higher incidence of BPD. Interestingly, however, the study did show that the disorder was less prevalent in Americans with Asian or Central/South American heritage, suggesting that personality disorder varies not only between cultures but also within.

In addition Coid *et al.* (2006) found differing levels of prevalence even within Western culture when conducting research on UK personality disorder prevalence. They used a structured clinical interview for DSM-IV Axis II disorders in 626 persons aged 16–74 years in households across England, Scotland and Wales in a two-phase survey. The weighted prevalence of personality disorder was 4.4 per cent (95% CI: 2.9–6.7). The prevalence of borderline personality disorder was, however, far lower than that found in the US by Grant *et al.* (2008) at around 0.7 per cent and ASPD at around 1.2 per cent. This a number similarly supported by Torgerson *et al.* (2001) who found prevalence of BPD to again be around the level of 0.7 per cent and ASPD around 1.3 per cent within Norwegian society. What these studies begin to highlight is increasingly relevant variance within Western culture

and the population of a country than simply just a Western and Eastern divide. Raffi and Malik (2010) highlight cultural difference of personality diagnosis within a single culture, evidencing how personality disorder prevalence appears to vary depending on clinical sub-group. Using a cross-sectional survey of a sample of 6,531 psychiatric inpatients collected over a 2-year period (2007–2009), respondents were divided into one of two categories: white British and black minority ethnic. Within this sample 273 patients (4.2%) were diagnosed with personality disorder, 23 (8.4%) were black and minority ethnic patients and 250 (91.6%) were white British patients. The most common diagnosis was BPD (184 cases). From these figures black patients appear far less likely to be diagnosed with a personality disorder. Results suggest an underdiagnosis within the clinical practice building on growing evidence that the way in which psychological distress is presented, perceived and interpreted differs between individuals from different cultures. It proposes that different cultures develop different responses and mechanisms for coping with psychological distress. The study also highlights that cultural and racial stereotyping are common in the context of assessing and diagnosing personality disorder adding another confounding factor for cross-cultural presentation of personality disorder.

Given the previous evidence stating the effect of 'culture clash' on mental development (Caldwell-Harris and Ayçiçegi, 2006) one would expect the incidence of personality disorder to be higher within black minority ethnic and other immigrant groups. In fact the inverse is seen with personality disorder diagnosis lower within non-indigenous groups. The literature struggles to fully suggest why this may occur. Racial and cultural bias in psychiatric assessment and subsequent diagnosis is one proposed theory (Raffi and Malik, 2010). With an increase incidence of schizophrenia reported in immigrant groups (Cantor-Graae, and Selten, 2005), are the symptoms of ASPD and BPD being misdiagnosed within immigrant and minority groups?

Role of Environment in Personality Disorder Development

As previously mentioned, individuals with characteristics who fit well in a given environment adapt better and have healthier psychological development (Caldwell-Harris and Ayçiçegi, 2006). Such a concept is demonstrated in areas of behavioural genetics where the roles of both socio-cultural and socio-economic environment are evidenced to have a modifying effect on the psychological development of personality disorder.

The relationship itself is bi-directional, suggesting that genotype can influence an individual's decision to expose themselves to certain environments, how that individual experiences the environment and the degree of influence that certain environments exert. This is referred to in the literature as a gene–environment correlation (Dick, 2005). Gene–environment correlations have been shown specifically for the development of antisocial behaviour in children as a result of negative parenting, with the child having a genetic propensity for being antisocial, antisocial parents who may parent badly and the child evoking negative responses from others (Larsson *et al.* 2008). It is likely that such an explanation could also be applied to the 'goodness of fit' interaction between culture and personality. The theory could be taken further to provide an evolutionary perspective on how cultural values and norms have developed over time.

In addition, genetic personality temperament and environment do not just correlate but there also appears to be a modifying effect in what is specifically named within the field as gene–environment interaction. Overview of research using a variety of experimental designs including twin studies, molecular genetics and magnetic resonance imaging (MRI) shows traits present in personality disorder such as high levels of callous unemotional traits are modified by environmental influence (Viding and McCrory, 2012). Meta-analysis of such gene–environment interactions shows repeated statistical significance for a specific interaction between mono-amine oxidase A (MAOA) and childhood maltreatment with the risk of later development of ASPD (Taylor and Kim-Cohen, 2007). These results indicate that the type of environment an individual is exposed to in fact can modify the genetically predisposed expression of personality disorder.

Whilst the above study looks specifically at immediate familial environment it stands to reason the results could generalize to an individual's cultural environmental experience. As evolutionary psychologists would argue the universal reason for personality traits is to aid survival. 'The derivation of behaviour is prone to expression under certain environmental conditions.' Whilst usually associated with high levels of mortality (NICE, 2009) the development of

antisocial behaviour would be beneficial for individuals with ASPD or BPD given a developmental socio-cultural background of potential stress and deprivation (Fabrega, 2006).

The Health-Seeking Behaviour of Personality-Disordered Patients

It has been suggested that the word 'illness' stands for 'what the patient feels when he goes to the doctor', and 'disease' for 'what he has on the way home from the doctor's office' (Helman, 1998). With the exception of users of psychotherapy services, in Western society, it is unusual for someone to visit a doctor complaining of personality difficulties. The label of 'personality disorder' is more usually 'earned' as a result of displaying certain 'dysfunctional personality traits' to the doctor, such as a repeated need for 'excessive reassurance', or 'demanding' and 'manipulative' behaviour. (Arguably the diagnosis may have as much to do with the personality of the clinician as it does with that of the patient!) Unlike other mental and physical disorders, the diagnosis will rarely be shared with the patient, as there is no specific 'treatment'. However, the doctor may record the diagnosis in the case notes and will certainly make a mental note of the difficult encounter. Indeed, there is substantial evidence to show that the diagnosis is frequently made in psychiatric settings, where prevalence rates of personality disorder may be as high as 30–40 per cent (de Girolamo and Reich, 1993). General practitioners are frequently able to identify their 'heartsink' patients, although the extent to which this term overlaps with personality disorder remains unexplored. Personality disorder is also a common diagnosis among so-called 'revolving-door patients' (Saarento *et al.*, 1997). Such patients are defined by their frequent use of health services. However, in this context, the diagnosis seems to add little to the treatment plan, as the patient's difficult behaviour, i.e. frequent use of services, is merely reformulated as a symptom of their underlying psychopathology, i.e. a personality disorder. Perhaps a more informed approach is to attempt to disentangle the patient's specific needs (e.g. psychological symptoms, such as feelings of hopelessness) rather than merely arriving at the rather unhelpful diagnosis of personality disorder – a diagnosis which may only serve to engender therapeutic nihilism.

Smith (1990) in a small-scale study gave a 40 item Narcissistic Personality Inventory to 14 Asian, 58 Caucasian and 16 Hispanic American women attending college. The Asian group comprised Chinese, Japanese, Filipino and Vietnamese women, thereby illustrating cultural heterogeneity, whereas Hispanic women were primarily of Mexican descent. Mean narcissism scores for Asian women were dramatically lower than those for Caucasian women, especially on authority, exhibitionism, superiority and vanity. The cultural norms, which expect these women to be submissive, may be playing a role here. Bearing in mind that numbers are small and attending college, it is difficult to generalize these findings. However, these findings indicate that there may well be cultural differences in personality traits. Lasch (1979) had noted an increase in trend of narcissism in the USA in the 1970s.

Borderline personality disorder (BPD) is characterized by impulsive behaviour, repetitive parasuicide, affective instability and unstable intimate relationships. Paris (1996a) argues that BPD is sensitive to socio-cultural context and is probably less frequent in traditional societies. Patients in traditional societies are said to have more classical neurotic symptoms and fever behavioural ones (Murphy, 1982) which could be explained by family structure and kinship patterns which may not encourage expression of emotion. Thus, conversion systems may be more prevalent in traditional societies. Antisocial personality disorder (ASPD) is seen rarely in East Asian societies (Hwu et al., 1989) and Japan (Sato and Takeichi, 1993). Paris (1996b) argues that the societies which have lower rates of ASPD are more cohesive socially, which makes the development of antisocial pathology less likely. It is possible that the notion of shame and bringing dishonour especially to the family are strong deterrents. Antisocial pathology shares a common dimension of impulsivity with BDP, but related to concept of the self the impulsive behaviour will differ against the individual self or social self. Antisocial personality disorder is reported more commonly in males and BPD in females, and therefore it is likely that the two conditions are somehow variants of the same personality type and their different behaviour manifestations reflect the effects of gender (Paris, 1994) but may also be linked with gender roles and gender role expectations. Paris (1996a) also emphasizes that the prevalence of the most characteristic symptom of BPD – repetitive parasuicide – shows a sensitivity to cultural context. Furthermore, there is

the suggestion that BPD is becoming more common in North America (Millon, 1993). The risk factors for BPD include trauma, emotional neglect, family dysfunction and parental separation or loss (Paris, 1994). Millon (1993) hypothesizes that borderline pathology emerges under conditions of rapid social change and in the presence of breakdown of community norms and values. This will fit in with a potential increase of the condition in ego-centric or individualistic societies and is less likely to occur in socio-centric or collective societies. Paris (1996a, b) suggests that children growing up in dysfunctional families in traditional societies have more opportunities (or likelihood) to buffer the effects of negative experiences, thus the extended or joint family may absorb some of the trauma. Those children who make attachments outside the nuclear family are less likely to develop responses to pathology in their parents (Kaufman et al., 1979). Thus extended family members in collectivist societies may provide role models and support. It is also likely that collectivist societies reward those behaviours which are associated with group cohesion and discourage behaviours which are associated with individualism.

In her comments on the observations of Paris (1996a), Miller (1996) focuses on the heterogeneity of individuals within cultures. She indicates that comparable disorders may exist in other cultures. All cultures contain some individuals who perceive themselves to be unable to meet what is expected of them, and how the resultant distress is expressed differs across cultures, as does the response to it. Miller illustrates this by indicating that feeling good and the pursuit of happiness as a constitutional right is common in the US, whereas despair may have different meanings.

Treatment and Prognosis

The cultural difficulties within psychiatric assessment and diagnosis of personality disorder may also reflect within the current difficulty in successfully treating personality disorder. Despite changes in NICE guidelines (2009) addressing clinician's negative attitudes towards personality disorder, especially with regard to treatment neglect, recent evidence suggests these attitudes still exist.

Chartonas and colleagues (2016), using Lewis and Appleby's (1988) questionnaire Attitudes to Personality Disorder Questionnaire (APDQ), block randomized

166 psychiatric trainees in the UK to receive one of four case vignettes (varied by diagnosis and ethnic group) comparing BPD and depression. Seventy-six responses showed attitudes towards personality disorder appeared more negative than with depression and with significantly less sense of purpose when working with personality disorder. In sub-group analysis, only the white British patient group was there significantly more negative attitudes to personality disorder (Chartonas et al., 2016). The results indicate that personality disorder prevalence has negative impact on attitude, treatment and perceived prognosis for psychiatrists working with such patients in comparison to other psychopathologies. The lower effect of negative attitude in ethnic groups could again demonstrate the underdiagnoses and recognizing of personality disorder symptoms in individuals of black minority ethnic backgrounds as found by Raffi and Malik (2010).

One proposed reason for such attitudes could be due to the inability to fully treat the symptoms of personality disorder with medication. Martean and Evans (2014) using a qualitative design again in the UK explored the experiences of general and forensic psychiatrists within the National Health Service (NHS). Data was obtained through semi-structured interviews (with a sample size of 11) transcribed and analysed using thematic analyses. Results showed powerful relational effects and lack of available treatments resulted in psychiatrists feeling helpless, with a decrease in their confidence as a doctor and feeling a pressure to prescribe unnecessarily, not only to provide a solution to symptoms but also to prevent conflict and preserve the doctor–patient relationship.

Difficulty within treatment may in part be due to the medical approach to treatment as guided by usual psychiatric diagnosis. Medicalization of symptoms, in particular in North America, can be seen as a Western cultural response to mental illness and in particular culturally sensitive 'externalized' (Mulder et al., 2011) behaviours. In non-Western cultures such deviations from cultural norms would require civil and familial modes of resolution rather than medical intervention (Watters, 2010). In following with this line of thought it is psychosocial treatments that gain the most evidence base in terms of positive personality disorder treatment outcomes within the current clinical guidelines (NICE, 2009).

Evidence for cognitive-behavioural therapy (CBT) and psychoanalytical intervention for personality disorder has been found within cross-Western societies including the US (Leichsenring and Leibing, 2003) and more recently a combined CBT psychoanalytic intervention, mentalization based therapy (MBT) within the UK found benefits for patients with comorbid BPD and ASPD in the reduction of anger, hostility, paranoia, frequency of self-harm/suicide attempts, and improvement of negative mood, general psychiatric symptoms, interpersonal problems, and social adjustment (Bateman et al., 2016). However, within the current UK mental health system patients diagnosed with BPD and ASPD often do not receive the level of psychosocial support they require (NICE, 2009), and even less so within minority cultural groups, such as black patients under-represented in psychotherapy services and are thus less likely to be offered psychological therapy for personality disorder (Raffi and Malik, 2010).

When looking at the DSM-5 and its ability to provide cross-cultural diagnostic criteria for which similar clinical interventions can then be applied, we must acknowledge that whilst it is a global framework the manual establishes universal definitions for disorders without fully acknowledging cross-cultural variation. Cultural psychiatrists looking specifically at this issue will note key issues such as non-Western illness categories being omitted or consigned to a glossary on 'culture-bound' syndromes but in contrast, Western diagnoses such as eating disorders are deemed universal, highlighting the bias. In addition most evidence the DSM relies upon is through studies conducted for short periods in Western, middle-class, educated young people often without comorbidities. These results are then generalized to other populations. Aggarwal (2013) highlights the DSM's hesitation in treating findings from cultural psychiatry and the social sciences with the same authority accorded to 'evidence' from medicine as one of its key flaws.

In response to such criticism the literature suggests considering a shift to the dimensional classification of personality disorder in response to the failures with the DSM's diagnostic categories and integrating psychiatric with personality structure research being conducted by psychology (Widiger and Trull, 2007). By integrating normal and abnormal conceptualization of personality classification (Widiger and Costa, 2012) and understanding the DSM categories as extreme maladaptive variants of the FFM, the advantages of switching to such a conceptualization benefit both assessment and measuring of treatment outcomes.

Assessment could be carried out based on psycho-metric measures of the five personality traits to see which are at abnormal levels with psychosocial intervention focusing on positive outcome measures at the targeted personality dimension addressed as needing treatment (Widiger and Presnall, 2013).

When reviewing the current literature for the cross-cultural differences in personality disorder, specifically cluster B antisocial and borderline types, we see interesting differences in presentation. Not surprisingly cultural variations in particular differing traditional collectivist or socio-centric and modern individualistic/ego-centric societies alter this presentation. With personality disorder diagnosis highest in the US (Grant *et al.*, 2008) and not diagnostically classified in Chinese culture (Yang *et al.*, 2000) research suggests that 'culture shock' in relation to having a personality style which conflicts with the values of society is associated with higher levels of personality disorder aetiology (Caldwell-Harris and Ayçiçegi, 2006). This is in keeping with evidence from behavioural genetics showing the modifying effect of environment on genetic trait expression of personality traits, particularly antisocial behaviour (Viding and McCrory, 2012)

Cultural variation in presentation not only differentiates between rates of prevalence in Western and Eastern societies but also for the assessment and diagnosis of personality disorder between cultural groups within a society (Raffi and Malik, 2010). Immigrants show lower levels of personality diagnosis than indigenous groups, throwing into question a personality 'goodness of fit' cultural explanation. When exploring cultural variations using large samples through meta-analysis or alternative personality measuring criteria, stable, cross-culturally generalizable factors have been found (Mulder *et al.* 2011). Such findings raise current concerns with culturally biased diagnostic criteria with researchers calling for a more unified dimensional-based categorization system to reduce cross-cultural bias and improve identification of varied presentation of personality disorder based on environmental factors such as culture (Aggarwal, 2013; Jani *et al.* 2016).

Adopting a trait-based classification system for the use of personality disorder diagnosis is proposed, with many researchers suggesting the Five Factor Model (Costa and McCrae, 1998) due to its level of cross-cultural validity and links with explaining pathological personality traits as the combination of environmental influence on genetic propensity. The five traits, openness, agreeableness, conscientiousness, neuroticism and extroversion, have been shown to correlate with each personality disorder profile which in turn has led to the belief they could be used as both cross-cultural diagnostic criteria and psychosocial treatment outcome measures (Widiger and Presnall, 2013).

A Need to Redefine Personality Variation in the Social Context?

The political–economic approach (Ackerknecht, 1943) within medical anthropology attempts to recontextualize disease in a broader social setting. In western countries over the past 50 years, there has been a progressive 'medicalization' of social problems and everyday life. As Ackerknecht (1943) observed 'one of the characteristic mental traits of our culture is the labelling of phenomena with psychiatric diagnoses', and tragically 70 years on in many settings this continues to be the case. Doctors have found themselves increasingly concerned with the 'diagnosis' and treatment of socially unacceptable behaviours. It should be emphasized that the medical profession has not merely been a passive participant in the process of medicalization. Indeed, psychiatrists have often exacerbated the process by invoking 'biopsychosocial' explanations for many of society's problems. As Frankenberg (1980) notes, such explanations may serve a convenient function in advanced capitalist societies where 'making conflicts social is too threatening'.

Currently in the UK and, in part, fuelled by these explanations, there is an expectation that psychiatrists should be able to prevent serious violence. A recent series of highly publicized crimes committed by people with personality disorders has heightened anxiety about violent crime. This has prompted the UK government to respond with a proposal for new legislation, which would include the 'indeterminate reviewable detention' and compulsory treatment of people who have a 'dangerous severe personality disorder' (Hansard, 1999). The government's proposals have provoked angry debate within the medical profession, although broad professional consensus about the utility of the diagnosis antisocial personality disorder is lacking.

Antisocial personality disorder is heavily over-represented among low social classes (Kessler *et al.*, 1994) and individuals with the disorder invariably report histories of childhood abuse and neglect –

phenomena which have been shown to be strongly associated with poverty. Quite apart from the fact that violence is as much a comment on the society in which we live, and not a medical disorder, it would seem that if enacted, the proposed legislation could result in the further marginalization of an already disadvantaged section of our society. If there was ever a need to 'make disease social', it is in the arena of antisocial personality disorder.

Conclusions

From an anthropological perspective, it has been shown that there are substantial problems with the diagnosis of personality disorder. The term does not adequately meet the criteria for a 'disease' and may be misapplied with potentially dangerous consequences. In addition, little data exists to demonstrate that these disorders occur outside Western cultures. Further research is needed. From an anthropological perspective, there appears to be a particular need to explore the illness narratives of people who have been given the diagnosis. If certain universal themes were to emerge from these narratives, this might then lend some support for the current Western psychiatric classification of these disorders. Finally, it must be emphasized that deviancy is a relative social construct and not an absolute fixed entity. From a political economic perspective, a plea has been made to redefine personality variation within its proper social context.

References

Aberle, D. F., Cohen, A. K., Davis, A., Levy, M. and Sutton, F. X. (1960). The functional prerequisites of a society. *Ethics*, **60**, 100–111.

Ackerknecht, E. (1943). Psychopathology, primitive medicine and primitive culture. *Bulletin of the History of Medicine*, **14**, 30–67.

Aggarwal, N. K. (2013). From DSM-IV to DSM-5: an interim report from a cultural psychiatry perspective. *The Psychiatrist Online*, **37**(5), 171–174.

American Psychiatric Association (2013). *Diagnostic and Statistical Manual of Mental Disorders*, 5th edn. Washington DC: American Psychiatric Association.

Balaratnasingam, S. and Janca, A. (2017). Culture and personality disorder: a focus on indigenous Australians. *Current Opinion in Psychiatry*, **30**, 31–35.

Bandura, A. and Walters, R. E. (1963). *Social Learning and Personality Development*. New York: Holt, Rinehart and Winston.

Barron, D., Swami, V., Towell, T., Hutchinson, G., Morgan, K. D. (2015). Examination of the factor structure of the Schizotypal Personality Questionnaire among British and Trinidadian adults. *BioMed Research International*, 258275.

Bateman, A., O'Connell, J., Lorenzini, N., Gardner, T. and Fonagy, P. (2016). A randomised controlled trial of mentalization-based treatment versus structured clinical management for patients with comorbid borderline personality disorder and antisocial personality disorder. *BMC Psychiatry*, **16**(1), 304.

Benedict, R. F. (1934). Anthropology and the abnormal. *Journal of General Psychology*, **10**, 59–82.

Caldwell-Harris, C. L. and Ayçiçegi, A. (2006). When personality and culture clash: the psychological distress of allocentrics in an individualist culture and idiocentrics in a collectivist culture. *Transcultural Psychiatry*, **43**(3), 331–361.

Cantor-Graae, E. and Selten, J. P. (2005). Schizophrenia and migration: a meta-analysis and review. *American Journal of Psychiatry*, **162**(1), 12–24.

Chartonas, D., Kyratsous, M., Dracass, S., Lee, T. and Bhui, K. (2016). Personality disorder: still the patients psychiatrists dislike? *BJPsych Bulletin*, **41**(1), 12–17.

Chen, Y., Nettles, M. E., Chen, S. W. (2009). Rethinking dependent personality disorder: comparing different human relatedness in cultural contexts. *Journal of Nervous and Mental Disease*, **197**(11), 793–800.

Cheung, F. M., van de Vijver, F. J., Leong, F. T. (2011). Toward a new approach to the study of personality in culture. *American Psychologist*, **66**, 593–603.

Child, J. I. (1968). Personality in culture. In *Handbook of Personality Theory and Research*, ed. E. F. Borgatta and W. W. Lambert. Chicago: Rand McNally.

Church, A. T. (2000). Culture and personality: toward an integrated cultural trait psychology. *Journal of Personality*, **68**(4), 651–703.

Coid, J., Yang, M., Tyrer, P., Roberts, A. and Ullrich, S. (2006). Prevalence and correlates of personality disorder in Great Britain. *The British Journal of Psychiatry*, **188**(5), 423–431.

Costa, P. T., Jr and Widiger, T. A. (1994). *Personality Disorders and the Five-Factor Model of Personality*. Washington DC: American Psychological Association.

De Girolamo, G. and Reich, J. H. (1993). *Personality Disorders*. Geneva: WHO.

Dick, D. M. (2005). Gene–Environment Correlation. In *Encyclopedia of Statistics in Behavioural Science*, ed. B. Everitt and D. Howell. Chichester: John Wiley & Sons, Ltd.

Eisenberg, L. (1977). Disease and illness: distinctions between professional and popular ideas of sickness. *Culture, Medicine and Psychiatry*, **1**, 9–23.

Fabrega, H. (2006). Why psychiatric conditions are special: an evolutionary and cross-cultural perspective. *Perspectives in Biology and Medicine*, **49**(4), 586–601.

Fonseca-Pedrero, E., Compton, M. T., Tone, E. B., Ortuño-Sierra, J., Paino, M., Fumero, A., Lemos-Giráldez, S. (2014). Cross-cultural invariance of the factor structure of the Schizotypal Personality Questionnaire across Spanish and American college students. *Psychiatry Research*, **220**, 1071–1076.

Ford, M. R. and Widiger, T. A. (1989). Sex bias in the diagnosis of histrionic and antisocial personality disorders. *Journal of Consulting and Clinical Psychology*, **57**, 301–305.

Frankenberg, R. (1980). Medical anthropology and development: a theoretical perspective. *Social Science and Medicine*, **14**(B), 197–207.

Geertz, C. (1975). *The Interpretation of Cultures*. London: Hutchinson.

Grant, B. F., Chou, S. P., Goldstein, R. B. *et al.* (2008). Prevalence, correlates, disability, and comorbidity of DSM-IV borderline personality disorder: results from the Wave 2 National Epidemiologic Survey on Alcohol and Related Conditions. *The Journal of Clinical Psychiatry*, **69**(4), 533.

Hansard (1999). 15 February: columns 601–603.

Helman, C. G. (1998). Doctor–patient interactions. In *Culture, Health and Illness*. Oxford: Heinemann-Butterworth.

Henderson, D. K. (1939). *Psychopathic States*. New York: W. W. Norton.

Horan, J. M., Brown, J. L., Jones, S. M., Aber, J. L (2014). Assessing invariance across sex and race/ethnicity in measures of youth psychopathic characteristics. *Psychological Assessment* **27**, 657–68.

Hwu, H. G., Yeh, E. K. and Change, L. Y. (1989). Prevalence of psychiatric disorders in Taiwan defined by the Chinese Diagnostic Interview Schedule. *Acta Psychiatrica Scandinavica*, **79**, 136–147.

Jani, S., Johnson, R. S., Banu, S. and Shah, A. (2016). Cross-cultural bias in the diagnosis of borderline personality disorder. *Bulletin of the Menninger Clinic*, **80**, 146–165.

Kaplan, M. (1983). A woman's view of DSM-III. *American Psychologist*, **38**, 786–792.

Kaufman, A. S., Wood, M. M. and Swan, W. W. (1979). Dimensions of problem behaviours of emotionally disturbed children as seen by their parents and teachers. *Psychology in the Schools*, **16**, 207–217.

Kendell, R. E. (1975). The concept of disease and its implications for psychiatry. *British Journal of Psychiatry*, **127**, 305–315.

Kessler, R. C. (1994). The national comorbidity survey of the United States. *International Review of Psychiatry*, **6**(4), 365–376.

Kessler, R. C., McGonagle, K. A., Zao, S. *et al.* (1994). Lifetime and 12-month prevalence of DSM-III-R psychiatric disorders in the United States: results from the National Comorbidity Survey. *Archives of General Psychiatry*, **51**, 8–19.

Koch, J. L. A. (1891). *Die Psychopathischen Minderwerigkeiten*. Dorn: Ravensburg.

Larsson, H., Viding, E., Rijsdijk, F. V. and Plomin, R. (2008). Relationships between parental negativity and childhood antisocial behaviour over time: a bi-directional effects model in a longitudinal genetically informative design. *Journal of Abnormal Child Psychology*, **36**(5), 633–645.

Lasch, C. (1979). *The Culture of Narcissism: American Life in an Age of Diminishing Expectations*. New York: W. W. Norton.

Le Vine, R. L. (1973). *Culture, Behaviour and Personality*. London: Hutchinson.

Lewis, G. and Appleby, L. (1988). Personality disorder: the patients psychiatrists dislike. *British Journal of Psychiatry*, **153**, 44–49.

Loranger, A. W., Sartorius, N., Andreoli, A. *et al.* (1994). The International Personality Disorder Examination (IPDE). The World Health Organization/Alcohol, Drug Abuse and Mental Health Administration International Pilot Study of Personality Disorders. *Archives of General Psychiatry*, **51**, 215–224.

Maudsley, H. (1868). *A Physiology and Pathology of Mind*, 2nd edn. London: Macmillan.

McCrae, R. R. and Costa, P. T., Jr (1999). A five-factor theory of personality. *Handbook of Personality: Theory and Research*, **2**, 139–153.

McCrae, R. R., Costa, P. T., Del Pilar, G. H., Rolland, J. P. and Parker, W. D. (1998). Cross-cultural assessment of the five-factor model: the revised NEO personality inventory. *Journal of Cross-Cultural Psychology*, **29**(1), 171–188.

McCrae, R. R., Costa, P. T., Jr, Ostendorf, F., Angleitner, A., Hřebíčková, M., Avia, M. D. and Saunders, P. R. (2000). Nature over nurture: temperament, personality, and life span development. *Journal of Personality and Social Psychology*, **78**(1), 173.

Mellsop, G., Varghese, F. T. N., Joshua, S. and Hicks, A. (1982). Reliability of Axis II of DSM-III. *American Journal of Psychiatry*, **139**, 1360–1361.

Miller, J. D., Maples, J. L., Buffardi, L. *et al.* (2015). Narcissism and United States' culture: the view from home and around the world. *Journal of Personality and Social Psychology*, **109**, 1068–1089.

Miller, S. G. (1996). Borderline personality disorders in cultural context: commentary on Paris. *Psychiatry*, **59**, 193–195.

Millon, T. (1993). Borderline personality disorder: a psychosocial epidemic. In *Borderline Personality Disorder: Aetiology and Treatment*, ed. J. Paris. Washington DC: American Psychiatric Press, pp. 197–210.

Morice, R. (1979). Personality disorder in transcultural practice. *Australian and New Zealand Journal of Psychiatry*, **13**, 293–300.

Morris, B. (1994). *Anthropology of the Self*. London: Pluto Press.

Murphy, H.B.M. (1982). *Comparative Psychiatry*. New York: Springer.

Nuckolls, C. W. (1992). Toward a cultural history of the personality disorders. *Social Science and Medicine*, **35**, 37–47.

Paris, J. (1994). *Borderline Personality Disorder: A Multidimensional Approach*. Washington DC: American Psychiatric Press.

Paris, J. (1996a). Cultural factors in the emergence of borderline pathology. *Psychiatry*, **59**, 185–192.

Paris, J. (1996b). *Social Factors in the Personality Disorders: A Biopsychosocial Approach to Aetiology and Treatment*. Cambridge: Cambridge University Press.

Paris, J. (1997). Antisocial and borderline personality disorders: two aspects of the same psychopathology. *Comprehensive Psychiatry*, **38**, 237–242.

Paris, J. (1998). Personality disorders in sociocultural perspective. *Journal of Personality Disorders*, **12**(4), 289–301.

Paris, J. and Lis, E. (2013). Can sociocultural and historical mechanisms influence the development of borderline personality disorder? *Transcultural Psychiatry* **50**, 140–151.

Pinel, P. (1801). *Traité médico-philosophique sur l'alienaition mentale*. Paris: Richard, Caille et Ravier.

Pritchard, J. C. (1835). *A Treatise on Insanity*. London: Sherwood, Gilbert and Piper.

Raffi, A., and Malik, A. (2010). Ethnic distribution of personality disorder. *The Psychiatrist*, **34**(1), 36–37.

Raza, G. T., DeMarce, J. M., Lash, S. J., Parker, J. D. (2014). Paranoid personality disorder in the United States: the role of race, illicit drug use, and income. *Journal of Ethnicity in Substance Abuse*, **13**, 247–257.

Rolland, J. P. (2002). The cross-cultural generalizability of the five-factor model of personality. In *The Five-Factor Model of Personality across Cultures*, ed. R. McCrae and J. Allik, New York: Springer, pp. 7–28.

Rossier, J., Ouedraogo, A., Dahourou, D., Verardi, S., de Stadelhofen, F. M. (2013). Personality and personality disorders in urban and rural Africa: results from a field trial in Burkina Faso. *Frontiers in Psychology*, **11**(4), 79.

Rush, B. (1812). *Medical Inquiries and Observations on the Diseases of the Mind*. Philadelphia: Kimber and Richardson.

Russell, D. (1995). *Woman, Madness and Medicine*. Oxford: Blackwell.

Ryder, A. G., Sun, J., Dere, J., Fung, K. (2014). Personality disorders in Asians: summary, and a call for cultural research. *Asian Journal of Psychiatry*, **7**, 86–88.

Ryder, A. G., Sunohara, M., Kirmayer, L. J. (2015). Culture and personality disorder: from a fragmented literature to a contextually grounded alternative. *Current Opinion in Psychiatry*, **28**, 404–405.

Saarento, O., Nieminen, P., Hakko, H., Isohanni, M. and Vaisanen, E. (1997). Utilization of psychiatric inpatient care among new patients in a comprehensive community-care system: a 3-year follow-up study. *Acta Psychiatrica Scandinavica*, **95**, 132–139.

Sato, T. and Takeichi, M. (1993). Lifetime prevalence of specific psychiatric disorders in a general medicine clinic. *General Hospital Psychiatry*, **15**, 224–233.

Saulsman, L. M. and Page, A. C. (2004). The five-factor model and personality disorder empirical literature: a meta-analytic review. *Clinical Psychology Review*, **23**(8), 1055–1085.

Schneider, K. (1923). *Die Psychopathischen Persönalichkeiten*. Berlin: Springer.

Schneider, K. (1958). *Psychopathic Personalities*. London: Cassell.

Schwartz, R. A. and Schwartz, I. K. (1976). Are personality disorders diseases? *Diseases of the Nervous System*, **86**, 613–617.

Shweder, R. A. and Bourne, E. J. (1984). Does the concept of the person vary cross-culturally? In *Culture Theory: Essays on Mind, Self, and Emotion*, ed. R. A. Shweder and R. A. LeVine, Cambridge: Cambridge University Press, pp. 158–200.

Silberschmidt, A., Lee, S., Zanarini, M., Schulz, S. C. (2015). Gender differences in borderline personality disorder: results from a multinational, clinical trial sample. *Journal of Personality Disorders*, **29**, 828–838.

Singleton, N., Meltzer, H., Gatward, R., Coid, J. and Deasy, D. (1998). *Psychiatric Morbidity among Prisoners in England and Wales*. ONS. London: Stationery Office.

Smith, B. M. (1990). The measurement of narcissism in Asian, Caucasian and Hispanic women. *Psychology Reports*, **67**, 779–785.

Szasz, T. (1972). *The Myth of Mental Illness: Foundations of a Theory of Personal Construct*. London: Granada Publishing.

Taylor, A. and Kim-Cohen, J. (2007). Meta-analysis of gene–environment interactions in developmental psychopathology. *Development and Psychopathology*, **19**(04), 1029–1037.

Torgersen, S., Kringlen, E. and Cramer, V. (2001). The prevalence of personality disorders in a community sample. *Archives of General Psychiatry*, **58**(6), 590–596.

Tyrer, P., Casey, P. and Ferguson, B. (1991). Personality disorder in perspective. *British Journal of Psychiatry*, **159**, 463–471.

Viding, E. and McCrory, E. J. (2012). Genetic and neurocognitive contributions to the development of psychopathy. *Development and Psychopathology*, **24**(03), 969–983.

Watters, E. (2010). *Crazy Like Us: The Globalization of the American Psyche*. New York: Simon and Schuster.

Widiger, T. A. and Costa, P. T. (2012). Integrating normal and abnormal personality structure: the five-factor model. *Journal of Personality*, **80**(6), 1471–1506.

Widiger, T. A. and Presnall, J. R. (2013). Clinical application of the five-factor model. *Journal of Personality*, **81**(6), 515–527.

Widiger, T. A., and Trull, T. J. (2007). Plate tectonics in the classification of personality disorder: shifting to a dimensional model. *American Psychologist*, **62**(2), 71–83.

WHO (1992). *The ICD-10 Classification of Mental and Behavioural Disorders: Clinical Descriptions and Diagnostic Guidelines*. Geneva: WHO.

Yang, J., McCrae, R. R., Costa, P. T., Yao, S., Dai, X., Cai, T. and Gao, B. (2000). The cross-cultural generalizability of Axis-II constructs: an evaluation of two personality disorder assessment instruments in the People's Republic of China. *Journal of Personality Disorders*, **14**(3), 249–263.

Zhou, X., Peng, Y., Zhu, X., Yao, S., Dere, J., Chentsova-Dutton, Y. E., Ryder, A. G. (2015). From culture to symptom: testing a structural model of 'Chinese somatization'. *Transcultural Psychiatry*, **53**, 3–23.

Culture and Obsessive–Compulsive Disorder

Antonio Ventriglio, Rubens Dantas and Dinesh Bhugra

Editors' Introduction

Like other psychiatric disorders, obsessive–compulsive disorder is one of those disorders in which the contents of the obsessional ruminations and compulsive rituals are very strongly influenced by culture, even though epidemiological data are not as strong as in many other psychiatric disorders. The management of the rituals and ruminations, especially if they are influenced by culture, has to be culturally moulded too. There is no doubt that the genetic aspects of aetiology and management using pharmacotherapy create problems of their own. Religious rituals and expectations may well contribute to persistence of obsessive–compulsive behaviours. The role of culture in encouraging purity in the context of food preparation is well described in anthropological and sociological literature and in some settings may well contribute to ritualistic behaviours.

In this chapter, Ventriglio et al. describe obsessive–compulsive disorder, body dysmorphic disorder, trichotillomania, skin picking disorder and hoarding. They go on to highlight the impact of religion and superstition on the aetiology of obsessive–compulsive disorders. They argue that, within each culture, there are concerns which are common even though a lack of epidemiological data across cultures makes comparisons difficult. These concerns may well contribute to specific contents of ruminations as well as compulsive behaviours. In addition, the contents also reflect religious ideas and themes. In some religious settings, hyperscrupulosity is noted, which may well be heightened in individuals with obsessive–compulsive disorder. Themes of dirt, purity, contamination and aggression are often culturally sanctioned. As cognitions vary across cultures, therefore specific thoughts related to rituals and compulsions will also differ. Similarly, superstition and perfectionism and responsibility have been linked together. It is possible that culturally sanctioned rituals may be seen as aberrant and abnormal if the individual is being assessed outside the context of their culture. Their normal

distress thus becomes abnormal and clinicians have a duty to ascertain whether these contents are part of the cultural make-up or are demonstrating real hardship and impairment of functioning. Assessing religious beliefs and cultural practices is an important first step in assessing patients with obsessive–compulsive disorder.

Introduction

Obsessive–compulsive disorders have been described across cultures although the presentations and symptoms may vary depending upon a number of psychological, social and cultural factors. Often associated with anxiety, obsessive–compulsive disorders tend to occur in both males and females. Cultural factors such as religious practices may well contribute to presentation and modification of various symptoms. Also associated are ethnicity, impulsivity, social class, educational status and other factors. In some cultures, symptoms related to obsessive–compulsive disorders are expected especially when part of religious rituals whereas in many others these become pathological.

Background

Obsessive–compulsive disorder (OCD) is a major anxiety disorder, and is well described in the literature (see de Silva and Rachman, 2004; Veale, 2014). It is characterized by unwanted, intrusive cognitions (thoughts, images, impulses) which are recurrent and persistent, and by compulsive behaviour that the person carries out – usually against their will – out of a strongly felt inner urge. These compulsive actions are mostly overt motor (e.g. repetitive hand washing, checking things, touching and arranging objects); but they can also be internal or covert (e.g. counting backwards from ten to one, silently saying a prayer a fixed number of times, conjuring up a visual image of a particular description).

Obsessions are recurrent, persistent thoughts, urges or images that are experienced as unwanted, intrusive whereas compulsions are repetitive behaviours or mental acts that an individual feels driven to perform in response to an obsession or according to rules that must be applied rigidly (American Psychiatric Association, 2013). In order to reach a clinical diagnosis of OCD the individual must experience either obsessions or compulsions. However, in a majority of cases the person has both, usually interlinked. The obsession generates discomfort and/or anxiety, which can be dissipated, albeit temporarily, by the successful completion of the compulsive behaviour. The obsession and/or the compulsion must cause distress and/or interfere with the person's life and activities in such a way that this warrants a diagnosis (APA, 2013). These stipulations are important, as many people have unwanted intrusive cognitions, and/or minor compulsive behaviours, which are neither distressing nor handicapping.

Some Historical Precursors

Some early writings contain accounts of behaviours and cognitions which today many would consider as constituting OCD (de Silva and Rachman, 2004). The early Buddhist text *Dhammapadatthakathā* describes a monk, Sammuñjani, who engaged in sweeping the monastery with a broom repeatedly. This took up most of his time and the activity took priority over everything else (see Burlingame, 1979).

The Japanese Zen master Hakuin (1685–1768) is reported to have suffered from serious obsessional thoughts and doubts as a young man. An even more influential religious figure in the West, Martin Luther (1483–1546), was tormented by severe intrusive cognitions, which took the form of doubts and blasphemous thoughts. One of his recurrent thoughts was whether he had confessed his sins fully and properly. He also had doubting thoughts that he might have carried out various sinful acts.

John Bunyan (1628–1688), the author of *The Pilgrim's Progress*, also suffered distressing obsessional thoughts of a blasphemous and malicious nature. One of his major fears was that, instead of words of praise for God, he might utter blasphemous words. He struggled hard to get rid of satanic ideas and thoughts renouncing God and Jesus, but achieved only occasional success in this endeavour. An illuminating passage in his autobiographical book, *Grace Abounding to the Chief of Sinners* published in 1666 (see Bunyan,

1998), describes one of his unwanted intrusive thoughts vividly:

> But it was neither my dislike of the thought, nor yet any desire and endeavour to resist it, that at the least did shake or abate the continuation of force and strength thereof; for it did always in almost whatever I thought, intermix itself with, in such sort that I could neither eat my food, stoop for a pin, chop a stick, or cast mine eye to look on this or that, but still the temptation would come, *Sell Christ for this, or Sell Christ for that; Sell him, Sell him.*

The English writer and lexicographer Samuel Johnson (1709–1784) had numerous worrying thoughts and evidently compulsive behaviours. These are noted in his biography written by his friend and companion Boswell. One such behaviour was to go out or in at a door or passage by a certain fixed number of steps from a certain point. If this went wrong, he would go back and start again. Boswell referred to this as 'another particularity' that Johnson had (Boswell, 1980).

The Danish philosopher Søren Kierkegaard (1813–1855) and Norwegian playwright Henrik Ibsen (1828–1906) have also been described to have had behaviours suggestive of obsessions and compulsions. The former is said to have kept 50 cups and saucers in his cabinet, each set in a different pattern. The latter evidently compulsively destroyed and rewrote his works, striving for a perfect end-product. He also is said to have taken an hour or more to get dressed in the morning (see Toates and Coschug-Toates (2002) for more detailed accounts).

Culture and OCD

It should be clear from the previous that obsessions and compulsions, and thus OCD, are not confined to one culture or one period of time. Obsessive–compulsive disorder is found in different parts of the world, and in different cultures. Clinical accounts of the disorder are available in the scientific literature and even in fiction from most Western cultures, as well as from many other parts of the world including India, Pakistan, Sri Lanka, Nepal, Hong Kong, Taiwan, Egypt, Singapore, Saudi Arabia and Turkey. The similarities of the OCD symptoms found in reports from these diverse cultures are remarkable. The basic characteristics of the disorder transcend cultures and eras.

However, OCD is not entirely free from cultural influences (de Silva and Rachman, 2004; Steketee *et al.*, 1991). There are several ways in which cultural factors play a significant part in this disorder. Before discussing these, however, it is useful to look at the prevalence of OCD in cultures and the question of whether these prevalence rates of OCD vary across cultures.

Prevalence of OCD in Different Cultures

Horwath and Weissman (2000) summarized that rates of obsessive–compulsive disorders and age of onset and comorbidities are similar across cultures, among adults and adolescents. The much cited Cross-National Collaborative Study (Weissman et al., 1994) investigated the lifetime prevalence of the disorder across several countries. Lifetime prevalence of OCD was approximately 2.3 per cent in the United States, Canada, Puerto Rico, Germany and New Zealand. The figure for Korea was slightly lower at 1.9, and for Taiwan less than one-third at 0.7. Data are also available from other, unrelated, studies. Figures comparable to those of the United States and Canada were found in Iceland by Stefansson (1993). On the other hand, investigations of ethnicity and OCD have yielded lower rates in African, Afro-Caribbean, and Asian groups in Britain (Meltzer et al., 1995), and in Australian aborigines (Jones and Horne, 1973). A low frequency of the disorder has also been reported for sub-Saharan Africa (German, 1972).

There is a suggestion that cultural differences have a clear impact on various cognitive variables (Yorulmaz and Işık, 2011). These authors compared three Turkish samples living in three countries and reported on the interrelationships between thought–action fusion, thought control strategies and OCD symptoms in three non-clinical samples. They studied those Turks who had returned to Turkey from Bulgaria comparing them with those living in Bulgaria with those who had not migrated and were settled in Turkey. They reported that worrying was a common factor. Those who had returned to Turkey were similar to Turks remaining in Bulgaria on a number of parameters. Yorulmaz et al. (2009) had previously compared Turks and Canadians and reported that among vulnerability factors in symptoms of obsessive–compulsive disorders some factors such as neuroticism and some meta-cognitions were common but Turkish participants often utilized worry and thought suppression in contrast with Canadians who utilized self-punishment more frequently.

Fontenelle et al. (2004) compared the symptoms of Brazilian individuals presenting with obsessive–compulsive disorders with international samples reported in the literature and revealed that the condition was commoner in females and had an early onset. They noted that a predominance of aggressive and religious obsessions was found only in Brazilian and Middle Eastern samples, respectively. There is no doubt that like all other conditions, cultures will influence the contents of rituals and behaviours. From Egypt, Okasha et al. (1994) reported a preponderance of male patients in their sample and pointed out that one-fifth of the subjects had a positive family history of obsessive-compulsive disorders. As noted by Fontenelle et al. (2004) the commonest reported obsessions were religious and contamination obsessions (60%) and somatic obsessions (49%). Common compulsions were repeating rituals (68%), cleaning and washing compulsions (63%), and checking compulsions (58%). Akhtar et al. (1978) had reported predominance of religious compulsions from India. However, fear of contamination and ritualistic washing have been reported from Iran (Ghassemzadeh et al., 2002) and from Singapore (Chia, 1996). Juang and Liu (2001) reported from Taiwan that the commonest obsession was about contamination and commonest compulsion was checking. Other common obsessions were about pathological doubt and need for symmetry. Two-fifths of subjects were also suffering from depression. As reported by Karno (1988) even within the same country the rates may well vary. This study showed that between 1.9 per cent and 3.3 per cent of the population reported obsessive–compulsive disorders. Mohammedi et al. (2004) reported similar figures from Iran with higher rates in females.

Wheaton et al. (2013) compared symptoms of obsessive–compulsive disorder in four groups: European Americans, African Americans, Asian Americans and Latino Americans. They reported that Asian Americans and African Americans experienced more contamination-related OCD symptoms than did European Americans. Asian Americans also reported higher levels of obsessive beliefs.

In a study from Mexico, based on clinical population, Nicolini et al. (1997) reported that obsessive-compulsive disorder in their group started earlier among males and aggression obsessions were related to later age of onset.

Weissman et al. (1994) noted that the contents of and predominance of obsessions or compulsions varies, though others have not proved this (Zor et al., 2010) which may be due to small numbers and it compares British patients with Israeli patients.

Interestingly, it has been shown from data from Japan that symmetry dimension was related to early age of onset whereas hoarding dimensions were associated with decreased functioning as well as treatment resistance (Matsunaga *et al.*, 2008). Matsunaga and Seedat (2007) emphasize that in spite of many features of cultural homogeneity, cultural factors do affect mood and impulse disorders even though the exact pathway of impact is not clear.

Comparing data from Costa Rica and the USA, Chavira *et al.* (2008) reported that rates of comorbidity were higher among the American sample though the set of symptoms appeared to be very similar though rates of obsessions and compulsions were higher among Americans.

It is difficult to draw definite conclusions from these studies, as sometimes different screening methods have been used. The use of diagnostic criteria to ascertain prevalent rates has also varied. While the work of the Cross-National Collaborative Study has made valuable strides in standardizing data collection methods and thus ensuring comparability across the countries studied, the overall picture does not offer a firm answer to the question as to whether there are significant differences among nations and cultures in the prevalence of OCD.

Common Concerns within Culture

People of a particular culture, or a particular era, have common concerns. These shared concerns tend to be reflected in the obsessions and compulsions found in that population. For example, obsessions and compulsions related to possible contamination by asbestos was a relatively common problem among OCD patients in the United Kingdom three decades ago. More common in recent years have been obsessions, and associated compulsions, with the theme of HIV/AIDS. Fernández de la Cruz (2015) noted that different ethnic minorities see obsessive–compulsive disorder in different ways and allow varying pathways into care. Furthermore, some groups see treatment barriers as the main reason for not seeking help.

The Influence of Religion

An aspect of human life which might be expected to have a bearing on a person's psychological well-being and mental health is religion. Key issues in this area have been well discussed in Bhugra (1996). As religion represents, and determines, some of one's

major beliefs and concerns, it is not surprising that clinical OCD reflects this. Many authors, including Rachman (2003), have emphasized this point. The content of the obsessions can reflect religious ideas or themes. Studies have also shown that OCD patients with clearly religious obsessions (cf. Martin Luther's and those of John Bunyan as noted earlier) tend to be significantly more religious than those who do not experience such obsessions.

A symptom commonly found in OCD patients is a heightened degree of scrupulosity (see de Silva and Rachman, 2004). Hyperscrupulosity has been noted in some religious persons in the Christian tradition, and priests have had to deal with 'parishioners who prayed excessively and who came to confessions far beyond what was justified by reality' (Worthington *et al.*, 2005: 184). The doubts and worries of Bunyan and Luther reflect this, as do the obsessional cognitions of some patients presenting at clinics today.

Several empirical studies investigating OCD in particular cultural settings have shown a link between the presentation of clinical OCD and religion. Studies in India have shown a preponderance of OCD with themes of dirt and contamination, and low frequency of obsessions with aggressive content, among Hindu patients. This is seen as reflecting the preoccupation with matters of purity and cleanliness, and the presence of a variety of purification rituals, in that culture (Akhtar, 1978; Akhtar *et al.*, 1978; Khanna and Channabavasanna, 1988). Chaturvedi (1993) has provided a discussion of the ways in which the Hindu culture can affect the presentation of OCD. For example, the 'ritualistic avoidances during menstruation in themselves may generate conflicts and precipitate obsessional behaviour or give content to an already existing obsessional illness' (Chaturvedi, 1993: 185). A report by Sharma (1968) has shown that the themes of obsessions in Nepal, a predominantly Hindu country, are often related to religious practices. In a study carried out in Egypt, it was found that both obsessions and compulsions showed the influence of the Muslim culture (Okasha *et al.*, 1994). Compared to British samples, the Egyptian sample had obsessions mostly linked to religious matters, and to cleanliness and contamination. Muslims are required to pray five times a day, preceded on each occasion by a ritualistic ablution. Strict fundamentalist Muslims may be required to perform complex ritualistic cleansing if they should touch a woman. How the concerns with cleanliness, and the ritualistic ways of achieving it, are reflected in the OCD symptoms of patients in this context is understandable. Maghoub and Abdel-Hafeiz (1991) found that in the Muslim culture of Saudi Arabia the themes of obsessions were more often related to religious practices than were evident in British OCD patients. A study from Israel (Greenberg and Witzum, 1994) looking at OCD symptoms in a sample of 34 patients found symptoms linked to religious practices in 13 of 19 ultra-orthodox Jewish patients, and in only 1 out of 15 non-ultra-orthodox Jewish patients. Judaism is one of many religions that demand cleanliness and exactness, inculcate the performance of rituals from childhood and view their non-performance as wrong or sinful. Rituals concerning cleanliness and exactness are the commonest presentations of OCD. Main topics of religious symptomatology included prayers, dietary practices, menstrual practices and cleanliness before prayer. These authors conclude that religion appears not to be a distinctive topic of OCD but a setting within which such symptoms may occur and may be seen as normal or abnormal. Raphael et al. (1996) also noted the adherence to religion by individuals with obsessive–compulsive disorders which may be a defence mechanism or a causative factor. Himle et al. (2012) compared African Americans and black Caribbeans on levels of religious involvement and presence of obsessive–compulsive disorder and reported that frequent attendance at religious services was negatively associated with obsessive–compulsive disorders and Catholic affiliations and religious coping were strongly associated with obsessive–compulsive disorder. In an interesting study from south London, Fernández de la Cruz et al. (2015) reported that when compared with the white population, black and ethnic minority individuals were more likely to seek help from religious healers for their obsessive–compulsive symptoms

In addition to influencing the content of obsessions and compulsions, there seems to be another way in which religion can influence OCD. Rachman (1997) has argued that normal intrusive cognitions, which most people experience, turn into clinical obsessions as a result of the significance the person attaches to their thoughts. Those with a strict religious background tend to attach a high degree of significance to some of their unwanted intrusions, in a way that most people do not. Blasphemous or sexual thoughts, for example, may cause a great deal of distress, and the thoughts are perpetuated through this

mechanism in those brought up in a strict religious background. Rachman (2003) has given several examples of this process. It seems that getting a 'bad' thought is perceived as sinful or immoral by these individuals; a thought about a 'bad' act (e.g. harming someone, unacceptable sexual behaviour) may be seen as sinful as the behaviour itself. This 'thought–action fusion' invests a great deal of significance to the thought which then becomes a persistent and recurrent obsession.

Sica et al. (2002a) investigated OCD symptoms and cognitions in three groups in Italy. These were: 54 Catholic nuns and friars, 47 lay Catholic persons who regularly attended church, and 64 students not particularly involved with religion. After controlling for anxiety and depression, the two religious groups scored higher than the students on measures of obsessionality, perfectionism, inflated responsibility, over-importance of thoughts and control of thoughts. Moreover, measures of control of thoughts and over-importance of thoughts were associated with OCD symptoms only in the religious subjects.

Comparisons of OCD Cognitions across Cultures

One recent study has examined the links between OCD cognitions and symptoms across different cultural groups. Kyrios et al. (2001) compared large, non-clinical, samples of Australian and Italian college students on several dimensions of OCD symptoms and cognitions. They focused on three dimensions of inflated responsibility (safety of others; blame and responsibility for faults and negative outcomes; need to control, hinder or compensate for negative outcomes), three dimensions of perfectionism (socially prescribed; self-orientated; other-orientated), and five symptom domains of OCD (impaired mental control; contamination; checking; urges/worries; overall obsessionality). The results suggested a greater association in the Australian sample between some specific cognitive domains (blame and personal responsibility for faults and negative outcomes, and self-oriented perfectionism) with the symptom domain scores. Their conclusion was that the Anglo-Celtic culture, represented by the Australian sample, might be more concerned about issues of personal control than the Italian culture.

A detailed review of this area has been given by Sica et al. (2002b). While stressing the need for further research, they conclude from their review of the available literature that a high involvement in religion seems to play a particular role in OCD psychopathology. They also emphasize that the influence of this factor on the aetiology is an open question which requires further examination.

Superstitions

Another phenomenon that is relevant in this context is superstition. Different cultures have distinctive superstitious beliefs and practices arising from them (Jahoda, 1969). There are not many empirical investigations of links between OCD and superstitions. In a pioneering study, Leonard et al. (1990) conducted semi-structured interviews about superstitions with 38 children with OCD, and with 22 matched controls. The parents also had semi-structured interviews about their child's developmental rituals (e.g. doing things in exactly the same way, games with elaborate rules). No differences were found between the two groups in the frequency of superstitions. However, the OCD patients were identified by their parents as having significantly more ritualized behaviours in childhood. In a questionnaire study, Frost et al. (1993) found that measures of superstition were correlated with overall compulsiveness, compulsive checking, perfectionism and responsibility. They were not, however, correlated with compulsive cleaning/washing. The correlations between superstition and the cognitive measures (perfectionism and responsibility) were larger than those between superstition and overt OCD symptoms. This suggests that superstitions might be associated more closely with obsessional thoughts than with compulsive behaviours. As the content of superstitious beliefs and related behaviours varies across cultures, it may be inferred that this is one way, albeit a minor one, by which cultural differences in OCD are determined.

In sum, there are several ways in which cultural factors play a role in OCD. These may be summarized as follows.

- Content of obsessions/compulsions may reflect common concerns within a culture.
- Obsessions/compulsions may be linked to religious beliefs and/or practices.
- Those with strict religious beliefs may be more prone to developing clinical obsessions, as a result of attaching high significance to unwanted intrusive thoughts.
- Superstitions prevalent in a culture may be reflected in the OCD symptoms in members of that culture.

Hoarding

The core feature of hoarding disorder is persistent difficulties discarding or parting with possessions, regardless of their actual value (APA, 2013). This is generally a long-standing difficulty and the underlying explanations include perceived utility and aesthetic value or for sentimental reasons. These individuals specifically save possessions, and discarding them causes distress. Thus hoarding may lead to cluttering making the place of living hazardous. Hoarding disorder is not secondary to any other condition. According to DSM-5 other common features include indecisiveness, perfectionism, procrastination, avoidance, difficulties in planning and organizing tasks and distractibility. More commonly seen among older males in the general population, females tend to demonstrate excessive acquisition and are more likely to be seen in clinical populations. The prevalence is 3–6 per cent among samples from the USA and Europe. There may be a family history suggesting a genetic component. Three-quarters of individuals will have a comorbid mood or anxiety disorder (major depression, social anxiety or social phobia and generalized anxiety disorder). In about a fifth there may be obsessive–compulsive disorder leading to help-seeking rather than for hoarding per se. Timpano et al. (2013) linked hoarding with impulsivity. They found that, undoubtedly, hoarding disorder is a serious psychiatric condition. Using impulsivity scales they noted that among their sample impulsivity was very strongly hoarding but more specifically with motor and attentional facets along with urgency. This study raises questions about the role impulsivity may play in other obsessive–compulsive behaviours.

Body Dysmorphic Disorder

Body dysmorphic disorder (BDD) is described in DSM-5 as part of the obsessive–compulsive disorders and it also appears in the draft version of ICD-11. The key diagnostic criteria for body dysmorphic disorder are a preoccupation with one or more perceived defects or flaws in physical appearance that are not observable to others or appear slight to others. During the course of the disorder the individual may have carried out repetitive behaviours or checks through looking at mirrors, excessive grooming, skin picking, reassurances which do not appear to work. As a result of this preoccupation they are distressed or have significant impairment in their functioning (APA, 2013).

According to DSM-5 the point prevalence of body dysmorphic disorder is 2.4 per cent among American adults and marginally higher in females. In Germany the rate is lower at 1.7 per cent. Not surprisingly, among patients attending dermatology clinics the rates are higher. The age of onset is 12–13 years and in a vast majority the onset would have been below the age of 18. More than half of the individuals are preoccupied by head and face, around 20 per cent with body and 15 per cent or so with arms and legs. About 7–10 per cent will be preoccupied with genitalia and around 7 per cent with skin and a small proportion with body smell. Body dysmorphic disorders in adolescents can lead to high levels of suicidal thoughts and acts and affect academic performance as well as cause social withdrawal.

Males may well have more preoccupation with penis size whereas females may focus more on facial features or in some cases breasts. Underdiagnosis may be due to individuals seeking help from non-medical sources or when seen among adolescents may well be seen as normal concerns and preoccupation when they are individualizing and establishing their own identity. Body dysmorphic disorder has been reported across cultures. For example, in Japan this is known as *shubo-kyofu* (translated as the phobia of a deformed body). This condition is under-researched and underdiagnosed so the exact prevalence across cultures is not well known. Further research is needed across cultures especially combining qualitative and quantitative concepts to have proper epidemiological and socio-cultural findings. Differential diagnosis must include anxiety, major depression, other obsessive–compulsive disorders and eating disorders among other conditions. Substance use disorders, social anxiety disorders and major depression may also occur as comorbidities.

Trichotillomania

As mentioned earlier, hair pulling or trichotillomania involves recurrent pulling out of one's hair leading to hair loss. This causes significant clinical distress and there are no underlying medical causes for hair loss. The individual may well attempt repeatedly to decrease or stop hair pulling. More common in females, annual prevalence is between 1 and 2 per cent of the adult population and, although seen across cultures, the exact rates are not known. Often starting at puberty, it may wax and wane over years if untreated. Major depressive disorders and excoriation may accompany trichotillomania.

Excoriation (Skin Picking Disorder)

Skin picking disorder shows recurrent skin picking leading to skin lesions and repeated attempts to decrease or stop the act. Like other conditions described here, it causes considerable distress and is not attributable to other conditions (APA, 2013). Prevalence in general population is around 1.5 per cent and often much more common in females and starts with puberty or development of acne. Although reported across cultures, there is not enough epidemiological evidence to establish rates across cultures.

Implications for Clinical Practice

Considering these links, clinicians have to be aware of several implications for clinical practice. Some of these are noted later. It is possible that the culturally accepted and sanctioned rituals that a person performs may be seen as aberrant or even pathological if the person lives among people of a very different culture. The person may become distressed, and be referred for help, simply as a result of being perceived as abnormal by others from the same cultural background. Clinicians need to ascertain carefully whether the apparent symptoms are merely part of one's cultural make-up, and/or whether they cause real impairment of functioning or genuine distress.

In the overall assessment of a patient referred for therapy, the clinician needs to make a careful assessment of the patient's religious/cultural beliefs and practices. Indeed, it is clear from the literature that in all cases of psychiatric disorder these factors have potential relevance (e.g. Koenig and Larson, 2001), and assessing these will enable the clinician to get a full understanding of the presenting symptoms, including an understanding not only of the significance the patient attaches to them but also the degree of distress. It will also guide and enable the clinician in negotiating realistic treatment goals with the patient.

In terms of actual therapy, there is a small but increasingly important literature about the role of cultural factors. With increasing migration and globalization there is a potential danger that individual clinicians may not take into account cultural and especially religious factors. It has been shown that the religious coping that a person learns from his/her culture often has relevance in the clinical picture, and that clinicians need to pay serious attention to this (e.g. Pargement, 1997). Several authors have also argued that clinicians should have sensitivity to cultural issues as well as cultural competence. For example, Witztum and Buchbinder (2001) have described culture-sensitive therapy with religious Jews, while Juthani (2001) has highlighted cultural–religious parameters that are relevant in the treatment of Hindu patients.

Specifically in relation to OCD, Rachman (2003, 2006) has argued, and provided evidence, for the use of carefully planned cognitive tactics to enable the patient to understand the link between their obsessions and religious concerns in cases where the obsessional problems are related to, or caused by, religious ideas. Cognitive treatment of religious obsessions, Rachman says, is also helped by elucidating the exacerbating effects of low mood. Under such circumstances, help, assistance and advice of a religious authority or counsellor can be very productive in engaging with the patient and leading to clarification and comfort, while supporting the psychological therapy. A case example given by Rachman (2003) is worth citing here. The patient was a 43-year-old practising Catholic. As a child he had been given a bible that contained a disturbing picture of the devil. Soon after that he began to have intrusive thoughts and images about the devil. He tried to neutralize these by praying, and by repeating the sentence 'I love God and God alone.' During the treatment he was helped to make the connection between his religious obsessions and his other obsessions, which were about harming. This led to a reinterpretation of his 'blasphemy' as one manifestation of a psychological disorder, i.e. OCD. He made good progress and reported decreasing frequency of the religious obsessions. The distress and interference caused by them also declined significantly. With further therapy he showed a shift in his beliefs about religious obsessions, and felt that God would not want him to suffer. To quote; 'We reviewed the adaptive implications of changing the meaning of his religious obsessions, and then spent the remainder of the sessions introducing the idea of . . . thought–action fusion. He felt that this played a role in his reluctance to challenge his harm obsessions, and agreed to begin to challenge the negative meaning placed upon ambiguous events or incidences' (Rachman, 2003: 72).

Another implication for therapy relates to the greater significance attributed to personal control and responsibility in some cultures than in others. If the preliminary findings on this, noted earlier from Italian and Australian samples (Kyrios et al., 2001), are replicated in subsequent research, it would be plausible to argue that cognitive reappraisals encouraged in the psychological therapy of OCD could profitably take into account these cultural factors. Cognitions, which will be changed using cognitive-behavioural therapy (CBT), will be culturally influenced. Therefore, the clinicians must explore normative religious rituals and cultural explanations for this prior to commencing any intervention. For body dysmorphic disorder, cognitive behaviour therapy has been used effectively.

There is also the general issue of whether, in a given culture, there is a preference for psychological therapy over pharmacological treatment, or vice versa. While a therapist treating OCD will wish to use the best treatment for each patient's presentation, the latter's ability and willingness to accept and comply with the treatment will, to some degree at least, be influenced by his culture's attitude to the therapy.

Finally, there is the question of using, in the treatment of OCD, therapeutic strategies that may be derived from various cultural traditions especially among those with religious obsessions and rituals. Rachman (2006) has discussed the religious tactics that are used for dealing with certain types of OCD problems. In the Judaeo-Christian tradition, these include: prayers, pardons, offerings, disclosure, confessions, repentance and so on. Religious persons suffering from OCD often report that they resort to some of these in order to combat their obsessions. Such strategies may well be considered for incorporation into clinical treatment approaches, with the proviso that their efficacy is properly evaluated. The general points on religious coping made by Pargement (1997) and others have similar implications.

A further specific example is the relevance of Buddhist strategies in this area, which has been discussed by de Silva (1985, 2001). The discourse *Vitakkasaṇṭhāna Sutta* of the *Majjhima Nikāya* deals with the control of unwanted, intrusive cognitions which particularly hinder one's meditative efforts. When unwanted, unwholesome cognitions occur during meditation, one is advised to use one of five strategies in order to eliminate them. The techniques are further elaborated and explained in the commentary *Papañcasūdanī*. A summary of these is given here:

1. *Switch to an opposite or incompatible thought.* The first is to reflect on an object which is associated with thoughts which are the opposite of the unwanted thought. This means that if the unwanted cognition is associated with lust, one should think of something promoting lustlessness; if it is associated with hatred, one should think of something promoting loving kindness; and if it is something associated with delusion or confusion, one should think of something promoting clarity. This exercise of switching to a thought that is incompatible with the unwanted one, 'like carpenter getting rid of a coarse peg with a fine one', is said to help eliminate the unwanted intrusion.

2. *Ponder on the disadvantages: 'scrutinize the peril'.* If, however, the unwanted thought still keeps rising, one is advised to ponder on the perils and disadvantages of the thought. This would help one to immediately rid one's self of the thought in question, 'like the case of a young man or woman, who is eager to look nice and clean, would be revolted and disgusted if he/she finds the carcass of a snake, dog or human being round his neck and would immediately cast it aside'.

3. *Ignore and distract.* If that too fails, the technique of ignoring the unwanted thought is recommended. One is to strive not to pay attention, 'like a man who closes his eyes or looks in another direction in order to avoid seeing a visual object that he does not wish to see'. It is suggested that various distracting activities may be used in order not to pay attention, or dwell on, the unwanted cognition. These include: recalling of a doctrinal passage one has learned, concentrating on actual concrete objects, or indeed some unrelated physical activity, like darning a worn out part of one's robe.

4. *Reflect on the removal of the sources of the thought.* If the unwanted cognition still persists, then a further strategy is recommended; this is to reflect on the removal or stopping of the sources of the target thought. This is explained with the analogy of a man walking briskly who ask himself 'Why am I walking briskly?' and then slows down his pace as he sees no reason to walk briskly; then reflects on his walking and stops and stands; then reflects on his standing and sits down; and finally reflects on sitting, and then lies down.

5. *Control with forceful effort.* If the fourth strategy, too, fails then a fifth method is advocated, which is to forcefully restrain and dominate the mind, 'with clenched teeth and tongue pressed hard against palate'. This use of effort is linked to 'a strong man holding, restraining and dominating a weaker man'. One is to use the 'effort of one part of the mind to control another'.

The recommendation is, very clearly, to use these five strategies in a hierarchical way. Each of the five is to be resorted to if the preceding one fails. This is compared to the progressive use of five weapons in a battle. The bow is to be used first, if the bow breaks, use the spear and then the sword, etc.

Interestingly, many of these are very similar to strategies used in present-day cognitive-behaviour therapy (e.g. thought-switching, thought-stopping, covert sensitization). These similarities have been discussed in detail elsewhere (de Silva, 1985, 2001). Cognitive-behaviour therapy has also been shown to be helpful in cases of body dysmorphic disorders. Antidepressants such as clomipramine and fluoxetine have been shown to work well (Mataix-Cols *et al.* 2015; Phillips 2005; Wilhelm *et al.* 2013).

Early Buddhist texts offer a further technique which has relevance to the treatment of obsessions. In present-day therapy, satiation/habituation training is commonly used. The patient is advised to expose himself/herself to the unwanted thought repeatedly and/or for prolonged periods (de Silva and Rachman, 2004). This is similar to aspects of the mindfulness meditation advocated in the *Satipatthāna Sutta* of the *Majjhima Nikāya*. In developing mindfulness or awareness of one's thoughts, which is part of the overall mindfulness training, one is advised to be alert to all cognitions that arise, including unwanted ones. If and when an unwanted thought arises, one is to face it directly and continuously, rather than try to get rid of it. The thought then loses its salience and the chances of its persistence and/or recurrence diminish (see de Silva, 1985).

These Buddhist techniques can be incorporated into the treatment of obsessions in OCD patients – indeed, as noted earlier, the modern parallels of some of them are already widely in use. The use of these with Buddhist patients, with the explicit acknowledgement that they are part of the Buddhist tradition, may well enhance therapeutic compliance, as they will not be seen as alien. It is, however, important that their efficacy is evaluated in the clinical context.

As alluded to earlier, the relationship between pharmacotherapy and psychotherapy is complex. Furthermore, as described elsewhere in this volume (see Chapter 33), the role of psychopharmacology across different ethnic groups and cultures must include knowledge of differing pharmacodynamics and pharmacokinetics. These changes in metabolism of drugs are influenced by genetic and ethnic factors as well as factors to do with lifestyle, such as smoking and dietary factors. Although anti-depressant medication has been used, there appears to be some evidence that one antidepressant medication is significantly more effective than another for the treatment of OCD (Murphy and Pigott, 1990; Pigott, 1996). For example, tricyclic antidepressants and monoamine oxidase inhibitors have been ineffective for patients with OCD (see Pigott and Seay, 1997), but clomipramine, fluvoxamine, fluoxetine, sertraline and paroxetine have all demonstrated efficacy in patients with OCD. Most studies indicate that 60–80 per cent of patients with OCD receiving adequate response will respond to serotonin response inhibitors (STIs such as sertraline, clomipramine, fluoxetine, fluvoxamine and paroxetine). Pigott and Seay (1997) observe that determining the most effective medication for an individual with OCD continues to represent a very lengthy process. Another complicating factor in managing OCD is its comorbidity with depression, which is equally culturally influenced. The chances of medication failing are linked with comorbid conditions such as personality disorder, social phobia and with presence of soft neurological signs. Comorbid depression and presence of bizarre or fixed obsessional beliefs are not associated with poor outcome (Pigott and Seay, 1997). Treatment of OCD that combines behaviour therapy with antidepressant medication is used often, though the outcome is not always better (McLeod, 1997).

Brakoulias *et al.* (2016) studied national prescribing practices in obsessive–compulsive disorder across seven countries and reported that selective serotonin reuptake inhibitors (SSRIs) were most commonly used (73.5 per cent), but their use ranged from 59 per cent in Australia to 96 per cent in Japan. Clomipramine use varied from 5 per cent in Japan and South Africa to 26 per cent in India and Italy. Atypical antipsychotic use ranged from 12 per cent in South Africa to 50 per cent in Japan. These findings suggest that availability of certain medications and guidelines may play a role in prescription patterns.

Equally importantly prospective studies are required to determine the cultural, pharmacokinetic and pharmacodynamic factors which will affect compliance as well as acceptance across cultures.

Conclusions

Religion and religious practices are an integral part of cultures and in understanding rituals related to obsessive thoughts and compulsive behaviour. There is little doubt that obsessive–compulsive disorders appear across cultures. However, the contents of the thoughts and types of behaviours may be associated with religious rituals and leading to what is acceptable and what is not acceptable specifically in the context of culture. It is critical that clinicians are sensitive to cultural variations and what is seen as normal and what is abnormal whether it is the severity or contents. An ongoing dialogue with the religious and community leaders as sources of information and potential co-therapist must be remembered. Using illustrative techniques from different religions increases the acceptability of the services and therapeutic techniques.

Acknowledgements

This chapter is dedicated to the memory of Padmal de Silva, who contributed to the chapter in the first edition and passed away in 2008.

References

Akhtar, S. (1978). Obsessional neurosis, marriage, sex and personality: some transcultural comparisons. *International Journal of Social Psychiatry*, 24, 164–166.

Akhtar, S., Wig, N., Varma, N. *et al.* (1978). Sociocultural and clinical determinants of symptomatology in obsessional neurosis. *International Journal of Social Psychiatry*, 24, 157–162.

American Psychiatric Association (2013). *Diagnostic and Statistical Manual of Mental Disorders*, 5th edn. Washington DC: APA.

Bhugra, D. (ed.) (1996). *Psychiatry and Religion: Context, Consensus and Controversies*. London: Routledge.

Boswell, J. (1980). *Life of Johnson*. Oxford: Oxford University Press (originally published in 1791).

Brakoulias, V., Starcevic, V., Belloch, A. *et al.* (2016). International prescribing practices in obsessive–compulsive disorder (OCD). *Human Psychopharmacology: Clinical and Experimental*, 31(4), 319–324.

Bunyan, J. (1998). *Grace Abounding to the Chief of Sinners.* Oxford: Oxford University Press (originally published in 1666).

Burlingame, E. W. (1979). *Buddhist Legends* (translation), Part 3. London: Pali Text Society (originally published in 1921).

Chaturvedi, S. K. (1993). Neurosis across cultures. *International Review of Psychiatry,* 5, 179–191.

Chavira, D., Garrido, H., Bagnarello, M., Azzam, A., Reus, V. and Mathews, C. (2008). A comparative study of obsessive–compulsive disorder in Costa Rica and the United States. *Depression and Anxiety,* 25(7), 609–619.

Chia, B. H. (1996). A Singapore study of obsessive compulsive disorder. *Singapore Medical Journal,* 37, 402–406.

de Silva, P. (1985). Early Buddhist and modern behavioral strategies for the control of unwanted intrusive cognitions. *Psychological Record,* 35, 437–443.

de Silva, P. (2001). A psychological analysis of the Vittakkasaṇṭhāna Sutta. *Buddhist Studies Review,* 18, 65–72.

de Silva, P. and Rachman, S. (2004). *Obsessive-Compulsive Disorder: The Facts,* 3rd edn. Oxford: Oxford University Press.

Fernández de la Cruz, L., Kolvenbach, S., Vidal-Ribas, P. et al. (2015). Illness perception, help-seeking attitudes, and knowledge related to obsessive–compulsive disorder across different ethnic groups: a community survey. *Social Psychiatry and Psychiatric Epidemiology,* 51(3), 455–464.

Fontenelle, L., Mendlowicz, M., Marques, C. and Versiani, M. (2004). Trans-cultural aspects of obsessive-compulsive disorder: a description of a Brazilian sample and a systematic review of international clinical studies. *Journal of Psychiatric Research,* 38(4), 403–411.

Frost, R. O., Krause, M. S., McMahon, M. J., Peppe, J., McPhee, A. E. and Holden, M. (1993). Compulsivity and superstitiousness. *Behaviour Research and Therapy,* 31, 423–425.

German, G. A. (1972). Aspects of clinical psychiatry in sub-Saharan Africa. *British Journal of Psychiatry,* 121, 461–479.

Ghassemzadeh, H., Mojtabai, R., Khamseh, A., Ebrahimkhani, N., Issazadegan, A. and Saif-Nobakht, Z. (2002). Symptoms of obsessive–compulsive disorder in a sample of Iranian patients. *International Journal of Social Psychiatry,* 48(1),20–28.

Greenberg, D. and Witzum, E. (1994). The influence of cultural factors on obsessive–compulsive disorder: religious symptoms in a religious society. *Israel Journal of Psychiatry and Related Sciences,* 31, 211–220.

Himle, J., Taylor, R. and Chatters, L. (2012). Religious involvement and obsessive compulsive disorder among African Americans and Black Caribbeans. *Journal of Anxiety Disorders,* 26(4), 502–510.

Horwath, E. and Weissman, M. (2000). The epidemiology and cross-national presentation of obsessive compulsive disorder. *Psychiatric Clinics of North America,* 23(3), 493–507.

Jahoda, G. (1969). *The Psychology of Superstition.* London: Penguin.

Jones, I. H. and Horne, D. J. (1973). Psychiatric disorders among aborigines of the Australian Western Desert. *Social Science and Medicine,* 7, 219–228.

Juang, Y. and Liu, C. (2001). Phenomenology of obsessive-compulsive disorder in Taiwan. *Psychiatry and Clinical Neurosciences,* 55(6), 623–627.

Juthani, N. V. (2001). Psychiatric treatment of Hindus. *International Review of Psychiatry,* 13, 125–130.

Karno, M. (1988). The epidemiology of obsessive-compulsive disorder in five US communities. *Archives of General Psychiatry,* 45(12), 1094.

Khanna, S. and Channabavasanna, S. M. (1988). Phenomenology of obsessions in obsessive-compulsive neurosis. *Psychopathology,* 20, 23–28.

Koenig, H. G. and Larson, D. B. (2001). Religion and mental health: evidence of an association. *International Review of Psychiatry,* 13, 67–78.

Kyrios, M., Sanavio, E., Bhar, S. and Liguori, L. (2001). Associations between obsessive–compulsive phenomena, affect and beliefs: cross-cultural comparisons of Australian and Italian data. *Behavioural and Cognitive Psychotherapy,* 29, 409–422.

Leonard, H. L., Goldberger, E. L., Rapoport, J. L., Cheslow, D. L. and Swedo, S. E. (1990). Childhood rituals: normal development or obsessive–compulsive symptoms? *Journal of American Academy of Child and Adolescent Psychiatry,* 29, 17–23.

McLeod, D. R. (1997). Psychosocial treatment of OCD. *International Review of Psychiatry,* 9, 119–132.

Maghoub, M. O. and Abdel-Hafeiz, H. B. (1991). Patterns of obsessive–compulsive disorder in eastern Saudi Arabia. *British Journal of Psychiatry,* 158, 840–842.

Mataix-Cols, D. et al. (2015). A pilot randomized controlled trial of cognitive–behavioural treatment for adolescents with body dysmorphic disorder. *Journal of the American Academy of Child and Adolescent Psychiatry,* 54(11), 895–904.

Matsunaga, H. and Seedat, S. (2007). Obsessive-compulsive spectrum disorders: cross-national and ethnic issues. *CNS Spectrums,* 12(05), 392–400.

Matsunaga, H., Maebayashi, K., Hayashida, K., Okino, K., Matsui, T., Iketani, T., Kiriike, N. and Stein, D. (2008). Symptom structure in Japanese patients with obsessive-compulsive disorder. *American Journal of Psychiatry,* 165(2), 251–253.

Meltzer, H., Gill, B. and Petticrew, M. (1995). *Surveys of Psychiatric Morbidity in Great Britain, Report No. 1. The Prevalence of Psychiatric Morbidity among Adults Living in Private Housing*. London: Office of Population Censuses and Surveys.

Mohammadi, M., Ghanizadeh, A., Rahgozar, M. *et al.* (2004). Prevalence of obsessive–compulsive disorder in Iran. *BMC Psychiatry*, 4, 2.

Murphy, D. and Pigott, T. (1990). A comparative examination of a role for serotonin in obsessive compulsive disorder, panic disorder and anxiety. *Journal of Clinical Psychiatry*, 51, 53–58.

Nicolini, H., Orozco, B., Gluffra L. *et al.* (1997). Age of onset, gender and severity in obsessive compulsive disorder: a study on Mexican population. *Salud Mental*, 20, 1–4.

Okasha, A., Saad, A., Khalil, A., El-Dawla, A. and Yehia, N. (1994). Phenomenology of obsessive-compulsive disorder: a transcultural study. *Comprehensive Psychiatry*, 35, 191–197.

Pargement, K. I. (1997). *Psychology of Religion and Coping: Theory, Research, and Practice*. New York: Guilford Press.

Phillips, K. A. (2005). *The Broken Mirror: Understanding and Treating Body Dysmorphic Disorder*. New York: Oxford University Press.

Pigott, T. A. (1996). Where the serotonin selectivity story begins? *Journal of Clinical Psychiatry*, 57, 11–20.

Pigott, T. and Seay, S. (1997). Pharmacotherapy of obsessive compulsive disorder. *International Review of Psychiatry*, 9, 133–147.

Rachman, S. (1997). A cognitive theory of obsessions. *Behaviour Research and Therapy*, 35, 793–802.

Rachman, S. (2003). *The Treatment of Obsessions*. Oxford: Oxford University Press.

Rachman, S. (2006). *Fear of Contamination: Assessment and Treatment*. Oxford: Oxford University Press.

Raphael, F., Rani, S., Bale, R. and Drummond, L. (1996). Religion, ethnicity and obsessive–compulsive disorder. *International Journal of Social Psychiatry*, 42(1), 38–44.

Sharma, B. P. (1968). Obsessive compulsive neurosis in Nepal. *Transcultural Psychiatric Research Review*, 5, 38–41.

Sica, C., Novara, C. and Sanavio, E. (2002a). Religious and obsessive–compulsive cognitions and symptoms in an Italian population. *Behaviour Research and Therapy*, 40, 813–823.

Sica, C., Novara, C., Sanavio, E., Dorz, S. and Coradeschi, D. (2002b). Obsessive compulsive disorder cognitions across cultures. In *Cognitive Approaches to Obsessions and Compulsions: Theory, Assessment, and Treatment*, ed. R. O. Frost and G. Steketee. Oxford: Pergamon.

Stefansson, J. G. (1993). The lifetime prevalence of anxiety disorders in Iceland as estimated by the United States National Institute of Mental Health Diagnostic Interview Schedule. *Acta Psychiatrica Scandinavica*, 88, 29–34.

Steketee, G., Quay, S. and White, K. (1991). Religion and guilt in OCD patients. *Journal of Anxiety Disorders*, 5, 359–367.

Timpano, K., Rasmussen, J., Exner, C., Rief, W., Schmidt, N. and Wilhelm, S. (2013). Hoarding and the multi-faceted construct of impulsivity: a cross-cultural investigation. *Journal of Psychiatric Research*, 47(3), 363–370.

Toates, F. and Coschug-Toates, O. (2002). *Obsessive-Compulsive Disorder*, 2nd edn. London: Class Publishing.

Veale, D. (2014). Obsessive–compulsive disorder. *British Medical Journal*, 348: g2183.

Weissman, M. M., Bland, R. C., Canino, G. J. *et al.* (1994). The cross national epidemiology of obsessive-compulsive disorder. *Journal of Clinical Psychiatry*. 55 (suppl. 3), 5–10.

Wheaton, M., Berman, N., Fabricant, L. and Abramowitz, J. (2013). Differences in obsessive–compulsive symptoms and obsessive beliefs: a comparison between African Americans, Asian Americans, Latino Americans, and European Americans. *Cognitive Behaviour Therapy*, 42(1), 9–20.

Wilhelm, S., Philips, K., Steketee, G. (2013). *Cognitive Behavioural Therapy for Body Dysmorphic Disorder: A Treatment Manual*. New York: Guilford Press.

Witztum, E. and Buchbinder, J. T. (2001). Strategic culture sensitive therapy with religious Jews. *International Review of Psychiatry*, 13, 117–124.

Worthington, E. L., O'Connor, L. E., Berry, J. W., Sharp, C., Murray, R. and Yi, E. (2005). Compassion and forgiveness: implications for psychotherapy. In *Compassion: Conceptualisations, Research and Use in Psychotherapy*, ed. P. Gilbert. London: Routledge.

Yorulmaz, O. and Işık, B. (2011). Cultural context, obsessive–compulsive disorder symptoms, and cognitions: a preliminary study of three Turkish samples living in different countries. *International Journal of Psychology*, 46(2), 136–143.

Yorulmaz, O., Gençöz, T. and Woody, S. (2009). Vulnerability factors in OCD symptoms: cross-cultural comparisons between Turkish and Canadian samples. *Clinical Psychology and Psychotherapy*, 17(2), 110–121.

Zor, R., Fineberg, N., Hermesh, H., Asigo, G., Nelson, S., Agha, H., Ellam, J. (2010). Are there cross-country differences in motor behavior of obsessive compulsive disorder. *CNS Spectrums*, 15, 445–455.

Chapter 25

Culture and Eating Disorders

Anne E. Becker

Editors' Introduction

Eating disorders are not a new phenomenon but until relatively recently they were largely confined to more developed countries. However, as a result of the rise of globalization and social media and other factors in cultures-in-transition, these disorders are beginning to appear in cultures where they were until now relatively unknown. In this chapter, Becker describes the underlying concepts of body image, satisfaction with body shape and aesthetic ideals, arguing that all of these are culturally mediated. She points out that in turn, these contribute to social values and norms that underwrite pressures to be thin and body dissatisfaction which elevate risk for eating disorders. However, local cultural preferences and practices are fluid and change in response to social and cultural factors. These are increasingly influenced by a number of social factors such as globalizing commerce, media and communications. Inevitably these social norms are not localized and respond to changes in the use of media and interconnectedness which may not be confined to local geographies and may cross geographical boundaries. Although there is well-established historical and cultural variation in eating disorder prevalence, eating disorders increasingly have a global distribution. However, studies examining treatment outcomes for eating disorders outside high-income populations are sparse. The lack of epidemiologic and clinical trial data within populations in the global south remain an important lacuna in the scientific literature. Becker points out various ways forward in answering research questions. Cultures around the globe are in transition as a result of globalization, industrialization – rapid in some cases and consequent urbanization which is changing support and expectations in attitudes towards urban living. This needs to be understood in the mediation and distribution of eating disorders.

Introduction

Both historical and cross-cultural variations in the presentation and global epidemiology of eating disorders have illuminated socio-cultural contextual factors in their pathogenesis and maintenance (e.g. Gordon, 1990; Habermas, 2005) in addition to biological and psychological vulnerabilities that contribute to their multi-factorial aetiology. Other observational and experimental data also support socially and culturally mediated risk and presentation. Indeed, as one of the very few mental illnesses at one time conceptualized as culture-bound to North America and Western European populations (Weiss, 1995), anorexia nervosa (AN) has excited intellectual discourse in cultural psychiatry for several decades. Eating disorders have animated academic inquiry in part because, to borrow from Levi-Strauss's famous statement, 'they are good to think [with]' (see Levi-Strauss, 1966). That core symptoms of eating disorders – e.g. those relating to dietary intake and body image disturbance – are dimensional and best interpreted against local social norms, underscores their cultural relativity. Moreover, the meta-story of the emergence first of anorexia nervosa, next of bulimia nervosa (BN), and then binge-eating disorder, with additional presentations on the nosologic horizon is also a vivid illustration of the social construction of illness.

Whereas this intellectual unpacking of eating disorders has been informative as an exemplar of the cultural mediation of illness presentation, experience, and pathogenesis – it has also occasionally diverted attention from the more pragmatic and exigent implications of their protean manifestations. Not least of these is the low prioritization and neglect of the eating disorder population in low-resource regions of the world. Even in high-income countries, moreover, cultural models that inform clinical decision-making or patient help-seeking have very real impacts on the lived experience and social course of illness. Eating disorders frequently remain undetected, even in clinical settings and a sizeable percentage of individuals with an eating disorder do not access specialty care for a variety of reasons. This poor access to care results in ethnic disparities in service utilization in the US. Eating disorders are associated with substantial medical morbidity and early mortality, yet effective treatments are available (Becker *et al.*, 1999). Impeded access to quality care is thus highly consequential.

Cultural Mediation of Body Image and Eating Disorder Risk

Abundant evidence supports the cultural mediation of body image and, by extension and relevant to eating disorders, the valuation of a particular bodily aesthetic as well as body satisfaction. The ethnographic record provides robust documentation of cultural diversity in embodied experience, bodily practices and dietary norms. Cross-cultural variation in body practices includes piercings, tattoos, skin bleaching, hair-dying, and depilation, as well as body-shape manipulation ranging from foot-binding to breast augmentation. Cultural variation in weight management ranges from fattening practices in the South Pacific (Pollock, 1995) to the billion dollar diet industry in the US (Becker, 2013). In addition, there has been remarkable variability in body-shape ideals across geographically and culturally diverse regions, notwithstanding some interesting commonalities (Furnham and Alibhai, 1983; Becker, 1995; Anderson-Fye, 2004; Swami *et al.*, 2010). Social norms for body weight and aesthetic ideals, of course, are heterogeneous even within national populations and also vary by numerous dimensions of social identity, including occupation (Garner and Garfinkel, 1980), ethnicity (e.g., Rubin *et al.*, 2003; Brown *et al.*, 2009), and gender (Pope *et al.*, 2000).

Changes in body size ideals over time within particular societies also provide a striking illustration of their plasticity. A notable example is the migration of American body-shape preferences for women from plump or corpulent in the early twentieth century to slender circa 1920 (Brumberg, 1988). These changes were later followed by a fluctuating preference for curvaceous and tubular body shapes, represented in print and other visual media (Silverstein *et al.*, 1986; Garner *et al.*, 1980). The salience of these ideals could be traced to social values and changes in the built and technological environment that, in turn, were anchored to shifting economic and political contexts (Brumberg, 1988). Both body size and dietary practices serve as markers of social identity and prestige in many societies, but the specific meanings are closely tied to the local contexts. For example, in the setting of late Western capitalism, the body became a locus of personal cultivation (Turner, 1984). Notwithstanding their fluidity, at the historical moment that body aesthetic ideals approached a more slender shape, they were also increasingly easily ratified and reified within communities with shared access to visual media (see Bordo, 1993).

Longitudinal ethnographic and other data from Fiji provide an illustration of both cultural mediation of body size ideals as well as their plasticity over time. Among *iTaukei* Fijians (a small-scale population indigenous to Fiji), the traditional cultural preference for larger body size embodied both a dense social network as well as potential to contribute labour to the community. Prior to the widespread electrification of residential villages and introduction of broadcast television, *iTaukei* cultural practices had reflected values placed on capacity to care for children, family members, community leaders and guests. However, the preference shifted toward a more slender shape over the past several decades as infrastructural developments brought electricity and televised media to rural areas. Concomitant with these changes, disordered eating attitudes and behaviours appeared to emerge and become more prevalent in Fiji (Becker, 1995; Becker *et al.*, 2002; Becker, 2004; Becker *et al.*, 2011), just as eating disorders had in the US in the second half of the twentieth century.

Social and Cultural Mediation of Eating Disorder Risk

The eating disorders have multifactorial aetiology, and can best be understood as disorders that are bio-socially mediated. A distinguished scientific literature began to set forth evidence linking a cultural premium on thinness to disordered eating in the 1980s (Garner *et al.*, 1980; Striegel-Moore *et al.*, 1986). Given the understanding that the valuation of thinness was culturally mediated, this linkage aligned with available evidence in the 1980s that eating disorders were prevalent in some westernized societies while being rare in regions with historically different cultural traditions. Over the ensuing years, evidence has continued to accrue that internalization of a thin ideal, body dissatisfaction and disordered eating are causally linked (Stice and Shaw, 1994; Stice, 2002). Two key theoretical models – the 'dual-pathway model of bulimic pathology' (Stice, 2001) and the 'tripartite influence model of body image and eating disturbance' (van den Berg *et al.*, 2002) – that relate socioculturally mediated body weight ideals to the pathogenesis of eating disorders via body dissatisfaction have particular empirical traction. Each of these models, moreover, invokes the social influences of family, peers and the media on valuation of thinness. Given the dynamic nature of social norms for body size as well as the expanding reach of media access, these models are consistent with changes over time in eating disorder risk within particular cultures and regions.

Insofar as each of these aetiologic models relates body dissatisfaction to attitudes and practices that elevate risk, they support a common pathway for the pathogenesis of eating disorders. Regional data from disparate cultural settings, including populations in France, Hungary, Australia, Japan and China, suggest that linkages described by the Tripartite Influence Model apply across a wide variety of cultural settings; however, regional differences identified also have important implications for local adaptation of interventions (Chen *et al.*, 2007; Yamamiya *et al.*, 2008; Rodgers *et al.*, 2011; Papp *et al.*, 2013). These models are also consistent with both cross-cultural and historical variation in eating disorders prevalence, given that body shape ideals, commentary about weight, and agency over weight-loss behaviours are mediated by local social norms, cultural values and related environmental constraints. These models also fit with evidence supporting increasing prevalence of eating disorders in certain social settings (defined variously by socio-economic strata) with increasing exposure to global commerce and media via access to communications technology. There is robust documentation of the relation between media exposures and body dissatisfaction (e.g. Groesz *et al.*, 2002; Grabe *et al.*, 2008; Levine and Murnen, 2009). Hence, increasing global access to media can at least partially account for the broad diffusion of values and practices that once seemed culturally particular to Western youth culture (Gerbasi *et al.*, 2014). Moreover, new social media amplify exposure to images and ideas that also confer risk (Perloff, 2014; Mabe *et al.*, 2014; Rodgers *et al.*, 2016) and may further augment diffusion of exposures related to eating pathology.

Culture Change and Risk for Eating Disorders

Numerous studies have examined eating disorder risk in populations undergoing social and economic transition or transnational migration. These data have raised the question of whether acculturation per se elevates risk for eating disorders, or whether the new exposure to specific values, images, and ideas originating from historically Western societies confers risk. The former builds upon the 'stress-diathesis' model (Fabrega, 1969) by posing questions germane to the turbulence, cognitive dissonance, and transgenerational tensions that arise during urban or transnational migration (e.g. Furnham and Husain, 1999; Nasser *et al.*, 2001). However, evidence that acculturation has a heterogeneous relation to eating pathology (Becker *et al.*, 2010a) suggests a complex interplay of social transition, resilience and outcomes. For example, evidence supports that local cultural resources and values, such as collectivism, may provide some resilience to eating disorders or shape their presentation and social course (Becker, 1995; Littlewood, 1995; Bhugra *et al.*, 2000; Lee *et al.*, 2003; Becker and Thomas, 2015). Nonetheless, the accrued literature supports the relation between a 'culture of modernity' and eating pathology (Lee, 1996). This relation is supported by both the emergence of eating disorders over the twentieth century in post-industrialized westernized countries as well as the evidence that exposure to Western cultural traditions and values – and notably, the valuation of thinness and individual achievement – aligns with the increasingly broad distribution of eating disorders across diverse regions.

Phenomenologic Diversity in Presentation of Disordered Eating

In addition to cultural mediation of local norms and ideals for dietary practices, body size and weight, there is also evidence of culturally particular patterning of symptom presentation. Of these variants, the best documented in the scientific literature has been a presentation first described in Hong Kong by Lee and colleagues as 'non-fat phobic anorexia nervosa' (NFP-AN) (Lee *et al.*, 1993). This presentation resembles conventional AN, including the clinical features of low weight and refusal to maintain an adequate dietary intake, but is distinguished by the absence of the intense fear of weight gain or becoming 'fat' that is its hallmark. Lee and colleagues argued that the rationales for food refusal observed in patients with NFP-AN mapped onto locally salient cultural meanings (Lee *et al.*, 2001). Over two decades, Lee and colleagues documented that the proportion of patients presenting with NFP-AN decreased as the proportion presenting with conventional AN increased, closely paralleling ongoing cultural change in Hong Kong (Lee *et al.*, 2010). Over this period of time fat phobia as a rationale for food refusal became increasingly relevant in Hong Kong. Non-fat phobic anorexia nervosa was subsequently identified in other regions of Asia as well as globally (Becker *et al.*, 2009b).

Another example of a culture-specific phenotypic variant of an eating disorder has been described in Fiji, where a study combining narrative and survey data demonstrated a high prevalence of purging behaviour among school-going adolescent *iTaukei* girls ($n = 523$). A latent profile analysis of the 222 study participants (42%) who self-reported purgative use or purging to manage weight in the past month showed two distinctive profiles, one typified by conventional vomiting to lose weight and the other by herbal purgative use. Whereas the two profiles were each associated with significantly greater eating disorder psychopathology (as measured by the Eating Disorders Examination-Questionnaire; EDE-Q), than among study participants who did not purge at all, the subsample characterized by herbal purgative use had significantly higher associated distress and impairment (as measured by the Clinical Impairment Assessment; CIA) than those who reported purging consistent with a more bulimia nervosa-like presentation (Thomas *et al.*, 2011).

Over the past several decades, the narrative fixing anorexia nervosa – and other eating disorders – to a particular cultural setting or social stratum has gradually been rewritten to accommodate evidence of their very broad distribution across geographically and socially diverse populations. On the one hand, evidence supports that risk for eating disorders has increased in the setting of cultural transition that accompanies transnational or urban migration and modernization. On the other hand, there is also evidence that eating disorders may not be fully visible in clinical settings and epidemiological studies. In this respect, failure to encompass culture-specific presentations of eating disorders may have unfortunate consequences. The examples of phenotypes seen in China and Fiji raise questions about whether local presentations of eating disorders elsewhere in the global south are detected and measured sufficiently well with classification tools developed for populations residing in Europe and North America. Poor capture of local variation may result in non-detection both in clinical settings as well as underestimates of the prevalence and health burdens of eating disorders at a population level.

Implications of Cultural Variation in Eating Disorders for Diagnostic Assessment and Intervention

Diagnostic assessment of eating disorders in research settings should ensure that self-report measures are valid within the local social context. Although a number of these eating disorder assessments have been translated and validated across several language and social contexts, the majority have been developed for populations within predominantly English-speaking, high-income countries.

Even when assessments are carefully translated into local vernacular languages, conceptual translation may be misaligned. Limited comprehension of idiomatic and symptom-specific terms as well as discrepancies in factor structure have also been noted (Choudry and Mumford, 1992). For example, Le Grange and colleagues (2004) have described how the meaning of 'self-starvation' was interpreted differently than intended in standardized self-report assessment of eating disorders in black South African secondary school students. The discrepancy, which artificially inflated scores indicating greater eating pathology, was only revealed during subsequent debriefing interviews. Conversely, Lee and colleagues (2002) reported findings suggesting that use of the conventional cut-point for the 26-item Eating Attitudes Test (EAT-26) in Hong Kong potentially resulted in misclassification of cases as non-cases. In addition to adaptation of eating disorder assessments to the local cultural context of symptoms, norms, and idiomatic language as well as subsequent validation (e.g. Becker *et al.*, 2010c; Becker *et al.*, 2010d), two--stage screening for diagnostic ascertainment is recommended. However, even in the context of an interview, diagnostic ascertainment of an eating disorder requires local contextualization of patient experience, attitudes, behaviours and response styles since eliciting disclosure of behaviours that run counter to norms centred on collectivism and filial piety may be especially challenging in some cultural contexts (e.g. Ma, 2007c; Becker and Thomas, 2015). Especially since some symptoms of anorexia nervosa and bulimia nervosa do not always manifest physically, clinical detection may be dependent upon the affected individual's capacity to formulate attitudes and behaviours as a clinical problem and/or willingness to disclose them (Becker *et al.*, 2009a).

An excellent tool for conducting a patient-centred psychiatric interview is the Cultural Formulation Interview (Weiss, 1995; APA, 2013), which structures questions that elicit information about explanatory models, social identities, help-seeking preferences, concerns about the patient–clinician relationship, and stigma that are relevant to diagnostic ascertainment and therapeutic engagement. Finally, revision of the DSM-IV criteria for the eating disorders in DSM-5 (APA, 2013), included changes that result in fewer cases being classified within the residual category (Machado *et al.*, 2013). This residual category for the eating disorders was formerly the most common presentation in clinical settings, but even the changes in DSM-5 do not encompass an exhaustive list of heterogeneous presentations (Fairburn and Cooper, 2011). Nonetheless, new criteria that encompass a greater diversity of presentations can be beneficial in rendering such cases more clinically visible.

Similarly, therapeutic interventions developed for eating disorders in westernized populations may not be transferable without local adjustment. In particular, the psychosocial therapies such as cognitive-behavioural therapy (CBT), interpersonal therapy (IPT), and family-based treatment (FBT) that have strong support for effectiveness require additional empirical evaluation for effectiveness in social contexts where family and social relationships as well as the triggers and meanings of dietary restriction and weight management may differ. For example, the assumptions upon which deployment of CBT and FBT are premised (e.g. that overvalued ideas about body shape underpin eating disorders or who typically has authority over meals), require evaluation and quite likely adjustments for the local contexts. For example, Ma (2007b) reported the uptake of family therapy upon referral (only 20 per cent of 25 families referred) in Shenzhen, China was low when compared with uptake in nearby Hong Kong. She discussed a number of cultural practices, values, and expectations that may make family therapy unappealing in the Chinese context. For instance, she described how the Chinese practice of *guanxi*, relating to relationship building, had likely motivated parents' attempts to cultivate a relationship with the therapist, and thereby had undermined establishing trust with the patient (Ma, 2007b). Likewise, conflict resolution during family therapy could be thwarted by local values emphasizing allegiance to family that result in a patient's avoiding statements that could cause parents to lose face (*mianzi*) (Ma, 2008). These and local expectations of a therapist's role as 'expert' illustrate elements of the local context that could fruitfully be addressed, in part, by making adjustments that respond to the local context and providing psychoeducation (Ma, 2007b; Ma, 2007c; Ma, 2008). On the other hand, local social contexts may offer novel approaches to engage patients in therapeutic work. For example, Ma described how filial piety – as a Confucian value underscoring a child's obligatory responsibilities to parents in the Chinese context – could be tapped as a resource in motivating recovery from AN (Ma, 2007a). Finally, given the heterogeneity of eating disorder presentations – both within the residual diagnostic category and across diverse social contexts – and the dearth of clinical trials for these kinds of presentations, a strategy for adapting treatments to local contexts will be a necessary and fruitful area for future research.

Social Barriers to Care

Individuals with an eating disorder often go without clinical detection. There is, moreover, evidence of ethnic disparities in access to treatment (Cachelin and Striegel-Moore, 2006; Marques *et al.*, 2011). These disparities may result, in part, from culture-specific barriers that influence help-seeking for mental illness and attach stigma for engaging in behaviours or attitudes that are perceived to depart from social norms (e.g. Becker *et al.*, 2010b). There are additional social barriers to treatment utilization that differentially impact some ethnic minority and low-income populations, including accessibility to specialized mental healthcare, affordability of medication or opportunity cost for attending sessions, and low mental health literacy about eating disorders as serious mental illnesses. There is also evidence of clinician bias, including ethnicity-based stereotypes of

Table 25.1 Percentage of global school-based health surveys including questions about disordered eating and attitudes by region

Region(s)	Number of countries with surveys*	Number (and per cent) of surveys which address nutrition and dietary intake	Number (and per cent) of surveys which address eating disorders
Africa	21	21 (100%)	2 (9.5%)
Americas	34	33 (97.1%)	5 (14.7%)
Southeast Asia	10	10 (100%)	1 (10%)
Europe	2	1 (50%)	0 (0%)
Eastern Mediterranean	19	19 (100%)	4 (21.1%)
Western Pacific	22	22 (100%)	0 (0%)
Total	108	106 (98.1%)	12 (11.1%)

Note * For countries with multiple surveys, only the most recent survey was used and counted.
Data from: World Health Organization (2016). Global school-based student health survey (GSHS) implementation. Geneva, Switzerland: WHO Headquarters. Available from www.who.int/chp/gshs/country/en/ (accessed 16 August 2016).

risk for eating disorders and detection or referral bias (Gordon *et al.*, 2002; Becker *et al.*, 2003; Becker *et al.*, 2010b) that may impede access to treatment. In addition to social barriers to care for eating disorders, Ma (2007a) identified poverty as the trigger to an eating disorder in two cases of low-income patients. Each of these young women described having inadequate money for school lunches; this resulted in weight loss for one of them and she then experienced her slimness as a 'secondary gain'. Another described the cycle of hunger followed by binge eating upon her return home from school (Ma, 2007a).

In this respect, it is essential to highlight and redress social barriers to treatment for individuals with an eating disorder. Social barriers also include the low prioritization of eating disorders on the public-health agenda in many regions; this low prioritization helps to perpetuate a cycle of neglect wherein both the disorders and their associated health and social burdens continue to have poor visibility (Becker and Thomas, 2015). Two examples of this neglect are the frequent absence of eating disorder screening in nationally representative epidemiologic studies in low- and middle-income countries (LMICs) and the comparatively infrequent inclusion of eating

disorders screening questions among LMICs that implement the World Health Organization's (WHO) Global School-based Health Survey (GSHS; WHO, 2016) as a surveillance tool for health risk behaviours among school-going adolescents (Table 25.1). For instance, whereas over 98 per cent of the most recent GSHS surveys conducted in 108 countries included questions that addressed nutrition and dietary intake, only 11 per cent included screening questions for eating disorders. This low percentage is disappointing given that the WHO had identified eating disorders as a global adolescent mental health priority (WHO, 2003).

Global Distribution of Eating Disorders and Associated Health Burdens

Although there are a large number of studies that report prevalence of eating disorders attitudes and behaviours in community or clinic-based samples, there remain comparatively few nationally representative samples of eating disorders prevalence assessed by interviews outside the global north. Notable examples include a handful of studies using similar methodology and making diagnostic assessment with the

Composite International Diagnostic Interview (CIDI; see Table 25.2). Moreover, we could identify no incidence study of eating disorders outside high-income nations. Although epidemiologic surveys such as the CIDI rely upon conventional presentations of eating disorders, this standardized assessment facilitates some cross-national comparison. These data are consistent with globally broad distribution of eating disorders in the populations surveyed. It is noteworthy that whereas reported prevalence estimates for BN fell under 2 per cent in the majority of studies, three exceptions included an urban Brazilian population, Māori, and other Pacific Islanders residing in New Zealand where the lifetime prevalence of BN in adults was 2.0, 2.4 and 3.9 per cent, respectively (Baxter et al., 2006; Foliaki et al., 2006; Kessler et al., 2013). Very few LMICs were surveyed, however.

The Global Burden of Disease (GBD) study data, first published in the 1990s, were instrumental in advancing comparison of the premature mortality and disability associated with various health conditions, across both types of disorders and geographies. Indeed, the development of the health metrics, disability-adjusted life years (DALYs) and years lived with disability (YLDs) rendered visible for the first time the considerable health burdens associated with the mental disorders (Becker and Kleinman, 2013). That eating disorders were not encompassed in the originally published estimates further underscores their marginality on the global health agenda, even within the already marginalized field of mental health. Although the estimates generated for this study for eating disorders, like many other disorders, are based on imperfect and incomplete data, they nonetheless provide fresh and informative perspectives on the global landscape of eating disorders. In particular, these data challenge the conventional scientific narrative that had situated the relevance of eating disorders in the global north while fortifying evidence of their presence and impacts in the global south (Thomas et al., 2016). A comparison of DALYs per 100,000 caused by eating disorders demonstrates that *rates* are highest in regions of western Europe, the Americas, Australia, and New Zealand, generally high-income countries in the global north (IHME, 2015). However, an examination of annual per cent increases in DALYs per 100,000 across countries introduces a new storyline. These data support that while annual per cent change over the past two decades shows a decline across regions of the global north

where eating disorders are more prevalent, they appear to have increased in regions of the global south. Moreover, the 'hot spots' for the steepest annual per cent increases over this same time period include subnational and national regions in Africa, Asia and the Middle East (IHME, 2015; Thomas et al., 2016). Likewise, whereas the per cent YLDs caused by eating disorders of total YLDs in the developing world is 0.2% (0.14–0.28%) and slightly lower than the per cent YLDs in the developed world (0.36%; 0.29–0.44%), the 2013 rate of change in this metric reflects an increase in the developing world (+0.25%) and a decrease in the developed world (−0.44%) (IHME, 2015).

The changing narrative of global distribution of health burdens caused by eating disorders also supports and illustrates how the prevalence of eating disorders may be fluid and dynamic over time. Although it is certainly possible that some of the increased prevalence reflects better detection of eating disorders, evidence of annual per cent DALYs increases in some regions over the past two decades in regions of the global south supports that eating disorders may be emerging there. Epidemiologic data, although still quite sparse in some regions of the world, are also consistent with increasing prevalence. These data both demonstrate the growing global footprint and health relevance of eating disorders beyond the boundaries of high-income countries with historically Western cultural traditions. This diffusion is, at the same time, consistent with models linking certain socio-cultural factors and exposures to elevated risk for eating disorders.

Finally, the shifting understanding of the cultural mediation and distribution of eating disorders may also reflect cultural factors influencing the generation of scientific knowledge. Relatedly, high impact psychiatric journals have been critiqued for the under-representation of over 90 per cent of the world's population in published papers (Patel and Kim, 2007). For eating disorders, this perpetual neglect undermines a well-informed and scientifically broad understanding of phenotypes, risk factors and course. Whereas, it is understandable that eating disorders research activity and public-health prioritization country by country would align with the local prevalence and health impacts vis-a-vis other health and mental health priorities, there has been a striking lack of recognition of the enormous proportional share of the global health

Table 25.2 A cross-national comparison of lifetime prevalence of eating disorders using the CIDI[1]

Nation	Sample size[2]	Representativeness	Age range (yrs)	Anorexia nervosa[3]	Bulimia nervosa	Binge-eating disorder
Global North						
Europe						
Belgium (Kessler et al., 2013)	518	National	18+	NR[4]	1.0 ±0.5%	1.2 ±0.4%
France (Kessler et al., 2013)	466	National	18+	NR	0.7 ±0.4%	1.7 ±0.8%
Germany (Kessler et al., 2013)	658	National	18+	NR	0.3 ±0.1%	0.5 ±0.2%
Italy (Kessler et al., 2013)	900	National	18+	NR	0.1 ±0.1%	0.7 ±0.3%
Netherlands (Bijl et al., 1998)	7,076	National	18–64	1.0 ±0%	0.6 ±0.1%	NR
Netherlands (Kessler et al., 2013)	540	National	18+	NR	0.9 ±0.5%	0.9 ±0.5%
Northern Ireland (Kessler et al., 2013)	1,432	National	18+	NR	0.5 ±0.1%	1.5 ±0.3%
Portugal (Kessler et al., 2013)	509	National	18+	NR	0.8 ±0.3%	2.4 ±0.6%
Romania (Kessler et al., 2013)	2,357	National	18+	NR	0.0 ±0.0%	0.2 ±0.0
Spain (Kessler et al., 2013)	1,057	National	18+	NR	0.7 ±0.4%	0.8 ±0.3%
Switzerland (Mohler-Kuo et al., 2016)	10,038	National	15–60	0.7% (0.6–0.9)	1.7% (1.4–1.9)	1.6% (1.3–1.8)
Antipodes						
New Zealand (Kessler et al., 2013)	7,312	National	16+	NR	1.3 ±0.1%	1.9 ±0.2%
New Zealand (Browne et al., 2009)[5]	12,992	Nationwide sample, from New Zealand Mental Health Survey, which included oversampling of self-identified minority ethnic groups, with Māori (n = 2,457) and Pacific (n = 2,236) people and mixed Māori and Pacific (n = 138) people in NZ	16+	0.6% (0.4–0.8)	1.3% (1.1–1.5)	
New Zealand (Baxter et al., 2006)	2,595	Nationwide sample, from New Zealand Mental Health Survey, of Māori people and Māori and Pacific identity in New Zealand	16+	0.7% (0.2–1.6)	2.4% (1.8–3.2)	
New Zealand (Foliaki et al., 2006)	2,236	Nationwide sample, from New Zealand Mental Health Survey, of Pacific people in New Zealand	16+	NR	3.9% (2.7–5.5)	
North America						
United States (Kessler et al., 2013)	2,980	National	18+	NR	1.0 ±0.2%	2.6 ±0.3%
United States (Taylor et al., 2007)	5,191 adults (1,170 adolescents not described here)	Nationally representative sample of African Americans (n = 3,570) and Caribbean blacks (n = 1,621) in US	18+	0.17 ±0.07%	1.49 ±0.20%	1.66 ±0.24%
United States (Alegria et al., 2007)	2,554	Nationally representative sample of Latino Americans, consisting of ethnic sub-groups: Puerto Rican (n = 495), Mexican (n = 868), Cuban (n = 577), and other (n = 614) 2,554 English and Spanish-speaking Latinos (overall response rate 75.5%) from the four major subethnic groups: 868 Mexicans, 495 Puerto Ricans, 577 Cubans, and 614 other Latinos	18+	0.08 ±0.07%	1.61 ±0.33%	1.92 ±0.33%

Table 25.2 (cont.)

Nation	Sample size[2]	Representativeness	Age range (yrs)	Anorexia nervosa[3]	Bulimia nervosa	Binge-eating disorder
United States (Nicdao et al., 2007)	2,095	Nationally representative sample of Asian Americans, consisting of ethnic sub-groups: Chinese (n = 600), Filipino (n = 508), Vietnamese (n = 520), and other (n = 467)	18+	0.08 ±0.05%	1.09 ±0.31%	2.04 ±0.35%
Asia						
Korea (Cho et al., 2007)	6,275	National	18–64	0.2 ±0.1%	0.0 ±0.0%	NR
Global South						
Brazil (Kessler et al., 2013)	2,942	Sao Paulo, Brazil	18+	NR	2.0 ±0.2%	4.7 ±0.3%
Colombia (Kessler et al., 2013)	1,217	All urban areas	18+	NR	0.4 ±0.1%	0.9 ±0.2%
Mexico (Kessler et al., 2013)	1,236	All urban areas	18+	NR	0.8 ±0.2%	1.6 ±0.4%

Notes:

[1] All studies used versions of the Composite International Diagnostic Interview (CIDI). Kessler et al., 2013, Mohler-Kuo et al., 2016, Browne et al., 2006, Hudson et al., 2007, Taylor et al., 2007, Alegria et al., 2007 and Nicdao et al., 2007 used versions of the World Health Organization (WHO) CIDI. Cho et al., 2007 used the Korean version of the CIDI.

[2] Sample sizes listed here reflect the number assessed for eating disorders, if only assessed within a subsample (e.g., Kessler et al., 2013). Methods for describing prevalence estimates within probability subsamples included weighting and are described elsewhere (e.g., see Kessler et al., 2013; Heeringa et al., 2008).

[3] Results are reported with standard errors, except for Mohler-Kuo et al., 2016 and Browne et al., 2009, which use 95% confidence intervals.

[4] Not reported for this subsample.

[5] Kessler et al., 2013; Browne et al., 2009; Baxter et al., 2006; and Foliaki, et al., 2006 reported results from the New Zealand Mental Health Survey. Thus samples overlap among these studies. Kessler's sample only consists of participants who were assessed for presence of bulimia nervosa and binge eating disorder in the survey.

burden resulting from eating disorders contributed by two countries in Asia – India and China. Although each of these countries has a comparatively low rate of disability-adjusted life years per 100,000 caused by eating disorders, they also comprise two of the three countries with the largest absolute share of DALYs caused by eating disorders. Although their proportionally high contributions are driven by the massive size of their populations and eating disorders contribute only a small percentage of DALYs to the overall health burdens within each of these countries, their contributions to global DALYs caused by eating disorders are very high (Thomas *et al.*, 2016). The high numbers contributed have important relevance for scientific research to advance understanding of both aetiology and therapeutic interventions, especially when the absolute numbers of cases are low in other regions. Arguably even more important, if our collective scientific understanding of eating disorders is based only upon data from populations that are not representative of the global population, we miss important scientific and advocacy opportunities.

References

Alegria, M., Woo, M., Cao, Z., Torres, M., Meng, X., Striegel-Moore, R. (2007). Prevalence and correlates of eating disorders in Latinos in the United States. *International Journal of Eating Disorders*, **40**, S15–S21.

American Psychiatric Association (2013). *Diagnostic and Statistical Manual of Mental Disorders DSM-5*, 5th edn. Washington DC: American Psychiatric Association.

Anderson-Fye, E. P. (2004). A 'Coca-Cola' shape: cultural change, body image, and eating disorders in San Andres, Belize. *Culture, Medicine and Psychiatry*, **28**(4), 561–595.

Baxter, J., Kingi, T. K., Tapsell, R., Durie, M., McGee, M. A. (2006). Prevalence of mental disorders among Māori in Te Rau Hinengaro: the New Zealand Mental Health Survey. *Australian and New Zealand Journal of Psychiatry*, **40**, 914–923.

Becker, A. E. (1995). *Body, Self, and Society: The View from Fiji*. Philadelphia: University of Pennsylvania Press.

Becker, A. E. (2004). Television, disordered eating, and young women in Fiji: negotiating body image and identity during rapid social change. *Culture, Medicine and Psychiatry*, **28**(4), 533–559.

Becker, A. E. (2013). Resocializing body weight, obesity, and health agency. In *Reconstructing Obesity: The Meaning of Measures and the Measures of Meanings*, ed. Megan

B. McCullough and Jessica A. Hardin. New York; Oxford: Berghahn Books, pp. 27–48.

Becker, A. E. and Kleinman, A. (2013). Mental health and the global agenda. *New England Journal of Medicine*, **369**(1), 66–73.

Becker A. E. and Thomas J. J. (2015) Eating pathology in Fiji: phenomenologic diversity, visibility, and vulnerability. In *Revisioning Psychiatry: Cultural Phenomenology*, ed. L. Kirmayer, R. Lemelson, C. Cummings. Cambridge: Cambridge University Press, pp. 515–543.

Becker A. E., Grinspoon S. K., Klibanski A., Herzog D. B. (1999). Eating disorders. *New England Journal of Medicine*, **340**, 1092–1098.

Becker, A. E., Burwell, R. A., Herzog, D. B., Hamburg, P. and Gilman, S. E. (2002). Eating behaviours and attitudes following prolonged exposure to television among ethnic Fijian adolescent girls. *The British Journal of Psychiatry*, **180**(6), 509–514.

Becker, A. E., Franko, D. L., Speck, A., and Herzog, D. B. (2003). Ethnicity and differential access to care for eating disorder symptoms. *International Journal of Eating Disorders*, **33**(2), 205–212.

Becker, A. E., Eddy, K. T. and Perloe, A. (2009a). Clarifying criteria for cognitive signs and symptoms for eating disorders in DSM-V. *International Journal of Eating Disorders*, **42**(7), 611–619.

Becker, A. E., Thomas, J. J., and Pike, K. M. (2009b). Should non-fat-phobic anorexia nervosa be included in DSM-V? *International Journal of Eating Disorders*, **42**(7), 620–635.

Becker, A. E., Fay, K., Agnew-Blais, J., Guarnaccia, P. M., Striegel-Moore, R. H. and Gilman, S. E. (2010a). Development of a measure of 'acculturation' for ethnic Fijians: methodologic and conceptual considerations for application to eating disorders research. *Transcultural Psychiatry*, **47**(5), 754–788.

Becker, A. E., Hadley Arrindell, A., Perloe, A., Fay, K. and Striegel-Moore, R. H. (2010b). A qualitative study of perceived social barriers to care for eating disorders: perspectives from ethnically diverse health care consumers. *International Journal of Eating Disorders*, **43**(7), 633–647.

Becker, A. E., Thomas, J. J., Bainivualiku, A. *et al.* (2010c). Adaptation and evaluation of the Clinical Impairment Assessment to assess disordered eating related distress in an adolescent female ethnic Fijian population. *International Journal of Eating Disorders*, **43**(2), 179–186.

Becker, A. E., Thomas, J. J., Bainivualiku, A. *et al.* (2010d). Validity and reliability of a Fijian translation and adaptation of the Eating Disorder Examination Questionnaire. *International Journal of Eating Disorders*, **43**(2), 171–178.

Becker, A. E., Fay, K. E., Agnew-Blais, J., Khan, A. N., Striegel-Moore, R. H. and Gilman, S. E. (2011). Social network media exposure and adolescent eating pathology in Fiji. *The British Journal of Psychiatry*, **198**(1), 43–50.

Bhugra, D., Bhui, K. and Gupta, K. R. (2000). Bulimic disorders and sociocentric values in north India. *Social Psychiatry and Psychiatric Epidemiology*, **35**(2), 86–93.

Bijl, R. V., Ravelli, A., van Zessen, G. (1998). Prevalence of psychiatric disorder in the general population: results of the Netherlands Mental Health Survey and Incidence Study (NEMESIS). *Social Psychiatry and Psychiatric Epidemiology*, **33**(12), 587–595.

Bordo, S. (1993). *Unbearable Weight: Feminism, Western Culture, and the Body*. Oakland, CA: University of California Press.

Brown, M., Cachelin, F. M. and Dohm, F. A. (2009). Eating disorders in ethnic minority women: a review of the emerging literature. *Current Psychiatry Reviews*, **5**(3), 182–193.

Browne, M. A. O., Wells, E. J., Scott, K. M., McGee, M. A., The New Zealand Mental Health Survey Research Team. (2009). Lifetime prevalence and projected lifetime risk of DSM-IV disorders in Te Rau Hinengaro: the New Zealand Mental Health Survey. *Australian and New Zealand Journal of Psychiatry*, **40**(10), 865–874.

Brumberg, J. J. (1988). *Fasting Girls: The Emergence of Anorexia Nervosa as a Modern Disease*. Cambridge, MA: Harvard University Press.

Cachelin, F. M. and Striegel-Moore, R. H. (2006). Help seeking and barriers to treatment in a community sample of Mexican American and European American women with eating disorders. *International Journal of Eating Disorders*, **39**(2), 154–161.

Chen, H., Gao, X. and Jackson, T. (2007). Predictive models for understanding body dissatisfaction among young males and females in China. *Behaviour Research and Therapy*, **45**(6), 1345–1356.

Cho, M. J., Kim J. K., Jeon, H. J., *et al.* (2007). Lifetime and 12-month prevalence of DSM-IV psychiatric disorders among Korean adults. *Journal of Nervous and Mental Disease*, **195**(3), 203–210.

Choudry, I. Y. and Mumford, D. B. (1992). A pilot study of eating disorders in Mirpur (Pakistan) using an Urdu version of the Eating Attitudes Test. *International Journal of Eating Disorders*, **11**(3), 243–251.

Fabrega, H. (1969). Social psychiatric aspects of acculturation and migration: a general statement. *Comprehensive Psychiatry*, **10**(4), 314–326.

Fairburn, Christopher G. and Cooper, Zafra (2011). Eating disorders, DSM-5 and clinical reality. *The British Journal of Psychiatry*, **198**(1), 8–10.

Foliaki, S. A., Kokaua, J., Schaaf, D. and Tukuitonga, C. (2006). Twelve-month and lifetime prevalences of mental disorders and treatment contact among Pacific people in Te Rau Hinengaro: the New Zealand Mental Health Survey. *Australian and New Zealand Journal of Psychiatry*, **40**, 924–934.

Furnham, A. and Alibhai, N. (1983). Cross-cultural differences in the perception of female body shapes. *Psychological Medicine*, **13**(04), 829–837.

Furnham, A., and Husain, K. (1999). The role of conflict with parents in disordered eating among British Asian females. *Social Psychiatry and Psychiatric Epidemiology*, **34**(9), 498–505.

Garner, D. M. and Garfinkel, P. E. (1980). Socio-cultural factors in the development of anorexia nervosa. *Psychological Medicine*, **10**(04), 647–656.

Garner, D. M., Garfinkel, P. E., Schwartz, D. and Thompson, M. (1980). Cultural expectations of thinness in women. *Psychological Reports*, **47**(2), 483–491.

Gerbasi, M. E., Richards, L. K., Thomas, J. J., Agnew-Blais, J. C., Thompson-Brenner, H., Gilman, S. E. and Becker, A. E. (2014). Globalization and eating disorder risk: peer influence, perceived social norms, and adolescent disordered eating in Fiji. *International Journal of Eating Disorders*, **47**(7), 727–737.

Gordon, K. H., Perez, M. and Joiner, T. E. (2002). The impact of racial stereotypes on eating disorder recognition. *International Journal of Eating Disorders*, **32**(2), 219–224.

Gordon, R. A. (1990). *Anorexia and Bulimia: Anatomy of a Social Epidemic*. Cambridge, MA: Basil Blackwell.

Grabe, S., Ward, L. M. and Hyde, J. S. (2008). The role of the media in body image concerns among women: a meta-analysis of experimental and correlational studies. *Psychological Bulletin*, **134**, 460–476.

Groesz, L. M., Levine, M. P. and Murnen, S. K. (2002). The effect of experimental presentation of thin media images on body satisfaction: a meta-analytic review. *International Journal of Eating Disorders*, **31**(1), 1–16.

Habermas, T. (2005). On the uses of history in psychiatry: diagnostic implications for anorexia nervosa. *International Journal of Eating Disorders*, **38**(2), 167–182.

Heeringa, S. G., Wells, J. E., Hubbard, F., Mneimneh, Z., Chiu, W. T. and Sampson, N. (2008). Sample designs and sampling procedures. In *The WHO World Mental Health Surveys: Global Perspectives on the Epidemiology of Mental Disorders*, ed. R. C. Kessler and T. B. Üstün. New York, NY: Cambridge University Press, pp. 14–32.

Hudson, J. I., Hiripi, E., Pope, H. G., Kessler, R. C. (2007). The prevalence and correlates of eating disorders in the National Comorbidity Survey Replication. *Biological Psychiatry*, **61**(3), 348–358.

Institute for Health Metrics and Evaluation (IHME) (2015). GBD Compare. Seattle, WA: IHME, University of Washington, Available from http://vizhub.healthdata .org/gbd-compare/ (accessed 28 July 2016).

Kessler, R. C., Berglund, P. A., Chiu, W. T. *et al.* (2013). The prevalence and correlates of binge eating disorder in the World Health Organization World Mental Health Surveys. *Biological Psychiatry*, 73(9), 904–914.

Lee, S. (1996). Reconsidering the status of anorexia nervosa as a Western culture-bound syndrome. *Social Science and Medicine*, 42(1), 21–34.

Lee, S., Ho, T. P. and Hsu, L. K. G. (1993). Fat phobic and non-fat phobic anorexia nervosa: a comparative study of 70 Chinese patients in Hong Kong. *Psychological Medicine*, 23, 999–1017.

Lee, S., Lee, A. M., Ngai, E., Lee, D. T. and Wing, Y. K. (2001). Rationales for food refusal in Chinese patients with anorexia nervosa. *International Journal of Eating Disorders*, 29(2), 224–229.

Lee, S., Kwok, K., Liau, C. and Leung, T. (2002). Screening Chinese patients with eating disorders using the Eating Attitudes Test in Hong Kong. *International Journal of Eating Disorders*, 32(1), 91–97.

Lee, S., Chan, Y. L. and Hsu, L. G. (2003). The intermediate-term outcome of Chinese patients with anorexia nervosa in Hong Kong. *American Journal of Psychiatry*, 160(5), 967–972.

Lee, S., Ng, K. L., Kwok, K. and Fung, C. (2010). The changing profile of eating disorders at a tertiary psychiatric clinic in Hong Kong (1987–2007). *International Journal of Eating Disorders*, 43(4), 307–314.

Le Grange, D., Louw, J., Breen, A. and Katzman, M. A. (2004). The meaning of 'self-starvation' in impoverished black adolescents in South Africa. *Culture, Medicine and Psychiatry*, 28(4), 439–461.

Levine, M. P. and Murnen, S. K. (2009). 'Everybody knows that mass media are/are not [pick one] a cause of eating disorders': a critical review of evidence for a causal link between media, negative body image, and disordered eating in females. *Journal of Social and Clinical Psychology*, 28(1), 9–42.

Levi-Strauss, C. (1966). *The Savage Mind*. Chicago: University of Chicago Press.

Littlewood, R. (1995). Psychopathology and personal agency: modernity, culture change and eating disorders in South Asian societies. *British Journal of Medical Psychology*, 68(1), 45–63.

Ma, J. L. (2007a). Living in poverty: a qualitative inquiry of emaciated adolescents and young women coming from low-income families in a Chinese context. *Child and Family Social Work*, 12(2), 152–160.

Ma, J. L. (2007b). Journey of acculturation: developing a therapeutic alliance with Chinese adolescents suffering from eating disorders in Shenzhen, China. *Journal of Family Therapy*, 29(4), 389–402.

Ma, J. L. (2007c). Meanings of eating disorders discerned from family treatment and its implications for family

education: the case of Shenzhen. *Child and Family Social Work*, 12(4), 409–416.

Ma, J. L. (2008). Patients' perspective on family therapy for anorexia nervosa: a qualitative inquiry in a Chinese context. *Australian and New Zealand Journal of Family Therapy*, 29(01), 10–16.

Mabe, A. G., Forney, K. J. and Keel, P. K. (2014). Do you 'like' my photo? Facebook use maintains eating disorder risk. *International Journal of Eating Disorders*, 47(5), 516–523.

Machado, P. P., Gonçalves, S. and Hoek, H. W. (2013). DSM-5 reduces the proportion of EDNOS cases: evidence from community samples. *International Journal of Eating Disorders*, 46(1), 60–65.

Marques, L., Alegria, M., Becker, A. E. *et al.* (2011). Comparative prevalence, correlates of impairment, and service utilization for eating disorders across US ethnic groups: implications for reducing ethnic disparities in health care access for eating disorders. *International Journal of Eating Disorders*, 44(5), 412–420.

Moher-Kuo, M., Schnyder, U., Dermota, P., Wei, W., Milos, G. (2016). The prevalence, correlates, and help-seeking of eating disorders in Switzerland. *Psychological Medicine*, 22, 1–10.

Nasser, M., Katzman, M. and Gordon, R. A. (eds) (2001). *Eating Disorders and Cultures in Transition*, Hove, UK: Psychology Press.

Nicdao, E. G., Hong, S., Takeuchi, D. T. (2007). Prevalence and correlates of eating disorders among Asian Americans: results from the National Latino and Asian American Study. *International Journal of Eating Disorders*, 40, S22–S26.

Papp, I., Urbán, R., Czeglédi, E., Babusa, B. and Túry, F. (2013). Testing the tripartite influence model of body image and eating disturbance among Hungarian adolescents. *Body Image*, 10(2), 232–242.

Patel, V. and Kim, Y. R. (2007). Contribution of low- and middle-income countries to research published in leading general psychiatry journals, 2002–2004. *The British Journal of Psychiatry*, 190(1), 77–78.

Perloff, R. M. (2014). Social media effects on young women's body image concerns: theoretical perspectives and an agenda for research. *Sex Roles*, 71(11–12), 363–377.

Pollock, N. J. (1995). Cultural elaborations of obesity-fattening practices in Pacific societies. *Asia Pacific Journal of Clinical Nutrition*, 4, 357–360.

Pope, H., Phillips, K. A., and Olivardia, R. (2000). *The Adonis Complex: The Secret Crisis of Male Body Obsession*. Simon and Schuster.

Rodgers, R., Chabrol, H. and Paxton, S. J. (2011). An exploration of the tripartite influence model of body dissatisfaction and disordered eating among Australian and French college women. *Body Image*, 8(3), 208–215.

Rodgers, R. F., Lowy, A. S., Halperin, D. M. and Franko, D. L. (2016). A meta-analysis examining the influence of pro-eating disorder websites on body image and eating pathology. *European Eating Disorders Review*, **24**(1), 3–8.

Rubin, L. R., Fitts, M. L. and Becker, A. E. (2003). 'Whatever feels good in my soul': body ethics and aesthetics among African American and Latina women. *Culture, Medicine and Psychiatry*, **27**(1), 49–75.

Silverstein, B., Perdue, L., Peterson, B. and Kelly, E. (1986). The role of the mass media in promoting a thin standard of bodily attractiveness for women. *Sex Roles*, **14**(9–10), 519–532.

Stice, E. (2001). A prospective test of the dual-pathway model of bulimic pathology: mediating effects of dieting and negative affect. *Journal of Abnormal Psychology*, **110**(1), 124.

Stice, E. (2002). Risk and maintenance factors for eating pathology: a meta-analytic review. *Psychological Bulletin*, **128**(5), 825.

Stice, E. and Shaw, H. E. (1994). Adverse effects of the media portrayed thin-ideal on women and linkages to bulimic symptomatology. *Journal of Social and Clinical Psychology*, **13**(3), 288–308.

Striegel-Moore, R. H., Silberstein, L. R. and Rodin, J. (1986). Toward an understanding of risk factors for bulimia. *American Psychologist*, **41**(3), 246.

Swami, V., Frederick, D. A., Aavik, T. *et al.* (2010). The attractive female body weight and female body dissatisfaction in 26 countries across 10 world regions: results of the International Body Project I. *Personality and Social Psychology Bulletin*, **36**(3), 309–325.

Taylor, J. Y., Caldwell, C. H., Baser, R. E., Faison, N. and Jackson, J. S. (2007). Prevalence of eating disorders among blacks in the National Survey of American Life. *International Journal of Eating Disorders*, **40**, S10–S14.

Thomas, J. J., Crosby, R. D., Wonderlich, S. A., Striegel-Moore, R. H. and Becker, A. E. (2011). A latent profile analysis of the typology of bulimic symptoms in an indigenous Pacific population: evidence of cross-cultural variation in phenomenology. *Psychological Medicine*, **41**(01), 195–206.

Thomas, J. J., Lee, S. and Becker, A. E. (2016). Updates in the epidemiology of eating disorders in Asia and the Pacific. *Current Opinion in Psychiatry*, **29**(6), 354–362.

Turner, B. S. (1984). *The Body and Society* (vol. **24**). Oxford: Blackwell.

Van den Berg, P., Thompson, J. K., Obremski-Brandon, K. and Coovert, M. (2002). The Tripartite Influence model of body image and eating disturbance: a covariance structure modeling investigation testing the mediational role of appearance comparison. *Journal of Psychosomatic Research*, **53**(5), 1007–1020.

Weiss, M. G. (1995). Eating disorders and disordered eating in different cultures. *Psychiatric Clinics of North America*, **18**, 261.

World Health Organization (2003). *Caring for Children and Adolescents with Mental Disorders*. Geneva: World Health Organization.

World Health Organization (2016). Global school-based student health survey (GSHS) implementation. Geneva, Switzerland: WHO Headquarters. Available online from www.who.int/chp/gshs/country/en/ (accessed 16 August 2016).

Yamamiya, Y., Shroff, H. and Thompson, J. K. (2008). The tripartite influence model of body image and eating disturbance: a replication with a Japanese sample. *International Journal of Eating Disorders*, **41**(1), 88–91.

Child and Adolescent Psychiatric Disorders

Nisha Dogra, Panos Vostanis and Niranjan Karnik

Editors' Introduction

Cultures determine patterns of child rearing and how a child's world view is formed. Although developmental stages may well be similar, it is inevitable that geography, poverty and other social determinants (including nutrition) determine how a child develops into a young adult. Furthermore, how the adolescent or the young person develops into adulthood. It is well recognized that a majority of mental illnesses in adulthood start below the age of 24. Hence, it is important to understand developmental aspects of the individual. However, it must also be recognized that development continues over the lifetime and does not end at adolescence. In this chapter, Dogra *et al.* describe and explore the notions of childhood and the differing views about children. These authors then go on to explain these factors and their relationship with child mental health. They discuss some theoretical perspectives and challenges in collecting and comparing data about child mental health problems in different cultures and contexts. Dogra *et al.* show that general trends of the prevalence of child mental health problems vary across cultures and societies. This variation may reflect many things. This could be due to actual variation in rates or in the context of using culturally inappropriate assessment tools. Dogra *et al.* particularly offer a brief look at common and/or serious disorders in childhood and adolescence. They do not identify the ways in which culture and mental health are linked as that has been described elsewhere in this volume but they highlight key additional factors which need to be taken into account in child mental health. They remind us that consideration of culture and the social world where the individual grew up and is currently living is important in understanding what children and young people need in the psychiatric context. It is essential to consider cultural norms and how these norms and symptoms are perceived within the context in which they present. Dogra *et al.* emphasize that families should be seen as

unique within the wider culture, which influences child-rearing patterns.

Introduction

Before focusing on culture and the psychiatric disorders of childhood, there is a need to consider the views of children in different cultures. We then discuss some theoretical perspectives and challenges in collecting and comparing data about child mental health problems in different cultures and contexts. There is then a section on general trends of the prevalence of child mental health problems largely from international reviews. It is not within the scope of this chapter to review the prevalence of all disorders of childhood so the focus is a brief look at common and/ or serious disorders. Treatment approaches are also not discussed here as they are covered in the companion Chapter 39. As this is a textbook about culture and mental health we will not in this chapter identify the different ways in which culture and mental health are linked but only highlight which additional factors need to be taken into account for child mental health. We begin by considering how children are viewed.

Views of Children and Childhood

The ways that children are perceived within any given culture are important, as they influence how children are understood and prioritized within any society. Culture is itself determined by many ideas that change over time. Culture itself is dynamic and ever evolving in any society. Conceptualizing childhood can therefore be quite a complex task. The term childhood is non-specific but has generally been used to refer to the range of years in human development in different contexts. In developmental terms, the notion of childhood refers to the period between infancy and adulthood (often defined as between 0 and 18 years of age). As theories about childhood have changed, arguments have been put forward that childhood is a sociological

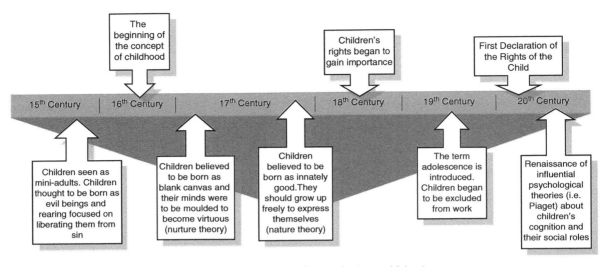

Figure 26.1 A timeline in the history of childhood (permission kindly given by Sage publishers)

concept, rather than being a natural phenomenon; and this is why our understanding of childhood and its components is subject to the changing values, definitions and expectations within any society (for example Corsaro, 2011). That is to say that the concept of childhood evolves in response to societal changes, and that the perspectives of society change in response to new ideas or findings. Concepts of developmental age as opposed to chronological age, and the meanings given to these age related groupings, are neither fixed nor universal. Developmental age (the age at which a child functions) may also differ from the child's chronological equivalent. Whilst aspects (such as gross motor, fine motor) of child development are universal, social and emotional development will vary widely across different groups – that is, what is expected and considered appropriate from children will vary, depending on the context.

Children and adults share the same status of personhood, as they have civil, political, social and economic rights, which in theory enable them to practise their citizenships. Yet, legally, children are not considered citizens, in as far as they do not have the right to vote and their rights are limited by age, and in many societies, children are not afforded the freedom to make choices about their own lives. Most countries have signed up to international agreements such as the United Nations Convention on the Rights of the Child (1989). This defines a child as 'every human being below the age of eighteen'. Beyond this age,

they are not vulnerable solely on age grounds. However, the implications and applications of the same piece of legislation vary widely by country.

Figure 26.1 (from O'Reilly *et al.*, 2013) shows how the views of children have changed significantly in the UK over the last few centuries. The views and details will differ in different cultures and those cultures viewed as more 'modern' will accord children greater value, although again what this means in practice differs.

Theoretical Perspectives

The contexts previously mentioned are important when considering all psychiatric disorders, but particularly those that do not have a predominantly organic basis. Falicov (1995) identified four theoretical perspectives to harmonize systemic theory with culture. These were:

- Ethnic focused: This stresses that families differ, but assumes that diversity is primarily due to ethnicity. It focuses on the commonality of thoughts, behaviours, feelings, customs and rituals that are perceived as belonging to a particular ethnic group.
- Universalist: Families are more alike than they are different. Hence, universalist rules are thought to apply to all families.

- Particularist: Families are more different than they are alike. No generalizations are possible, as each family is unique.
- Multidimensional: This goes beyond a unidimensional definition of culture and ethnicity, and aims at a more comprehensive and complex definition of culture that embraces other potential variables.

For the purpose of this chapter, the perception of culture as a multidimensional entity with a social constructionist bias is central. Age is only one aspect of the way that culture influences the role of children. The differences in the way that female children are perceived compared to male children can have fundamental influences on how their needs and wishes are interpreted. Within the human rights legislation, there is a move to view all children as having fundamental rights. Although it is implied that these rights stretch beyond cultural boundaries, attitudes to gender that exist across different cultures are not usually acknowledged. Most of the research discussed in this chapter has focused on ethnicity or nationality which is often used as a proxy for ethnicity. Few have considered the intersectionality between different variables, for example culture and gender.

There is also the issue that children do not often present themselves to child and adolescent mental health services, and the context of the family is even more crucial than when considering adults. Families and the expectations that different cultures place on them change, as do the roles of children within them. There is now more diversity than ever in what constitutes a family. As if this was not complicated enough there are also significant methodological challenges when collecting and comparing data. Furthermore, important factors to be aware of are the views of the clinician about children, family and culture. Societies are not homogeneous and overcoming the difficulties this puts on researching child mental health problems presents challenges discussed in the following.

Methodological Challenges in Identifying and Comparing Mental Health Problems

There are significant challenges to undertaking research in child mental health. We begin by considering the use of classifications and culture. Rousseau *et al.* (2008) reviewed the literature on culture and

DSM-IV classification in child psychiatry, using attention deficit hyperactivity disorder (ADHD) as an example of how diagnostic categories can be influenced by cultural issues. They argue that, whilst diagnostic categories are viewed as universally applicable, variation in prevalence rates supports the hypothesis of at least a partial role for social and cultural factors in the diagnostic process. The authors conclude that clinicians need to be aware of how culture may influence the diagnostic process in child psychiatry. We would argue this is relevant to all clinical care, and that clinicians need to be aware of their own perspectives and how these influence their interpretation of symptoms and presentations across different contexts (Karnik and Dogra, 2010). Clinician perspectives may account for the fact that black and native Hawaiian youth were more likely than white youth to be diagnosed with disruptive behavioural disorders (Nguyen *et al.*, 2007). Hispanic and black youth were less likely than white youth to be diagnosed with depression, black, Hispanic and native Hawaiian youth were rated as exhibiting less internalizing behaviour problems than white children. These were the findings when age, gender, functional impairment and socioeconomic status had been controlled for. Canino and Alegria (2008) reviewed empirical studies to present evidence in favour of or against a universalist or relativistic view of child psychiatric disorders and found that cross-cultural data on outcomes was unequivocal. They concluded that the cross-cultural validity of the criteria and diagnosis of child disorders may vary drastically depending on the disorder, but empirical evidence that attests for the cross-cultural validity of diagnostic criteria for each childhood disorder is lacking.

Lehti *et al.* (2016) examined the association between parental immigration and the diagnosis of ADHD in offspring in Finland. The likelihood of being diagnosed with ADHD was significantly increased among children of two immigrant parents and children of an immigrant father. The association between parental migration and ADHD was strongest among fathers born in sub-Saharan Africa or Latin America and among mothers born in sub-Saharan Africa, North Africa and the Middle East. The authors concluded that their findings of increased rates amongst children of immigrants may be because of increased exposure to environmental risk factors, difference in the use of health services or challenges in diagnosis of immigrants' children. However, migration impacts on children through a range of factors (Dogra *et al.*, 2011).

The tools used to collect data are increasingly standardized but there is variation in how those completing them interpret the information from them. Many studies have used standardized instruments (predominantly, the long established US-developed Child Behaviour Checklist; Achenbach, 1991). More recently, the UK-developed Strengths and Difficulties Questionnaire (SDQ; Goodman, 2001) has been used to establish broad rates of morbidity from varying sources of information (usually parents, sometimes teachers and, in some studies, adolescents, as neither self-report form is available for the less cognitively able pre-adolescent children) (e.g. Heyerdahl *et al.*, 2004; Kashala *et al.*, 2005). Despite the cross-cultural validation of these instruments, the differences between such designs has resulted in varying prevalence rates of mental health problems, and usually an overestimate of disorders. These methodological difficulties are more pronounced in pre-school children (Prior *et al.*, 1999). Studies with two-stage designs, i.e. using first-stage screening and second-stage interviewing methods, have addressed such difficulties, particularly those that have recently used the same or adapted diagnostic instruments. Heiervang *et al.* (2008) reported that Norwegian children had lower SDQ scores on all problem scales (emotional, behavioural, hyperactive and peer relationship) according to parents as well as teachers. Interviews found that the Norwegian prevalence of externalizing disorders (behavioural and hyperactivity) was about half that found in Britain, whereas rates of emotional disorders were similar. Lower Norwegian questionnaire scores for externalizing problems appear to reflect real and substantial differences between the two countries. By contrast, lower questionnaire scores for emotional problems seem to reflect under-reporting/under-recognition by Norwegian adults, and not a genuinely lower prevalence of emotional disorders. This illustrates that cross-cultural differences in psychopathology based only on questionnaire data may be misleading. Nevertheless, careful use of questionnaire and interview data can focus mental health research on cross-cultural variations likely to reflect genuine health differences. However, even two stage studies will be impacted on by how diagnostic criteria are interpreted in a particular context. That said, whatever the limitations and challenges, there is increasing evidence that children

and young people have significant rates of mental health problems across different cultures. There appear to be more similarities than differences and we will explore some worldwide data after a brief look at the part religion may play. Data to establish prevalence rates may include data from children and/or parents making the process even more complex.

Dogra *et al.* (2012) argued for the need for better research evidence on the prevalence of child mental health problems in minority ethnic groups, service utilization patterns, and barriers to service access. The terms ethnicity, race and migration are often imprecisely defined and how these are used may influence the research outcomes. Sampling techniques for national surveys have constrained the statistical power in estimating prevalence rates of child mental health problems in minority ethnic groups, as children from different cultures may be combined for sampling convenience.

The Impact of Religion on Child Mental Health

Although religion and culture are not the same, they are often closely related. Religion cannot necessarily be separated from all the other factors (such as family factors, culture as discussed earlier, peer relationships etc.) which may also be aetiological factors for the development of child mental health problems. Children may identify a religious affiliation without actually being religious, that is they are associating with the cultural aspects (the rituals and customs) of the religion as opposed to the beliefs. Rew and Wong (2006) systematically reviewed the relationships among religiosity, spirituality, health attitudes and health behaviours in adolescents. Most of the studies showed that measures of religiosity/spirituality had positive effects on health attitudes and behaviours. They concluded that the variety of studies and measures indicate that religiosity and spirituality may be important correlates of adolescent health attitudes and behaviours. Although the majority of the studies reviewed were well designed, there was no consistency in the theoretical bases and operational definitions of religiosity/spirituality phenomena making it difficult to draw conclusions or identify implications for practice. However, religion may be potentially harmful to young people's mental health (this may be especially true when the young person's perspective differs from the family and/or their values and preferences go against the religion ideals as this is likely to cause tensions within the family).

Patterns and Prevalence of Child Psychiatric Morbidity across Different Cultural and Ethnic Groups

The last 30 years have seen a substantial amount of child psychiatry epidemiological research, with indications of a gradual rise in psychiatric disorders in young life, accounting for changes in diagnostic criteria and research methods (Collishaw *et al.*, 2004). However, there has been relatively limited evidence on the nature and severity of mental health problems and disorders in non-Western child populations, and in non-white ethnic groups within Western societies. We review some of these studies here.

As Kieling *et al.* (2011) identify, the assessment of the mental health needs of children and adolescents is complex, encompassing epidemiological data gathering and comparisons of data from different areas which can be challenging. They compared prevalence rates for low- and middle-income countries (LMIC) and disadvantaged communities in high-income countries. Although there is less research, epidemiological studies of the prevalence of childhood and adolescent mental health problems in LMIC show that such problems are common. Kieling *et al.* (2011) report on a systematic review of original studies in non-referred samples from LMIC that showed prevalence of about 10–20 per cent in most of the 16 surveys identified, which is consistent with earlier studies. However, the range varied widely from 1.81 to 39.4 per cent. As the authors identify the cultural context in which the mental health problems occur is important. The way different cultural and environmental factors coexist lead to difficulties in making comparisons across different contexts.

Bor *et al.* (2014) reviewed 19 studies that explored mental health problems of toddlers, children and adolescents. Seventeen studies examined internalizing problems, and 11 studies examined externalizing problems. A majority (14 of 19) were carried out in Europe with one in Australia, one in the USA and two in China). For both children and toddlers, recent cohorts in comparison to previous cohorts did not exhibit worsening of mental health symptoms and nor did externalizing problems in adolescents. However, the majority of studies report an increase in internalizing

problems in adolescent girls with less clear evidence for boys. Collishaw's review (2015) also reflects this.

Polanczyk *et al.* (2015) conducted a systematic review of prevalence studies of mental disorders investigating community samples of children and adolescents and used standard assessment methods to diagnose using DSM or ICD. Their review incorporated 41 studies from 27 countries from every world region. The worldwide prevalence of mental health disorders was 13.4% with rates for anxiety at 3.4%, depression 2.6%, ADHD at 3.4% and any disruptive disorder at 5.7%. On this basis, they conclude that mental health problems affect a significant number of young people across the globe, which remains consistent whichever way you view the studies. However, it is less clear how risk factors across different contexts play out. The worldwide data may be usefully compared with data from the US (Merikangas *et al.*, 2010) which found anxiety disorders were the most common condition (31.9%), followed by behaviour disorders (19.1%), mood disorders (14.3%), and substance use disorders (11.4%), with approximately 40% of participants with one class of disorder also meeting criteria for another class of lifetime disorder. The overall prevalence of disorders with severe impairment and/or distress was 22.2% (11.2% with mood disorders, 8.3% with anxiety disorders, and 9.6% behaviour disorders). The median age of onset for disorder classes was earliest for anxiety (6 years), followed by 11 years for behaviour, 13 years for mood, and 15 years for substance use disorders. Merikangas *et al.* (2010) reported that mood and anxiety disorders were more prevalent among females whereas males had higher rates of behaviour and substance use disorders. Rates of mood and substance use disorders were higher among older adolescents. There were few racial/ethnic differences in the major classes of mental disorders, with the exception of increased rates of anxiety disorders and lower rates of substance use disorder among non-Hispanic black adolescents compared with non-Hispanic white adolescents, and higher rates of mood disorders among Hispanic adolescents compared with non-Hispanic white adolescents. After adjusting for family factors, there were four significant interactions for other disorders: (1) the prevalence of mood disorders was higher in white adolescents in homes with higher levels of parental education than that in black and Hispanic adolescents; (2) rates of substance use disorders increased more dramatically with age for males than females; (3) sex differences in substance use disorders were largest for black adolescents compared with other ethnic groups; and (4) increased rates of substance use disorders were observed among Hispanic adolescents whose parents were divorced. However, rates were decreased among black adolescents whose parents were never married or divorced. Collishaw (2015) argues that the evidence that shows that the increasing rates of child mental health problems are related to real change and not merely changes in how rates are recorded or how data is collected. It appears as though over the last decade that rates of externalizing disorders are relatively stable but that internalizing disorders have increased.

The number of factors that influence the development and presentation of child mental health problems remains consistent and newer research continues to show the strong link between child mental health and social factors including culture. Hussein et al. (2012) identified a range of factors for Pakistani children that were consistent with factors identified in other parts of the world. There are a number of interrelated factors involved, which all possibly play a part in the presentation of child mental health problems, such as adjustment to a different society and socioeconomic deprivation (Boardman et al., 2015; Froehlich et al., 2007), experience of racism and discrimination (Tumaini et al., 2009; Williams and Mohammed, 2009; Paradies et al., 2006), impact of past trauma and immigration and forced migration (Vostanis, 2014; Dogra et al., 2011; Fazel et al., 2012 respectively), war (Thabet and Vostanis, 2012), cultural influences on symptom presentation (Fishman and Fishman, 1999), perceptions of mental health and mental illness (Gulliver et al., 2010; Reinke et al. 2011), different thresholds of reporting problems (Baio, 2012), changing family structures and parenting and gender expectations, sense of identity and self-esteem within a marginalized societal group (Fazel et al. 2012. Paradies (2006) and Fazel et al. (2012) highlight the methodological challenges, which resonate with those discussed above.

Evidence on the prevalence of disorders within different ethnic groups in Western populations is still somewhat limited although there is now data from the US as discussed earlier. The studies in this section were not national surveys but specific population samples. Dogra et al. (2012) studied the prevalence rates of mental health problems in ethnic Indian adolescents in England and compared those with matched white adolescents living in the same areas. A cross-sectional survey with oversampling of Indian adolescents aged 13–15 years was used to overcome the sampling issues identified above. This study found that ethnically Indian adolescents living in England had lower rates of all types of mental health problems and substance misuse than white adolescents did. This was consistent with a study by Goodman et al. (2010), which showed that Indian children are more likely to be protected against externalizing problems. These rates were also consistent with those among indigenous adolescents of a similar age in India (Pillai et al. 2008). Although the proportion of problems and their gender associations were similar to the white population (higher rates of emotional problems for girls and higher rates of conduct problems for boys), as established by Green et al. (2005) and Ravens-Sieberer et al. (2008), rates were significantly lower for all problems, apart from eating disorders.

Van Oort et al. (2007) found that internalizing problems in childhood was a strong predictor for the development of disparities in educational attainment in migrant Turkish families compared with their Dutch counterparts. They argued that prevention or treatment of internalizing problems among Turkish girls would probably contribute to the prevention of educational disparities. Van Oort et al. (2007) also found that Turkish migrant adolescents reported more problems that Dutch children. Similarly, Zwirs et al. (2006) concluded that, in comparison to Dutch boys, Moroccan and Turkish boys were more likely to display problem behaviours and had higher impairment scores.

Future research needs to focus on specific questions related to these variables and probably take a more multidimensional theoretical perspective. Research needs to establish the impact of the variables and their relationships on overall child psychiatric morbidity, as well as specific conditions. It also needs to account for societies, which are changing rapidly and changing patterns of migration. Although not all types of child psychiatric disorders could be covered within this chapter, the major types of disorders are briefly discussed in relation to cultural issues. Whilst there continues to be epidemiological research looking at prevalence rates more broadly, the impact of culture through investigation of specific populations in a multidimensional way is generally less well researched. We now move to look briefly at major disorders and differences across different cultures although research is somewhat limited.

Schizophrenia

Although hallucinations in children and adolescents are relatively common, schizophrenia is not. Psychotic symptoms in children and adolescents are diagnostically non-specific, occurring in a wide range of functional psychiatric and organic brain disorders (e.g. affective disorders, autistic spectrum disorder, substance-use-related psychosis and temporal-lobe epilepsy).

Kelleher et al. (2012) conducted a systemic review on psychotic symptom prevalence in children aged 9–12 years and adolescents aged 13–18 years. Nineteen studies were found with a median prevalence of psychotic symptoms in the younger age group at 17 per cent and 7.5 per cent for adolescents. They identify these rates as being higher than for adults. However, most of those with psychotic symptoms. Bartels-Velthuis et al. (2009) found that auditory hallucinations in younger children had only a minor association with psychopathology but this increased as children approached middle adolescence. Scott et al. (2009) studying Australian adolescents aged 13–17 reported rates of 8.4 per cent. They found hallucinations were more associated with depression and more prevalent in those who had used cannabis. Again, they make the point that hallucinations in children are often not related to psychopathology.

Depression

Depression occurs in 1 per cent of older children, which rises to 4 per cent in adolescence (higher in girls). Children have non-specific symptoms, such as physical complaints, irritability and withdrawal, while adolescents present with adult-like symptoms. Young people with depression often have comorbidity with anxiety, behavioural problems or eating disorders.

Despite several studies in this area, the impact of cultural factors on the presentation and aetiology of depression is inconclusive. Stewart et al. (2002) found similar prevalence rates and cognitive patterns in Hong Kong and the US, but a different symptom profile, with Hong Kong adolescents reporting more fatigue/loss of energy, and less irritability. Similarly, Fleitlich-Bilyk and Goodman (2004) found similar depression rates in Brazil and the UK. Others questioned whether depression is less prevalent among certain ethnocultural groups (e.g. Chinese Americans), because of socially approved mechanisms that protect them from stressors (Chen et al., 1998), or cultural differences in the expression of grief (Murray-Parkes, 1998).

Anxiety Disorders

The presentation of anxiety disorders is broadly similar to that of adults, with the notable exception of separation-anxiety disorders. Anxiety is identified as the commonest mental health problem of young people through several studies as cited previously. There is less evidence on underlying culture-related mechanisms. Meltzer et al. (2008) found that for children's fears, the most marked associations were fears of the dark, loud noises, imagined supernatural beings in younger children and fear of animals in girls and all non-white groups. They concluded that children's fears differ in nature across different ethnic groups and that culturally mediated beliefs, values and traditions may play a role in the expression of different fears. Culturally, girls may also be encouraged to articulate their fears whereas boys may be discouraged from expressing fear.

In contrast, separation-anxiety disorders are more likely to be affected by culture-related attachment and child-rearing factors (Thabet et al., 2000). Cultural and societal concepts of acceptable child-rearing practices (i.e. for how long an infant or toddler may share the parents' bed or room, if at all), will impact on the perceptions of normal or dysfunctional parent–child separation, across different settings.

Dyregrov and Yule (2006) reported that more girls than boys qualify for the diagnosis of post-traumatic stress disorder, while boys show higher rates of behaviour symptoms. In adolescence, there is often a sense of foreshortened future in line with their understanding of long-term perspectives, as well as the social ramifications of trauma.

Eating Disorders

Swanson et al. (2011) examined the prevalence and correlates of eating disorders in a large, representative sample of US adolescents. Lifetime prevalence estimates of anorexia nervosa, bulimia nervosa, and binge-eating disorder were 0.3, 0.9 and 1.6 per cent, respectively. Significant ethnic differences emerged for bulimia nervosa, with Hispanic adolescents reporting the highest prevalence; there was a trend toward ethnic minorities reporting more binge eating disorders, while non-Hispanic white adolescents tended to report more anorexia nervosa. Measures of socio-economic status, including parental education, household income, and parental/surrogate marital status, were not significantly associated with any eating disorder presentation. The majority of respondents with an eating disorder met criteria for at least one other lifetime DSM-IV disorder across the lifetime.

Swanson et al. (2012) also found that the lifetime prevalence of binge-eating disorder was 1.6 per cent in Mexico and 2.2 per cent among Mexican Americans. Compared with Mexicans in families with migrants, risk for binge-eating disorder was higher in US-born Mexican Americans with two US-born parents. Among respondents reporting binge eating, onset in the US compared with Mexico was not associated with prevalence of further eating disorder symptoms. Migration from Mexico to the US is associated with an increased risk for binge-eating disorders that may be partially attributable to non-specific influences on internalizing disorders. Among respondents reporting binge eating in either country, similar levels of further symptoms were endorsed, suggesting some cross-cultural generalizability of criteria.

At 8 per cent, there was no significant difference in the rates of possible eating disorders between the British Indian and British white adolescents in the study by Dogra et al. (2013). This, however, was considerably less than identified in a German study of 1,895 young people aged between 11 and 17 years, which found that 29 per cent girls and 14 per cent of boys scored beyond the normal threshold (Herpertz-Dahlmann et al. 2008). The figures from the Dogra study suggest that there may be less discrepancy between white and Indian groups than was previously identified (for example Jennings et al., 2005). Mellor et al. (2009) investigated body dissatisfaction and body change behaviours among a sample of 529 Malaysian high school students (103 Malays, 344 Chinese and 82 Indians), who completed a set of measures in classroom settings. Chinese girls were more dissatisfied with their bodies than Chinese boys were, but no gender difference was found for

Malay and Indian participants. Girls were more likely to engage in behaviours to lose weight, and boys were more likely to engage in behaviours to increase muscle. Thomas et al. (2002) found high eating symptoms in Asians and Muslims and for mixed-race young women than among white or African Caribbean subjects. These were also associated with low self-esteem and depressed mood, as was having only one parent in employment. The findings suggest that effects of cultural and socio-economic stresses on eating disorders may be mediated through depressed mood and low self-esteem.

Substance-Use Disorders

An epidemiological survey in north-east India (Chaturvedi and Mahanta, 2004) found high prevalence of substance use (tobacco at 30.9%, alcohol at 30% and opium at 4.8%). The prevalence varied across location, gender, race, age, education and occupation. Certain tribes had high alcohol use related to strong cultural beliefs. Average age of initiation of alcohol use at 12.4 years was significantly lower than tobacco at 17.6 years, and opium at 23.3 years. Obe and Wibberley (2002) found that, whilst patterns of substance use and misuse amongst Asians may be similar in many ways to those for the general population, they occur within a different cultural context. The higher use of substances in boys compared to girls, found in the Indian and white groups by Dogra et al.'s (2013) study reflects the same pattern as identified previously in that boys reported higher rates of substance misuse. However, rates were higher in the white group, which is also consistent with earlier work (for example, Karlsen et al., 1998).

Sami youth showed less risk-taking behaviour as substance and drug use than the Norwegian majority (Kvernmo, 2004). Sami adolescents growing up in Sami dominated areas have a strong bicultural identification, are practising more Sami cultural behaviour and have better mental health compared to Sami peers in marginal Sami areas. This suggests that a strong sense of cultural identity may only be an issue in marginal areas when it may be difficult to express the sense of identity.

Self-Harm

The lifetime prevalence of deliberate self-harm in adolescence has been found to be between 2 and 3.5

per cent in studies from Europe, and much higher in the United States (about 9%). It increases with age, is more common in females (3:1) and low socio-economic groups, and is often precipitated by arguments with family, friends or partner.

Madge *et al.* (2008) reported deliberate self-harm is a widespread yet often hidden problem in adolescents, especially females, which shows both similarities and differences internationally through a study of seven countries with self-report data from over 30,000 adolescents. Self-harm was more than twice as common among females as males and, in four of the seven countries, at least one in ten females had harmed herself in the previous year. Additional young people had thought of harming themselves without doing so. More males and females in all countries except Hungary cut themselves than used any other method, most acts took place at home, and alcohol and illegal drugs were not usually involved. The most common reasons given were 'to get relief from a terrible state of mind' followed by 'to die', although there were differences between those cutting themselves and those taking overdoses. Through a systematic review, Muehlenkamp *et al.* (2012) also concluded that non-suicidal self-injury and deliberate self-harm have a comparable prevalence in studies with adolescents from different countries.

Neurodevelopmental Disorders

Part of the increasing prevalence of child mental health disorders has been an improvement in their recognition. Attention deficit disorders and autistic spectrum disorders (ASD) have emerged over the past three decades as a significant issue for child psychiatrists in the US and Europe (Collishaw 2015). The prevalence rate for attention deficit/hyperactivity disorder (ADHD) was between 3 and 7 per cent (American Psychiatric Association and APA Task Force on DSM-IV; APA 2000). Outside the US, prevalence rates are lower which may reflect diagnostic differences rather than true prevalence differences. Collishaw (2015) cites research from across different countries that has found evidence of a continuing increase in the diagnosis of ASD. Elsabbagh *et al.* (2012) through a systematic review reported a median prevalence of 62 per 10,000 but as high as 1 in 100 in Sweden and the United States. It is likely that the differences result from a combination of different factors including cultural contexts, understandings

and expectations. As discussed earlier, Lehti *et al.* (2016) found increased rates of ADHD in children of immigrants but in another study (Lehti *et al.*, 2015) they found children whose parents are both immigrants have a significantly lower likelihood of being diagnosed with ASD than those with two Finnish parents. Again, they conclude that the difference may be accounted for by differential service use.

Conclusions

As in all other psychiatric specialties, consideration of culture and the social world is important in understanding individuals who present with psychiatric symptomatology. With children and young people, it is also necessary to consider how these are perceived within the context they present, as this varies from culture to culture and from family to family. Whilst over the last two decades research in this area has increased, there is still limited evidence on the nature and severity of mental health problems and disorders in non-Western child populations and in non-white ethnic groups within Western societies. However, the prevalence of child mental health disorders appears to be increasing worldwide particularly for internalizing disorders.

References

Achenbach, T. (1991). *Manual for the Child Behaviour Checklist/4–18*. Burlington, VT: University of Vermont.

Baio, Jon (2012). Prevalence of autism spectrum disorders: Autism and Developmental Disabilities Monitoring Network, 14 Sites, United States 2008. *Morbidity and Mortality Weekly Report. Surveillance Summaries*, **61**(3), 1–19.

Bartels-Velthuis, A., Jenner J., van de Willige, G., van Os, J. and Wiersma, D. (2009). Prevalence and correlates of auditory vocal hallucinations in middle childhood. *British Journal of Psychiatry*, **196**, 41–46, doi: 10.1192/bjp.bp.109.065953.

Boardman, J., Dogra, N. and Hindley, P. (2015). Mental health and poverty in the UK: time for change. *BJPsych International* **12**, 27–28.

Bor, W., Dean, A.J., Najam, J. and Hayatbakhsh, R. (2014). Are child and adolescent mental health problems increasing in the 21st century? A systematic review. *Australian and New Zealand Journal of Psychiatry*, **48**, 606–616.

Canino, G. and Alegría, M. (2008). Psychiatric diagnosis: is it universal or relative to culture? *Journal of Child Psychology and Psychiatry*, **49**, 237–250.

Chaturvedi, H. and Mahanta, J. (2004). Sociocultural diversity and substance use pattern in Arunachal Pradesh, India. *Drug and Alcohol Dependency*, **74**, 97–104.

Chen, I., Roberts, R. and Aday, L. A. (1998). Ethnicity and adolescent depression: the case of Chinese Americans. *Journal of Nervous and Mental Disease*, **186**, 623–630.

Collishaw, S. (2015). Annual research review: secular trends in child and adolescent mental health. *Journal of Child Psychology and Psychiatry*, **56**, 370–393.

Collishaw, S., Maughan, B., Goodman, R. and Pickles, A. (2004). Time trends in adolescent mental health. *Journal of Child Psychology and Psychiatry*, **45**, 1350–1362.

Corsaro W. (2011). *The Sociology of Childhood*, 3rd edn. California: Pine Forge Press.

Dogra, N., Karim, K. and Ronzoni, P. (2011). Migration and its effects on child mental health. In *Migration and Mental Health*, ed. D. Bhugra and S. Gupta. Cambridge: Cambridge University Press, pp. 196–208.

Dogra, N., Singh, S., Svirydzenka, N. and Vostanis, P. (2012). Prevalence of mental health problems in children and young people from ethnic minority groups: the need for targeted research. *British Journal of Psychiatry*, **200**, 265–267.

Dogra, N., Svirydzenka, N., Dugard, P., Singh, S. P. and Vostanis, P. (2013). The characteristics and rates of mental health problems among Indian and white adolescents in two English cities. *British Journal of Psychiatry*, **203**, 44–50.

Dyregrov, A. and Yule, W. (2006). A Review of PTSD in children. *Child and Adolescent Mental Health*, **11**, 176–184, doi: 10.1111/j.1475–3588.2005.00384.

Elsabbagh, M., Divan, G., Koh, Y.-J. et al. (2012). Global prevalence of autism and other pervasive developmental disorders. *Autism Research*, **5**, 160–179.

Falicov, C. (1995). Training to think culturally: a multidimensional comparative framework. *Family Process*, **34**, 373–388.

Fazel, M., Reed, R. V., Panter-Brick, C. and Stein, A. (2012). Mental health of displaced and refugee children resettled in high-income countries: risk and protective factors. *The Lancet*, **379**, 266–282.

Fishman, S. and Fishman, R. (1999). Cultural influences on symptom presentation in childhood. *Journal of the American Academy of Child and Adolescent Psychiatry*, **38**, 782–783.

Fleitlich-Bilyk, B. and Goodman, R. (2004). Prevalence of child and adolescent psychiatric disorders in Southeast Brazil. *Journal of the American Academy of Child and Adolescent Psychiatry*, **43**, 727–734.

Froehlich, T., Lanphear, B., Epstein, J., Barbaresi, W., Katusic, S., Kahn, R. (2007). Prevalence, recognition, and treatment of attention-deficit/hyperactivity disorder in a national sample of US children. *Archives of Pediatric and Adolescent Medicine*, **9**, 857–864.

Goodman, R. (2001). Psychometric properties of the Strengths and Difficulties Questionnaire. *Journal of the American Academy of Child and Adolescent Psychiatry*, **40**, 1337–1345.

Goodman, A., Patel, V., Leon, D. (2010). Why do British Indian children have an apparent mental health advantage? *The Journal of Child Psychology and Psychiatry*, **51**, 1171–1183.

Green, H., McGinnity, A., Meltzer, H., Ford, T. and Goodman, R. (2005). *Mental Health of Children and Young People in Great Britain*. Norwich: ONS/HMSO; Basingstoke: Palgrave Macmillan.

Gulliver, A., Griffiths, K. and Christensen, H. (2010). Perceived barriers and facilitators to mental health help-seeking in young people: a systematic review. *BMC Psychiatry*, **10**, 113.

Heiervang, E., Goodman, A. and Goodman, R. (2008). The Nordic advantage in child mental health: separating health differences from reporting style in a cross-cultural comparison of psychopathology. *Journal of Child Psychology and Psychiatry*, **49**, 678–685.

Herpertz-Dahlmann, B., Wille, N., Holling, H., Vloet, T. and Ravens-Sieberer, U. (2008). BELLA study group. Disordered eating behaviour and attitudes, associated psychopathology and health related quality of life: results of the BELLA study. *European Child and Adolescent Psychiatry*, (Suppl 1) **17**, 82–91.

Heyerdahl, S., Kvernmo, S. and Wichstrom, L. (2004). Self-reported behavioural/emotional problems in Norwegian adolescents from multiethnic areas. *European Child and Adolescent Psychiatry*, **13**, 64–72.

Hussein, S., Vostanis, P. and Bankart, J. (2012). Social and educational risk factors for child mental health problems in Karachi, Pakistan. *International Journal of Mental Health and Culture*, **5**, 1–14.

Jennings, P., Forbes, D., McDermott, B., Juniper, S. and Hulse, G. (2005). Acculturation and eating disorders in Asian and Caucasian Australian adolescent girls. *Psychiatry and Clinical Neurosciences*, **59**, 56–61.

Karlsen, S., Rogers, A. and McCarthy, M. (1998). Social environment and substance misuse: a study of ethnic variations among inner London adolescents. *Ethnicity and Health*, **3**, 265–273.

Karnik, N. and Dogra, N. (2010). The cultural sensibility model for children and adolescents: a process oriented approach. *Child and Adolescent Psychiatric Clinics of North America*, **19**, 719–738.

Kashala, E., Elgen, I., Sommerfelt, K. and Tylleskar, T. (2005). Teacher ratings of mental health among schoolchildren in Kinshasa, Democratic Republic of Congo. *European Child and Adolescent Psychiatry*, **14**, 208–215.

Kelleher, I., Connor, D., Clarke, M. C., Devlin, N., Harley, M. and Cannon, M. (2012). Prevalence of psychotic symptoms in childhood and adolescence: a systematic review and meta-analysis of population-based studies. *Psychological Medicine*, **9**, 1–7.

Kieling, C., Baker-Henningham, H., Belfer, M., Conti, G., Ertem, I., Omigbodun, O., Rohde, L.A., Srinath, S., Ulkuer, N. and Rahman, A. (2011). Child and adolescent mental health worldwide: evidence for action. *The Lancet*, **378**, 1515–1525.

Kvernmo, S. (2004). Mental health of Sami youth. *International Journal of Circumpolar Health*, **63**, 221–224.

Lehti, V., Cheslack-Postava, K., Gissler, M., Hinkka-Yli-Salomäki, S., Brown, A. S. and Sourander, A. (2015). Parental migration and Asperger's syndrome. *European Child and Adolescent Psychiatry*, **24**, 941–948.

Lehti, V., Chudal, R., Suominen, A., Gissler, M. and Sourander, A. (2016). Association between immigrant background and ADHD: a nationwide population-based case control study. *Journal of Child Psychology and Psychiatry*, **57**(8), 967–975, doi: 10.1111/jcpp.12570.

Madge, N., Hewitt, A., Hawton, K. *et al.* (2008). Deliberate self-harm within an international community sample of young people: comparative findings from the Child and Adolescent Self-harm in Europe (CASE) study. *Journal of Child Psychology and Psychiatry*, **49**, 667–677.

Mellor, D., McCabe, M., Ricciardelli, L., Yeow, J., Daliza, N. and Hapidzal, N. (2009). Sociocultural influences on body dissatisfaction and body change behaviors among Malaysian adolescents. *Body Image*, **6**, 121–128.

Meltzer, H., Vostanis, P., Dogra, N., Doos, L., Ford, T. and Goodman, R. (2008). Children's specific fears. *Child: Care, Health and Development*, **35**(6), 781–789.

Merikangas, K., He, J., Burstein, M., Swanson, S., Avenevoli, S., Cui, L. and Swendsen, J. (2010). Lifetime prevalence of mental disorders in US adolescents: results from the national comorbidity study – adolescent supplement (NCS-A). *Journal of the American Academy of Child and Adolescent Psychiatry*, **49**, 980–989.

Muehlenkamp, J. J., Claes, L., Havertape, L. and Plener, P. L. (2012). International prevalence of adolescent non-suicidal self-injury and deliberate self-harm. *Child and Adolescent Psychiatry and Mental Health*, **6**, 10.

Murray-Parkes, C. (1998). Understanding grief across cultures. *Psychiatry in Practice*, Winter Issue, 5–8.

Nguyen, L., Huang, L. N., Arganza, G. F. and Liao, Q. (2007). The influence of race and ethnicity on psychiatric diagnoses and clinical characteristics of children and adolescents in children's services. *Cultural Diversity and Ethnic Minority Psychology*, **13**, 18–25.

Obe, K. and Wibberley, C. (2002). Young Asians and drug use. *Journal of Child Health Care*, **6**, 51–59.

O'Reilly, M., Ronzoni, P. and Dogra, N. (2013). *Research with Children*. London: Sage.

Paradies, Y. (2006) A systematic review of empirical research on self-reported racism and health. *International Journal of Epidemiology*, **35**, 888–901.

Pillai, A., Patel, V., Cardozo, P., Goodman, R., Weiss, H. A. and Gracy, A. (2008) Non-traditional lifestyles and prevalence of mental disorders in adolescents in Goa, India. *BJPsych*, **192**, 45–51.

Polanczyk, G. V., Salum, G. A., Sugaya, L. S., Caye, A. and Rohde, L. A. (2015). Annual research review: a meta-analysis of the worldwide prevalence of mental health disorders in children and adolescents. *Journal of Child Psychology and Psychiatry*, **56**, 345–365.

Prior, M., Sanson, A. and Oberklaid, F. (1999). Psychological disorders and their correlates in an Australian community sample of preadolescent children. *Journal of Child Psychology and Psychiatry*, **40**, 563–580.

Ravens-Sieberer, U., Wille, N., Erhart, M., *et al.* the BELLA study group (2008). Prevalence of mental health problems among children and adolescents in Germany: results of the BELLA study within the National Health Interview and Examination survey. *European Child and Adolescent Psychiatry* (Suppl 1) **17**, 22–33.

Reinke, W., Stormont, M., Herman, K., Puri, R., Goel, N. (2011) Supporting children's mental health in schools. *School Psychology Quarterly*, **26**, 1–13.

Rew, L. and Wong, Y. J. (2006). A systematic review of associations among religiosity/spirituality and adolescent health attitudes and behaviors. *Journal of Adolescent Health*, **38**, 433–442.

Rousseau, C., Measham, T. and Bathiche-Suidan, M. (2008). DSM IV, culture and child psychiatry. *Journal of the Canadian Academy of Child and Adolescent Psychiatry*, **17**, 69–75.

Scott, J., Martin, M., Bor, W., Sawyer, M., Clark, J. and McGrath, J. (2009). The prevalence and correlates of hallucinations in Australian adolescents: results from a national survey. *Schizophrenia Research*, **107**, 179–185.

Stewart, S. M., Lewinsohn, P., Lee, P. *et al.* (2002). Symptom patterns in depression and 'subthreshold' depression among adolescents in Hong Kong and the United States. *Journal of Cross Cultural Psychology*, **33**, 559–576.

Swanson, S., Crow, S., Le Grange, D., Swendsen, J. and Merikangas, J. (2011). Prevalence and correlates of eating disorders in adolescents: results from the national comorbidity survey replication adolescent supplement. *Archives of General Psychiatry*, **68**, 714–723.

Swanson, S. A., Borges, G., Benjet, C., Aguilar-Gaxiola, S., Medine-Mora, M. E. and Brelau, J. (2012). Change in binge eating and binge eating disorder associated with migration from Mexico to the US. *Journal of Psychiatric Research*, **46**, 31–37.

Thabet, A. A. and Vostanis, P. (2012). Impact of political violence and trauma in Gaza on children's mental health and types of interventions: a review of research evidence in a historical context. *International Journal of Peace and Developmental Studies*, 2, 214–218.

Thabet, A. A., Stretch, D. and Vostanis, P. (2000). Child mental health problems in Arab children: application of the Strengths and Difficulties Questionnaire. *International Journal of Social Psychiatry*, 46, 266–280.

Thomas, C., James, A. and Bachmann, M. (2002). Eating attitudes in English secondary school students: influences of ethnicity, gender, mood, and social class. *International Journal of Eating Disorders*, 31, 92–96.

Tumaini, R., Coker, M., Elliott, D., Kanouse, J., Grunbaum, D., Schwebel, M., Gilliland, J., Tortolero, S., Peskin, M. and Schuster, M. (2009). Perceived racial/ethnic discrimination among fifth-grade students and its association with mental health. *American Journal of Public Health*, **99**, 878–884.

United Nations Convention on the Rights of the Child (1989). Conventions on the rights of the child. London: UNICEF. Available at www.unicef .org.uk/Documents/Publication-pdfs/UNCRC_PRES S200910web.pdf (accessed 19 June 2016).

Van Oort, F., Van der Ende, J., Crijnen, A., Verhulst, F., Mackenbach, J. and Joung, I. (2007). Ethnic disparities in mental health and educational attainment: comparing migrant and native children. *International Journal of Social Psychiatry*, 53, 514–525.

Vostanis, P. (2014). *Helping Children and Young People Who Experience Trauma: Children of Despair, Children of Hope*. London: Radcliffe Publishing.

Williams, D. R. and Mohammed, S. A. (2009). Discrimination and racial disparities in health: evidence and needed research. *Journal of Behavioral Medicine*, 32, 20–47.

Zwirs, B., Burger, H., Schulpen, T. and Buitelaar, J. (2006). Different treatment thresholds in non-Western children with behavioral problems. *American Academy of Child and Adolescent Psychiatry*, 45, 476–483.

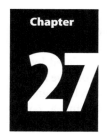

Culture and Schizophrenia

Thomas Stompe and David Holzer

Editors' Introduction

Over the decades as our understanding of schizophrenia has progressed, it has become clearer that the symptoms of the condition and indeed the syndrome are seen across all cultures although actual rates may vary. There have been arguments and debates which suggest some universal features and others unique to some cultures. Stompe and Holzer in this chapter describe some of the phenomena and their commonalities. It is inevitable that cultures affect not only the contents of hallucinations and delusions but also actual presentations. As has been noted elsewhere especially by Jablensky in his chapter in this volume, cross-epidemiological studies set out by the WHO highlighted common features and offered an indication of actual rates. There is no doubt that schizophrenia is a complex disorder which should be seen as a syndrome. It is also notable that presentation of different subtypes of schizophrenia such as hebephrenic or catatonic types are becoming rare. Reasons for this variation are not always clear, Stompe and Holzer remind us that schizophrenia is both universal and homogeneous of all major mental disorders. It may show similar epidemiological patterns and phenomenological features across all cultures. They go on to argue that these large WHO studies may have set the applicable comparable standards but the research on comparing psychotic symptoms in schizophrenia across cultures has shown that reality is somewhat more complicated. Like other psychiatric illnesses, culture has a major impact on prevalence and outcome of schizophrenic disorders, as well as on their occurrence and their psychopathology and presentations in health services. Stompe and Holzer argue passionately that despite the fact that many facets of the way in which culture influences mental disorders remain unknown, in the era of globalization, cultural knowledge and sensitivity are essential qualities of professionals treating migrants as well as native-born mentally ill patients.

Introduction

The phenomenology of what we nowadays call schizophrenia has been recognized in almost all cultures. The first systematic descriptions of this disease can be found since the beginning of the nineteenth century. In 1899 Kraepelin combined different clinical pictures, characterized by early age of onset and a chronic and deteriorating course, under the term dementia praecox (Kraepelin, 1899). To emphasize the occurring cognitive impairment and the concept of the splitting of psychic processes, Eugen Bleuler introduced the term schizophrenia (Bleuler, 1911). In current diagnostic criteria DSM-IV and DSM-IV-TR, schizophrenia is defined by a group of characteristic positive, negative, psychomotor and disorganized symptoms, deterioration in social, occupational or interpersonal relationships and continuous signs of the disturbance for at least 6 months (APA, 1994, 2000).

Culture and the Epidemiology of Schizophrenia

Varying incidence and prevalence rates define the 'epidemiological landscape' of a disease. Meta-analysing 161 studies on the incidence of schizophrenia from 33 countries, McGrath et al. (2004) found a median value of 15.2 (7.7–43.0) of new cases per 100,000 population. However, compared to somatic diseases like diabetes or cancer, the incidence of schizophrenia is very similar across populations (Saha et al., 2006). Reviewing and meta-analysing 188 studies from 46 countries, the calculated median value for lifetime prevalence was 4.0 (1.6–12.1) per 1,000 population (Saha et al. 2005). The prevalence estimates for 'least developed' countries (median = 2.62) were significantly lower ($P = 0.02$) than those from 'emerging' (median = 4.69) and from developed sites (median = 3.30). These prevalence rates confirm the results of authors like Torrey et al. (1974), who investigated the prevalence of schizophrenia in traditional cultures like Papua New Guinea. In the mountain districts the prevalence rate was between 0.03 and 0.19 per 1,000 population, in the coast districts with a longer tradition of contacts with Australians and Europeans the rates were significantly higher (0.38 and 0.77 per 1,000).

Culture and the Outcome of Schizophrenia

One of the most striking findings of the World Health Organization (WHO) International Pilot Study of Schizophrenia (IPSS) conducted in the 1960s and 1970s was the more favourable outcome for patients in the developing world (Jablensky, 1987, 2000; Leff et al., 1992; Sartorius et al., 1986). The original IPSS consisted of 1,202 patients with a PSE (present state examination) diagnosis of schizophrenia drawn from China, Columbia, Czechoslovakia, Denmark, India, Nigeria, the United Kingdom, the United States, and the Union of Soviet Socialist Republics. The 5-year follow-up showed a broad heterogeneity and a more favourable outcome of the disorder in the developing countries. This result was confirmed by the following cross-cultural studies organized and performed by the WHO: the Determinants of Outcome of Severe Mental Disorder (DOSMeD; e.g. Edgerton and Cohen, 1994) and the International Study of Schizophrenia (ISoS; e.g. Hopper and Wanderling, 2000). The aim of the DOSMeD project was to identify all persons suffering from the first onset of schizophrenia in 13 catchment areas located in 10 different countries over a period of 2 years. Like with the IPSS, the most important finding of this research was the existence of consistent and marked differences in the prognosis of schizophrenia between the centres of developed countries and the centres of developing countries (Craig et al., 1997; Edgerton and Cohen, 1994; Jablensky et al., 1992). A series of further studies in India continued the programme of the IPSS. In a multicentre study in Lucknow, Vellore and Madras of 323 early-course schizophrenic patients (modified Feighner's criteria) the authors found a 66 per cent remission rate at 2-year follow-up (Verghese et al., 1993). Comparable with a similar study conducted in Columbia (Leon, 1989), there was only a 2 per cent suicide rate, and 40 per cent of patients were employed at 2 years. In a second Indian research project, the Madras Longitudinal Study, both positive and negative symptoms showed a significant decline

at the end of 10 years. Sixty-seven per cent of the sample showed a good pattern of course, leading to partial or complete recovery (Thara et al., 1994; Thara, 2004). In a Nigerian study stimulated by the IPSS, Ohaeri (1993) conducted a retrospective follow-up of 142 patients meeting the research diagnostic criteria (RDC) for schizophrenia. During a 7-year follow-up, 50.7 per cent achieved a good outcome and 23.9 per cent a moderate outcome. An acute onset followed by an episodic course with rapid remission in response to treatment was typical. In a 1-year follow-up of 56 patients with schizophrenia from Trinidad, Bhugra found low poor-outcome rates of 19 per cent (Bhugra et al., 1996). Although most studies showed a favourable prognosis of course and outcome of schizophrenic psychoses in developing countries, this result as well as the possible reasons were discussed as being highly controversial (e.g. Patel et al., 2006; Williams 2003). Patel et al. (2006) pointed at methodological limitations of the three WHO cross-national studies, but also mentioned the lack of evidence on the socio-cultural factors, which apparently contribute to the better outcome.

Culture and the Rate of Schizophrenia Subtypes

Kraepelin performed the first study on schizophrenia in traditional cultures by investigating psychotic patients in Java (Kraepelin 1904a, b). He found all classical clinical features of dementia praecox, however, with different accentuations and frequencies. Initial depression was rare, the psychosis usually started with confusion and agitation; auditory hallucinations, thought influence and hypochondriac delusions played a minor role; delusions were seldom systematized, negativistic stupor was rare (Jilek, 1995).

The first systematic investigation on schizophrenia subtypes in different cultures was carried out by Murphy in the 1960s (Murphy, 1982). Catatonic subtypes were rare among Euro-Americans, hebephrenic subtypes occurred more often in Japanese and Okinawan, and the simple subtype occurred in Asian patients.

The IPSS was a milestone for our knowledge of the cultural distribution of schizophrenic subtypes (WHO, 1973). Schizophrenic patients, 811 from nine centres (Washington, London, Aarhus, Prague, Moscow, Cali, Agra, Ibadan and Taipei), were subclassified according to the ICD-9 criteria of schizophrenia subtypes (Table 27.1).

Table 27.1 The frequency (in %) of schizophrenia subtypes according to ICD-9 in the International Pilot Study of Schizophrenia

	Simple	Hebephrenic	Catatonic	Paranoid	Acute	Latent	Residual	Schizoaffective	Other specified	Unspecified
Washington	4.1	–	1.0	52.6	15.5	2.1	6.2	15.5	–	3.1
London	2.0	9.0	3.0	75.0	1.0	–	1.0	8.0	–	1.0
Aarhus	11.3	22.6	3.8	52.8	–	5.7	–	1.9	1.9	–
Prague	6.6	3.9	–	47.4	5.3	2.6	2.6	26.3	3.9	1.3
Moscow	–	–	16.9	14.3	18.2	–	6.5	44.2	–	–
Agra	4.0	3.0	21.7	14.9	9.9	–	–	16.8	3.0	26.7
Cali	2.0	19.8	12.9	19.8	28.7	3.0	5.9	6.9	–	1.0
Taipei	1.2	34.9	3.5	41.8	4.7	–	–	9.3	–	3.5
Ibadan	5.8	7.5	8.3	40.8	4.2	–	–	21.7	2.5	9.2

Source: WHO (1973)

The largest diagnostic sub-group in the total sample was paranoid schizophrenia with 39.8 per cent. It accounted for 75 per cent of all patients in London, 53 per cent in Aarhus and Washington, and more than 40 per cent in both Ibadan and Taipei. The hebephrenic subtype was assigned in 10.6 per cent of all patients, with the highest rates in Cali and Taipei; 10.6 per cent were classified as catatonic schizophrenia, with the highest rates in the centres of the developing countries (Agra, Cali, Ibadan). In a transcultural study on schizophrenia, the International Study on Psychotic Symptoms (ISPS) organized by the Vienna International Research Group on Cultural Psychiatry, DSM-IV criteria were applied.

Similar to the IPSS, in most of the investigated sites paranoid schizophrenia was the most frequent subtype (19–90 per cent), only in Nigeria was schizo-affective disorder diagnosed more often (see Table 27.2). In contrast to the findings of studies on schizophrenic subtypes conducted in Africa during the last century (Murphy, 1982), the rate of catatonic subtypes was very similar in all sites. This may be due to DSM-IV criteria of catatonic schizophrenia, a problem which was discussed in detail (Stompe et al., 2002, 2005). While Austria, Georgia and Pakistan show the highest rates of chronic patients (residual and disorganized type), the African countries are characterized by higher rates of acute forms, especially schizoaffective (Nigeria and Ghana) and schizophreniform disorders (Nigeria).

Culture and Psychotic Symptoms in Schizophrenia

Contents of Delusions

For the contents of delusions, the personal and cultural system of values of an individual is of particular importance. For example, delusions of grandeur can hardly be found in village communities where it is regarded as reprehensible and dangerous to strive for a given social level (Pfeiffer, 1994; Stompe et al., 1999). While religious delusions and delusional guilt are primarily found in societies with a Christian tradition, these contents are infrequent in Islamic, Hindu or Buddhist societies (Kala and Wig, 1982; Kim et al., 2001; McLean et al. 2014; Murphy, 1967; Ndetei and Vadher, 1984a; Stompe et al., 1999, 2006; Tateyama et al., 1998). However, recent studies have shown that traditional religious beliefs occur also in delusions and hallucinations of Chinese patients with

schizophrenia (Yip, 2003). These and similar results point at the difficulties of distinguishing between religious illness concepts and true religious delusions, especially in schizophrenic patients from non-Western countries (Stompe 2014).

Table 27.3 shows the 1-year prevalence of delusional themes reported by schizophrenic patients of the ISPS. Independent of culture, persecution was the most common delusional theme in all sites, followed by grandeur. Pakistan, the only pure Islamic country, showed a pattern of delusional contents remarkably different from the other sites with Christian majorities: low rates of religious delusions, delusions of grandeur and delusions of guilt (Stompe et al., 2006). Religious delusions occurred only as persecution by demons or possession by Djins (Stompe et al., 1999). In contrast to the African countries religious grandiosity ('being an angel or a prophet', etc.) was not reported by Pakistani patients. Taking into account the different rates of delusional contents in Pakistan and the West African countries, one has to conclude that the distinction 'developed' vs 'developing' countries is an oversimplification with less explanatory value.

Hallucinations

The first large study about the frequency of different kinds of hallucinations in a cross-cultural investigation was conducted in the 1960s (Murphy et al., 1963). One of the central findings was that visual hallucinations as well as tactile hallucinations occurred most frequently in patients from Africa and the Near East. Nearly 20 years later, Ndetei and Vadher (1984c) carried out a cross-cultural study including patients with schizophrenia from nine ethnicities admitted to a London hospital. The authors found higher rates of both auditory and visual hallucinations in non-European patients compared to English and continental Europeans. To investigate the impact of the culture of origin and the environmental influence of the second home, Suhail and Cochrane (2002) compared a sample of patients from Pakistan living in their home country, with a sample of Pakistanis, who immigrated to Great Britain, and with patients of white British origin. Patients living in Pakistan reported visual hallucinations and also visualizations of spirits or ghosts statistically significantly more often compared with the two British groups. Acoustic hallucinations were significantly less frequent in the Pakistani group than in both British groups. These findings underline

Table 27.2 The frequency of schizophrenia subtypes according to DSM-IV

	Disorganized	Catatonic	Paranoid	Residual	Indifferent	Schizoaffective	Schizophreniform	Brief psychotic
Austria (N = 350)	3.7	7.4	70.9	10.4	3.0	4.7	–	–
Poland (N = 80)	5.0	3.6	88.8	–	–	2.5	–	–
Lithuania (N = 73)	1.4	4.1	90.4	–	–	–	4.1	–
Georgia (N = 74)	10.8	8.1	50.0	17.6	–	11.2	1.4	–
Pakistan (N = 103)	23.3	2.9	43.7	13.6	16.5	–	–	–
Nigeria (N = 324)	6.3	6.3	18.8	2.1	10.4	29.2	27.1	–
Ghana (N = 76)	6.6	6.6	40.8	3.9	1.3	35.5	2.6	2.6

Source: International Study on Psychotic Symptoms; N = 1,080

Table 27.3 Frequency of occurrence of contents of delusions in schizophrenia during the last year by culture

	Austria (N = 350)	Poland (N = 80)	Lithuania (N = 73)	Georgia (N = 74)	Pakistan (N = 103)	Nigeria (N = 324)	Ghana (N = 76)
Persecution	82.1	90.0	98.6	66.2	91.3	77.1	98.7
Grandeur	43.5	41.3	42.5	37.8	10.7	41.7	64.5
Religion	34.7	33.8	30.1	32.4	7.8	37.5	51.3
Hypochondria	17.4	28.8	23.3	3.4	4.9	14.2	27.6
Guilt	13.8	18.8	24.7	5.4	1.0	10.4	9.2
Poisoning	10.7	31.3	32.9	32.4	16.5	29.2	39.5
Apocalypse	8.3	12.5	32.9	2.7	1.0	18.8	9.2
Descent	4.7	12.5	15.1	25.7	–	8.3	10.5
Being Loved	5.5	11.3	4.1	12.2	–	6.3	9.2
Jealousy	2.2	1.3	5.2	6.8	1.9	6.3	2.6

Source: International Study on Psychotic Symptoms; N = 1,080

Table 27.4 Frequency of occurrence of hallucinations in schizophrenia during the last year by culture

	Austria (N = 350)	Poland (N = 80)	Lithuania (N = 73)	Georgia (N = 74)	Pakistan (N = 103)	Nigeria (N = 324)	Ghana (N = 76)
Audible	64.7	83.8	82.2	71.6	72.8	85.2	90.8
Visual	38.0	45.0	37.0	9.5	3.9	45.8	53.9
Coenesthetic	35.0	28.8	31.5	20.3	23.3	18.8	48.7
Gustatory	3.6	8.8	13.7	14.0	–	8.3	6.6
Olfactory	8.3	10.0	12.3	6.8	–	8.3	1.3
Tactile	5.0	7.5	11.0	8.1	2.9	14.6	6.6

Source: International Study on Psychotic Symptoms; N = 1,080

the major importance of the immediate environment on the phenomenology of hallucinations compared with the influence of culture.

Significant differences in the frequencies of several kinds of hallucinations were found in our study (Table 27.4). The prevalence of visual hallucinations in developing countries was inhomogeneous (Bauer *et al.*, 2011). As to be expected, in every country, auditory hallucinations showed the highest prevalence. In line with the literature, visual hallucinations were most frequently reported by West African patients (Nigeria, 45.8 per cent; Ghana, 53.9 per cent); the rate for Pakistanis was only 3.9 per cent. As mentioned earlier, the distinction of 'developing' and 'developed' countries seems not to be meaningful. To explain these different rates, one has to separately scrutinize the cultural tradition and the socialization pattern of each country.

Schneider's First Rank Symptoms (FRS)

Critical of the theoretical complexity of Bleuler's approach to defining schizophrenia, Schneider introduced the concept of 'nuclear' or 'first-rank' symptoms (FRS; Schneider, 1992). They include psychotic phenomena like delusional perceptions, audible thoughts, thought broadcasting, thought insertion, thought withdrawal, commenting and dialogue voices, made volition and somatic passivity. The pathognomonicity of the FRS has been challenged, while their frequency was primarily dependent on the cultural context. The frequency of the FRS in general has been found to be low in a number of non-Western countries: 56.5 per cent in Saudi Arabia (Zarrouk, 1978), 35 per cent in India (Radhakrishnan *et al.*, 1983), 25 per cent in Sri Lanka (Pela, 1982), 26.7 per cent in Malaysia (Salleh, 1992), between 31 and 43 per cent among

Table 27.5 Frequency of occurrence of first-rank symptoms in schizophrenia during the last year

	Austria (N = 350)	Poland (N = 80)	Lithuania (N = 73)	Georgia (N = 74)	Pakistan (N = 103)	Nigeria (N = 324)	Ghana (N = 76)
Delusional perception	81.5	90.0	69.9	81.1	54.4	72.9	81.1
Audible thoughts	16.0	21.3	13.7	6.8	21.3	33.3	28.1
Thought broadcast	13.5	21.3	8.2	21.6	11.7	43.8	32.4
Thought insertion	35.0	37.5	34.2	28.4	26.2	41.7	36.2
Thought withdrawal	10.2	18.8	11.0	5.4	7.8	12.5	14.0
Commenting voices	31.4	70.0	41.1	56.8	43.7	56.3	52.8
Dialogue voices	19.6	48.8	21.9	52.2	28.2	47.9	52.8
Made volition	23.4	17.5	13.7	19.5	9.7	18.8	21.4
Somatic passivity	15.4	30.0	37.0	5.4	20.4	6.3	14.0

Source: International Study on Psychotic Symptoms; *N* = 1,080

non-Western immigrant groups in England (Ndetei and Vadher, 1984b). On the other hand, a study from Nigeria reported 60.3 per cent FRS (Gureje and Bamgboye, 1987).

These differences could be due to different definitions of the single symptoms and to the time under study, because the FRS are not as stable as delusional contents. However, they could also reflect true cultural differences. In the ISPS, patients with schizophrenia were asked about the 1-year prevalence of FRS.

At least one FRS across the regions was registered between 100 per cent (Nigeria), 97.3 per cent (Georgia), 96.3 per cent (Poland), 90.4 per cent (Lithuania), 90.3 per cent (Austria), 83.5 per cent (Pakistan), and 81.6 per cent (Ghana).

The frequency of the single FRS varied remarkably in the sub-samples (see Table 27.5). Those FRS associated with disturbances of the ego-boundaries (audible thoughts, thought broadcast, and thought insertion) most frequently occur in both West African countries. The acoustic first-rank hallucinations were also most common in Nigeria and in Ghana; however, they were also very often reported in Poland and in Georgia. Somatic passivity was most frequent in Poland and in Lithuania. The rates for delusional perception exceeded the numbers found in other studies to a large extent. This may be due to the fact that this phenomenon is part of the symptomatology of acute psychotic episodes and very rare in subacute or chronic states.

Conclusions

Schizophrenia is often considered to be the most universal and homogeneous of all major mental disorders, showing roughly the same epidemiological patterns and phenomenological features in all cultures. However, the large WHO studies and the research on psychotic symptoms in schizophrenia have shown that reality is somewhat more complicated. Culture has a major impact on prevalence and outcome of schizophrenic disorders, as well as on their occurrence and their psychopathology. Despite the fact that many facets of the way in which culture influences mental disorders are still unknown, large parts of the scientific community agree that, in the era of globalization, cultural knowledge and sensitivity are essential qualities of professionals treating foreign as well as native-born mentally ill patients.

References

American Psychiatric Association (1994). *Diagnostic and Statistical Manual of Mental Disorders*, 4th edn. Washington DC: American Psychiatric Association.

American Psychiatric Association (2000). *Diagnostic and Statistical Manual of Mental Disorders*, 4th edn. Text Revision. Washington DC: American Psychiatric Association.

Bauer, S. M., Schanda, H., Karakula, H. *et al.* (2011) Culture and the prevalence of hallucinations in schizophrenia. *Comprehensive Psychiatry*, 52, 319–325.

Bhugra, D., Hilwig, M., Hossein, B. *et al.* (1996). First-contact incidence rates of schizophrenia in Trinidad and one-year follow-up. *British Journal of Psychiatry*, **169**, 587–592.

Bleuler, E. (1911). *Demetia praecox oder die Gruppe der Schizophrenien*. Leipzig: Deuticke.

Craig, T. J., Siegel, C., Hopper, K., Lin, S. and Sartorius, N. (1997). Outcome in schizophrenia and related disorders compared between developing and developed countries. A recursive partitioning re-analysis of the WHO DOSMD data. *British Journal of Psychiatry*, **70**, 229–233.

Edgerton, R. B. and Cohen, A. (1994). Culture and schizophrenia: the DOSMD challenge. *British Journal of Psychiatry*, **164**, 222–231.

Gureje, O. and Bamgboye, E. A. (1987). A study of Schneider's first-rank symptoms of schizophrenia in Nigerian patients. *British Journal of Psychiatry*, **150**, 868–870.

Hopper, K. and Wanderling, J. (2000). Revisiting the developed versus developing country distinction in course and outcome in schizophrenia: results from ISoS, the WHO collaborative follow-up project. International Study of Schizophrenia. *Schizophrenia Bulletin*, **26**, 835–846.

Jablensky, A. (1987). Multicultural studies and the nature of schizophrenia: a review. *Journal of the Royal Society of Medicine*, **80**, 162–167.

Jablensky, A. (2000). Epidemiology of schizophrenia: the global burden of disease and disability. *European Archives of Psychiatry and Clinical Neuroscience*, **250**, 274–285.

Jablensky, A., Sartorius, N., Ernberg, G. *et al.* (1992). Schizophrenia: manifestations, incidence and course in different cultures. A World Health Organization ten-country study. *Psychological Medicine. Monograph Supplement*, **20**, S1–S97.

Jilek, W. G. (1995). Emil Kraepelin and comparative socio-cultural psychiatry. *European Archives of Psychiatry and Clinical Neuroscience*, **245**, 231–238.

Kala, A. K. and Wig, N. N. (1982). Delusions across cultures. *International Journal of Social Psychiatry*, **28**, 185–193.

Kim, K., Hwu, H., Zhang, L. D. *et al.* (2001). Schizophrenic delusions in Seoul, Shanghai and Taipei: a transcultural study. *Journal of Korean Medical Science*, **16**, 88–94.

Kraepelin, E. (1899). *Ein kurzes Lehrbuch für Studirende und Aerzte. Sechste, Vollstandig Umgearbeitete Auflage*, Leipzig: Barth.

Kraepelin, E. (1904a). Vergleichende Psychiatrie. *Zentralblatt für Nervenheilkunde und Psychiatrie*, **27**, 433–437.

Kraepelin, E. (1904b). Psychiatrisches aus Java. *Zentralblatt für Nervenheilkunde und Psychiatrie*, **27**, 468–469.

Leff, J., Sartorius, N., Jablensky, A., Korten, A. and Ernberg, G. (1992). The International Pilot Study of Schizophrenia: five-year follow-up findings. *Psychological Medicine*, **22**, 131–145.

Leon, C. A. (1989). Clinical course and outcome of schizophrenia in Cali, Colombia: a 10-year follow-up study. *Journal of Nervous and Mental Disease*, **177**, 593–606.

McGrath, J., Saha, S., Welham, J., El Saadi, O., MacCauley, C. and Chant, D. (2004). A systematic review of the incidence of schizophrenia: the distribution of rates and the influence of sex, urbanicity, migrant status and methodology. *BMC Medicine*, **28**, 13.

McLean, D., Thara, R., John, S., Barrett, R., *et al.* (2014). DSM-IV 'criterion A' schizophrenia symptoms across ethnically different populations: evidence for differing psychotic symptom content or structural organization? *Culture, Medicine and Psychiatry*, **38**, 408–426.

Murphy, H. B. M. (1967). Cultural aspects of the delusion. *Studium Generale*, **11**, 684–692.

Murphy, H. B. M. (1982). *Comparative Psychiatry*. Berlin and Heidelberg, New York: Springer.

Murphy, H. B. M., Wittkower, E. D., Fried, J. and Ellenberger, H. A. (1963). Cross-cultural survey of schizophrenic symptomatology. *International Journal of Social Psychiatry*, **10**, 237–249.

Ndetei, D. M. and Vadher, A. (1984a). Frequency and clinical significance of delusions across cultures. *Acta Psychiatrica Scandinavica*, **70**, 73–76.

Ndetei, D. M. and Vadher, A. (1984b). A cross-cultural study of the frequencies of Schneider's first rank symptoms of schizophrenia. *Acta Psychiatrica Scandinavica*, **70**, 540–544.

Ndetei, D. M. and Vadher, A. (1984c). A comparative cross-cultural study of the frequencies of hallucinations in schizophrenia. *Acta Psychiatrica Scandinavica*, **70**, 545–549.

Ohaeri, J. U. (1993). Long-term outcome of treated schizophrenia in a Nigerian cohort. Retrospective analysis of 7-year follow-ups. *Journal of Nervous and Mental Disease*, **181**, 514–516.

Patel, V., Cohen, A., Thara, R. and Gureje, O. (2006). Is the outcome of schizophrenia really better in developing countries? *Revista Brasileira de Psiquiatria*, **28**, 149–152.

Pela, O. A. (1982). Cultural relativity of first-rank symptoms in schizophrenia. *International Journal of Social Psychiatry*, **28**, 91–95.

Pfeiffer, W. M. (1994). *Transkulturelle Psychiatrie*, 2nd edn. Stuttgart and New York: Thieme.

Radhakrishnan, J., Mathew, K., Richard, J. and Verghese, A. (1983). Schneider's first rank symptoms – prevalence, diagnostic use and prognostic implications. *British Journal of Psychiatry*, **142**, 557–559.

Saha, S., Chant, D., Welhalm, J. and McGrath, J. (2005). A systematic review of the prevalence of schizophrenia. *PLoS Medicine*, **2**, 413–433.

Saha, S., Welham, J., Chant, D. and McGrath, J. (2006). Incidence of schizophrenia does not vary with economic status of the country: evidence from a systematic review. *Social Psychiatry and Psychiatric Epidemiology*, **41**, 338–340.

Salleh, M. R. (1992). Specificity of Schneider's first-rank symptoms for schizophrenia in Malay patients. *Psychopathology*, **25**, 199–203.

Sartorius, N., Jablensky, A., Korten, A. *et al.* (1986). Early manifestations and first-contact incidence of schizophrenia in different cultures. A preliminary report on the initial evaluation phase of the WHO Collaborative Study on determinants of outcome of severe mental disorders. *Psychological Medicine*, **16**, 909–928.

Schneider, K. (1992). *Klinische Psychopathologie*, 14th edn. Stuttgart: Thieme.

Stompe, T. (2014) Verhexung und Besessenheit im Wahn westafrikanischer Schizophreniekranker. *Schweizer Archiv für Neurologie und Psychiatrie*, **165**, 17–24.

Stompe, T., Friedmann, A., Ortwein, G. *et al.* (1999). Comparison of delusions among schizophrenics in Austria and in Pakistan. *Psychopathology*, **32**, 225–234.

Stompe, T., Ortwein-Swoboda, G., Ritter, K., Schanda, H. and Friedmann, A. (2002). Are we witnessing the disappearance of catatonic schizophrenia? *Comprehensive Psychiatry*, **3**, 167–174.

Stompe, T., Ortwein-Swoboda, G., Ritter, K., Marquart, B. and Schanda, H. (2005). The significance of classification systems for the fluctuation of schizophrenic subtypes during the last century. *Comprehensive Psychiatry*, **46**, 433–439.

Stompe, T., Bauer, S., Ortwein-Swoboda, G. *et al.* (2006). Delusions of guilt: the attitude of Christian and Islamic confessions towards Good and Evil and the responsibility of men. *Journal of Muslim Mental Health*, **1**, 43–56.

Suhail, L. K. and Cochrane, R. (2002). Effect of culture and environment on the phenomenology of delusions and hallucinations. *International Journal of Social Psychiatry*, **48**, 126–138.

Tateyama, M., Masahiro, A., Kamisada, M., Hashimoto, M., Bartels, M. and Kasper, S. (1998). Transcultural study of schizophrenic delusions. Tokyo versus Vienna and Tübingen. *Psychopathology*, **31**, 59–68.

Thara, R. (2004). Twenty-year course of schizophrenia: the Madras Longitudinal Study. *Canadian Journal of Psychiatry*, **49**, 564–569.

Thara, R., Henrietta, M., Joseph, A., Rajkumar, S. and Eaton, W. W. (1994). Ten-year course of schizophrenia: the Madras Longitudinal Study. *Acta Psychiatrica Scandinavica*, **90**, 329–336.

Torrey, E. F., Torrey, B. and Burton-Bradley, B. G. (1974). The epidemiology of schizophrenia in Papua New Guinea. *American Journal of Psychiatry*, **131**, 567–573.

Verghese, A., John, J. K., Rajkumer, S., Richard, J., Sethi, B. B. and Trivedi, J. K. (1993). Factors associated with the course and outcome of schizophrenia in India: results of a two-year multicentre follow-up study. *British Journal of Psychiatry*, **163**, 535–541.

Williams, C. C. (2003). Re-reading the IPSS research record. *Social Science Medicine*, **56**, 501–515.

World Health Organization (WHO) (1973). *Report of the International Pilot Study of Schizophrenia*, vol. 1. Geneva: World Health Organization.

Yip K.-S., (2003) Traditional Chinese religious beliefs and superstitions in delusions and hallucinations of Chinese schizophrenic patients. *International Journal of Social Psychiatry*, **49**, 97–111.

Zarrouk, E. T. (1978). The usefulness of first rank symptoms in diagnosis of schizophrenia in a Saudi Arabian population. *British Journal of Psychiatry*, **132**, 571–578.

Chapter

28

Disorders of Ageing across Cultures

Ajit Shah

Editors' Introduction

Globally, people are living longer as standards of hygiene are improving and infectious diseases are becoming treatable. Levels of nutrition are also improving. However, the likelihood of people living longer has brought likelihood of increasing rates of psychiatric disorders in the older age populations. These include paraphrenias, depression and dementias in particular. In addition, physical comorbidity contributes to increasingly complex needs of patients as well as their carers and families. In this chapter, Shah highlights that not only the proportion of elderly in the general population across the globe is increasing due to increased life expectancy but in developed countries the proportion of those over the age of 80 years is also increasing which brings with it clear challenges in managing normal ageing but also psychiatric illnesses of old age. He reminds us that there has been a clear paucity of epidemiological and clinical information on mental illness in older people from many low- and middle-income countries and ethnic minorities in developed countries. However, studies are now emerging. Shah describes and examines cultural issues pertaining to the epidemiology, clinical presentation, help-seeking and diagnosis with specific focus on dementia and depression, the two main mental disorders in old age. There is often a degree of confusion in diagnosis between depression presenting as pseudo-dementia and dementia especially in many minority communities. He also goes on to describe schizophrenia and other disorders seen in old age. There is no doubt that an understanding of additional cross-cultural aspects of behavioural and psychological signs and symptoms of dementia is critical. These cultural factors and variations may often precipitate a clinical presentation. Shah describes the newly developed epidemiological transition hypothesis of dementia in some detail.

Introduction

The proportion of older people in the general population is increasing in developing and developed countries due to increased life expectancy and reduced mortality (Oeppen and Vaupel, 2002). Moreover, the population of the elderly from ethnic minority groups in developing countries, including the United Kingdom (UK) (Shah et al., 2005a; Zarate-Escudero and Shah, 2013) and the United States (Markson, 2003), is also increasing. Furthermore, there is a paucity of epidemiological and clinical information on mental illness amongst older people from developing countries and ethnic minority groups within developed countries (Subedi et al., 2004; Shah et al., 2005b; Zarate-Escudero and Shah, 2013), but studies are emerging. Cultural issues pertaining to epidemiology, clinical presentation and diagnosis are examined with the main focus on depression and dementia, the two most prevalent mental disorders in old age.

Demography

International and Some National Trends

The number of those over 65 years worldwide is predicted to increase from 50 million in 1990 to 1 billion in 2025 (Desjarlais et al., 1995), an increase of 100 per cent. Moreover, 72 per cent of those aged over 60 years will be living in developing countries by 2025 (Levkoff et al., 1995). In developed countries, there is a particular increase in the size of the oldest-old group (80+ years) (Jeune and Skythe, 2001; Shah, 2007a; Christensen et al., 2009).

Calculations from the 2011 census data for England and Wales indicated that the proportion of ethnic minority individuals over the age of 65 years has progressively increased from 3 per cent in 1991 to 8 per cent (Zarate-Escudero and Shah, 2013). Closer political and economic union with Europe may also lead to increased migration of elderly people between neighbouring countries (e.g. English elderly retiring to Spain, France or Italy). In the US, the elderly population in ethnic groups, including African Americans, Hispanic, Asians and Pacific Islanders, is also predicted to increase (Mui *et al.*, 2003). The proportion of non-Caucasians in the US is predicted to increase from 10 per cent to 20 per cent by 2050 (Markson, 2003).

Implications of these Demographic Changes

The two most common mental disorders in old age are dementia and depression. The prevalence of dementia doubles every 5.1 years after the age of 60 (Jorm *et al.*, 1987; Hofman *et al.*, 1991). Thus, with the increase in the elderly population (particularly those over 80 years), the absolute number of dementia sufferers will increase worldwide. The World Alzheimer's Report (Alzheimer's Disease International, 2015) noted that in 2015 there were 46.8 million dementia sufferers worldwide and this is predicted to increase to 74.7 million by 2030. Prevalence rates of up to 15 per cent have been reported for depression in those aged over 65 years, and this will also result in a worldwide increase in the absolute number of cases of depression. Moreover, suicide rates also increase with ageing in many countries (Shah, 2007b), and the impending demographic changes may lead to an increase in the actual numbers of suicide in older people.

Concept of Multiple Jeopardy

Older people from ethnic minority groups with mental disorder face multiple difficulties (Rait *et al.*, 1996). The concept of age- and race-related disadvantages was originally described as double jeopardy (National Urban League, 1964; Dowd and Bengston, 1978). A model of triple jeopardy was developed by adding sexism (Palmore and Manton, 1973) and social deprivation (Norman, 1985). A model of multiple disadvantages due to ageism, racism, gender disparities, restricted access to health and welfare services, internal ethnic divisions and class struggle was subsequently developed (Boneham, 1989).

Epidemiology

There are methodological difficulties with epidemiological studies of mental disorders in older people from different ethnic groups, including the definitions of age and ethnicity, diagnostic issues, and the paucity of validated screening and diagnostic instruments.

Age

Epidemiological studies in developed countries have traditionally focused on those over the age of 60 or 65 years. Some ethnic groups, particularly from developing countries, have a shorter life expectancy, retire early and assume the role of an elder at a younger age (Rajkumar *et al.*, 1997). Therefore, a younger age cut-off (40 to 55 years) has been used in some studies of UK ethnic groups (Barker, 1984; McCallum, 1990; Manthorpe and Hettiaratchy, 1993) and in some developing countries (Yu *et al.*, 1989; Zhang *et al.*, 1990; Ganguli *et al.*, 1995; Vas *et al.*, 2001). Similarly, old age has officially been defined to commence at the age of 50 years for indigenous Australians (Commonwealth Department of Health, Housing and Community, 1991). Moreover, there are difficulties in ascertaining the precise age in some ethnic groups (Chandra *et al.*, 1994; Rajkumar and Kumar, 1996; Rait and Burns, 1997).

Race, Culture and Ethnicity

Race, culture and ethnicity are often erroneously used interchangeably. Race is a phenomenological description based on physical appearance (Bhopal, 1997). Culture refers to shared features which bind individuals together into a community. The definition and identification of ethnicity is problematic (McKenzie and Crowcroft, 1996; Pringle and Rothera, 1996) because it includes aspects of race and culture, and other characteristics including traditions, language, religion, upbringing, nationality and ancestral place of origin (Rait and Burns, 1997). It is also a personal expression of identity influenced by life experience and place of habitation, and is dynamic and changes over time (Senior and Bhopal, 1994). A useful working definition of ethnic minority individuals is 'those with a cultural heritage distinct from the majority population' (Manthorpe and Hettiaratchy, 1993). This definition is appropriate in countries like the UK where the indigenous population forms the majority. However, it creates difficulties in countries like Australia, United States and New Zealand where the indigenous population is a minority.

Table 28.1 Difficulties with epidemiological studies

Difficulties	References
Ascertainment of age	Rait *et al.*, 1997
Illiteracy	Lindesay *et al.*, 1997a, b
Innumeracy	Prince *et al.*, 2003
Small sample sizes	Rait and Burns, 1997; Bhatnagar and Frank, 1997. Lindesay, 1998
Inappropriate sample frames	Richards, 1997; Richards and Brayne, 1996; McCracken *et al.*, 1997
Low response rate	Woo *et al.*, 1994; Bhatnagar and Frank, 1997; Lindesay *et al.*, 1997b; McCracken *et al.*, 1997
Refusal to participate	Bhatnagar and Frank, 1997
Lack of valid tools to identify and quantify mental illness	Lindesay, 1998; Shah, 1998
Lack of comparisons with indigenous population	Bhatnagar and Frank, 1997
Amalgamation of heterogeneous groups of ethnic elders	Bhatnagar and Frank, 1997; McCracken *et al.*, 1997; Livingston and Sembhi, 2003
Assumption that general practices' data are accurate	Bhatnagar and Frank, 1997; Lindesay *et al.*, 1997a,b; McCracken *et al.*, 1997

Table 28.2 Cultural factors complicating diagnosis

Cultural factors	Studies
Communication difficulties	George and Young, 1991; Shah, 1992, 1997a, b; Livingston and Sembhi, 2003
Taboo topics	Shah, 1992
Stigma attached to mental illness	Barker, 1984; Livingston *et al.*, 2002
Bias and prejudice of clinicians	Solomon, 1992
Institutional racism	Solomon, 1992
Unfamiliarity with symptoms of mental illness by relatives	Manthorpe and Hettiarachy, 1993
Illness being viewed as a function of old age	Redelinghuys and Shah, 1997

Other Methodological Issues

There is a paucity of epidemiological studies of mental disorders among ethnic minority elders in a given country (and studies of indigenous populations usually exclude ethnic minority subjects who do not speak the principal language) and of older people from developing countries. Moreover, they are fraught with difficulties listed in Table 28.1.

Diagnostic Difficulties

Mental disorders are difficult to identify among ethnic elders (George and Young, 1991) and in older people in non-Western cultures because of culture-related factors listed in Table 28.2, which complicate diagnosis. A further issue is the paucity of suitable screening and diagnostic instruments (Shah, 1998). For example,

cognitive tests for dementia standardized in one ethnic group may not be appropriate for another ethnic group because they are influenced by factors listed in Table 28.3; similar factors apply to screening or diagnostic instruments for other mental disorders (Lindesay, 1998). Also, screening instruments, like the 15-item version of the Geriatric Depression Scale (GDS-15) (Sheikh and Yesavage, 1986), have sometimes been erroneously used as diagnostic instruments (Lee *et al.*, 1993, 1994; Woo *et al.*, 1994; Liu *et al.*, 1997).

Cognitive Tests

Cognitive tests using the discrepancy between age and date of birth (Bhatnagar and Frank, 1997; McCracken *et al.*, 1997) may disadvantage older people born in rural areas with poor birth registration facilities, and those who have altered age and date of birth to facilitate migration (Rait *et al.*, 1997). Culture-specific questions (e.g. about royalty or politicians) are also problematic (Bhatnagar and Frank, 1997; McCracken *et al.*, 1997), although these can be modified (e.g. to dates of independence of the country of origin) (Chandra *et al.*, 1994; Rait *et al.*, 1997). Differing concepts of orientation in time and place in different cultures (Escobar *et al.*, 1986; Ganguli *et al.*, 1995; Lindesay *et al.*, 1997b) and preferential use of the Western or traditional calendar (Kua, 1992; Bhatnagar and Frank, 1997; Lindesay *et al.*, 1997b; Rait *et al.*, 1997) can influence performance.

Table 28.3 Factors affecting cognitive tests

Factors	Studies
Culture	Gurland et al., 1992; Chandra et al., 1994; Teresi et al., 1995; Livingston and Sembhi, 2003; Prince et al., 2003; Ramirez et al., 2006
Education	Chandra et al., 1994; Teresi et al., 1995; Stewart et al., 2003; Kim et al., 2003a, b; Livingston and Sembhi, 2003; Prince et al., 2003; Sjahir et al., 2001; Ramirez et al., 2006; Kochhann et al., 2010; Kumar et al., 2014
Language	McCracken et al., 1997; Livingston and Sembhi, 2003; Prince et al., 2003; Ramirez et al., 2006
Literacy skills	Chandra et al., 1994; Kabir and Herlitz, 2000; Livingston and Sembhi, 2003; Prince et al., 2003
Numeracy skills	Prince et al., 2003
Sensory impairments	Lindesay et al., 1997b
Unfamiliarity with test situations	Chandra et al., 1994; Richards and Brayne, 1996
Socio-economic status	Kumar et al., 2014
Anxiety	Lindesay, 1998

Expression of Depression and Other Emotional Symptoms

Depression and other emotional disorders may present with different clinical features in different ethnic groups (Baker et al., 1995; Abas, 1996; Abas et al., 1996, 1998; Lindesay, 1998; Shah, 1999; Livingston and Sembhi, 2003). Emotional expression, including depression, in different cultures is influenced by several overlapping concepts including the context of disclosure, vocabulary and language of emotional expression, selective expression of emotions and definition of self (Lindesay, 1998). Gender, age, family relationship, professional status and religious background can influence the disclosure of distress (Lindesay, 1998) and some examples are illustrated. Females among African Americans and Hispanics express more depressive symptoms (Mui, 1993). Religious denomination can modify the type of depressive symptoms in old age; for example, among Dutch Calvinists depressed subjects scored highly for vegetative symptoms (Braam et al., 2000). Among Koreans, attending religious activities is protective towards depression (Hahn et al., 2004). In many communities, including Korean Americans, those with poor health, experience of adverse life events, dissatisfaction of help received from the family and with few friends may develop depression with a poor quality of life (Mui, 2008).

The vocabulary and language to express emotions across cultures are variable (Abas, 1996; Abas et al., 1996, 1998; Lindesay, 1998; Shah, 1999; Bhugra and Mastrogianni, 2004). Equivalent vocabulary to express emotions in different languages may not be present (Lindesay, 1998; Shah, 1999). Furthermore, styles of expressing biological and physical symptoms of emotional disorders including anxiety and depression may be different in different cultures (Abas, 1996; Abas et al., 1996, 1998; Lindesay, 1998). Depressed mood and feelings of sadness are prevalent in some cultures and somatic symptoms and pain in other cultures (Lindesay, 1998; Lindesay et al., 1997b; Livingston et al., 2002). Semi-rural Indian subcontinent origin elders may not regard depression and anxiety as mental illnesses and may perceive them as bodily illnesses with symptoms like fatigue, aches and pains, weakness, tiredness and other physical symptoms (Bhatnagar, 1997); they may consult doctors with physical symptoms or consult traditional healers like *hakims* and *vaids*, the latter having no boundary between physical and psychological scenarios (Bhatnagar, 1997). Somatic symptoms including sinking feelings in the stomach, attacks of hot and cold feelings, attacks of blushing, pains in the head, pains in the chest and pains in the stomach were more common among UK Gujarati elders than indigenous elders in a population-based study (Lindesay et al., 1997a). The possibility of depression should be considered if Indian-subcontinent elders present with persistent low energy, bodily aches and pains, and gas in the abdomen (Bhatnagar, 1997). Among elderly depressed Cypriots in London, somatic symptoms were more prevalent than in indigenous elders (Livingston et al., 2002). Older Turkish and Moroccan migrants to the Netherlands also present with somatic symptoms (Spijker et al., 2004). However, somatic symptoms should be seen in parallel with, rather than an alternative to, expression of distress (Lindesay, 1998). Older African Caribbeans in the

UK rarely use the terms 'sad' or 'unhappy' to describe emotional distress, but they use other terms including 'being low spirited', 'fed up' and 'weighed down' (Baker *et al.*, 1995; Abas, 1996; Abas *et al.*, 1996, 1998). Korean elders in the US express emotions of depression symbolically or physically (Pang, 1998). For example, dysphoria was expressed as a symptom somewhere between a bodily symptom and an emotional symptom as 'melancholia has been absorbed in my body'. A recent review concluded that somatic symptoms are a common presentation of depression across the world (Bhugra and Mastrogianni, 2004), particularly in older people.

Lindesay (1998) divided the definition of self into an egocentric concept in Western cultures and a socio-centric concept in many non-Western cultures (Lindesay, 1998). Individuals in the socio-centric model express emotional distress in terms of its impact on relationships with others (Lindesay, 1998). Elders in the Hindu tradition are expected to disengage themselves of worldly economic, social and domestic responsibility and adopt a greater spiritual role (Shah, 1988; Ganguli *et al.*, 1999), and feelings of contentment, disengagement and peacefulness are considered more desirable than feelings of excitement and enthusiasm (Ganguli *et al.*, 1999). Also reflection is considered more appropriate than novelty seeking (Ganguli *et al.*, 1999). This may lead to false positive responses and erroneously higher scores on standard depression-measurement instruments, and has been observed during the development of Hindi and Chinese Geriatric Depression Scales (GDS) (Mui, 1996; Ganguli *et al.*, 1999). For example, on the Chinese GDS, the item on staying at home may result in a false-positive response because elderly Chinese may consider staying at home a privilege and they may perform useful duties of looking after the grandchildren (Mui, 1996). For similar reasons, the most prevalent items on the Hindi GDS including 'diminished clarity of thinking', 'dropping many of the previous interests and activities', 'memory problems', 'feelings of worthlessness', 'boredom' and 'difficulty starting new projects' may result in false-positive responses (Ganguli *et al.*, 1999). This has prompted modification of items on standard depression screening instruments. For example, in the 15-item Chinese GDS (Mui, 1996), also considered suitable for other Asian elders in the US (Mui *et al.*, 2003), items of 'getting restless and fidgety', 'worry about the future', 'feel down hearted and blue', 'get upset about little things' and 'feel like crying' have replaced items of 'feel helpless', 'prefer to stay at home', 'wonderful to be alive', 'full of energy', 'situation hopeless' (Mui, 1996; Mui *et al.*, 2003). The item 'are you hopeful about the future?' in the Turkish version of GDS-30 (Ertan and Eker, 2000) was problematic because the concept of hope was viewed as economic and social expectation in their personal life and most subjects gave an answer in favour of depression. This item was therefore modified to a question expecting a positive response 'are you pessimistic about the future'. The Korean version of the 30-item GDS (Jung *et al.*, 1997) was mainly developed from the original English version (Yesavage *et al.*, 1983), but items from Zung Self Rating Depression Scale (Zung, 1965), Beck Depression Scale (Beck *et al.*, 1961), the Minnesota Multiphasic Personality Inventory Depression Scale (Hathaway and McKinley, 1943), and the Centre for Epidemiologic Studies Depression Rating Scale (CES-D) (Radloff and Teri, 1986) were added to include somatic symptoms excluded in the GDS because somatic symptoms are frequent among depressed Korean elders. The Japanese version of the 15-item GDS (Niino *et al.*, 1991) revealed that symptoms of 'not full of energy', 'felt helpless', 'memory worse than other people's' and 'preferred to stay at home' were most prevalent in Japanese post-stroke patients (Schreiner *et al.*, 2001).

Other Disorders

A Turkish study of the clinical features of late-onset schizophrenia reported that Turkish patients do not have nihilistic delusions, delusions of poverty or guilt, delusions of erotomania, thought withdrawal, thought insertion and thought broadcasting and very late-onset schizophrenia patients do not have grandiose and mystic delusions (Alici-Evcimen *et al.*, 2003). A study of first presentation with psychosis in old age in Singapore observed that 89 per cent had persecutory delusions, and the symptom profile was similar to that in Western countries except social isolation and partition delusions were less prominent (Tan and Seng, 2011). A longitudinal study of symptoms of schizophrenia revealed no relationship between improvement in the core symptoms of schizophrenia and cognition except motor speed independent of age and ethnicity (Hughes *et al.*, 2001). Cognitive impairment in several domains was more severe amongst

Egyptians with late-onset schizophrenia when compared to healthy older people (Radwan *et al.*, 2014).

Symptom profile across different ethnic groups for other functional mental disorders, including neurotic disorders, and personality disorders in old age has not been critically studied.

Development and Validation of New Diagnostic and Screening Instruments

Both screening and diagnostic instruments that account for the influence of factors discussed above need development. Either new instruments can be developed, or existing instruments can be adapted. In general, the second option has been widely adopted (Hall *et al.*, 1993; Chandra *et al.*, 1994, 1998; Ganguli *et al.*, 1995, 1999; Rait *et al.*, 1997), although one study developed a culturally sensitive screening instrument for emotional distress among older UK African Caribbeans afresh (Abas, 1996; Abas *et al.*, 1996, 1998). There are two formal approaches: a Delphi panel of experts from the culture of interest or a more widespread consultation technique. The Delphi panel method can use structured or semi-structured interviews, questions or vignettes (Rait *et al.*, 1997). The consultation approach involves professionals and/or lay members working closely, sometimes focusing on separate issues initially, and later sharing them (Rait *et al.*, 1997); this approach has been successfully used in developing a depression screening instrument for African Caribbean elders in London (Abas, 1996; Abas *et al.*, 1996, 1998). Either method should examine each item on the instrument for cultural relevance, translation, adaptation and modification with the aim of producing a culture-fair, education-free and analogous instrument (Hall *et al.*, 1993; Chandra *et al.*, 1994, 1998; Graves *et al.*, 1994; Richards and Brayne, 1996; Richards, 1997; Mui *et al.*, 2001; Steis and Schrauf, 2009). Newly developed instruments should have comparable meaning, difficulty, familiarity and salience.

Translation and back-translation by separate groups of bilingual translators is absolutely necessary to ensure accuracy of translation (Brislin, 1970; Katzman *et al.*, 1988; Yu *et al.*, 1989; Chandra *et al.*, 1994; Lindesay *et al.*, 1997b). Bilingual translators can also ensure that the meaning and significance of the items are preserved as much as possible (Lindesay

et al., 1997b); this could also be achieved by the Delphi panel if the panel members originate from the same culture. Translation should ensure content, semantic, technical, criterion and conceptual equivalence with the parent version of the scale for each and every item (Flaherty *et al.*, 1988; Rait *et al.*, 1997; Steis and Schrauf., 2009). Several rounds of field pre-testing (Chandra *et al.*, 1994; Ganguli *et al.*, 1995) followed by pilot field testing to determine the distribution of scores (Chandra *et al.*, 1994; Ganguli *et al.*, 1996; Rait *et al.*, 2000a, b; Sjahrir *et al.*, 2001; Stewart *et al.*, 2001, 2002; Steis and Schrauf, 2009) and their ability to discriminate between mental disorders of different severity (Chandra *et al.*, 1994; Lindesay *et al.*, 1997b) are essential. Newly developed instruments should have their psychometric properties rigorously evaluated and they should be similar to the parent version (Shah and Lindesay, 2000).

Validation against a gold-standard diagnosis of the specific mental disorder is needed where the newly developed instrument is to be used for screening or diagnostic purposes (Shah and Lindesay, 2000; Livingston and Sembhi, 2003). Standardized clinical interview can be used as the gold standard, although the diagnostic accuracy of the 'gold-standard' measure is often difficult to evaluate (Shah *et al.*, 1998). One useful method of validating such instruments for dementia is by serial follow-up of dementia cases, whereupon true dementia cases are likely to demonstrate continuing cognitive decline (Shah *et al.*, 1998). Presence of functional impairment is a necessary prerequisite for the diagnosis of dementia in ICD-10 and DSM-IV. This is problematic because of major conceptual difficulties in the definition and measurement of functional impairment across different cultures (Chandra *et al.*, 1994; Pollit, 1996; Richards and Brayne, 1996), although measurement instruments have been developed a priori in illiterate populations (Fillenbaum *et al.*, 1999) and in other populations in developing countries (Jitapunkul *et al.*, 1994). Translated versions of the Geriatric Mental State Examination (GMS) (Copeland *et al.*, 1976) have been used among older Asians, Chinese, Somali, Afro-Caribbean and British blacks in Liverpool (Blakemore and Boneham, 1994; McCracken *et al.*, 1997), Indian subcontinent elders in Bradford (Bhatnagar and Frank, 1997), Chinese in Taiwan (Tsang *et al.*, 2002), and among respondents from India, China and Southeast Asia, Africa, Latin America and the Caribbean (Prince *et al.*, 2003).

Information from the CAMDEX interview and the Consortium to Establish a Registry for Alzheimer's Disease (CERAD) interview (Morris *et al.*, 1989) have been used by a panel of physicians to make consensus DSM-III-R diagnosis of dementia among Cree Indians and English-speaking Canadians (Hall *et al.*, 1993).

Available Diagnostic and Screening Instruments for Dementia

As illustrated in Table 28.4, the Mini Mental State Examination (MMSE) (Folstein *et al.*, 1975) has been developed in several different languages. However, comparisons between these different versions are problematic, as not all studies have followed a rigorous procedure for the development of screening instruments, and/or evaluated the psychometric properties adequately. Individual items of the MMSE may perform differently in different populations because they may be influenced by age (Sjahir *et al.*, 2001; Kumar

Table 28.4 MMSE in different languages

Language	Reference
Chinese	Serby *et al.*, 1987; Katzmann *et al.*, 1988; Salmon *et al.*, 1989; Yu *et al.*, 1989; Xu *et al.*, 2003
Korean	Park and Kwon, 1990; Park *et al.*, 1991
Finnish	Salmon *et al.*, 1989
Italian	Rocca *et al.*, 1990
Yoruba (Nigeria)	Hendrie, 1992
Spanish	Escobar *et al.*, 1986; Anzola-Perez *et al.*, 1996
Thai	Phanthumchida *et al.*, 1991
Cree (Canadian Indians)	Hall *et al.*, 1993
Hindi	Ganguli *et al.*, 1995; Rait *et al.*, 2000a
Punjabi	Rait *et al.*, 2000a
Urdu	Rait *et al.*, 2000a
Bengali	Rait *et al.*, 2000a
Bangla	Kabir and Herlitz, 2000
Malyalum	Shaji *et al.*, 1996
Gujarati	Lindesay *et al.*, 1997b; Rait *et al.*, 2000a
Sinhalese	De Silva and Gunatilake, 2002

et al., 2014), education (Sjahir *et al.*, 2001; Ramirez *et al.*, 2006; Kochhann *et al.*, 2010; Kumar *et al.*, 2014), race and ethnicity (Ramirez *et al.*, 2006), socio-economic status (Kumar *et al.*, 2014) and whether English is the subject's first language or not (Ramirez *et al.*, 2006). Moreover, differing MMSE cut-off scores for screening for possible dementia may be need in different cultural groups for different educational levels (Kochhann *et al.*, 2010). However, there was no difference in the performance of English and Farsi versions of the MMSE when administered to bilingual Iranian Americans (Davoudzadeh, 2010).

A number of other cognitive screening tests for dementia have been developed for use in different cultures. The abbreviated Mental Test Score (Quereshi and Hodkinson, 1974) has been developed in several Asian languages, and in English for use among African Caribbeans in the UK (Rait *et al.*, 1997; Rait *et al.*, 2000a, 2000b). The Alzheimer's Disease Assessment Scale (Rosen *et al.*, 1984) has been developed in Korean (Youn *et al.*, 2002). The MMSE, selected items from the CERAD neuropsychological test battery (Morris *et al.*, 1989) and the CAMCOG component of the CAMDEX interview (Roth *et al.*, 1986) have been evaluated in older African Caribbean people (Richards and Brayne, 1996; Richards *et al.*, 2000). Orientation items of the MMSE, selected items of the CERAD battery and the clock drawing test have been evaluated in African Caribbean elders and normative data is available (Stewart *et al.*, 2001). An approach involving the use of three instruments (the GMS, the CIS-D and the ten-word list-learning task from the CERAD battery appropriately translated into native languages) and an algorithm derived from these instruments has been shown to have high specificity and sensitivity in the diagnosis of dementia in culturally diverse populations from several countries including India, China and Southeast Asia, Africa, Latin America and the Caribbean (Prince *et al.*, 2003). A large cross-national study across 26 centres in India, China, Latin America and Africa demonstrated good psychometric properties for GMS-AGECAT in the diagnosis of dementia, and this could be improved with locally appropriate modifications (Prince *et al.*, 2004). A six-item Rowlands Universal Dementia Assessment Scale has been successfully evaluated for use among several ethnic groups in Australia (Storey *et al.*, 2004). A Japanese version of the Addenbrookes Cognitive Examination Revised version has been developed with good evidence of reliability and validity on several parameters (Kawata *et al.*, 2012). The Chula Mental Test, developed for Thai elderly by selecting and adapting items from several existing screening tests, has been shown to reduce the influence of illiteracy on scores (Jitapunkul *et al.*, 1996).

The Community Screening Interview for Dementia (CSI-D), with a cognitive test for the subject and an informant history, has been developed for use among Cree Indians in Canada (Hall *et al.*, 1993, 2000), English speaking Canadians (Hall *et al.*, 1993, 2000; Hendrie *et al.*, 1993) and Yoruba Nigerians in Ibadan (Hendrie *et al.*, 1995; Hall *et al.*, 2000), African Americans in Indianapolis (Hall *et al.*, 2000), Jamaicans (Hall *et al.*, 2000) and in study populations in India, China and Southeast Asia, Africa, Latin America and the Caribbean (Prince *et al.*, 2003). The Alzheimer's Disease Risk Questionnaire (Brietner and Folstein, 1984), which obtains information on history of cognitive impairment among first-degree relatives, has been translated into Chinese and Spanish, and has been administered by bilingual workers (Silverman *et al.*, 1992). The Informant Questionnaire on Cognitive Decline in the Elderly (IQCODE) (Jorm *et al.*, 1991) has been developed for use in illiterate Chinese populations (Fuh *et al.*, 1995).

Available Diagnostic and Screening Instruments for Depression

As illustrated in Table 28.5, the 30-item GDS (GDS-30) (Yesavage *et al.*, 1983) and the 15-item GDS (GDS-15) (Sheikh and Yesavage, 1986) have been evaluated in a number of languages and ethnic groups. However, comparison between these different versions is problematic, as not all studies have followed a rigorous procedure for development of the GDS, and/or evaluated the psychometric properties adequately. Moreover, there is differential item functioning in the GDS in different ethnic groups, as was shown in Singapore (Broekman *et al.*, 2007). Because a considerable number of elderly Chinese in Hong Kong are illiterate, a standardized version of the Chinese version of 15-item GDS was developed, and this version was found to be better than the directly translated versions of 15-item GDS (Wong *et al.*, 2002). The 15-item GDS, Even Briefer Assessment Scale for depression (Allen *et al.*, 1994) and a single question (Do you often feel sad or depressed?) were

Table 28.5 Geriatric Depression Scale in different languages and ethnic groups

Language and ethnic group	Reference
GDS-30:	
Korean	Jung *et al.*, 1997; Jang *et al.*, 2001; Bae and Cho, 2004
Turkish	Ertan and Eker, 2000
Hong Kong Chinese	Chan, 1996
Singapore Chinese	Lim *et al.*, 2000
Nigeria	Sokoya and Bayewu, 2003
Hindi	Ganguli *et al.*, 1999
Spanish in Spain	Izal and Montorio, 1993
Spanish in Mexican Americans	Espino *et al.*, 1996
GDS-15:	
UK African Caribbeans	Rait *et al.*, 1999
Hong Kong Chinese	Lee *et al.*, 1993, 1994
Greek	Fountoulakis *et al.*, 2014
Japanese	Niino *et al.*, 1991
Korean	Bae and Cho, 2004
Chinese, Japanese, Indian, Korean and Filipino migrants to US	Mui *et al.*, 2003
Israel heterogeneous ethnic groups	Cwikel and Ritchie, 1988
African Americans	Baker *et al.*, 1993
Spanish in Mexican Americans	Baker *et al.*, 1993
Native Americans	Ferraro, 1997

successfully evaluated among elderly Singaporean Chinese (Lim *et al.*, 2000). A comparative study of the short version of the GDS between older Koreans and Americans reported good reliability, but observed the concept of depression to vary in the two groups despite efforts to ensure that the questionnaire in both languages was equivalent (Jang *et al.*, 2001). The 15-item GDS developed for use with older Chinese in Canada observed a four-factor model with negative mood, positive mood, inferiority, and disinterested and uncertainty (Lai *et al.*, 2005); these characteristics were thought to be linked to migration. The GDS (Bae and Cho, 2004) and 15-item GDS (Bae and Cho, 2004; Fountoulakis *et al.*, 2014) have been successfully evaluated for use in older people in Korea and Greece. A meta-analysis of 26 studies demonstrated that there are language differences in the factor structure of the GDS leading to the recommendation that this should be considered in the administration of the GDS and the interpretation of the findings (Kim *et al.*, 2013).

Three depression screening instruments including the 15-item GDS, Brief Assessment Schedule Cards (Adshead *et al.*, 1992) and Caribbean Culture Specific Screen (Abas *et al.*, 1998) for UK African Caribbean elders were successfully evaluated against a 'gold-standard' diagnosis of depression on the GMS (Rait *et al.*, 1999). All three instruments showed satisfactory sensitivity and specificity in detecting depression in older Jamaicans with little difference between the three scales. The CCSS was developed 'a priori' by ascertaining terminology used to describe emotional distress using various techniques described earlier (Abas *et al.*, 1996). In general, lower cut-off scores have been suggested on some scales like the GDS for African Caribbeans in the UK (Abas *et al.*, 1998). Both the GDS-30 and GDS-15 have been used to measure depressive symptoms (Tsai *et al.*, 2005), screen for depression (Tsai *et al.*, 2005) and erroneously to diagnose depression (Lee *et al.*, 1993, 1994; Woo *et al.*, 1994; Liu *et al.*, 1997).

The Zung self-rating depression scale (Zung, 1965) has been developed and used to identify depressive symptoms in a rural Japanese population (Ambo *et al.*, 2001). The Symptoms of Anxiety and Depression Scale (Bedford *et al.*, 1976) was developed in Gujarati, Somali and Bengali and was used to measure the prevalence of depression in convenience samples of elderly Gujarati (Ebrahim *et al.*, 1991), Somali (Silveira and Ebrahim, 1995) and Bengali (Silveria and Ebrahim, 1995) in London. The Short Care Interview (Gurland *et al.*, 1984) has been developed and used to evaluate depression in UK elders born in Cyprus, Africa and the Caribbean (Livingston *et al.*, 2002). A Nigerian version of the Self-Reporting Questionnaire has been developed (Abiodun, 1989).

The ICD-10 (WHO, 1992) diagnosis (unclear if clinical or research version) of depression has been used among Nigerians (Sokoya and Baiyewu, 2003; Uwake, 2000a, b). The DSM-III-R (American Psychiatric Association, 1987) diagnosis of depression has been used among elders in India (Jhinghan *et al.*,

2001) and Hong Kong (Liu *et al.*, 1997). The GMS has been developed and used to diagnose depression in the following elderly groups: UK Asians in Hindi (Bhatnagar and Frank, 1997); United Arab Emirates in Arabic (Ghubash *et al.*, 2004); Chinese (Chen *et al.*, 2004); Korean (Kim *et al.*, 2004); and Nigerian (Sokoya and Baiyewu, 2003; Uwake, 2000a, b). The concordance between the GMS and clinical diagnosis was high in the Hindi and Chinese versions (Bhatnagar and Frank, 1997; Chen *et al.*, 2004); the same was the case with the Nigerian GMS and ICD-10 diagnosis of depression (Sokoya and Baiyewu, 2003). A large cross-national study across 26 centres in India, China, Latin America and Africa demonstrated good psychometric properties for GMS-AGECAT in the diagnosis of depression (Prince *et al.*, 2004). The factor structure of CES-D was similar in older Chinese and Dutch individuals: somatic complaints, depressed affect, positive affect and interpersonal problems (Zhang *et al.*, 2011). Another study of Chinese older people reported good psychometric properties for the 10- and 20-item CES-D (Cheng and Chan, 2005). A Turkish and an Arabic version of the CES-D has been effectively evaluated for use among older Turkish and Moroccan migrants to the Netherlands (Spijker *et al.*, 2004).

Prevalence of Mental Disorders around the World

A recent review of prevalence studies of dementia in African and Asian countries including Nigeria, South Africa, India, Sri Lanka, Israel, Singapore, China, Hong Kong, Taiwan, Korea and Japan reported prevalence rates in the range 0–13.2% (median 4%) (Shah *et al.*, 2005b). In general, the prevalence rates were lower than in Western countries. However, there were notable exceptions including South Africa (Ben Arie *et al.*, 1983), Singapore (Lim *et al.*, 2003), Korea (Park *et al.*, 1994; Woo *et al.*, 1998; Kim *et al.*, 2003a) and Japan (Yamada *et al.*, 1999), where the prevalence rates were similar to Western countries. The prevalence of DSM-IV dementia in a large study across India, China and Latin America ranged from 0.3% in rural India to 6.3% in Cuba, but using the 10/66 algorithm the prevalence was higher and more consistent across sites ranging from 5.6% in rural China to 11.7% in the Dominican Republic (Llibre Rodriguez *et al.*, 2008). However, the 10/66 criteria do not take into account the functional disability required in DSM-IV, although the 10/66 algorithm diagnoses were associated with high levels of disability. Almost universally, the prevalence of dementia increased with age, and generally it was higher in women. This is consistent with integrated analysis of the world literature indicating that the prevalence of dementia doubles every 5.1 years after the age of 60 years (Jorm *et al.*, 1987; Hofman *et al.*, 1991). The prevalence of Alzheimer's disease is generally lower and the prevalence of vascular dementia is generally higher in Asian countries than in Western countries (Hasegawa *et al.*, 1986; Shibayama *et al.*, 1986; Li *et al.*, 1989).

There is a paucity of prevalence studies of depression from developing countries. The prevalence of depression in older people in Peru, Mexico and Venezuela ranged from 26 to 36 per cent depending on the criteria used (Gueraa *et al.*, 2009), but was much higher than low single figures using DSM-IV or ICD-10 criteria. Moreover, in a comparative study across ten countries in three continents, the prevalence of combined anxiety and depression comorbidity was between 0.9 and 4.2 per cent (Prina *et al.*, 2011). The prevalence of depression using ICD-10 and EURO-D ranged between 0.3–13.8% and 1.0% and 38.6% respectively across nine countries on three continents (Guerra *et al.*, 2016); the prevalence was particularly high in the Dominican Republic and rural India. Moreover, the prevalence of depression appears to vary depending on the criteria or instruments used (Guerra *et al.*, 2016). Prevalence rates for depression in the elderly in Singapore (Kua, 1992), the UK (Shah, 1992), the US (Blazer and Williams, 1980; Gurland *et al.*, 1983; Weismann *et al.*, 1988), Australia (Kay *et al.*, 1985; Henderson *et al.*, 1993) and Finland (Kivela *et al.*, 1988) of up to 5.7%, 15%, 15.5%, 16% and 26% respectively, have been reported.

Prevalence of Mental Disorders among Ethnic Elders in the UK and Other Countries

The prevalence of dementia among elders from different ethnic groups in the UK is generally similar to that amongst indigenous elders (Bhatnagar and Frank, 1997; Lindesay *et al.*, 1997b; McCracken *et al.*, 1997). The prevalence of depression amongst ethnic elders, in general, was similar to that amongst indigenous elders.

A population-based study from Bradford, using the Hindi version of the GMS administered to Indian subcontinent elders, reported a prevalence rate of 7 per cent for dementia (Bhatnagar and Frank, 1997). However, using a clinician's diagnosis of dementia, the prevalence was only 4 per cent, and there was poor agreement between the diagnoses by these two methods. The same study reported a prevalence of 20 per cent for depression and 2 per cent for anxiety neurosis; the concordance for depression with clinical diagnosis was high, but poor for neurosis.

A two-stage population-based study from Leicester, using a Gujarati MMSE administered by trained personnel in Gujarati, and a clinical interview and an ad hoc translated version of the CAMDEX and the SCAN interviews administered by a Gujarati-speaking psychiatrist, found prevalence rates of 0 per cent and 20 per cent in the 65–74 and 75+ years age groups respectively (Lindesay *et al.*, 1997b). This study included a comparison group of indigenous elders and the prevalence of dementia was higher in the Gujaratis, although this was not statistically significant. The stability of the diagnosis of dementia was confirmed at 27-month follow-up by another Gujarati-speaking psychiatrist using similar diagnostic techniques (Shah *et al.*, 1998). This study reported prevalence rates of 22%, 1% and 4% for agoraphobia, simple phobia and panic attacks (Lindesay *et al.*, 1997a); simple phobias were less prevalent in the ethnic minority group. Although the prevalence of depression was not measured, depression scores were not different between the Gujaratis and indigenous elders.

A population-based study from Liverpool of African, Caribbean, Asian, Chinese and Middle Eastern elders used the GMS either in English or an ad hoc translation during interview (McCracken *et al.*, 1997). The prevalence of dementia in English-speaking individuals of black African, black Caribbean, black other, Chinese and Asian origin were 8%, 8%, 2%, 5% and 9%, respectively, similar to the 3% found in the indigenous population. Prevalence in the black African and Chinese who did not speak English was 27% and 21%, respectively. These higher prevalence figures among non-English speakers may be an artefact of communication and translation difficulties. The prevalence of depression amongst black African, black Caribbean, Chinese and Asian groups was 19%, 16%, 13% and 15%, respectively (McCracken *et al.*, 1997) and these figures are comparable to indigenous elders (Shah, 1992). Lack of social contact was thought to be an important risk factors for developing depression (McCracken *et al.*, 1997).

A population-based study in Islington used the Short-CARE (Gurland *et al.*, 1984) in those born in the UK, Ireland, Cyprus, Africa and the Caribbean (Livingston *et al.*, 2001). The prevalence of dementia on those born in the UK, Ireland, Cyprus, and Africa and the Caribbean was 10%, 3.6%, 11.3% and 17% respectively. Logistic regression analysis revealed that living in a residential home, age, being African or Caribbean and years of education were the only significant predictors of dementia. The prevalence of depression in those born in the UK, Ireland, Cyprus, and Africa and the Caribbean was 18%, 16.5%, 28% and 14%, respectively. Logistic regression analysis revealed that needing help with functional activities, being female and subjective ill health were significant predictors of depression.

Studies in the US have reported higher prevalence of dementia among African Americans (Still *et al.*, 1990; Heyman *et al.*, 1991; Gurland *et al.*, 1995, 1999; Perkins *et al.*, 1997) and Hispanics (Perkins *et al.*, 1997; Gurland *et al.*, 1995, 1999). A higher prevalence of vascular dementia among African Americans may be associated with a higher prevalence of strokes and hypertension in this group (Heyman *et al.*, 1991; Perkins *et al.*, 1997). The prevalence of depression in older Mexican Americans was 30 per cent (Gonzalez *et al.*, 2001); degree of acculturation was an important predictor of depression.

Turkish and Moroccan immigrants over the age of 55 years in Holland had a prevalence of 34 per cent and 62 per cent, respectively, compared to Dutch (Van der Wurff *et al.*, 2004). Lower income and physical illness were predictors for depression. Nearly 40 per cent of older Korean migrants to the United States had significant depression (Lee *et al.*, 2005); perceived health status, education, positive support from the family and family relationships predicted depression, but the degree of acculturation did not.

Although there are no population-based studies of late-onset schizophrenia, the first contact incidence rate of late-onset schizophrenia (aged 60 and over) among African Caribbeans in London was significantly higher than in indigenous older people (Reeves *et al.*, 2001; Mitter *et al.*, 2004); this was not the case for older Bangladeshi people (Mitter *et al.*, 2004). The incident contact rate for African Caribbean men and women was 172 and 323 per 100,000 population, respectively (Reeves *et al.*, 2001).

Behavioural and Psychological Signs and Symptoms of Dementia

Behavioural and psychological symptoms of dementia (BPSD) (i.e. non-cognitive symptoms) including disorders of behaviour, mood, thought content, perception and personality change (Foli and Shah, 2000) have been poorly studied in developing countries and among ethnic minority groups in a given country (Jitapunkul *et al.*, 1996; Shah and Dighe-Deo, 1998). Data on BPSD among different ethnic groups are emerging (Shah and Mukherjee, 2000; Shah *et al.*, 2005c).

An Indian study reported that the prevalence of one or more BPSD in a convenience sample of dementia sufferers was 96.6 per cent, and was higher in Alzheimer's disease and Lewy body dementia than in vascular dementia (Shaji *et al.*, 2009). These findings were similar to those observed in another Indian study (Pinto and Seethalaksmi, 2006). Moreover, the prevalence of paranoid delusions, hallucinations, activity disturbance, aggressiveness, diurnal rhythm disturbance, affective disturbance and anxiety and phobias was 66%, 41%, 66%, 52%, 45%, 45% and 24% respectively (Shaji *et al.*, 2009). The delusional types were: people are stealing things (48%); home is not one's home (35%); abandonment (17%); infidelity (7%); paranoia (45%) and others (24%) (Shaji *et al.*, 2009). Levels of care-giver distress were associated with levels of BPSD and delusions, activity disturbance and aggressiveness were considered to be the most troublesome symptoms (Shaji *et al.*, 2009). The prevalence of at least one BPSD among dementia sufferers in a population-based study in Tanzania was 88% and reduced to 51% for three or more BPSD features (Paddick *et al.*, 2015); anxiety (47%), agitation/aggression (39%), night time disturbance (35%), irritability (33%) and depression (33%) were the most prevalent symptoms. In a community sample from Nigeria depression and distress were more prevalent in those with dementia compared to those with normal cognition (Baiyewu *et al.*, 2012). A population-based study in Mexico reported that depression (47.8%), irritability (37.2%) and sleeplessness (34.4%) were the most prevalent (Acosta-Castillo *et al.*, 2012). Severity of dementia was associated with the frequency of delusions, hallucinations, agitation, depression, euphoria, apathy, disinhibition, irritability and aberrant motor behaviours (Acosta-Castillo *et al.*, 2012). Anxiety, depression and sleep disorders were associated with care-giver distress (Acosta-Castillo *et al.*, 2012). Another Mexican study reported that the prevalence of BPSD was higher among dementia suffers in urban areas compared to rural areas, and affective symptoms, anxiety and irritability were the most prevalent (Rodriguez-Agudelo *et al.*, 2011).

A study of BPSD from 17 developing countries (*n* = 555) observed the prevalence to be 71% (Ferris *et al.*, 2004); the prevalence of depression syndrome, anxiety neurosis and paranoid psychosis were 44%, 14% and 11% respectively. Moreover, anxiety neurosis and paranoid psychosis predicted care-giver strain (Ferris *et al.*, 2004). A comparative study of BPSD among Chinese in Hong Kong and Taiwan and Caucasians in the US with Alzheimer's disease reported anxiety and delusions were more prevalent in the Chinese than the Caucasians and appetite changes and apathy were less prevalent (Chow *et al.*, 2002). Scores on a measure of BPSD were higher among referrals to a Korean psychogeriatric service than those in the UK (Shah *et al.*, 2004). All individual BPSD scores were higher among Koreans other than aggression (Shah *et al.*, 2004), and this was sustained when Alzheimer's disease and vascular dementia were examined separately (Shah *et al.*, 2005d). The prevalence and severity of BPSD were similar amongst Indian-origin and indigenous dementia sufferers admitted to an English day hospital (Haider and Shah, 2004); the only difference was the lower scores on the symptom of anxiety and phobia among those of Indian origin.

Instruments measuring BPSD have been formally developed in languages spoken in developing countries like Nigeria (Baiyewu *et al.*, 2003), Taiwan (Fuh *et al.*, 2001) and Korea (Shah *et al.*, 2004, 2005d). However, the prevalence and types of BPSD across different countries may vary because of differing methodologies and measurements used and genuine differences influenced by cultural factors.

Epidemiological Transition Hypothesis Model for Dementia

There is wide variation in the prevalence of dementia across different countries as discussed in an earlier section. These variations may be explained by differing methodologies used in different studies. However, as prevalence is a function of incidence and duration of illness, some of the variation may be due to differing incidence and differing duration of illness, particularly in cross-national studies using identical methodology (Chandra *et al.*, 1998; Hendrie *et al.*, 1995; Prince *et al.*, 2012). As dementia is a progressive disorder and recovery being unlikely, the duration of survival after the onset of dementia can represent duration of the illness. Thus, the prevalence of dementia is a function of the incidence and the duration of survival after the onset of dementia.

This model was based on several theoretical assumptions:

- Different countries will be at different stages of development within the model.
- Each country would sequentially progress through the hypothetical four stages over time with progress in socio-economic development.
- Both socio-economic status and the prevalence of dementia can be dichotomized into two groups: high and low.
- Dementia is considered as a unitary diagnosis rather than a label for a heterogeneous group of disorders.

This hypothetical model, whereby the relationship between socio-economic status (plotted on the *x*-axis) and the prevalence of dementia (plotted on the *y*-axis) follows an inverted U-shaped curve (although, as discussed later in the fourth stage, this may not necessarily be the case).

Stage 1 Low Prevalence and Low Socio-Economic Society Stage

Societies with low socio-economic status have poorly developed healthcare services (Shah, 2007c, 2009; Jacob *et al.*, 2007; Jacob, 2008; Shah *et al.*, 2008; Shah and Bhat, 2008a, b). Poorly developed healthcare services may mediate an increase in child mortality rates by being unable to provide primary preventative measures for diseases in childhood (e.g. immunization programmes) and general population mortality rates due to reduced treatment for diseases that are directly related to low socio-economic status (e.g. infectious diseases) (Suh and Shah, 2001). This will reduce life expectancy; there was a positive linear relationship between societal socio-economic status measured by gross national domestic product (GDP) and life expectancy (Shah *et al.*, 2008; Shah, 2007c). Given that dementia is an age-related disorder, reduced life expectancy will result in fewer people reaching the age of increased risk for developing dementia. Additionally, selective survival of those at reduced risk of dementia in old age, due to genetic or constitutional factors, may further compound this trend (Suh and Shah, 2001). Moreover, there is evidence that in societies with low socio-economic status, adversity early in life affords a protective effect on suicides later in life (Seiden, 1981; McIntosh, 1984; Lindesay, 1991); it is possible that similar protective mechanisms may operate in dementia. These factors could lead to a low incidence of dementia in societies with low socio-economic status. Some of the lowest figures for the incidence of dementia have been reported in India (Chandra et al., 2001) and Nigeria (Hendrie et al., 2001). Studies from Brazil (Nitrini et al., 2004) and China (Li et al., 1991) also reported low incidence rates. Similarly, the 10/66 incidence studies, using similar methodology across all studied countries, and when using the less controversial DSM-IV diagnosis of dementia, reported low incidence for dementia in several Latin American countries and China (Prince et al., 2012).

The poorly developed health and social care services (Shah, 2007c, 2009; Jacob et al., 2007; Jacob, 2008; Shah et al., 2008; Shah and Bhat, 2008a, b) in low socio-economic countries reduces life expectancy (Shah et al., 2008; Shah, 2007c). This impact is likely to be even greater among those with dementia. Mortality rates in dementia were increased in Nigeria and Brazil over 5 year and 3 year follow-up respectively (Nitrini et al., 2005; Perkins et al., 2002). They were also increased in China and several Latin American countries (Prince et al., 2012), and these mortality rates were higher than in developed countries (Dewey and Saz, 2001).

The combination of low incidence and shorter duration of survival after the onset of dementia will lead to a low prevalence of dementia. Very low prevalence rates for dementia have been reported in India (Chandra et al., 1998; Vas et al., 2001) and Nigeria (Hendrie et al., 1995). Studies from Brazil (Nitrini et al., 2004) and China (Li et al., 1991) also reported low prevalence rates. Similarly, the 10/66 studies, using identical methodology across the studied countries and when using the less controversial DSM-IV diagnosis of dementia, also reported very low prevalence rates in several developing countries: urban Peru, 3.1%; rural Peru, 0.4%; rural Mexico, 2.2%; rural China, 2.4%; urban India, 0.9%; and rural India, 0.8% (Llibre Rodriguez et al., 2008). The

authors concluded that the DSM-IV prevalence of dementia, when compared with pooled European data, was less than a quarter in India, about half in China and about four-fifths in Latin America. Moreover, the prevalence rates were particularly low in rural areas. Such a society could be labelled as a low prevalence and low socio-economic society.

Stage 2 High Prevalence and Low Socio-Economic Society Stage

With improvement in the socio-economic status of countries, the degree of development of health and social care services will also improve (Zhang, 1998; Shah, 2007c, 2009; Jacob et al., 2007; Shah et al., 2008; Shah and Bhat, 2008a, b). This improvement in health and social care services may facilitate reduction in child mortality rates because of improved ability to provide primary preventative measures for diseases in childhood (e.g. immunization programmes) and general population mortality rates related to poor treatment of diseases that are directly related to low socio-economic status (e.g. infectious diseases) (Suh and Shah, 2001). This will lead to an increase in life expectancy; there was a positive linear relationship between societal socio-economic status measured by GDP and life expectancy (Shah et al., 2008; Shah, 2007c). This, in turn, will result in greater number of subjects reaching the age of increased risk for dementia. Moreover, the effects of selective survival of those at reduced risk of dementia in old age, due to genetic or constitutional factors, will be weakened (Suh and Shah, 2001). This will lead to an increase in the incidence of dementia. The wide variation in the incidence of dementia using the less controversial DSM-IV diagnosis across different Latin American countries and between urban and rural areas within the same country in the 10/66 study (Prince et al., 2012) suggests that, even in socio-economically less developed countries, improvement in socio-economic status is associated with an increase in the incidence of dementia. Furthermore, this improvement in health and social care is likely to increase the duration of survival after the onset of dementia. There was heterogeneity between mortality rates across different developing countries and between rural and urban sites in the 10/66 study (Prince et al., 2012). This heterogeneity suggests that, even within socio-economically less developed countries, improvement in socio-economic status is associated with reduced mortality in dementia. Both these factors will tend to increase the prevalence of dementia. The increased prevalence of dementia, comparable to that in developed countries, in some Indian studies (Rajkumar and Kumar, 1996, Rajkumar *et al.* 1997; Shaji *et al.*, 2005), Sri Lanka (De Silva *et al.*, 2003), and in some Latin American countries in the 10/66 prevalence studies (Llibre Rodriguez *et al.*, 2008) suggests that there may be an association between improved socio-economic status and increasing prevalence of dementia. Such a society could be labelled as a high prevalence and low socio-economic society.

Stage 3 High Prevalence and High Socio-Economic Society Stage

As societies develop they are likely to change from being socio-economically less developed to being socio-economically more developed. Further improvement in health and social care services may facilitate further reductions in child mortality rates because of improved ability to provide primary preventative measures for diseases in childhood (e.g. immunization programmes) and general population mortality rates due to treatment of diseases that are directly related to low socio-economic status (e.g. infectious diseases) (Suh and Shah, 2001). This will lead to further increase in life expectancy. This, in turn, will result in an increasing number of subjects reaching the age of increased risk for dementia. This will also weaken any effect of selective survival of those at reduced risk of dementia due to constitutional or genetic factors. Thus, the incidence of dementia will increase. The incidence rate for DSM-III-R dementia was higher in the Eurodem study (pooled data from Denmark, France, the Netherlands and United Kingdom) (Launer *et al.*, 1999) compared to those for DSM-IV dementia in the 10/66 study (Prince *et al.*, 2012). Furthermore, the improvement in the availability of health and social care is likely to increase the duration of survival after the onset of dementia. Relatively recent studies from high-income countries have reported higher survival duration than two decades ago (Williams *et al.*, 2006; Xie *et al.*, 2008). Both these factors will tend to increase the prevalence of dementia. The prevalence of dementia in high-income countries is generally higher than in low-income countries (Hendrie *et al.*, 1995; Llibre Rodriguez *et al.*, 2008). The prevalence of DSM-IV dementia in a pooled study of 12 European countries (Lobo *et al.*, 2000)

was higher than that observed in Latin America, India and China in the 10/66 study (Llibre Rodriguez *et al.*, 2008). Comparatively high prevalence rates in Europe were also reported in another pooled study of 23 European data sets (Hofman *et al.*, 1991). Such a society could be labelled as a high prevalence and high socio-economic society. It is likely that most high-income countries are currently at this stage of epidemiological transition because of reasons discussed under the next sub-heading.

Stage 4 Variable Prevalence and High Socio-Economic Society Stage

Theoretically, in socio-economically well developed societies, due to improved health and social care leading to further reduction in child mortality rates and increase in life expectancy, greater numbers of people would reach the age of increased risk for dementia, and consequently lead to a higher incidence of dementia. This improvement in health and social care would also increase the duration of survival after the onset of dementia. Thus, the prevalence of dementia would increase further. However, the picture in socio-economically very well developed societies is complex because such societies are much more likely to have developed primary preventative strategies. For example, in England and Wales there is a national dementia strategy, which incorporates many aspects of primary prevention; similar strategies have been developed in several high-income countries. Also, primary, secondary and tertiary prevention programmes for hypertension, heart disease, cerebrovascular disease and diabetes are much more likely to be established in socio-economically well developed countries; these are also likely to reduce the incidence of dementia further. Thus, the incidence of dementia may be reduced further by improved efforts to control the risk factors for dementia and enhance the protective factors for dementia. For example, the prevalence of dementia was a third less, despite an increase in the prevalence of stroke, in a Swedish birth cohort of 85 years olds compared to a birth cohort of 85 year olds from 20 years before (Skoog, 2012). At the same time, better provision of health and social care and advances in medical care may increase the duration of survival after the onset of dementia. In this scenario, the incidence of dementia and duration of survival after the onset would have opposite effects on the prevalence of dementia. Thus, the relative balance between the amount of reduction in the incidence and the amount of increase in the duration of survival after the onset would determine whether the prevalence would decrease, remain the same or increase. Such a society could be labelled as a variable prevalence and high socio-economic society. This last stage for dementia differs significantly from the last stage for elderly suicides as the prevalence of dementia may not continue to decline. It is unlikely that there are any countries at this stage of epidemiological transition in dementia.

Conclusions

Although studies have emerged in recent years, there remains a paucity of studies of clinical features and clinical presentation of mental illness in ethnic elders in a given country and in many other cultures; hence, there is an urgent need to conduct studies to examine these areas. Such studies should be coupled with development of clinical services with an evaluative component for the effectiveness of the clinical services.

References

Abas, M. (1996). Depression and anxiety among older Caribbean people in the UK: screening, unmet need and the provision of appropriate services. *International Journal of Geriatric Psychiatry*, **11**, 377–382.

Abas, M., Phillips, C., Richards, M., Carter, J. and Levy, R. (1996). Initial development of a new culture-specific screen for emotional distress in older Caribbean people. *International Journal of Geriatric Psychiatry*, **11**(12), 1097–1103.

Abas, M., Phillips, C., Carter, J., Walker, S., Banerjee, S. and Levy, R. (1998). Culturally sensitive validation of instruments in older African-Caribbean people living in south London. *British Journal of Psychiatry*, **17**, 249–254.

Abiodun, O. A. (1989). Sensitivity and validity of the Self Reporting Questionnaire (SRQ) in a primary health centre in a rural community in Nigeria. *Psychopathologie Africaine*, **XXII**, 89–94.

Acosta-Castillo, G. I., Luisa Sosa, A., Orozco, R., Borges, G. (2012). Neuropsychiatric symptoms in older adults with dementia and their relationship to disease severity. *Revista de Investigacion Clinica*, **64**, 354–363.

Adshead, G., Cody, D. and Pitt, B. (1992). BASDEC: a novel screening instrument for depression in elderly medical inpatients. *British Medical Journal*, **305**, 397.

Alici-Evcimen, Y., Ertan, T. and Eker, E. (2003). Case series with late-onset psychosis hospitalised in a geriatric psychiatry unit in Turkey: experience of 9 years. *International Psychogeriatrics*, **15**, 69–72.

Allen, N., Ames, D., Ashby, D., Bennetts K., Tuckwell, V. and West, C. (1994). A brief sensitive screening instrument for depression in late life. *Age and Ageing*, **23**, 213–218.

Alzheimer's Disease International (2015). World Alzheimer Report 2015. The Global Impact of Dementia: an analysis of prevalence, incidence, cost and trends. Available online at www.alz.co.uk/research/WorldAlzheimerReport2015.pdf (accessed 3 March 2016).

Ambo, H., Meguro, K., Ishizaki, J. *et al.* (2001). Depressive symptoms and associated factors in a cognitively normal elderly population: the Tajiri Project. *International Journal of Geriatric Psychiatry*, **16**, 780–788.

American Psychiatric Association (1987). *Diagnostic and Statistical Manual of Mental Disorders*, 3rd revised edn. Washington DC: American Psychiatric Association.

Anzola-Perez, E., Bangdiwala, S. I., De Llano, G. B. *et al.* (1996). Towards community diagnosis of dementia: testing cognitive impairment in older persons in Argentina, Chile and Cuba. *International Journal of Geriatric Psychiatry*, **11**, 429–438.

Bae, J. N. and Cho, M. J. (2004). Development of the Korean version of the Geriatric Depression Scale and its short form among elderly psychiatric patients. *Journal of Psychosomatic Research*, **57**, 297–305.

Baiyewu, O., Smith-Gamble, V., Akinbiyi, A. *et al.* (2003). Behavioural and caregiver reaction of dementia as measured by the neuropsychiatric inventory in Nigerian community residents. *International Psychogeriatrics* **15**, 399–409.

Baiyewu, O., Unverzagt, F. W., Ogunniyi, A., Smith-Gamble, V. *et al.* (2012). Behavioural symptoms in community-dwelling elderly Nigerians with dementia, mild cognitive impairment and normal cognition. *International Journal of Geriatric Psychiatry*, **27**, 931–939.

Baker, F. M., Espine, D. V., Robinson, B. H. and Stewart, B. (1993). Assessing depressive symptoms in African American and Mexican elders. *Clinical Gerontologist*, **14**, 15–29.

Baker, F. M., Parker, D. A., Wiley, C., Velli, S. A. and Johnson, J. T. (1995). Depressive symptoms in African-American medical patients. *International Journal of Geriatric Psychiatry*, **19**, 9–14.

Barker, J. (1984). *Research Perspectives on Ageing: Black and Asian Old People in Britain*, 1st edn. London: Age Concern Research Unit.

Beck, A. T., Ward, C. H., Mendelson, M., Mock, J. and Erbaugh, J. (1961). An inventory for measuring depression. *Archives of General Psychiatry*, **4**, 53–63.

Bedford, A., Foulds, G. A. and Sheffield, B. F. (1976). A new personal disturbance scale. *British Journal of Social and Clinical Psychology*, **15**, 387–394.

Ben-Arie, O., Swartz, L., Teggin, A. F. and Elk, R. (1983). The coloured elderly in Cape Town – a psychosocial, psychiatric and medical community survey. Part II Prevalence of psychiatric disorders. *South African Medical Journal*, **64**, 1056–1061.

Bhatnagar, K. S. (1997). Depression in South Asian elders. *Geriatric Medicine*. February, 55–56.

Bhatnagar, K. S. and Frank, J. (1997). Psychiatric disorders in elderly from the Indian subcontinent living in Bradford. *International Journal of Geriatric Psychiatry*, **12**, 907–912.

Bhopal, R. (1997). Is research into ethnicity and health racist, unsound or unimportant science? *British Medical Journal*, **314**, 1751–1756.

Bhugra, D. and Mastrogianni, A. (2004). Globalisation and mental disorder. *British Journal of Psychiatry*, **184**, 10–20.

Blakemore, K. and Boneham, M. (1994). *Age, Race and Ethnicity: A Comparative Approach*. Buckingham: Open University Press.

Blazer, D. and Willians, C. D. (1980). Epidemiology of dysphoria and depression in an elderly population. *American Journal of Psychiatry*, **137**, 439–444.

Boneham, M. (1989). Ageing and ethnicity in Britain: the case of elderly Sikh women in a Midlands town. *New Community*, **15**, 447–459.

Braam, A. W., Sonnenberg, C. M., Beekman, A. T. F., Deeg, D. J. H. and Van Tilburg, W. V. (2000). Religious denomination as a symptom formation factor of depression in older Dutch citizens. *International Journal of Geriatric Psychiatry*, **15**, 458–466.

Brietner, J. C. S. and Folstein, M. (1984). Familial Alzheimer's dementia: a prevalent disorder with specific clinical features. *American Journal of Psychiatry*, **14**, 63–80.

Brislin, R. (1970). Back-translation for cross-cultural research. *Journal of Cross-Cultural Psychology*, **1**, 185–216.

Broekman, B. F. P., Nyunt, S. Z., Niti, M., *et al.* (2007). Differential item functioning of the Geriatric Depression Scale in an Asian population. *Journal of Affective Disorders*, **108**, 285–290.

Chan, A. C. (1996). Clinical validity of the Geriatric Depression Scale (GDS): Chinese version. *Journal of Ageing and Health*, **8**, 238–253.

Chandra, V., Ganguli, M., Ratcliff, G. *et al.* (1994). Studies of the epidemiology of dementia: comparison between developed and developing countries. *Aging, Clinical and Experimental Research*, **6**, 307–321.

Chandra, V., Ganguli, M., Pandav, R., Johnston, J., Belle, S. and DeKosky, S. T. (1998). Prevalence of Alzheimer's and other dementias in rural India: the Indo-US study. *Neurology*, **51**, 1000–1008.

Chandra, V., Pandav, R. and Dodge, H. H. (2001). Incidence of Alzheimer's disease in a rural community in India: the Indo-US study. *Neurology*, **57**, 985–989.

Chen, R., Hu, Z., Qin, X., Xu, X. and Copeland, J. (2004). A community-based study of depression in older people in Hefei, China – the GMS-AGECAT prevalence, cross validation and socio-economic correlates. *International Journal of Geriatric Psychiatry*, **19**, 407–413.

Cheng, S. T. and Chan, A. C. M. (2005). The centre for epidemiologic studies depression scale in older Chinese: thresholds for long and short forms. *International Journal of Geriatric Psychiatry*, **20**, 465–470.

Chow, T. W., Liu, C. K., Fuh, J. L. *et al.* (2002). Neuropsychiatric symptoms of Alzheimer's disease differ in Chinese and American patients. *International Journal of Geriatric Psychiatry*, **17**, 22–28.

Christensen, K., Doblhammer, G., Rau, R. and Vaupel, J. W. (2009). Ageing populations: the challenges ahead. *The Lancet*, **374**, 1196–1208.

Commonwealth Department of Health, Housing and Community (1991). *Aged Care Reform Strategy Mid-Term Review 1990–1991 Report*. Canberra: Australian Government Publishing Service.

Copeland, J. R. M., Kelleher, M. J., Kellett, J. M. *et al.* (1976). A semi-structured interview for the assessment of diagnosis and mental state in the elderly. The Geriatric Mental State Schedule. 1. Development and reliability. *Psychological Medicine*, **6**, 439–449.

Cwikel, J. and Ritchie, K. (1988). The short GDS: evaluation in a heterogenous multilingual population. *Clinical Gerontologist*, **8**, 63–79.

Davoudzadeh P (2010). The Mini-Mental State Examination in Iranian Americans. MA thesis available online at http://sdsu-dspace.calstate.edu/bitstream/handle/10211.10/278/Davoudzadeh_Pega.pdf?sequence=1 accessed 7 March 2016.

De Silva, H. A. and Gunatilake, S. B. (2002). Mini Mental State Examination in Sinhalese: a sensitive test to screen for dementia in Sri Lanka. *International Journal of Geriatric Psychiatry*, **17**, 134–139.

De Silva, H. A., Gunatilake, S. B. and Smith, A. D. (2003). Prevalence of dementia in a semi urban population in Sri Lanka: reports from a regional survey. *International Journal of Geriatric Psychiatry*, 711–715.

Desjarlais, R., Eisenberg L., Good, B. and Klienman, A. (1995). *World Mental Health Problems and Priorities in Low Income Countries*. Oxford: Oxford University Press.

Dewey, M. and Saz, P. (2001). Dementia, cognitive impairment and mortality in persons aged 65 and over living in the community: a systematic review of the literature. *International Journal of Geriatric Psychiatry*, **16**, 751–761.

Dowd, J. J. and Bengston, V. L (1978). Aging in minority populations: an examination of double jeopardy hypothesis. *Journal of Gerontology*, **3**, 427–436.

Ebrahin, S., Patel, N., Coats, M. *et al.* (1991). Prevalence and severity of morbidity among Gujarati Asian elders: a controlled comparison. *Family Practice*, 8, 57–62.

Ertan, T. and Eker, E. (2000). Reliability, validity, and factor structure of the Geriatric Depression Scale in Turkish elderly: are there different factor structures for different cultures. *International Psychogeriatrics*, 12, 163–172.

Escobar, J. I., Burnham, A., Karno, M. *et al.* (1986). Use of the Mini-Mental State Examination (MMSE) in a community population of mixed ethnicity. *Journal of Nervous and Mental Diseases*, 174, 607–614.

Espino, D. V., Bedolla, M. A., Perez, M. and Baker, F. M. (1996). Validation of the Geriatric Depression Scale in an elder Mexican American population: a pilot study. *Clinical Gerontologist*, 16, 55–67.

Ferraro, F. R. (1997). Geriatric Depression Scale short form (GDS-SF) performance in native American elderly adults. *Clinical Gerontologist*, 18, 52–55.

Ferris, C. P., Ames, D., Prince, M. *et al.* (2004). Behavioural and psychological symptoms of dementia in developing countries. *International Psychogeriatrics*, 16, 441–459.

Fillenbaum, G. G., Chandra, V., Ganguli, M. *et al.* (1999). Development of an activities of daily living scale to screen for dementia in an illiterate rural population in India. *Age and Ageing*, 28, 161–168.

Flaherty, J. A., Gaviria, F. M., Pathak, D. *et al.* (1988). Developing instruments for cross-cultural psychiatric research. *Journal of Nervous and Mental Diseases*, 176, 257–263.

Foli, S. and Shah, A. K. (2000). Measurement of behaviour disturbance, non-cognitive symptoms and quality of life. In *Dementia*, ed. J. O'Brien, D. Ames, and A. Burns. London: Arnold, pp. 87–100.

Folstein, M. F., Folstein, S. E. and McHugh, P. R. (1975). 'Mini Mental State': a practical method for grading the cognitive state of patients for the clinician. *Journal of Psychiatric Research*, 12, 189–198.

Fountoulakis, K. N., Tsolaki, M., Lacovides, A., Yesavage, J., O'Hara, R., Kazis, A., Lerodiakonou, C. (2014). The validation of the short form of the Geriatric Depression Scale (GDS) in Greece. *Aging Clinical and Experimental Research*, 11, 367–372.

Fuh, J. L., Teng, E. L., Lin, K. N. *et al.* (1995). The informant questionnaire on cognitive decline in the elderly (IQCODE) as a screening tool for dementia for a predominantly illiterate Chinese population. *Neurology*, 45, 92–96.

Fuh, J. L., Liu, C. K., Mega, M. S., Wang, S. J., Cummings, J. L. (2001). Behavioral disorders and caregivers' reaction in Taiwanese patients with Alzheimer's disease. *International Psychogeriatrics*, 13, 121–128.

Ganguli, M., Ratcliff, G., Chandra, V. *et al.* (1995). A Hindi version of the MMSE: development of a cognitive screening instrument for a largely illiterate rural population of India. *International Journal of Geriatric Psychiatry*, 10, 367–377.

Ganguli, M., Chandra, V., Gilby, J. E. *et al.* (1996). Cognitive test performance in a community-based nondemented elderly sample in rural India: the Indo-US cross-national dementia epidemiology study. *International Psychogeriatrics*, 8, 507–524.

Ganguli, M., Dube, S., Johnston, J. M., Pandav, R., Chandra, V. and Dodge, H. H. (1999). Depressive symptoms, cognitive impairment and functional impairment in a rural elderly population in India: a Hindi version of the Geriatric Depression Scale (GDS-H). *International Journal of Geriatric Psychiatry*, 14, 807–820.

George, J. and Young, J. (1991). The physician. In *Multicultural Health Care and Rehabilitation of Older People*, ed. A. J. Squires. London: Edward Arnold.

Ghubash, R., El-Rufaie, O., Zoubeidi, T., Al-Shbol, Q. M. and Sabri, S. M. (2004). Profile of mental disorder among the elderly United Arab Emirates population: socio-economic correlates. *International Journal of Geriatric Psychiatry*, 19, 344–351.

Gonzalez, H. M., Haan, M. N., Hinton, L. (2001). Acculturation and the prevalence of depression in older Mexican Americans: baseline results of the Sacramento area Latino study on Ageing. *Journal of American Geriatric Society*, 49, 948–953.

Graves, A. B., Larson, E. B., White, L. R., Teng, E. L. and Homma, A. (1994). Opportunities and challenges in international collaborative epidemiological research of dementia and its subtypes. Studies between Japan and the US. *International Psychogeriatrics*, 6, 209–223.

Guerra, M., Ferri, C. P., Sosa, A. L., *et al.* (2009). Late-life depression in Peru, Mexico and Venezuela: the 10/66 population-based study. *British Journal of Psychiatry*, 195, 510–515.

Guerra, M., Prina, A. M., Ferri, C. P., *et al.* (2016). A comparative cross-cultural study of the prevalence of late life depression in low and middle income countries. *Journal of Affective Disorders*, 190, 362–368.

Gurland, B., Copeland, J., Kuriansky, J., Kelleher, M., Sharpe, L. and Dean, L. L. (1983). *The Mind and Mood of Ageing*. London: Croom Helm.

Gurland, B., Golden, A., Teresi, J. A. *et al.* (1984). The Short-Care. An efficient instrument for the assessment of depression and dementia. *Journal of Gerontology*, 39, 166–169.

Gurland, B. J., Wilder, D. E., Cross, P. *et al.* (1992). Screening scales for dementia: towards reconciliation of conflicting cross-cultural findings. *International Journal of Geriatric Psychiatry*, 7, 105–113.

Gurland, B., Wilder, D., Cross, P. *et al.* (1995). Relative rates of dementia by multiple case definitions, over two prevalence periods in three sociocultural groups. *American Journal of Geriatric Psychiatry*, 3, 6–20.

Gurland, B., Wilder, D., Lantigua, R. et al. (1999). Rates of dementia in three ethnoracial groups. *International Journal of Geriatric Psychiatry*, **14**, 481–493.

Hahn, C., Yang, M., Yang, M., Shih, C. and Lo, H. (2004). Religious attendance and depressive symptoms among community dwelling elderly in Taiwan. *International Journal of Geriatric Psychiatry*, **19**, 1148–1154.

Haider, I. and Shah, A. K. (2004). A pilot study of behavioural and psychological signs and symptoms of dementia in patients of Indian sub-continent origin admitted to a dementia day hospital in the United Kingdom. *International journal of Geriatric Psychiatry*, **19**, 1195–1204.

Hall, K. S., Hendrie, H. C., Britain, H. M. et al. (1993). The development of dementia screening interview in two distinct languages. *International Journal of Methods in Psychiatric Research*, **3**, 1–28.

Hall, K. S., Gao, S., Emsley, C. L. et al. (2000). Community screening interview for dementia (CIS D): performance in five disparate study sites. *International Journal of Geriatric Psychiatry*, **15**, 521–531.

Hasegawa, K., Homma, A. and Imai, Y. (1986) An epidemiological study of age-related dementia in the community. *International Journal of Geriatric Psychiatry*, **1**, 45–55.

Hathaway, S. R. and McKinley, J. C. (1943). *The Minnesota Multiphasic Personality Scale*. Minneapolis: University of Minnesota.

Henderson, A. S., Jorm, A. F., MacKinnon, A. et al. (1993). The prevalence of depressive disorders and the distribution of depressive symptoms in later life: a survey using draft ICD-10 and DSM-III-R. *Psychological Medicine*, **23**, 719–729.

Hendrie, H. (1992). Indianapolis–Ibadan dementia project. In 'Multi-National Studies of Dementia' (symposium abstract), ed. J. D. Curb and A. B. Graves. *Gerontologist* **32** (Suppl. 2), 219.

Hendrie, H., Hall, K. S., Pillay, N. et al. (1993). Alzheimer's disease is rare in the Cree. *International Psychogeriatrics*, **5**, 5–15.

Hendrie, H. C., Osuntokun, B. O. and Hall, K. S. (1995). Prevalence of dementia in two communities: Nigerian Africans and African Americans. *American Journal of Pschiatry*, **152**, 1485–1492.

Hendrie, H. C., Ogunniyi, A. and Hall, K. S. (2001). Incidence of dementia and Alzheimer's disease in two communities: Yoruba residing in Ibadan, Nigeria and African Americans residing in Indianopolis, Indiana. *Journal of the American Medical Association*, **285**, 739–747.

Heyman, A., Fillenbaum, G. and Prosnitz, B. (1991). Estimated prevalence of dementia among elderly black and white community residents. *Archives of Neurology*, **48**, 594–598.

Hofman, A., Rocca, W. A., Brayne, C. et al. (1991). The prevalence of dementia in Europe: a collaborative study of 1980–1990 findings. *International Journal of Epidemiology*, **20**, 736–748.

Hughes, C., Kumari, V., Soni, W., Das, M., et al. (2001). Longitudinal study of symptoms and cognitive function in schizophrenia. *Schizophrenia Research*, **59**, 137–146.

Izal, M. and Montorio, I. (1993). Adaptation of the Geriatric Depression Scale in Spain: a preliminary study. *Clinical Gerontologist*, **13**, 83–91.

Jacob, K. S. (2008). The prevention of suicide in India and the developing world: the need for population-based strategies. *Crisis*, **29**(2), 102–106.

Jacob, K. S., Sharan, P., Mirza, I. et al. (2007). Global mental health 4. Mental health systems in countries: where are we now? *The Lancet*, **370**, 1061–1077.

Jang, Y., Small, B. J., Haley, W. E. (2001). Cross-cultural comparability of the Geriatric Depression Scale: comparison between older Koreans and older Americans. *Ageing and Mental Health*, **5**, 31–37.

Jeune, B. and Skytthe, A. (2001). Centenarians in Denmark in the past and the present. *Population: An English Selection*, **13**, 75–94.

Jhinghan, H. P., Sagar, R. and Pandey, R. M. (2001). Prognosis of late-onset depression in the elderly: a study from India. *International Psychogeriatrics*, **13**, 51–61.

Jitapunkul, S., Kamolratanakul, P., Ebrahim, S. (1994). The meaning of activities of daily living in a Thai elderly population: development of a new index. *Age and Ageing*, **23**, 97–101.

Jitapunkul, S., Lailert, C., Worakul, P. et al. (1996). Chula Mental Test: a screening test for elderly people in less developed countries. *International Journal of Geriatric Psychiatry*, **11**(8), 715–720.

Jorm, A. F., Korten, A. E. and Henderson, A. S. (1987). The prevalence of dementia: a quantitative integration of the literature. *Acta Scandinavica Psychiatrica*, **76**, 465–479.

Jorm, A. F., Scott, R., Cullen, J. S. et al. (1991). Performance of Informant Questionnaire on Cognitive Decline in the Elderly (IQCODE) as a screening test for dementia. *Psychological Medicine*, **21**, 785–790.

Jung, I. K., Kwak, D. I., Joe, S. H. and Lee, H. S. (1997). A study of standardization of Korean form of Geriatric Depression Scale (KGDS). *Korean Journal of Geriatric Psychiatry*, **1**, 61–72.

Kabir, Z. H. and Herlitz, A. (2000). The Bangla adaptation of mini-mental state examination (BMASE): an instrument to assess cognitive function in illiterate and literate individuals. *International Journal of Geriatric Psychiatry*, **15**, 441–450.

Katzman, R., Zhang, M., Qu, Q. Y. et al. (1988). A Chinese version of the Mini-Mental State Examination: impact of illiteracy in a Shanghai dementia survey. *Journal of Clinical Epidemiology*, **41**, 971–978.

355

Kawata, K. H. D. S., Hashimoto, R., Nishio, Y. *et al.* (1985) The prevalence of dementia and depression among the elderly living in the Hobart community: the effect of diagnostic criteria on prevalence rates. *Psychological Medicine*, **15**, 771–788.

Kawata, K. H. D. S., Hashimoto, R., Nishio, Y., Hayashi, A. *et al.* (2012). A validation study of the Japanese Version of the Addenbrooke's Cognitive Examination – Revised. *Dementia and Geriatric Cognitive Disorders Extra*, **2**, 29–37.

Kim, G., DeCoster, J., Huang, C. H., Bryant, A. N. (2013). A meta-analysis of the factor structure of the Geriatric Depression Scale (GDS): the effect of language. *International Psychogeriatrics*, **25**, 71–81.

Kim, J., Jeong, I., Chun, J. H. *et al.* (2003a). The prevalence of dementia in a metropolitan city of South Korea. *International Journal of Geriatric Psychiatry*, **18**, 617–622.

Kim, J., Stewart, R., Prince, M. *et al.* (2003b). Diagnosing dementia in a developing nation: an evaluation of the GMS-AGECAT algorithm in an older Korean population. *International Journal of Geriatric Psychiatry*, **18**, 331–336.

Kim, J., Stewart, R., Shin, I., Yoon, J. and Lee, H. (2004). Lifetime urban/rural residence, social support and late-life depression in Korea. *International Journal of Geriatric Psychiatry*, **19**, 843–851.

Kivela, S. L., Pahkala, K. and Laippala, P. (1988). Prevalence of depression in an elderly population in Finland. *Acta Psychiatrica Scandinavica*, **78**, 401–413.

Kochhann, R., Varela, J. S., Lisboa, C. S. D. M., Lorena, M. and Chaves, F. (2010). The Mini Mental State Examination Review of cutoff points adjusted for schooling in large southern Brazilian sample. *Dementia Neuropsychologia*, **4**, 35–41.

Kua, E. H. (1992). A community study of mental disorders in elderly Singaporean Chinese using the GMS-AGECAT package. *Australia and New Zealand Journal of Psychiatry*, **25**, 502–506.

Kumar, S., Tiwari, S. C., Tripthi, R. K. and Pandey, N. M. (2014). Socio-economic status has bearing on Mini-Mental State Examination among Indians. *Journal of Geriatric Mental Health*, **2**, 90–93.

Lai, D. W. L, Fung, T. S., Yuen, C. T. Y. (2005). The factor structure of a Chinese version of the Geriatric Depression Scale. *International Journal of Psychiatry in Medicine*, **35**, 137–148.

Launer, L. J., Andersen, K. and Dewey, M. E. (1999). Rates and risk factors for dementia and Alzheimer's disease: results from EURODEM pooled analysis. EURODEM Incidence Research Group and work Groups. *Neurology*, **52**, 78–84.

Lee, H. C. B., Chiu, H. F. K., Kwok, W. Y., Leung, C. M., Kwong, P. K. and Chung, D. W. S. (1993). Chinese elderly and the short form GDS: a preliminary study. *Clinical Gerontologist*, **14**, 37–42.

Lee, H. C. B., Chiu, H. F. K. and Kwong, P. P. K. (1994). Cross-validation of the Geriatric Depression Scale short form in the Hong Kong elderly. *Bulletin of the Hong Kong Psychological Society*, **32**, 72–77.

Lee, H. Y., Moon, A., Knight, B. G. (2005). Depression among elderly Korean immigrants. *Journal of Ethnic and Cultural Diversity in Social Work*, **13**, 1–26.

Levkoff, S. E., MacArthur, I. W. and Bucknail, J. (1995). Elderly mental health in the developing world. *Social Science and Medicine*, **41**, 983–1003.

Li, G., Shen, Y. C., Chen, C. H. *et al.* (1989). An epidemiological survey of age-related dementia in an urban area of Beijing. *Acta Psychiatric Scandinavica*, **79**, 557–563.

Li, G., Shen, Y. C., Chen, C. H., Zhau, Y. W., Li, S. R., Lu, M. (1991). A three-year follow-up study of age-related dementia in an urban area of Beijing. *Acta Psychiatrica Scandinavica*, **83**, 99–104.

Lim, P. P., Ng, L. L., Chiam, P. C., Ong, P. S., Ngui, F. T., Sahadevan, S. (2000). Validation and comparison of three brief depression scales in an elderly Chinese population. *International Journal of Geriatric Psychiatry*, **15**(9), 824-830.

Lim, P. P. J., Ng, L. L., Chiam, P. C., Ong, P. S., Ngui, F. T. and Sahadevan, S. (2003). Validation and comparison of three brief depression rating scales in an elderly Chinese population. *International Journal of Geriatric Psychiatry*, **15**, 824–830.

Lindesay, J. (1991). Suicide in the elderly. *International Journal of Geriatric Psychiatry*, **6**, 355–361.

Lindesay, J. (1998). The diagnosis of mental illness in elderly people from ethnic minorities. *Advances in Psychiatric Treatment*, **4**, 219–226.

Lindesay, J., Jagger, C., Hibbert, M. J., Peet, S. M. and Moledina, F. (1997a). Knowledge, uptake and availability of health and social services among Asian Gujarati and white elders. *Ethnicity and Health*, **2**, 59–69.

Lindesay, J., Jagger, C., Mlynik-Szmid, A. *et al.* (1997b). The Mini-Mental State Examination (MMSE) in an elderly immigrant Gujarati population in the United Kingdom. *International Journal of Geriatric Psychiatry*, **12**, 1155–1167.

Liu, C. Y., Wang, S. J., Teng, J. L. *et al.* (1997). Depressive disorders among older residents in a Chinese rural community. *Psychological Medicine*, **27**, 943–949.

Livingston, G. and Sembhi, S. (2003). Mental health of the ageing immigrant population. *Advances in Psychiatric Treatment*, **9**, 31–37.

Livingston, G., Leavey, G., Kitchen, G. *et al.* (2001). Mental health of migrant elders: the Islington study. *British Journal of Psychiatry*, **179**, 361–366.

Livingston, G., Leavey, G., Kitchen, G. *et al.* (2002). Accessibility of health and social services to immigrant elders: the Islington study. *British Journal of Psychiatry*, **180**, 369–374.

Llibre Rodriguez, J. J., Ferri, C. P., Acosta, D. *et al.* (2008). Prevalence of dementia in Latin America, India, and China: a population-based cross-sectional survey. *The Lancet*, **372**, 464–474.

Lobo, A., Launer, L. J., Fratiglioni, L. *et al.* (2000). Prevalence of dementia and major sub-types in Europe. A collaborative study of population-based cohorts. Neurologic Diseases in the Elderly Research Group. *Neurology*, **54**, S4–S9.

Manthorpe, J. and Hettiaratchy, P. (1993). Ethnic minority elders in Britain. *International Review of Psychiatry*, **5**, 173–180.

Markson, E. W. (2003). *Social Gerontology Today. An Introduction*. Los Angeles: Roxbury Publishing.

McCallum, J. A. (1990).*The Forgotten People: Carers in Three Minority Commmunities in Southwark*. London: King's Fund Centre.

McCracken, C. F. M., Boneham, M. A., Copeland, J. R. M. *et al.* (1997). Prevalence of dementia and depression among elderly people in black and ethnic groups. *British Journal of Psychiatry*, **171**, 269–273.

McIntosh, J. L. (1984). Components of the decline in elderly suicides: suicide in young old and old old by race and sex. *Death Education*, **8**, 113–124.

McKenzie, K. and Crowcroft, N. S. (1996). Describing race, ethnicity and culture in medical research: describing the groups is better than trying to find a catch all name. *British Medical Journal*, **312**, 1051.

Mitter, P. R., Krishnan, S., Bell, P., Steward, R., Howard, R. J. (2004). The effect of ethnicity and gender on first contact rates for schizophrenia-like psychosis in Bangladesh, black and white elders in Tower Hamlets, London. *International Journal of Geriatric Psychiatry*, **19**, 286–290.

Morris, J., Heyman, A., Mohs, R. *et al.* (1989). The consortium to establish a registry for Alzheimer's disease (CERAD). Part 1. Clinical and neuropsychological assessment of Alzheimer's disease. *Neurology*, **39**, 1159–1165.

Mui, A. C. (1993). Self-reported depressive symptoms among black and Hispanic frail elders: a sociocultural perspective. *Journal of Applied Gerontology*, **12**, 170–187.

Mui, A. C. (1996). Geriatric Depression Scale as a community screening instrument for elderly Chinese immigrants. *International Psychogeriatrics*, **8**, 445–458.

Mui, A. C. (2008). Stress, coping and depression among elderly Korean immigrants. *Journal of Human Behaviour in the Social Environment*, **3**, 281–299.

Mui, A. C., Burnette, D., Mei, C. L. (2001). Cross-cultural assessment of depression: a review of the CES-D and GDS. *Journal of Mental Health and Ageing*, **7**, 137–164.

Mui, A. C., Kang, S., Chen, L. M. and Domanski, M. D. (2003). Reliability of the geriatric depression scale for use among elderly Asian immigrants in the USA. *International Psychogeriatrics*, **15**, 253–271.

National Urban League (1964). *Double Jeopardy: The Older Negro in America Today*. New York: NUL.

Niino, N., Imaizumi, T. and Kawakai, N. (1991). A Japanese translation of the Geriatric Depression Scale. *Clinical Gerontologist*, **10**, 85–86.

Nitrini, R., Caramelli, P., Herrera, E. *et al.* (2004). Incidence of dementia in a community-dwelling Brazilian population. *Alzheimer's Disease and Associated Disorders*, **18**, 241–246.

Nitrini, R., Caramelli, P., and Herrera, E. (2005). Mortality from dementia in a community-dwelling Brazilian population. *International Journal of Geriatric Psychiatry*, **20**, 247–253.

Norman, A. (1985). *Triple Jeopardy: Growing Old in a Second Homeland*. London: Centre for Policy on Ageing.

Oeppen, J. and Vaupel, J. W. (2002). Broken limits to life expectancy. *Science*, **296**, 1029–1031.

Paddick, S. M., Kisoli, A., Longdon, A. *et al.* (2015). The prevalence and burden of behavioural and psychological symptoms of dementia in rural Tanzania. *International Journal of Geriatric Psychiatry*, **30**, 815–823.

Palmore, E. and Manton, K. (1973). Ageism compared to racism and sexism. *Journal of Gerontology*, **28**, 363–369.

Pang, K. Y. C. (1998). Symptoms of depression in elderly Korean immigrants: narration and healing process. *Culture, Medicine and Psychiatry*, **22**, 93–122.

Park, J. H. and Kwon, Y. C. (1990). Modification of the Mini-Mental State Examination for use in the elderly in a non-Western society. Part 1: Development of the Korean version of Mini-Mental State Examination. *International Journal of Geriatric Psychiatry*, **5**, 381–387.

Park, J. H., Park, Y. N. and Ko, H. J. (1991). Modification of the Mini Mental State Examination for use with the elderly in a non-Western society. Part II: Cut-off points and their diagnostic validities. *International Journal of Geriatric Psychiatry*, **6**, 875–882.

Park, J. H., Ko, H. J., Park, Y. N. and Jung, C. (1994). Dementia among the elderly in a rural Korean community. *British Journal of Psychiatry*, **164**, 796–801.

Perkins, P., Annegers, J. F., Doody, R. S. *et al.* (1997). Incidence and prevalence of dementia in older adults in low and middle income countries: findings from 10/66 study. *Psychological Medicine*, **41**, 2047–2056.

Perkins, A. S., Hui, S. L., Ogunniyi, A. *et al.* (2002). Risk of mortality for dementia in a developing country: the Yoruba in Nigeria. *International Journal of Geriatric Psychiatry*, **17**, 566–573.

Phanthumchinda, K., Jitapunkul, S., Sitthi-Amorn, C. *et al.* (1991). Prevalence of dementia in an urban slum population in Thailand: validity of screening methods. *International Journal of Geriatric Psychiatry*, 6, 639–646.

Pinto, C. and Seethalaksmi, R. (2006). Behavioural and psychological symptoms of dementia in an Indian population: comparison between Alzheimer's disease and vascular dementia. *International Psychogeriatrics*, 18, 87–93.

Pollit, P. (1996). Dementia in old age: an anthropological perspective. *Psychological Medicine*, 26, 1061–1074.

Prina, A. M., Ferri, C. P., Guerra, M., Bryane, C., Prince, M. (2011). Prevalence of anxiety and its correlates among older adults in Latin America, India and China: cross-cultural study. *British Journal of Psychiatry*, 199(6), 485–491.

Prince, M., Acosta, D., Chiu, H. et al. (2003). Dementia diagnosis in developing countries: a cross-cultural validation study. *The Lancet*, 361, 909–917.

Prince, M., Acosta, D., Chiu, H. et al. (2004). Effects of education and culture on the validity of the Geriatric Mental State and its AGECAT algorithm. *British Journal of Psychiatry*, 185, 429–436

Prince, M., Acosta, D., Ferri, C. P. et al. (2012). Dementia incidence and mortality in middle income countries, and associations with indicators of cognitive reserve: a 10/66 Dementia Research Group population-based cohort study. *The Lancet*, 380(9836), 50–28.

Pringle, M. and Rothera, I. (1996). Practicality of recording patient ethnicity in general practice: descriptive intervention study and attitude survey. *British Medical Journal*, 312, 1080–1082.

Qureshi, K. N. and Hodkinson, H. M. (1974). Evaluation of a ten-question mental test in institutionalised elderly. *Age and Ageing*, 3, 152–157.

Radloff, L. S. and Teri, l. (1986). Use of the Centre for Epidemiological Studies depression scale for older adults. *Clinical Gerontologist*, 5, 119–137.

Radwan, D. N., Dalia, H. A., Elmissiry, A. A., Elbanouby, M. M. (2014). Cognitive and functional impairment in Egyptian patients with late-onset schizophrenia versus elderly healthy controls. *Middle East Current Psychiatry*, 21, 28–37.

Rait, G. and Burns, A. (1997). Appreciating background and culture: the South Asian elderly and mental health. *International Journal of Geriatric Psychiatry*, 12, 973–977.

Rait, G., Burns, A. and Chew, C. (1996). Age, ethnicity and mental illness: a triple whammy. *British Medical Journal*, 313, 1347.

Rait, G., Morley, M., Lambat, I., Burns, A. (1997). Modification of brief assessments for use with elderly people from the South Asian sub-continent. *Ageing and Mental Health*, 1, 356–363.

Rait, G., Burns, A., Baldwin, R. et al. (1999). Screening for depression in African-Caribbean elders. *Family Practice*, 16, 591–595.

Rait, G., Burns, A., Baldwin, R. et al. (2000a). Validating screening instruments for cognitive impairment in older South Asians in the United Kingdom. *International Journal of Geriatric Psychiatry*, 15, 54–62.

Rait, G., Morley, M., Burns, A. et al. (2000b). Screening for cognitive impairment in older African-Caribbeans. *Psychological Medicine*, 30, 957–963.

Rajkumar, S. and Kumar, S. (1996). Prevalence of dementia in the community: a rural–urban comparison from Madras, India. *Australian Journal on Ageing*, 15, 9–13.

Rajkumar, S., Kumar, S. and Thara, R. (1997). Prevalence of dementia in a rural setting: a report from India. *International Journal of Geriatric Psychiatry*, 12, 702–707.

Ramirez, M., Terisi, J. A., Holmes, D., Gurland, B., Lantigua, R. (2006). Differential item functioning (DIF) and the Mini-Mental State Examination (MMSE). Overview, sample and issues of translation. *Medical Care*, 44, S95–S106.

Redelinghuys, J. and Shah, A. K. (1997). The characteristics of ethnic elders from the Indian subcontinent using a geriatic psychiatry service in west London. *Ageing and Mental Health*, 1, 243–247.

Reeves, S. J., Sauer, J., Stewart, R., Granger, A. and Howard, R. (2001). Increased first contact rates for very late onset schizophrenia-like psychosis in African and Caribbean born elders. *British Journal of Psychiatry*, 179, 172–174.

Richards, M. (1997). Cross-cultural studies of dementia. In *Advances in Community Care. Chromosomes to Community Care*, ed. C. Holmes and R. Howard. Petersfield: Wrightson Biomedical.

Richards, M. and Brayne, C. (1996). Cross-cultural research into cognitive impairment and dementia: some practical experiences. *International Journal of Geriatric Psychiatry*, 11, 383–387.

Richards, M., Brayne, C., Dening, T. et al. (2000). Cognitive function in UK community dwelling African Caribbean and white elders: a pilot study. *International Journal of Geriatric Psychiatry*, 15, 621–630.

Rocca, W. A., Bonaiuto, S., Lippi, A. et al. (1990). Prevalence of clinically diagnosed Alzheimer's disease and other dementing disorders. A door-to-door survey in Appigano, Macerata Province, Italy. *Neurology*, 40, 626–631.

Rodriguez-Agudelo, Y., Solis-Vivanco, R., Acosta-Castillo, I., Garcia-Ramirez, N., Rojas-de-la-Torres, G. and Sosa, A. L. (2011). Neuropsychiatric symptoms in older adults with and without dementia in urban and rural regions. Results of the 10/66 Dementia Research Group in Mexico. *Revista de Investigacion Clinica*, 63, 382–390.

Rosen, W. G., Mohs, R. C. and Davis, K. L. (1984). A new rating scale for Alzheimer's disease. *American Journal of Psychiatry*, 141, 1356–1364.

Roth, M., Tym, E., Mountjoy, C. Q. et al. (1986). CAMDEX: a standardised instrument for diagnosis of mental disorder in the elderly with special reference to the early detection of dementia. *British Journal of Psychiatry*, **149**, 698–709.

Salmon, D. P., Reikkinen, P. J., Katzmman R. *et al.* (1989). Cross-cultural studies of dementia: a comparison of the Mini-Mental State Examination performance in Finland and China. *Archives of Neurology*, **46**, 769–772.

Schreiner, A. S., Morimoto, T. and Asano, H. (2001). Depressive symptoms among post-stroke patients in Japan: frequency distribution and factor structure. *International Journal of Geriatric Psychiatry*, **16**, 941–949.

Seiden, R. H. (1981). Mellowing with age: factors affecting the non-white suicide rate. *International Journal of Ageing and Human Development*, **13**, 265–284.

Senior, P. A. and Bhopal, R. (1994). Ethnicity as a variable in epidemiological research. *British Medical Journal*, **309**, 327–330.

Serby, M., Chou, J. C. and Franssen, E. H. (1987). Dementia in an American Chinese nursing home population. *American Journal of Psychiatry*, **144**, 811–812.

Shah, A. K. (1992a). *The Prevalence and Burden of Psychiatric Disorders. A Report to the Department of Health*. London: Institute of Psychiatry.

Shah, A. K. (1997a). Interviewing mentally ill ethnic minority elders with interpreters. *Australian Journal on Ageing*, **16**, 220–221.

Shah, A. K. (1997b). Straight talk. Overcoming language barriers in diagnosis. *Geriatric Medicine*, **27**, 45–46.

Shah, A. K. (1998). The psychiatric needs of ethnic minority elders in the UK. *Age and Ageing*, **27**, 267–269.

Shah, A. K. (1999). Difficulties experienced by a Gujarati psychiatrist in interviewing elderly Gujaratis in Gujarati. *International Journal of Geriatric Psychiatry*, **14**, 1072–1074.

Shah, A. K. (2007a). Demographic changes among ethnic minority elders in England and Wales. Implications for development and delivery of old age psychiatry services. *International Journal of Migration, Health and Social Care*, **3**, 22–32.

Shah, A. K. (2007b). The relationship between suicide rate and age: an analysis of multinational data from the World Health Organization. *International Psychogeriatrics*, **19**(6), 1141–1152.

Shah, A. K. (2007c). The importance of socio-economic status of countries for mental disorders in old age: a development of an epidemiological transition model. *International Psychogeriatrics*, **19**, 785–787.

Shah, A. K. (2009). The relationship between socio-economic status and mental health funding, service provision and national policy: a cross-national study. *International Psychiatry*, **6**, 44–46.

Shah, A. K and Bhat, R. (2008a). The relationship between elderly suicide rates and mental health funding, service provision and national policy: a cross-national study. *International Psychogeriatrics*, **20**, 605–615.

Shah, A. K and Bhat, R. (2008b). Are elderly suicide rates improved by increased provision of mental health service resources? *International Psychogeriatrics*, **20**, 1230–1237.

Shah, A. K. and Dighe-Deo, D. (1998). Elderly Gujaratis and psychogeriatrics in a London psychogeriatric service. *Bulletin of the International Psychogeriatric Association*, **14**, 12–13.

Shah, A. K. and Lindesay, J. (2000). Cross-cultural issues in the assessment of cognitive impairment. In *Dementia*, ed. J. O'Brien, D. Ames and A. Burns. London: Arnold, pp. 217–232.

Shah, A. K. and Mukherjee, S. (2000). Cross-cultural issues in the measurement of behavioural and psychological signs and symptoms of dementia (BPSD). *Ageing and Mental Health*, **4**, 244–252.

Shah, A. K., Lindesay, J. and Jagger, C. (1998). Is the diagnosis of dementia stable over time among elderly immigrant Gujaratis in the United Kingdom (Leicester)? *International Journal of Geriatric Psychiatry*, **13**, 440–444.

Shah, A. K., Ellanchenny, N., Suh, G. H. (2004). A comparative study of behavioural and psychological signs and symptoms of dementia in patients with dementia referred to psychogeriatric services in Korea and the United Kingdom. *International Psychogeriatrics*, **16**, 219–236.

Shah, A. K., Oommen, G. and Wuntakal, B. (2005a). Cultural aspects of dementia. *Psychiatry*, **4**, 103–106.

Shah, A. K., Lindesay, J. and Nnatu, I. (2005b). Cross-cultural issues in the assessment of cognitive impairment. In *Dementia*, ed. A. Burns, J. O'Brien, and D. Ames. London: Arnold, pp. 147–164.

Shah, A. K., Dalvi, M. and Thompson, T. (2005c). Behavioural and psychological signs and symptoms of dementia across cultures: current status and the future. *International Journal of Geriatric Psychiatry*, **20**, 1187–1195.

Shah, A. K., Ellanchenny, N., Suh, G. H. (2005d). A comparative study of behavioural and psychological symptoms of dementia in patients with Alzheimer's disease and vascular dementia referred to psychogeriatric services in Korea and the United Kingdom. *International Psychogeriatrics*, **17**, 207–219.

Shah, A. K., Bhat, R., MacKenzie, S. and Koen, C. (2008). A cross-national study of the relationship between elderly suicide rates and life expectancy and markers of socio-economic status and healthcare status. *International Psychogeriatrics*, **20**, 347–360.

Shah, C. (1988). *Jainism in North India*. Delhi: Sagar Publishing House.

Shaji, S., Promodu, K., Abraham, T., Jacob, R. K. and Verghese, A. (1996). An epidemiological study of dementia in a rural community in Kerala, India. *British Journal of Psychiatry*, **168**, 747–80.

Shaji, S., Bose, S. and Verghese, A. (2005). Prevalence of dementia in an urban population in Kerala, India. *British Journal of Psychiatry*, **186**, 136–140.

Shaji, K. S., George, R. K., Prince, M., Jacob, K. S. (2009). Behavioural symptoms and caregiver burden in dementia. *Indian Journal of Psychiatry*, **51**, 45–49.

Sheikh, J. A. and Yesavage, J. (1986). Geriatric Depression Scale (GDS). Recent findings and development of a shorter version. *Clinical Gerontologist*, **5**, 165–173.

Shibayama, H., Kashara, Y., Kobyashi, H. *et al.* (1986). Prevalence of dementias in a Japanese elderly population. *Acta Psychiatrica Scandinavica*, **74**, 144–151.

Silveira, E. and Ebrahim, S. (1995). Mental health and health status of elderly Bengalis and Somalis in London. *Age and Ageing*, **24**, 474–480.

Silverman, J. M., Li, G., Schear, S. *et al.* (1992). A cross-cultural family history study of primary progressive dementia in relatives of non-demented elderly Chinese, Italians, Jews and Puerto Ricans. *Acta Psychiatrica Scandinavica*, **85**, 211–217.

Sjahrir, H., Ritarwan, K., Tarigan, S., Rambe, A. S., Lubis, I. D. and Bhakti, I. (2001). The Mini-Mental State Examination in healthy individuals in Medan, Indonesia by age and educational level. *Neurology Journal of Southeast Asia*, **6**, 19–22.

Skoog, I. (2012). Vascular factors and dementia in the oldest old. Abstract presented at the Brain Ageing and Dementia in Developing Countries Symposium. Nairobi, Kenya, December.

Sokoya, O. O. and Baiyewu, O. (2003). Geriatric depression in Nigerian primary care attenders. *International Journal of Geriatric Psychiatry*, **18**, 506–510.

Solomon, A. (1992). Clinical diagnosis among diverse populations: a multicultural perspective. *Family in Society: The Journal of Contemporary Human Services*, June, 371–377.

Spijker, J., van der Wurff, F. B., Poort, E. C., Smits, C. H. M., Verhoeff, A. P., Beekman, A. T. F. (2004). Depression in first generation labour migrants in Western Europe: the utility of the Centre for Epidemiologic Studies Depression Scale (CES-D). *International Journal of Geriatric Psychiatry*, **6**, 538–544.

Steis, M. R. and Schrauf, R. W. (2009). A review of translations and adaptations of the Mini-Mental State Examination in languages other than English and Spanish. *Research in Gerontological Nursing*, **2**, 214–224.

Stewart, R., Richards, M., Brayne, C. *et al.* (2001). Cognitive function in UK community-dwelling African Caribbean elders: normative data for a test battery. *International Journal of Geriatric Psychiatry*, **16**, 518–527.

Stewart, R., Johnson, J., Richards, M., Brayne, C., Mann, A. and Medical Research Council Cognitive Function and Ageing Study (2002). The distribution of Mini-Mental State Examination scores in an older UK African Caribbean population compared to MRC CFA study norms. *International Journal of Geriatric Psychiatry*, **17**, 745–751.

Stewart, R., Kim, J., Shin, I. *et al.* (2003). Education and the association between vascular risk factors and cognitive function: a cross-sectional study in older Koreans with cognitive impairment. *International Psychogeriatrics*, **15**, 27–36.

Still, C. N., Jackson, K. L., Brandes, D. A. *et al.* (1990). Distribution of major dementias by race and sex in South Carolina. *Journal of South Carolina Medical Association*, **86**, 453–456.

Storey, J. E., Rowland, J. T. J., Conforti, D. A. and Dickson, H. G. (2004). The Rowlands Universal Dementia Assessment Scale (RUDAS): a multicultural cognitive assessment scale. *International Psychogeriatrics*, **16**, 13–31.

Subedi, S., Tausing, M., Subedi, J., Broughton, C. L., Williams-Blangero, S. (2004). Mental illness and disability among elders in developing countries. *Journal of Ageing and Health*, **16**, 71–87.

Suh, G. H. and Shah, A. (2001). A review of the epidemiological transition in dementia – cross-national comparisons of the indices related to Alzheimer's disease and vascular dementia. *Acta Psychiatrica Scandinavica*, **104**, 4–11.

Tang, L. L., Seng, K. H. (2011). First presentation psychosis among the elderly in Singapore. *Singapore Medical Journal*, **53**, 463–467.

Teresi, J. A., Golden, R. R., Cross, P. *et al.* (1995). Item bias in cognitive screening measures: comparisons of elderly white, Afro-American, Hispanic and high and low education subgroups. *Journal of Clinical Epidemiology*, **4**, 473–483.

Tsai, Y., Chung, J. W. Y., Wong, T. S. K. and Huang, C. (2005). Comparison of the prevalence and risk factors for depressive symptoms among elderly nursing home residents in Taiwan and Hong Kong. *International Journal of Geriatric Psychiatry*, **20**, 315–321.

Tsang, H., Chong, M. and Cheng, T. A. (2002). Development of the Chinese version of the Geriatric Mental State Schedule. *International Psychogeriatrics*, **14**, 219–226.

Uwakwe, R. (2000a). The pattern of psychiatric disorders among the aged in a selected community in Nigeria. *International Journal of Geriatric Psychiatry*, **15**, 355–362.

Uwakwe, R. (2000b). Psychiatric morbidity in elderly patients admitted to non-psychiatric wards in a general/teaching hospital in Nigeria. *International Journal of Geriatric Psychiatry*, **15**, 346–354.

Van Der Wurff, F. B., Beekman, A. T., Dijkshoorn, H. *et al.* (2004). Prevalence and risk factors for depression in elderly Turkish and Moroccan migrants in the Netherlands. *Journal of Affective Disorders*, **83**, 33–41.

Vas, C. J., Pinto, C., Panikker, D. et al. (2001). Prevalence of dementia in an urban Indian population. *International Psychogeriatrics*, **13**, 439–450.

Weissman, M. M., Leaf, P. L., Tischler, G. L. et al. (1988). Affective disorders in five United States communities. *Psychological Medicine*, **18**, 141–153.

Williams, M. M., Xiong, C., Morris, J. C. and Galvin, J. E. (2006). Survival and mortality differences between dementia with Lewy bodies vs Alzheimer's disease. *Neurology*, **67**, 1935–1941.

Wong, M. T. P., Ho, T. P., Ho, M. Y., Yu, C. S., Wong, Y. H. and Lee, S. Y. (2002). Development and inter-rater reliability of a standardised verbal instruction manual of the Chinese Geriatric Depression Scale short form. *International Journal of Geriatric Psychiatry*, **17**, 459–463.

Woo, J., Ho, S. S., Lau, J. et al. (1994). The prevalence of depressive symptoms and predisposing factors in an elderly Chinese population. *Acta Psychiatrica Scandinavica*, **89**, 8–13.

Woo, J. I., Lee, J. H., Yoo, K. et al. (1998). Prevalence estimation of dementia in a rural area of Korea. *Journal of the American Geriatric Society*, **46**, 983–987.

World Health Organization (1992). *The ICD-10 Classification of Mental and Behavioural Disorders. Clinical Descriptions and Diagnostic Guidelines*. Geneva: World Health Organization

Xie, J., Brayne, C. and Matthews, F. (2008). Survival times in people with dementia: analysis from population based cohort study with 14 year follow-up. *British Medical Journal*, **336**, 258

Xu, G., Meyer, J. S., Huang, Y. et al. (2003). Adapting Mini-Mental-State Examination for dementia screening among illiterate or minimally educated elderly Chinese. *International Journal of Geriatric Psychiatry*, **18**, 609–616.

Yamada, M., Sasaki, H., Mimori, Y. et al. (1999). Prevalence and risks of dementia in the Japanese population: RERF's adult health study of Hiroshima subjects. *Journal of the American Geriatric Society*, **47**, 189–195.

Yesavage, J. A., Brink, T. L., Rose, T. L. et al. (1983). Development and validation of a geriatric depression scale: a preliminary report. *Journal of Psychiatric Research*, **17**, 37–49.

Youn, J. C., Lee, D. Y., Kim, K. W. et al. (2002). Development of the Korean version of Alzheimer's Disease Assessment Scale (ADAS-K). *International Journal of Geriatric Psychiatry*, **17**, 797–803.

Yu, E. S. H., Liu, W. T., Levy, P. et al. (1989). Cognitive impairment among elderly adults in Shanghai, China. *Journal of Gerontology*, **44**, S97–106.

Zarate-Escudero, S. and Shah, A. K. (2013). The needs of ethnic minority individuals with dementia. *Neurodegenerative Disease Management*, **3**, 291–294.

Zhang, B., Fokkema, M., Cuijpers, P., Li, J., Smits, N., Beekman, A. (2011). Measurement invariance of the centre for epidemiological studies depression scale (CES-D) among Chinese and Dutch elderly. *BMC Medical Research Methodology*, **11**, 74, doi: 10.1186/1471-2288-11-74.

Zhang, J. (1998). Suicide in the world: toward a population increase theory of suicide. *Death Studies*, **22**, 525–539.

Zhang, M., Katzman, R., Salmon, D. et al. (1990). The prevalence of dementia and Alzheimer's disease in Shanghai, China: Impact of age, gender, and education. *Annals of Neurology*, **27**, 428–437.

Zung, W. W. K. (1965). A self-rating depression scale. *Archives of General Psychiatry*, **12**, 63–70.

Chapter

29

Traumascape

An Ecological–Cultural–Historical Model for Extreme Stress

Joop T. V. M. de Jong and Devon Hinton

Editors' Introduction

Refugees, asylum seekers and immigrants may well experience various traumas during their move to new countries. In addition, they may have suffered different types of loss and these factors may contribute to psychiatric illnesses. There is no doubt that people will deal with these stresses and stressors in different ways and not all go on to develop illnesses. There may be factors related to social support, individual resilience, and welcome in the new countries. De Jong and Hinton in this chapter explain the ecological utility of the concept of post-traumatic stress disorder (PTSD) as well as its validity from a cross-cultural and historical perspective. They then go on to address the issue of medicalization and politicization of this diagnosis. There is no doubt that disasters – be they man-made or natural – contribute to the likelihood of developing stresses, but different cultures posit different loci of control which in turn will determine how these acts are seen, experienced and explained. De Jong and Hinton utilize a syndemic model indicating that exposure to trauma may well contribute to depression, substance abuse, domestic inter-personal violence, and child neglect. Furthermore, they describe the concept of traumascape as enabling the clinician and researcher alike to explore and describe how traumatic distress interacts with political, historical, religious and cultural factors that inevitably will be influenced by cultural and individual means of coping. In situations of man-made or natural disasters, if masses of people are affected, the role of the media, rescuers, emergency services, political will and action at local, regional, national or international levels are important as these agencies determine the focus, the size and the nature of assistance for a group of survivors. Other factors identified by de Jong and Hinton include (geo)political, voter-dependent or populistic considerations, which determine whether international attention and

funding will be directed at terrorism, human rights or child rights, governance, gender-based or domestic violence, former combatants, or child soldiers. Mental health professionals have to bear in mind that these geopolitical and other forces often overrule their epidemiological, clinical, human rights, evidence based or cost-effectiveness considerations. De Jong and Hinton argue that in this regard there is no difference between the two World Wars and more recent disasters, genocides or refugee flows.

Introduction

Over the past decades psychiatry and psychology have seen intense debates about trauma and post-traumatic stress disorder (PTSD) in different cultural contexts. This chapter will first summarize these debates, which in our opinion focus on three major topics: (1) ecological utility, (2) validity from a cross-cultural and historical perspective, and (3) medicalization and politicization. We then introduce three concepts that help to reflect on the ongoing PTSD and culture debate. We think that these three concepts simultaneously may further the disciplines of cultural psychiatry and psychology. The three concepts are syndemics, dynamic networks and traumascape, which we will first briefly explain.

Syndemics refers to two or more enmeshed and mutually enhancing health problems that, working together, contribute to an excess disease burden in a specific population (Singer, 1994, 2007). The focus in a syndemic approach is on how social and economic inequity (e.g. poverty, poor access to healthcare, gender inequity, stigma) gives rise to clusters of interacting epidemics in vulnerable populations and how such clustering reinforces the social and environmental problems of such populations. A syndemic approach counters the biomedical focus on diseases as entities that can be studied out of context. Some examples of syndemics involving mental health problems are the tripartite clustering of substance abuse, violence, and AIDS (SAVA) among various disadvantaged populations (Singer, 1996; Singer *et al.*, 2006), the clustering of depression and diabetes among Mexican immigrant women in Chicago (Mendenhall, 2012), or the malnutrition and depression syndemic among welfare recipients in the USA (Heflin, Siefert and Williams, 2005). Exposure of populations to trauma, both in man-made or natural disaster conditions often plays a pivotal role in syndemics of depression, substance abuse, domestic violence and child neglect. We refer to these syndemics as *traumasyndemics*.

The second concept, dynamic networks, regards psychopathology as interactions between symptoms (Kendler *et al.*, 2011; Borsboom *et al.*, 2011; 2013; Wigman *et al.*, 2015). In the network approach, our habitual focus *on* symptoms in DSM or ICD shifts to the dynamics *between* symptoms. This enables us to abandon concepts of Western or non-Western disorders and to disentangle what is universal and what is particular or local in studying psychopathology. Dynamic networks may provide detailed illustrations of how human beings in different cultural contexts react to trauma. In the near future, dynamic networks will help us to empirically test and study looping processes within and across cultures. These dynamic networks include catastrophic cognitions. Hinton and Good (2009; 2016a, b) describe how ethnopsychologies and ethnophysiologies specific to given cultures and local cultural illness syndromes may lead to heightened attention to particular symptoms (hypersemiotized symptoms) and lead to 'catastrophic cognitions', resulting in bio-attentional looping processes that produce a trauma-based illness reality. For example, fear of having certain complaints, symptoms or a particular disorder or syndrome will increase psychological and somatic distress, which in turn will worsen the psychological and somatic distress, bringing about even more fear of having the symptoms or a disorder (such as a cultural syndrome). Dynamic networks is an innovative approach to empirically test these bio-attentional looping processes.

The third concept, the *traumascape*, helps us to understand how local socio-cultural contexts influence local peoples' lives under duress, paying particular attention to the interaction of local and global frames of understanding, with an eye to social and economic forces and the pragmatics of care. Traumascape is a concept inspired by the social theorist Appadurai

(1996) and can be defined as 'the systemic dynamics of local and international representations and actions around extreme stress' (de Jong, 2007). Appadurai used the suffix 'scape' – for example, in technoscape, mediascape, ethnoscape – as a framework for examining the 'new global cultural economy as a complex, overlapping, disjunctive order that cannot any longer be understood in terms of existing centre–periphery models'.[1] The concept of a traumascape enables us to describe how traumatic distress interacts with historical, political, religious and cultural factors. On a local level it helps us to grapple with the complexity of resilience and resources that individuals may access to make sense of and recover from trauma, including treatment, religious and ritual traditions. An individual or community in low-income or middle-income countries (LMIC) has access to different resources in terms of healing, mental health professionals, or evidence based and culturally appropriate treatments than a person in high-income countries (HIC). On an international and global level individuals and those offering support in disaster situations or complex humanitarian emergencies increasingly interact with macro socio-ecological forces that have far-reaching consequences for those who are exposed to extreme stress.

In this chapter we will first review the culture and PTSD debate from these three perspectives. The final part of the chapter amplifies on the traumascape model as a general analytic framework and emphasizes a life course view of trauma, aiming to show culture's impact in the context of extreme trauma on trauma symptomatology and its relation with wider social, political, historical and religious factors. (Also see Chapter 42.)

The Culture and PTSD Debate

Despite many variations of the ongoing and at times vehement discussions and polemics, in our opinion the culture and PTSD debate can be subsumed under three perspectives. We distinguish issues related to (1) ecological utility, (2) validity from a cross-cultural and historical perspective, and (3) medicalization and politicization.

---

[1] The historian Tumarkin (2005) uses the word 'traumascape' for a landscape marked by the need of people to build memorials at sites where massive deaths happened. She regards traumascapes not simply as locations of tragedies and trauma, but also as mediators between the living and the dead. Our concept of traumascape has a wider bearing.

Ecological Utility

In research we use the concept of ecological validity as 'the extent to which the conclusions of a study can be generalized to the settings in which the phenomenon naturally occurs' (Bernal *et al.*, 1995). Here we consider ecological utility as the extent to which the concept of PTSD can be generalized to settings in which traumatic distress occurs in the sense of capturing salient aspects of trauma-related experiencing.[2]

For example, certain PTSD symptoms or other trauma-caused symptoms may be locally interpreted in terms of certain ethnopsychologies and ethnophysiologies and those symptoms may be attributed to certain cultural syndromes. Not capturing the full spectrum of experiencing has been called 'category truncation' (Hinton and Good, 2016a, b), resulting in a lack of 'experiential validity', the neglect of experience-near categories.[3] These are aspects that determine ecological validity and ecological utility, which we discuss more fully below.

Context and culture influence how people delineate between 'normal' and 'abnormal' (Helman, 2007). Definitions of mental disorders are embedded in how people view the world and conceptualize personhood (Kleinman and Good, 1985). This leads to important variations in how people express that they are unhappy and distressed, for example by using 'cultural idioms of distress' (common modes of expressing distress within a culture or community); or by using 'cultural syndromes' (a coherent set of symptoms and aetiology), also defined as 'a widely recognized prototypical ailment that encompasses a fuzzy set of associations coalescing around one or more core cultural symbols' (Nichter, 2010). The DSM-5 refers to idioms of distress and cultural syndromes as 'cultural concepts of distress', defined as the 'ways that cultural groups experience, understand, and communicate suffering, behavioural problems, or troubling thoughts and emotions' (APA, 2013). Idioms of distress (IODs) and cultural syndromes may occur concurrently with other expressions of psychopathology, they may overlap with internationally known ICD or DSM diagnostic constructs, or they may be more or less unique locally

salient symptom clusters. In other words, an idiom can be indicative of a psychopathological state, but certainly should not be considered as always indicative. This may lead to diagnostic errors. Either a clinician can miss a diagnosis such as PTSD because associated features of idioms and cultural syndromes are most prominent, or the associated features can be overlooked because of the presence of the diagnosis of, for example, PTSD.

We illustrate cultural concepts of distress with a few examples of the two largest refugee groups currently in the world, Syrians (4.9 million) and Afghani (2.7 million) (UNHCR, 2016). Hassan *et al.* (2015) describe that Syrian Arabic has a range of idioms to indicate general distress ('heaviness in the heart, cramps in the guts' and other complaints); one idiom is *habit qalbi*, 'failing or crumbling of the heart' corresponding to the somatic reaction of sudden fear; *atlan ham*, referring to anticipated anxiety and worry. The syndrome *halat ikti'ab* resembles depression with concepts such as brooding, darkening of mood, aches and a gloomy outlook, and may be accompanied by a variety of medically unexplained somatic symptoms and fatigue, as well as signs of social isolation and not talking much. Lack of resources and financial hardship is often referred to as *al ayn bassira wal yadd kassira*, 'the eye sees but the hand is short or cannot reach'. Expressions often used by Syrians to express helplessness are: *mafi natija*, 'there is no use'; *hasis hali mashlol*, 'I feel like I'm paralysed'. Kurdish similarly has a wide range of expressions and idioms.

Among Afghans in Kabul various idioms were identified such as *jigar khun* 'bloody liver', which occurs in the wake of a strongly painful event in a person's life, or after chronic stress; *asabi* 'being nervous'; and *fishar*, an internal state of emotional pressure and/or agitation, or conversely, of very low energy and motivation (Miller *et al.*, 2006; Omidian and Miller, 2006). Ventevogel (2016: 258) described several idioms among Afghans in Nangarhar: *waswasi*, constant worry, thinking a lot, social isolation and repetitive actions; *wahmi*, unreasonable fear, easily being frightened and frightening dreams; *peyran*, being possessed by spirits with pseudo seizures and a variety of somatic complaints. Here is a description of an Afghan female refugee expressing the IOD *deltangi*:

> The space that occupies my heart becomes smaller (*delam tang meshad* or *deltangi*), and I feel that someone stops my breath. I am restless and I walk back

---

[2] One might also use the concept of 'external validity', see later.

[3] Put another way, here we are examining the content validity of the PTSD construct in respect to trauma experiencing, that is, the extent to which the concept of PTSD captures local ways of experiencing trauma-related distress in a particular ecological context (Hinton and Good, 2016b).

and forth. It seems that my heart vibrates and then I have a shortness of breath and I start crying, and when it is over I feel quiet (*oram*). If I do not cry this will continue and I will feel stuffy. This will lead to the restlessness, and my speech falters.

(Delawar, 2016)

Ecological utility not only plays a role when idioms of distress or cultural syndromes are possible diagnostic confounders. A meta-analysis by Steel *et al.* (2009) estimated that 13–25 per cent of refugees resettled in high-income countries (HIC) suffer from PTSD. But one may question the utility of a PTSD-diagnosis if it is highly comorbid: another meta-analysis, also among adult refugees in HIC, showed that 71 per cent of those diagnosed with depression also had PTSD, and that 44 per cent of those diagnosed with PTSD also had depression (Fazel *et al.* 2005). In addition, the response to trauma includes not just PTSD and depression, but also somatic symptoms, bereavement, anxiety, panic attacks, acting out and substance abuse. Several authors have been raising questions about whether these are comorbid disorders or whether they should be incorporated into a broader post-traumatic stress *syndrome* instead of a post-traumatic stress *disorder*. They feel that the term 'post-traumatic stress syndrome' better conveys the sense of the lived, contextualized experience of trauma than does the narrower term PTSD; it better describes the lived experience of illness than does the disease concept PTSD (Eisenberg 1977; Hinton and Good, 2016a).

Another aspect of ecological utility is that in many LIC and MIC, PTSD may occur after traumatic distress, but other expressions of psychopathology may be much more prevalent, socially manifest or prominent, as is also the case with idioms and cultural syndromes. This happens predominantly around phenomena of dissociation, that is, a lack of integration of personal memory or identity (Spiegel *et al.*, 2011). Mental health professionals tend to regard dissociative disorders as real, spontaneous alterations in brain states that reflect basic neurobiological phenomena, or alternatively as fragments of one's self, 'unconscious' conflicts, subpersonalities or 'alters'. Anthropologists prefer to interpret dissociation as imaginary, socially constructed role performances dictated by interpersonal expectations, power dynamics and cultural script, or as discursive processes of attributing action and experience to agencies other than the self. Anthropologists often refer to dissociation as an IOD (Seligman and Kirmayer, 2008; de Jong and Reis, 2013). Around the globe the use of

trance and dissociation expressing distress and traumatic events is omnipresent. Hundreds of millions of people in the Americas and parts of Africa use dissociation on a regular basis in Pentecostal or apostolic churches, expressing a range of hassles going from worries, to 'thinking too much', to traumatic stress. In the largest centre of religious and ritual healing in India, Balaji, thousands of visitors per year go into trance during their healing process. Moreover, there are hundreds of such ritual healing temples and *durghas* around India (Satija *et al.*, 1981; Kakar, 1983; Dwyer, 2003; Basu, 2009; Pakaslahti, 2009; Sax and Weinhold, 2010; Thirthalli *et al.*, 2016). Around the globe healers use dissociation on a daily base during their diagnostic divination of patients in distress.

Dissociation has also been described in various post-conflict settings in, for example, Mozambique, Uganda, Rwanda, Burundi, Nepal and Sri Lanka, at times in combination with fugue states or psychogenic seizures (Geffray, 1990; Allen 1991; Wilson, 1992; Perera, 2001; van Ommeren *et al.*, 2001; Honwana, 2003; van Duijl *et al.*, 2005; Baines, 2007; Gobodo-Madikizela and van der Merwe, 2009; Hagengimana and Hinton, 2009; Tol *et al.*, 2009; Igreja *et al.*, 2010; Reis, 2016; Ventevogel, 2016). De Jong and Reis (2013) coined the term 'collective trauma processing' to describe mass possession trance in Guinea Bissau as an indigenous way to process the horrendous traumatic stress in an African post-war context where mental health professionals were virtually absent. Epidemic expressions of anxiety also take place in LMIC and HIC. 'Mass hysteria', mass psychogenic illness or medically unexplained illness tends to occur in connection with distress caused by exams or other stressors in schools, environmental pollution, work conditions, exposure to toxins or exposure to nuclear fallout; for example, syndromes among war veterans, the *cola-affaire* in Belgium, or satanic sects. Another example is the *yao yan* or 'salt hysteria' when large numbers of Chinese wanted to buy salt that was thought to protect them against the fallout after the Fukushima disaster in Japan. One may regard these often relatively brief epidemics as another form of processing traumatic stress or more common distress (Bartholomew and Sirois, 2000; de Jong and Colijn, 2010: 410).

In short, PTSD lacks ecological utility in certain respects because trauma results in multiple cultural syndromes and idioms of distress. Trauma experiencing is depicted by other expressions of distress that are culturally more relevant, more salient and prominent, and that often play a dominant role in help-seeking pathways. Just determining PTSD presence is to commit an error of category truncation. It is obvious that the co-occurrence of PTSD with other expression of distress and of psychopathology is closely related to the second topic of the PTSD and culture debate, that is, the validity of PTSD.

Construct Validity from a Cross-Cultural and Historical Perspective

Cross-Cultural Evidence

A core problem in psychiatry is the lack of validity of currently used ICD and DSM diagnoses, which are not based on empirical evidence but on clinical consensus, leading to arbitrary boundaries and much overlap between diagnoses (Kendell, 1989). In cross-cultural work we often assume that a diagnostic category that is valid in one culture is also valid in another culture without first (re)testing its construct validity, resulting in what Kleinman (1980) called a 'category fallacy'. Validity is a multidimensional concept including measurement reliability, construct validity, diagnostic, content and criterion-related validity, as well as statistical, internal and external validity (van Ommeren, 2003). The debate about PTSD and culture mainly focuses on the cross-cultural validity of the PTSD construct. A seminal review by Hinton and Lewis-Fernández (2011) concluded that

> substantial evidence of cross-cultural validity of PTSD was found, but that issues concerning symptom complexes critical to diagnosis, including the cross-cultural salience of avoidance and numbing symptoms, the importance of local cultural interpretations as shaping symptomatology, the place of somatic symptoms, and the overlap or comorbidity of PTSD, anxiety disorders, and depressive disorders require further empirical research.

Symptom clusters described by DSM-5 for PTSD are found around the globe, although the rates vary. Even in studies with over a thousand variables, the PTSD construct appeared to be a recognizable diagnostic entity in a variety of cultures (Algerians, Cambodians, Afghanis, Bhutanese, Ethiopians, Tibetans, Sri Lankans) without secondary benefits such as disability allowances, and often without a notion of words such as trauma or PTSD (de Jong, 2005a). Although biomarkers for PTSD have not been definitively identified, some

DSM-PTSD criteria may constitute a stable cross-cultural core trauma response (Hinton and Lewis-Fernández, 2011). As one example, supporting the cross-cultural validity of the reactivity criteria, Kinzie et al. (1998) demonstrated more physiological (e.g. heart rate) reactivity to trauma-related themes in Cambodian refugees with PTSD as compared to those without PTSD. As another example, an orthostatic challenge (i.e. rising from sitting to standing) that provoked dizziness, Cambodian refugees experienced flashbacks, some full reliving in type (i.e. there was a multisensorial reliving of the trauma event), and this was highly associated with receiving a diagnosis of PTSD (Hinton et al., 2010). This finding supports the theory that flashbacks are part of a universal biological response to trauma that may be triggered by trauma cues (e.g. dizziness as an encoder of trauma memory). Other support for the validity of PTSD across cultures are studies that examined the factor structure of PTSD symptoms across cultural settings, showing that most of the findings differ little from what is found in Western samples, although the prevalence might differ across countries (Fawzi et al., 1997; Sack et al., 1997; Norris et al., 2001a, b; Palmieri et al., 2007; Lim et al., 2009; Yufik and Simms 2010; Karam et al., 2014). Based on these considerations, Osterman and de Jong (2007) proposed to end the debate about the validity of the diagnosis of PTSD, asserting that the disorder appears to be a universal reaction to severe stressors that has transcultural diagnostic validity.

That the PTSD diagnosis has cross-cultural diagnostic validity obviously does not mean that trauma reactions around the globe are identical, as indicated by the concept of ecological utility. Contributing to the variation in trauma experiencing, the local conception of mental conditions caused by 'traumatic events' frequently vary considerably from PTSD, as demonstrated in Gambia (Fox, 2003), Rwanda (Bolton, 2001), among Darfuri refugees in Chad (Rasmussen et al., 2011), or among Cambodian refugees in the USA (Hinton and Good 2016a, b).

Culture influences local phenomenologies of post-trauma experiences, local illness vocabularies, mental and bodily experience (the local ethnopsychology and ethnophysiology), attention to particular symptoms, and practices aimed at reducing these symptoms. As another example of variation in trauma experiencing, somatic symptoms are not in the DSM-5 or ICD-11 criteria for PTSD but are a common reaction to trauma in many cultural contexts. The reasons for certain somatic symptoms being so prominent in the trauma presentation of a certain group are multifactorial. They range from the nature of the trauma event; to the encoding of certain trauma memories in terms of somatic sensations; to great chronic arousal and frequent panic owing to a biological recalibration of the nervous system; to catastrophic cognitions about somatic symptoms such as attribution to certain cultural syndromes; to the symptoms being prominent in local metaphors used to express dysphoria, resulting in metaphor-guided somatization; to the role of certain somatic symptoms as an idiom of distress in the culture in question. For example, among Cambodian refugees, a particular cultural syndrome is one reason dizziness and several other somatic symptoms are prominent: the syndrome referred to as 'khyâl attacks' gives rise to multiple catastrophic cognitions about somatic symptoms, creating a hypervigilant surveying of the body for them, particularly for dizziness (a key indicator of a khyâl attack), in multiple situations said to trigger the khyâl attacks, such as engaging in worry or standing up (Hinton et al., 2012; 2013a). Other symptoms and symptom complexes common in many traumatized populations but that are not in the DSM-5 criteria are sleep paralysis (Hinton et al. 2005; de Jong, 2005b), and other phenomena we referred to before such as substance abuse and acting out (externalizing) behaviours, complicated bereavement, cultural syndromes, multiple anxiety disorders (panic disorder, panic attacks, generalized anxiety disorder), a rapid induction of distress, arousal, and somatic symptoms, and the 'thinking a lot' complex (what is essentially a hypercognizing complex) (Hinton and Good, 2016a, b).

Cross-cultural variation in the experiencing of trauma disorder may be greater in the context of complex trauma in that the multiple symptoms of the disorder may give rise to a wide range of local cultural interpretations and local practices and responses. Complex trauma can refer to experiencing prolonged trauma while in a state of vulnerability, such as when young, or when subject to multiple stresses. The term complex PTSD often refers to the clinical picture that may result from complex trauma, due to many causes: the nature and severity of traumatic experience including war, civil conflict, torture; duration of the trauma; age the trauma occurs and developmental effects; genetic vulnerability; current levels of stress; experiences involving pervasive loss of control over aversive consequences. The term also may refer specifically to the complexity of the clinical picture, including specific symptoms, characterized

by a recalibration of the nervous system to a state of hyperreactivity to a wide range of stimuli, such as to noises or visual reminders of the trauma, and by poor regulation of negative emotion, such as anger. This hyperreactivity to stimuli and poor emotion regulation result in the frequent experiencing of symptoms such as anger, anxiety and somatic symptoms (Bryant, 2012; Resick et al., 2012; Hinton and Good, 2016a, b). Regarding Complex PTSD or DESNOS (Disorders of Stress not Otherwise Specified) de Jong et al. (2005) found a range of symptoms other than PTSD symptoms that can be found or elicited in different cultures. Also, the complexity of trauma-related disorder may be related not only to trauma severity and vulnerability to trauma but also to other important variables, namely, to the social response such as stigma associated with the traumatizing events and with the induced symptoms, and to cultural interpretation of particular trauma-related symptoms (Bryant, 2010; Hinton and Good, 2016a, b).

Historicity Evidence

The historicity debate on PTSD also addresses validity, but from a transhistorical perspective. Since initial nineteenth-century descriptions in the scientific literature of conditions that resemble what we now call PTSD, there has been controversy about PTSD's validity as a psychiatric condition. Debate has continued over the past 150 years about its core symptoms and behavioural manifestations. Moreover, there has been an ongoing debate about whether PTSD and its associated symptoms are psychological or neurological, and whether or not PTSD and mild traumatic brain injury (mTBI) are distinct entities or overlapping conditions (Boehnlein and Hinton, 2016).

The historical critique became more prominent when Young (1995) wrote that 'PTSD is a culture-derived diagnosis that only existed in the late 20th century'. McNally (2016: 117–135) writes that views such as Young's often incite anger among traumatologists because he seems to unmask PTSD as an artefact, a product of culture, not nature. This might not be such a problem if he were considering also other anxiety disorders that do not imply the moral categories of innocent victim and perpetrator. Yet when someone develops PTSD, there is almost always someone or something to blame for the suffering. Traumatologists seemingly presuppose that to assert the artefactual character of PTSD delegitimizes the suffering of victims.

Traumatologists have sought to rebut social constructionist interpretations of PTSD in three ways (McNally, 2016). First, they have adduced biological data in support of the claim that PTSD is a natural kind. Yehuda and McFarlane (1997) said, 'biological findings have provided objective validation that PTSD is more than a politically or socially motivated conceptualization of human suffering'. Of note, even neurobiologists often think that factors such as lack of social support, continued adversity, or inability to make sense of the traumatic event, are more important (see, e.g., Brewin *et al.* 2000; Shalev, 2007). Second, traumatologists have successfully conducted cross-cultural studies seeking to test whether PTSD occurs in non-Western societies, as we mentioned before. Third, traumatologists have sought to identify instances of PTSD throughout history. Many have argued that syndromes, such as shell shock in World War I and battle fatigue in World War II, were really PTSD under different names. Jones *et al.* (2003) in their study of UK service men who had fought in wars from 1854 onwards, support the hypothesis that some of the characteristics of PTSD, such as intrusion and avoidance, are culture-bound and that earlier conflicts showed a greater emphasis on somatic symptoms. Shay (1991) on the contrary suggested that elements of the post-traumatic stress disorder could be identified in Homer's *Iliad*. Ben-Ezra (2003) asserts that the symptoms of nightmares, sleep disturbances, and increased anxiety have not changed in 4,000 years. The symptoms reported in a family trapped in the Bergemoletto avalanche have been quoted as evidence for the disorder's existence in the mid eighteenth century (Parry-Jones and Parry-Jones, 1994). Dean (1997) identified symptoms of PTSD in the accounts of veterans of the American Civil War. Trimble (1985) concluded that 'this relatively common human problem has been known for many hundreds of years, although under different names'. These various labels each have had implications for diagnosis and treatment, and also broader social implications in regard to disability, along with the social perception of disability and associated stigma (Kugelmann, 2009).

McNally (2016: 120) further argues that a failure to detect PTSD throughout history is not necessarily fatal to claims about its validity. There are genuine disease entities that do not appear transhistorically despite their worldwide prevalence today. One example is schizophrenia. A comprehensive search of historical, medical, and fictional literature in Greek and Roman antiquity uncovered clear descriptions of epilepsy, alcoholism, mania, delirium, and social phobia, but no descriptions of schizophrenia (Evans *et al.*, 2003). In fact, few, if any, convincing descriptions of schizophrenia appear prior to the nineteenth century (Hare, 1988). Schizophrenia is seemingly a disease of recent origin whose prevalence increased throughout the nineteenth-century Western world, remaining rare elsewhere until the twentieth century. Hence, there is an asymmetry in how we interpret the historical data. Recognizing a syndrome throughout time supports its validity, whereas noting its recent appearance does not necessarily undermine such claims. Some genuine diseases are of recent vintage. McNally (2016: 130) wonders what are the implications of these findings for the historicity of PTSD. He mentions that understanding PTSD from a historical perspective may be especially challenging if what counts as traumatic varies as a function of context, a theme we will discuss further on. For example, people whose understanding of trauma has been shaped by the horrors of the holocaust during World War II are unlikely to be much affected by the stressors that can cause PTSD today. Perhaps one unfortunate consequence of the otherwise undeniable benefits of modernity is diminished resilience.

One may conclude that – as has been described for other expressions of psychopathology – that the symptoms of trauma-related disorder change over time and that a historical era, to some extent, expresses itself in an idiosyncratic way in the presentation of individual suffering. Depending on the conceptualization of mind, body and vulnerabilities and the effect of 'trauma' in a certain historical period, one would expect variations in the salience of certain PTSD symptoms, and trauma-related symptoms more broadly. But one would expect 'PTSD' symptoms to be present, although not necessarily emphasized in experience and presentation.

Politicization and Medicalization

To understand the debate on politicization and medicalization we first cite Parsons' sociological theory. Parsons (1952) asserted that societies tend to transform social problems into individual problems and thus tend to conceal their sociogenesis. Once a social problem is transformed into an individual problem, the individual cannot be blamed, while simultaneously being expected to find a solution: the 'sick role' exempts the ill individual from certain responsibilities and offers care and concern. When the individual has accepted this 'sick role', suffering is regarded as a medical instead of a social problem, and therefore de-politicized. Parsons also asserted that people would never choose collectively for sickness as a way of dealing with frustrating aspects of the social system, because sickness is defined as an undesirable condition. One recent example may help to put Parsons' theory in a different perspective. The Gulf War syndrome caused veterans to fear that exposure to fumes and toxic substances might cause bodily harm, when in fact those symptoms resulted from anxiety and depression; as a result, veterans often came to reframe psychological distress as the Gulf War syndrome, a kind of 'toxic neurasthenia' (Jones and Wessely, 2005), which one may regard as an idiom of distress or cultural syndrome. In contrast with Parsons' theory, the former combatants collectively chose sickness. Moreover, once their suffering was labelled as a medical instead of a social problem, it was not de-politicized as Parsons claimed. On the contrary, the Gulf War syndrome resulted in heated debates e.g. in the political and military arenas. The example also illustrates another ambiguity. Medical anthropology handles dichotomies to classify how societies attribute responsibility for disease or sickness. For example, Young (1976) distinguished externalizing and internalizing aetiologies. However, the Gulf War syndrome shows that aetiological interpretations are often much more complex, both among former combatants and among professionals. Reis (1992) therefore proposed to distinguish two types of aetiological interpretations, 'centripetal' and 'centrifugal'. During her work in Africa she realised that people often interpret disease or predicaments with a sliding scale combining both personal-type and environmental-type aetiological considerations. It is interesting that meta-analyses of psychotherapy in HIC produce similar insights into the role of environmental factors. For example, Asay and Lambert (1999) ascribed 30% of the variance in psychotherapy to universal therapist variables, 15% to placebo, 15% to technique, and *40% to contextual variables*. All psychotherapy, psychiatry, and public mental health are inherently socio-cultural–ecological processes.

Another level of critique of the PTSD category involves its 'dangerous potential for medicalizing human suffering; that is, for reducing the social and moral implications of traumatizing events, such as war or genocide, to a strictly professional, even biological, set of consequences'. This critique suggests that, by emphasizing the 'reality' of PTSD as

a universal biopsychological category, research on PTSD may have unintentionally and paradoxically helped decrease social and moral responsiveness to these events (Hinton and Lewis-Fernández, 2011). For example, Breslau (2004) states:

> The expansion of PTSD into the international health arena thus involves complicity and interdependence between promoters of the disorder as a privileged window onto human suffering and local actors advancing political agendas on the global stage. PTSD can function in this way because of the symbolic power of medical science ... PTSD offers scientific credibility to claims of victimization, while political actors provide contexts for expanding the purview of PTSD.

In a similar vein, Pupovac (2004) writes:

> War trauma is influenced by contemporary Anglo-American emotionology ..., which tends to pathologise ordinary responses to distress, including anger related to survival strategies ... international therapeutic governance pathologises war affected populations as emotionally dysfunctional and problematizes their right to self-government, leading to extensive external intervention. However, international therapeutic governance may be detrimental to postwar recovery as well as legitimizing a denial of self-government.

Some authors participating in this debate emphasize the aspect of medicalization and refer to mental health as a 'trauma industry' and PTSD as a tool to pathologize whole societies:

> for the vast majority of survivors posttraumatic stress is a pseudo condition, a reframing of the understandable suffering of war as a technical problem to which short-term technical solutions like counselling are applicable. These concepts aggrandize the Western agencies and their 'experts' who from afar define the condition and bring the cure. There is no evidence that war-affected populations are seeking these imported approaches, which appear to ignore their own traditions, meaning systems, and active priorities.
> (Summerfield, 1999)

For Summerfield (2001), the extension of notions of trauma and PTSD to non-Western societies represents forms of psychological imperialism that 'risk an unwitting perpetuation of the colonial status of the non-Western mind'.

It might be a bit easy to argue that Hippocrates, Pasteur, Semmelweis, Freud or any medical or psychiatric practitioner can be accused of promoting the power of medical science or the industry, of self-aggrandizement, of pathologizing ordinary responses to distress, and of dealing with pseudoconditions. To some extent many of us will agree and be able to spontaneously provide some poignant examples. Yet, we think this form of reasoning is based on false premises and contrary to a basic ethical principle, *no nocere*, do not harm. Why? First, earlier on in this chapter we argued that PTSD can easily be distinguished as a relevant construct in large data sets collected among survivors in (post-)conflict societies who rarely had a notion of the concept of (post-traumatic) stress, and who did not receive any benefit derived from such a label. Calling PTSD a pseudocondition is a vast underestimation of the suffering it entails. An extensive literature shows that individuals who develop PTSD often experience impaired role functioning and reduced life-course opportunities due to a higher incidence of a range of somatic disorders, poor educational attainment, unemployment, marital instability and disability (Kessler, 2000; Alonso et al., 2013). The likelihood of experiencing particular types of violence and trauma varies by sex, age, ethnicity and sexual orientation, and is often increased in humanitarian crises such as protracted wars and armed conflicts. Pseudocondition thus is a misnomer.

Second, PTSD is depicted as 'a window onto human suffering and actors advancing political agendas', and as part of a 'trauma industry', 'pathologizing ordinary responses to distress'. But in fact the 'PTSD industry' tells the contrary: it tells people that PTSD is a *normal* reaction to extreme stress, even though that reaction may affect them badly. It is far from a 'trauma industry' promoting the benefits of pharmaceutical companies. On the contrary, survivors hear that most people spontaneously get over extreme stress, and that only a relatively small group of about 12–20 per cent develop PTSD (Yehuda and McFarlane, 1995; Breslau and Kessler, 2001). Shalev (2007) even defines PTSD as a disorder of recovery because most persons who suffer initial experiences characteristic of PTSD, recover in a natural way. The latest WHO guidelines for management of acute stress, PTSD, and bereavement advice that individual or group CBT-T (trauma-focused CBT), EMDR (eye movement desensitization and reprocessing) or stress management should be considered, and that medication should *not* be offered as the first line of treatment, either for adults or children (Tol et al., 2014). The word 'trauma industry' also suggests that money is pumped into some kind of business, but that is an unfounded presupposition (Tol et al., 2011b).

Third, in humanitarian emergencies one does find that mental health and psychosocial issues do play a role and are spontaneously mentioned by the population (without 'advancing political agendas', promoting a 'trauma industry', or 'pathologizing ordinary responses to distress'). The most prominent problems mentioned are economic aspects (such as poverty, loss of goods and houses), health aspects (increase in prevalence of diseases and malnutrition), but without being probed, people also clearly indicate social aspects (weakening of mechanisms for social support and conflict resolution) and psychological aspects (sadness, grief) (de Jong, 2011; Ventevogel, 2016). This discredits the notion that issues related to psychological well-being would not be prioritized by people in Africa or Asia, or would represent externally imposed categories (Summerfield, 1999; Fernando, 2014). Studies with populations in the African Great Lakes Region also found that mental and psychosocial issues are considered a real concern and are perceived as embedded within larger socio-cultural phenomena (Bolton, 2001; Horn, 2009; Tankink et al., 2010). Survivors prioritize loss-related problems, such as depression, trauma and grief, followed by severe mental disorder and then alcohol and drug use. This is highly relevant given these discussions around the significance of post-traumatic stress disorder in post-war contexts, with a minority arguing that this is the key issue for war affected populations (Neuner, 2010; Neuner et al., 2014), and a large majority opposing that view and emphasizing the role of daily stressors and ongoing adversity as the major contributor to mental health problems (Silove et al., 1997; Steel et al., 1999; de Jong et al., 2001; de Jong, 2002; Bhui et al., 2003; Laban et al. 2008; IASC, 2010; Miller and Rasmussen, 2010; Song et al. 2015; Ventevogel, 2016). Most experts are of the opinion that mental health and psychosocial programmes should aim at a wide range of mental health issues, and not merely one condition.

The critics also do not seem to be aware of the basics of public health, the preventive discipline including social science aiming at 'prolonging life and promoting health through the organized efforts and informed choices of society, organizations (public and private), communities and individuals' (Winslow, 1920). Most experts agree that public mental health is the way to address conflict-related psychosocial problems in LIC, for example because the major determinants of violence play at an (inter)national level, and because mental health professionals are often virtually absent, especially in those areas of the world that are harshly hit by political violence (e.g. Middle East, Great Lake area in Africa, West Africa) (de Jong *et al.*, 2015). Scholars do study a variety of psychological problems and psychiatric disorders among groups such as combatants, children, women, or first- or second-generation survivors of genocides such as the Holocaust, the Khmer Rouge or the Armenian genocide. In addition to conducting research, researchers indeed 'try to advance political agendas on the global stage'. That is what public health aims at, 'organizing efforts in the society and among public and private organizations'. They certainly try to influence political agendas on all levels to increase respect for human, social and cultural rights, to decrease new wars and ongoing armed conflicts, or to prevent torture, rape, domestic violence, femicide or yet another genocide (de Jong, 2005a, 2010).

In sum, the proponents of the critique of politicization and of medicalization – in line with Parsons – argue that there is widespread tendency to individualize a social problem as in the case of PTSD. But their critique seems to miss the mark. They are unaware of the socio-contextual approach of virtually all (inter)national agencies that are active in the field. With their sweeping and rather paranoid statements that are devoid of facts and figures they side with current populistic discourse that is *en vogue* in politics. They devalue social science that in our view is a fundamental discipline in addressing the consequences of mass violence. Their stereotype that 'psychological imperialism risks an unwitting perpetuation of the colonial status of the non-Western mind' exposes a more serious problem: their idea that all trauma treatment is flawed, is a post-colonial guise of stating that non-Westerners are psychologically less sophisticated, reminiscent of the colonial literature of the less developed frontal lobes of non-Westerners. Their unfounded accusations serve to legitimize the withdrawal of scarce resources for the development of mental health and psychosocial services among those who need it most.

Three Analytic Optics to Study Trauma

Syndemics

As indicated earlier, syndemics refers to two or more enmeshed and mutually enhancing health problems that, working together, contribute to an excess disease burden in a specific population (Singer, 1994; 2007). Complex emergencies and political violence often take place when a combination of social determinants or risk factors prevails: faulty governance, lack of democracy, inequality and inequity, marginalization of groups according to ethnic and religious identity, and health and nutritional indicators per se (Staub, 2011; de Jong, 2010). To a large extent these very same social determinants produce ill health, resulting, for example, from a low priority of health to impaired access to health and education (Daar *et al.*, 2007; Collier, 2008; Collins *et al.*, 2011; WHO, 2011). The interconnection and interaction of these risk factors damage social, physical and human capital in conflict-related countries; hamper their economic development during and after the conflict; and contribute to an excess burden of social, psychological and medical problems (Stewart *et al.*, 2001). The syndemics of risk factors cause and maintain underdevelopment, poverty, weakened political states, corruption, socio-economic inequalities, and the struggle over access to resources that characterize the areas of protracted conflicts around the world. The deterioration of services creates a vicious circle of reduced access to services, increased morbidity, mortality and disability, and widespread discontent that engenders further conflict or that creates refugee flows. Structural violence and disadvantage – poverty, low socio-economic class, lack of support – create the traumasyndemics of suffering and vulnerabilities of the population. Most mental health professionals are aware of the linkage between poverty and common mental disorders (Patel and Kleinman, 2003). Social inequalities increase the risk of disorders such as depression, alcohol and substance use, and stress-related disorders. Social factors are paramount in the aetiology of many mental disorders ('social causation') and conversely these mental disorders have negative socio-economic consequences and may contribute to continuing impoverishment ('social drift') (Lund *et al.*, 2011).

Therefore, it is no surprise that over the past decade public-health approaches to political violence and mass trauma have been promoted and developed. Preventive strategies from the realm of public health can restore the balance between risk and protective factors. Prevention rests on a few generic public-health principles that can be applied both to 'violence' and 'disorder': uncovering knowledge about violence and disorder and reacting early to signs of trouble; using a comprehensive approach to alleviate risk factors that trigger or maintain violent conflict or disorder; addressing the underlying root causes of violence and disorder; and implementing, monitoring and evaluating interventions that appear promising (de Jong 2010; 2011; de Jong et al., 2015). One can translate risk and protective factors into multisectoral, multi-modal and multilevel preventive interventions involving the economy, governance, diplomacy, the military, human rights, agriculture, health and education (de Jong, 2010). One can develop a preventive framework mapping the complementary fit among the actors while engaging in preventive, rehabilitative and reconstructive interventions. In other words, a mental health professional can contribute to relieving the stress of trauma and war while providing treatment or tertiary prevention in a public-health pyramid. While realizing the impact limitations, they may contribute to restoring the fabric of an individual or a family destroyed by major socio-economic and political forces. They will be aware of macro-politics and its impact on their patients, but they need not be a politician or diplomat. Neither should they be accused of unwittingly medicalizing the local group or of self-aggrandizing, of pathologizing war-affected populations as emotionally dysfunctional, or of enriching the pharma industry. They may provide a modest contribution to unravelling and decreasing the mutually enhancing health problems involved in traumasyndemics.

Syndemics may also help us to understand some other problems of working with trauma patients. Where to start – both in complex emergency settings and in a consultation room – when there are so many problems simultaneously? For example, when we see a refugee, do we first help to stabilize and normalize their living situation, help to get a refugee status, discuss the worries about the family back home, address the cultural bereavement, or rather start with a psychotherapeutic intervention such as CBT, EMDR or NET (narrative exposure therapy)? When

people are suffering in virtually every domain of life caught in traumasyndemics of social and psychological problems, is it appropriate to speak of a disorder such as PTSD? And when people are long-term exposed to chronic stress, due to political violence, or pervasive family and sexual violence, is the concept of PTSD adequate or should we aim at managing the disabling condition, complex PTSD?

Dynamic Networks

As mentioned before as well as in several chapters in this textbook, one of the greatest problems of cultural psychiatry is the problem of validity and of the universality of psychiatric nosology. Over the past years, when the USA's National Institute of Mental Health (NIMH) distanced itself from the DSM-5, the NIMH director wrote, 'Diagnosis has confounded psychiatry for the past century, with the DSM approach enhancing diagnostic reliability (ensuring that clinicians use the same term in the same way), but not validity' (Insel, 2015). The NIMH launched the Research Domain Criteria (RDoC) project to transform diagnosis by incorporating genetics, imaging, cognitive science and other levels of information to lay the foundation for a new classification system. But in view of previous miracles expected from genetic or biological approaches, one may seriously wonder how many decades the RDoC project will take, whether biomarkers will indeed result in the advent of 'precision medicine' in psychiatry, and whether the hoped for innovative diagnostic and treatment techniques will be accessible and affordable in large areas around the globe.

Over the past years, two global surveys (Evans et al., 2013; Reed et al., 2013) showed that both psychiatrists and psychologists prefer more flexible and conceptual diagnostic guidelines, with fewer categories, giving more scope for clinical judgement and cultural variation. We already saw that a core problem for scientific research has been the lack of validity of currently used ICD and DSM diagnoses, which are not based on empirical evidence but on clinical consensus, leading to arbitrary boundaries and much overlap between diagnoses. In addition, over the past few decades, dysphoric emotional states that are often tied to life circumstances and socio-economic factors have been progressively reframed as mental disorders (Horwitz, 2007). A second related problem lies in the syndrome approach commonly used for categorizing patients, which results in a great deal of heterogeneity among patients with the same diagnosis (Kendell and Jablensky, 2003; Widiger and Samuel, 2005).[4] A third issue that bedevils psychiatric epidemiology in complex humanitarian emergencies is to what extent the measured mental distress represents true psychopathological states and to what extent mental distress is a transient reaction to major stress factors (Horwitz, 2007).

Simultaneously, a radical different approach to psychopathology is developing. This innovative approach, dynamic networks, regards psychopathology as interactions between symptoms (Kendler *et al.*, 2011; Borsboom *et al.*, 2011; 2013; Wigman *et al.*, 2015). In the network approach, our habitual focus *on* symptoms in DSM or ICD shifts to the dynamics *between* symptoms. The network approach is interested in the longitudinal course of symptoms, either in terms of symptom reduction or aggravation, and in the trajectory of the symptom patterns. It wonders what comes first, what next, and to what degree? It aims at a dimensional classification. Clinicians with vast clinical experience may have insight in symptom trajectories of their patients, but in ICD and DSM the thrust of diagnosis is counting symptoms and assessing if they meet a (culturally variable) threshold and fit a categorical category. Dynamic networks look at the feedback loops between causal factors (i.e. the reciprocal influences between symptoms over time, one symptom causing another e.g. sleeplessness causing fatigue causing apathy/depression; or anxiety causing paranoia causing delusional thinking causing psychosis).

Why is this interesting for cultural psychiatry and for the study of trauma?

A dimensional network approach elicits a sliding scale of local complaints (such as vernacular complaint terms, idioms of distress, cultural syndromes) and other symptom domains (e.g. depression, anxiety, cognitive limitations) across diagnostic categories or spectrum disorders, for example, for affective disorders, obsessive behaviour, stress-induced disorders, and psychotic spectrum disorders (cf. Barlow, 1988; Krueger, 1999; Dutta *et al.* 2007; Helzer *et al.*, 2007; Van Os *et al.*, 2010). It encourages study of change in dynamic networks through time, such as how local and vernacular symptoms that belong to the realm of IODs and cultural syndromes become more serious psychopathology; or to study when does suffering – in the form of local IODs – become a medical problem, a condition needing medical intervention? Dynamic networks may help mental health professionals to conceptualize the development of mental illness as a gradual transition from normalcy to perceived deviancy in a specific socio-cultural context, rather than relying on predetermined cut-points and thresholds that raise questions of validity and results in sometimes extremely skewed prevalence rates in cross-cultural epidemiological studies (de Jong, 2014), for example, the range of PTSD of 0–99 per cent in conflict affected populations (Steel *et al.*, 2009).

Another intriguing aspect is that dynamic networks allow for the interdisciplinary use of qualitative methods such as in-depth ethnography or more rapid anthropological appraisals, with quantitative techniques to generate a new phenomenology that may reinvent psychiatry. The longitudinal perspective on the development or resolution of complaints, symptoms and syndromes opens the door to new methods of personal (idiographic), ecological and digital self-quantification. For example, experience sampling or momentary assessment technologies can help to capture daily life by installing an application on a smartphone allowing monitoring of psychological experiences (e.g. mood), behaviours (eating, intake of substances), environment (stress, company), and activities (work, study, leisure) over time (Myin-Germeys *et al.*, 2009). These innovative approaches promise an epistemological and methodological breakthrough in the perennial universalism–relativism debate because they allow us to generate culturally and ecologically meaningful categories of psychopathology. It may help us to transcend the methodological hurdle to first conduct complex preparatory qualitative research of collecting vernacular indigenous symptoms and compare them with internationally recognized psychiatric nosologies such as DSM or ICD (de Jong, 2014).

Regarding the study of trauma, dynamic networks may provide detailed illustrations of how human beings in different cultural contexts react to traumatic distress. Dynamic networks will help us to empirically test and study looping processes within and across

---

[4] This problem of heterogeneity applies to most psychiatric diagnoses. It also applies to the heterogeneity of factors causing someone to manifest psychological problems. One wonders why Young and Breslau (2015) position PTSD in a special position amidst other diagnoses when they also examine the historical origins of the PTSD concept and argue that it is a heterogeneous entity because the supposed cause (a trauma) is so variable and at times almost non-existent, or even imagined (Hinton and Good, 2016a, b).

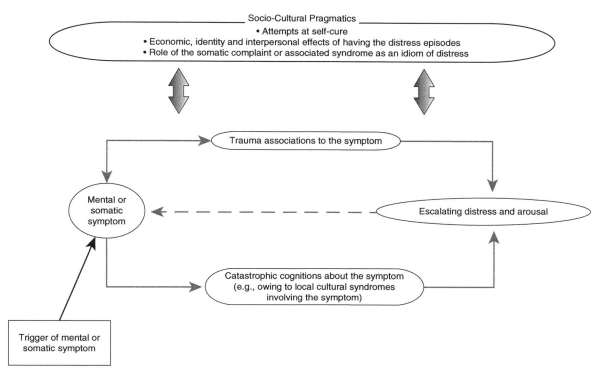

Figure 29.1 A multiplex model of the generation of trauma related disorder

cultures. Based on clinical observations and surveys, Hinton *et al.* (for reviews, see Hinton and Good, 2016b; Hinton and Simons, 2015) elicited and conceptualized a variety of feedback loops that describe the interaction between ethnopsychologies and ethnophysiologies and evolving symptom patterns. These multiplex models show how trauma-related disorder not only involves a dynamic interaction of symptoms but also dimensions of distress. A multiplex model for trauma-related disorder is shown in Figure 29.1.

So for example, worry may trigger symptoms like anger, poor concentration. and somatic symptoms, and then these symptoms may give rise to catastrophic cognitions (the meaning of symptoms in terms of local cultural syndromes) and trauma recall (e.g. arousal and somatic symptoms as encoding trauma memories). Next increasing arousal and even panic may result, and soon there may be an escalation of distress by looping processes. In this scenario, there are GAD-type processes (e.g. worry), panic-disorder processes (catastrophic cognitions), PTSD processes (e.g. anger and trauma recall), and panic attacks, and there are other dimensions, such as somatic symptoms. It is also a symptom–interaction model. Such a

causal network model illustrates that often there are not discrete disorders – or symptoms – but interactive ones. In the model focusing on worry, social context is also emphasized: local concerns such as poverty give rise to worry that then unleashes the various processes, which loop and multiply and generate trauma-syndemics. When the local processes of dealing with the induced symptoms are added to the multiplex model, a sense of certain aspects of the local trauma-scape emerges (see the following section). Seen more broadly, there is looping of symptoms, dimensions of disorder, and local means of response to symptoms. Through a more dynamic and ecological view of disorder a truer understanding of the local experiencing of trauma-related disorder emerges, which also highlights potential points of intervention. (On a dynamic network depiction of the syndrome 'thinking a lot', found in many cultures, see Hinton *et al.*, 2016a, b.)

Traumascape

Traumascape refers to the systemic dynamics of local and international representations and actions around extreme stress (de Jong, 2007). Every society represents individual or collective traumatic events or historic episodes in specific ways. The narratives of events and of survivors figure in public memorials, commemorative holidays and rituals, television and visual arts, newspapers, books and state rhetorics. Traumascape is a concept enabling us to describe how traumatic distress interacts with political, historical, religious and cultural factors. In situations of mass trauma or disaster a cascade of events determined by the media, international organizations such as the United Nations, (non)governmental organizations, funders and health professionals, often determines the focus, the size and the nature of assistance for a group of survivors. Selective reporting and media hypes – possibly triggered by an iconic picture as seen in pictures of child migrants and victims in the Syrian conflict – in parallel with (geo) political, voter-dependent or populistic considerations determine whether migration, terrorism, human rights or child rights, governance, gender-based or domestic violence, former combatants or child soldiers, are the main concern of the international community. And, subsequently, whether attention will go to a specific region, to certain disasters or calamities, or specific groups of survivors, possibly to the detriment of other catastrophic events. In this regard there is no difference between the two World Wars and more recent disasters, genocides or refugee flows.

Similarly, from a local perspective, (inter)national helpers may feel they have to build 'trauma awareness' explaining the concepts of trauma or PTSD using ICD or DSM criteria. The local survivors may get quickly conditioned through looping processes to mould distress into symptoms of PTSD instead of expressing their distress via local idioms or syndromes. On the other hand, local inhabitants may perceive sudden PTSD symptoms as extremely frightening. Nightmares may be given a spiritual interpretation. They may interpret symptoms as flashbacks or intrusive memories as the beginning of a 'mental disease' causing them to wander around as people with chronic afflictions due to the fact that their culture has no sophisticated classification that might help them differentiate the prognoses of different illnesses. In our opinion it is important that mental health professionals are aware of the meta-forces driving these local and global dynamics around trauma. Earlier in this chapter we mentioned the rather fact-free statements pervading the politicization and medicalization debate of trauma. We regard those discourses, theoretically

relevant to the humanitarian field, as part of the traumascape. Moreover, mental health professionals are accustomed to think that epidemiological figures, evidence-based and cost-effective considerations guide their professional field (for efficacy overviews, see Foa et al., 2009; Friedman et al., 2014; Tol et al. 2014; for asylum seekers and refugees see Slobodin and de Jong, 2014, 2015). But we should realise that the dynamics of the traumascape often overrule what health professionals regard as rational. This may not surprise those among us who wonder about populistic and dangerous or even 'thanatophilic' ('death wish') political forces as Freud would call them, in today's world.

Traumascape as an Ecological–Cultural–Historical Model for Extreme Stress

In this chapter we used several concepts that show the profoundly ecological aspects of trauma, which is shown in Figure 29.2. We proposed to look beyond classical person-centred PTSD models. Traumasyndemics and the traumascape underline the importance of social and interpersonal factors. We mentioned the role of contextual actors in explaining the effects of psychotherapy. Measures of social support are among the best predictors of PTSD according to two meta-analyses. In addition, the social interpersonal realm – such as a partner's or relatives' reactions to the trauma – comprises powerful mechanisms that can either prevent or cause PTSD-related suffering in the individuals (Brewin et al., 2000; Ozer et al., 2003). Investigating childhood trauma, Charuvastra and Cloitre (2008) reviewed research findings that pointed to the importance of attachment behaviours for short-term and long-term outcomes of trauma. Social affects accompanying post-traumatic cognitive changes are shame and guilt. Horowitz (2007) highlighted revenge as being a composite of social affects that include anger at perpetrators, frustration about the injustices of the world, and a belief that no rescuer can be trusted.

In the remaining part of this chapter we therefore present a model for understanding and studying the interaction between extreme stress, the individual, social ecology, history, politics and culture. The model has four objectives. The first is to provide a transdisciplinary framework for scholars to study these complex interactions. The second

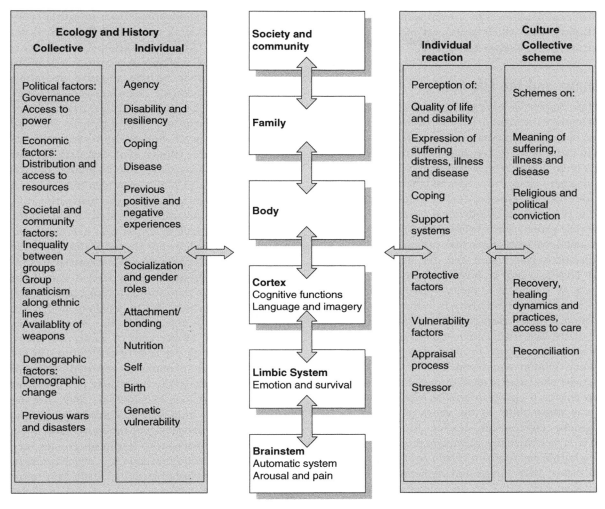

Figure 29.2 An ecological–cultural–historical model for extreme stress

objective is to provide some illustrations from around the globe testifying how survivors make sense of and recover from trauma. The third is to provide a public-health framework that can be translated into preventive interventions, policies and practices. Political violence and complex humanitarian emergencies do not remain within national boundaries and are push factors that drive migration and contribute to multiracial societies. Therefore, the fourth objective is in line with the aim of this book: inviting professionals to become interculturally competent, either in working with asylum seekers, refugees or immigrants, or in crossing borders.

Our ecological–cultural–historical model for extreme stress presents the person as part of a hierarchy of organizational levels. The person is first presented as an organism composed of interrelated parts of the central nervous system and the body, then on to the level of the family and, finally, the community and society (see Figure 29.2). From a wider ecological perspective, the person is enveloped and interacts with corresponding historical, political and economic processes and domains. In the different domains we distinguish a *collective* and an *individual* dimension. We realize that this distinction is artificial because the gist of our argument throughout this chapter is that they closely interact with each other. However, we believe that for transdisciplinary scholars it is helpful from a methodological point to be able to distinguish at

377

which ecological level they want to focus their data collection, and which multilevel models are most appropriate to analyse those data.[5]

Trauma and the Life Course

In this chapter we have emphasized dynamic models and levels of interaction. Here we consider the importance of studying trauma across the life course. Earlier on in this chapter we concluded that the symptoms of post-traumatic stress – as in many other psychiatric syndromes – change over time and that a historical era, to some extent, expresses itself in an idiosyncratic way in the presentation of individual suffering. This idiosyncratic process starts before birth when individuals are equipped with genes that promote resiliency or vulnerability (see Figure 29.2, the heading 'Ecology and History', and subheading 'Individual'). A key aspect of trauma is a biology-generated emotional and somatic hyper-reactivity in response to negative emotions. Among other effects, this results in ruminative states like worry, frequent bouts of anger and reactivity in response to external reminders of the trauma (Hinton and Good, 2016a, b). The hyper-reactivity may begin in utero through intergenerational mechanisms: if a pregnant woman experiences trauma, it may cause shifts in the genes of the foetus by epigenetic mechanisms, leading to psychobiology-driven hyper-reactivity, seemingly preparing the child for a hostile environment (Heim et al., 2000; Yehuda and Bierer, 2009; Binder and Nemeroff, 2010; Sherin and Nemeroff, 2011). So an individual's life history starts in utero with the interaction between a person's genetic make-up and the environment. A traumasyndemic that affects vulnerability to stress has been identified by Caspi et al. (2003). Individuals who carry two copies of the short allele of 5-HTTLPR – serotonin transporter gene – are at greater risk of depression at higher levels of stress and trauma exposure when compared with a person carrying one or two copies of the long allele. Most people of European descent carry the high-risk allele and are at higher risk of depression. However, studies show that carriers only develop depression if they are exposed to stressful and traumatic events, especially early in life. The same short

allele also is associated with greater amygdala activity, which is associated with PTSD (Munafo et al., 2008). The 5-HTTLPR short allele polymorphism is further associated with greater cortisol release to social stressors that include negative appraisals (Way and Taylor, 2010). There are genetic differences in other components of the hypothalamic pituitary adrenal axis and cortisol pathway that also appear to confer psychological risk versus resilience in the face of trauma (Binder et al., 2008). In a review by Caspi and colleagues (2010), 44 studies of GxE interaction for 5-HTTLRP were identified; nine of these studies examined childhood maltreatment as the environment stressor (Kohrt et al., 2015). Of the 44 studies in the review, 89 per cent had been conducted in HIC such as the United States, Australia and New Zealand. The only other countries including populations not of European descent were Japan (one study), Korea (two studies), China (one study), and Taiwan (one study), but they did not study child maltreatment. Of note, while the Asian studies represented only 11 per cent of studies reviewed, they represented 33 per cent of associations in the opposite direction of commonly reported pattern in the literature; that is, the long allele posed greater risk than the short allele (Zhang et al., 2009). Among the 5-HTTLRP studies, the Taiwanese sample showed a greater frequency of the short–short allele combination compared with European groups; they also carry an extra-long variant (XL), which is rare in European groups (Goldman et al., 2010). This raises questions about whether risk and resilience alleles may operate differently across cultural settings. Ultimately, one must be cautious in making any causative claims about ethnic differences in genetic polymorphisms, as there is more variation within ethnic and racial groups than between groups (Brown and Armelagos, 2001). Rather than focusing on static group differences, a life history approach will likely be the key to unlocking group and individual differences in PTSD. Yehuda (2009: 63) concludes her review of PTSD and cortisol biology by calling for more attention to 'developmental issues, the longitudinal course of the disorder, and individual differences that affect these processes'. The diversity of findings point toward multiple possible pathways to PTSD and a need for better evaluation of personal, contextual and cultural differences that may be reflected in biological differences (Kohrt et al., 2015).

Birth itself can be a risk factor, especially in war or disaster circumstances, where often poor prenatal

---

[5] For example, Wardenaar and de Jonge (2013) propose multimode principal component analysis and (mixture)-graphical modelling as promising techniques to solve the basic and enduring problem that classifications are heterogeneous clinical descriptions rather than valid diagnoses.

and perinatal care are compounded by the collapse of the public healthcare sector. Famine, starvation, nutritional deficiency, consanguineous marriages, environmental health hazards, postnatal brain infections (cerebral malaria, meningitis, parasites), head trauma, diarrhoeal diseases and respiratory infections may further negatively influence cognitive and bodily development both in utero and later in life. Family disruption, parental illness and death, possibly aggravated by the AIDS pandemic, can affect attachment, bonding, separation and socialization and contribute to anxiety, depression, PTSD, attachment disorders of childhood, and antisocial, borderline or traumatic personality development (such as complex PTSD). Difficult living conditions such as poor nutrition, hygiene and healthcare may lead to developmental problems in children. Excessive numbers of infants are born with congenital abnormalities, which probably result from maternal malnutrition during early foetal development. Developmental milestones are often significantly delayed, as shown e.g. among Afghan children (Prasad, 2006).

Psychosocial well-being of children can be affected by traumatic events and by daily stressors. Traumatic stressors may include war-related events, but also daily stressors: social and economic hardships in everyday life, related to physical ill health, malnutrition, crowding, unemployment, low wages, illiteracy and gender-based discrimination including domestic violence, community-level violence not directly related to war, social isolation and barriers to equitable access to health, educational and vocational resources (De Berry 2008; Panter-Brick *et al.* 2009; Ventevogel, 2016).

Thus, the call from public-health advocates for a population-based, youth-focused model, which explicitly integrates mental health with other health and welfare initiatives in low- and middle-income countries (Patel *et al.*, 2007a) is highly relevant. In short, prior to the onset or during episodes of political violence, the individual may be exposed to positive or negative life experiences that may either contribute to resiliency and post-traumatic growth, or to further vulnerability later in life. Post-traumatic growth manifests itself in an increased appreciation for life, more meaningful interpersonal relationships, an increased sense of personal strength, changed priorities, and a richer existential and spiritual life (Tedeschi and Calhoun, 2004; Aldwin and Levinson, 2004). The interaction of individual and ecological sources of resiliency, vulnerability and growth factors may result in a proneness to disorder and the development of disability. Alternatively, it may result in a more or less diversified repertoire of coping skills and generation of resources. This may, in turn, influence the ability of the individual to display agency and to survive in an adverse environment.

Culture, Trauma Symptoms and the Trajectory of Recovery

In the previous sections we have discussed that culture has important impacts on trauma symptoms and the trajectory of recovery. Within current models of stress in psychology and psychiatry, cultural factors modulate the relationship between the events, moderators, mediators and outcomes. Here, some examples of the influence of culture on an individual will be presented by following common stress models with a cultural lens (de Jong, 2002, 2004, 2007). Stress models primarily distinguish traumatic stressors as independent variables being appraised by an individual and resulting in psychological and psychiatric problems moderated and mediated by a range of protective and vulnerability factors, as well as other intervening variables. Common psychological disorders or more serious mental disorders are regarded as dependent variables, that in turn affect functioning, quality of life, personality growth or disability. Although these models have universal applicability, they can be enriched when we obtain more insight into the transformation of its components by the work of culture.

The Traumatic Stressor, Protective and Vulnerability Factors, Coping, Social Support and Expression of Distress and Disability

The DSM-5 (APA, 2013) narrowed the definition of what counts as a qualifying traumatic stressor.[6] But the perception of threat as traumatic varies across individuals and across cultures. One may even doubt if stressors are ever traumatic per se and argue that an event can only become traumatic after appraisal (as

---

[6] For one to qualify for indirect exposure to trauma, a person must learn that a close friend or family member has died violently or accidentally or has survived a threat to his or her life. Moreover, exposure to trauma via television or other electronic media no longer qualifies the viewer as a trauma survivor unless the exposure concerns the viewer's occupation (e.g. viewing scenes of carnage for an emergency personnel worker).

was mentioned in the DSM stressor criterion). For instance, was the premeditated loss of thousands of people on a single day on the ancient battlefields perceived as traumatic, and did this differ for those ordering the battle or the individuals surviving it? There is ongoing debate about the question whether the loss of a child is a universal stressor. Based on our experience with mothers across cultures who heard about the (impending) death of their child, we tend to regard the confrontation with the death of a child as a universal traumatic event. Similarly, Einarsdóttir (2004) argues that, despite high infant mortality, there is no normalization of child death among the Papel in Guinea Bissau. Our views contrast that of Schepers-Hughes (1992), who stated that high-infant mortality in Brazil protects mothers from suffering as compared to countries with low-infant mortality. In our view the mothers' wording of their previous loss during an anthropological encounter reflects a useful defence mechanism that may differ from their deep suffering when their child died. In contrast to the death of a child in Africa, the death of an older loved person who has children and some accumulated wealth is typically acceptable in sub-Saharan African cultures, since it is believed that the deceased will travel to the realm of the ancestors and occupy an intermediary position between the living and the dead.

A similar debate exists regarding loss of wealth. Higher levels of socio-economic status and education before forcible displacement are associated with worse mental health outcomes (Porter and Haslam, 2005). However, adult Tibetans did not perceive the loss of their personal possessions as traumatic, but rather the desecration of their religious symbols by the Chinese (Terheggen et al., 2001).

Both problem-focused and emotion-focused coping are influenced by culture and locality. When a Middle Eastern family realizes that a female member (wife, sister, daughter) is flirting with a man, the event can be devastating to the family honour and result in revenge killing. It is the culture-bound appraisal of the flirting, regarded as innocent in other cultures, which evokes emotions that result in culturally prescribed action. If a man thus loses control of female family members, his *namus* is lost in the eyes of the community and he has to cleanse his (and his family's) honour. This is often done by abortion, murder, or forced suicide or immolition. This example illustrates how coping, protective and vulnerability factors can depend on cultural context. The concept of honour may function as a protective factor in the context of Middle Eastern cultures by promoting endogamy, chasteness and peaceful coexistence of families and clans. The culturally prescribed revenge killing related to the appraisal of loss of honour can result in positive coping in the Middle East, while the same behaviour may be a negative coping style resulting in social exclusion or imprisonment in a Western multicultural setting. Likewise, war veterans or former combatants may have developed coping styles that are appropriate in conflict areas but that may be far less appropriate when they return home from a combat mission. Or refugees needing asocial coping styles to deal with deprivation or human traffickers, styles that do not always fit their country of arrival. Once coping strategies and resources are identified and understood, preventive interventions may be developed. These interventions often regard multilevel and multisectoral approaches involving, for example, health, education, justice, rural or community development, as well as economic, social and cultural rights.

Grief is an essential task of survivors and provides another example of the influence of culture on coping. There are several dimensions distinguishing cultures regarding grief and bereavement. High-income countries use concepts such as grief counselling or terminal care. In contrast, in LIC, people's attention is especially focused on varying supernatural beliefs (a) that the dead communicate with the living, (b) that other people's supernatural abilities such as witchcraft can cause death, (c) that the ghost of the deceased will take revenge if one does not complete proper rituals for the deceased, for example, in cases of suicide or homicide as often happens in conflict settings or ethnic cleansing, (d) that verbalizing the name of the deceased is dangerous, (e) that a newborn is a reincarnation of a deceased person, (f) that hearing or seeing the deceased person is normal, and (g) that tie-breaking customs are useful to cope with loss (de Jong and Van Schaik, 1994; Hinton et al., 2013b; Irish et al., 1993; Parkes et al., 1997; Rosenblatt et al., 1976). Anger toward the deceased is another difference in grief between African, African Caribbean and Euro-American cultures. The common Christian habit is to encourage saying nothing but good about the dead, possibly hindering the expression of negative feelings toward the dead. In African and African Caribbean cultures, the expression of emotions such as anger towards the deceased is often permitted in a ritual context. This may be done in a benign and mocking way, since the family needs the help of the deceased who just rose to the status of ancestor, to cope with life. Later, this ancestor may transmit messages through an elected person whom we might regard as hallucinating but who in the local culture is often perceived to be called to become a healer. Nevertheless, local culture often deals in a ruthless way with that same anger and despair by accusing the living of causing the death of a family member. The accusation of magic manipulation may involve parents being accused of the death of their own child thus impeding a normal grief process. It seems that the anger caused by death is expressed in a highly ambivalent way. Both the deceased and his or her family members or co-villagers may become the target of a witchcraft or sorcery accusation. The accusation may correspond with pre-death conflicts or be in line with structural tensions such as that between generations, sexes, co-wives or differences in wealth (de Jong and Reis, 2013).

As mentioned before, the nature of the *expression* or the *presentation* of distress and suffering in response to threats also varies across cultures. Working in postwar circumstances in West Africa, presentation of PTSD symptoms was rare, while patients regularly presented stiff or contracting catatonic bodies, accompanied by bouts of shouting and twisting movements of body parts. These expressions were local idioms of distress in the guise of dissociative reactions reminiscent of scenes of 1890s Salpêtrière. From a cross-cultural perspective, it is interesting that one often still comes across expressions of psychopathology in low- and middle-income countries that have gradually disappeared in the West over the past 100 years. The expression of feelings, often related to abuse or repression of women, greatly varies and evolves over time, resulting in dissociative states such as classical 'hysteric' attacks, spirit possession, conversion (blindness, aphonia), or psychogenic convulsive attacks. An additional problem in diagnosing psychopathology across cultures is that the reactions to trauma are often expressed in narratives that express distress along with explanatory models. Moreover, these narratives are often intertwined with the cultural transitions and losses that confront the survivors resulting in acculturative stress, culture shock and cultural bereavement (Eisenbruch, 1984).

In low-income settings families are often the main provider of social support, social capital and mental well-being. As such, families are a protective factor when a person is confronted with extreme stress. Norris and Kaniasty (1996) showed that, after mass trauma, initial periods of a high degree of social support are followed by a quick deterioration of the

support system under the pressure of overuse and the need for individuals to get on with their lives. This problem is compounded when many adults die due to war or AIDS, or when families seek refuge in the houses of other family members, turning a large extended family into a vulnerability factor (de Jong, 2004: 166).

Another relevant cross-cultural domain is the careful interpretation of concepts such as dysfunction, disability, impairment or quality of life. This may happen when researchers apply the WHO Disability Assessment Schedule (WHO DASII) or the WHO International Classification of Functioning, Disability and Health (WHO ICF) across cultures, among adults or youth (de Jong and van Ommeren, 2002; Jordans *et al.*, 2009; Tol *et al.*, 2011a; Tol *et al.*, 2010; Von Korff *et al.*, 2008). The United Nations (2006) explicitly defines disability not as the attribute of a person, but as a product of the interaction of people with functional impairments and environmental factors, including social support. Likewise, population attributable risk proportion (PARP), and disability-adjusted life years (DALYs) are measures of illness burden in global health. The global health movement and health economists use DALYs as a metric allowing for direct comparisons between interventions.[7] DALYs are often mentioned to illustrate the importance of the burden of the mental, neurological, or substance misuse (MNS) disorders that constitute 13 per cent of the global burden of disease, surpassing both cardiovascular disease and cancer (Collins *et al.*, 2011; Patel *et al.*, 2007b; WHO, 2006). However, DALYs – and the same applies to PARP – are often used as if they are carved in stone; as if they are definitive indicators of health or mental health status, whereas they should be considered only as rough measures of various conditions. One of the methodological questions associated with these measures is how to weigh the degree to which a person suffers from a particular disability or disorder, taking age, gender and socio-cultural context into account. Minor differences in parameter choices may change the number of DALYs associated with a condition by a few per cent or by as much as a factor of two

---

[7] The DALY gauges the disvalue of health conditions by the number of years of life lost due to the condition plus the number of years lived with disability multiplied by a number representing the severity of the disability. The PARP can be interpreted as the proportion of instances of the outcome that would not have occurred in the absence of the predictor disorders.

(Glassman and Chalkidou, 2012). Moreover, like other forms of 'hard evidence' focused on individual outcomes, the DALY does not address the syndemics of disability's impact on a household or community, or the interplay with socio-economic factors or often occurring comorbidities of physical and mental conditions. A mixed methods approach may help researchers assess the interpersonal, cultural, and temporal variation of the disability metrics by engaging the perspective of those who suffer from a condition (de Jong, 2014). In other words, most (in)dependent and intervening variables in current stress models are heavily influenced by the work of culture.

The individual level of perceiving and dealing with threats interacts with the collective level of the traumascape. The collective level operates its influence through schemata defined as structured cognitive representations of sets of rules of human populations. Culture-based schemata are part of the traumascape. Schemata are dynamic and provide a means for cultural prototypes to be revised as a function of individual experience (Rumelhart et al., 1986; Chemtob, 1996). We will limit ourselves to schemes related to recovery and healing, and to religious and political conviction.

Schemes on Recovery and Healing

Psychiatrists and psychologists tend to apply cognitive or other psychotherapeutic interventions based on Western concepts of autonomy and individualization. This may be out of place among patients with other views of the ego and the self, living in collective, socio-centric societies that promote interdependency. In these cultures, Western interventions promoting assertiveness or autonomy may be perceived as selfish. On the other hand, Western professionals may diagnose interdependency or taking others' opinions into account as a tendency towards dependent or avoidant traits or a personality disorder. Two major impediments to the implementation of appropriate psychosocial and mental healthcare programmes are the Janus faces of stigma and dogma. Stigma schemes around deviant behaviour may be a major impediment to develop interventions in the local culture. Stigma may shift over time. For example, in the past decade stigmatizing witchcraft accusations in Africa have shifted to children who at times were killed, because they allegedly machinated the plight of the local population. Dogma about the appropriateness of certain interventions among helpers may equally influence the local traumascape. For example,

Western helpers may have non-founded views about the effectiveness of all kinds of interventions, ranging from culturally non-adapted versions of EMDR, CBT, family interventions or testimony methods to new-age therapies. Or, they may cherish religious, proselytizing or other dogmas that are incompatible with the world views or the problems of those they want to assist. Over the last decade, a major step forward has been the development of a series of guidelines and books on providing psychosocial and mental healthcare by the UN, WHO, consortia of NGOs and professional societies. These guidelines are obligatory reading for anyone who wishes to enter the 'trauma field', due to the heterogeneity of traumatic events, the lack of empirical support for specific interventions, or the need for adaptations of interventions to local needs and culture (de Jong and Clarke, 1996; de Jong, 2002; Weine et al., 2002; Green et al., 2003; Eisenman et al., 2006; IASC, 2007, 2015; WHO, 2013).

A global expert panel gained consensus on empirically supported intervention principles that cover the period for several months after a disaster (Hobfoll et al., 2007). The principles consist of schemes of recovery and healing.

1. Safety on an individual, family, group and community level to prevent situations where reminders contribute to an ongoing sense of exaggerated fear. It includes safety from bad news and rumours (Bryant, 2006; Ehlers and Clark, 2000).

2. Calming of extreme emotions through interventions such as breathing retraining, muscle relaxation or mindfulness, through a 'normalization' of stress reactions by survivor education about reactions, and by fostering positive emotions including joy and humour.

3. A sense of self and community efficacy, reinforced by practising increasingly difficult situations in which increments of success build to a reality-based appraisal of efficacy which supports calming as well.

4. Connectedness, increasing appropriate knowledge, providing social support activities such as problem-solving, sharing of experience and emotional understanding, and mutual instruction about coping. Research indicates that social support is related to better emotional well-being and recovery. Therefore, interventions have to identify those who lack social support and who are socially isolated and promote social support

networks in communities (de Jong, 2002). Tangible support is often of critical importance in community mental health interventions. In India, for example, advice by community health workers about women's shelters and legal rights was found to be as essential an element of an intervention for severely depressed women as the use of antidepressants (Chatterjee *et al.*, 2008). However, one has to remain sensitive to the potential for social undermining based on racial, ethnic and tribal divisions.

5. Hope or the expectation that a positive future outcome is possible. Hope for most people in the world has a religious connotation and is not action-orientated (Antonovsky, 1979). Hope is often ambivalent, for example when children are expected to advance the economic situation of a household, thus bearing the burden of such expectations. In LMIC where a whole generation has endured human rights violations or war (e.g. Afghanistan, Burma, Burundi, Cambodia, Kashmir, Tibet, Sri Lanka, Vietnam, Angola, Sudan), people often seem to have hope-inspired internal resources that are beyond the imagination of many middle-class Westerners.

Political and Religious Conviction

Political and religious convictions are equally part of the traumascape and moderate the processing of distress. Political conviction can mediate grief or mourning, as has been described in, for example, Gaza (Qouta, 2000; Qouta and El-Sarraj, 2002; de Jong, 2004). Similarly to Albanian Kosovar families, Middle Eastern groups including adherents of terrorism, often regard their deceased family members as martyrs. These views can, on the one hand, alleviate loss, while, on the other hand, complicate the mourning process since the family that is applauded for having given a martyr for the common cause may find it difficult to sense its loss and express its grief. A child soldier may be regarded as a human-rights violator, or, alternatively, as a hero who helps his family to survive in harsh economic times. A rehabilitation programme must formulate its objectives and interventions depending on the child soldier's local context. For instance, vocational skills training appeared to be a suitable strategy to reintegrate child soldiers in Burundi but not in northern Uganda where their newly acquired skills were already widely available in the local economy.

The effect of trauma can be mediated by religious convictions, such as the role of karma in Buddhism in Asia, explaining, for example, the plight of the Cambodian people under the Khmer Rouge regime as the punishment for previously generated karma, or by divine persecution during the Holocaust (Abramson, 2000; Van de Put and Eisenbruch, 2002). Or in Africa or the Caribbean, deceased ancestors are often considered to continue to play an active role in the lives of their offspring, and maintaining a good reciprocal relationship is therefore considered important. In many countries, when it is impossible to do mortuary rites for a person (e.g. burial or cremation rites) because the body was never found, or person's whereabouts remain unknown, the mourning process can be disturbed (Hinton *et al.*, 2013b). The spirits of the dead who are not properly buried can cause all kinds of misfortune.

Conclusion

As we have described, culture-based schemata and practices have a profound effect on the trajectory of trauma. From prehistoric times onwards cultures have developed coping strategies to deal with extreme stress. Each era and culture expresses the consequences in semantics, explanatory models, and idioms of distress, and develops ways of healing that fit its cosmology. Ever-changing traumascapes show that there are universal similarities and major differences that constitute the 'human' responses to trauma. In this chapter, the concepts of traumasyndemics and the traumascape were presented as theoretical concepts to explore the complex global and local interactions among vital systems that determine how an individual, a society, and a culture respond to emergencies that make up the daily life of many. Other key concepts were also presented like that of network models and that of content and experiential validity. The traumascape model (Figure 29.2) presented in this chapter provides a framework for scholars to study the dynamic interactions of culture, history, social ecology and politics. The factors described in the model contribute to the understanding of vulnerability and resiliency of population groups and individuals. The components of the model will guide us in describing the variety of expressions of human suffering and the way cultures, and individual and families within those cultures, try to cope. The model may also guide us to develop policies and practices and effective interventions to deal with extreme stress.

References

Abramson, H. (2000). The esh kodesh of rabbi Kalonimus Kalmish Shapiro: a Hasidic treatise on communal trauma from the Holocaust. *Transcultural Psychiatry*, 37(3), 321–335.

Aldwin, C. M. and Levinson, M. R. (2004). Posttraumatic growth: a developmental perspective. *Psychological Inquiry*, 15(1), 19–52.

Allen, T. (1991). Understanding Alice: Uganda's holy spirit movement in context. *Africa*, 61, 370–400.

Alonso, J., Chatterji, S., He, Y. (2013). The burdens of mental disorders. In *Global Perspectives from the WHO World Mental Health Surveys*, ed. J. Alonso, S. Chatterji, Y. He. New York: Cambridge University Press.

American Psychiatric Association (2013). *Diagnostic and Statistical Manual of Mental Disorders: DSM-5*. Washington DC: AMA.

Antonovsky, A. (1979). *Health, Stress and Coping*. San Francisco: Jossey-Bass.

Appadurai, A. (1996). *Modernity at Large: Cultural Dimensions of Globalization*. Public Worlds Volume 1. Minneapolis: University of Minnesota Press.

Asay, T. R. and Lambert, M. J. (1999).The empirical case for the common factors in therapy: quantitative findings, in *The Heart and Soul of Change: What Works in Therapy*, ed. M. A. Hubble, B. L. Duncan and S. D. Miller, Washington DC: American Psychological Association, pp. 23–55.

Baines, E. K. (2007). The haunting of Alice: local approaches to justice and reconciliation in northern Uganda. *The International Journal of Transitional Justice*, 1, 91–114.

Barlow, D. H. (1988). *Anxiety and its Disorders*. New York, NY: Guilford.

Bartholomew, R. and Sirois, F. (2000). Occupational mass psychogenic illness: a transcultural perspective. *Transcultural Psychiatry*, 37, 495–524.

Basu, H. (2009). Contested practices of control: psychiatric and religious mental health care in India. *Curare*, 32(1+2), 28–39.

Ben-Ezra, M. (2003). Flashbacks and PTSD. *The British Journal of Psychiatry*, 183, 75.

Bernal, G., Bonilla, J., Bellido, C. (1995). Ecological validity and cultural sensitivity for outcome research: issues for the cultural adaptation and development of psychosocial treatments with Hispanics. *Journal of Abnormal Child Psychology*, 23, 1, 67–82.

Bhui, K., Abdi, A., Abdi, M., Pereira, S., Dualeh, M., Robertson, G., Sathyamoorthy, G. and Ismail, H. (2003). Traumatic events, migration characteristics and psychiatric symptoms among Somali refugees. *Social Psychiatry and Psychiatric Epidemiology*, 38, 35–43.

Binder, E. B. and Nemeroff, C. B. (2010). The CRF system, stress, depression and anxiety: insights from human genetic studies. *Molecular Psychiatry*, 15, 574–588.

Binder, E. B., Bradley, R. G., Wei Liu, M. P. *et al.* (2008). Association of FKBP5 polymorphisms and childhood abuse with risk of posttraumatic stress disorder symptoms in adults. *Journal of the American Medical Association*, 299(11), 1291–1305.

Boehnlein, J. K. and Hinton, D. E. (2016). From shell shock to PTSD and traumatic brain injury: a historical perspective on responses to combat trauma. In *Culture and PTSD: Trauma in Historical and Global Perspective*, ed. D. E. Hinton and B. J. Good. Pennsylvania: University of Pennsylvania Press, pp. 161–176.

Bolton, P. (2001). Local perceptions of the mental health effects of the Rwandan genocide. *Journal of Nervous and Mental Disease*, 189, 243–248.

Borsboom, D., Cramer, A. O. J., Schmittmann, V. D., Epskamp, S., Waldorp, L. J. (2011). The small world of psychopathology. *PloS One*, 6(11), e27407.

Borsboom, D. and Cramer, A. O. J. (2013). Network analysis: an integrative approach to the structure of psychopathology. *Annual Review of Clinical Psychology*, 9, 91–121.

Breslau, Joshua (2004). Cultures of trauma: anthropological views of posttraumatic stress disorders in international health. *Culture, Medicine and Psychiatry*, 28(2), 113–126.

Breslau, Naomi and Kessler, Ronald C. (2001). The stressor criterion in DSM-IV posttraumatic stress disorder: an empirical investigation. *Biological Psychiatry*, 50, 699–704.

Brewin, C. R., Andrews, B. and Valentine, J. D. (2000). Meta-analysis of risk factors for posttraumatic stress disorder in trauma-exposed adults. *Journal of Consulting and Clinical Psychology*, 68(5), 748–766.

Brown, Ryan A. and Armelagos, George J. (2001). Apportionment of racial diversity: a review. *Evolutionary Anthropology*, 10(1), 34–40.

Bryant, R. A. (2006). Cognitive behavior therapy: implications from advances in neuroscience. In *PTSD: Brain Mechanisms and Clinical Implications*, ed. N. Kato, M. Kawata and R. K. Pitman. Tokyo: Springer, pp. 255–270.

Bryant, R. A. (2010). The complexity of complex PTSD. *American Journal of Psychiatry*, 167, 879–881.

Bryant, R. A. (2012). Simplifying complex PTSD: comment on Resick *et al. Journal of Traumatic Stress*, 25, 252–253.

Caspi, A., Sugden, K., Moffitt, T. E et al. (2003). Influence of life stress on depression: moderation by a polymorphism in the 5-HTT gene. *Science*, 301(5631), 386–389.

Caspi, Avshalom, Hariri, Ahmad, R., Holmes, Andrew, Uher, Rudolf and Moffitt, Terrie E. (2010). Genetic sensitivity to the environment: the case of the serotonin transporter gene and its implications for studying complex diseases and traits. *American Journal of Psychiatry* **167**(5), 509–527.

Charuvastra, A. and Cloitre, M. (2008). Social bonds and posttraumatic stress disorder. *Annual Review of Psychology*, **59**, 301–328.

Chatterjee, S., Chowdhary, N., Pednekar, S. *et al.* (2008). Integrating evidence-based treatments for common mental disorders in routine primary care: feasibility and acceptability of the MANAS intervention in Goa, India. *World Psychiatry*, 7, 39–46.

Chemtob, C. M. (1996). Posttraumatic stress disorder, trauma and culture. In *International Review of Psychiatry*, ed. F. Mak and C. Nadelson, vol. II. Washington DC: American Psychiatric Press, pp. 257–292.

Collier, Paul (2008). Global policies for the bottom billion. In *A Progressive Agenda for Global Action*. London: Policy Network, pp. 141–150.

Collins, P. Y., Patel, V., Joestl, S. S., March, D., Insel, T. R., Daar, A. S. (2011). Grand challenges in global mental health. *Nature*, **475**, 27–30.

Daar, A. S., Singer, P. A., Persad, D. L. *et al.* (2007). Grand challenges in chronic non-communicable diseases. *Nature*, 450, 494–496.

Dean, E. T. (1997). *Shook over Hell: Post-Traumatic Stress, Vietnam, and the Civil War.* Cambridge, MA: Harvard University Press, pp. 101–114.

De Berry, J. (2008). The challenges of programming with youth in Afghanistan. In *Years of Conflict: Adolescence, Political Violence and Displacement*, ed. J. Hart. New York: Berghahn, pp. 209–229.

De Jong, J. T. V. M. (2002).Trauma, war, and violence: *Public Mental Health in Socio-Cultural Context.* New York, NY: Kluwer Academic.

De Jong, Joop T. V. M. (2004). Public mental health and culture: disasters as a challenge to Western mental health care models, the self, and PTSD. In *Broken Spirits: The Treatment of Asylum Seekers and Refugees with PTSD*, ed. John P. Wilson and Boris Drozdek. New York: Brunner/Routledge Press, pp. 159–179.

De Jong, J. T. V. M. (2005a). Deconstructing critiques on the internationalization of PTSD. *Culture, Medicine and Psychiatry*, **29**, 361–370.

De Jong, Joop T. V. M. (2005b). Cultural variation in the clinical presentation of sleep paralysis. *Transcultural Psychiatry*, **42**(1), 78–92.

De Jong, J. T. V. M. (2007). Traumascape: an ecological–cultural–historical model for extreme stress. In *Textbook of Cultural Psychiatry*, ed. D. Bhugra and K. Bhui. Cambridge: Cambridge University Press, pp. 347–364.

De Jong, J. T. V. M. (2010). A public health framework to translate risk factors related to political violence and war into multilevel preventive interventions. *Social Science and Medicine*, **70**, 71–79.

De Jong, J. T. V. M. (2011). (Disaster) public mental health. In *Trauma and Mental Health: Resilience and Posttraumatic Disorders*, ed. D. J. Stein, M. J. Friedman, C. Blanco. London: Wiley-Blackwell, pp. 217–262.

De Jong, J. T. V. M. (2014). Challenges of creating synergy between global mental health and cultural psychiatry. *Transcultural Psychiatry*, **51**(6), 806–828, doi: 10.1177/1363461514557995.

De Jong, J. T. V. M. and Clarke, L. (eds) (1996). Mental Health of Refugees. World Health Organization, Geneva. Available online at http://whqlibdoc.who.int/hq/1996/a49374.pdf. (Available in, e.g. Arabic, Dutch, English, French, Khmer, Nepali, Portuguese, Spanish, Tamil, Tigrinha.)

De Jong, J. and Colijn, S. (2010). *Handboek culturele psychiatrie en psychotherapie*. Utrecht: de Tijdstroom.

De Jong, J. T. V. M. and Reis, R. (2010). Kiyang-yang, a West-African post-war idiom of distress. *Culture, Medicine and Psychiatry*, **34**(2), 301–321.

De Jong, J. T. V. M. and Reis, R. (2013). Collective trauma processing: dissociation as a way of processing postwar traumatic stress in Guinea Bissau. *Trancultural Psychiatry*, **50**(5) 644–661.

De Jong, J. T. V. M., and van Ommeren, M. H. (2002). Toward a culture-informed epidemiology: combining qualitative and quantitative research in transcultural contexts. *Transcultural Psychiatry*, **39**, 422–433.

De Jong, J. T. V. M. and Van Schaik, M. M. (1994). Cultural and religious aspects of coping with trauma after the Bijlmer disaster (in Dutch). *Tijdschrift voor Psychiatrie*, **36**(4), 291–304.

De Jong, J. T. V. M., Komproe, I. H., van Ommeren, M., El Masri, M., Araya, M., Khaled, N., van de Put, W. and Somasundaram, D. (2001). Lifetime events and posttraumatic stress disorder in four postconflict settings. *Journal of the American Medical Association*, **286**(5), 555–562.

De Jong, Joop T., Komproe, Ivan H., Spinazzola, Joseph, van der Kolk, Bessel A. and van Ommeren, Mark H. (2005). DESNOS in three postconflict settings: assessing cross-cultural construct equivalence. *Journal of Traumatic Stress*, **18**, 13–21.

De Jong, J. T. V. M., Berckmoes, L. H., Kohrt, B. A., Song, S. J., Tol, W. A., Reis, R. (2015). A public health approach to address the mental health burden of youth in situations of political violence and humanitarian emergencies. *Child and Family Disaster Psychiatry*, **17**(7), doi: 10.1007/s11920-015-0590-0.

Delawar, A. (2016). Personal research communication.

Dutta, R., Greene, T., Addington, J., McKenzie, K., Phillips, M., and Murray, R. M. (2007). Biological, life course, and cross-cultural studies all point toward the value of dimensionaland developmental ratings in the classification of psychosis. *Schizophrenia Bulletin*, **33**, 868–876.

Dwyer, G. (2003). *The Divine and the Demonic. Supernatural Affliction and its Treatment in North India.* London: Routledge Curzon.

Ehlers, A. and Clark, D. M. (2000). A cognitive model of PTSD. *Behaviour Research and Therapy*, **38**, 319–345.

Einarsdóttir, J. (2004). *Tired of Weeping. Mother Love, Child Death, and Poverty in Guinea Bissau*, 2nd edn. Wisconsin: University of Wisconsin Press.

Eisenberg, L. (1977). Disease and illness: distinctions between professional and popular ideas of sickness. *Culture, Medicine and Psychiatry*, **1**, 9–23.

Eisenbruch, M. (1984). Cross-cultural aspects of bereavement: I, II. A conceptual framework for comparative analysis. *Culture, Medicine and Psychiatry*, **8**(3), 283–309 and (4) 315–347.

Eisenman, D. P., Green, B. L., de Jong, J. *et al.* (2006). Guidelines on mental health training of primary care providers for trauma exposed populations. *Journal of Traumatic Stress*, **19**(1), 5–17.

Evans, Katie, McGrath, J. and Milns, R. (2003). Searching for schizophrenia in ancient Greek and Roman literature: a systematic review. *Acta Psychiatrica Scandinavica*, **107**, 323–30.

Evans, S. C., Reed, G. M., Roberts, M. C., Esparza, P., Watts, A. D., Mendonca Correia, J., Saxena, S. (2013). Psychologists' perspectives on the diagnostic classification of mental disorders: results from the WHO-IUPsyS Global Survey. *International Journal of Psychology*, **48**(3), 177–193.

Fazel, M., Wheeler, J., Danesh, J. (2005). Prevalence of serious mental disorder in 7000 refugees resettled in Western countries: a systematic review. *The Lancet*, **365**, 1309–1314.

Fernando, S. (2014). *Mental Health Worldwide: Culture, Globalization and Development.* Basingstoke: Palgrave Macmillan.

Foa, Edna B., Keane, Terence M., Friedman, Matthew J. and Cohen, Judith A. (eds) (2009). *Effective Treatments for PTSD: Practice Guidelines from the International Society for Traumatic Stress Studies.* New York: Guilford Press.

Fox, S. H. (2003). The Mandinka nosological system in the context of post-trauma syndromes. *Transcultural Psychiatry*, **40**, 488–506.

Friedman, Matthew J., Keane, Terence M. and Resick, Patricia A. (2014). *Handbook of PTSD: Science and Practice.* New York: Guilford Press.

Geffray, C. (1990). *La Cause des armes au Mozambique. Anthropologie d'une guerre civile.* Paris: Karthala.

Glassman, A. and Chalkidou, K. (2012). Priority-setting in health: building institutions for smarter public spending.

Center for Global Development. Available online at www.cgdev.org/publication/priority-setting-health-building-institutions-smarter-public-spending (accessed August 2 2017).

Gobodo-Madikizela, P. and van der Merwe, C. (2009). *Memory, Narrative, and Forgiveness: Perspectives on the Unfinished Journeys of the Past.* Newcastle upon Tyne: Cambridge Scholars.

Goldman, Noreen, Glei, Dana A., Lin, Yu-Hsuan and Weinstein, Maxine (2010). The serotonin transporter polymorphism (5-HTTLPR): allelic variation and links with depressive symptoms. *Depression and Anxiety* **27**(3), 260–269.

Green, B., Friedman, M., Jong, de J. *et al.* (eds) (2003). *Trauma Interventions in War and Peace: Prevention, Practice, and Policy.* New York: Plenum-Kluwer.

Hagengimana, Athanase, and Hinton, Devon E. (2009). Ihahamuka, a Rwandan syndrome of response to the genocide: blocked flow, spirit assault, and shortness of breath. In *Culture and Panic Disorder*, ed. Devon E. Hinton and Byron J. Good. Stanford, CA: Stanford University Press, pp. 205–229.

Hare, Edward (1988). Schizophrenia as a recent disease. *British Journal of Psychiatry*, **153**, 521–531.

Hassan, G., Kirmayer, L. J., Mekki-Berrada A. *et al.* (2015). *Culture, Context and the Mental Health and Psychosocial Wellbeing of Syrians: A Review for Mental Health and Psychosocial Support Staff Working with Syrians Affected by Armed Conflict.* Geneva: UNHCR.

Heflin, C. M., Siefert, K., Williams, D. R. (2005). Food insufficiency and women's mental health: findings from a 3-year panel of welfare recipients. *Social Science and Medicine*, **61**(9), 1971–1982.

Heim, Christine, D., Newport, Jeffrey, Heit, Stacey *et al.* (2000). Pituitary, adrenal and autonomic responses to stress in women after sexual and physical abuse in childhood. *Journal of the American Medical Association*, **284**, 592–597.

Helman, C. G. (2007). *Culture, Health and Illness*, 5th edn. London: Hodder Arnold.

Helzer, J. E., Kraemer, H. C., Krueger, R. F., Wittchen, H. U., Sirovatka, P. J. and Regier, D. A. (2007). *Dimensional Approaches in Diagnostic Classifications. Refining the Research Agenda for DSM-5.* Arlington, VA: American Psychiatric Association.

Hinton, D. E. and Good, B. J. (eds) (2009). *Culture and Panic Disorder.* Palo Alto, CA: Stanford University Press.

Hinton, D. E. and Good, B. J. (eds) (2016). *Culture and PTSD: Trauma in Historical and Global Perspective.* Pennsylvania: University of Pennsylvania Press.

Hinton, D. E., and Good, B. J. (2016). The culturally sensitive assessment of trauma: eleven analytic perspectives, a typology of errors, and the multiplex models of distress generation. In *Culture and PTSD:*

Trauma in Historical and Global Perspective, ed. D. E. Hinton and B. J. Good. Pennsylvania: University of Pennsylvania Press, pp. 50–113.

Hinton, Devon E. and Lewis-Fernández, Roberto (2011). The cross-cultural validity of posttraumatic stress disorder: implications for DSM-5. *Depression and Anxiety*, **28**, 783–801.

Hinton, D. E. and Simons, N. (2015). Somatization, anxiety disorders (GAD, panic disorder, and PTSD), and the arousal complex in cultural context: the multiplex model and the cultural neuroscience of anxiety disorders. In *Revisioning Psychiatry: Cultural Phenomenology, Critical Neuroscience, and Global Mental Health*, ed. L. J. Kirmayer, R. Lemelson and C. Cummings. Cambridge: Cambridge University Press, pp. 343–374.

Hinton, Devon E., Pich, Vuth, Chhean, Dara, Pollack, Mark H. and McNally, Richard J. (2005). Sleep paralysis among Cambodian refugees: association with PTSD diagnosis and severity. *Depression and Anxiety*, **22**, 47–51.

Hinton, D. E., Hofmann, S. G., Orr, S. P. *et al.* (2010). A psychobiocultural model of orthostatic panic among Cambodian refugees: flashbacks, catastrophic cognitions, and reduced orthostatic blood-pressure response. *Psychological Trauma: Theory, Research, Practice and Policy*, **2**, 63–70.

Hinton, Devon E., Hinton, Alexander L., Eng, Kok-Thay and Choung, Sophearith (2012). PTSD and key somatic complaints and cultural syndromes among rural Cambodians: the results of a needs assessment survey. *Medical Anthropology Quarterly*, **29**, 147–154.

Hinton, Devon E., Kredlow, Alexandra M., Pich, Vuth, Bui, Eric and Hofmann, Stefan G. (2013a). The relationship of PTSD to key somatic complaints and cultural syndromes among Cambodian refugees attending a psychiatric clinic: the Cambodian somatic symptom and syndrome inventory (SSI). *Transcultural Psychiatry*, **50**, 347–370.

Hinton, D. E., Peou, S., Joshi, S., Nickerson, A. and Simon, N. (2013b). Normal grief and complicated bereavement among traumatized Cambodian refugees: cultural context and the central role of dreams of the deceased. *Culture, Medicine and Psychiatry*, **37**, 427–464.

Hinton, D. E., Reis, R. and de Jong, J. T. (2016a). The 'thinking a lot' idiom of distress and PTSD: an examination of their relationship among traumatized Cambodian refugees using the 'Thinking a Lot' Questionnaire. *Medical Anthropology Quarterly*, **29**, 357–380.

Hinton, D. E., Reis, R., de Jong, J. T. (2016b). A transcultural model of the centrality of 'thinking a lot' in psychopathologies across the globe and the process of localization: a Cambodian refugee example. *Culture, Medicine and Psychiatry*, **40**(4), 570–617.

Hobfoll, S. E., Watson, P., Bell, C. C., *et al.* (2007). Five essential elements of immediate and mid-term mass trauma intervention: empirical evidence. *Psychiatry*, **70**(4), 283–315.

Honwana, A. (2003). Undying past: spirit possession and the memory of war in southern Mozambique. In *Magic and Modernity: Interfaces of Revelation and Concealment*, ed. B. Meyer and P. Pels. Stanford, CA: Stanford University Press, pp. 60–80.

Horn, R. (2009). Coping with displacement: problems and responses in camps for the internally displaced in Kitgum, northern Uganda. *Intervention*, 7, 110–129.

Horowitz, M. J. (2007). Understanding and ameliorating revenge fantasies in psychotherapy. *The American Journal of Psychiatry*, **164**(1), 24–27.

Horwitz, A. V. (2007). Distinguishing distress from disorder as psychological outcomes of stressful social arrangements. *Health*, **11**, 273–289.

IASC (2007). *IASC Guidelines on Mental Health and Psychosocial Support in Emergency Settings*. Geneva: IASC.

IASC (2010). *IASC Guidelines on Mental Health and Psychosocial Support in Emergency Settings*. Geneva: IASC.

IASC Reference Group for Mental Health and Psychosocial Support (2015). *Review of the Implementation of the IASC Guidelines on Mental Health and Psychosocial Support in Emergency Settings*. Geneva: IASC.

Igreja, V., Dias-Lambranca, B., Hershey, D. A., Racin, L., Richters, A. and Reis, R. (2010). The epidemiology of spirit possession in the aftermath of mass political violence in Mozambique. *Social Science and Medicine*, **71**, 592–599.

Insel, T. (2015). Director's Blog. Available online at www.nimh.nih.gov/about/director/bio/publications/psychiatric-epidemiology.shtml accessed 5 November, 2015.

Irish, D. P., Lundquist, K. F. and Nelsen, V. J. (eds) (1993). *Ethnic Variation in Dying, Death and Grief: Diversity in Universality*. Washington DC: Taylor and Francis.

Jones, E., and Wessely, S. (2005). *Shell Shock to PTSD: Military Psychiatry from 1900 to the Gulf War*. Hove, East Sussex: Psychology Press.

Jones, E., Hodgins Verrmaas, R., McCartney, H. *et al.* (2003). Flashbacks and post-traumatic stress disorder: the genesis of a 20th-century diagnosis. *British Journal of Psychiatry*, **182**, 158–163.

Jordans, M. J. D., Komproe, I. H., Tol, W. A. and de Jong, J. T. V. M. (2009). Screening for psychosocial distress amongst war affected children: cross-cultural construct validity of the CPDS. *Journal of Child Psychology and Psychiatry*, **4**, 514–523.

Kakar, S. (1983). *Shamans, Mystics and Healers. A Psychological Enquiry into India and its Healing Traditions*. Oxford: Oxford University Press.

Karam, E. G., Friedman, Matthew J., Hill, Eric D. *et al.* (2014). Cumulative traumas and risk thresholds: 12-month PTSD in the World Mental Health (WMH) Surveys. *Depression and Anxiety*, **31**(2), 130–142.

Kendell, R. E. (1989). Clinical validity. *Psychological Medicine*, **19**, 45–55.

Kendell, R. and Jablensky, A. (2003). Distinguishing between the validity and utility of psychiatric diagnoses. *American Journal of Psychiatry*, **160**, 4–12.

Kendler, K., Zachar, P., Craver, C. (2011). What kinds of things are psychiatric disorders? *Psychological Medicine*, **41**(6), 1143.

Kessler, R. C. (2000). Posttraumatic stress disorder: the burden to the individual and to society. *Journal of Clinical Psychiatry*, **61**(suppl 5), 4–12.

Kinzie, J. D., Denney, D., Riley, C. *et al.* (1998). A cross-cultural study of reactivation of posttraumatic stress disorder symptoms: American and Cambodian psychophysiological response to viewing traumatic video scenes. *Journal of Nervous and Mental Disorders*, **186**, 670–676.

Kleinman, A. M. (1980). *Patients and Healers in the Context of Culture*. Berkeley: University of California Press.

Kleinman, A. and Good, B. (eds) (1985). *Culture and Depression. Studies in the Anthropology and Cross-Cultural Psychiatry of Affect and Disorder*. Berkeley: University of California Press.

Kohrt, Brandon A., Worthman, Carol M. and Upadhaya, Nawaraj (2015). Karma to chromosomes: studying the biology of PTSD in a world of culture. In *Culture and PTSD: Trauma in Global and Historical Perspective*, ed. D. Hinton and B. Good. Philadelphia, PA: University of Pennsylvania Press, pp. 307–333.

Krueger, R. F. (1999). Structure of common mental disorders. *Archives of General Psychiatry*, **56**, 921–926.

Kugelmann, Robert (2009). The irritable heart syndrome in the American Civil War. In *Culture and Panic Disorder*, ed. Devon E. Hinton and Byron J. Good. Palo Alto, CA: Stanford University Press, pp. 85–112.

Laban, C. J., Komproe, I. H., Gernaat, H. P. E., de Jong, J. T. V. M. (2008). The impact of a long asylum procedure on quality of life, disability and physical health in Iraqi asylum seekers in the Netherlands. *Social Psychiatry and Psychiatric Epidemiology*, **43**, 507–515.

Lim, Hyun-Kook, Woo, Jong-Min, Kim, Tae-Suk *et al.* (2009). Reliability and validity of the Korean version of the impact of event scale – revised. *Comprehensive Psychiatry*, **50**(4), 385–90.

Lund, C., De Silva, M., Plagerson, S., *et al.* (2011). Poverty and mental disorders: breaking the cycle in low-income and middle-income countries. *The Lancet*, **378**, 1502–1514.

McNally, R. J. (2016). Is PTSD a transhistoric phenomenon? In *Culture and PTSD: Trauma in Historical and Global Perspective*, ed. D. E. Hinton and B. J. Good. Pennsylvenia: University of Pennsylvenia Press, pp. 117–135.

Mendenhall, E., Fernandez, A., Adler N., Jacobs, E. A. (2012). Susto, coraje, and abuse: depression and beliefs about diabetes. *Culture, Medicine and Psychiatry*, **36**, 480–492.

Miller, K. E. and Rasmussen, A. (2010). War exposure, daily stressors, and mental health in conflict and post-conflict settings: bridging the divide between trauma-focused and psychosocial frameworks. *Social Science and Medicine*, **70**, 7–16.

Miller, K. E., Omidian, P., Quraishy, A. S. *et al.* (2006). The Afghan symptom checklist: a culturally grounded approach to mental health assessment in a conflict zone. *American Journal of Orthopsychiatry*, **76**, 423–433.

Munafo, Marcus R., Brown, Sarah M. and Hariri, Ahmad R. (2008). Serotonin transporter (5-HTTLPR) genotype and amygdala activation: a meta-analysis. *Biological Psychiatry* **63**(9), 852–857.

Myin-Germeys, I., Oorschot, M., Collip, D., Lataster, J., Delespaul, P., van Os, J. (2009). Experience sampling research in psychopathology: opening the black box of daily life. *Psychological Medicine* **39**, 1533–1547.

Neuner, F. (2010). Assisting war-torn populations: should we prioritize reducing daily stressors to improve mental health? Comment on Miller and Rasmussen (2010). *Social Science and Medicine*, **71**, 1381–1384.

Neuner, F., Schauer, M. and Elbert, T. (2014). On the efficacy of narrative exposure therapy: a reply to Mundt *et al. Intervention*, **12**, 267–278.

Nichter, M. (2010). Idioms of distress revisited. *Culture, Medicine and Psychiatry*, **34**, 401–416.

Norris, F. H. and Kaniasty, K. (1996). Received and perceived social support in times of stress: a test of the Social Support Deterioration Deterrence Model. *Journal of Personality and Social Psychology*, **71**, 498–511.

Norris, Fran H., Perilla, Julia L., Ibanez, Gladys E. and Murphy, Arthur D. (2001a). Sex differences in symptoms of posttraumatic stress: does culture play a role? *Journal of Traumatic Stress*, **14**(1), 7–28.

Norris, Fran H., Perilla, Julia L., Ibanez, Gladys E. and Murphy, Arthur D. (2001b). Postdisaster stress in the United States and Mexico: a cross-cultural test of the multicriterion conceptual model of posttraumatic stress disorder. *Journal of Abnormal Psychology*, **110**(4), 553–563.

Omidian, P. and Miller, K. (2006). Addressing the psychosocial needs of women in Afghanistan. *Critical Half*, **4**, 17–22.

Osterman, Janet E. and de Jong, Joop T. V. M. (2007). Cultural issues and trauma. In *Handbook of PTSD: Science and Practice*, ed. Matthew J. Friedman, Terence

M. Keane and Patricia A Resick. New York: Guilford, pp. 425–446.

Ozer, E. J., Best, S. R., Lipsey, T. L. and Weiss, D. S. (2003). Predictors of posttraumatic stress disorder and symptoms in adults: a meta-analysis. *Psychological Bulletin*, **129**, 52–73.

Pakaslahti, A. (2009). Health-seeking behaviour for psychiatric disorders in north India. In *Psychiatrists and Traditional Healers: Unwitting Partners in Global Mental Health*, ed. Mario Incayawar, Ronald Wintrob and Lise Bouchard. Oxford: Wiley-Blackwell, pp. 149–166.

Palmieri, Patrick A., Marshall, Grant N. and Schell, Terry L. (2007) Confirmatory factor analysis of posttraumatic stress symptoms in Cambodian refugees. *Journal of Traumatic Stress*, **20**(2), 207–216.

Panter-Brick, C., Eggerman, M., Gonzalez, V. and Safdar, S. (2009). Violence, suffering, and mental health in Afghanistan: a school-based survey. *The Lancet*, **374**, 807–816.

Parkes, C. M., Laungani, P. and Young, B. (eds) (1997). *Death and Bereavement across Cultures*. London: Routledge.

Parry-Jones, B. and Parry-Jones, W. L. L. (1994). Post-traumatic stress disorder: supportive evidence from an eighteenth century natural disaster. *Psychological Medicine*, **24**, 15–27.

Parsons, T. (1952). *The Social System*. London: Tavistock.

Patel, V. and Kleinman, A. (2003). Poverty and common mental disorders in developing countries. *Bulletin of the World Health Organization*, **81**, 609–615.

Patel, V., Flisher, A. J., Hetrick, S. and McGorry, P. (2007a). Mental health of young people: a global public-health challenge. *The Lancet*, **369**, 1302–1313.

Patel, V., Araya, R., Chatterjee, S. *et al.* (2007b). Treatment and prevention of mental disorders in low-income and middle-income countries. *The Lancet*, **370**, 991–1005.

Perera, S. (2001). Spirit possessions and avenging ghosts: stories of supernatural activity as narratives of terror and mechanisms of coping and remembering. In *Remaking a World: Violence, Social Suffering and Recovery*, ed. V. Das, A. Kleinman, M. Lock, M. Ramphele and P. Reynolds. Berkeley: University of California Press, pp. 157–200.

Porter, M. and Haslam, N. (2005). Predisplacement and post-displacement factors associated with mental health of refugees and internally displaced persons: a meta-analysis. *Journal of the American Medical Association*, **294**(5), 602–612.

Prasad, A. N. (2006). Disease profile of children in Kabul: the unmet need for health care. *Journal of Epidemiology and Community Health*, **60**, 20–23.

Pupavac, V. (2004). War on the couch. the emotionology of the new international security paradigm. *European Journal of Social Theory*, **7**, 149–170.

Qouta, S. (2000). *Trauma, Violence and Mental Health: The Palestinian Experience*. Published doctoral dissertation, Vrije Universiteit, Amsterdam.

Qouta, S. and El-Sarraj, E. (2002). Community mental health as practiced by the Gaza community mental health programme. In *Trauma, War and Violence: Public Mental Health in Socio-cultural Context*, ed. Joop T. V. M. de Jong, New York: Plenum/Kluwer, pp. 317–337.

Rasmussen, A., Katoni, B., Keller, A. S. and Wilkinson, J. (2011). Posttraumatic idioms of distress among Darfur refugees: Hozun and Majnun. *Transcultural Psychiatry*, **48**, 392–415.

Reed, G. M., Roberts, M. C., Keeley, J., Hooppell, C., Matsumoto, C., Sharan, P., Medina-Mora, M. E. (2013). Mental health professionals' natural taxonomies of mental disorders: implications for the clinical utility of the ICD-11 and the DSM-5. *Journal of Clinical Psychology*, **69**(112), 1191–1212.

Reis, R. (1992). Het ziektestempel in Swaziland: parsons in Afrika [The label of disease in Swaziland: parsons in Africa]. *Antropologische Verkenningen*, **11**(3), 27–43.

Reis, R. (2016). Children's idioms of distress. In *The Routledge Handbook of Medical Anthropology*, ed. L. Manderson, E. Cartwright and A. Hardon. London: Routledge, case study 2.1, pp. 36–42.

Resick, Patricia A., Bovin, Michelle J., Calloway, Amber L. *et al.* (2012). A critical evaluation of the complex PTSD literature: implications for DSM-5. *Journal of Traumatic Stress*, **25**, 241–251.

Rosenblatt, P. C., Walsh, R. P. and Jackson, D. A. (1976). *Grief and Mourning in Cross-Cultural Perspective*. New Haven, CT: HRAF Press.

Rumelhart, D. E., Smolensky, P., McClelland, J. L. *et al.* (1986). Schemata and sequential thought processes in PDP models. In *Parallel Distributed Processing: Explorations in the Microstructure of Cognition*, ed. J. L. McClelland and D. E. Rumelhart. Cambridge, MA: MIT Press, pp. 7–57.

Sack, William H., Seeley, John R. and Clarke, Gregory N. (1997) Does PTSD transcend cultural barriers? A study from the Khmer adolescent refugee project. *Journal of the American Academy of Child and Adolescent Psychiatry*, **36**(1), 49–54.

Satija, D., Singh, C. D., Nathawat, S. S., Sharma, V. (1981). A psychiatric study of patients attending Mehandipur Balaji temple. *Indian Journal of Psychiatry*, **23**(3), 247–250.

Sax, W. S. Weinhold, J. (2010). Rituals of possession. In *Ritual Matters: The Dynamics of Change and Stability*, ed. Christiane Brosius and Ute Husken, Delhi: Routledge, pp. 236–252.

Schepers-Hughes, N. (1992). *Death without Weeping: the Violence of Everyday Life in Brazil*. Berkeley: University of California Press.

389

Seligman, R. and Kirmayer, L. J. (2008). Dissociative experience and cultural neuroscience: narrative, metaphor and mechanism. *Culture, Medicine, and Psychiatry*, **32**, 31–64.

Shalev, Arieh Y. (2007). PTSD: a disorder of recovery? In *Understanding Trauma: Biological, Clinical and Cultural Perspectives*, ed. Laurence Kirmayer, Robert Lemelson and Mark Barad. New York: Cambridge University Press, pp. 207–224.

Shay, J. (1991). Learning about combat stress from Homer's *Iliad*. *Journal of Traumatic Stress*, **4**, 561–579.

Sherin, Jonathan E., and Nemeroff, Charles B. (2011) Post-traumatic stress disorder: the neurobiological impact of psychological trauma. *Dialogues in Clinical Neuroscience*, **13**(3), 263–278.

Silove, D., Sinnerbrink, I., Field, A., Manicavasagar, V. and Steel, Z. (1997). Anxiety, depression and PTSD in asylum-seekers: associations with premigration trauma and post-migration stressors. *British Journal of Psychiatry*, **170**, 351–357.

Singer, M. C. (1995). Beyond the ivory tower: critical praxis in medical anthropology. *Medical Anthropology Quarterly*, **9**, 80–106.

Singer, M. (1996). A dose of drugs, a touch of violence, a case of AIDS: conceptualizing the SAVA syndemic. *Free Inquiry in Creative Sociology*, **24**(2), 99–110.

Singer M. C. (2009). *Introduction to Syndemics: A Critical Systems Approach to Public and Community Health*. San Francisco: Wiley.

Singer, M., Erickson. P. I., Badiane, L., Diaz, R., Ortiz, D., Abraham, T. and Nicolaysen, A. M. (2006). Syndemics, sex and the city: understanding sexually transmitted diseases in social and cultural context. *Social Science and Medicine*, **63** 2010–2021.

Slobodin, O. and de Jong, J. T. (2014). Mental health interventions for traumatized asylum seekers and refugees: what do we know about their efficacy? *International Journal of Social Psychiatry*, **61**(1), 17–26, pii:0020764014535752.

Slobodin, O. and de Jong, J. T. V. M. (2015). Family interventions in traumatized immigrants and refugees: a systematic review. *Transcultural Psychiatry*, **52**(6), 723–742, doi: 10.1177/1363461515588855.

Smith Fawzi, Mary Catherine, Pham, Thang, Lin, Lien, Nguyen, Tho Viet, Ngo, Dung, Murphy, Elizabeth and Mollica, Richard F. (1997). The validity of posttraumatic stress disorder among Vietnamese refugees. *Journal of Traumatic Stress*, **10**(1), 101–108.

Song, S. J., Kaplan, C., Tol, W., Subica, A., and de Jong, J. (2015). Psychological distress in torture survivors: pre- and post-migration risk factors in a US sample. *Social Psychiatry and Psychiatric Epidemiology*, **50**(4), 549–560.

Spiegel, D., Loewenstein, R. J., Lewis-Fernandez, R., Sar,V., Simeon, D., Vermetten, E., Cardeña, E. and Dell, P. F. (2011). Dissociative disorders in DSM-5. *Depression and Anxiety*, **28**, E17–E45.

Staub, E. (2011). *Overcoming Evil*. New York: Oxford University Press.

Steel, Z., Silove, D., Bird, K., McGorry, P. and Mohan, P. (1999). Pathways from war trauma to posttraumatic stress symptoms among Tamil asylum seekers, refugees, and immigrants. *Journal of Traumatic Stress*, **12**, 421–435.

Steel, Z., Chey, T., Silove, D., Marnane, C., Bryant, R. A. and van Ommeren, M. (2009). Association of torture and other potentially traumatic events with mental health outcomes among populations exposed to mass conflict and displacement: a systematic review and meta-analysis. *Journal of the American Medical Association*, **302**, 537–549.

Stewart, F., Cindy, H., and Michael, W. (2001). Internal wars: an empirical overview of the economic and social consequences. In *War and Underdevelopment: The Economic and Social Consequences of Conflict*, vol. **1**, ed. F. Stewart, and V. Fitzgerald. Oxford: Oxford University Press, pp. 67–103.

Summerfield, D. (1999). A critique of seven assumptions behind psychological trauma programmes in war affected areas. *Social Science and Medicine*, **48**, 1449–1462.

Summerfield, D. (2001). The invention of post-traumatic stress disorder and the social usefulness of a psychiatric category. *British Medical Journal*, **322**, 95.

Tankink, M., Ventevogel, P., Ntiranyibagira, L., Ndayisaba, A. and Ndayisaba, H. (2010). Situation and needs assessment of mental health and psychosocial support in refugee camps in Tanzania, Rwanda and Burundi. Unpublished report: HealthNet TPO.

Tedeschi, R. G. and Calhoun, L. G. (2004). Posttraumatic growth: conceptual foundations and empirical evidence. *Psychological Inquiry*, **15**(1), 1–18.

Terheggen, M. A., Stroebe, M. S. and Kleber, R. J. (2001). Western conceptualizations and Eastern experience: a cross-cultural study of traumatic stress reactions among Tibetan refugees in India. *Journal of Traumatic Stress*, **14**(2).

Thirthalli, J., Zhou, L., Kumar, K., *et al.* (2016). Traditional, complementary, and alternative medicine approaches to mental health care and psychological well-being in India and China. *The Lancet Psychiatry*, **3**(7), 660–672, doi: 10.1016/S2215-0366(16)30025-6.

Tol, W. A., Jordans, M. J. D., Reis, R., and de Jong, J. T. V. M. (2009). Ecological resilience: working with child-related psychosocial resources in war-affected communities. In *Treating Traumatized Children: Risk, Resilience, and Recovery*, ed. D. Brom, R. Pat-Horenczyk and J. Ford. London: Routledge, pp. 164–182.

Tol, W. A., Reis, R., Susanty, D., and de Jong, J. T. V. M. (2010). Communal violence and child psychosocial well-being: qualitative findings from Poso, Indonesia. *Transcultural Psychiatry*, **47**(1), 112–135.

Tol, W. A., Komproe, I. H., Jordans, M. J., Susanty, D. and de Jong, J. T. V. M. (2011a). Developing a function impairment measure for children affected by political violence: a mixed methods approach in Indonesia. *International Journal for Quality in Health Care*, **23**(4), 375–383.

Tol, W. A., Barbui, C., Galappatti, A., Silove, D., Betancourt, T. S., Souza, R., Golaz, A., van Ommeren, M. (2011b). Mental health and psychosocial support in humanitarian settings: linking practice and research. *The Lancet*, **378**, 1–10.

Tol, W. A., Barbui, C., Bisson, J., *et al.* (2014). World Health Organization guidelines for management of acute stress, PTSD, and bereavement: key challenges on the road ahead. *PLoS Med* **11**(12), e1001769, doi: 10.1371/journal.pmed.1001769.

Trimble, M. R. (1985). Post-traumatic stress disorder: history of a concept. In *Trauma and its Wake: The Study and Treatment of Post-Traumatic Stress Disorder*, ed. C. R. Figley. New York: Brunner/Mazel, p. 5.

Tumarkin, M. (2005). *Traumascapes: The Power and Fate of Places Transformed by Tragedy*. Carlton: Melbourne University Press.

United Nations (2006). *Convention on the Rights of Persons with Disabilities*. New York: United Nations High Commissioner for Refugees.

UNHCR (2016). *Global Strategy Implementation Report*. Geneva: United Nations High Commissioner for Refugees.

Van de Put, W. A. C. M. and Eisenbruch, M. (2002). The Cambodian experience. In *Trauma, War and Violence: Public Mental Health in Socio-cultural Context*, ed. J. T. V. M. de Jong. New York: Plenum/Kluwer: pp. 93–157.

Van Duijl, M., Cardena, E., and de Jong, J. T. V. M. (2005). The validity of DSM-IV dissociative disorders categories in south-west Uganda. *Transcultural Psychiatry*, **6**, 219–241.

Van Ommeren, M. (2003). Validity issues in transcultural epidemiology. *British Journal of Psychiatry*, **182**, 376–378.

Van Ommeren, M., Sharma, B., Komproe, I., Poudyal, B., Sharma, G. K., Cardeña, E., de Jong, J. T. V. M. (2001). Trauma and loss as determinants of medically unexplained epidemic illness in a Bhutanese refugee camp. *Psychological Medicine*, **31**(7), 1259–1267.

Van Os, J., Kenis, K. and Rutten, B. B. F. (2010). The environment and schizophrenia. *Nature*, **468**, 203–212.

Ventevogel, P. (2016). Borderlands of mental health: explorations in medical anthropology, psychiatric epidemiology and health systems research in Afghanistan and Burundi, PhD thesis, Amsterdam: University of Amsterdam.

Von Korff, M., Crane, P. K., Alonso, J., Vilagut, G., Angermeyer, M. C., Bruffaerts, R., Ormel, J. (2008). Modified WHO DAS-II provides valid measure of global disability but filter items increased skewness. *Journal of Clinical Epidemiology*, **61**, 1132–1143.

Wardenaar, K. J., and de Jonge, P. (2013). Diagnostic heterogeneity in psychiatry: towards an empirical solution. *BMC Medicine*, **11**, 201. Available from www.biomedcentral.com/1741%2D7015/11/201.

Way, Baldwin M., and Taylor, Shelley E. (2010). The serotonin transporter promoter polymorphism is associated with cortisol response to psychosocial stress. *Biological Psychiatry*, **67**(5), 487–492.

Weine, S., Danieli, Y., Silove, D., van Ommeren, M., Fairbank, J. A. and Saul, J. (2002). Guidelines for international training in mental health and psychosocial interventions for trauma exposed populations in clinical and community settings. *Psychiatry*, **65**, 156–164.

WHO (2012). Social determinants of health report. Geneva: WHO.

WHO (2013). *Building Back Better: Sustainable Mental Health Care after Disaster*. Geneva, Switzerland: WHO.

Widiger, T. A. and Samuel D. B. (2005). Diagnostic categories or dimensions? A question for the diagnostic and statistical manual of mental disorders – fifth edition. *Journal of Abnormal Psychology*, **114**, 494–504.

Wigman, J. T. W., van Os, J., Borsboom, D., *et al.* (2015). Exploring the underlying structure of mental disorders: cross-diagnostic differences and similarities from a network perspective using both a top-down and a bottom-up approach. *Psychological Medicine*, **45**(11), 2375–2387, doi: 10.1017/S0033291715000331.

Wilson, K. B. (1992). Cults of violence and counter-violence in Mozambique. *Journal of Southern African Studies*, **18**, 531–582.

Winslow, C. (1920). The untilled fields of public health. *Science New Series*, **51**(1306), 23–33.

Yehuda, Rachel (2009). Status of glucocorticoid alterations in post-traumatic stress disorder. *Annals of the New York Academy of Sciences*, **1179**, 56–69.

Yehuda, Rachel and Bierer, Linda M. (2009). The relevance of epigenetics to PTSD: implications for the DSM-5. *Journal of Traumatic Stress* **22**(5), 427–434.

Yehuda, Rachel and McFarlane, Alexander C. (1995). Conflict between current knowledge about posttraumatic stress disorder and its original conceptual basis. *American Journal of Psychiatry*, **152**, 1705–1713.

Yehuda, Rachel and McFarlane, Alexander C. (1997). Introduction. In *Psychobiology of Posttraumatic Stress Disorder*, ed. Rachel Yehuda and Alexander

C. McFarlane. New York: New York Academy of Sciences, pp. xi–xv.

Young, A. (1976). Internalizing and externalizing medical belief systems: an Ethiopian example. *Social Science and Medicine*, **10**, 147–156.

Young, Allan (1995). *The Harmony of Illusions: Inventing Post-Traumatic Stress Disorder*. Princeton, NJ: Princeton University Press.

Young, A. and Breslau, N. (2015). What is 'PTSD'? The heterogeneity thesis. In *Culture and PTSD: Trauma in Historical and Global Perspective*, ed. D. E. Hinton and B. J. Good. Pennsylvania: University of Pennsylvania Press, pp. 135–155.

Yufik, Tom, and Simms, Leonard J. (2010). A meta-analytic investigation of the structure of posttraumatic stress disorder symptoms. *Journal of Abnormal Psychology*, **119**(4), 764–776.

Zhang, Kerang, Xu, Qi, Xu, Yong *et al.* (2009). The combined effects of the 5-HTTLPR and 5-HTR1A genes modulates the relationship between negative life events and major depressive disorder in a Chinese population. *Journal of Affective Disorders*, **114**(1–3), 224–231.

Chapter 30

Sexual Dysfunction across Cultures

Dinesh Bhugra, Antonio Ventriglio and Gurvinder Kalra

Editors' Introduction

Sexual activity is both for pleasure and procreation. Therefore the impact of sexual dysfunction on individuals and their relationships can be dramatic. There is no doubt that sexual dysfunction is seen across cultures, ethnic groups and societies even though its actual presentation may well differ according to cultural norms. The gender roles and role expectations also influence how sexual activity and sexual dysfunction are seen and how help is sought. Societies have been described as sex positive (where sex is seen as a pleasurable activity) or sex negative. Thus, within sex-positive societies, sexual activity is more likely to be for pleasure, whereas in sex-negative societies, sex is more for procreative purposes and less for personal pleasure. Therefore the expectations of the individuals and their partners will vary too. In this chapter, Bhugra *et al.* provide an overview of some epidemiological findings of sexual dysfunctions in the West and selected cultures. Epidemiological data across cultures are often scanty. From cultures and societies, where sex is seen purely for procreative purposes, it is possible that women are more likely to be referred via gynaecologists and obstetricians and in many traditional cultures may have already used alternative and complementary therapies. This inevitably will affect their motivation for treatment. Delays in seeking help and simultaneous use of other therapies may complicate matters further. The authors indicate that prevalence of sexual dysfunction will depend upon a number of factors, most of which are environmental and social. Placing sexual dysfunction and its management in the cultural context means that the outcome can be improved. The affective states and cognitive schema also vary across cultures, thereby making the task of the therapist more difficult.

Introduction

Sex is one of the basic universal human instincts and it can be argued that over the centuries and with the shift of societies from traditional to less traditional and more modern models may see moving sexual functioning varying from procreation to pleasure. Different cultures in different time spans have looked upon sex and sexual behaviour in different tones and shades, sometimes with fear, sometimes as magico-religious experience. An inherent danger in studying sexual behaviour across historical periods is the real or potential inaccuracy of the data (Bullough, 1972). These data are often descriptive and occasionally epidemiological, whereas the attitudes to sex and sexual behaviour and psychosexual dysfunction change according to prevalent social norms and mores and whether sexuality is controlled by the state.

Early writers made assumptions about the function of the sexual act but had to use religious texts, which are one of the richest sources of information on the topic of sexual behaviour (Bhugra and de Silva, 1995). The assumptions about the sexual act and its purpose have been greatly influential (Bullough, 1976) in human functioning and expectations, perhaps because they had been immortalized in the religious canon. These deeply ingrained assumptions did not change dramatically, although with the advent of new religions and religious coda some modifications occurred. There is little doubt that sexuality is defined within a specific cultural setting and depends greatly on socialization (Bullough, 1976; Gregersen, 1986; Segal *et al.*, 1986; Bhugra and de Silva, 1993). There is little doubt that a large number of cultures have different sets of standards regarding sexual behaviour across genders. The more powerful gender in a society, i.e. the male, secures control of the social institutions thereby shaping gender roles in ways that accord themselves greater sexual privilege (Reiss, 1986). Male and female patterns of sexual behaviour and sexual orientation are socially learnt with genetic encoding. Heterosexual coitus is the most prevalent sexual behaviour for a vast majority of individuals in any given society, although the societies define what is deviant and what is normal (Ford and Beach 1951; Segal *et al.*, 1986; Bhugra 1997). Bullough (1976) notes that societies accepted or tolerated other (other than heterosexual) behaviour only after the tribe had perpetuated itself and perhaps did not face a threat of annihilation.

The variations in sexual behaviour have been studied more extensively over the last 70 years or so. Unwin (1934) reported on a cross-cultural study, which tested the relationship between sexual expression and cultural achievement from nearly 80 countries. The literature by anthropologists such as Malinowski (1927) and Mead (1977) among others indicates the role and function of sexuality and sexual behaviour played in different societies.

In this chapter we discuss the relationship between culture and sexual dysfunction. Although we touch on cultures' differences related to homosexuality and paraphilias, the focus in this chapter remains on prevalence and presentation of sexual dysfunction relying on epidemiological data across cultures. The management strategies are presented in Chapter 40.

Role of Culture in Sexual Dysfunction

Until relatively recently, the study of sexual medicine was seen as exotic and prosaic, and the religious and social observations referred to the subject extensively. There are crucial factors which determine any individual's patterns of sexual behaviour and norms. The types of sexual dysfunction can generally be divided across the two genders into the phases of sexual desire, sexual arousal, act itself and post-coital period. Among both males and females, sexual desire and sexual arousal can be raised or decreased. The act of orgasm for males can lead to premature or delayed ejaculation and anorgasmia in females. Post-coitally, both males and females can experience pain either at the time of ejaculation or orgasm. Among females, vaginismus can be seen as another sexual dysfunction. There are, of course, various so-called culture-bound syndromes, which influence sexual performance or performance anxiety, such as *dhat* or semen-loss anxiety (these are further discussed in Chapter 14). It must be recognized that these are strongly influenced by cultures though not confined to specific cultures as previously thought.

Cultures themselves have been described as sex positive or sex negative (Bullough, 1976). He argues persuasively that sex-positive cultures saw the phenomenon of sex as life affirming and pleasurable, whereas sex-negative cultures saw the act as procreative. He further suggests that this pleasure is influenced by gender roles and in (some) sex-positive cultures sexual pleasure is meant to be experienced by males and this is what dictates how society defines pleasure. In addition, he highlights the role of education and experience, along with how folklore, music, dance and arts influence societies, which in turn influence these forms.

In ancient India, several erotic classics and sex manuals existed and these described various sexual acts for pleasure at great length, along with sex aids. The existence of these classics indicates clearly that the ancient inhabitants were not scared of sex compared with their contemporary Western counterparts, and the themes of strong approval of sex appear early in Hindu history (Bullough, 1976). The text of *Kamasutra* distils the sensual pleasure – the *kama*, which is one of the key human goals or ideals in Hinduism. Magical spells to bind and seduce potential lovers and to hurt potential competitors by inducing impotence are described in the Hindu scriptures – the Vedas (Bhugra and de Silva, 1995).

Meyer (1971) highlights that, in some of these scriptures and texts, sexual pleasure is directed by getting two people (usually in a marital state) together on certain nights at certain times with the right ambience, food and drink. *Kamasutra* describes love as being one of four types – acquired by continual habit resulting from imagination; from belief or from the perception of external objects. To enhance one's attractiveness to potential consorts, unguents and potions along with amulets are recommended. Virility can be increased and the use of aids to increase the girth and/or length of the penis are described. Artificial penises (akin to dildoes) with studs, and organized to fit the vagina, were described which could be used in conjunction with, or in place of, the penis. Sexual intercourse was a crucial part of the male/female relationship and males had to be aware of the different phases of functioning in different parts of life. Ayurvedic texts described the formation of semen in stages and emphasized that diet, individual personality traits and season affect the production of semen (Thakkur, 1974; Bhugra and Buchanan, 1989; Bhugra, 1992). In addition, semen was of eight varieties, and at least ten different herbs could be used for increasing semen production. Syed (1999) notes that although the *Kamasutra* did not describe the female Gräfenberg zone and female ejaculation, other ancient

Indian texts such as *Pañcasayaka* (eleventh century), *Jayamangala* (Yaśodhara's commentary on the *Kamasutra* from the thirteenth century), the *Ratirahasya* (thirteenth century), as well as *Smaradipika* and *Anangaranga* (*c.* sixteenth century) describe both the Gräfenberg zone and female ejaculation.

Male impotence, according to Ayurvedic texts, could result from old age, excessive semen loss, penile conditions and dietary causes, along with emotional problems such as anger, grief, fear, apprehension, drunkenness and jealousy. Bhugra and Buchanan (1989) point out that some early writers note primary impotence to result from genetic factors and features of anticipatory and performance anxiety. King (1994) also noted descriptions of impotence in poetry. As part of the positive attitudes towards sex, transvestism was described. Although male aspects of pleasure have been described perhaps more extensively, not surprisingly as a result of more patriarchal attitudes, female desire and pleasure were noted to be greater than those of males, and for females this pleasure depended upon education, experience, physical type and stimuli that aroused her. Hindu texts also emphasized the coexistence of the male and the female in each individual, and the two could function well depending upon a number of external factors.

The Chinese, too, saw the world in dualistic terms, bur rather than focusing on the conflict between the spiritual and the material they looked to the inherent unity of the opposing forces. For example, heaven was masculine and the earth feminine. The clouds were the vaginal secretion allowing the heavenly sperm, the rain, into the earth (womb), from the union of which all life force came. The two forces of *yin* and *yang*, respectively, earth and heaven, moon and sun, male and female, came together in sexual union, which is essential to achieve harmony as well as a happy and healthy life. Seasonal illnesses could be lodged in either *yin* or *yang* and any imbalance could produce serious difficulties in functioning. Each time a man had intercourse, he was to try to absorb as much *yin* from the woman as possible, but without giving up any of his *yang* (Bullough, 1976). Buddhist principles, Confucian thought and Mongol conquest all played their part in modifying Chinese philosophy. Later, sex became a secret act which, although sacred, was not to be talked about publicly. Humidity, heat, liver and kidney disease and energy depletion were seen as causes of impotence (Xu, 1990).

Aristotle described animals as those reproducing by sexual means, by asexual means and by spontaneous generation. His teachings could be responsible for seeing the female as a passive receptacle to the male desire and the fact that marriage was seen as being for procreation and not (even) for companionship (Bullough, 1976). Yet early Greeks and Romans also appeared to have manuals on sex (King, 1994).

Early Christians changed the attitudes towards sex in the West. This again may reflect a need for the newly formed Christian tribe to survive and thrive in their early stages. Bullough (1976) argues that the subjugation of the body along with attainment of perfection through renunciation may have contributed to negative attitudes. Early Christianity saw justification of sexual intercourse between male and female in marriage and for procreation only. Celibacy was the highest good and goal, and sex was simply animal lust allowed only within the boundaries of marriage.

Although Biblical references to erectile failure (Rosen and Leiblum, 1992) and in Greek mythology (Johnson, 1968) existed, in the Middle Ages the causation was seen as demonic possession and witchcraft. Additional factors, which may have influenced the Christian attitudes towards sex, included the merging of religion and state, and the dissonance in state proclamations and individual experiences contributed further to this change. Sexual acts of masturbation, sodomy and fellatio became offences and everything that medieval people feared came to have sexual connotations and overtones (Bullough, 1976).

This broad overview emphasizes that attitudes towards sex, sexuality and sexual behaviour are influenced by a number of factors, including religion and its interpretations. Trying to turn sexual medicine and mores into science rather than art may have further contributed to these perhaps more negative attitudes (Foucault, 1981).

Homosexuality across Cultures

There needs to be a recognition that sexual orientation is innate and sexual behaviour is both learnt and opportunistic whereas sexual fantasy can be much broader. Although same-sex behaviours have been described across all societies and cultures across different times (Bullough, 1979), the response to such an act or behaviour varies across cultures. Often innate orientation and actual act can be confused hence often emphasis in many countries on conversion therapy. The legal proscription on same-sex behaviour further helps such behaviour to go underground, with no clear evidence of its prevalence.

In ancient Hindu texts and literature, same-sex attraction has been described fully (Bullough, 1979; Vanita and Kidwai, 2000; Vanita, 2005). These interpretations have to be seen in the context of the prevalent cultural mores when, as noted earlier, sex was seen as a pleasurable activity. Both genders were noted to have indulged in same-sex behaviours. The sex aids described in *Kamasutra* enable both men and women to have same-sex relationships, indicating that such behaviour was available.

Hinsch (1990) noted that in China 'In many periods homosexuality was widely accepted and even respected, had its own formal history and had a role in shaping Chinese political conventions and spurring artistic creations.' In ancient China, like in ancient Rome and Greece, kings were allowed to keep male sex partners. In ancient Greece, the role of same-sex relationships was well noted and described (Bullough, 1979). The availability of such behaviour was accepted not as a phase but as part of the bisexual nature of man.

In Christianity, however, as part of the sexual repertoire, same-sex behaviour was frowned upon and individuals were discouraged from practising it. These attitudes remained fairly static over several hundred years and different Christian groups still argue against same-sex behaviour, citing Biblical sources (see also Vanita, 2005). Removal of homosexuality as a mental illness from DSM-III reflected changing attitudes to same-sex behaviour, although in some national classificatory systems, for example, in Indonesia and in Egypt, homosexuality still remains as a mental illness in the classification systems whereas in 2001 it was removed from the Chinese classification system (CPS, 2001).

The range of sexual dysfunctions experienced by homosexual men and women are broadly the same as those experienced by heterosexual men and women. However, some additional factors may affect these. They may not seek help because of perceived or real homophobia which may also contribute to associated anxiety and depression. Other factors may include the fact that they may not have 'come out' and belonging to specific gay subculture within that may further contribute to distress. Factors related to 'coming out' (telling others about sexual orientation) will influence help-seeking and will be affected by cultural attitudes, which will dictate when and how to come out to others.

Paraphilias across Cultures

Paraphilias have been recognized historically. These are referred to as sexual deviations or sexual variations and distinguished from psychosexual dysfunction reflect a problem of sexual preference and/or direction of one's sexual desire (de Silva, 1995). Those individuals whose sexual interests are of a paraphilic nature are also referred to as 'sexual minorities' (Money, 1984; Wilson, 1987; Bancroft, 1989). Exhibitionism, voyeurism, sadomasochism and paedophilia are some of the common paraphilias. The data on cross-cultural prevalence of paraphilias are scanty because in many societies many of the paraphilias are illegal acts. There is a hypothetical possibility that, in societies where the sex act is seen as mainly procreative, the prevalence of paraphilias may be lower. Another key difficulty in identifying the rates of paraphilias in any given population is that often these do not come into contact with services at all, largely because if the individuals and their partners are satisfied, unless there is a problem, they would not be identified as such. Most of the clinical presentations may be associated with legal problems. Paraphilias are multifaceted problems and any assessment may need to take into account factors such as deviant arousal, anxiety, skills deficits, gender-role identity problems (Gudjonsson, 1986). There appear to be references to some paraphilias such as voyeurism, bestiality, exhibitionism and necrophilia in the Bible (Aggrawal, 2009). Herdt (1987) found that, in the Sambia tribe in New Guinea, young men are expected to perform fellatio with older men as a rite of passage. Transvestism and transgender have different cultural connotations. In countries such as India, transgendered individuals such as *hijras* have cultural value and importance. They will be invited to dance at weddings and also at the birth of a son. Similarly, *berdache* have a social role. In Thailand, ladyboys function as entertainers and the societal stigma towards such individuals is rare. Dressing up can be seen as fashionable or fetishistic, depending upon the individual society where such a behaviour is acceptable or enjoyable (transgenderism is further discussed in detail in Chapter 41).

The management of paraphilias is discussed in Chapter 40. However, it must be emphasized that the role of the sex act, availability of fetishistic objects and the societal attitudes to such behaviour all play a key role in the way paraphilias present are treated and the outcome following interventions.

Sexual Jealousy across Cultures

Jealousy itself is a complex emotion and arouses very strong feelings in the individual who is experiencing it and also in those who are observing it. Morbid jealousy is a type of sexual jealousy related to a sense of fear that the partner is having affairs and there is an imminent threat of loss of relationship, irrespective of the truth of the matter. This is, in turn, associated with own self-worth and health of our relationships in terms of sexual fidelity (Clanton and Smith 1977). Jealousy is an emotion that covers the threat of potential loss to a rival and is experienced as fear of loss, anger over betrayal and/or insecurity (Hupka 1984, Mathes et al., 1985; Mathes, 1991). A universal social function of jealousy is the protection of marriage. Motives for jealousy are a product of the culture and vary according to social organizations, economic, political and legal systems and patterns of kinship (Hunter and Whitten, 1976). Hupka et al. (1985), in a cross-cultural study of jealousy, found that socialist nations had lower levels of jealousy. Following globalization and changes in many countries, it will be interesting to repeat this study. Schlegal (1972) studied 66 matrilineal societies and found that, where men have minimal authority over women, adultery of wives was less likely to be punished than where husbands or the brothers had the power. Studying 92 cultures from the Human Relations Area file, Hupka and Ryan (1990) found that severity of reactions to jealousy increased with importance of pair bonding, emphasis on personal ownership of property and limited possibilities of sexual gratification (which may reflect low self-worth). The assessment of any individual with sexual dysfunction must take cultural factors and sexual jealousy and paraphilias into account.

Epidemiology of Sexual Dysfunction

Johnson et al. (1994), in a detailed survey of sexual attitudes and lifestyles in the UK, studied 18,876 individuals who were randomly selected for interviews and completed these interviews. For younger men aged 16–19, the mean age for first sexual intercourse was 17, 3 years earlier than among those who were aged 55–59. For women too this dropped to 14 from 16 for women in similar age groups. Racial and ethnic differences demonstrated that those of Bangladeshi, Pakistani and Indian origin were much less likely to report sexual intercourse under the age of 16, whereas this was more likely in black men and women. The median age for first sexual intercourse for men was higher for Asian groups and lower for blacks in comparison with whites. Religion too played a role in this very complex interaction. Respondents belonging to the Church of England or other Christian Churches (excluding the Roman Catholic Church) were less likely to do so. Factors reportedly associated with first intercourse included curiosity, peer experience, being drunk. A total of 6.8 per cent of men reported that they had paid for sex with a woman at some time in their life and 1.8 per cent had done so within the last 5 years. The frequency of heterosexual sex (defined as acts of oral, vaginal and anal intercourse) showed a very wide variability as measured by the number of occasions in the previous 4 weeks, with a very small proportion of the population reporting a very high frequency of sexual contact. Not surprisingly, age was closely related to the number of acts, with frequency peaking in the mid-20s and thereafter a gradual decline more marked for women than for men. The number of sexual sessions decreased the longer the relationship lasted. Over 93 per cent of respondents were attracted exclusively to people of the opposite sex and a similar proportion also reported exclusively heterosexual experiences. Homosexual behaviour was reported by 6.1% of men and 3.4% of women when asked about any homosexual experience ever, and 1.1% of men and 0.4% of women reported having had a homosexual partner in the past year.

Melman and Gingell (1999) identified over 400 studies which looked at erectile dysfunction and impotence in epidemiological and pathophysiological studies, and confirmed that prevalence of sexual dysfunction of all degrees was seen in 52 per cent of males aged 40–70 with even higher rates with an increase in age. The quality of life was influenced by erectile dysfunction and risk factors such as medication, smoking, ageing, chronic illness, all of which played a role.

Using data recorded between 1987 and 1996 from health insurance agencies, a sample of 124,917 men and women in Germany were studied. Aged between 20 and 60 years attending hospital services showed a prevalence of 0.1 per cent of sexual disturbances (Geyer *et al.*, 2001). These are contact rates rather than true prevalence, but indicate that there are multiple factors, including physical illness, which must be taken into account. The relationship between ageing and sexuality is important, but most studies tend to exclude older adults. In an unusual study in Australia, Dennerstein *et al.* (2001) recruited 438 Australian born women aged 45 to 55 who were menstruating at base line. Of these, 197 were studied further, with a focus on menopausal transition. Compared with two control groups, these authors found that sexual responsivity declined significantly.

Comparing cultural and biological factors regarding sexual health and marital satisfaction in Germany and the USA, Mazur *et al.* (2002) noted that sexuality declined with age, and neither testosterone levels nor psychological depression could explain levels of sexuality. Sexual health and marital satisfaction were related to sexuality among Americans but not Germans. They concluded that, in both cultural settings, the wife's sexual desire, the subject's ability to maintain an erection and the subject's imagination/fantasy may play a role. Thus, the relationship between ageing and sexual function is multilayered and complex.

Cognitive functioning is strongly influenced by culture. Audu (2002) noted among infertile Nigerian women the presence of a number of sexual problems. Reporting on data from 97 infertile women using questionnaires to ascertain frigidity (*sic*), 78 per cent of the sample acknowledged with 58 per cent admitting to dyspareunia. Nearly one-fifth had difficulties in arousal and the same proportion had difficulties in reaching orgasm. The study reflects that sexual dysfunction is related to infertility and the sources of data collection influence reported prevalence. Skinner *et al.* (2002) found that Bangladeshi men were six times (12%) more likely to have sexual dysfunction compared with women, although the data was collected from a genito-urinary clinic. Syphilis was commoner in Bangladeshi men compared with controls.

Bancroft *et al.* (2003) studied 987 white or black African American women aged 20 to 85 years to measure stress about sex. Using a telephone – audio-computer – assisted self-interviewing with the response rate of 53 per cent, these authors applied weighting to increase the representativeness of the sample. A total of 22 per cent of women reported marked stress about the sexual relationship and/or

their own sexuality. The best prediction of sexual distress were marks of general emotional well-being and emotional relationship with the partner during sexual activity. Physical aspects of sexual response in women, including arousal, vaginal lubrication and orgasm, were reported as poor predictors. In general, the authors felt that predictors of distress did not fit well with the DSM-IV criteria for the diagnosis of sexual dysfunction in women. There are conceptual problems in using terms such as distress and dysfunction and comparing these. And these results indicate that there are several additional issues in sexual dysfunction which need to be identified. The low response rate does have its problems; however, the strength of this study lies in the inclusion of African American women as a group.

In order to describe the demographics, presenting problems and physical laboratory investigations in women presenting with vulvo-vaginal disorders, Hansen *et al.* (2002) studied medical records of all cases who presented to the clinic between 1996 and 1999 with vulvar problems. Of 322 women identified, 94 per cent were Caucasians and 64 per cent married. A majority (73%) reported at least one vaginal delivery. Common symptoms reported were vulvar pains (87%), dyspareunia (76%), itching (37%) and skin changes (18%). Prevalent diagnosis included Bartholin fossa pain, vulvar vestibulitis, restriction and fissuring of posterior labial commissure, vulvodynia and pelvic floor dysfunction. The authors emphasize the heterogeneity of the sample as well as the problems and recommend that physical causation must be ruled out prior to a diagnosis being made.

The rates of sexual problems and their prevalence in women depend upon a number of factors, including the source of the sample, method of data collection and measures for clinical identification of diagnosis. In a population-based study, Kadri *et al.* (2002) studied 728 women in an epidemiological study from Casablanca. These were aged 20 and over. Using the DSM-IV criteria for diagnosis of sexual dysfunction, 27 per cent were found to have a lifetime or 6-month prevalence of sexual dysfunction. Their most common finding was that of hypoactive sexual disorder. Age, financial dependency, number of children and sexual harassment were positively associated with these symptoms. Interestingly, in spite of their awareness of these symptoms, only 17 per cent had sought help for their symptoms, suggesting cultural bias in help-seeking or the inability to know from where to seek help. This is also likely to be affected by how much the affected individual is bothered by the sexual (dys)function as was observed by Namiki *et al.* (2008) who noted that Japanese men were less likely than American men to be bothered by sexual function.

On the other hand, Kantor *et al.* (2002) reported that prevalence of complete erectile dysfunction was 36 per cent in a sample of 268 subjects (out of 334 who were approached in primary-care settings). At the same time, they noted that the prevalence of current depression was 12 per cent and concomitant depression and erectile dysfunction was 5 per cent. Using logistic regression, these authors found that current depressive symptoms were not associated with moderate or complete erectile dysfunction. A similar study using somewhat different methods of reporting from 1250 males in Thailand showed that age was not a significant factor contributing to prevalence of erectile disorder, but diabetes and hypertension were (Kongkanand, 2000). The sample was collected from four sites around the Bangkok metropolitan area, again indicating that there are both similarities and differences in prevalence and association of erectile dysfunction across different nations and different cultures. In a recent study from Mumbai, India by Kalra *et al.* (2015), premature ejaculation was the most common sexual dysfunction seen in male patients presenting with sexual dysfunction to a psychiatric outpatient clinic while depression was seen only in 16 per cent of the respondents. In another similar study from a South Indian rural population, Sathyanarayana *et al.* (2015) found erectile dysfunction to be the most common sexual dysfunction in men presenting with sexual problems and hypoactive sexual desire disorder to be the most common sexual dysfunction in the women presenting with such problems. Anxiety and depression are the common mental illnesses seen in other socio-cultural groups as well such as working class Pathans in an industrial area of Karachi, Pakistan (Khan and Ahmed, 1990). Such depressive symptoms are often linked to erectile dysfunction through decreased sexual activity and the dissatisfaction that is caused by the inability to lead a healthy sexual life (Nicolosi *et al.*, 2004).

In a Belgian study, it was reported that, of 799 men who were interviewed, 60 per cent complained of erectile difficulties (Mak *et al.*, 2002). An age stratified random sample of the male population aged between 40 and 70 years were interviewed, using standardized assessment questionnaires. Of the 799 men (a participation rate of 38%), 10% reported severe, 25% moderate and 27% mild erectile dysfunction; only 38% reported no problems. Age and absence of sexual activity were the strongest predictors of erectile dysfunction. Other correlates included depression, absence of physical activity and other physical health problems. Among women attending a menopause clinic, Nappi *et al.* (2002) studied 355 subjects aged 46 to 60. The study, based in Italy, used visual analogue scales. The authors reported that 30 per cent of subjects complained of pain during sexual intercourse and 22 per cent complained of low libido and lack of sexual desire, both of which increase with age and years since menopause. Reduction of sexual pleasure/satisfaction was common with age, but was more frequent the longer the time since menopause. By examining the intensity of sexual symptoms according to the presence of other complaints, the authors concluded that physical, psychological and genital well-being significantly affects the components of sexual responses after the menopause. They suggest that lack of fitness, urogenital symptoms, negative self-image and depressive symptoms were commoner in women with sexual complaints. They recommended using a comprehensive approach to assessment of female health around menopause; thus cultural factors may play a less active role in physical aspects of female sexual dysfunction, but not necessarily in seeking help.

The relationship between sexual dysfunction and marriage is multi-factored. Duration of marriage, expectations of marriage, romantic perceptions, couple communication, sexual satisfaction within marriage all may play a role. Litzinger and Gordon (2005) examined relationships among couple communication, sexual satisfaction and marital satisfaction in 387 married couples and noted that there was a significant interaction between communication and sexual satisfaction. If couples are good at constructive communication, sexual satisfaction does not contribute to marital satisfaction. However, poor communication but good sexual satisfaction leads to greater marital satisfaction compared to a poor sexually satisfying relationship. Thus they inferred that communication and sexual satisfaction independently predict marital satisfaction. It is also likely that the relationship between sexual and marital problems is much closer for men than for women with the specific male sexual dysfunctions of erectile dysfunction and premature ejaculation playing a much larger role in marital discord than the female dysfunctions of anorgasmia and vaginismus (Rust *et al.*, 1988). It is thus important to consider sexual dysfunction as a disease of the couple and hence the couple as a whole must be treated (Pacheco Palha and Lourenco, 2011).

Liu (2003) raised an interesting question about whether the quality of marital sex increases or decreases with marital duration. Although several studies in the past had highlighted that a decrease takes place, empirical data are lacking. This study examines theoretically as well as empirically the alteration in quality of marital sex in relation to duration of marriage. Theoretically, two effects may influence the change of quality in marital sex: the effect of diminishing marginal utility (the marginal utility of consuming goods or services diminishes as the consumption of those goods or services increases), and the effect of investment in the marriage – specific human capital (including the 'partner-specific' skills that enhance the enjoyment of marital sex and the knowledge about the spouse's sexual preferences, desires and habits). The quality of marital sex could either increase or decrease, depending upon which effect is dominant. Liu used the data from the National Roles and Social Life Survey and found that marital duration did have a small negative effect on the quality of marital sex.

In the Indian subcontinent too, cultural values see sexual adequacy, particularly in males, as the benchmark of masculinity, virility, personal adequacy and fulfilment (Kulhara and Avasthi, 1995). The prevalence of sexual dysfunctions in hospital-based psychiatric clinic populations is said to vary from 9.2 to 13 per cent (Nakra *et al.*, 1977; Bagadia *et al.*, 1972). However, these are likely to be an underestimate because the prevalence in the patient population really depends upon the clinics from which the data are collected, along with what measures are used to ascertain sexual dysfunction. Bagadia *et al.* (1972) had collected their sample from a psychiatric clinic where they recruited 551 patients, of whom 339 had a sexual problem as a presenting complaint. Of these, the researchers were unable to evaluate 81 patients, and complete assessment was possible on 258 patients. The assessments included physical examination and Rorschach test. Of the sample, 119 were married and in this group 48% of the sample reported impotence, 35% reported premature ejaculation and 44% reported passage of semen in the urine. In the 139

unmarried patients, the commonest complaint was that of nocturnal emission (65% of the sample) and nearly half (44%) complained of passage of semen in the urine. All the patients had a diagnosed psychiatric condition with anxiety being the commonest, followed by neurotic depression. In addition to the sampling problems, the study did not present the data on Rorschach test and did not explore or standardize definitions of nocturnal emission, passage of semen, etc. Nakra *et al.* (1977, 1978) reported from a psychiatric clinic in north India that 9.2% of all patients attending had impotency (*sic*) problems – impotence being the commonest (reported in 35% of the sample), followed by premature ejaculation (reported by 25% of the sample). Interestingly, the spouses were either indifferent or unhelpful, thereby indicating the female expectations of the relationship. Three-quarters of the sample had practised masturbation and 43 per cent reported guilt as a result of this. Adolescent homosexual contact was acknowledged by 16% of the patients. Kar and Varma (1978), reporting on a sample of psychiatric patients, noted that 48% of the patients (*n* = 72) had failed to perform on their honeymoon, compared with 19% of sex-matched controls. In another clinical sample, Kumar *et al.* (1983) observed that in patients with neurosis, sexual frequency and satisfaction both dropped significantly. Avasthi *et al.* (1994) reported that 30% of cases recruited from a general hospital had erectile dysfunction and 12% had premature ejaculation, though in 45% of the cases these two were combined. Avasthi *et al.* (1995) studied 464 cases (96% male) in a sexual dysfunction clinic and 30.4% had clinical diagnosis of erectile dysfunction followed by a combination of erectile dysfunction and premature ejaculation in 26.5% of cases. Among females, vaginismus, dyspareunia and lack of sexual desire were common presenting complaints. In the Indian context, lack of privacy is often associated with premature ejaculation (Nag, 1972).

From Turkey, Uguz *et al.* (2004) reported that prevalence and types of sexual dysfunction were broadly similar to those reported from the West.

In South Asians in Leicester, Bhugra and Cordle (1986, 1988) found that male partners often spoke on behalf of their female partners. The referrals were more likely to be from secondary care. Shaeer *et al.* (2003) found that 57.4% of men attending a primary care clinic in Nigeria had erectile dysfunction, whereas in Egypt 63.6% of men and in Pakistan

80.8% of men (aged 35–70) reported so. Older age, diabetes, peptic ulcer, prostate disease, depression-related symptoms and caffeine intake were independently associated with increased prevalence of moderate to complete erectile dysfunction. In an unusual study exploring the attitudes and experiences of psychoanalysts regarding their patients in the USA, Canada and Australia, Doidge *et al.* (2002) found that mood disorder, anxiety disorder, sexual dysfunction and personality disorder were the commonest reasons for analysands seeking help. Although the numbers are small and response rates poor, the data clearly indicate that neuroses still form the bulk of the psychoanalysts' workload.

In another interesting study, Mirone *et al.* (2002) reported on men using a free phone call service on information on erectile dysfunction in Italy between 1993 and 1997. Each subject calling was asked if he was affected by erectile dysfunction and, if so, whether he had discussed it with a doctor or partner. Of a total of 12,761 callers, 7,265 (57%) acknowledged that they had discussed it with their partner. Not surprisingly, the longer the duration of the problem, the more likely the subject was to discuss this with his partner. Only 48 per cent of subjects had duration less than 6 months and for 60 per cent of those the duration was longer than 3 years. Similarly, only 50 per cent had discussed it with a physician, but in those subjects with duration of erectile dysfunction of less than 6 months, only one-third had informed their physician. If the duration was longer than 3 years, the proportion rose to 58 per cent. However, the authors do not clarify the quality or duration of partnerships. It is likely that those who were in a short-term or transient relationship may not have discussed it with their partners, but the evidence of the difficulty would be clear in any sexual activity.

Sexual deviance is often used as a term for individuals whose sexual preferences or mores do not fall into mainstream sexual behaviour. However, this remains a pejorative term so that, by definition, a negative value is being expressed. Bancroft (1989) suggests using sexual minority behaviour as a term. Paraphilia is the current preferred term in psychiatric literature.

Gagnon and Simon (1967) classified sexual deviance as normal, subcultural or individual deviance. Normal deviance includes behaviour such as masturbation, oral sex and premarital intercourse which, legally or socially proscribed in some parts of the world, is practised by large numbers of people, thereby

Table 30.1 Types of deviance and socio-cultural and biological influences

	Cultural influence	Biological influence
Normal deviance masturbation	+ + +	+
Oral sex	+ + +	?
Premarital sex	+ + +	?
Subcultural deviance fetishism	+	?
Sadomasochism	+	?
Transsexualism	?	+ +
Individual deviance exhibitionism	?	
Incest	?	?

falling within the statistical norm. Subcultural deviance is associated with particular subcultures (for example, homosexual) and will include categories of fetishism, sadomasochism, transvestism and transsexualism. These are often consensual behaviours, and their incidence is difficult to establish because individuals may not acknowledge these patterns and may well not seek help. Table 30.1 illustrates some of the diagnostic categories with possible aetiological factors divided into socio-cultural and biological factors and their possible impact.

Sexual Variance in Society and History by Bullough (1976) provides a classic account of sexual variance and society across different time periods, religions and geographical areas. He argues that male and female patterns of sexual orientation and behaviour (i.e. sex roles) are attributable to acquired learning, and therefore, to social and cultural factors. For example, Ford and Beach (1951) found that there was a wide variation in sexual behaviour in people and cultures and, although there are many similarities, there existed differences too. Different societies, for instance, have had widely different rules and attitudes about masturbation but, regardless of whether the attitude was one of approval or condemnation, at least some adults in all or nearly all societies appear to have masturbated. In the Indian study on male sexual dysfunction by Kalra *et al.* (2015), a minor 10% of the respondents denied having masturbated at all in their youth with about 14% having been prohibited by their parents or other elders from masturbating at some point in time and another 8% having received some sort of punishment for being caught during the act of masturbation. It is likely that cultural notions of high importance that are given to semen may frighten some men into developing a sense of doom and intense physical weakness if a single drop of semen is lost (Buchanan and Bhugra, 1989, Sumathipala *et al.*, 2004). This may lead to a sense of guilt after masturbation in these men thus any interventions in self-pleasure need to take this into account.

For nearly every human society, sexual intercourse is usually preceded by some degree of sensory stimulation and is often accompanied by stimulation, often visual or tactile. Visual stimulation is often of the individual partner, but sometimes this stimulation is related to a body part or part of clothing in achieving sexual excitement. Among societies where a minimum of such activity is carried out, it is possible that fetishistic sexual activity may well be lower. In the absence of concrete data, it is difficult to ascertain whether individual fetishistic behaviours are affected by the proliferate nature of the society or the sociocentrism of the individual. Within each culture and society, there are variations, too, both in preintercourse stimulation and foreplay. Some couples may well practise elaborate forms of genital manipulation, whereas others who may have bad feelings about sex or their partner may wish to skip the preliminaries. Breast stimulation and kissing as forms of sexual stimulation are more or less restricted to the human species, whereas preliminary stimulation of genital organs has a more ancient phylogenetic origin (Ford and Beach, 1951).

Sexual Attraction

There are few, if any, universal standards of sexual attractiveness. The physical characteristics, which are regarded as sexually stimulating, vary appreciably from one society to another as from one individual to another. In most societies, the physical beauty of the female receives more explicit consideration than that of the male. This may go some way towards explaining why men get turned on by objects. These selected female traits include plump body build, small ankles, elongated labia majora, large clitoris or pendulous breasts.

In some societies, bestiality is tolerated (even though seen as unnatural, silly and disgusting, and inferior to normal sexual activity) in the absence of more appropriate sexual behaviour. Such contact is often seen as inadequate and is sometimes allowed for teenage males. There are at least four societies in which animal contacts are practised and do not meet with condemnation (Ford and Beach, 1951). Such a variation reflects the influence of learning and social channelization.

Similarly, adult masturbation is tolerated in some societies and encouraged in others, but the double standards in response to male and female masturbation remain. The relative infrequency of adult masturbation in some societies is said to be the result of socialization (Ford and Beach, 1951). In societies which are restrictive in their attitudes to sex, teenagers may suppress their sexual desire but it is unlikely that no sexual activity takes place. Where boys are less carefully watched than girls, it appears that youths are able to circumvent the barriers. In semi-restrictive societies, formal prohibitions exist but are apparently not very serious, and are not enforced. Sexual experimentation may take place in secrecy, but without incurring punishment. Permissive societies have a permissive and tolerant attitude towards sex expression in childhood. In restrictive societies, girls are expected to remain virgins until marriage, whereas in the other two types, such expectations if they exist at all are not obvious. Actual sexual behaviour develops somewhat more rapidly in certain societies than in others.

Culture and Behaviour

Intracultural and intercultural behaviours are affected to a degree by learning behaviours. With increasing globalization, industrialization and the spread of global media, very few societies and cultures have been left isolated. The attitudes of a society towards certain sexual activities and behaviours are key factors in the way individuals adopt and enjoy a passive or an active role in the sexual relationship. The emphasis on the feminine means that females are encouraged not to take the lead in sexual intercourse and to be passive; they are less likely to experience clear-cut sexual orgasm. Although some patterns of sexual behaviour are reflexive incorporation of painful stimulation (sadomasochistic activity), the culturally accepted patterns of pre-coital play and the type of response to such stimulation are strongly influenced by learning. In societies where sexual excitement is associated with the experience of being scratched or bitten, these feelings become eroticized, and it is possible that limited or no enjoyment occurs without such actions. Similar foreplay techniques in other cultures may not produce similar results.

Paraphilias across Cultures

The knowledge, and especially that of prevalence, of paraphilias in normal population across cultures is severely limited. Although a fetish is defined as a magic erotic or love icon, its existence across cultures is by no means confirmed in the sense that individuals can out-perform sexually in its presence. Of the four paraphilias to be considered here, fetishism is probably quite common, although the rates are derived from those who attend clinics. There is general agreement that fetishism is rare in women. The principal categories of sexual signal or stimulus have been considered by Bancroft (1989). These are a part of the body or an intimate extension of the body, e.g. a piece of clothing and a source of specific tactile stimulation. The determinants of fetishism are many, and social learning theory must be seen to play an important role. There is virtually no literature reporting fetishism from non-industrialized countries. It is possible that, because of a lack of resources, individuals do not seek help, because two key reasons for seeking help are legal (once an individual has been in trouble with the law) or personal. As legal systems vary across societies, it is possible that such help-seeking is not encouraged in legal circles. At a more personal level, it is probable that the first or only port of call may be either an alternative practitioner or a primary-care physician, without the individual ever reaching a psychiatric clinic. The second possibility is that the rates are genuinely low because the society's expectations of a male are to procreate, without any underlying notions of pleasure for the self or the partner.

Bancroft (1989) argues that a majority of fetishes can be understood as an extension of the loved one which acquires special importance if there are other factors or causes of anxiety blocking the development of a more appropriate sexual relationship. Under these circumstances, it makes sense that, in societies where sexual love may have amorphous meaning and the individual's concept of the self is socio-centric rather than ego-centric, the likelihood of

being attracted to high heels, leather, rubber or boots may be low. In cases where fetishes are extremely bizarre and cannot be understood as extensions of the body, but are more likely to be associated with some neurological abnormality such as temporal-lobe epilepsy, the stimulus may be random, and it is possible that cases may occur across cultures. As discussed, sadomasochistic behaviour is more likely to occur across cultures especially if it develops as part of sexual foreplay and individuals accept it.

Of the two remaining paraphilias, transvestism and transexualism are quite interesting. Cross-dressing occurs in most societies and throughout history, and is also less likely to be a true paraphilia. Bhugra and de Silva (1996) postulate that, for uniforms to work as a fetish or individuals to dress in uniforms for sexual performance can be a reflection of fashion or fantasy. The sexual significance of cross-dressing is incredibly complex. Bancroft (1989) divides this group into four types: the fetishistic transvestite, the transsexual, the double-role transvestite and the homosexual transvestite. The sexual relationships of cross-dressers vary accordingly.

In their cross-cultural study of the sexual thoughts of children, Goldman and Goldman (1982) found that 55 per cent of boys and 9.5 per cent of girls expressed aversion to their biological sex. This reaction peaked in adolescence, with 30 per cent of 13-year-old boys in Australia and 20 per cent in the USA expressing such feelings which, by contrast, were virtually absent in Sweden. Bancroft (1989) suggests that, the more rigid the sex role stereotypes in a society, the greater the likelihood of this gender dysphoria. Thus, rigid expectations could produce anxiety and insecurity about gender identity, for which transsexual ideas would offer one method of coping. Consequently, Australia has a greater number of transsexuals seeking help than Sweden. Similarly, Australian gay males see themselves as more strongly feminine than their counterparts in Sweden (Ross et al., 1981; Ross, 1983).

The heterogeneity of sexual behaviour and societies in which they occur suggests that males are more likely to have fetishistic tendencies and that the development of sexual identity is dictated by social and cultural factors, thereby producing variation in rates of different fetishistic behaviours.

Several authors (Caplan, 1987; Herdt, 1990a, b; Herdt and Stoller, 1990) have argued that intersexes may not be discomfited by issues of sex and gender identity. Yet across cultures this identity may not

403

conform to that coinciding with the Western binary mode of gender assignment. Herdt (1990b), in contrast to the Western notion of binary gender (male vs female), calls for a three-sex code system because some societies are more flexible about the fit between gender identity and gender classification and emphasize the social context, ideology, socialization and gender development. Such an individual in this cultural milieu is neither a man nor a woman, nor a man wanting to be a woman (or vice versa), but belongs to a distinct third category. Other similar categories based on social and cultural categories have been described (David and Whitten, 1987). Jacobs and Roberts (1989) suggest that (even) three genders may not be enough to capture the complexity of the ethnographic material. Different gender designations are reflected in some Latin American settings (Parker, 1991).

It must be emphasized that gender identity may not bear any relation to sexual arousal. Sexual identity, cross-dressing and sexual orientation are not on a direct continuum but discrete independent categories (Callender and Kochens, 1986). There remain several problems in this classification and, as noted, the binary model is not necessarily applicable to many other societies.

Conclusions

Although the epidemiological data are scanty, there is enough clinical evidence to suggest that sexual dysfunction is present across all societies and cultures. However, the prevalence of patients presenting to clinics varies dramatically. This may be due to a number of factors. Furthermore, the role of the female sex in the act, their needs and desires are often ignored completely. The prevalence of various types of sexual dysfunction when confirmed is likely to lead to a clear understanding of treatment needs and accurate service planning.

The role of paraphilias, transgender, homosexuality, bisexuality and morbid jealousy also varies across cultures. Cultures determine and define what is normal and what is deviant and are therefore likely to develop pathways into care for psychosexual dysfunction. There is an urgent need for further exploration of social, biological, anthropological and psychological factors in the genesis and perpetuation of sexual dysfunctions and their management. The type of society and culture and the emphasis it places on the role of the sex act is important in understanding how patients and their

partners present and how they accept help. Patients in sex-positive societies may have higher levels of paraphilias and yet may readily seek help for their sexual dysfunction, whereas for sex-negative societies the reasons may be an urgent need for procreation rather than for pleasure. It must be emphasized that individual societies and cultures are not static and their characteristics may shift between sex-positive, sex-negative and sex-neutral status. Under these circumstances, the individual attitudes may also shift and their engagement in any therapeutic endeavour may become difficult.

Acknowledgements

This chapter is dedicated to the memory of Padmal de Silva, who contributed to the chapter in the first edition and passed away in 2008.

References

Aggrawal, A. (2009). References to the paraphilias and sexual crimes in the Bible. *Journal of Forensic and Legal Medicine*, **16**, 109–114.

Audu, B. M. (2002). Sexual dysfunction among infertile Nigerian women. *Journal of Obstetrics and Gynaecology*, **22**, 655–657.

Avasthi, A., Basu, D., Kulhara, P. and Bannerjee, S. T. (1994). Psychosexual dysfunction in Indian male patients. *Archives of Sexual Behaviour*, **23**, 685–695.

Avasthi, A., Arora, A., Kulhara, P. and Bannerjee, S. T. (1995). A study of psychosexually disordered patients attending a special clinic. *Archives of Indian Psychiatry*, **4**, 92–96.

Bagadia, V. N., Dave K. P., Pradhan, P. V. and Shah, L. P. (1972). A study of 258 male patients with sexual problems. *Indian Journal of Psychiatry*, **14**, 143–151.

Bancroft, J. (1989). *Human Sexuality and its Problems*. Edinburgh: Churchill Livingstone.

Bancroft, J., Loftus, J. and Long, J. S. (2003). Distress about sex: a national survey of women in heterosexual relationships. *Archives of Sexual Behaviour*, **32**, 193–208.

Bhugra, D. (1992). Psychiatry in ancient Indian texts. *History of Psychiatry*, **3**, 167–186.

Bhugra, D. (1997). Experiences of being a gay man in urban India: a descriptive study. *Sexual and Marital Therapy*, **12**(4), 371–375.

Bhugra, D. and Buchanan, A. (1989). Impotence in ancient Indian texts. *Sexual and Marital Therapy*, **4**, 87–92.

Bhugra, D. and Cordle, C. (1986). Sexual dysfunction in Asian couples. *British Medical Journal*, **292**, 11–112.

Bhugra, D. and Cordle, C. (1988). Sexual dysfunction in Asian couples: a case controlled study. *Sexual and Marital Therapy*, **3**, 69–75.

Bhugra, D. and de Silva, P. (1993). Sexual dysfunction across cultures. *International Review of Psychiatry*, **5**, 243–252.

Bhugra, D. and de Silva, P. (1995). Sexual dysfunction and sex therapy: an historical perspective. *International Review of Psychiatry*, **7**, 159–166.

Bhugra, D. and de Silva, P. (1996). Uniforms: fact, fashion, fantasy and fetish. *Sexual and Marital Therapy*, **11**, 393–406.

Buchanan A,. and Bhugra D (1989). Impotence in ancient Indian texts: implications for modern diagnosis. *Sexual and Marital Therapy*, **4**(1), 87–91.

Bullough, V. (1972). Sex in history: a virgin field. *Journal of Sex Research*, **8**, 101–116.

Bullough, V. (1976). *Sexual Variance in Society and History.* Chicago: University of Chicago Press.

Bullough, V. (1979). *Homosexuality.* Buffalo: New American Library.

Caplan, P. (ed.) (1987). *The Cultural Construction of Bisexuality.* London: Tavistock.

Chinese Psychiatric Society (CPS) (2001). *The Chinese Classification of Mental Disorders* (3rd edn [CCMD-3]) Shandong: Shandong Publishing House of Science and Technology [in Chinese].

Clanton, G. and Smith, L. G. (1977). *Jealousy.* Englewood Cliffs, NJ: Prentice Hall.

David, D. L. and Whitten, R. G. (1987). The cross-cultured study of human sexuality. *Annual Review of Anthropology*, **16**, 69–98.

De Silva, P. (1995). Paraphilias and sexual dysfunction. *International Review of Psychiatry*, **7**, 225–230.

Dennerstein, L., Dudley, E. and Burger, H. (2001). Are changes in sexual functioning during midlife due to ageing or menopause? *Fertility and Sterility*, **76**, 456–460.

Doidge, N., Simon, B., Brauer, L. *et al.* (2002). Psychoanalytic patients in the US, Canada and Australia. *Journal of American Psychoanalytical Association*, **50**, 575–614.

Ford, C. S. and Beach, F. A. (1951). *Patterns of Sexual Behaviour.* New York: Harper.

Foucault, M. (1981). *The History of Sexuality.* Harmondsworth: Penguin.

Gagnon, J. and Simon, W. (1967). *Sexual Deviance.* New York: Harper and Row.

Geyer, S., Haltenhof, H. and Peter, R. (2001). Social inequality in the initialisation of in and outpatient treatment of non psychotic/non organic disorders: study with health insurance data. *Social Psychiatry and Psychiatric Epidemiology*, **36**, 373–380.

Goldman, R. and Goldman, J. (1982). *Children's Sexual Thinking.* London: Routledge and Kegan Paul.

Gregersen, E. (1986). Human sexuality in cross-cultural perspective. In *Alternative Approaches to the Study of Sexual Behaviour*, ed. D. Byrne and K. Kelly. Hillsdale, NJ: LEA.

Gudjonsson, G. H. (1986). Sexual variations: assessment and treatment in clinical practice. *Sexual and Marital Therapy*, **1**, 191–212.

Hansen, A., Carr, K. and Jenssen, J. (2002). Characteristics and initial diagnosis in women presenting to referral centre for vulvovaginal disorders in 1996–2000. *Journal of Reproductive Medicine*, **47**, 854–860.

Herdt, G. H. (1987). *The Sambia: Ritual and Gender in New Guinea.* Belmont, CA: Wadsworth.

Herdt, G. H. (1990a). Mistaken gender. *American Anthropologist*, **92**, 433–446.

Herdt, G. H. (1990b). Development discontinuities and sexual orientation across cultures. In *Homosexuality/ Heterosexuality*, ed. D. McWhirter. New York: Oxford University Press.

Herdt, G. H. and Stoller, R. (1990). *Intimate Communications.* New York: Columbia University Press.

Hinsch, B. (1990). *Passions of the Cut Sleeve: The Male Homosexual Tradition in China.* Berkeley, CA: University of California Press.

Hunter, D. and Whitten, P. (1976). *Encyclopaedia of Anthropology.* New York: Harper and Row.

Hupka, R. (1984). Jealousy: compound emotion or label for a particular situation? *Motivation and Emotion*, **8**, 141–155.

Hupka, R. and Ryan, J. M. (1990). The cultural contribution to jealousy: cross-cultural aggression in sexual jealousy situation. *Behaviour Science Research*, **24**, 51–71.

Hupka, R., Brunk, B., Falns, G. *et al.* (1985). Romantic jealousy and romantic envy: a seven nation study. *Journal of Cross-Cultural Psychology*, **16**, 423–446.

Jacobs, S. and Roberts, C. (1989). Sex, sexuality, gender, and gender variance. In *Gender and Anthropology*, ed. S. Morgan. Washington DC: American Anthropological Association.

Johnson, A., Wadsworth, J., Wellings, K. and Field, J. with Bradshaw S. (1994) *Sexual Attitudes and Lifestyles.* Oxford: Blackwell Scientific.

Johnson, J. (1968). *Disorders of Sexual Potency in the Male.* New York: Pergamon.

Kadri, N., McHichi, A. and McHakra, T. S. (2002). Sexual dysfunction in women: population-based epidemiological study. *Archives of Women and Mental Health*, **5**, 59–63.

Kalra, G., Kamath, R., Subramanyam, A. and Shah, H. (2015). Psychosocial profile of male patients presenting with sexual dysfunction in a psychiatric outpatient department in Mumbai, India. *Indian Journal of Psychiatry*, **57**, 51–58.

Kantor, J., Bilker, W., Glasser, D. and Margolis, D. (2002). The prevalence of erectile dysfunction and active depression: an analytical cross-sectional study of general medical patients. *American Journal of Epidemiology*, **156**, 1035–1042.

Kar, G. C. D. and Varma, L. P. (1978). Sexual problems of married male mental patients. *Indian Journal of Psychiatry*, **20**, 365–370.

Khan, M. F., and Ahmed, S. H. (1990). Potency disorder among Pathans. *The Journal of the Pakistan Medical Association*, **40**, 12–14.

King, H. (1994). Sowing the field: Greek and Roman sexology. In *Sexual Knowledge, Sexual Science: The History of Attitudes to Sexuality*, ed. R. Porter and M. Teich. Cambridge: Cambridge University Press.

Kongkanand, A. (2000). Prevalence of erectile dysfunction in Thailand: Thai erectile dysfunction Epidemiological Study Group. *International Journal of Andrology* (Supplement), **2**, 77–80.

Kulhara, P. and Avasthi, A. (1995). Sexual dysfunction on the Indian subcontinent. *International Review of Psychiatry*, **7**, 231–240.

Kumar, S., Agarwal, A. K. and Trivedi, J. K. (1983). Neurosis and sexual behaviour in men. *Indian Journal of Psychiatry*, **25**, 190–197.

Litzinger, S. and Gordon, K. C. (2005). Exploring relationships among communication, sexual satisfaction, and marital satisfaction. *Journal of Sex and Marital Therapy*, **31**, 409–424.

Liu, C. (2003). Does quality of marital sex decline with duration? *Archives of Sexual Behaviour*, **32**, 55–60.

Mak, R., De Backer, G., Kornitzer, M. and De Meyer, J. (2002). Prevalence and correlates of erectile dysfunction in a population based study in Belgium. *European Urology*, **41**, 32–38.

Malinowski, B. (1927). *Sex and Repression in Savage Society*. London: Routledge and Kegan Paul.

Mathes, E. W. (1991). A cognitive theory of jealousy. In *The Psychology of Jealousy and Envy*, ed. P. Salovey. New York: Guilford Press, pp. 52–78.

Mathes, E. W., Adams, H. E. and Danes, R. M. (1985). Jealousy: loss of relationship: rewards, loss of self-esteem, depression, anxiety and anger. *Journal of Personality and Social Psychology*, **48**, 1552–1561.

Mazur, A., Mueller, U., Krause, W. and Booth, A. (2002). Causes of a sexual decline in ageing married men: Germany and America. *International Journal of Impotence Research*, **14**, 101–106.

Mead, M. (1977). Jealousy: primitive and civilized. In *Jealousy*, ed. G. Clanton and L. G. Smith. Englewood Cliffs, NJ: Prentice Hall, pp. 115–128.

Melman, A. and Gingell, J. C. (1999). The epidemiology and pathophysiology of erectile dysfunction. *Journal d'Urologie*, **161**, 5–11.

Meyer, J. J. (1971). *Sexual Life in Ancient India*. New Delhi: Motilal Banarasi Dass.

Mirone, V., Gentile, V., Zizzo, G. *et al.* (2002). Did men with erectile dysfunction discuss their condition with partner and physicians? A survey of men attending a free call information service. *International Journal of Impotence Research*, **14**, 256–258.

Money, J. (1984). Paraphilias: phenomenology and classification. *Journal of Applied Behavioural Analysis*, **12**, 377–389.

Nag, M. (1972). Sex culture and fertility: India and the United States. *Current Anthropology*, **13**, 231–237.

Nakra, B. R. S., Wig, N. N. and Varma, V. K. (1977). A study of male potency disorders. *Indian Journal of Psychiatry*, **19**, 13–18.

Nakra, B. R. S., Wig, N. N. and Varma, V. K. (1978). Sexual behaviour in the adult north Indian male. *Indian Journal of Psychiatry*, **20**, 178–182.

Namiki, S., Kwan, L., Kagawa-Singer, M., Saito, S., Terai, A., Satoh, T., Baba, S., Arai, Y. and Litwin, M. S. (2008). Sexual function reported by Japanese and American men. *Journal of Urology*, **179**, 245–249.

Nappi, R., Verde, J., Polanti, F., Genazzani, A. and Zara, C. (2002). Self reported sexual symptoms in women attending menopause clinic. *Gynecologic and Obstetric Investigation*, **53**, 181–187.

Nicolosi, A., Moreira, E. D., Jr, Villa, M., and Glasser, D. B. (2004). A population study of the association between sexual function, sexual satisfaction and depressive symptoms in men. *Journal of Affective Disorders*, **82**, 235–243.

Pacheco Palha, A. and Lourenço, M. F. (2011). Psychological and cross-cultural aspects of infertility and human sexuality. *Advances in Psychosomatic Medicine*, **31**, 164–183.

Parker, R. (1991). *Bodies, Pleasures and Passions*. Boston: Beacon Press.

Reiss, I. L. (1986). *Journey into Sexuality: An Exploratory Voyage*. Englewood Cliffs, NJ: Prentice Hall.

Rosen, R. and Leiblum, S. (1992). Erectile disorders: an overview of historical trends and clinical perspectives. In *Erectile Disorders: Assessment and Treatment*, ed. R. C. Rosen and S. R. Leiblum. New York: Guilford Press.

Ross, M. W. (1983). Societal relationships and gender roles in homosexuals. *Journal of Sex Research*, **19**, 273–288.

Ross, M. W., Walinder, J., Lindstrom, B. and Thuwe, I. (1981). Cross-cultural approaches to transsexualism: a comparison between Sweden and Australia. *Acta Psychiatrica Scandinavica*, **63**, 75–82.

Rust, J., Golombok, S. and Collier, J. (1988). Marital problems and sexual dysfunction: how are they related? *The British Journal of Psychiatry*, **152**, 629–631.

Sathyanarayana Rao, T. S., Darshan, M. S. and Tandon, A. (2015). An epidemiological study of sexual disorders in south Indian rural population. *Indian Journal of Psychiatry*, **57**, 150–157.

Schlegal, A. (1972). *Male Dominance and Female Autonomy: Domestic Authority in Matrilinear Societies*. New Haven, CT: HRAF Press.

Segal, M. H., Dasen, P. R., Berry, J. W. and Poortinga, Y. H. (1986). *Human Behaviour in Global Perspective*. New York: Pergamon.

Shaeer, K. Z., Osegbe, D., Siddiqui, S. H., Razzaque, A., Glasser, D. and Jaguste, V. (2003). Prevalence of erectile dysfunction and its correlates among men attending primary care clinics in three countries. *International Journal of Impotence Research*, **15**, S8–S14.

Skinner, C., Saulsbury, N. and Goh, B. (2002). Sexually transmitted infections in Bangladeshi residents in the UK: a case-control study. *Sexually Transmitted Infections*, **78**, 120–122.

Sumathipala, A., Siribaddana, S. H., and Bhugra, D. (2004). Culture-bound syndromes: the story of *dhat* syndrome. *British Journal of Psychiatry*, **184**, 200–209.

Syed, R. (1999). Knowledge of the 'Gräfenberg zone' and female ejaculation in ancient Indian sexual science. A medical history contribution. *Sudhoffs Archives*, **83**, 171–190.

Thakur, G. G. (1974). *Introduction to Ayurveda: The Science of Life*. New York: ASJ Publishers.

Uguz, S., Soylu, L., Diler, R. S. and Evlice, Y. (2004). Psychosocial factors and sexual dysfunctions: a descriptive study in Turkish males. *Psychopathology*, **37**, 145–151.

Unwin, J. D. (1934). *Sex and Culture*. Oxford: Oxford University Press.

Vanita, R. (2005). *Love's Rite: Same Sex Marriage in India and the West*. New Delhi: Penguin India.

Vanita, R. and Kidwai, S. (2000). *Same-Sex Love in India: Readings from Literature and History*. New York: St Martin's Press.

Wilson, G. (1987). *Variant Sexuality: Research and Theory*. London: Croom Helm.

Xu, S. (1990). Treatment of impotence by Chinese herbal medicine. In *Sexuality in Asia*, ed. M. Ling and L. S. Lam. Hong Kong: Hong Kong College of Psychiatry.

Chapter 31

Therapist–Patient Relationships and Culture

Digby Tantam

Editors' Introduction

In any type of psychotherapy the possibility for improvement or change is founded on the actual relationship in the treatment setting between the participants and the psychotherapist. As culture provides the values with which all individuals start out in life, cultural fit between client and therapist is important. Ethnic matching of therapist and the patient raises ethical and moral issues. Having set the scene on the theme of culture and psychotherapy, in this chapter Tantam deals with therapist–patient interaction and expectations of the patients from the therapeutic encounter. There is a distinction between a patient's expectations at the beginning of the encounter and as therapy progresses these expectations change. Expectations will be influenced by previous experience (whether of counselling, which may actually increase the likelihood of continuing with treatment or other treatments). The expectations that therapists carry with them are also important and these depend upon a number of factors, including their own cultures and their experiences with members of other cultures. Therapeutic alliance may not itself be therapeutic. Its impact is most likely to be on preventing premature discontinuation. The alliance begins with the fit between client's expectations and therapist's provision. One important expectation of the client is that their values will be understood and respected. The world views of both the therapist and the patient have to have some common values so that therapeutic work can begin. Cultures have unique and common values and some values which are common to other cultures. Similarly, between the therapist and the patient there will be common values and unique values. Empathy as a process by which the thoughts, feelings and emotions of an individual can be understood is a key component of the therapeutic encounter. Becoming more culturally aware of and therein becoming sensitive to and meeting patient's expectations and dealing with patients in an empathic and compassionate manner will improve therapeutic engagement and outcome.

Introduction

Sir William Osler is often taken as the pattern of the physician, a doctor who was variously described by his famous pupil Cushing as 'one of the most greatly beloved physicians of all time' (Bliss, 1999). One of his more famous patients was the American poet, Walt Whitman. Whitman was his patient between 1896 and 1890 when he was living in Camden, New Jersey and Osler was Professor of Clinical Medicine at the University of Pennsylvania. They shared the same view about the importance of personal care. Osler is often quoted as saying that the doctor should understand the patient with the disease, and not the disease. Whitman put it more prosaically: in a conversation between a customer and a shoemaker whether a shoe fits 'the fellow who wears the shoes always knows' (quoted in Hookman, 1995). Despite this, Whitman was not altogether pleased with Osler's care. He was upset that Osler seemed less interested in his patients than in academic medicine. He was bothered when Osler did not visit when he had said that he would. Most upsetting of all was Osler's breezy manner (he was an inveterate practical joker, having once quipped that as people's creativity diminished with age, they may as well be chloroformed at 60). Whitman wrote:

> I confess I do not wholly like or credit what he says – I do not fancy the jaunty way in which he seems inclined to dismiss the troubles. Still, that may all be a part of his settled policy – I do not object to cheer. I don't know if it's from getting down to hard pan or is a theory, but whatever, Osler pursues it . . . Still, I know my own condition – don't need him to tell me about that – can't be fooled. (Martens, 1997)

Whitman had had a stroke and Osler, presumably, had nothing specifically therapeutic to offer but believed that his determination to be optimistic would be helpful.

Further on in the article from which this information was taken, Martens goes on to consider the effect on Osler of World War I, in which he had lost his only son, and the subsequent influenza pandemic and compares it with Whitman's own experiences of being a nurse in the American Civil War. Osler himself referred to the effects in his presidential address to the Classical Association: 'If survived, a terrible infection, such as confluent smallpox, seems to benefit the general health. Perhaps such an attack through which we have passed may benefit the body cosmic.' Osler goes on to sketch a new order, and a revival of old medical values. Osler quotes approvingly from Hippocrates, whom he describes as the 'father of medicine' extolling 'the love of humanity associated with the love of his craft! – philanthropia and philotechnia – the joy of working joined in each one to a true love of his brother' (Osler, 1920).

Philanthropia and philotechnia do not always go hand in hand, but most doctors and patients alike would agree with the views attributed to Hippocrates, that they should do so in medicine and, a fortiori, in psychiatry. Or, to put it in contemporary language, the relationship between patient and doctor should be based on an alliance between them, as both Whitman and Osler thought.

The Therapeutic Alliance

There is considerable evidence that a good therapeutic alliance is associated with better outcomes: in the treatment of anorexia nervosa (Oyer et al., 2016; Rienecke et al., 2016), depression (Carter et al., 2015; Cooper et al., 2016), substance abuse and psychosis (Berry et al., 2016), people preoccupied with suicide (Gysin-Maillart et al., 2016) to name only some conditions. Breakdowns of the therapeutic alliance, on the other hand, lead to a loss of hopefulness about therapy (Bartholomew et al., 2016).

Bordin (1979) proposed that the therapeutic alliance had three elements: agreement on goals, assignment of tasks, and the development of bonds. There has been extensive research trying to pin these down further but without success. Attention has therefore turned to how an alliance is established, and how it can be re-established ('repaired') after 'ruptures' (Dixon et al., 2016). Focusing on 'ruptures' may be particularly important when clients have had repeated

previous experience of relationships going wrong (Gersh et al., 2017).

One criticism of this 'negotiation' model of the therapeutic alliance is that it presupposes shared cultural norms, notably that of compliance to professionals by clients (Doran, 2016). I have previously suggested (Tantam, 2002) that congruence of values, along with a focus on the client's preoccupying concern and an emotional flavour that is palatable to the client, is an essential contributor to the treatment alliance (see also Chapter 34).

Value Congruence

Empirical research has supported my hypothesis that value incongruence undermines the therapeutic alliance (Hogan et al., 2016). But it may be difficult for clinicians to recognize their own values and their incongruence with those of their clients. Cultural competence training may sensibilize clinicians to these issues that can apply even when dealing with clients from one's country and sharing one's own language (Fantini, 2016). One particularly challenging issue is the extent to which the client's family members or community have a say in their treatment that should be addressed (Henry and Baghdadli, 2016).

World View, Values and Emotions

World view is an Anglicization of the original German 'Weltanschauung', a term to which Freud dedicated a paper (Freud, 1933) in which he castigated what he described as the infantile Weltanschauung of religion. Indeed, he rejected the idea of having a Weltanschauung at all, inasmuch as he considered it to be a 'comprehensive hypothesis, a construction, therefore, in which no question is left open and in which everything in which we are interested finds a place'. He goes on to say that 'It is easy to see that the possession of such a Weltanschauung is one of the ideal wishes of mankind' (Freud, 1933: 92). Freud's view of Weltanschauung was no doubt coloured by the Nazi's annexation of the term, and by his long-standing concerns with social control, and in particular religious control, and its repressive effect. Sociologists have provided some support for the phenomenon, although giving it a different explanation. For example, Pike (1986) describes the severe penalties for voting against the majority, for allowing a child to have a tonsillectomy rather than to be traditionally healed, or for committing a shameful act in Mixtec society. He concludes that social rejection and gossip are used to extrude all such people because they challenge the Mixtec world view. From the anthropologist's point of view 'Public approval versus public disapproval can help focus attention on the values of that society and on the mechanisms of enforcement of those values' (Pike, 1986: 3048).

Freud's account is that people cleave to a world view for emotional reasons; Pike's that they subscribe to one imposed on them by their culture in order to maintain their status within the society whose culture it is.

One possible reason for the discrepancy is the differing focus of psychoanalysis, with its emphasis on emotion, and linguistics, with its emphasis on cognition. Pike was focusing on those beliefs which act as values, Freud on what I shall call in this chapter emotional flavour. Both are, as Dr Sayar and I shall argue in Chapter 34, elements of culture but transmitted differently. Emotional learning occurs at the parent's knee, as a result of discussions as soon as the child can talk about emotions (Mancuso and Sarbin, 1998) and perhaps even earlier, as a result of modelling. Learning about values occurs later, and involves an element of systematic instruction (Prencipe and Helwig, 2002).

Values and Expectations

Culture can, as we shall consider in more detail in Chapter 34, be mapped by its effects on the values, norms and artefacts of a society or social group. Rokeach (1973: 5) defines a value as 'an enduring belief that a specific mode of conduct or end state of existence is personally or socially preferable'. This definition is itself based on Kluckhohn's (1951: 395) definition of values as 'conceptions of the desirable means and ends of action'.

Kelly and Strupp (1992) used the Rokeach scale, based on this definition, to evaluate to what extent values determine outcome. They hypothesized that similarity of ideological values, and dissimilarity of lifestyle values, would correlate with a good outcome.

Unexpectedly, they found that many values did not change or even became less congruent to those of the therapist. These were wisdom, social values (equality, freedom, national security, a world of peace and a world of beauty), intellectuality and logicality, cleanliness, politeness and responsibility. There were values that changed, however, including most of the personal goals (valuing a comforting and an exciting life, family security, health, inner harmony, mature love, pleasure, salvation, self-respect, a sense of accomplishment and social recognition) and competency values (including ambition, broad-mindedness, capability, courage, imagination and independence).

A belief in salvation seemed different to the other values. Patients who had a conviction about salvation had a poor outcome with therapists who did not have this belief and who were not willing to respect it in clients.

Many other studies support this finding. Patients or clients who have strong religious convictions tend, or so it seems, to explain psychological distress in terms of their spiritual health. Therapists who are not willing to work in these terms cannot get on terms with them at all (Schultz-Ross and Gutheil, 1997). Unfortunately, as the earlier quotation from Freud indicates, psychotherapy has often set itself up as a rival to spirituality and religion. As a result, many people from cultures where spirituality continues to be an important and everyday part of life choose spiritual healers or priests for help, rather than psychotherapists (Kelm, 2006). Spirituality is especially important for people of colour in the US (Cervantes and Parham, 2005) and may be one reason why the uptake and outcome of psychotherapy is particularly low in that group.

Kelly and Strupp (1992) found that an adequate degree of similarity of values, or values matching, was required for good outcome. Too little similarity increased the risk of drop-out (and probably also reduced the likelihood of a person seeking therapy at all). However, leaving aside the particular value of salvation, it did not seem to matter which particular values were similar, almost as if values are like a Velcro sheet – enough similarity, enough contact at any point of the sheet, and there is some adhesion between patient and service.

Culture and Values

Cultures, by definition, are defined by their unique values. A therapist and a patient within the same culture are likely therefore to share values that are part of that culture, and to have a basis for the kind of adhesion or, to use another analogy, value matching that increases the chance of a therapeutic relationship being developed.

Cross-cultural therapy, on the other hand, places therapist and patient in a situation in which cross-cultural overlap is reduced. Therefore, finding enough of an overlap between values for the therapeutic relationship requires effort or skill. Guidelines published by the American Psychological Association (APA) on 'Multicultural Education, Training, Research, Practice, and Organizational Change for Psychologists' (American Psychological Association, 2003) take this into consideration. The APA points out that the previously accepted 'colour-blind' approach in which therapists try to ignore any ethnic, cultural and linguistic differences that may exist between themselves and their clients should be abandoned. Although colour blindness might reduce overt racism or stigmatization, it also means that therapists do not actively explore their own and their patients' values and therefore do not seek out points of overlap.

The APA recommends a 'culture-centred' approach to psychological practice. Psychologists are encouraged 'to use a "cultural lens" as a central focus of professional behaviour. In culture-centred practices, psychologists recognize that all individuals, including themselves, are influenced by different contexts, including the historical, ecological, socio-political, and disciplinary' (APA, 2003: 380). The 'cultural lens' or the 'culture-centred approach' are devices by which psychologists or therapists can try to transcend their own culturally determined viewpoint or world view. The authors of the guidelines review a substantial amount of relevant literature and propose three strategies for doing this. The first and 'most critical' is for the therapist to become more aware of their own attitudes and values and not assume that these simply reflect how the world is, or how it has to be. The second and third strategies are 'effort and practice in changing the automatically favorable perceptions of in-group and negative perceptions of out-group' by increased contact with members of other cultural groups, particularly with individuals of equal status whose perspective one can take, and with whom one can empathize.

Treatment Expectations

Empirical studies have avoided taking either the patient's or the therapist's viewpoint, and instead enquired about patient's expectations, how they match with those of the therapist, and how they relate to outcome. Expectations are influenced by previous experience, and it is therefore not surprising that previous experience of counselling significantly reduces the odds ratio of unilateral treatment termination vs other reasons for termination. However, counterintuitively, previous experience of counselling also reduces the odds ratio of mutually agreed termination (Corning *et al.*, 2004) as against termination for external reasons or continuing in therapy. The anomaly arises because the predictors of reason for termination change as treatment progresses (in this study, after session eight). Treatment, and treatment aims, become more personal and the factors that influence treatment adherence change. We will consider these later effects in the following section, on therapist–patient interaction.

In another study, of child and adult mental health services, problem improvement, environmental obstacles, and dissatisfaction with treatment were the reasons most often cited for dropping out. However, all the patients who dropped out rated their therapists as being less satisfactory than did the patients who were continuing in treatment or who had completed by mutual agreement (Pekarik, 1992).

What Do Patients Expect from Therapists?

Therapists have many times been the subject of documentaries, films, novels and other texts. Few people in a Western culture consult a therapist without some expectations of what they will find. Many of these accounts tend to emphasize therapists' human frailties (Gabbard, 2001) but they also shape expectations and these seem generally positive, with the expectations of psychological therapies being more positive than those for psychiatric treatment generally (Noble *et al.*, 2001). Studies of cultures which are less exposed to the Hollywood film might provide more information about naive expectations of therapists and therapies. These studies, too, also throw light on one of the important issues in cross-cultural psychotherapy provision: to what extent can traditional Western psychotherapy meet the needs of people from different cultures, and different ethnic groups whose expectations of help may be very different from those of Westerners.

In one such study, in Holland, 82 Turkish and 58 Moroccan attenders at a community mental health centre were interviewed and asked about their satisfaction with their therapists. Ethnic matching (see later) was only weakly associated with satisfaction, which was mainly determined by perceived clinical competence, and compassion. There were two elements to compassion: shared world view and empathy (Jeroen, 2004).

Empathy and Intersubjectivity

Goldie (2003: 195) defines empathy as 'a process or procedure by which a person *centrally imagines the narrative* (the thoughts, feelings, and emotions) of another person' (italics in original). In order to be able to do this imagining, a person needs access to another person's feelings and this is provided directly through a process of emotional contagion. Preston and de Waal (2002: 4) in an influential review define empathy in terms of emotional contagion or at least in terms of a more general process by which 'attended perception of the object's state automatically activates the subject's representations of the state, situation, and object, and that activation of these representations automatically primes or generates the associated autonomic and somatic responses, unless inhibited'.

It is the inhibition of empathy that is of particular interest in the so-called empathy disorders (Tantam, 1995), but empathy training of clinicians has focused on the later process of imagining what it would be like to be a person experiencing a particular feeling.

There is, however, an intermediate stage in the development of empathy which occurs in later infancy when infants are acquiring prosocial behaviour (Eisenberg, 2003) and learning to control their own emotions. This socialization process leads children to inhibit emotions that are not considered acceptable by a member of their family, by the family in general, or in their culture. This learning also extends to the child's empathic, emotional responses to others. Empathic responses which correspond to emotions that the child has learnt to inhibit are also inhibited (Eisenberg *et al.*, 1991b). The process may apply particularly to negative emotions. Children whose negative emotions – anger, fear or sadness – are contained by their families without being rejected appear to be more able to empathize with another child showing negative emotion (Eisenberg *et al.*, 1991a; Eisenberg *et al.*, 1994).

Describing these changes as the result of processes makes them seem more determinate than they probably are. I prefer to think of emotional development as consisting of something akin to aesthetic appreciation, in which development consists in finding greater emotional complexity and

nuancing in events, objects, relationships or people (Tantam, 2003) as a result of repeated experience and co-experience, and not as a result of deliberation. This account is consistent with that of the psychoanalysts who have added considerably to the conceptual tools which can be applied to emotional development (Tantam, 1996). Fairbairn, for example, describes in object-relation theory terms how some emotional responses can become inhibited because they are ones that have consistently elicited rejection by a carer; or to use my terms, emotions that are associated with rejection are likely to become unpalatable to the child, and therefore emotional flavours to be avoided (Tantam, 1996).

Learning to empathize more with others is, I would say, not only a cognitive exercise, of imagining more fully what it would be like to have that emotion, but also an aesthetic/affective accommodation to previously unpalatable emotional flavours.

Ethnic Matching

In a previous study of patients who drop out of community mental health treatment, Tantam and Klerman (1979) found that patients who did not keep even their first appointment had sometimes come to the clinic, walked in and then walked out again. These individuals said that they simply did not like the feel of the place. I would now say that the emotional flavour of our community mental health centre was unpalatable to these potential patients. One reason may have been that many of them were Hispanic, whilst our clinic staff were predominantly white. Maybe in the 30 seconds in which they made up their minds whether or not to make themselves known to the receptionist, these potential patients had seen all these white faces or some kind of white emotional flavour, and found it unpalatable.

One possible answer to this is to 'ethnically match': to provide patients with therapists of their own ethnicity. This obviously presents practical problems as there simply may not be enough suitably trained therapists of a relevant ethnicity. It also fails to address the other cultural elements which may lead to unpalatability, such as age, gender, dress code, language, class and so on.

There are two strong arguments in favour of ethnic matching. The first is that the no-show rate for mental health-related appointments can be as high as 50 per cent. If a proportion of these no-shows are, in fact, people for whom the therapy offered is emotionally unpalatable and if a proportion of this is due to the lack of ethnic matching, then ethnic matching is a way of increasing the accessibility of services.

The other argument is that the unpalability of the emotional flavour of the therapist or the therapy may also influence early drop-out rates, which are particularly high in some ethnic-minority groups accessing white-dominated services, at least in the US. There is a considerable accumulation of evidence for an exposure effect in psychotherapy: the longer people choose to remain in therapy, the more likely they are to benefit. Compliance may be affected by factors other than choice. For example, many recent studies of psychotherapy in the US have been of outpatients receiving psychotherapy as part of the treatment of their substance misuse. Attendance at psychotherapy sessions may, for them, be linked to avoiding gaol or receiving methadone maintenance. However, in a situation where there is free choice, persistence in treatment is directly, and drop-out rate is inversely, linked to outcome.

Despite the theoretical support for the value of ethnic matching, a recent review (Karlsson, 2005: 117) concludes that 'there is little evidence that ethnic matching leads to better outcomes or greater satisfaction of psychotherapy'. One reason may be that the patients who did not enter treatment at all are excluded from the evaluations reviewed. Another may be the practical problems already alluded to, and also considered in this review. Another may be that what matters in the therapeutic relationship is the match between therapist and patient, and matching ethnicity cannot guarantee this nor can a lack of matching on ethnicity be assumed to be a lack of any match. However, perhaps the most important reason that ethnic matching is not effective is that psychotherapy is a human process, in which people adjust. If the patient and the therapist can both accommodate to each other – an accommodation that involves both a respect for other values, and the ability to learn to like new emotional flavours – then ethnic matching may not be important.

Therapist Interaction

The ability of therapists to reach out to their patients, either emotionally or by being able to understand and respect their values, is only one facet of therapeutic success. Close relationships of all kinds can only be maintained if there is a device for managing negative emotion which spills over into the relationship itself,

as it usually will sooner or later. Men may remain friends over long periods by avoiding areas of possible disagreement (Duck, 1995), but the consequence is a lack of intimacy which is inimical to psychotherapy.

The link between drop-out from therapy and outcome might seem tautologous. It might seem that people continue to attend psychotherapists whilst they are rewarded by an improvement until that reward falls below the cost of attendance, and then they stop. This explanation, though, is based on the presumption that psychotherapy provides continuous incremental improvements after each session. Studies of psychotherapy over time do not often fit this model. There are sudden breakdowns in the therapeutic relationship and sudden gains, improvement is typically seen after a latency period, and there is an optimal treatment dose which differs for different treatment outcomes, exceeding which can result in a poorer outcome. More importantly, there are substantial differences between therapists, which are reflected in the greater likelihood for therapists who have poorer effectiveness to have their patients drop out (Lambert and Ogles, 2004). Clients who are predicted to have a poor prognosis have as good an outcome as those who are predicted to have a good prognosis if they complete the course of therapy – but, of course, many more of them drop out, which is what makes for their poor prognosis (Tantam, 2002; Wampold, 2001).

Training in cultural competence is designed to increase cultural awareness. The methods are considered elsewhere in this book. In one study, even brief cultural-awareness training resulted in a reduction of the proportion of African American clients dropping out of treatment with therapists who had been trained (Wade and Bernstein, 1991). Cultural awareness does not just apply to making a relationship with the patient in the first place, although this is important, but also managing negative emotion and challenges to personal values. Cultural competency therefore does not just apply to being warm and friendly. It also extends to being able to use culturally appropriate means of resolving conflict and negativity.

Humanities, Again

Travel and wide reading are long prescriptions for developing knowledge and sympathy for other peoples and other cultures. Whilst the APA guidelines seemed mainly to be focused on encouraging psychologists to work more with people from cultures other than their own, they could have referred to these values of an earlier age, values which Osler himself espoused.

However, there was a further element in Osler's humanity which did not come from his eclectic reading, nor from his experience of practice in both North America and Europe: his empathy. This, according to Martens (1997), was something that Osler conspicuously displayed only late in his career. He gives the example of Osler giving a rose to the mother of an influenza victim that Osler had been treating, and contrasts this with the breezy manner that he had shown to Whitman earlier in his career.

We can speculate that the loss of his own child made it possible for Osler to empathize with another bereaved parent. But more generally, we can speculate that an experience of emotional upheaval, in which our accustomed emotions and emotional reactions no longer seem to apply, may be one route by which therapists and physicians become more open to their patients' own emotional uncertainties and upheavals. This is certainly one of the contentions of the wounded-healer movement (Jackson, 2001).

However, there is the further requirement on the therapist that they have the ability to repair breaches in the therapeutic relationship when they occur. This certainly requires an awareness and respect for the values of the patient, as well as empathy for them. But is also requires a degree of emotional steadiness, sometimes termed the capacity for containment, by psychoanalysts.

Travel, with its own small attendant desperations, and reading, with its opportunity to identify with heroes and heroines stricken by circumstance, might in lesser ways also increase our capacity to empathize. Both travel and reading can certainly open our eyes to other values, and other world views. Can they help to increase our capacity for containment?

Perhaps they can, but only if we have the perspicacity to know that, when we visit a place that has a powerfully negative effect on us, or when we throw down a book in disgust or anger, that is the place or the book that we should persevere with. Perseverance is, however, effortful. Not only does it provoke cognitive dissonance, but it requires us to accustom ourselves to previously unpalatable emotional flavours. Doing that requires a degree of emotional comfort.

Becoming more culturally aware, and therefore more effectively meeting and working with our patients' expectations, as well as interacting with our patients in a manner that satisfies them and us,

requires effort too. But we can only expend this if we have reserves. If what patients want from us is compassion – and that is what one previously quoted cross-cultural study has suggested (Jeroen, 2004) – then the heart of compassion has its own beat. The compassion of the therapist has its diastole in which care and comfort has to be taken in, as well as its systole. Perhaps, like Osler, we might keep some books on our bedside table that can provide comfort and refuge as well as stimulation and challenge and in both of these ways increase our compassion.

References

American Psychological Association (2003). Guidelines on multicultural education, training, research, practice, and organizational change for psychologists. *American Psychologist*, **58**, 377–402.

Bartholomew, T. T., Gundel, B. E. and Scheel, M. J. (2016). The relationship between alliance ruptures and hope for change through counseling: a mixed methods study. *Counselling Psychology Quarterly*, 1–19, doi:10.1080/09515070.2015.1125853.

Berry, K., Gregg, L., Lobban, F. and Barrowclough, C. (2016). Therapeutic alliance in psychological therapy for people with recent onset psychosis who use cannabis. *Comprehensive Psychiatry*, **67**, 73–80, doi:10.1016/j.comppsych.2016.02.014.

Bliss, M. (1999). William Osler at 150. *Canadian Medical Association Journal*, **161**, 831–834.

Bordin, E. (1979). The generalizability of the psychoanalytic concept of the working alliance. *Psychotherapy: Theory, Research and Practice*, **16**, 252–260.

Carter, J. D., Crowe, M. T., Jordan, J., McIntosh, V. V. W., Frampton, C. and Joyce, P. R. (2015). Predictors of response to CBT and IPT for depression; the contribution of therapy process. *Behaviour Research and Therapy*, **74**, 72–79, doi:10.1016/j.brat.2015.09.003.

Cervantes, J. M. and Parham, T. A. (2005). Toward a meaningful spirituality for people of color: lessons for the counseling practitioner. *Cultural Diversity and Ethnic Minority Psychology*, **11**, 69–81.

Cooper, A. A., Strunk, D. R., Ryan, E. T., DeRubeis, R. J., Hollon, S. D. and Gallop, R. (2016). The therapeutic alliance and therapist adherence as predictors of dropout from cognitive therapy for depression when combined with antidepressant medication. *Journal of Behavior Therapy and Experimental Psychiatry*, **50**, 113–119, doi:10.1016/j.jbtep.2015.06.005.

Corning, A. F. and Malofeeva, E. V. (2004). The application of survival analysis to the study of psychotherapy termination. *Journal of Counseling Psychology*, **51**, 354–367.

Dixon, L. B., Holoshitz, Y. and Nossel, I. (2016). Treatment engagement of individuals experiencing mental illness: Review and update. *World Psychiatry*, **15**(1), 13–20, doi:10.1002/wps.20306.

Doran, J. M. (2016). The working alliance: where have we been, where are we going? *Psychotherapy Research*, **26**(2), 146–163, doi:10.1080/10503307.2014.954153.

Duck, S. (1995). *Human Relationships: An Introduction to Social Psychology*. London: Sage.

Eisenberg, N. (2003). Prosocial behavior, empathy, and sympathy. In *Well-Being: Positive Development over the Life Course*, ed. M. H. Bornstein, L. Davidson, C. Keyes and K. Moore. Mahwah, NJ: Lawrence Erlbaum Associates, Publishers, pp. 253–265.

Eisenberg, N., Fabes, R. A., Schaller, M., Carlo, G. and Miller, P. A. (1991a). The relations of parental characteristics and practices to children's vicarious emotional responding. *Child Development*, **62**(6), 1393–1408.

Eisenberg, N., Fabes, R. A., Schaller, M. *et al.* (1991b). Personality and socialization correlates of vicarious emotional responding. *Journal of Personality and Social Psychology*, **61**, 459–470.

Eisenberg, N., Fabes, R. A., Nyman, M. *et al.* (1994). The relations of emotionality and regulation to children's anger-related reactions. *Child Development*, **65**, 109–128.

Fantini, Alvino and Tirmizi, Aqeel, (2006). Exploring and assessing intercultural competence. *World Learning Publications*. **1**. http://digitalcollections.sit.edu/world learning_publications/1.

Freud, S. (1933). A philosophy of life. In *New Introductory Lectures on Psycho-analysis*, ed. J. Strachey. London: Allen & Unwin.

Gabbard, G. O. (2001). Psychotherapy in Hollywood cinema. *Australasian Psychiatry*, **9**, 365–369.

Gersh, E., Hulbert, C. A., McKechnie, B., Ramadan, R., Worotniuk, T. and Chanen, A. M. (2017). Alliance rupture and repair processes and therapeutic change in youth with borderline personality disorder. *Psychology and Psychotherapy: Theory, Research and Practice*, **90**(1), 84–104, doi:10.1111/papt.12097.

Goldie, P. (2003). *The Emotions*. Oxford: Oxford University Press.

Gysin-Maillart, A. C., Soravia, L. M., Gemperli, A., and Michel, K. (2016). Suicide ideation is related to therapeutic alliance in a brief therapy for attempted suicide. *Archives of Suicide Research*, **21**(1), 113–126, doi:10.1080/13811118.2016.1162242.

Henry, V., and Baghdadli, A. (2016). How sociocultural aspects influence health and mental health care: a case study on a young gypsy girl with autism. *Archives de Pediatrie*, **23**(6), 599–602, doi:10.1016/j.arcped.2016.03.014.

Hogan, L. R., Callahan, J. L. and Shelton, A. J. (2016). A matter of perception: patient and therapist value

differences impact working alliance and outcome. *Revista Argentina de Clinica Psicologica*, **25**(1), 5–16.

Hookman, P. (1995). A comparison of the writings of Sir William Osler and his exemplar, Sir Thomas Browne. *Bulletin of the New York Academy of Medicine*, **72**(1), 136–150.

Jackson, S. W. (2001). The wounded healer. *Bulletin of the History of Medicine*, **75**, 1–36.

Jeroen, W. K. (2004). A need for ethnic similarity in the therapist–patient interaction? Mediterranean migrants in Dutch mental-health care. *Journal of Clinical Psychology*, **60**, 543–554.

Karlsson, R. (2005). Ethnic matching between therapist and patient in psychotherapy: an overview of findings, together with methodological and conceptual issues. *Cultural Diversity and Ethnic Minority Psychology*, **11**, 113–129.

Kelly, T. A. and Strupp, H. H. (1992). Patient and therapist values in psychotherapy: perceived changes, assimilation, similarity, and outcome. *Journal of Consulting and Clinical Psychology*, **60**, 34–40.

Kelm, M.-E. (2006). Wilp Wa'ums: colonial encounter, decolonization and medical care among the Nisga'a. *Social Science and Medicine*, **59**, 335–349.

Kluckhohn, C. (1951). Values and value orientations in the theory of action. In *Toward a General Theory of Action*, ed. T. Parsons and E. Shils. Cambridge, MA: Harvard University Press.

Lambert, M. and Ogles, B. M. (2004). The efficacy and effectiveness of psychotherapy. In *Berger and Garfield's Handbook of Psychotherapy and Behavior Change*, ed. M. J. Lambert and B. M. Ogles, 5th edn. New York: John Wiley, pp. 139–193.

Mancuso, J. C. and Sarbin, T. R. (1998). The narrative construction of emotional life: developmental aspects. In *What Develops in Emotional Development?*, ed. M. F. Mascolo. New York, NY: Plenum Press, pp. 297–316.

Martens, P. (1997). War, Walt Whitman, and William Osler. *Literature and Medicine*, **16**, 210–225.

Noble, L., Douglas, B. and Newman, S. (2001). What do patients expect of psychiatric services? A systematic and critical review of empirical studies. *Social Science and Medicine*, **52**, 985–998.

Osler, W. (1920). *The Old Humanities and the New Science*. Boston: Houghton Mifflin Co.

Oyer, L., O'Halloran, M. S. and Christoe-Frazier, L. (2016). Understanding the working alliance with clients diagnosed with anorexia nervosa. *Eating Disorders*, **24**(2), 121–137, doi:10.1080/10640266.2015.1034050.

Pekarik, G. (1992b) Relationship of clients' reasons for dropping out of treatment to outcome and satisfaction. *Journal of Clinical Psychology*, **48**, 91–98.

Pike, K. (1986). Mixtec social 'credit rating': the particular versus the universal in one emic world view. *Proceedings of the National Academy of Sciences, USA*, **83**, 3047–3049.

Prencipe, A. and Helwig, C. C. (2002). The development of reasoning about the teaching of values in school and family contexts. *Child Development*, **73**, 841–856.

Preston, S. D. and de Waal, F. B. M. (2002). Empathy: its ultimate and proximate bases. *Behavioral and Brain Sciences*, **25**, 1–72.

Rienecke, R. D., Richmond, R. and Lebow, J. (2016). Therapeutic alliance, expressed emotion, and treatment outcome for anorexia nervosa in a family-based partial hospitalization program. *Eating Behaviors*, **22**, 124–128, doi:10.1016/j.eatbeh.2016.06.017.

Rokeach, M. (1973). *The Nature of Human Values*. New York: Free Press.

Schultz-Ross, R. A. and Gutheil, T. G. (1997). Difficulties in integrating spirituality into psychotherapy. *Journal of Psychotherapy Practice and Research*, **6**, 130–138.

Tantam, D. (1995). Empathy, persistent aggression and antisocial personality disorder. *Journal of Forensic Psychiatry*, **6**, 10–18.

Tantam, D. (1996). Fairbairn. In *150 Years of British Psychiatry*, ed. G. Berrios and H. Freeman. London: Athlone Press.

Tantam, D. (2002). *Psychotherapy and Counselling in Practice*. Cambridge: Cambridge University Press.

Tantam, D. (2003). The flavour of emotions. *Psychology and Psychotherapy: Theory, Research and Practice*, **76**, 23–45.

Tantam, D. and Klerman, G. (1979). Patient transfer from one clinician to another and dropping-out of outpatient treatment. *Social Psychiatry*, **14**, 107–113.

Wade, P. and Bernstein, B. (1991). Culture sensitivity training and counselor's race. *Journal of Counseling Psychology*, **38**, 9–15.

Wampold, B. (2001). *The Great Psychotherapy Debate*. New Jersey: Lawrence Erlbaum.

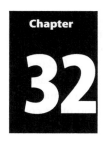
Developing Effective Mental Health Services for Multicultural Societies

Harry Minas

Editors' Introduction

There are major challenges ahead when planning services for multicultural societies due to a number of reasons. These include variety of minority groups, languages, educational and economic status, etc. In this chapter Minas points out that in multicultural societies the development of mental health services that are responsive, accessible, culturally appropriate and effective, should not be an add-on or an afterthought. Separate services for minority groups will bring with them another set of issues. Obviously close attention to issues of cultural competence is not and should not be seen as a distraction from the 'core business' of mental health services. It should be seen as good clinical practice. Minas argues that cultural competence is more important now than at any other time in the past in a world where more and more countries are becoming multi-ethnic and multicultural, it is critical that healthcare professionals learn and are indeed trained to respond to the needs of the populations they serve which may well include increased numbers of traumatized asylum seekers and refugees. Taking into account these cultural variations should be at the heart of mental healthcare and services. It is entirely possible; as Minas reminds us, knowledge about culture, migration and mental health may well be limited, partial or inconsistent, but there is enough known about how to provide equitable culturally acceptable services to enable informed policy development. In these days of access to the Internet there is no reason not to explore knowledge in developing the right type of services and service planning which must be evaluated regarding satisfaction and outcome. Minas suggests that while working through the process of reforming services so that they are capable of meeting the needs of a culturally diverse society the clinicians and service providers as well as policy makers must ensure that services are flexible and responsive to the needs of all members of the community.

Introduction

Throughout human history wars and revolutions, the formation and fragmentation of empires, the partition and collapse of states, colonial wars and postcolonial civil disorder, epidemics, droughts and crop failures, natural disasters and economic collapses have produced population movements on a grand scale (Minas, 2001a). The modern era is not exempt from such troubles and has experienced unprecedented movements of people due to the same reasons. In 2005 (UNHCR, 2007) the number of 'people of concern' to UNHCR was 19.2 million, an increase from 17 million the previous year. In 2015 there were 65.3 million people who had been forcibly displaced: 40.8 million internally displaced, 21.3 million refugees and 3.2 million asylum seekers. Almost 30 per cent of refugees are children (United Nations High Commissioner for Refugees, 2016). The conflict in Syria alone has resulted in an unprecedented flight from danger with, in July 2016, more than 4.8 million registered refugees and many more millions internally displaced. Germany has accepted more than 1 million Syrian refugees, while 2.7 million UNHCR-registered Syrian refugees are in Turkey. While UNHCR has estimated that USD5.5 billion is required in 2016 to support Syrian refugees only USD1.3 billion has been received. The failed military coup in Turkey in July 2016 and the draconian government response have increased the level of uncertainty for refugees as well as for the general Turkish population.

In the previous edition of this book I wrote the following: 'In our own time, the so-called war on terror and the political doctrine of unilateralism and preemption will play out in unpredictable and probably disastrous ways, as is happening in Iraq.'

Unfortunately this observation has been borne out by events. In 2014, 20,030 civilians died in violent incidents in Iraq, and 16,115 in 2015 (Conflict Casualties Monitor, 2016). The Chilcot Inquiry into the UK's 'invasion and full-scale occupation' of the sovereign state of Iraq was scathing in its conclusions (Chilcot, 2016). It has been persuasively argued that the military adventure in Iraq by a hastily assembled Western coalition of forces, and the catastrophic aftermath of this invasion and occupation, created the conditions for the rise of so-called 'Islamic State' (Barton, 2016) which has carried out and inspired multiple terrorist atrocities primarily in the Middle East but also in Western countries. In 2016 alone, terrorist attacks resulting in mass casualties have occurred in France, Belgium, Germany and Turkey. While these incidents have captured attention in the West, in 2015 and 2016 deaths from terrorist incidents perpetrated by several groups and by individuals in the Middle East, Africa and Asia have been 50 times those in Europe and the Americas.

In addition to the consequences of conflict the pressures of globalization (structural adjustment, technological change, the globalization of work and trade liberalization), environmental degradation, and the increasing economic non-viability of rural life in villages and towns everywhere will continue to produce massive movements of people from rural areas to the mega-cities and across borders. There are more than 100 million rural migrants in cities in China, with a great number in the mega-cities such as Shanghai where industrial development has been most rapid and jobs are to be found. There is rising concern about structural inequities and mental health problems experienced by many internal rural-to-urban migrants in China and elsewhere (Lin *et al.*, 2011) and the 150 million international labour migrants, 55 per cent of whom are female (International Labour Organization, 2016). Among the most troublesome global developments, for social stability and for population mental health, is the ever-increasing gap between rich and poor and the relentless concentration of wealth in the hands of a very small proportion of the world's population (Stiglitz, 2015).

Given the scale and nature of people movements and the complex interplay of the drivers of such movements it may become increasingly difficult to maintain the distinction between refugees who are subject to political oppression and violence and are protected by international agreements and those who are not – economic and environmental 'refugees'. Poverty and unemployment have resulted in large numbers of temporary labour migrants (International Labour Organization, 2016). People-trafficking is among the most profitable forms of illegal trade. A number of countries have come to rely on remittances from their nationals working abroad and other countries rely on illegal migrants to do work that their own citizens prefer not to do. Patterns of migration, voluntary and forced, are very fluid. Many of the former colonial powers have experienced a massive influx of immigrants from their former colonies in North and sub-Saharan Africa, Asia, the Caribbean and elsewhere. Concern about the scale and sources of migration has been a major factor in the rise of nationalist movements and right-wing political groupings in many Western countries. It was perhaps the defining factor in the June 2016 decision by referendum of the UK to leave the European Union.

The mental health of immigrants and refugees will continue to be shaped by the nature of pre- and post-migration experiences.

Ethnic and cultural diversity is a prominent feature of most nations, developed and developing. Even nations that are generally thought of as ethnically and culturally homogeneous, such as China and Vietnam, are in fact ethnically and culturally diverse, with multiple minority ethnic groups. These minorities, like minorities everywhere, experience many disadvantages and sometimes discrimination and abuse of rights. Although a major focus of transcultural psychiatry has been the mental health of immigrants and refugees, there are of course many forms of cultural diversity, other than the ethnic and linguistic diversity characteristics of immigrants and refugees, that must be considered in relation to population mental health and culturally appropriate mental health services. The mental health of indigenous populations is now receiving increased attention (Kirmayer and Brass, 2016). An example of diversity that is of increasing importance is diversity in sexual orientation. Lesbian, gay, bisexual, trans-sexual and intersex (LGBTI) communities and individuals have for centuries been subject to discrimination, social exclusion and abuse. Debate continues concerning whether homosexuality is a diagnosable mental disorder and subject to 'treatment'. In many countries homosexuality is illegal and punishable by imprisonment, corporal punishment and, in some countries, the death penalty. It is clear that negative societal responses to diverse sexual orientations greatly increase the risk of mental disorder and of suicide.

All forms of cultural diversity confront nations with numerous challenges (Kymlicka, 1995) and raise important questions concerning national identity, the legitimate role of government, distribution of resources, acceptable and unacceptable cultural practices, and the purposes, structure and operation of social institutions. Although I will focus in this chapter on cultural diversity that is the product of migration I would suggest that the principles outlined for development of effective mental health services for multicultural societies are relevant for mental health system responses to all kinds of population diversity.

Effective and Equitable Services

Mental health systems are on the front line in dealing with the mental health consequences of pre-migration trauma, migration and the rigours of settlement in a new country. Even in those countries where multiculturalism is broadly accepted by government and the majority of the population, health systems have been slow to organize themselves in ways that would enable them to meet the wide diversity of needs in multicultural populations.

More than 20 years ago several authors (Minas, 1991; Sue, *et al.*, 1991; Bhui *et al.*, 1995; Minas *et al.*, 1996) set out their views concerning the key features of equitable and effective mental health services for culturally diverse societies. These are still relevant. They have not yet been comprehensively achieved in any country. One such set of defining characteristics of an effective and equitable mental health system for multicultural societies is shown in Box 32.1.

While some conceptions of effective and equitable mental health systems (Minas *et al.*, 1996) have influenced, or have been incorporated into, policies (Multicultural Mental Health Australia, 2004, National Mental Health Commission, 2014) and mental health service standards (Australian Health Ministers, 1997), they remain aspirations, have not been integrated into general reform processes, and have had limited impact on the operation of mental health services (Fernando, 2005). Failure to fund and to implement even clearly stated policy intent in relation to multicultural mental health appears to be common (Minas *et al.*, 2007; Minas *et al.*, 2013).

Although many service models that focus on the particular needs of a diverse society, and other

---

BOX 32.1 Some defining characteristics of an effective and equitable mental health service

1. The mental health service needs of the community are jointly defined by consumers, carers, the community and service providers.
2. The types of services offered, their location and the skills of professionals, are all issues that are determined by the needs of the community to be served.
3. Service agencies recognize that it is their responsibility to develop the capacity to effectively meet diverse needs.
4. Service agencies respond appropriately to religious, cultural and communication needs of service recipients as well as to direct clinical needs.
5. Those who may require the service:
   5.1. know of its existence;
   5.2. regard it as being appropriate to their needs;
   5.3. can gain easy and timely access to the service;
   5.4. can communicate adequately with service providers;
   5.5. can gain access to the full range of services which are appropriate to their needs; and
   5.6. are treated with respect and without prejudice.
6. Outcome indicators demonstrate that the service is achieving the clinical and other goals of service providers and recipients.
7. The quality of outcome is not determined or substantially influenced by factors such as English language fluency or membership of any particular ethnic or social group.
8. Community, and consumer and carer, representatives are involved in the continuing evaluation, and redesign where necessary, of the service.

Source: modified from Minas *et al.* (1996)

---

initiatives such as professional training, have been proposed, and in some instances implemented, there are few examples of adequate evaluation of their effectiveness (Ziguras *et al.*, 2000; Bhui *et al.*, 2007; Minas *et al.*, 2013). The information that would need to be collected, sources of data and required methods for demonstrating effectiveness of services in a multicultural society have been outlined in four domains in which change is essential: (1) improvements in clinical interaction; (2) organizational adaptations in the clinical context; (3) relationship between health facilities and ethnic communities; and (4) relations between relevant elements of the health system (de Jong and van Ommeren, 2005).

Because of the great variety of political, economic and cultural contexts and histories within which mental health systems have developed and currently operate, there can be no single 'best practice' model of mental health services for multicultural societies. There are now some good accounts of things that have been tried in a variety of countries (Bhugra, 1997; Bäärnhielm *et al.*, 2005; Fernando, 2005; Ganesan and Janze, 2005; Lo and Chung, 2005). My intention in this chapter is to present a general outline of an approach that is likely to achieve positive system change. One should expect that the specific shape and content of services that emerge from the application of such an approach will differ according to the contexts in which they develop.

Mental Health System Reform

Mental health services that are of appropriate scope and reach, and that are adequately supported and resourced, cannot be developed in the absence of enabling national, regional and local agency policies. These are not just health policies. Economic and social policies are just as important for mental health. Policies may have negative or positive impacts on the mental health of immigrant and refugee populations. For example, Australia's immigration policy of mandatory detention of asylum seekers arriving by boat is actively producing serious and long-term mental health problems among asylum seekers subjected to this oppressive regime (Newman and Steel, 2008; Coffey *et al.*, 2010; Newman *et al.*, 2013), and substantially increasing the risk of suicide. The process of improving mental health systems so that they are capable of providing high quality services to multicultural populations is best seen as part of the broader process of continuing health-system reform. An example of a broad social policy that is likely to have substantial positive impact on the health and well-being of persons with mental disorders is the National Disability Insurance Scheme, recently introduced in Australia (Reddihough *et al.*, 2016). If adequately implemented, this programme is likely to be of great importance in the field of mental health

(Salvador-Carulla and Einfeld, 2014; Williams and Smith, 2014) although it is not primarily a health or mental health programme. Roberts and his colleagues (2004) have articulated an approach to health-system reform that can serve as a useful framework for thinking about how to develop mental health services for culturally diverse societies. A central requirement for reform is an understanding of the policy cycle, the components of which are (1) problem definition, (2) diagnosis of the causes of problems, (3) policy development, (4) political decision, (5) implementation and (6) evaluation. Acting to bring about reform requires an understanding of the levers for change that can be used to bring about the necessary changes. The approach is grounded in the recognition that health-sector reform occurs within a variety of ethical and political contexts.

Ethical Foundations

Any effective health system response to population diversity must be based on firm ethical foundations. Throughout the past two centuries, the period during which the discipline and practice of psychiatry have been developed (Cohen *et al.*, 2014), there are innumerable examples of abuse of the rights of persons with mental illness in the community (Minas and Diatri, 2008) and in mental health institutions of various kinds (Minas 2009; Cohen *et al.*, 2016; Cohen and Minas, 2017). As a minimal ethical stance the human rights abuses experienced by persons with mental illness must be eradicated (Irmansyah *et al.*, 2009; Puteh *et al.*, 2011; Cohen *et al.*, 2016; Cohen and Minas, 2017).

The theory of justice elaborated by Rawls (1971, 1993) requires that the most disadvantaged in the population are accorded priority in the framing of political and social arrangements (e.g. mental health policy, allocation of funds, health-system design and operation, training of clinicians) that are intended to ensure justice. Basic institutions and social arrangements are inherently unjust if they result in systematic disadvantage accruing to some minority sections of the population (Minas, 2001b). Where systematic disadvantage exists, specific attention needs to be paid to redressing such disadvantage by according priority to the needs of such groups (Barry, 1990) and, where necessary, making particular arrangements to meet needs that cannot be met by existing health-system arrangements (Kymlicka, 1995).

The Rawlsian notion of justice as fairness requires that a primary goal of health systems, and of health-system reform, is equity. Individuals should be able to attain their full health potential regardless of age, gender, race or socio-economic circumstances. Some unequal distributions of health between groups may be considered unavoidable (e.g. genetic disorders) or, if avoidable, nevertheless fair and acceptable (e.g. mountain climbers breaking limbs). Inequities in health (unequal distribution of health status, access to healthcare, or potential for future good health between social groups) arise when disparities in health status between groups defined by gender, socio-economic status, or ethnicity are avoidable, unacceptable and unfair. 'From an ethical perspective, inequities are intrinsically repugnant; disproportionate suffering offends our innate sense of justice and presents a strong case for limiting it wherever possible' (Evans and Norris, 2000). Lack of evidence due to inadequate support for necessary research renders inequities invisible (Minas *et al.*, 2013).

Stakeholder Analysis and Engagement

At the very beginning of any process of health-system reform it is essential to carry out stakeholder analysis (Roberts *et al.*, 2004) and to engage key stakeholders in relevant elements of the process, from agenda setting and problem definition, through problem diagnosis, policy development, political decision-making, implementation and evaluation. It is necessary to identify the groups and individuals that have a legitimate interest in the process, and in the possible outcomes of the process. Particularly at the stages of political decision-making (Caldas de Almeida *et al.*, 2014), implementation and evaluation, it is vital to assess the political resources and the possible roles of different stakeholders in the political process so as to understand their relative power over the policy issues under consideration. The current position of the various stakeholders on the proposed policy, and the intensity of their commitment to the position, will indicate where support and opposition are likely to come from and the likely force of such support and opposition. When the stakeholder analysis is complete, the proposer of the reform, in consultation with relevant stakeholders, is in a position to develop possible solutions to identified problems and a political strategy that will increase the probability of political acceptability of the proposed reform.

Problem Definition

A major impediment to improving mental health services for multicultural societies is the general lack of clarity in problem definition and the lack of agreed processes for allocating priority to different problem areas. A large part of this is due to lack of data (Minas *et al.*, 2013) and inconsistent research findings from different geographic regions, from different health systems, and in relation to different communities. There are several possible reasons for the inconsistency of findings (Minas, 2001b). These may include a wide variation in the demographic, cultural and migration profiles of the groups being studied; variation in the national and regional mental health service systems in which the work has been carried out; and major methodological difficulties in cross-cultural mental health research (Bhui and Bhugra, 2001), such as lack of common definitions of the populations being studied and problems with the concept of ethnicity, problems in sampling ethnic communities, lack of cross-culturally reliable and valid research instruments (Jacob *et al.*, 1997, Bhui and Bhugra, 2001), problems associated with cross-cultural diagnosis, lack of generally acceptable methods for studying culturally derived concepts of mental illness, and wide variations in clinical presentation across cultural groups and health systems. The collection and analysis of health status, health service use, and outcomes data is critical to the task of eliminating inequity (Minas *et al.*, 2013). The lack of adequate health information about cultural minority groups renders invisible the inequities that do exist. Box 32.2 shows a list of commonly identified problems.

Such a general listing of problems is of limited usefulness to policy-makers, service system designers and implementers in a programme of health-system reform. While such a list may be a necessary beginning to indicate the need for action, it is too broad and unfocused for the purpose of guiding specific action. To remedy all the problems listed would require major new research strategies and funding arrangements, large-scale community education programmes, education and training of all existing mental health clinicians and students in undergraduate and postgraduate programmes, a substantial increase in numbers of mental health interpreters in those health systems where they already exist and the creation and funding of a new discipline where they do not, new forms of participation for consumers, carers

BOX 32.2 Commonly identified problems

- Insufficient information about virtually all relevant aspects of mental health of ethnic minority communities.
- Insufficient data on prevalence of mental illness and mental health problems in specific ethnic communities, and a frequent failure to include adequate samples of cultural minority groups in large-scale epidemiological studies.
- Lack of knowledge by clinicians and health agencies of the needs of ethnic communities.
- Differing, and poorly understood, cultural conceptions of health and illness and of treatment and care.
- Poor access to service agencies and to the full range of services – particularly the psychotherapies and rehabilitation and social support services – with an inadequate understanding of the factors responsible for underutilization.
- Poor quality of services.
- Poor clinical and social outcomes.
- High levels of stigma in ethnic communities.
- Inadequate participation by ethnic consumers, carers and communities in policy-making, service design and evaluation, and service reform.
- Inadequate knowledge and skills of clinicians, and inadequate provision of education and training programmes in transcultural mental health.
- Lack of appropriate connectedness of the different components of health systems, and of health systems with broader social systems.
- Failure of mental health promotion and illness prevention programmes to reach ethnic (particularly non-English speaking) communities.
- Significant communication barriers (linguistic and cultural) between clinicians and (non-English speaking) consumers and their families, and inadequate access to skilled interpreters.
- Inadequate information about the quality of interpreting services when they are available.
- Inadequate information on the factors which constitute risks for mental disorders in ethnic minority communities, preventing targeted programmes for vulnerable groups and the development of tailored programmes that address special needs of these groups.
- Inadequate understanding of the factors that influence treatment-seeking decision-making.
- Inadequate support for carers (family and friends) of ethnic minority people (Chisholm *et al.*, 2016) with mental illness.

and communities, and much more. Such wholesale renovations of health systems simply do not occur. Effective and sustainable reform can only occur in manageable chunks, usually in chunks that can be achieved in an electoral cycle. Would-be reformers must be passionate and persistent but they must also be focused, realistic and patient.

Some health-sector planners argue that all one needs to identify problems are good data. But this is not how the world operates. Many reforms move ahead without good data. Many well-documented problems are ignored in reform programmes. Any policy decision must rely, implicitly and explicitly, on both science and ethics (Roberts *et al.*, 2004).

It is likely to be strategically useful to focus on problems that: (1) indicate poor health-system performance with undesirable health-system outcomes; (2) are associated with substantial economic costs of inaction; (3) are agreed by key stakeholders to be important; and (4) there is a reasonable expectation that feasible, affordable and politically acceptable solutions can be found. In many examples of national mental health system reform and in increasing the level of attention paid to mental health compelling information about the economic consequences of inaction has been decisive (Chisholm *et al.*, 2016). From the extensive list of problems in Box 32.2 it might be useful to focus on one or more of the following critically important health-system problems that require attention:

- lack of adequate information about virtually all aspects of the mental health of ethnic minority communities;
- poor access to service agencies and to the full range of services;
- poor clinical and social outcomes.

Identifying the Causes of Mental Health System Problems

Having settled on one or more important problems as the focus for reform, the task is then to identify the reasons for, or the causes of, these problems. Let us take inequitable access to services as an example. The various domains of accessibility (Minas *et al.*, 1996) include:

Visible Accessibility

Potential users must be aware of the existence of the service. Non-English-speaking communities or black and ethnic minorities generally do not have access to adequate information about available services.

Physical Accessibility

Geographic location, availability of transport, etc. Ethnic minority communities may live in deprived parts of cities, or on the outskirts of cities, where mental health services are generally less available.

Procedural Accessibility

The use of particular procedures (e.g. a requirement to complete registration forms in English) may deter some potential service users, as will the characteristics of reception areas and the linguistic and cultural skills of reception staff.

Economic Accessibility

Services outside the financial capabilities of potential users are inaccessible. Costs include direct cost of the service, transport and child-minding costs, lost income from work, etc. Immigrant and refugee communities are likely to have lesser economic means, and may be less likely to have private health insurance than the general community, so that fee-for-service mental health systems are less accessible.

Psychological Accessibility

Aspects of the service that do not conform with expectations and psychological needs will deter use. For example, high levels of stigma associated with mental illness and psychiatric treatment will deter access to mental health services.

Cultural Accessibility

Services that do not accommodate, as far as possible, the potential user's preferred language, values, beliefs and behavioural norms will deter access. Services that are perceived as discriminatory will be avoided.

Problems in each of these different domains of accessibility have different causes and will require different solutions. For the mental health system in general, or for a particular service agency and particular communities, which of these domains of accessibility are most problematic and need to be most urgently addressed? Is it all components of the service system that are inaccessible or only some? For example, frequently lack of access is less of a problem for inpatient services and more of a problem for psychological and rehabilitation services that are more language-dependent.

Clarifying causes of major problems in health-system outcomes will be the basis for the development of policy options designed to reduce or eliminate the problems.

Development of Policy Options

As the causes of problems are identified it becomes possible to identify possible options for their solution. This option development process is an essential component of policy formulation. Roberts and his colleagues (2004) suggest that, once plausible policy solutions have been developed for identified problems, reform proposals must have three characteristics in order to be accepted: (1) implementability; (2) political feasibility; and (3) political controllability. A policy that, for whatever reason, cannot be implemented is useless. Most policies are not implemented at all or not as intended (Minas *et al.*, 2007). Faithful implementation of policies is the exception. The policy proposal must be political acceptable. It must be seen by political decision-makers as dealing with important, clearly defined problems, as politically feasible (e.g. acceptable to powerful interest groups) and affordable. Finally, the implementation of the policy must be politically controllable. It will not lead to a runaway increase in costs, or create new institutions or arrangements that are not sufficiently accountable and that are difficult to control.

Political Decision-Making

Transcultural psychiatry has developed in different directions in different countries due to the varying demographic composition of populations, and particular histories and the varied cultural and political commitments of different nations (Kirmayer and Minas, 2000). Countries such as Australia and Canada, that have explicit national policies of multiculturalism that explicitly value cultural diversity and enable cultural maintenance as well as assisting cultural integration and social inclusion, take a different view of the political status of ethnic minorities than do countries such as France, where the republican model of integration privileges the values and interests of the state over the values and interests of ethnic minorities. In France no specific epidemiological studies of immigrant and refugee populations have been carried out. This absence of epidemiological data mirrors political unwillingness, at the national level in France, to treat the health problems of immigrants and refugees outside the general healthcare system. Thus no national policy for the prevention and treatment of psychiatric illness aimed at these groups has been pursued by the state. Only a few independent initiatives have been undertaken to create centres offering psychiatric care for immigrants and refugees (Fassin and Rechtman, 2005).

By contrast, in Australia, national mental health policy (Australian Health Ministers, 1992) and the national mental health service standards (Australian Health Ministers, 1997) specify the obligation of mental health services to be cognizant of, and to respond appropriately to, the diverse needs of a culturally diverse population. Specific national policies have been developed to improve the quality and accessibility of services for a culturally diverse population (Multicultural Mental Health Australia, 2004). State health departments support specialist transcultural mental health units and services for survivors of trauma and torture that are responsible for improving the quality of mental health services for immigrant and refugee communities.

The political context, which is different in every country, is of course crucially important in the process of policy-making and in the process of political decision-making. While in general mental health has moved up the list of health priorities over the past several decades (Kleinman et al., 2016; Patel et al., 2016), there are major differences across countries in the extent to which mental health, and the provision of high quality mental health services, is seen as a political priority.

Attempts to develop effective mental health systems for multicultural societies in the absence of adequate political analysis are bound to fail (Caldas de Almeida et al., 2014). Political strategies need to be developed that take into account the players (individuals and groups who are involved in the reform process and who may facilitate or derail the intended reform), the relative power of each player in the political process, the positions taken by each player (support or opposition), the intensity of commitment to the position, and the perception of the proposed policy, including the definitions of problems and proposed solutions, and the consequences for each player of implementation of the policy (Roberts et al., 2004).

Implementation and Evaluation

Most policies, including policies intended to improve the mental health situation of immigrant and refugee communities in multicultural societies, fail to be implemented (Ziguras, 1997; Minas et al., 2007;

Minas et al., 2013). It may be that this is due to inadequate preparation during previous phases of the policy development cycle. It may be due to the fact that there are always competing health-system priorities. A particular deficiency in attempts to develop equitable mental health systems for multicultural societies is the lack of adequate economic analysis (both the downstream costs of failing to develop such systems and the estimated economic benefits of developing equitable mental health systems) of the kind that have been so influential in the national mental health reform arena (Hickie et al., 2006) and in increasing attention to global mental health (Chisholm et al., 2016). However, it is important to remember that implementation is difficult, particularly when the new system requires new skills, new ways of working, new patterns of relationships, and shifts in the relative power of professionals and consumers, and of the different professional disciplines. It is also a common experience that pilot programmes are very difficult to sustain (Fernando 2005) and to scale up to a level where they have a system-wide impact. Very few transcultural mental health programmes have been evaluated. Those that have been adequately evaluated have frequently demonstrated considerable benefits (Ziguras et al., 2000; Kirmayer et al., 2003; Ziguras et al., 2003).

Leadership for Mental Health System Development

A critical ingredient in developing mental health for multicultural societies is leadership. The policy development process outlined previously requires leadership in multiple domains and at multiple levels that is clear-sighted, focused and sustained over time. Bringing about major change in social institutions, such as the substantial reform of the Australian mental health system (Thornicroft and Betts, 2002; Whiteford et al., 2002; Hickie et al., 2005; Whiteford and Buckingham, 2005; National Mental Health Commission, 2014), solves some problems and creates others (Mental Health Council of Australia, 2005; Senate Select Committee on Mental Health, 2006). The essence of leadership is bringing about change in complex systems (Minas, 2005). Mental health systems are complex in the everyday sense of being complicated, and in the more formal sense of being complex adaptive systems. Regardless of the composition of complex adaptive systems (e.g. physical, biological, ecological, organizational systems), they share a number of crucial properties, including multiple levels of organization, open boundaries, rule sets or control parameters that determine the state of the system at any point in time, adaptation and structural coupling, self-organization, emergence, and non-linear causality (Plsek and Greenhalgh, 2001; Plsek and Wilson, 2001; Wilson *et al.*, 2001). The behaviours of agents in the system are governed by rule sets. The settings, or values, of these rules are the system's control parameters. In human systems, such as health service organizations, the actions of agents (clinicians, managers, hospitals, community mental health centres, NGOs, academic departments, ministries of health) are governed by laws and regulations, and cultural values, beliefs and commitments.

It is now recognized that improving quality of care involves improving whole systems around the clinician–patient interaction and that a key task for quality improvement is the creation of an environment in which excellence in clinical care will flourish (Callaly *et al.*, 2005). The interactions within a complex adaptive system are more important than the discrete actions of the component parts. Clinical governance aims to facilitate multidisciplinary teamwork, partnerships and cooperative working practices. Productive or generative relationships occur when interactions produce new and valuable capabilities that are not possible through individual action of the parts (Plsek and Wilson, 2001).

Progress toward goals that are desirable but difficult to achieve can occur through applying to the system a few simple, flexible rules, sometimes referred to as *minimum specifications* (Minas, 2005). While the tendency in policy implementation and management is to specify in great detail what is to be done at all levels of the system, taking a *minimum specifications* approach makes clear what is essential and irreducible and leaves room for creativity and innovation. They encourage discussion about how they are to be achieved, thereby increasing connectedness and facilitating shared views of what is to be done. If minimum specifications focus on system-wide targets, they encourage generative relationships and the emergence of solutions that are relevant to local conditions. The concept of minimum specifications is being applied to the redesign of healthcare in the United Kingdom (Plsek and Wilson, 2001). An example (Box 32.3) of such a set of minimum specifications, or criteria for a high-performance mental

health system, is contained in the Victorian Strategy for Safety and Quality in Public Mental Health Services (Metropolitan and Aged Care Services Division, 2004) and the Commonwealth document *National Action to Improve the Quality of Mental Health Services* (AHMAC National Mental Health Working Group Information Strategy Committee, 2005). I have added some questions that may be asked in relation to the existing mental health system that may be used to determine whether even a well-performing mental health system is performing equally well for everyone, including immigrant and refugee communities. The answers to these questions will identify both problems and things that are being done well. The setting of minimum specifications (e.g. principles, values, outcomes), and the task of securing the commitment of all players to the achievement of the specifications, is a critical step in development of more appropriate mental health services.

Making changes in one of these nine areas will generally result in (perhaps unintended) changes in one or more of the other areas. For example, measures to improve safety and reduce risk may result in a negative impact on the cultural appropriateness of the service. Improving cultural appropriateness may in itself reduce risk and improve safety.

That best practices are so slow to be adopted throughout health systems is frequently attributed to resistance to change. If resistance is seen as the reason, then the solution is to battle against and to overcome resistance, wherever it is to be found. However, in complex adaptive systems, behaviour follows attractors in the system. Understanding where the attractors in the system are is part of the art of health-system reform. Understanding how a change in system parameter settings can shift the system from the current inadequate state to a more desirable one is a key task of leadership for change. An example of such control parameter change is the creation of financial incentives, linked to training, for the purpose of encouraging general practitioners to take a greater interest in acquiring psychiatric treatment skills and to take the time to apply these to people with mental illness in their practice (Hickie and Groom, 2002; Minas, 2005).

Standards and guidelines encourage uniformity. This is desirable when we are improving the reliability in application of technical interventions, such as drug prescribing. However, in a system that is far from

BOX 32.3 Health-system performance

How well is the health system performing in delivering quality health actions to improve the health of all the population? Is it the same for everyone? Are some sub-groups systematically disadvantaged?

Criterion	Description	Questions
Effective	Care, intervention or action achieves desired outcome.	• Are outcomes the same for immigrant and refugee communities as for the general population?
Appropriate	Care/intervention/action provided is relevant to the client's needs and based on established standards.	• Are the needs of different immigrant and refugee communities well understood and are they appropriately met? • Are there established standards that are relevant and applicable to ethnic minority communities?
Efficient	Achieving desired results with most cost-effective use of resources.	• Is the best use possible being made of the resources and skills of the mental health system, e.g bilingual/ bicultural clinicians? • Are the wrong things being done efficiently?
Responsive	Service provides respect for persons and is client orientated and includes respect for dignity, confidentiality, participation in choices, promptness, quality of amenities, access to social support networks, and choice of provider.	• Are services respectful of cultural and religious commitments? • Do ethnic consumers/carers/communities participate in policy-making, service design and evaluation, service management structures? • Do ethnic minority consumers feel discriminated against or marginalized?
Accessible	Ability of people to obtain healthcare at the right place and right time irrespective of income, physical location and cultural background.	• Is access to services based on needs that are well understood? • Is there equitable access to services by all communities?
Safe	The avoidance or reduction to acceptable limits of actual or potential harm from healthcare management or the environment in which healthcare is delivered.	• Are incidences of violence, self-harm, suicide the same for ethnic patients as for the general population of patients? • Does the service have the capacity to carry out accurate risk assessment in cross-cultural clinical situations? • Are families appropriately engaged in risk reduction, particularly when the ill person is discharged from the service?
Continuous	Ability to provide uninterrupted, coordinated care or service across programmes, practitioners, organizations and levels over time.	• Is continuity of care (number and frequency of consultations and admissions, drop-outs from services, etc.) the same or different for ethnic community service users as for the general population of service users? • If so, what are the reasons for these differences?

BOX 32.3 (cont.)

Criterion	Description	Questions
Capable	An individual's or service's capacity to provide a health service based on skills and knowledge.	• Do clinical and other health service staff have the necessary knowledge and skills for effective cross-cultural practice? • Is the service organized in a way that ensures its capacity to provide effective and acceptable services? Does the service actively seek to employ bilingual and bicultural clinical and other staff in areas where these skills are most valuable?
Sustainable	System or organization's capacity to provide infrastructure such as workforce, facilities and equipment, and be innovative and respond to emerging needs	• Is the service adequately staffed? • Does it have the necessary facilities where they are most required? • Does the service carry out evaluation and research and evaluation that will inform continuing improvement? • Does the service develop and then drop pilot programmes rather than scaling up those programmes that have been shown to be successful?

Source: modified from (AHMAC National Mental Health Working Group Information Strategy Committee, 2005)

perfect and looking to continually improve, there is merit also in encouraging diversity, of fostering creativity and accepting locally relevant structures and processes rather than seeking to impose a stifling uniformity. Variation and diversity are core features of any complex evolving system. The importance of biodiversity to the health of the biosphere is now well understood. The importance of cultural diversity in social systems is less well understood and less accepted. Diversity in service systems, such as the mental health system, and to a certain extent in clinical practice, tends to be regarded with suspicion. This is a critical error, one that can have a very negative impact on the continuing evolution of the service system.

A key component of any minimum specifications approach to leadership for system change is the clear and explicit articulation of the values that will underpin everything else that occurs in the system. It is also critically important that, as far as possible, values are shared by all who are involved in the change agenda.

Values are deeply held views that act as guiding principles for individuals and organizations. When they are declared and followed they are the basis of trust. When they are left unstated they are inferred from observable behaviour. When they are stated and not followed trust is broken (Pendleton and King, 2002).

In a complex system leadership is required, and is often displayed, at all levels of the system. We do not know what are all the relevant control parameters, and can generally not predict with any certainty the impact of changing those control parameters that we can change – such as increasing or reducing money flowing to certain parts of the system or to the overall system, creating new community mental health teams with new responsibilities and ways of working, and increasing the participation of consumers, carers and communities in decision-making processes.

It is increasingly clear that, in thinking of mental health systems as complex adaptive systems, and of leadership for change in such systems, command and control styles of leadership are dead. An analogy for the changes that are occurring in our mental health systems is to be found in economics. In mental health we are doing the equivalent of moving from a command economy to a market economy, with all of the uncertainty and risk that such a move entails.

Conclusions

The need to develop effective and equitable mental health systems for multicultural societies is now on the agenda in many developed countries. A summary of the key steps in this process is offered in Box 32.4. The lessons that have been learned in general health-system reform need to be applied more systematically to the task of improving mental health services for culturally diverse populations. In addition, the insights that have come from the study of complex systems can be useful to us in framing an approach that is applicable in a very wide range of political, economic and cultural contexts. A complex systems perspective on leadership suggests that a clear definition of minimum specifications for the system be developed, and a readiness for flexible, context-dependent, emergence of the details of the

system is likely to ensure that the details (which determine whether a system is functional or not) are more likely to be relevant to local needs and circumstances.

In multicultural societies the development of mental health services that are responsive, accessible, culturally appropriate and effective, should not be an add-on or an afterthought. Attention to issues of cultural competence is not a distraction from the 'core business' of mental health services and is more important than at any time in the past in a world where more and more countries are having to respond to the needs of increasingly diverse populations, including the greatly increased numbers of traumatized asylum seekers and refugees. Whether cultural considerations and other forms of population diversity are part of the fundamental character of the mental health system is a test of the extent to which a society values justice and equity. Even though knowledge about culture, migration and mental health is partial and sometimes inconsistent, there is enough known about how to provide equitable culturally acceptable services to enable informed policy development and service planning, implementation and evaluation. Working through the process of reforming services so that they are capable of meeting the needs of a culturally diverse society will have the direct benefit of making those services more flexible and responsive to the needs of all members of the community.

BOX 32.4 Developing effective and equitable mental health systems for multicultural societies

1. Carry out stakeholder analysis and engage stakeholders in the process of service development.
2. Agree on the set of minimum specifications for the services. Ensure that these are firmly based on clear ethical foundations.
3. Evaluate current services in relation to the minimum specifications (de Jong and van Ommeren, 2005).
4. Clearly define a small number of important problems that are focused on system outcomes, then analyse the causes – and the causes of causes.
5. Decide where action is required, and is likely to be effective, and set priorities.
6. Carry out political analysis and review stakeholder analysis in the light of what needs to be done.
7. Ensure that policy proposals (proposed solutions to problems) are capable of implementation, politically feasible and politically controllable.
8. Decide which are the most important system parameters, and which system parameters are most amenable to change, in the current political and service system circumstances.
9. Act collectively, decisively and with clarity of purpose.

References

AHMAC National Mental Health Working Group Information Strategy Committee (2005). *National Action to Improve the Quality of Mental Health Services: A Summary of Activity 1992–2003*. Canberra: Commonwealth Department of Health and Ageing.

Australian Health Ministers (1992). *National Mental Health Policy*. Canberra: Australian Government Publishing Service.

Australian Health Ministers (1997). *National Standards for Mental Health Services*. Canberra: Commonwealth Department of Health and Family Services.

Bäärnhielm, S., Ekblad, S., Ekberg, J. and Ginsburg, B. E. (2005). Historical reflections on mental health care in Sweden: the welfare state and cultural diversity. *Transcultural Psychiatry*, **42**(3), 394–419.

Barry, B. (1990). *Political Argument*. Berkeley: University of California Press.

Barton, G. (2016). Out of the ashes of Afghanistan and Iraq: the rise and rise of Islamic State. Available online at https://theconversation.com/out-of-the-ashes-of-afghanistan-and-iraq-the-rise-and-rise-of-islamic-state-55437 (accessed 29 July 2016).

Bhugra, D. (1997). Setting up psychiatric services: cross-cultural issues in planning and delivery. *International Journal of Social Psychiatry*, **43**(1), 16–28.

Bhui, K. and Bhugra, D. (2001). Methodological rigour in cross-cultural research. *British Journal of Psychiatry*, **179**, 269.

Bhui, K., Christie, Y. and Bhugra, D. (1995). The essential elements of culturally sensitive psychiatric services. *International Journal of Social Psychiatry*, **41**(4), 242–256.

Bhui, K., Warfa, N., Edonya, P., McKenzie, K. and Bhugra, D. (2007). Cultural competence in mental health care: a review of model evaluations. *BMC Health Services Research*, 7, 15.

Caldas de Almeida, J. M., Minas, H. and Cayetano, C. (2014). Generating political commitment for mental health system development. In *Global Mental Health: Principles and Practice*, ed. V. Patel, H. Minas, M. Prince and A. Cohen. New York: Oxford University Press.

Callaly, T., Arya, D. and Minas, H. (2005). Quality, risk management and governance in mental health: an overview. *Australasian Psychiatry*, **13**(1), 16–20.

Chilcot, J. (2016). The Iraq Inquiry. Statement by Sir John Chilcot: 6 July 2016. London: p. 12.

Chisholm, D., Sweeny, K., Sheehan, P., Rasmussen, B., Smit, F., Cuijpers, P. and Saxena, S. (2016). Scaling-up treatment of depression and anxiety: a global return on investment analysis. *Lancet Psychiatry*, **3**(5), 415–424.

Coffey, G. J., Kaplan, I., Sampson, R. C. and Tucci, M. M. (2010). The meaning and mental health consequences of long-term immigration detention for people seeking asylum. *Social Science and Medicine*, **70**(12), 2070–2079.

Cohen, A. and Minas, H. (2017). Global mental health and psychiatric institutions in the 21st century. *Epidemiology and Psychiatric Sciences*, **26**(1), 4–9.

Cohen, A., Patel, V. and Minas, H. (2014). A brief history of global mental health. In *Global Mental Health: Principles and Practice*, ed. V. Patel, H. Minas, A. Cohen, M. Prince. New York: Oxford University Press, pp. 3–26.

Cohen, A., Chatterjee, S. and Minas, H. (2016). Time for a global commission on mental health institutions. *World Psychiatry*, **15**(2), 116–117.

Conflict Casualties Monitor. (2016). Iraq Body Count: Iraq 2015 – A Catastrophic Normal. Available online at www.iraqbodycount.org/analysis/numbers/2015/ (accessed 29 July 2016).

De Jong, J. T. and van Ommeren, M. (2005). Mental health services in a multicultural society: interculturalization and its quality surveillance. *Transcultural Psychiatry*, **42**(3), 437–456.

Evans, T. and Norris, A. (2000). Policy-oriented strategies for health equity. In *Efficient, Equity-Oriented Strategies for Health: International Perspectives, Focus on Vietnam*, ed. P. M. Hung, I. H. Minas, Y. Liu, G. Dahlgren and W. Hsiao. Melbourne: Centre for International Mental Health.

Fassin, D. and Rechtman, R. (2005). An anthropological hybrid: the pragmatic arrangement of universalism and culturalism in French mental health. *Transcultural Psychiatry*, **42**(3), 347–366.

Fernando, S. (2005). Multicultural mental health services: Projects for minority ethnic communities in England. *Transcultural Psychiatry*, **42**(3), 420–436.

Ganesan, S. and Janze, T. (2005). Overview of culturally-based mental health care in Vancouver. *Transcultural Psychiatry* **42**(3), 478–490.

Hickie, I. B. and Groom, G. (2002). Primary care-led mental health service reform: an outline of the Better Outcomes in Mental Health Care initiative. *Australasian Psychiatry*, **10**, 376–382.

Hickie, I. B., Groom, G. L., McGorry, P. D., Davenport, T. A. and Luscombe, G. M. (2005). Australian mental health reform: time for real outcomes. *Medical Journal of Australia*, **182**(8), 401–406.

Hickie, I. B., Davenport, T. A. and Luscombe, G. M. (2006). Mental health expenditure in Australia: time for affirmative action. *Australian and New Zealand Journal of Public Health*, **30**(2), 119–122.

International Labour Organization (2016). Labour migration. Available online at www.ilo.org/global/topics/labour-migration/lang-en/index.htm (accessed 29 July 2016).

Irmansyah, I., Prasetyo, Y. A. and Minas, H. (2009). Human rights of persons with mental illness in Indonesia: more than legislation is needed. *International Journal of Mental Health Systems*, **3**(1), 14.

Jacob, K. S., Bhugra, D. and Mann, A. H. (1997). The validation of the 12-item General Health Questionnaire among ethnic Indian women living in the United Kingdom. *Psychological Medicine*, **27**(5), 1215–1217.

Kirmayer, L. J. and Brass, G. (2016). Addressing global health disparities among Indigenous peoples. *The Lancet*, **388**(10040), 105–106.

Kirmayer, L. J. and Minas, H. (2000). The future of cultural psychiatry: an international perspective. *Canadian Journal of Psychiatry*, **45**(5), 438–446.

Kirmayer, L. J., Groleau, D., Guzder, J., Blake, C. and Jarvis, E. (2003). Cultural consultation: a model of mental health service for multicultural societies. *Canadian Journal of Psychiatry*, **48**(3), 145–153.

Kleinman, A., Estrin, G. L., Usmani, S., Chisholm, D., Marquez, P. V., Evans, T. G. and Saxena, S. (2016). Time for mental health to come out of the shadows. *The Lancet*, **387**(10035), 2274–2275.

Kymlicka, W. (1995). *Multicultural Citizenship: A Liberal Theory of Minority Rights*. Oxford: Clarendon Press.

Lin, D., Li, X., Wang, B., Hong, Y., Fang, X., Qin, X. and Stanton, B. (2011). Discrimination, perceived social inequity, and mental health among rural-to-urban migrants in China. *Community Mental Health Journal*, **47**(2), 171–180.

Lo, H.-T. and Chung, R. C. Y. (2005). The Hong Fook experience: working with ethnocultural communities in Toronto. *Transcultural Psychiatry*, **42**(3), 457–477.

Mental Health Council of Australia (2005). *Not for Service: Experiences of Injustice and Despair in Mental Health Care in Australia*. Canberra: Mental Health Council of Australia.

Metropolitan and Aged Care Services Division (2004). *Victorian Strategy for Safety and Quality in Public Mental Health Services: 2004–2008*. Melbourne: Victorian Government Department of Human Services.

Minas, H. (2001a). Migration, equity and health. In *International Cooperation in Health*, ed. M. McKee, P. Garner and R. Stott. Oxford: Oxford University Press, pp. 151–174.

Minas, H. (2001b). Service responses to cultural diversity. In *Textbook of Community Psychiatry*, ed. G. Thornicroft and G. Szmukler. Oxford: Oxford University Press, pp. 193–206.

Minas, H. (2005). Leadership for change in complex systems. *Australasian Psychiatry*, **13**(1), 33–39.

Minas, H. (2009). Mentally ill patients dying in social shelters in Indonesia. *The Lancet*, **374**(9690), 592–593.

Minas, H. and Diatri, H. (2008). Pasung: physical restraint and confinement of the mentally ill in the community. *International Journal of Mental Health Systems*, 2(1), 8.

Minas, H., Lambert, T., Boranga, G. and Kostov, S. (1996). *Mental Health Services for Immigrants: Transforming Policy into Practice*. Canberra: Australian Government Publishing Service.

Minas, H., Klimidis, S. and Kokanovic, R. (2007). Depression in multicultural Australia: policies, research and services. *Australia and New Zealand Health Policy*, 4(1).

Minas, H., Kakuma, R., Too, L. S. *et al.* (2013). Mental health research and evaluation in multicultural Australia: developing a culture of inclusion. *International Journal of Mental Health Systems*, 7(1), 23.

Minas, I. H. (1991). Inequalities in mental health care based on language and culture. Submission to the Human Rights and Equal Opportunity Commission National Inquiry Concerning the Human Rights of People with Mental Illness.

Multicultural Mental Health Australia (2004). *Framework for the Implementation of the National Mental Health Plan 2003–2008 Multicultural Australia*. Canberra: Department of Health and Ageing, Health Priorities and Suicide Prevention Branch.

National Mental Health Commission (2014). *Contributing Lives, Thriving Communities. Report of the National Review of Mental Health Programmes and Services. Volume 1: Strategic Directions, Practical Solutions 1–2 years*. Sydney: National Mental Health Commission.

Newman, L. K. and Steel, Z. (2008). The child asylum seeker: psychological and developmental impact of immigration detention. *Child and Adolescent Psychiatric Clinics of North America*, **17**(3), 665–683.

Newman, L., Proctor, N. and Dudley, M. (2013). Seeking asylum in Australia: immigration detention, human rights and mental health care. *Australasian Psychiatry*, **21**(4), 315–320.

Patel, V., Chisholm, D., Parikh, R. *et al.* (2016). Addressing the burden of mental, neurological, and substance use disorders: key messages from Disease Control Priorities, 3rd edition. *The Lancet*, **387**(10028), 1672–1685.

Pendleton, D. and King, J. (2002). Values and leadership. *British Medical Journal*, **325**, 1352–1355.

Plsek, P. E. and T. Greenhalgh (2001). Complexity science: the challenge of complexity in health care. *British Medical Journal* **323**(7313), 625–628.

Plsek, P. E. and Wilson, T. (2001). Complexity, leadership, and management in healthcare organisations. *British Medical Journal*, **323**(7315), 746–749.

Puteh, I., Marthoenis, M. and Minas, H. (2011). Aceh Free Pasung: releasing the mentally ill from physical restraint. *International Journal of Mental Health Systems*, 5, 10.

Rawls, J. (1971). *A Theory of Justice*. Cambridge, MA: Harvard University Press.

Rawls, J. (1993). *Political Liberalism*. New York: Columbia University Press.

Reddihough, D. S., Meehan, E., Stott, N. S., Delacy, M. J. and Australian Cerebral Palsy Register (2016). The National Disability Insurance Scheme: a time for real change in Australia. *Developmental Medicine and Child Neurolology*, **58**(Suppl 2), 66–70.

Roberts, M. J., Hsiao, W., Berman, P. and Reich, M. R. (2004). *Getting Health Reform Right: A Guide to Improving Performance and Equity*. New York: Oxford University Press.

Salvador-Carulla, L. and Einfeld, S. (2014). Mental illness and the National Disability Insurance Scheme: lessons from Europe. *Australian and New Zealand Journal of Psychiatry*, **48**(5), 482–484.

Senate Select Committee on Mental Health (2006). *A National Approach to Mental Health: From Crisis to Community*. Canberra: Parliament House, Commonwealth of Australia.

Stiglitz, J. E. (2015). *The Great Divide: Unequal Societies and What We Can Do About Them*. New York: W. W. Norton and Company Inc.

Sue, S., Fujino, D. C., Hu, L., Takeuchi, D. T. and Zane, N. W. S. (1991). Community mental health services for ethnic minority groups: a test of the cultural responsiveness hypothesis. *Journal of Consulting and Clinical Psychology*, **59**, 533–540.

Thornicroft, G. and Betts, V. (2002). *International Mid-Term Review of the Second National Mental Health Plan for Australia*. Canberra: Mental Health and Special Programs Branch, Department of Health and Ageing.

United Nations High Commissioner for Refugees (2007). *2006 Global Trends: Refugees, Asylum-Seekers, Returnees, Internally Displaced and Stateless Persons*. Geneva: United Nations High Commissioner for Refugees.

United Nations High Commissioner for Refugees (2016). *UNHCR Global Trends: Forced Displacement in 2015*. Geneva: United Nations High Commissioner for Refugees.

Whiteford, H. A. and Buckingham, W. J. (2005). Ten years of mental health service reform in Australia: are we getting it right? *Medical Journal of Australia*, **182**(8), 396–400.

Whiteford, H., Buckingham, B. and Manderscheid, R. (2002). Australia's National Mental Health Strategy. *British Journal of Psychiatry*, **180**, 210–215.

Williams, T. M. and Smith, G. P. (2014). Can the National Disability Insurance Scheme work for mental health? *Australian and New Zealand Journal of Psychiatry*, **48**(5), 391–394.

Wilson, T., Holt, T. and Greenhalgh, T. (2001). Complexity and clinical care. *British Medical Journal*, **323**(7314), 685–688.

Ziguras, S. (1997). Implementation of ethnic health policy in community mental health centres in Melbourne. *Australian and New Zealand Journal of Public Health*, **21**, 323–328.

Ziguras, S., Stuart, G., Klimidis, S., Minas, H., Lewis, J., Pennella, J. and Jackson A. (2000). *Evaluation of the Bilingual Case Management Program*. Melbourne: Victorian Transcultural Psychiatry Unit.

Ziguras, S., Klimidis, S., Lewis, J. and Stuart, G. (2003). Ethnic matching of clients and clinicians and use of mental health services by ethnic minority clients. *Psychiatric Services*, **54**(4), 535–541.

Cross-Cultural Psychopharmacotherapy

Chee H. Ng and Chad A. Bousman

Editors' Introduction

Prescribing medication for many psychiatric disorders is a common therapeutic approach across the globe. However, pharmacokinetics and pharmacodynamics of various drugs vary across cultures due to a number of biological, social and psychological reasons. Due to metabolic reasons there are commonly recognized cross-cultural variations in therapeutic response to medication. It is inevitable that rates of prescription of medication will vary across all countries. Ng and Bousman suggest that the practice of extrapolating results from psychopharmacological studies conducted in mostly Western settings for application in other cultures is problematic and a 'one size fits all' approach is clearly not suitable. The recent push towards drug trials being conducted in many countries in Asia brings with it additional problems in that whether doses established there will work elsewhere in the world? Other complicating factors include increasing population diversity as a consequence of globalization and migration. Therefore, clinicians are much more likely to be treating patients of divergent backgrounds more frequently and need to be aware of cultural differences in response to medication. Ng and Bousman remind us that essential differences in pharmacotherapy across diverse ethnic and cultural groups are increasingly being recognized in clinical psychiatric practice. Various important and complex factors must be considered in cross-cultural psychopharmacology. Pharmacogenetic data have also revealed considerable ethnic differences and will influence treatment decisions in terms of the drug selection, dose titration, and the prediction of side effects. However, the impact of dietary factors, lifestyle such as smoking and alcohol use, obesity, systemic and cultural variables on drug response must also be taken into account using an integrated bio-socio-cultural approach to psycho-pharmacotherapy. Psychopharmacogenomics may further assist in identifying fast and slow metabolizers in order to manage patients appropriately. To

understand the role of culture and ethnic factors in pharmacotherapy requires the consideration of multiple dimensions that encompass both the biological and socio-cultural diversity of the individual patient.

Introduction

Globally, it is standard practice to use psychotropic medications to treat psychiatric disorders to reduce symptoms and disability, and to prevent relapses. The World Health Organization (WHO) has listed psychotropic medications for treating mental disorders in the WHO Model List of Essential Medicines (2015). These include efficacious, safe and cost-effective medicines needed for a basic healthcare system to treat priority conditions such as psychotic, mood, anxiety, obsessive–compulsive and substance use disorders.

Cross-cultural variations in psychotropic responses have long been recognized in clinical practice, anecdotal reports, surveys and systematic clinical studies. In recent decades, psychotropic medication has rapidly spread across the world, including to developing countries. However, the practice of extrapolating results from psychopharmacological studies conducted in mostly Western settings for application in other cultures is problematic and a 'one size fits all' approach is clearly not suitable. Furthermore, a trend toward increased population diversity and globalization worldwide suggests clinicians will be treating patients of divergent backgrounds more frequently and as such cannot afford to ignore, or be ignorant of, the role of ethnicity and culture in routine practices (Yu et al., 2007).

To understand the role of culture and ethnic factors in pharmacotherapy requires the consideration of multiple dimensions that encompass both the biological and socio-cultural diversity of the individual patient. The integration of these relevant issues in clinical practice however lags far behind the rapid advances of pharmacotherapeutics and the availability of a growing armamentarium of new psychotropic drugs. In the contemporary era, as we move towards a personalized medicine approach, understanding the ethnic and cultural factors and their interactions with biological variations has become even more crucial.

Psychopharmacology and Cultural Variations

There are important ethnic variations in dosage requirements, response, and tolerability of psychotropic medications. Such variations between cultural and ethnic groups in drug responses reflect the differences in drug pharmacokinetics and pharmacodynamics, which are mediated by both genetic and non-genetic factors (Ng et al., 2004). Pharmacodynamics refers to action of the drug at the target organ site which corresponds to drug efficacy, toxicity and other effects, while pharmacokinetics refers to the physiological handling of the drug (encompassing absorption, distribution, metabolism and excretion). To date, pharmacokinetic processes, particularly metabolism, have been viewed as the most significant factor in inter-individual differences in drug response, although pharmacodynamic processes are receiving increased attention.

The variations in psychotropic response seen across ethnicities and cultures highlights the biological and cultural diversities in the real world practice of clinical psychopharmacotherapy. Although traditionally it is common in psychiatry to derive an idiographic formulation to understand the psychosocial uniqueness of each individual patient, the biological diversity between individuals is often neglected (Lin and Smith, 2000). When it comes to drug therapy, psychiatrists frequently shift to a unidimensional view of the patient and apply a categorical approach to prescribing medications (e.g. diagnostic subtypes to response, compliance/non-compliance, responder/non-responder, etc.). On the other hand, clinicians are increasingly aware of the differences between drugs, even within the same class of antidepressants, for example SSRIs. Yet, there tends to be an underlying assumption that the biology of the recipients is more or less the same. Clearly this is not the case with emerging evidence of both inter-individual and inter-ethnic differences in pharmacological response.

Although previous studies have found differences in dosing and response to tricyclic antidepressants and neuroleptic drugs between Caucasian, Asians and other ethnic groups, the findings have generally been mixed (Pi and Gray, 1998). More recent studies involving novel antidepressants and antipsychotics have likewise emerged, which also reveal significant inter-ethnic differences in selective serotonin reuptake inhibitors (SSRIs) such as sertraline (Ng et al., 2006) and atypical antipsychotics such as clozapine (Ng et al., 2005). However, methodological weaknesses in ethno-psychopharmacology studies have largely undermined the field to clarify whether differential response to psychotropic medication across ethnic groups truly exists, and whether these differences are principally biologically based or a result of socio-cultural factors. These limitations include low sample sizes, lack of rigorous designs, inadequate definition of ethnic group, lack of integration with genetic data, and lack of control for physical, dietary and environmental variables (Ng, 2008).

Caution nonetheless needs to be exercised in making assumptions regarding genetic expression within ethnic groups. Differences between ethnic or racial groups may be less significant than genetic variations within each group. Stereotypes, on the basis of ethnicity alone, may be misleading as even within the same ethnic group there are marked inter-individual differences in metabolism (Lin and Smith, 2000). Concerns have been raised about the validity of pharmacotherapy based solely on racial differences (Schwartz, 2001). Specific knowledge of both genotype and phenotype profile together with dietary and lifestyle factors may be necessary to accurately predict individual metabolic function. Nevertheless, ethnicity remains a useful and important clinical consideration in pharmacotherapy and should be considered in a manner similar to assessing other variables such as age, gender, hepatic/renal function, weight and physical status in tailoring individual dosage of medication.

Pharmacogenetics and Ethnic Variations

Genetic variations impact on both pharmacokinetics and pharmacodynamics, which are responsible for cross-ethnic and inter-individual differences in drug response (Yu et al., 2007).

Pharmacokinetic Factors

The metabolism of most psychotropic drugs, principally involves the oxidation phase mediated by the cytochrome P-450 (CYP450) isoenzymes. Overall, there are 57 CYP450 genes, 15 of which are involved in the metabolism of drugs in humans (Zanger et al., 2008). In psychiatry, CYP2D6, CYP2C19, CYP3A4, CYP1A2, and CYP2C9 are responsible for the metabolism of the majority of psychotropic drugs (Madhusoodanan et al., 2014). Genetic variations (e.g. deletions, duplications, point mutations) in these CYP450 genes can result in abolished, reduced, normal or enhanced enzyme activity (Padmanabhan, 2014). Based on these genetic variations, an individual's metabolic phenotype can be predicted. Individuals that carry two alleles that code for 'normal' enzyme function are classified as extensive or normal metabolizers (EMs), while those carrying two alleles that code for inactive or absent enzyme function are defined as poor metabolizers (PMs). Furthermore, individuals who carry one normal and one inactive/absent allele are classified as intermediate metabolizers (IMs) and those with gene duplications or multiplications are defined as ultra-rapid metabolizers (UMs). Importantly, the prevalence of EMs, IMs, PMs and UMs across different ethnic populations varies considerably (Ozawa et al., 2004; Gunes and Dahl, 2008; van Booven et al., 2010).

Perhaps the best-studied CYP450 enzymes in psychiatry are CYP2D6 and CYP2C19. CYP2D6 accounts for approximately 2 per cent of the total hepatic CYP450 content but is responsible for the metabolism of 20–30 per cent of all drugs, including all tricyclic antidepressants, most SSRIs, and about half of all antipsychotics (Padmanabhan, 2014). CYP2D6 is highly polymorphic with over 100 alleles (see the Human Cytochrome P450 Allele Nomenclature Committee website, www.cypalleles.ki.se), although only a handful of these are common. Importantly, these common alleles vary considerably between ethnicities. In fact, 5–10 per cent of Caucasians and 1–2 per cent of Asians are PMs based on CYP2D6 genotyping (Poolsup et al., 2000). The high prevalence of the CYP2D6*3 and *4 inactive alleles in Caucasians relative to Asians probably accounts for this difference. However, Asians are significantly more likely to carry the CYP2D6*10 allele which results in a decrease in enzyme function. The CYP2D6*10 allele makes up about 51–70 per cent of all CYP2D6 alleles in Asian populations, thus Asians overall have lower CYP2D6 activity (Bradford, 2002). Among Africans, the CYP2D6*17 'reduced activity' allele is significantly more common but this allele is almost non-existent in Asians or Caucasians. Similarly, the rates of CYP2D6 gene duplication and its corresponding UM phenotype vary widely across ethnicity. The frequency ranges from 1–2% in Caucasians, 7–10% in Mediterranean populations, 19% in Arabs, and up to 29% in East African populations (Teh and Bertilsson, 2012). Table 33.1 shows the distribution of the most common CYP2D6 variant alleles globally.

CYP2C19 accounts for approximately 2 per cent of the total hepatic CYP450 content and is particularly important in the metabolism of SSRIs. Individuals with two inactive alleles (*2/*2, *2/*3 or *3/*3) are considered CYP2C19 PMs; whereas, carriers of the CYP2C19*17 allele are predicted to have a UM metabolic phenotype. Genetic studies of CYP2C19 have found that 15–30% of certain Asian populations are PMs compared to 3–6% of Caucasians and 2–4% of Africans (Ng et al., 2004; Fricke-Galindo et al., 2016), contrary to what is observed for CYP2D6. This is most likely due to the high prevalence of the CYP2D6*2

Table 33.1 Major CYP2D6 allele frequencies (%) in major ethnic groups

CYP2D6 Allele	Enzyme activity	European	East Asian	African
*1	Normal	39.0	34.7	32.8
*2xn	Increased	1.2	0.4	1.6
*4	Inactive	18.0	0.5	3.4
*5	Inactive	2.8	5.2	6.1
*10	Decreased	2.9	42.7	6.8
*17	Decreased	0.4	0.01	20.0

Source: modified from (Hicks et al., 2015)

Table 33.2 Major CYP2C19 allele frequencies (%) in major ethnic groups

CYP2C19 Allele	Enzyme activity	European	East Asian	African
*1	Normal	62.1	58.0	36.4
*2	Inactive	14.6	29.0	14.2
*3	Inactive	0.6	8.5	0.8
*17	Increased	21.5	1.6	15.1

Source: modified from (Hicks *et al.* 2015)

and *3 alleles among Asians relative to other populations (Goldstein *et al.*, 1997). Table 33.2 shows the distribution of the most common CYP2C19 variant alleles in major ethnic groups.

Beyond the CYP450 system, ethnic variations in allelic frequencies associated with the function of other pharmacokinetic enzymes and transporters also exist, for instance N-acetyltransferase PM rates in Western populations is 38–50 per cent while in Asians and Eskimos is about 10–25 per cent (Grant *et al.*, 1990). The high rate of fast acetylators in Asians may have implications for the metabolism of drugs like nitrazepam, clonazepam and possibly phenelzine (Lin *et al.*, 1993). Furthermore, ethnic variation in allelic frequencies associated with the function of drug transporters such as p-glycoprotein (encoded by *ABCB1*) at the blood–brain barrier have also been identified (Baune *et al.*, 2010), and as such could have inter-ethnic implications for a number of psychotropic drugs that are p-glycoprotein substrates, many of which overlap with CYP3A4 substrates (Akamine *et al.*, 2012). Cross-ethnicity studies examining the genetic variation of non-CYP450 enzymes and drug transporters (e.g. p-glycoprotein) in relation to psychotropic drug efficacy and/or toxicity are warranted.

The collective genetic knowledge on pharmacokinetics suggests dose adjustments according to CYP450 genetic variation, particularly in CYP2D6 and CYP2C19, as well as non-CYP450 genes, may be required to account for inter-individual and inter-ethnic pharmacokinetic variation. In fact, the Clinical Pharmacogenetics Implementation Consortium (CPIC, see www.pharmgkb.org/page/cpic) has developed guidelines for dosing of SSRIs based on CYP2D6 and CYP2C19 genotypes (Hicks *et al.*, 2015), albeit the majority of the evidence favouring CYP2D6 and CYP2C19 based dosing adjustments is derived from studies of individuals of European descent. Refinement of these guidelines and the development of equivalent guidelines for psychotropic drugs relevant to psychiatry

practice (i.e. antipsychotics, antidepressants, anxiolytics, sedatives/hypnotics) will require more research related to pharmacokinetic genetic variation particularly in non-Caucasian populations.

Pharmacodynamic Factors

Genetic polymorphisms within genes encoding proteins/enzymes involved in neurotransmitter synthesis, reception, transport and degradation have been associated with variations in psychotropic drug response. Among these polymorphisms, the serotonin transporter linked-polymorphic region (5-HTTLPR) polymorphism is arguably the most studied pharmacodynamic variant in psychiatry. A number of studies have shown that depressed patients carrying the 5-HTTLPR long allele have greater response to SSRIs than those with the short allele (Pollock *et al.*, 2000; Ng *et al.*, 2013), although inconsistent results have been found, particularly in studies in Korean and Japanese depressed subjects. In fact, a recent cross-ethnic study showed 5-HTTLPR was associated with SSRI efficacy in an ethnicity-dependent manner (Bousman *et al.*, 2014). Caucasians with the long/long alleles but not long/short or short/short alleles had greater response and remission rates to escitalopram compared with Koreans. Notably, 19–29% of East Asians carry the 5-HTTLPR long allele compared to 72% of Africans and 57% of Caucasians (Goldman *et al.*, 2010). Thus, there is evidence for both inter-individual and inter-ethnic differences in SSRI response depending on 5-HTTLPR genotype. However, the 5-HTTLPR polymorphism is only one of many examples of pharmacodynamic-related polymorphisms with potential inter-individual and inter-ethnic differences in psychopharmacotherapy response. In fact, nearly all polymorphisms that have been shown to have a moderate or greater association with psychotropic drug response and/or adverse

Table 33.3 Allele frequencies of pharmacodynamics-related polymorphisms associated with psychopharmacotherapy efficacy and/or adverse effects across ethnic groups

Gene	Polymorphism*	Allele	European**	East Asian**	African**
SLC6A4	5-HTTLPR***	Long	57	19–29	72
HTR1A	rs6295	G	46	80	43
HTR2A	rs7997012	G	57	74	99
HTR2C	rs3813929	T	16	15	1
	rs1414334	C	15	1	49
DRD2	rs1800497 (TaqIA)	T (A1)	19	41	39
	rs1799978	C	6	18	17
COMT	rs4680 (Val158 Met)	A (Met)	50	28	28
GRIK4	rs1954787	T	47	17	90
FKBP5	rs4713916	G	68	79	94
MC4R	rs17782313	C	24	19	28
DPP6	rs6977820	T	31	24	82

Notes:

* Polymorphisms selected from the Pharmacogenomics Knowledgebase (pharmgkb.org) with at least a moderate level of association (Level 2B or greater), except 5-HTTLPR which is not listed on the PharmGKB website.

** Allelic frequency data was derived from the 1000 Genome Project (release 17, 1000genomes.org).

*** 5-HTTLPR allele frequencies based on Goldman *et al.* (2010).

effects have considerably different allelic frequencies across ethnicities (Table 33.3).

In summary, inter-individual and inter-ethnic differences in therapeutic and adverse effects of psychotropic drugs are largely determined by genetic factors. Recent advances in genotyping technology have shown utility in predicting individual metabolic phenotypes, risks for side effects and likelihood of drug response. Employing genotyping may optimize clinical response and prevent excessive adverse effects for individual patients from diverse backgrounds. Through systematic characterization of the nature and function of polymorphisms, genotype-guided pharmacotherapy could vastly improve the cost-effectiveness of the medication regime for individual patients across varied ethnic and cultural groups. In fact, there are over 20 commercial pharmacogenetic tests relevant to psychiatry worldwide that were developed and are marketed for that purpose (Bousman and Hopwood, 2016). However, most of these tests have yet to be adequately evaluated and those that have been evaluated have been limited to Caucasian populations. Larger studies of personalized psychopharmacology in diverse human populations are much needed (Murphy and McMahon, 2013).

Socio-Cultural Factors in Psychopharmacotherapy

Dietary habits and the use of traditional medicinal herbs, which are largely influenced by socio-cultural factors, have significant implications for pharmacotherapy. Culture may determine the type and amount of foods consumed, the way they are prepared and the exposure to environmental toxins or pesticides used in agriculture. Socially sanctioned behaviour may affect the level of consumption of alcohol, cigarettes, caffeine or illicit substances within a cultural group. In addition, local customs and traditions can influence the use of folk and alternative medicines as a preference or in addition to Western medicines.

Although pharmacokinetics is largely genetically driven, the expression of genes in pharmacokinetic pathways is often influenced by environmental and socio-cultural factors. Exposure to exogenous agents can either inhibit or induce the activity of drug metabolizing enzymes as well as drug transporters, thereby altering the drug pharmacokinetics (Padmanabhan, 2014). While CYP2D6 and CYP2D19 are largely under genetic control, the function of CYP1A2 and CYP3A4 appear to be highly sensitive to environmental influences such as diet, smoking, alcohol, pollutants and other substances. Thus, variations in diet and lifestyle that are common to a given ethnic group or culture can determine differences in drug response.

CYP3A4 appears to be sensitive to dietary effects, probably because of the high level of expression in the intestines and its extensive range of substrates (Harris et al., 2003). Flavonoid quercetin has been reported to decrease the metabolism of CYP3A4 substrates such as nifedipine. When nifedipine is combined with a flavonoid-rich diet, an increase in the frequency and severity of side effects may result (Palma-Aguirre et al., 1994). Similarly, CYP3A4 inhibitory effects can be found with citrus juices on nifedipine (Bailey et al., 1991) and with red wine on felodipine (Bailey et al., 2003), giving rise to an increase in drug bioavailability. In particular, flavonoid naringin found in grapefruit juice has been shown to inhibit CYP3A4 in the small intestine (Fuhr, 1998), leading to decreased metabolism of a number of CYP3A4 substrates. For example, the levels of cyclosporin, cisapride and felodipine can significantly increase in those taking grapefruit juice. Hence, patients only require a lower dose of medication when given grapefruit juice concomitantly, which could be a cost-effective strategy (Yee et al., 1995). These dietary interactions are of potential relevance when prescribing a number of antipsychotics (e.g. clozapine, risperidone), antidepressants (e.g. sertraline, venlafaxine), anxiolytics (e.g. diazepam) and sedatives/hypnotics (e.g. zaleplon) that are CYP3A4 substrates (Madhusoodanan et al., 2014).

Herbal products may interact with Western medicines through CYP3A4 induction or inhibition, potentially causing lack of efficacy or excessive side effects. Consumption of herbs varies across cultures and thus the probability of herb–drug interactions across culture should be carefully considered while prescribing CYP3A4 substrates. Hypericum (St John's wort) preparation has been demonstrated to alter CYP450 enzymes in vitro, which has led to several documented drug interactions in depression (Obach, 2000). These interactions suggest that the herb can induce CYP450 enzymes (CYP3A4 and possibly CYP2C9, CYP1A2 and p-glycoprotein transport) resulting in sub-therapeutic drug levels with potentially serious consequences. Studies have found a decreased serum concentration of CYP3A4 substrates such as antidepressants and benzodiazepines after administration of St John's wort (Mannel, 2004).

The CYP1A2 isoenzyme is highly inducible by a number of dietary factors, particularly smoking and certain foods (Carrillo et al., 1998). It is involved in the metabolism of many psychotropic medications, including atypical antipsychotics (e.g. clozapine and olanzapine) and antidepressants (especially fluvoxamine). Apart from smoking, cruciferous vegetables such as brussels sprouts, cabbage, broccoli, cauliflower and charcoal-broiled beef, can significantly induce CYP1A2 activity (Pantuck et al., 1979; Fontana et al., 1999). Similarly, a high-protein diet (in contrast to a high-carbohydrate diet) has been shown to significantly increase CYP1A2 activity (Kappas et al., 1976). However, among South Asians a study reported CYP1A2 activity was significantly lower compared to European populations and this could in part be explained by their 'heavy CYP1A2-inhibitor diet' such as coriander, cumin and grapefruit juice (Perera et al., 2012). Hence, variations in dietary and lifestyle habits across different cultural groups can influence metabolism of drugs and response.

Apart from environmental factors, cultural differences may also influence drug response through shaping attitudes towards medication prescribed for psychiatric disorders. In this regard, culturally based health beliefs or explanatory models of causative factors and treatment options can exert profound effects (Lin and Smith, 2000), such as the ability to recognize psychiatric symptoms and understand their cause and rationale for treatment. In turn, the physical and cognitive side effects of psychotropics are likely to result in negative attitudes and non-compliance (Awad, 1993). Furthermore, the attitudes in the patient's social network can influence both patient's behaviour and compliance (Mantonakis et al., 1985). Hence, the relationship between treatment attitudes and response is complex and consists of various dimensions including the subjective perception, expectations, general attitudes and insight.

Subjective experiences of medication (as opposed to direct pharmacological effects) are clinically important and should not be dismissed or regarded as non-specific. Negative subjective response to psychotropic medications has been associated with lack of adherence and poorer therapeutic outcome (Awad et al., 1995; Ng and Klimidis, 2008). Such correlation between early subjective response and treatment outcome has also been noted in depressed patients treated with antidepressants (Priebe, 1987). The impact of culturally specific attitudes towards Western medication on clinical outcomes has not been adequately studied particularly between ethnic groups. Studies into related concepts, such as placebo effects and the perception of adverse effects may shed light on the clinical impact of attitudinal differences.

The occurrence of placebo response remains largely underestimated and unexplored in Western medicine. The impact of symbolic healing is often neglected in clinical trials other than being regarded as a confounding factor. In general placebo response is predicted in at least a third of subjects in most clinical drug trials. Yet, the underlying mechanism is not well understood and has mostly been attributed to non-specific therapeutic elements such as the doctor–patient relationship or even to metabolic and other biological mechanisms (Lin and Smith, 2000). Multi-centre clinical drug trials involving numerous ethnic groups and cross-national comparisons suggest that there may be a higher placebo response rate in non-Caucasians (Escobar and Tuason, 1980). The expectations of drug effects are often shaped by the patient's cultural origin and past experiences, and may well play an important role in producing clinical effects of phamacotherapy, mediated through symbolic and social mechanisms.

In addition, there are cultural differences in the use and prescription of Western medicine and complementary medicines. In many settings, the use of a 'herbal medicine approach' is associated with expectation of rapid relief, few or no side effects, standard dose regime, simple switching process between medicine types, and that no change in the individual or family units is required. This is incongruent with the typical characteristics of Western psychopharmacotherapy, which include gradual improvement, notable side effects, individualized dosing, regular supervision and monitoring, and the need for patient education and combination biopsychosocial therapies over variable duration (Westermeyer, 1989). The majority of Chinese have been influenced by traditional Chinese medical concepts and practices (Lee, 1980), and it is commonly perceived that Western medicines are more potent and have greater adverse effects than herbal or traditional therapies. Neglect of cultural and biological aspects of phamacotherapy can lead to poor doctor–patient relationship, medication non-adherence, unsatisfactory response, and treatment failure. On the other hand, it has been shown that psychotropic prescribing practice varies widely across countries and regions (Udomratn and Ng, 2008), and this together with costs and availability of drugs, use of polypharmacy and health system factors are also important in understanding cross-cultural variation in drug response.

Conclusions

The differences in psychotropic response across ethnicities and cultures reflect the richness in both biological and cultural processes affecting the clinical response to psychotropic drugs. The current data indicates that variations in cross-cultural psychopharmacotherapy are both important and complex in clinical practice. This area remains under-studied, particularly involving novel psychopharmacological agents, which may have potential inter-ethnic differences. Pharmacogenetics, which exhibits significant ethnic variations, may help guide the clinicians to make treatment decisions in terms of the choice of psychotropics, strategies for titration, the optimal therapeutic dosage, and the prediction of likely side effects. However, the impact of dietary, lifestyle, systemic and cultural variables on drug response must also be taken into account. Such multifaceted diversity on pharmacotherapeutic response can be brought together in an integrated model as a basis for systematic research and clinical application (see Figure 33.1). To enable flexible individual tailoring of psychotropic drug therapy, evidence based

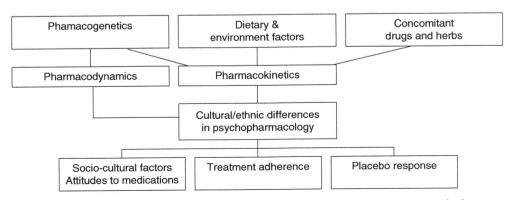

Figure 33.1 Variations in psychopharmacological response: influences of genetics, environment and culture

psychopharmacotherapy needs to be adapted to match both the biological and socio-cultural diversity of individual patients.

References

Akamine, Y., Yasui-Furukori, N., Ieiri, I. and Uno, T. (2012). Psychotropic drug–drug interactions involving P-glycoprotein. *CNS Drugs*, **26**(11), 959–973.

Awad, A. G. (1993). Subjective response to neuroleptics in schizophrenia. *Schizophrenia Bulletin*, **19**(3), 609–618.

Awad, A. G., Hogan, T. P., Voruganti, L. N. P. and Heslegrave, R. J. (1995). Patients' subjective experiences on antipsychotic medications: implications for outcome and quality of life. *International Clinical Psychopharmacology*, **10**(Suppl 3), 123–132.

Bailey, D. G., Spence, J. D., Munoz, C. and Arnold, J. M. O. (1991). Interaction of citrus juices with felodipine and nifedipine. *The Lancet*, **337**(8736), 268–269.

Bailey, D. G., Dresser, G. K. and Bend, J. (2003). Bergamottin, lime juice, and red wine as inhibitors of cytochrome P450 3A4 activity: comparison with grapefruit juice. *Clinical Pharmacology and Therapeutics*, **73**(6), 529–537.

Baune, B. T., Dannlowski, U., Domschke, K. *et al.* (2010). The interleukin 1 beta (IL1B) gene is associated with failure to achieve remission and impaired emotion processing in major depression. *Biological Psychiatry*, **67**(6), 543–549.

Bousman, C. A. and Hopwood, M. (2016). Commercial pharmacogenetic-based decision-support tools in psychiatry. *The Lancet Psychiatry*, **3**(6), 585–590.

Bousman, C. A., Sarris, J., Won, E. S. *et al.* (2014). Escitalopram efficacy in depression: a cross-ethnicity examination of the serotonin transporter promoter polymorphism. *Journal of Clinical Psychopharmacology*, **34**(5), 645–648.

Bradford, L. D. (2002). CYP2D6 allele frequency in European Caucasians, Asians, Africans and their descendants. *Pharmacogenomics*, **3**(2), 229–243.

Carrillo, J. A., Herraiz, A. G., Ramos, S. I., Benítez, J. (1998). Effects of caffeine withdrawal from the diet on the metabolism of clozapine in schizophrenic patients. *Journal of Clinical Psychopharmacology*, **18**(4), 311–316.

Escobar, J. I. and Tuason, V. B. (1980). Antidepressant agents – a cross-cultural study. *Psychopharmacology Bulletin*, **16**(3), 49–52.

Fontana, R. J., Lown, K. S., Paine, M. *et al.* (1999). Effects of a chargrilled meat diet on expression of CYP3A, CYP1A, and P-glycoprotein levels in healthy volunteers. *Gastroenterology*, **117**(1), 89–98.

Fricke-Galindo, I., Cespedes-Garro, C., Rodrigues-Soares, F. *et al.* (2016). Interethnic variation of CYP2C19 alleles, 'predicted' phenotypes and 'measured' metabolic phenotypes across world populations. *The Pharmacogenomics Journal*, **16**(2), 113–123.

Fuhr, U. (1998). Drug interactions with grapefruit juice. Extent, probable mechanism and clinical relevance. *Drug Safety*, **18**(4), 251–272.

Goldman, N., Glei, D. A., Lin, Y-H. and Weinstein, M. (2010). The serotonin transporter polymorphism (5-HTTLPR): allelic variation and links with depressive symptoms. *Depression and Anxiety*, **27**(3), 260–269.

Goldstein, J. A., Ishizaki, T., Kan, C. *et al.* (1997). Frequencies of the defective CYP2C19 alleles responsible for the mephenytoin poor metabolizer phenotype in various Oriental, Caucasian, Saudi Arabian and American black populations. *Pharmacogenetics*, **7**(1), 59–64.

Grant, D. M., Morike, K., Eichelbaum, M. and Meyer, U. A. (1990). Acetylation pharmacogenetics. The slow acetylator phenotype is caused by decreased or absent arylamine N-acetyltransferase in human liver. *The Journal of Clinical Investigation*, **85**(3), 968–972.

Gunes, A. and Dahl, M. L. (2008). Variation in CYP1A2 activity and its clinical implications: influence of environmental factors and genetic polymorphisms. *Pharmacogenomics*, **9**(5), 625–637.

Harris, R. Z., Jang, G. R. and Tsunoda, S. (2003). Dietary effects on drug metabolism and transport. *Clinical Pharmacokinetics*, **42**(13), 1071–1088.

Hicks, J. K., Bishop, J. R., Sangkuhl, K. *et al.* (2015). Clinical Pharmacogenetics Implementation Consortium (CPIC) guideline for CYP2D6 and CYP2C19 genotypes and dosing of selective serotonin reuptake inhibitors. *Clinical Pharmacology and Therapeutics*, **98**(2), 127–134.

Kappas, A., Anderson, K. E., Conney, Allan H. and Alvares, Alvito P. (1976). Influence of dietary protein and carbohydrate on antipyrine and theophylline metabolism in man. *Clinical Pharmacology and Therapeutics*, **20**(6), 643–653.

Lee, R. P. (1980). Perceptions and uses of Chinese medicine among the Chinese in Hong Kong. *Culture, Medicine and Psychiatry*, **4**(4), 345–375.

Lin, H. J., Han, C. Y., Lin, B. K. and Hardy, S. (1993). Slow acetylator mutations in the human polymorphic N-acetyltransferase gene in 786 Asians, blacks, Hispanics, and whites: application to metabolic epidemiology. *American Journal of Human Genetics*, **52**(4), 827–834.

Lin, K. M. and Smith, M. W. (2000). Psychopharmacotherapy in the context of culture and ethnicity. In *Ethnicity and Psychopharmacology*, ed. P. Ruiz. Washington DC: American Psychiatric Press, pp. 1–36.

Madhusoodanan, S., Velama, U., Parmar, J. *et al.* (2014). A current review of cytochrome P450 interactions of psychotropic drugs. *Annals of Clinical Psychiatry: Official*

Journal of the American Academy of Clinical Psychiatrists, **26**(2), 120–138.

Mannel, M. (2004). Drug interactions with St John's wort: mechanisms and clinical implications. *Drug Safety,* **27**(11), 773–797.

Mantonakis, J., Markidis, M., Kontaxakis, V. and Liakos, A. (1985). A scale for detection of negative attitudes towards medication among relatives of schizophrenic patients. *Acta Psychiatrica Scandinavica,* **71**(2), 186–189.

Murphy, E. and McMahon, F. J. (2013). Pharmacogenetics of antidepressants, mood stabilizers, and antipsychotics in diverse human populations. *Discovery Medicine,* **16**(87), 113–122.

Ng, C. H. (2008). Research directions in ethno-psychopharmacology. In *Ethno-Psychopharmacology: Advances in Current Practice,* ed. C. H. Ng, K. M. Lin, B. Singh and E. Chiu. New York, Cambridge University Press, pp. 169–176.

Ng, C. and Klimidis, S. (2008). Cultural factors and the use of psychotropic medications. In *Ethno-Psychopharmacology: Advances in Current Practice,* ed. C. H. Ng, K. M. Lin, B. Singh and E. Chiu. New York: Cambridge University Press, pp. 123–134.

Ng, C. H., Schweitzer, I., Norman, T., Easteal, S. (2004). The emerging role of pharmacogenetics: implications for clinical psychiatry. *The Australian and New Zealand Journal of Psychiatry,* **38**(7), 483–489.

Ng, C. H., Chong, S. A., Lambert, T. *et al.* (2005). An inter-ethnic comparison study of clozapine dosage, clinical response and plasma levels. *International Clinical Psychopharmacology,* **20**(3), 163–168.

Ng, C. H., Easteal, S., Tan, S. *et al.* (2006). Serotonin transporter polymorphisms and clinical response to sertraline across ethnicities. *Progress in Neuro-Psychopharmacology and Biological Psychiatry,* **30**(5), 953–957.

Ng, C., Sarris, J., Singh, A. *et al.* (2013). Pharmacogenetic polymorphisms and response to escitalopram and venlafaxine over 8 weeks in major depression. *Human Psychopharmacology,* **28**(5), 516–522.

Obach, R. S. (2000). Inhibition of human cytochrome P450 enzymes by constituents of St John's Wort, an herbal preparation used in the treatment of depression. *The Journal of Pharmacology and Experimental Therapeutics,* **294**(1), 88–95.

Ozawa, S., Soyama, A., Saeki, M. *et al.* (2004). Ethnic differences in genetic polymorphisms of CYP2D6, CYP2C19, CYP3As and MDR1/ABCB1. *Drug Metabolism and Pharmacokinetics,* **19**(2), 83–95.

Padmanabhan, S. (2014). *Handbook of Pharmacogenomics and Stratified Medicines.* London and San Diego: Academic Press.

Palma-Aguirre, J. A., Nava Rangel, J., Hoyo-Vadillo, C., *et al.* (1994). Influence of Mexican diet on nifedipine pharmacodynamics in healthy volunteers. *Proceedings of the Western Pharmacology Society,* **37**, 85–86.

Pantuck, E. J., Pantuck, C. B., Garland, W. A. *et al.* (1979). Stimulatory effect of brussels sprouts and cabbage on human drug metabolism. *Clinical Pharmacology and Therapeutics,* **25**(1), 88–95.

Perera, V., Gross, A. S. and McLachlan, A. J. (2012). Influence of environmental and genetic factors on CYP1A2 activity in individuals of South Asian and European ancestry. *Clinical Pharmacology and Therapeutics,* **92**(4), 511–519.

Pi, E. H. and Gray, G. E. (1998). A cross-cultural perspective on psychopharmacology. *Essential Psychopharmacology,* **2**, 233–262.

Pollock, B. G., Ferrell, R. E., Mulsant, B. *et al.* (2000). Allelic variation in the serotonin transporter promoter affects onset of paroxetine treatment response in late-life depression. *Neuropsychopharmacology: Official Publication of the American College of Neuropsychopharmacology,* **23**(5), 587–590.

Poolsup, N., Li Wan Po, A. and Knight, T. (2000). Pharmacogenetics and psychopharmacotherapy. *Journal of Clinical Pharmacy and Therapeutics,* **25**(3), 197–220.

Priebe, S. (1987). Early subjective reactions predicting the outcome of hospital treatment in depressive patients. *Acta Psychiatrica Scandinavica,* **76**(2), 134–138.

Schwartz, R. S. (2001). Racial profiling in medical research. *The New England Journal of Medicine,* **344**(18), 1392–1393.

Teh, L. K. and Bertilsson, L. (2012). Pharmacogenomics of CYP2D6: molecular genetics, interethnic differences and clinical importance. *Drug Metabolism and Pharmacokinetics,* **27**(1), 55–67.

Udomratn, P. and Ng, C. (2008). Outpatients prescribing practices in Asian countries. In *Ethno-Psychopharmacology: Advances in Current Practice,* ed. C. H. Ng, K. M. Lin, B. Singh and E. Chiu. New York: Cambridge University Press, pp. 135–143.

Van Booven, D., Marsh, S., McLeod, H. *et al.* (2010). Cytochrome P450 2C9-CYP2C9. *Pharmacogenetics and Genomics,* **20**(4), 277–281.

Westermeyer, J. (1989). Somatotherapies. In *Psychiatric Care of Migrants: A Clinical Guide,* ed. J. H. Gold. Washington DC: American Psychiatric Press, pp. 139–168.

World Health Organization (2016). WHO model list of essential medicines, 19th edn (cited 23 May 2016). Available online at www.who.int/medicines/publications/essentialmedicines/EML_2015_FINAL_amended_NOV2015.pdf?ua=1.

Yee, G. C., Stanley, D. L., Pessa, L. *et al.* (1995). Effect of grapefruit juice on blood cyclosporin concentration. *The Lancet*, **345**(8955), 955–956.

Yu, S. H., Liu, S. K. *et al.* (2007). Psychopharmacology across cultures. In *Textbook of Cultural Psychiatry*, ed. D. Bhugra and K. Bhui. Cambridge: Cambridge University Press.

Zanger, U. M., Turpeinen, M., Klein, K. and Schwab, M. (2008). Functional pharmacogenetics/genomics of human cytochromes P450 involved in drug biotransformation. *Analytical and Bioanalytical Chemistry*, **392**(6), 1093–1108.

Chapter 34

Psychotherapy across Cultures

Digby Tantam and Kemal Sayar

Editors' Introduction

Successful outcome in psychotherapy depends upon the core of therapeutic interaction and therapeutic alliance. This relationship relies on the characteristics of the therapist as well as the needs and non-specific factors attributed to the patient. Ethnic matching of patient and the therapist has already been discussed. In this chapter Tantam and Sayar emphasize that culture shapes all individuals, our world view and cognitions as well as behaviours. In many healthcare systems it is presumed wrongly that patients, especially those from minority communities, appear to have a culture and cultural base but the majority may not recognize this cultural bias. Tantam and Sayar argue that everyone lives in a world mediated by meaning and therefore influenced by shared language, beliefs and values which in turn are very strongly influenced by cultural values. This cultural impact on definitions of normality and abnormality, of justifiability or condemnation, and of how other people should and can change. They argue that all of this affects the practice of psychotherapy, and its accessibility by people from minority groups. Tantam and Sayar in this chapter provide a framework for considering the desiderata that potential clients use to determine whether they will require or even enter psychotherapy and whether they will see the process through. Furthermore, the authors note that there are ways in which psychotherapists can ensure that they minimize their own cultural barriers that can restrict uptake of therapy or hasten premature discontinuation. It is apparent that the broad therapeutic interventions of psychotherapy include a broad category of schools and methods which are used towards changing a patient's inner life through a specially constructed relationship between therapist and patient. It is important that the outcome of therapy should be agreed beforehand so that the therapist can work accordingly.

Introduction

Culture has been described in many ways. UNESCO's Declaration of Universal Cultural Diversity defined it as a 'set of distinctive spiritual, material, intellectual and emotional features of society or a social group, and that it encompasses, in addition to art and literature, lifestyles, ways of living together, value systems, traditions and beliefs'. Culture shapes how each of us acts, particularly when our actions are directed towards expression or communication rather than towards the performance of environmentally determined tasks. Culture therefore has a particular impact on that branch of psychiatry, psychotherapy, which is especially concerned with meaningful rather than causal connections between events (see also Chapter 1).

There are other, similar, influences. Each human language particularly affords its own way of articulating the world, and therefore tends towards some meanings rather than others. Many psychotherapists have stressed that how one says something alters what one says and, eventually, what one thinks. The use of 'self' to refer to what a person really is, which originates in English in the seventeenth century, gradually exerted a hold over psychology and psychotherapy in the later part of the twentieth century resulting in, as some have argued, a preoccupation with individuality ('self-development') and autonomy (self-determination). Sampson (1989) has argued that this is culturally divisive because it drains the meaning from intersubjective perspectives for which English has to resort to portmanteau expressions like 'self-in-other'.

English, with its plethora of, and reliance on, nouns also tends towards descriptions, which, as Schafer (1976) argued in his Freud Memorial lectures, are reifying. Expressions like 'the unconscious', 'the transference' or 'the libido' claim the same status as 'the appendix' or 'the blood pressure'. They also become shibboleths. A senior psychoanalyst once asked me, 'Do you believe in the unconscious?' as if he was asking me, 'Are you one of us?'

Schafer proposed replacing these terms as much as possible with verbs, or 'action language'. This would bring psychoanalysis closer to therapies like existential psychotherapy, which are concerned about the intentions that people have and how they realize them, not the processes to which they are subject.

Other concepts that are closely related to culture are 'class' or 'ethnicity'. (We prefer to use ethnicity rather than race because of the links of race with spurious and largely non-existent biological differences.) People have class and ethnic identities as they do cultural identities. There are class and ethnic, as well as cultural, values. There may be class and ethnic dialects. For the purposes of this chapter, we will deal with this overlap by considering culture as it applies to a class, an ethnic group, as well as a society. However, both class and ethnicity convey the importance of external circumstance in a way that culture does not.

Culture is something created, as its name indicates, out of the almost limitless capacity of human beings to weave a meaning around themselves. The weaving has both a warp and a woof, a synchronic and a diachronic or historical, element. But it is symbolic in that meaning does not have to cash out in any particular reality.

A person is immersed in a culture, but consigned to a class or an ethnic group. And membership of such a group is not purely symbolic. There are entailments. Class members have more or less status, social influence, health and opportunities for wealth creation depending on the class to which they have been assigned. Ethnicity may carry with it some of these entailments, but may also create expectations by others of personal characteristics that are associated with members of that ethnic group: Englishmen are, for example, supposedly cold and poor lovers, but make good policemen.

Religion is yet another closely related organizing principle in society. One can be born into a religion, but can also adopt it in a way that one cannot so easily adopt culture, class or ethnicity. However, religion is also an important element within culture, and the same religion may take distinct forms within different cultures: one need only think of the evangelical Pure Land Buddhism, open to everyone, and the Zen Buddhism whose exacting meditative practices confined it to a small but influential priesthood. There is a growing literature on religion and psychotherapy; we will not consider it separately here, but only in relation to culture.

Culture and Psychopathology

The substantial literature on 'culture-bound' disorders has been considered elsewhere in this book. There has been a shift from taking an alienated perspective, with weird culture-bound syndromes being carefully but distantly documented, to a recognition that there are few syndromes that are restricted to particular cultures, although there are many cultures that are known by their emblematic syndromes. The culture-bound syndromes discovered by colonizing Europeans in so-called primitive peoples, which reinforced European preconceptions of primitive beliefs and lack of self-control – *windigo*, for example, or *amok* – have given way to disorders associated with civilization, for example, neurasthenia in China, anorexia nervosa in Europe, and post-traumatic stress disorder in groups everywhere who have been caught up in conflict or disaster (see also Chapters 11 and 14).

It is worth noting that psychotherapies, too, have cultures, often with their own culture-bound syndromes. Some, like borderline personality disorder, have arisen in one psychotherapy culture – in this case, psychoanalysis – but have permeated other psychotherapy cultures, too. Others, like recovered-memory syndrome, have remained largely confined to the therapy culture, in this example feminist psychotherapy, in which they first emerged. Yet others, like battered-woman syndrome, have become accepted as a result of a particularly influential text, but their influence has subsequently waned (Rothenberg, 2002). What determines such 'cultural authority' has been discussed by Schudson (1989).

Twin Cultures

Western psychotherapists, and psychotherapy, typically draw on two cultural traditions which are so intertwined within what is called Western European thought that we cannot easily distinguish them, although from time to time intellectuals have called our attention to them. Dilthey (1883), himself influenced by Schleiermacher, distinguished between two kinds of understanding, *erklären* or explanation, which is, he said, proper to the *Naturwissenschaften* ('natural sciences') and *verstehen*, or 'meaning' which is appropriate to the *Geisteswissenschaften* (social sciences). C. P. Snow's famous distinction between the two cultures of the arts and the sciences refers to a similar distinction between fundamentally different holds on the world. More recently, the distinction has often been made in terms of 'causes' and 'reasons'. We have argued that an important difference between these two is that causes are, as Hume pointed out, events that are both constantly conjoined to, and precede, the events that are their consequences. Reasons are not constantly conjoined and may occur after the event, in which case they act as justifications (Tantam, 1999). But justifications have causal power, too, at least in the social world. In fact, one approach to psychotherapy that claims to be culture-free, the narrative approach, is based on the causal properties of reasons.

The Narrative Approach to Psychotherapy

Suppose you are being tried for assault. You have stopped another motorist and in a fit of road rage, have pulled him out of his car and punched him. Rage caused your actions and you tell the barrister that you could not really say what went through your mind before the action except that you felt a red mist come over you, and you 'just had to do it'. The barrister considers possible defences: perhaps you were undergoing some kind of ictally related episode. If you had been, you would have been able to argue that although you committed the act, the '*actus reus*' was undisputed, you did not know what you were doing because your brain was undergoing an electrical storm. In which case you would have had no '*mens rea*'. But in this case there was no evidence that epilepsy or any other automatism supervened. The assault was not caused by an external agency (as the law would see a disease of the brain), but by you. So the barrister turns their attention to mitigation. What can they say on your behalf that would reduce the sentence? They find that the other driver had overtaken you on the wrong side of the road (you were on a motorway) and had then swerved into your lane, narrowly missing hitting the near side and putting the passenger at risk. The passenger was your daughter who had started crying with fear and this had provoked you to a protective rage. The barrister finds a witness to say that the other driver had been drinking heavily at a wedding an hour before the assault.

The judge is moved by this account, and gives you a non-custodial sentence with a minimal period of community service. As it is a civil case, the judge splits the costs evenly between the two parties, so that the victim has to pay their own costs. The police decide to investigate the other party for dangerous driving. You

feel at least partly exonerated. The barrister's arguments in mitigation have had causal power. They have changed your emotions, other people's reactions to you, and have prompted a police investigation. The only odd causal property of reasons is that, as in this case, they may change past events, something that causes are never supposed to do. In this case, the assault, the event, had become a justified action rather than the wild action of a dangerously aggressive person as a result of a change in your reason for it.

Not all jurisdictions contemplate sentencing in this way. Many courts follow the Code of Hammurabi in fixing exact penalties to specified acts. Philosophers know this ethical system as 'act-utilitarianism'. Sharia law, as administered by Islamic clerics, may follow act utilitarianism according to this verse from the chapter in the Qur'an on consultation, 'The recompense for an injury is an injury equal thereto (in degree)' (42:40). The Surah al-Shura opens another complex ethical and legal issue: what injury can equal another injury, in degree. But it leaves out intention, or motive.

Inquiring about intentions is an essential element of many Western psychotherapies, and of the qualitative methods employed in research by many westernized psychotherapists. They contrast their focus on intentions with symptomatic approaches that embrace the medical model, for example the very successful family of therapies that apply learning theory or schema theory to the treatment of anxiety, depression and a variety of habit or behavioural disorders. There are many causal theories, other than these ones. Some are biological, for example those theories that see psychotherapy as a form of grooming and its effects as the result of released nonapeptides, or endogenous opioids. Other causal theories include those that posit evil forces that can cause harm to individuals or to society; theories of spirit possession; disorder as a punishment for failure to follow religious or cultural ordinances; or simply the effects of self-neglect or over-indulgence.

It is often assumed, although rarely tested, that a focus on causes springs from an overvaluing of the results of quantitative research, and an excessive preoccupation with the so-called medical model of symptoms and treatments. This is sometimes called, very broadly, 'positivism': a word coined by the philosopher Comte (1973 [1851]) although subsequently appropriated by the mathematically-orientated 'logical positivists'. Those Western psychotherapists who reject positivism often embrace the approaches of other cultures, particularly those of faraway places even though people resident in those places may themselves feel more comfortable with positivist approaches.

Religious Healing

An important tradition that has preceded psychotherapy everywhere in the world, and whose assumptions still interpenetrate it, is religious healing. People still turn to holy books for advice, guidance and solace. What they read, and what they focus on, is also subject to cultural shifts. One currently important focus is on forgiveness. This is enjoined in the Christian New Testament, in Buddhist scriptures such as the Dhammapada, and in the Qur'an, in which the Surah Al-Shura verse continues from the page quoted above with 'but whoever forgives and makes reconciliation, his reward is with Allah. Indeed, He likes not the wrong doers.'

Unglueing the Past

Forgiveness is only possible if one has given up thought of revenge. Thoughts of revenge, as opposed to campaigns or acts, keep on turning the past over and over. Forgiveness betokens moving on. The Qur'an's injunction to move on corresponds to what is arguably a transcultural principle in psychotherapy: leave the past behind. Nostalgia, regret, post-traumatic stress disorder, longings for justice or retribution, shame, lost love, and feeling let down by life, parents, the government, or the system are all examples of emotional attachment to the past that potentially blocks life in the present and the future (Tantam, 1998).

There are important factors that keep people locked into their past. They may be 'working things out'. They may feel the need to witness, to warn others, or right a wrong. But the most common reason might be not to let someone get away with something. People from every culture, like their cousins the chimps, are willing to take a smaller reward in order to penalize a con-specific who has taken an unfair advantage (Brosnan and de Waal, 2014).

Different cultures have different ways of dealing with this problem. Exorcism might be one way of divesting oneself of the evil spirit left over from the past. Reliance on an all seeing god to punish the evildoer on judgement day might also work, as might a rational calculation of the likely benefits of moving on. A psychotherapist who advocated relying on god to solve the problem will not appeal effectively to a client who has had the kind of experience that leaves them convinced that the world is unjust.

The Biological and the Psychological

Western psychotherapists have to be able to move between both kinds of explanation, both causes and reasons. They may, for example, tell a depressed patient that they are depressed because they have negative automatic thoughts (a presumed causal explanation) but also, in the same session, work with the patient's own account that they are depressed because they feel guilty at not having cared more for their eldest daughter who has now left home (a justification or post hoc explanation).

The success of causal explanations in the physical, biological and medical sciences has secured their pre-eminence over alternatives. This has had the consequence that other kinds of explanation have gone on to the defensive and even to a denial by some philosophers that there are important differences in kind between biological and cultural accounts (Luhrman, 2000; Gibbard, 2001). Some psychotherapists have tried to re-package as many of their traditional accounts as possible as if they are descriptions of causal processes. A more creative solution has been to argue for a multiplicity of explanations. Postmodernists have taken this process to the extreme of doubting the value of the science's application of testing for truth or refutation and so tried to reduce science to the status of being a colonial narrative of no particular intrinsic merit. However, one does not have to undermine causal explanation to allow a place for reasons; our culture has, as we noted at the beginning of this section, become almost casual in moving backwards and forwards between them.

We are used to there being several causes for one action, but also that each of these causes is interlinked, and that there is one causal sequence which will reproducibly produce the consequence whenever it occurs (we include here those causes which have their effects by influencing the state of reactivity of a system). By contrast, many independent reasons can be given for one action, and they are not necessarily linked. Some are only given once, or only given to one particular person, or group. All of this is legitimate, and we are used to it. A person may become addicted to heroin and tell his or her doctor that it was because heroin calmed them, tell his or her mother that it is because they have never properly recovered from the death of a younger sister, and pray to their God for strength to overcome the temptations of the Devil. It is clearly misconceived to ask which of these is the right explanation, although it may make sense to ask which is right for a particular situation. Since each of these reasons may have causal consequences in the future, it is also appropriate to ask what effect it will have to focus on one of these reasons or another.

Example

Deanna was a young woman with the ambition to become a musical artist but was inhibited by her lack of self-confidence and by a mild stammer. She was seeing a college counsellor for these problems, but there had been little progress. Then she watched a video biography of Jonathan Larson, the composer of *Rent*, a cult rock musical loosely based on Puccini's *La Boheme*. Larson conceived the idea of *Rent* when he was 29. He worked on the music and the lyrics until he was 32, when it had a studio performance, after which it was substantially revised. He continued to work in a diner to earn his keep, and composed during his free time. The first performance of the final version took place in 1996, when Larson was 35. Larson had chest pains during the final days of rehearsal, and was examined by a cardiologist who told him that he was fit and well, and that he was suffering from nerves. Following the triumphant dress rehearsal, Larson went home and collapsed and died in his kitchen when he was making a snack. A post-mortem showed that he had ruptured a thoracic aneurysm and that he had Marfan syndrome. The young woman was inspired by Larson emerging from obscurity to write a musical that has been staged in many countries of the world, successfully transferred to Broadway and, at the time of writing, had run continuously there for 10 years. She thought that she, too, could be like Larson. All it took was self-belief and hard work. Larson had a physical problem, like her, but he did not allow it to prevent him realizing his dream. She thought of him hanging on to life until he was sure that the dream had come true. She was so inspired that she told many of her friends. Some said that, if he had not worked so hard, he might have lived longer. Others said that, if he had not been so preoccupied with his musical, he might have paid more attention to his health, and perhaps then his Marfan syndrome would have been detected earlier. One friend said that she thought of it like a kind of pact with God:

he had paid with his life for the gift of one great creative act. Another, Fatema, said that he had been struck down for the immorality of his work, which had lionized the very people that this friend had been taught were evil doers.

Larson died as a result of a ruptured aortic aneurysm, and the cause of that happening was his Marfan syndrome. Deanna and all her friends accepted that as the cause. Knowing the cause has implications for medical practitioners and others, of course, but not really for these friends, unless they have, or know someone who has, Marfan syndrome. Knowing the reason for the death is much more important because it has moral significance, providing possible answers to such questions as, 'Is it sometimes better to die early and achieve something memorable than to die later, but to die as a nonentity?' However, Deanna and her friends did not agree about the reasons for Larson's death even though they agreed about the cause. Each of them assimilated the death into the cultural system of meanings that they already had or, if it would not be assimilated, making enough of a change in that system to accommodate it. Deanna herself made such a major accommodation that seeing the biography 'changed her life', to use her own words.

Cultural Tension and Identity

Deanna found it easy to accept that if you dreamed enough and were prepared to follow your dream, the dream would come true. The price to be paid for this did not matter. Her friend Fatema did not have the same value. In fact, she found it offensive. To have accepted Deanna's reason would have been to offend Fatema's values. Deanna, for her part, soon fell out with the friend who thought Jonathan had been punished. She realized that she had nothing in common with her any more.

Fatema identified herself as a member of a fundamentally religious culture. If pressed, she would have argued that the values expressed by any member of that culture were also her own, but she strongly identified with these two: that certain behaviours were unacceptable to God, and proscribed by scripture, and that presenting these practices without censoring them was, in itself, sinful. Deanna did not identify herself strongly with any culture, but did disidentify herself with these values of Fatema. She said that she was 'not the kind of person' to be so intolerant and 'bigoted'.

Personal identity is, like meaning, a common issue in psychotherapy, particularly longer-term psychotherapy. Identity issues include being 'somebody', coming to terms with being very different when intoxicated or under stress, having one's identity stolen or attached and dealing with opportunities to create virtual identities on the net or in fantasy games. Personal identity is determined by all the characteristics that enable us to distinguish one person from another, including their bank account number and their DNA. But John Locke's location of personal identity in consciousness (Locke, 1995) anticipated the principal modern usage of the term identity as a creation produced as a result of narration, particularly narration to oneself.

Fatema found the ideas of her culture about sin and censorship palatable and built them into her story of who she was and of what mattered to her. She identified with them. Deanna found them unpalatable, and rejected them and as a result also rejected Fatema. Had Deanna forced herself instead to hang on to Fatema's good opinion, and to talk disparagingly of Larson, it would have challenged not just Deanna's values, and the norms of her culture, but also her emotional investment in Larson as an inspiration.

Research evidence has consistently supported the power of cognitive dissonance in opinion change, although there are some cultural variations (Hoshino-Browne et al., 2005). If Deanna had aped Fatema's opinions, cognitive dissonance theory predicts that she would have tended to adopt them as her own. Deanna's emotional investment, her identification with Larson, counteracted this. She felt an aversion to pronouncing any negative opinion about Larson and had she tried to overcome this in order to maintain her relationship with Fatema, she might have said, as others do in a similar situation, that she felt dirty by having to say things that she did not believe.

Cultures provide us with values, norms and symbols, but these are not lacking in an affective content. Each is charged with an emotional flavour put there by our emotions at the time that we first encountered the value or the application of the norm or the symbol. Our identification with a culture is a product of the amount of overlap between our personal values, norms and symbols, and those of the culture, and the emotional flavour of these values, norms and symbols.

Asserting a cultural identity means championing the ideas of a culture but also holding on to the emotions with which those ideas are flavoured.

Providing psychotherapy across cultural boundaries means not only having to deal with the unfamiliarity and uncertainty created by novel ideas or situations, it also means dealing with the emotional flavour of the novelties. This is likely to be influenced by cultural transmission of emotional flavours. Given our preoccupation with the pressure of immigration, and in the aftermath of colonialism, other cultures, particularly those which are not economically dominant, are most likely to be viewed as potentially dangerous and the flavour of their ideas as unpalatable.

Moving between cultures, exercising what has come to be called cultural competence, involves therefore not just new learning but an emotional process of discovering the palatability of new values and norms. Psychotherapists who talk to colleagues working in a different modality even have to do this. For a psychoanalytic psychotherapist to be able to talk the same language as a cognitive-behavioural therapist may not be quantitatively as challenging as a white UK middle-class therapist finding a common language with a black African upper-class client, but it is not qualitatively different.

Could Hermeneutics Be a Common Ground for Psychotherapy?

Reasons are the answers we give to the questions, 'Why?' or 'What does it mean?' So long as we can give reasons for things, we can make sense of them and, if we can make sense of most of what happens to us, we can say that our lives have meaning. The potential universe of reasons is very large, but only a subset of them make sense to any particular person, and the membership of this subset is, or so some cultural anthropologists have argued, determined by the culture to which we belong. Christopher (2001: 116), for example, writes, 'From a hermeneutic point of view, culture is constituted by those shared meanings that make social life possible.'

Psychotherapists, too, have drawn on hermeneutic methods to collaborate with their clients in jointly discovering new meaning in the events of their client's lives (Lang, 1995). There is therefore a natural kinship in the methods of cultural anthropologists and psychotherapists in that both are interested in exploring meaning.

Culture provides us with the tools to create meaning, but it also limits the meaning that we can create, since each culture provides a different repertoire of tools. Most of us draw from several cultures. For many of us these different cultures are really subcultures of what constitutes our home culture and therefore our cultural toolboxes contain the same tools and the meaning that we place on our worlds is comparable. It is usual for each of them to have overlapping elements and no one can draw from all of human culture. As psychotherapy is a treatment based on shared meaning between patient(s) and therapist(s), the psychotherapist's culture and the client's culture have to overlap sufficiently for shared meaning to be possible (Qureshi, 2005).

Emic and Etic Elements of Culture

Part of the power of the scientific paradigm is that it claims to be universal and not culture-specific. Dropped stones fall after they are thrown everywhere in the world, with very few exceptions, and every world language has had to find a word like 'fall' to describe the effects of gravity. Culture has a very superficial effect on biology. So most biological descriptions are cultural universals or 'etic' (Pike, 1967). Kraepelin went to Java to find out if dementia praecox was present there as well as in Europe and found that it was, and concluded from this that it was a biological disease as well as a culturally defined illness. Although Javanese culture may not have recognized schizophrenia as a single entity at that time, as European culture had not before Kraepelin's description, the descriptor 'schizophrenia' is an 'etic' one because it maps on to the same state of affairs in Java as it does in Germany. Depression and anxiety are probably etic, too, but not 'love-sick' or 'relaxed' or 'borderline personality disorder'. These are only understandable in a particularly cultural context and are therefore 'emic'.

From the foregoing discussion it will be clear that reasons which add meaning after the event, values, norms and emotional flavours are 'emic' in that they apply only within particular cultures whereas causal explanations are 'etic'.

A psychiatrist who knows that substance X is likely to improve the condition of 80 per cent of her patients with schizophrenia knows this to be true irrespective of the patient's culture. Perhaps, though, substance X comes as a black tablet in which case Westerners might associate it with death, and be reluctant to take it. So the psychiatrist will have to discuss the colour and its significance with the patient, maybe explaining that it was manufactured by a new drug company in Tanzania, who chose black because among the Masai it is associated with prosperity. Even though psychiatrist X would like to prescribe medication without having to take any account of creed, colour or culture, she would be forced to take this into account, not on grounds of efficacy but on grounds of effectiveness. Only the patients that complied with treatment would benefit from it and compliance would be affected by emic factors, even if the effects of the drug would not.

Has Psychotherapy Developed Independently in Cultures Other than the Western European?

The 'drug metaphor' model of psychotherapy presumes that the treatment effects of psychotherapy are 'etic', and there is some evidence for this. Some of it comes from studies that compare apparently analogous healing practices in different parts of the world on the assumption that common factors may be 'etic' ones (Tantam, 1993; and see also Chapter 31).

Although studies like this contribute to the continuing search for the specific elements of psychotherapy, the non-specific, 'emic', factors are even more important than in other branches of psychiatry. So this kind of study may be less important than would seem at first sight. Such studies have an even larger drawback. They presume that psychotherapy occurs everywhere in the world in some form. But does it?

Preoccupying Concern

What happens when someone in Central Asia, or East Africa or Borneo, becomes depressed? Who do they turn to? This question immediately raises a difficulty: there may be no recognition of an illness called depression at all (Kleinman, 2004). The recognition of an illness affords a medical solution (similarly, the availability of doctors affords the perception of interpersonal problems as due to illness). It seems likely that, when a person first experiences physical or psychological symptoms of unease, when they first develop a concern that is relevant to psychotherapy, they find a reason for it. The commonest reason worldwide is spirit possession, followed closely by ill will or witchcraft. But other reasons might include misfortune due to actions undertaken at inauspicious times, the influence of the stars, family conflict, worries or stresses, failure to propitiate the deceased, too much alcohol or drugs, bad character, failure to fulfil spiritual or ceremonial duties, punishment for past sins or crimes, remorse, physical disorder, deficiency disease and trauma. Which reason is chosen will determine what help is sought out. Possible community resources are likely to include a friend, a family member, an elder, a priest, a traditional healer or a doctor. Although traditional healers are often considered the equivalent in many cultures of psychotherapists, they are more appropriately considered the equivalent of alternative and complementary practitioners in the West.

Each of the foregoing formulations of unease can be considered to have at its core a specific 'concern' or, to use Kleinman's term, an explanatory model. Frijda (1986: 100) defines a concern as 'the more or less enduring disposition to prefer particular states of the world. A concern is what gives a particular event its emotional meaning.' Elsewhere, it has been argued that psychotherapists who wish to gain the confidence of their patients must reach an agreement with their patients about the focus of therapy and that this must reflect the concern, the 'preoccupying concern', that is uppermost in the mind of the patient when seeking help (Tantam, 2002).

Choice of healer will depend on time and money costs, on reputation and on the importance of hedging one's bets. Many people in rural Zanzibar, for example, consult both the health centre and a traditional healer when a child is ill. But the choice of healer and healing method will also depend on whether the healer is expected to focus on the patient's preoccupying concern. Only those people who see their unease in terms of illness are likely to seek out a doctor or a mental health professional. How many people in the world do so is changing rapidly as education seems to bring with it an increased awareness of psychological and psychological factors affecting personal experience.

Ethnic Matching

One solution to the importance of matching patient expectation and psychotherapist behaviour is for patients to consult therapists who are from their same cultural group. It is difficult to know what a person's culture is until one gets to know them, and cultural matching is probably most important early on in the therapy or even before therapy begins, when the patient is selecting a therapist. Ethnic matching, which relies on demonstrable markers of ethnicity like name, skin colour, qualifications or neighbourhood, may be used as a proxy of cultural matching.

One definition of culture is that it creates the norms, the values and the artefacts in which, and by which, we live. Norms have an influential bearing on the dispositions, which, as noted in the previous section, generate the concerns that lead to therapy. That section dealt with the importance of matching the concerns of the patient with the concerns that the healing method highlights. It was noted that the concerns of psychotherapy include a preference for a 'state of the world', which accounts for unease by illness or disorder, and accounts for recovery by reference to mental or psychological explanations.

Congruent Values and Palatable Flavours

It has been previously suggested that treatment adherence, and therefore treatment effectiveness, also requires matching values and 'emotional flavours' (Tantam, 2002).

Values are culturally transmitted. So a congruence of values between patient and therapist is an important consequence of ethnic matching, and value incongruence is a significant barrier to cross-cultural psychotherapy.

Key values that have been described as being potential barriers are a focus on the psychological at the expense of the spiritual; an emphasis on independence and autonomy rather than interdependence and care for others; a focus on the individual rather than the family; and the expectation of instruction.

Values may be explicit. For example, patients from some cultures where a premium is placed on guidance may be confused to be told in the first session that their therapist will not be giving any specific advice.

Values may be implicit in administrative arrangements. Discouragement of family members being involved in psychotherapy may, for example, signal a depreciation of the value of the family as may asking patients not to discuss therapy outside the therapy hour.

Psychopathology also incorporates, and is influenced by, values. Diagnoses may implicitly communicate cultural assumptions. In the Muslim world, the absence of spiritual status from psychopathology is considered a weakness in Western orientated psychopathology, for example. In at least one former communist country, there has been a clear shift from group-orientated to individually orientated diagnostic labels, and consequently from group to individual treatments, following the abandonment of Marxist values and the assumption of consumerist ones (Leuenberger, 2002).

Not all values are constructive. Implicit values might include denigratory or racist ones. Patients may have stereotyped views of therapists, and therapists, too, may, without really being aware of this, consider people from other cultures to be unsophisticated, uncivilized or primitive. Peeling away the surface of expressed beliefs about other cultures might include values about the superiority of one's own culture's religious beliefs, or lack of them; about the psychological health or stability of people from one's culture; or about the lack of morality in other cultures.

Negative values may be communicated in many ways, not least by ignorance of what is important in another culture, for example, in relation to diet or religious observance or the manner of speaking to people of the other sex or of a different status.

Palatable Flavours

Therapists can learn to address their patients' concerns more effectively with brief training or through experience and so can have their eyes opened to the concerns of other cultures. Values may be harder to reveal or to address.

Challenging a value may feel like questioning a person's identity. However, regular case consultation, or supervision, by psychotherapists provides the opportunity of a safe and confidential environment in which issues like this can be addressed. There is a case for seeking out supervision with an experienced supervisor from another culture when working across cultures, since they are likely to be more aware of implicit racism.

The third factor in cultural matching, emotional flavour, is not so easily dealt with. Cultures live on in their artefacts. What makes artefacts so redolent of cultures is not usually their function, since most functions to which we put objects are culturally universal, but their accidental characteristics such as colour, decoration or embellishment. These accidental characteristics have an emotional flavour, which makes us like them, or want them, or fear them. Without necessarily seeing them, every psychotherapist is surrounded by artefacts that are redolent of their culture and its emotional flavour. The contents of our rooms, the presence or absence of paperwork or of a computer, whether our rooms are in a hospital or a domestic environment, the provenance of our

pictures and ornaments, the colour of the faces in other offices or in the waiting room: all of these give an immediate flavour.

Perhaps the single most important emotional flavour when it comes to psychotherapy is homeliness or, its converse, otherness. Freud (1919) in his paper on homeliness makes the interesting point that homely also means exclusive, because we try to confine our secret wishes and desires indoors. So, by creating a very homely environment, we may also be excluding those for whom it strongly signals the opposite. Heidegger (1927/1962) also sees homeliness as a kind of falling away from the anxiety that we inevitably feel when we open our eyes to the strangeness of our existence. Levinas (1995/1970) also argues for our willingness to embrace otherness.

Heimlichkeit – homeliness – is, we may conclude, a defensive position, which keeps threat out. Making our consulting rooms, our approaches, our theories and our therapeutic rituals highly emotionally flavoured, highly culturally specific one might say, probably also serves a defensive function. Those in the know feel privileged to be so, and comfortable to be in a familiar place. But the flavour is repugnant to others who are not in the privileged minority and keeps them away.

Empirical Findings

The conceptual status of many concepts in this field is so mutable that empirical studies are few and far between, and those that have been carried out have often had limited generalizability. There is no doubt, however, that a smaller proportion of the ethnic-minority groups in the UK and the US take up psychotherapy than the proportion of the white majority who do. There is also persuasive evidence that more patients from ethnic-minority groups drop out of treatment. People from every ethnic group appear to choose therapists of their own culture and probably some do not consult anyone if there is no therapist of their culture available. Increasing the cultural competence of therapists increases retention and therefore outcome.

In the UK, the government sponsored 'Improving Access to Psychological Treatment' (IAPT) treatment programme is now providing first line, but generally very basic, psychological treatment. A report in 2012 summarized statistics on the first 1 million patients treated. Patients declaring themselves to be from an ethnic minority were under-represented, as they had been from the onset of the service (IAPT, 2012).

Next Steps

A report on addressing some of the reasons that IAPT is not accessed by a higher proportion of people defining themselves as from an ethnic minority suggested that language, culturally appropriate services, and a lack of involvement in representation from the ethnic minority or minorities being targeted may all act as barriers (IAPT, 2009). Cultural appropriateness can be improved by representation, but also by cultural competency training for all of the practitioners providing services to a multicultural group.

We end this chapter with a closer consideration of culture in relation to psychotherapy.

Culture is described by Terry Eagleton (2016) as: (1) a body of artistic and intellectual work; (2) a process of spiritual and intellectual development; (3) the values, customs, beliefs and symbolic practices by which men and women live; or (4) a whole way of life. Culture and cultural factors play a distinct therapeutic role in the management of psychiatric disorders. Culture is the lens or template we use in constructing, defining, and interpreting everyday reality (Marsella and Yamada, 2010). Cultural considerations contribute to a better understanding of underlying pathology of psychiatric disorders and to the treatment of symptoms and maladaptive behaviours. Even when culture does not play a formal role as a therapeutic agent, cultural factors might exercise a protective and preventive function on individuals who are prone to psychiatric disorders and might mitigate the adverse impacts on patients and their surroundings. Therefore, psychotherapeutic communication between the therapist and the patient is a complex task that mandates cultural understanding and sensitivity, i.e. cultural competency.

In a psychotherapeutic intervention, the therapist and the patient are expected to attempt to understand each other's point of view (Jacob, 2013). However, as Jacob and Kuruvilla (2012) point out the challenge is to find a common psychotherapeutic language, which attempts to close the gap between the issues the patient has been facing and the therapist's skills. It is widely recognized that across cultures, any given conversation is dependent on context and circumstances. In some cultures, self-disclosure outside of certain socially prescribed contexts; i.e. directly discussing personal issues, is deemed inappropriate (Qureshi

and Collazos, 2011). Cultures with oral tradition emphasize the participants and the circumstances, rather than the semantic meaning (Ong, 1988). Nonverbal communication, tone of voice, body language or eye contact might change from one culture to another and might be interpreted differently in different contexts. Psychotherapy rests on a set of cultural assumptions, which are reflective of the age and ethos of a particular society. Euro-American psychotherapies reflect core ideas of expressive individualism, which encourage clients to talk openly about their emotions or relationships. Individual worth is measured in terms of psychological well-being, happiness, achievements or wealth and power. Many world cultures do not share these assumptions and some may indeed find explicit talk about relationships or private life potentially harmful. Endurance is emphasized and maturity is linked with resilience. Fragility and finitude of life may be accepted as givens and as Morita therapy of Japan suggests, 'acceptance of things as they are' might be regarded as chief goal in life. The natural world should not be subjugated to man's control and dependency needs, since respect for the sacred and relatedness with other fellow beings is the *sine qua non* of life. Eastern philosophies (i.e. Sufism or Buddhism) emphasize the inevitability of suffering, whereas in the age of global happiness culture, Western cultural tendency tries to end suffering and promote happiness. Giving no room for spirituality and deterministic explanations implicit in Western psychotherapies have been labelled as materialistic and reductionist by some critics and these have been contrasted with the holistic world views (Hoshmand, 2006). Psychotherapy is not a value-free enterprise. Which values a particular psychotherapy would foster is another question. Personal autonomy or social obligation? Individual freedom or social harmony? This choice will have immediate ethical repercussions as well as different measures of normality. Every community has its own notion of what a good life is and whatever constitutes the ethical behaviour. Imposing Western cultural concepts of the person as a healthy norm would be ignoring the cultural and historical currents behind those concepts. A meaning-centred, experience-near approach would prefer locating and understanding local cultures and selves in their own particular context. The therapist should also be wary of stereotyping a cultural community. For example, the Muslim community is quite heterogeneous and Muslims come from different ethnicities, national origins, socio-political histories, and cultural traditions. They show varying levels of adherence to religious values and hence the therapist should be able to consider these nuances (Amer and Jalal, 2012). The theoretical frame of Western psychology is considered to be largely secular and ethnocentric and in many instances it may contradict Islamic views on humankind (Haque, 2004). Many psychotherapy approaches are value laden, and in some cases they advocate principles that contradict the world views of Muslim clients (Shah, 2005). This may well be true for many practising clients from any different religion, be it Christianity, Judaism or Hinduism.

Cultural competence is defined as the 'ability of systems to provide care to patients with diverse values, beliefs and behaviours, including tailoring delivery to meet patient's social, cultural, and linguistic needs' (Betancourt et al., 2003). However, current approaches to cultural competence have been criticized for essentializing, commodifying and appropriating culture, leading to stereotyping and further disempowerment of patients (Kirmayer, 2012). Cultural safety concept has also been advocated alongside 'cultural responsiveness' (Sue et al., 1991) and 'cultural humility' (Tervalon and Murray-Garcia, 1998). Cultural safety implies 'creating a safe space for patients that is sensitive and responsive to their social, political, linguistic, economic and spiritual realities' (Kirmayer, 2012). So any actions demeaning and disempowering the cultural identity and well-being of an individual would be considered 'culturally safe'.

Given the increased diversity of human cultures in today's world, therapists need to be culturally competent. Cultural competence involves several therapist characteristics: cultural awareness including the sensitivity to the impact of one's values and biases on perceptions of the client, presenting problems, and the therapeutic relationship; knowledge of the client's cultural background, world view, and therapy expectations; and cultural skills, encompassing treatment (Sue et al., 1992). Knowledge about a culture does not always translate into cultural competence since it may form a kind of selective filter, where the patient's attitudes and ideas are filtered through a biased image that the therapist has of the patient's culture. Cultural awareness rather than mere knowledge is more effective and feasible in the development of a therapeutic relationship (Qureshi and Collazos, 2011). Hook et al. (2013) defined cultural humility as having an interpersonal stance that is other-oriented rather than being self-absorbed; by being

respectful; and by not feeling superior to the patient's cultural background and narrative. The client perceptions of their therapist's cultural modesty were positively associated with improvement in therapies (Hook et al., 2013). The therapist's willingness to engage in an exploration of her/his own racial and cultural prejudices, feelings, attitudes and beliefs contributes to the therapeutic process. This is especially important in psychotherapy, which has predominantly focused on the therapeutic needs of upper and middle class Europeans and Americans.

Ethnic matching has been proposed as a way of diminishing the cultural barriers between the therapist and the client. An initial positive alliance may be fostered with ethnic matching of the client and the therapist but this may also obscure the therapeutic process by disempowering the clinician (Guzder et al., 2014). Hybridity of the diasporic communities and the lack of shared cultural knowledge despite the same skin colour may lead to stereotyping and hence block communication and mutual understanding.

In the past, a feeling of life having meaning was supported by being immersed in a community, and people managed to live under the great tent of tradition. This protection has become tattered as so many of us have become exposed to so many different communities, and traditions. Psychotherapy has been called on to fill this niche (Paris, 2013). But contemporary psychotherapy continues to reflect the values of Western culture, with a persistent bias towards individualism (Sampson, 1998; Hoshmand, 2006; Griner and Smith, 2006). Self-control and self-efficacy are the most desired qualities of a human being in northern Europe with a long heritage of Protestantism (Kirschner, 1996). It is a stereotype of Western psychological discourse that the concept of self is given central importance (Rose, 1996). As Geertz (1984) observes, the idea of agency, emotion, and judgement being confined to a unique whole or self confined in one body is 'peculiar within the context of the world's cultures'. These attitudes continue to dominate many contemporary psychotherapy modalities, although not all. Existential therapy, for example, originates from a different tradition of 'intersubjectivity' with many similarities to the newer Buddhistically orientated 'third wave' cognitive therapies (Deurzen and Tantam, 2016).

In India, a person may be called a 'dividual'; who was constituted not by self-actualization and personal enterprise like individuals, but by exchanges of substances, especially foods, that created personal being. In this world view, persons are not autonomous and solitary individuals but permeable, absorbing the moral qualities of their families, their castes, and even their homes and villages (Lindholm, 2001). In Japan and other Asian societies, the self is located within a dense, pre-existent network of social obligations and hierarchical distinctions. Japanese socio-centrism is said to be manifested at every level of society. In the workplace, instead of being focused on maximizing profit, managers concern themselves with the contextual skills of maintaining sociability among colleagues; in therapy, the stress is on integration with society and maintaining relationships of dependency and protection, not, as seen in the West, with finding one's true self and asserting autonomy (Doi and Harbison, 1986; Lindholm, 2001). In many cultures, agency is not confined to one individual, but embedded in a nexus of social relationships (Kirmayer, 2007). Autonomy may not be the greatest aim in life. This might be openness, connectedness and permeability to others (Nedelsky, 1990).

Therapist self-disclosure on personal matters might be regarded as a violation of boundaries in the Western context, but its lack may equally be an obstacle in developing therapeutic alliance with non-Western patients. Greater transparency on the part of the therapist may foster alliance. Somatic metaphors are quite rich and they symbolize a wide array of emotional reactions in non-Western cultures. In the Middle East there are rich, poetic cultural resources in the form of imagery and language in describing mental distress. 'My heart is worried', 'my heart is anxious', 'my heart is wounded', 'my heart aches', 'chest tightness', 'ring around the chest', 'distress of the heart' are few of the idioms of distress that refer to the heart as the locus of emotional problems (Sayar and Kose, 2012). Punjabi women participating in a focus group in London recognized the English word 'depression' but the older ones used terms such as 'weight on my heart/mind' or 'pressure on the mind' (Bhugra, 1996). In a classical study, it was found that the meaning of sadness in Iranian Azerbaijan is somehow different from its meaning in the West. In Persian, sadness is associated with personal depth; a sad person is considered to be a thoughtful person (Good et al., 1984). Explicit talk about inner life may not be preferred in non-Western contexts, but metaphorical or indirect ways of putting distress into words are more frequent. Bringing the family into the session does not always mean that the patient is over dependent or enmeshed with the family, but rather a recognition that the family is a much valued social support system.

Additionally, open expression of interpersonal conflict and confrontation may not be valued in non-Western cultures; hence non-confrontation and social harmony might be viewed as paramount, resulting in suppression or containment of both interpersonal and internal conflict (Kirmayer, 2001). Lopez (1997) proposed a process model referred to as 'shifting cultural lenses'. He argued that 'the essence of cultural competence is moving between two cultural perspectives, that of the therapist and that of the client'. Here, the clinician accesses the client's cultural perspective and then integrates it within the clinician's own cultural perspective (Lakes et al., 2006). Most studies on culture and psychopathology examine culture as a fixed property of individuals and as something that only minorities and foreigners possess, as in the case of research examining culturally bound syndromes (Causadias, 2013). Apart from this, many theorists still regard culture as a solid and static entity unaffected by the flux of ideas, images and people across national borders. Actually migration and globalization result in hybridization and cultural assimilation so that cultural differences are not bound by geography or ethnic origin any more. Culture may rather be viewed as moving and dynamic (Hermans and Kempen, 1998). Culture is now an open-system shaped by forces of migration, hybridization, and creolization. Kirmayer (2006) emphasized how interaction between cultures ends up with hybridization/creolization in this 'run-away world' of globalization. Here, transforming identities and selves are constructed continually over time and under different circumstances.

Psychotherapy includes a broad category of interventions that aim to change a patient's inner life through a specially constructed relationship between therapist and patient. Most therapists would agree that a therapy that does not lead to any changes either noticeable by the patient or observable by significant others is to be regarded as a failure. Regrettably, this does not stop some doctors from continuing to prescribe variants of the same medication for years with the idea that one serotinergic antidepressant will be different from another, or psychotherapists from persevering to overcome 'resistance'. Frank and Frank (1991) viewed psychotherapy as a cultural healing practice with four essential components; a confiding therapeutic relationship with a culturally recognized/sanctioned healer, a context and/or setting distinguished from the ordinary, a rationale or myth providing a plausible explanation for the psychiatric disorder, and a ritual/intervention believed by both to be the effective means of restoring health.

According to Marsella and Yamada (2010), Western assumptions and practices might be relevant or accurate within a Western cultural context, but this does not mean they would also be relevant or accurate in other cultural contexts. Therefore, we must not mistake power or influence/dominance for accuracy. Cushman (1990) proposes the narrative of the self is constructed not just by the individual concerned but by the commonsense psychology to which that individual has been exposed, including the shared understandings within her/his culture of 'what it is to be human'. The self embodies what the culture believes as humankind's place in the cosmos; its limits, talents, expectations, and prohibitions. Hence according to Cushman, there are no universal, trans-historical selves, only local selves and no universal theories about the self but only local ones. Marsella and Yamada (2010) argue that our clinical knowledge and practice are not just shaped by science, but by social, political, and hegemonic considerations, including ethnic, class, and gender biases. Psychotherapists must be attuned to the existential issues facing their clients whatever their culture and geography. But the fear of war, of famine, of injustice, of abuse, of infant mortality, of disease and accident, and of homelessness may press particularly on those who are identified as non-Western. Being aware of these realities is an important element in cultural competence, too.

The basic strategy of generic cultural competence is to adopt an open, interested, respectful attitude toward the patient who may then be able to teach the therapist what the therapist needs to be able to understand the individual's mental problems and his/her autobiography against the larger social and cultural backdrop (Kirmayer, 2001). But as noted by Kirmayer, this may not be enough since sensitivity or knowledge does not always lead to an understanding of what therapies will be palatable and value congruent to any given patient. Intervention strategies should also take this into account, although not slavishly. For example, some Asian Americans prefer counsellors who provide structure, guidance, and direction rather than non-directedness in psychotherapeutic interventions. (Atkinson *et al.* 1978; Sue and Zane, 1987), but not all do.

In a recent meta-analysis, Benish *et al.* (2011) found that improved therapeutic outcomes emerged when the illness myth was adapted in a manner consistent with the client's world views. Myth adaptation that is compatible with the sufferer's own explanatory model fosters an essential resonance between the therapist and the client on the nature of illness and healing. In recent literature, the concept of the person as a distinct and continuous entity was regarded as part of modern Western culture. However, while the concept of person is in fact a socially derived category, it is crucial to examine the concepts of person as a cross-cultural phenomenon and go beyond the discussion of differences between them and look at the common ground in models of the person that relate to the shared experience of being a human.

Cushman (1995) criticizes the imbuing of psychotherapy with consumer culture and offering lifestyle solutions to clients who wish to be soothed the same way that they use consumption to fill their existential void. He proposes to think of psychotherapy as a moral discourse and cautions us to be wary of what types of stories it privileges and the nature of the cultural resources it offers. Psychotherapy is more than a science and the moral space in between the therapist and the client should be well addressed. The main therapeutic questions in the modern world centre around issues like what the good life is and how a person feels at home in this world. These are moral questions in broad sense, because morality faces questions not just for the right actions, but also questions like 'how may I live my life', 'what kind of a life is a life worth living?' (Guignon, 1993).

In sum, the recognition of the cultural components of psychotherapy would bring clarity to the therapeutic processes by fostering a thorough evaluation of the full range of external circumstances and possibilities. As more psychiatric disorders come to be understood at neurochemical level, the role of psychotherapy as a robust intervention might appear to wane in relative importance. However, the human interaction between a therapist and patient will always be relevant in the treatment of patients who suffer from mental and emotional disorders. This strengthens the notion that a multidimensional approach in psychotherapy should include the depth and breadth of cultural factors by establishing a culturally sensitive working relationship, realistic goals, and mitigation of harmful interactions. In this multicultural, globalized society therapy may serve as a vehicle for empowering clients to tell stories that cannot be told in ordinary life, those suppressed narratives that wait for their turn. Therapy 'can reflect the pluralistic cultural forces in a diverse world' and a therapeutic ethic of empowering, emancipatory, communitarian and culture sensitive approach could be endorsed (Hoshmand, 2001). As a moral conversation, therapy allows for many possibilities and criticizing our current cultural prescriptions for living is one of these. A self-critical attitude towards its ethnocentric biases and scotomata would pave the way for a more culturally safe and sensitive therapy. In this way both the client and the therapist may be invited to become cultural observers of each other through reflective conversation. Therapy is a mirror through which subtle, implicit and easily overlooked features of culture are reflected (Draguns, 2004). By equalizing the voice of the client with the therapist and not letting it become subordinated to the latter, we are creating a safe space of mutual recognition. This is to say that the therapist also has to be alert to whether she is properly heard and she should be aware of her own cultural blind spots. Locating the cultural mismatch only in the patient means ignoring the ways in which institutional practices may reflect cultural values of the dominant social groups and devalue, marginalize or exclude other groups (Kirmayer *et al.*, 2014). Psychotherapy 'as an instrument of culture' will acknowledge other cultural groups and their needs more, as it becomes more aware of its own inherent cultural biases and assumptions.

References

Amer, M. A. and Jalal, B. (2012). Individual psychotherapy/counseling. In *Counseling Muslims: Handbook of Mental Health Issues and Interventions*, ed. S. Ahmed and M. M. Amer: London: Routledge.

Atkinson, D. R., Maruyama, M. and Matsui, S. (1978). Effects of counselor race and counseling approach on Asian-Americans' perceptions of counselor credibility and utility. *Journal of Counseling Psychology*, 25, 76–83.

Benish, S. G., Quintana, S. and Wampold, B. E. (2011). Culturally adapted psychotherapy and the legitimacy of myth: a direct-comparison meta-analysis. *Journal of Counseling Psychology*, 58, 279–289.

Betancourt, J. R., Green, A. R., Carrillo, J. E. and Ananeh-Firempong, O. (2003). Defining cultural competence: a practical framework for addressing racial/ethnic disparities in health and health care. *Public Health Reports*, 118, 293–302.

Bhugra, D. (1996). *Psychiatry and Religion: Context, Consensus and Controversies*. New York, NY: Routledge.

Brosnan, S. F. and de Waal, F. B. M. (2014). Evolution of responses to (un)fairness. *Science*, 346(6207), 1251776.

Causadias, J. M. (2013). A roadmap for the integration of culture into developmental psychology. *Development of Psychopathology*, 25, 1375–1398.

Christopher, J. (2001). Culture and psychotherapy: toward a hermeneutic approach. *Psychotherapy: Theory, Research, Practice, Training*, 38, 115–128.

Comte, A. (1973 (1851)). *Containing the General View of Positivism and Introductory Principles*. New York: Burt Franklin.

Cushman, P. (1990). Why the self is empty: toward a historically situated psychology. *American Psychologist*, 45, 599–611.

Cushman, P. (1995). *Constructing the Self, Constructing America: A Cultural History of Psychotherapy*. Boston, MA: Da Capo Press.

Deurzen, E. van and Tantam, D. (2016). The phenomenology of mindfulness. *International Journal of Psychotherapy*, e-issue July 2016, 32–49.

Dilthey, W. (1883). *Introduction to the Human Sciences*. Princeton: Princeton University Press.

Doi, T. and Harbison, M. A. (1986). *The Anatomy of Self: The Individual versus Society*. Japan: Kodansha International Ltd.

Draguns, J. G. (2004). From speculation through description toward investigation: a prospective glimpse at cultural research in psychotherapy. In *Handbook of Culture, Therapy, and Healing*, ed. U. P. Gielen, J. M. Fish and J. G. Draguns. New Jersey: Lawrence Erlbaum Associates, Inc.

Eagleton, T. (2016). *Culture*. New Haven, CT: Yale University Press.

Frank, J. D. and Frank, J. B. (1991). *Persuasion and Healing: A Comparative Study of Psychotherapy*. London: Johns Hopkins Press.

Freud, S. (1919). The 'Uncanny'. *Imago*, 5, 1–21.

Frijda, N. (1986). *The Emotions*. Cambridge: Cambridge University Press.

Geertz, C. (1984). *The Interpretation of Cultures*. New York: Basic Books.

Gibbard, A. (2001). Living with meanings: a human ecology. *Proceedings and Addresses of the American Philosophical Association*, 75, 59–78.

Good, B. J., DelVecchio Good, M. and Moradi, R. (1984). The interpretation of Iranian depressive illness and dysphoric affect. In *Culture and Depression: Studies in the Anthropology and Cross-Cultural Psychiatry of Affect and Disorder*, ed. A. Kleinman and B. J. Good. Berkeley, CA: University of California Press.

Griner, D. and Smith, T. B. (2006). Culturally adapted mental health interventions: a meta-analytic review. *Psychotherapy: Theory, Research, Practice, Training*, **43**, 531–548.

Guignon, C. (1993). *Authenticity, Moral Values and Psychotherapy*. Cambridge: Cambridge University Press.

Guzder J., Shantanam-Martin R. and Rousseau, C. (2014). Gender, power and ethnicity in cultural consultation. In *Cultural Consultation: Encountering the Other in Mental Health Care*, ed. L. J. Kirmayer, J. Guzder and C. Rousseau. New York: Springer.

Haque, A. (2004). Psychology from the Islamic perspective: contributions of early Muslim scholars and challenges to contemporary Muslim psychologists. *Journal of Religion and Health*, **43**, 357–377.

Heidegger, M. (1927/1962). *Being and Time*. New York: Harper and Row.

Hermans, H. J. M. and Kempen, H. J. G. (1998). Moving cultures: the perilous problems of cultural dichotomies in a globalizing society. *American Psychologist*, **53**, 1111–1120.

Hook, J. N., Davis, D. E., Owen, J., Worthington, E. L. and Utsey, S. O. (2013). Cultural humility: measuring openness to culturally diverse clients. *Journal of Counseling Psychology*, **60**, 353–366.

Hoshino-Browne, E., Zanna, A. S., Spencer, S. J., Zanna, M. P., Kitayama, S. and Lackenbauer, S. (2005). On the cultural guises of cognitive dissonance: the case of Easterners and Westerners. *Journal of Personality and Social Psychology*, **89**, 294–310.

Hoshmand, L. T. (2001). Psychotherapy as an instrument of culture. In *Critical Issues in Psychotherapy*, ed. B. D. Slife, R. N. Williams and S. H. Barlow. Thousand Oaks, CA: Sage Publications.

Hoshmand, L. T. (2006). *Culture, Psychotherapy, and Counseling: Critical and Integrative Perspectives*. Thousand Oaks, CA: Sage Publications.

IAPT (2009). Black and Minority Ethnic (BME): Positive Practice Guide. Available online at www.iapt.nhs.uk/silo/files/black-and-minority-ethnic-bme-positive-practice-guide.pdf.

IAPT (2012). IAPT three-year report: the first million patients. Available online at www.iapt.nhs.uk/silo/files/iapt-3-year-report.pdf.

Jacob, K. S. (2013). Employing psychotherapy across cultures and contexts. *Indian Journal of Psychological Medicine*, **35**, 323–325.

Jacob, K. S. and Kuruvilla, A. (2012). Psychotherapy across cultures: the form–content dichotomy. *Clinical Psychology and Psychotherapy*, **19**, 91–95.

Kirmayer, L. J. (2001). Cultural variations in the clinical presentation of depression and anxiety: implications for diagnosis and treatment. *Journal of Clinical Psychiatry*, **62**, 22–28.

Kirmayer, L. J. (2006). Culture and psychotherapy in a creolizing world. *Transcultural Psychiatry*, **43**, 163–168.

Kirmayer, L. J. (2007). Psychotherapy and the cultural concept of the person. *Transcultural Psychiatry*, **44**, 232–257.

Kirmayer, L. J. (2012). Rethinking cultural competence. *Transcultural Psychiatry*, **49**, 149–164.

Kirmayer, L. J., Rousseau, C., and Guzder, J. (2014). The place of culture in mental health services. In *Cultural Consultation: Encountering the Other in Mental Health Care*, ed. L. J. Kirmayer, J. Guzder and C. Rousseau. New York: Springer.

Kirschner, S. (1996). *The Religious and Romantic Origins of Psychoanalysis: Individuation and Integration in Post-Freudian Theory*. Cambridge: Cambridge University Press.

Kleinman, A. (2004). Culture and depression. *New England Journal of Medicine*, **351**, 951–953.

Lakes, K., Lopez, S. R. and Garro, L. C. (2006). Cultural competence and psychotherapy: applying anthropologically informed conceptions of culture. *Psychotherapy: Theory, Research, Practice, Training*, **43**, 380–396.

Lang, H. (1995). Hermeneutics and psychoanalytically oriented psychotherapy. *American Journal of Psychotherapy*, **49**, 215–224.

Leuenberger, C. (2002). The end of socialism and the reinvention of the self: a study of the East German psychotherapeutic community in transition. *Theory and Society*, **31**, 255–280.

Levinas, E. (1995/1970). *Alterity and Transcendence*. New York: Columbia University Press.

Lindholm, C. (2001). *Culture and Identity: The History, Theory, and Practice of Psychological Anthropology*. Oxford: Oneworld Publications.

Locke, J. (1995). *An Essay Concerning Human Understanding*. Amherst, NY: Prometheus Books.

Lopez, S. R. (1997). Cultural competence in psychotherapy: a guide for clinicians and their supervisors. In *Handbook for Psychotherapy Supervision*, ed. C. E. Watkins. New York: Wiley.

Luhrman, T. (2000). *Of Two Minds: The Growing Disorder in American Psychiatry*. New York: Alfred A. Knopf.

Marsella, A. J. and Yamada, A. M. (2010). Culture and psychopathology: foundations, issues, directions. *Journal of Pacific Rim Psychology*, **4**, 103–115.

Nedelsky, J. (1990). Law, boundaries, and the bounded self. *Representations*, **30**, 162–189.

Ong, W. J. (1988). *Orality and Literacy: The Technologizing of the Word*. London: Methuen.

Paris, J. (2013). *Psychotherapy in an Age of Narcissism: Modernity, Science and Society*. New York, NY: Palgrave Macmillan.

Pike, K. (1967). *Language in Relation to a Unified Theory of Structure of Human Behavior*. The Hague: Mouton.

Qureshi, A. (2005). Dialogical relationship and cultural imagination: a hermeneutic approach to intercultural psychotherapy. *American Journal of Psychotherapy*, **59**, 119–135.

Qureshi, A. and Collazos, F. (2011). The intercultural and interracial therapeutic relationship: challenges and recommendations. *Pakistan Journal of Social and Clinical Psychology*, **3**, 3–20.

Rose, N. (1996). *Inventing Ourselves: Psychology, Power and Personhood*. New York, NY: Cambridge University Press.

Rothenberg, B. (2002). The success of the battered woman syndrome: an analysis of how cultural arguments succeed. *Sociological Forum*, **17**, 81–103.

Sampson, E. E. (1989). The Deconstruction of the Self. In *Texts of Identity*, ed. J. Shotter and K. Gergen. London: Sage, pp. 1–19.

Sampson, E. E. (1998). Establishing embodiment in psychology. In *The Body and Psychology*, ed. H. J. Stam. London: Sage.

Sayar, K. and Kose, S. (2012). Psychopathology and depression in the Middle East. *Journal of Mood Disorders*, **2**, 21–27.

Schafer, R. (1976). *A New Language for Psycho-Analysis*. New Haven, CT: Yale University Press.

Schudson, M. (1989). How culture works: perspectives from media studies on the efficacy of symbols. *Theory and Society*, **18**, 153–180.

Shah, A. (2005). Psychotherapy in vacuum or reality: secular or Islamic psychotherapy with Muslim clients. *International Journal for the Psychology of Religion*, **14**, 149–156.

Sue, D. W., Arredondo, P. and McDavis, R. J. (1992). Multicultural counseling competencies and standards: a call to the profession. *Journal of Multicultural Counseling and Development*, **20**, 64–88.

Sue, S. and Zane, N. (1987). The role of culture and cultural techniques in psychotherapy. *American Psychologist*, **42**, 37–42.

Sue, S., Fujino, D. C., Hu, L. T., Takeuchi, D. T. and Zane, N. W. (1991). Community mental health services for ethnic minority groups: a test of the cultural responsiveness hypothesis. *Journal of Consulting and Clinical Psychology*, **59**, 533–540.

Tantam, D. (1993). Exorcism in Zanzibar: an insight into groups from another culture. *Group Analysis*, **26**, 251–260.

Tantam, D. (1998). Meaning, cause and interpretation. In *Heart and Soul*, ed. C. Mace. London: Routledge.

Tantam, D. (2002). *Psychotherapy and Counselling in Practice*. Cambridge: Cambridge University Press.

Tervalon, M. and Murray-Garcia, J. (1998). Cultural humility versus cultural competence: a critical distinction in defining physician training outcomes in multicultural education. *Journal of Health Care for the Poor and Underserved*, **9**, 117–125.

Chapter 35

Psychological Interventions

Rachel Tribe and Aneta D. Tunariu

Editors' Introduction

In psychiatric and mental health services many psychological interventions are needed and indeed offered. These include behavioural interventions, cognitive, interpersonal and dialectic interpersonal therapies. Tribe and Tunariu in this chapter define psychological intervention as an act which usually leads to a change for an individual, family, group or community. Any psychological intervention should include a form of assessment and evaluation of its effectiveness as part of its design from the outset. They review the planning, use design, implementation and evaluation of psychological interventions within cultural psychiatry. They go on to describe various examples of where psychiatric and psychological knowledge and skills have been blended in non-traditional ways to deliver bespoke psychological interventions across different professional contexts. They illustrate these innovations using several of the interventions in domains which may not initially be viewed as within mainstream work for psychiatrists. Through these examples these authors show how innovation within cultural psychiatry can provide rich additional opportunities. It is inevitable that such approaches can then be used to develop the potential to benefit the well-being or mental health of groups or communities of people across different cultures. Tribe and Tunariu point out that psychological interventions can open up new and varied ways of using psychiatric skills and competencies outside the consulting room. These interventions can be used to benefit what have euphemistically been labelled 'hard to reach' groups. These authors use their own clinical experience to demonstrate how clinicians can work across cultures to improve recovery and resilience. Among examples, they illustrate well-being and resilience through a community organization to scale up knowledge around mental health, two projects with youth, the use of sport as a psychological intervention and a training intervention with academics working within a war zone.

Outline of Cultural Psychiatry

Cultural psychiatry has been defined as being 'concerned with understanding the impact of social and cultural differences and similarities on mental illness and its treatment' (Bhugra and Bhui, 2007: 1). Culture has been defined in various ways within the literature. Spencer-Oatey (2012) located numerous definitions including those which state that culture is both an individual and a social construct. It has also been defined in a range of ways including the following definition 'Culture refers to the cumulative deposit of knowledge, experience, beliefs, values, attitudes . . . is a collective programming of the mind that distinguishes the members of one group or category of people from another' (Texas, 2016: 1). It is a rich, if on occasions, nebulous concept and relates not just to issues of ethnicity, 'race' and religion but also to family, community, experience, history and values. It is a vibrant and changing phenomenon (Fernando, 2014). The way culture is considered has developed and evolved in high-income countries from the possibly well-intentioned but naive view of culture being something that was related to skin colour or religion and was frequently taken to refer to 'the other', or someone, or some aspect of that individual or group, that was viewed as different to the majority or dominant group 'norm'. This was frequently assumed to be the white Western (Sashidharan, 2001; Tribe, 2007) and often male perspective within the wider society and mainstream psychiatry (Condor, 1991).

This 'exoticization' and possibly racist discourse is beginning to give way to something more sophisticated. This understanding or discourse recognizes a range of diverse and varied ways of being and views of the world and also encourages clinicians in high-income countries to question their own cultural constructions and the limits of their generalizability. Culture is not a fixed entity but is dynamic and fluid and is influenced by a range of variables which include but are not limited to individual, familial and community meaning making

(Fernando, 2014; Tribe, 2014). It could be argued that all psychiatry should be cultural psychiatry, as every individual is affected by aspects of 'their' culture. In addition the cultural identity an individual develops or selects is multilayered and often supple and may be influenced throughout life by events and experiences.

In terms of psychiatry, culture may influence identity, behaviour, help-seeking behaviour, values, idioms of distress, explanatory health beliefs, recognized treatment and its perceived effectiveness. For example, the removal of symptoms versus adjusting to symptoms; as well as the notion and experience of recovery. Summerfield (2002: 248) notes that:

> The Diagnostic Statistical Manual (DSM) and the International Classifications of Diseases (ICD) are not, as some imagine, atheoretical and purely descriptive nosologies with universal validity. They are western cultural documents, carrying ontological notions of what constitutes a real disorder, epistemological ideas about what counts as scientific evidence, and methodological ideas as to how research should be conducted.

Views around culture and mental health will be held by the psychiatrist, service user and organization or health trust/employing organization and within the multidisciplinary team contained therein. These will all be present in the consulting room so cultural psychiatry is a fascinating and sophisticated process. How these diverse views and cultures are respected and viewed within psychiatry and psychological interventions is a complex issue, particularly when these issues all intersect within the frame of the professional culture of psychiatry and medicine. Therefore, how these are negotiated and considered within a psychological intervention provides a complex but rich range of opportunities.

What Is a Psychological Intervention?

The term intervention is often used to describe a reformulation, a hypothesis, a query or advice (which might on occasions be labelled as treatment) by the clinician during a clinical session. A psychological intervention is when an intervention strategy is developed, usually based on clinical information, available data, a needs analysis or an identified problem. The objective of a psychological intervention is usually to lead to a change for an individual, family, group or community. Any psychological intervention should include a form of assessment and evaluation of its effectiveness as part of its design from the outset.

Frameworks for psychological interventions normally include the following:

- Addressing a distinct issue, difficulty or problem which involves seeking solutions and resolutions.
- Defining clear objectives.
- Expanding a capacity which is potent in becoming an agent for change.
- Planning sustainability.
- Developing or expanding the change or resourcing programme or procedure at individual, community or group level (this may be potent for generating a domino effect change across communities or groups).
- Evaluation of the intervention should be built in from the outset.

Psychological Interventions in Different Professional Contexts

Psychological interventions in the loosest sense may be conducted by psychiatrists, psychologists, experts by experience, health or social care professionals or organizations as well as by charities, governments and others in partnership with service users, groups or communities. A variety of illustrations of diverse psychological interventions will be given in this chapter, some of which were conducted in the UK and some with colleagues from a range of countries. They typically involve work which foregrounds the importance of cultural diversity and sensitivity and which promotes social justice. Many of them draw upon and utilize the knowledge and skills developed within psychiatry and psychology and applies them in innovative ways or in less traditional or unusual contexts. The participants in these interventions come from a variety of groups, the interventions had a range of purposes, some people volunteered or were selected to attend and some were referred by government agencies or workers. They all were designed to benefit the well-being or the mental health of the participants, through developing knowledge, resilience, insight or psychological skills and understanding. Some of them may be viewed as being located outside the traditional remit of psychiatry. Although perhaps the remit can usefully be expanded; particularly in a time of austerity, recession and in a time of change and re-evaluation of the role of psychiatry nationally and internationally? There are considerable benefits and economies of scale to be found from working with groups or communities of people and in ways which benefit significant numbers of people. Psychological interventions may promote good mental health and well-being, develop relevant knowledge and expand life skills, challenge counterproductive behaviours or stereotypes, promote social justice and tackle stigmatization. Innovative psychological interventions are increasingly being used to good effect around the world, for example in Jamaica (Hickling, 2016); India (Chatterjee and Dasroy, 2016; Prashanth et al., 2016); Nicaragua (van der Geest, 2016) and in partnership working in Uganda (Hall et al., 2016). Many of these interventions are conducted by psychiatrists, others by psychologists or by other mental health professionals or by or in partnership with service users/experts by experience.

Illustrations of a Range of Psychological Interventions

Face-up and iNEAR: Two Resilience and Well-Being Programmes

A chief preoccupation of a psychological intervention, regardless of the professional context in which it takes place, is engendering change for an individual, a family, a group or a community. Traditional (clinical) psychological interventions involve structured interactions between professionals and clients typically informed by normative psychological knowledge with the aim of addressing and modifying cognition, emotional responses or behaviour towards a template of well-being conceived of as the absence of 'unwanted' symptoms. When used, for instance, as part of a solution-focused care programme for say, tacking anxiety related issues across a range of presenting problems not least mood disorders or sexual dysfunctions, it can offer positive results. When elements of the global intention which underpins the intervention's conception of change is closely examined, however, it highlights limitations not least in the form of missed opportunities. When change means in essence the task of repairing a 'deficit', an overarching (often latent) aspect of the human condition is bypassed; namely, the capacity for transformation through organic and creative participation for the sake of 'becoming' a deliberate agent as opposed to being 'mended' in some way in relation to a prescribed 'standard of normality' (Tunariu et al. 2017). This is a point of intersection where, perhaps, cultural psychiatry can look to apply its expertise towards developing innovative integrated

psychological interventions. Such integration would not only require attention to culture, discourse and social practices, but also to the benefits of integrating ideas and skills from across psychological disciplines – such as clinical, counselling, organizational, developmental coaching and existential psychology. Two such integrated psychological interventions are presented here: the Face-up and the iNEAR programmes.

The 'Face-up' psychological intervention was commissioned by the London Metropolitan Police and was designed and delivered by Boniwell and Tunariu (2010) in collaboration with the Young Foundation – a London-based charity. The aim was to assist the Metropolitan Police in their work with a group of up to 20 disenfranchised young men aged between 12 and 18 of various ethnic and socio-economic backgrounds. The young men were known to the police services in relation to repetitive antisocial behaviour, and typically disengagement from school, and a disruptive approach towards their family, their neighbours and the neighbourhood in general. The brief required a positive psychology programme with a strong developmental and restorative justice type ethos. A training guide and resources was also offered to re-run the programme in the future, potentially with programme 'graduates' as future facilitators.

The Face-up programme set out to facilitate:

1. greater flexibility of thinking: choice and decision-making;
2. stronger emotional resilience: self-regulation of emotions and behaviour;
3. reducing continued and persistent antisocial behaviour: impact awareness;
4. breaking down boundaries: increasing self-worth and visibility of future aspirations.

The three days of the intervention were structured in themed activities which addressed each of these objectives. A series of observational, interactional, experiential and reflexive exercises were included with the intention of enhancing young people's emotional intelligence, sense of ownership over their actions, decision-making skills, and greater knowledge of character/personality strengths and appreciation of relational resilience. From the onset the authors were mindful of person–activity fit as a marker for the successfulness of the intervention. In other words, we were mindful of the variety of psychological variables, sensitivities, preoccupations and resources that delineate the distinctiveness of each individual, and the need to optimize the impact of the Face-up activities towards the intended goal. The issue of person–activity fit was approached through looking to yield homogeneity by engineering conditions necessary to building a 'new' culture; a 'new' group to belong to in ways that a 'new' and positive identity could be creatively authored and rehearsed within the 'geographic' space of the Face-up. This required an impactful initial activity; something that could get the participants to buy-in, focusing their attention and engagement. In examining the self-narratives we requested and received from the participants as part of the product development phase, we noted that a collectively shared grievance was a strong sense of hurt and unfairness. Subsequently, we felt that the 'paper-man' activity would resonate with our participants. In a circle format, each participant was given a paper-man cutting and then instructed to tear it apart. The instruction was received as childish and pointless, yet also gently began to build up a common voice of the (new) group as distinct from the facilitators. As they each had agreed, as part of our contracting process, to fully partake at the programme, they each nonetheless reluctantly competed the task. The second instruction required participants to put back the paper-man to its original shape using an individually provided sticking tape. It too provoked a similar reaction. This time, however, they became both more curious and more serious. Importantly, as tension and uncertainty increased, this added impetus to the sense of 'us'/ the group. Chaos and collaboration emerged as these young men were looking for lost pieces of their paper-man on the floor, across the room. Laughter and industriousness to finish the task as promptly as possible strengthened the team spirit. Once each individual paper-man was restored as best as possible with the tape provided, the next instruction was delivered: 'Tear it apart once more.' Every attempt to do so now failed. Surprised by the instruction yet trying to comply, the group cried: 'We can't. It won't work.' The final instruction: 'Right. Now, in turn, tell the story of your paper-man.' As individual story telling progressed, the 'it happened to it/this imaginary paper-man' switched organically to 'they cannot break me again; I am stronger; I am now made in my image'. They got the point: the Face-up was about resilience – a capacity that we can each have and be expanded. Resilience in overdrive may be hiding a 'grandiose self' paradigm (Kohut, 1972) driven by a preoccupation to show 'never be dependent, and never feel lacking in any way' (Bromberg, 1983: 360) Most, if not all, of these young men have had life experiences beyond the maturity of

their age; and many presented an attitude of suspicion and caution; a 'heroic me' who needs no one's help. Devotedly negotiating challenges of working alone while longing for 'parental' holding the self tends to often encounter the other/the other's help with negativity – including, anger, mockery, self-righteousness, etc. The authors were sensitive to these potential complexities and used this to inform the approach to dealing with, for instance, the intersection of the real and borrowed selves. Within this developmental context, later activities focused on emotional intelligence and emotional resourcing were usefully nourished, and exercises addressing skills for and value of positive relationships, responsible citizenship, and positive future perspectives enabled. Moreover, each day of the programme began with a check-in, and ended with a check-out. This particular feature was on its own a gateway to achieving remarkable existential shifts for these young people. As one of them noted in our last check-out: 'There is no way back; there [is] only [a] way forward.'

One other exercise that was reported as particularly powerful by the Face-up participants was an exercise we called 'punch in/punch out emotions'. The first part of the exercise is to introduce to them two broad types of negative emotions (Tunariu, 2015); namely:

- 'Holding in' type of emotions. Some negative emotions such as shame; guilt; perceived betrayal; self-loathing are aimed towards ourselves. Having these emotions does not feel nice. It is as if we are 'punching in'. If we do not reflect on them, they can stop us from seeing the reality as it really is.
- 'Giving out' type of emotions. Some negative emotions such as anger; revenge; hatred; are aimed outwardly towards other people. It does not feel nice to be on the receiving end. It is as if we are 'punching out'. If we do not reflect on them, they can stop us from seeing the reality as it really is.

These descriptions serve to both normalize negative emotions and promote the need for action; namely, by indicating to the participants how we often cannot help having certain feelings but we can help by the way we understand what they are about; and we can help by responding to them with clarity, skill and sensitivity to others. Participants are then asked to write down as many 'punch in' or 'punch out' types of emotions as they can think of on post-it notes provided and place the notes on a designated wall. These are then discussed and unpacked by the group under the facilitator's guidance.

The 'punch in/punch out emotions' exercise was used for both programmes, Face-up and iNEAR (presented later) but with modifications responding to features specific to group composition and needs as well as the overall programme brief and objectives. For instance, the Face-up participants offered an overwhelming 'punch in' picture, more than twice the size of the 'punch out' picture with high frequency of reports of feeling 'invisible', unloved, rejected, betrayed. This was an important finding to share with the stakeholders to be used to inform their own planning of further work with the young men. The theme of feeling unseen and rejected is likely to have situated some of these young peoples' overt aggression, masked self-presentations, bravado, and position of 'attack and distrust first, just in case'; likewise, the theme of shame and the grinding effect of feeling inadequate. Reflecting on both these common themes helps us appreciate even more the participants' vulnerability of revealing themselves – a fear of being disliked, thus rejected once more; of being exploited or used, thus neglected once more; of being 'too much to handle', thus abandoned once more. We believe the Face-up programme has offered some valuable opportunities to 'internalise feelings of acceptance and kindness towards themselves' (Schimmenti, 2012: 206).

Each themed activity employed the group-facilitated permission-giving as a core platform to usher these young men's revealing, recognizing, and re-crafting self-views and value systems. Each was designed to last approximately 60 minutes; not too long yet enough time for 'new' realities/new boundaries of what really matters to emerge. Sobered and energized by what was being said, the young men began to *listen* to themselves and to their own stories as these were unfolding before them within a newly formed group and its associated culture. This made apparent how the content of the collective self often serves as a key 'motivational hub' for shifts and transformations to the individual self-system (Sedikides *et al.*, 2013). In summary, shared lived-experiences paired with a non-judgemental *witnessing* by others has, as intended, crystallized a 'new' group with a culture underpinned by authentic communication and relational empathy. It also offered recognition and delineation of individual selves within it for, as Winnicott (1958: 39) notes, 'It is a joy to be hidden, and disaster not to be found [out].'

The path to autonomy and authentic, mature self-concept is complex and wrought with challenges, ambivalence and vulnerability. It entails personal resilience. Identity formation is accelerated during the teenage years and remains an ongoing process in a (young) person's life as they search for a self-authored identity and synthesis of personal systems of value. Unsurprisingly the person-in-becoming is often vulnerable to strong reactions, confusions, resistance to perceived rigid authority, dis-alignment from the familiar as an over-compensation for the need to 'stand out' as unique. At the same time, there is the preoccupation to secure belonging to a group which is attributed with kudos, social influence and currency fit to render them a meaningful identity by association. Experiencing validation by others is an essential ingredient of effective group belonging and would typically involve feelings of acceptance and endorsements of individual contributions and achievements. Positive, non-judgemental, collaborative interventions during this process can open conversations, and unique opportunities for aiding development, self-efficacy, resilience, empathy, hope and meaning for the future (e.g. Boniwell and Tunariu, 2018). Amongst other things, greater resilience capacity can improve problem solving skills and increase creativity. Together with exposure to positive emotions, it has been found to also increase flexibility of thought, help combat learnt helplessness as well as depression and to catalyse greater academic achievements (e.g. Parks, and Schueller, 2014). The iNEAR is one such psychological intervention (Tunariu, 2015) and has resilience, emotional well-being and engaged citizenship at its heart. It constitutes a set of self-contained activities that can be usefully housed by a larger positive-education curriculum or to scaffold individual coaching interventions (Tunariu, 2017). The range of materials developed to support its activities are original yet embedded in research and some are adapted from relevant tool-oriented publications (e.g. MacConville and Rae, 2012; Corey and Corey, 2014). The programme addresses and fosters development across four core domains. Namely:

1. formation of positive identities;
2. emotion regulation, differentiation and modes of relating;
3. thinking blind-spots, creativity and malleability;
4. choice and choosing as an existential responsibility of the individual.

The focus is on *I* developing and owning:

N   New knowledge about myself.

E   Emotional resources and emotional intelligence.

A Awareness of values, of options, of choice.

R Responding with growth 'in spite of . . .'.

Each activity of the iNEAR aims to instigate existential moments in the workshop and so facilitate the subjective awareness and global positioning as a person within a common human condition. Each intended to offer an element of surprise, even if or especially if, the activity first appeared to be counterintuitive – as it would help mitigate against the 'pull of the familiar'; the tendency to deploy well-rehearsed narratives to make sense of new situations; and subsequently, allow space for forming new habits of thought.

The iNEAR programme has been piloted during terms times of 2016 at a school in south-east England with a sample of 350 young people aged 11 and 12. Unlike the Face-up, the iNEAR programme has had research evaluation inbuilt from the onset – involving university based ethical application and clearance. The results were published in the autumn of 2017. Preliminary analysis of data collected from these young people (via psychometric tests; sentence completion questionnaires and focus groups) confirms the following as good practice when designing and delivering a psychological intervention:

- Concept development: starting from the desired outcomes identify core 'concepts' (issues, psychological variables, phenomena, etc.) and map these onto the current thinking and research.

- Pinning down the intervention's professional intention: theories about change and the self–others system.

- Product development phase: requesting and receiving first-hand information about the concerns, dilemmas, needs and goals of the intended beneficiaries.

- Training development phase: run the same exercises with the intended trainers as part of the training process; this helps ensure fuller appreciation of concepts and intention of the programme as well as a welcomed personal resourcing.

- Choosing activities: activities organized around a theme informed by a clear set of objectives can ensure systematicity and rigour.

- Person–activity fit: look to maximize an activity's potential of resonating with as many as possible participants.

- Build in the research element from the onset.

Finally, the pilot supported the overreaching principle of iNEAR as transformation through participation kind of intervention. It made it obvious that its activities can serve as catalysts for change; and that this change follows a collective direction towards optimal functioning while at the same time, it remains necessarily unique and subjectively meaningful to each individual.

A Training Based Psychological Intervention with a Refugee Community Group: The Tamil Community Centre Based in London

Charities and voluntary organizations often support people from what have been labelled hard to reach communities and hidden populations such as ethnic minority communities (Bhugra and Gupta, 2011) as well as refugees and asylum seekers (Miller, 1999). People from these communities may be less likely to seek support from mainstream health and social services and their needs are often overlooked by commissioners of services and service providers (Mind, 2015). Evidence shows that there is disproportionally low access to mental healthcare for migrants (Lindert et al., 2012); refugees within primary care (Jones and Gill, 1998); vulnerable young people (de Antiss et al., 2009) and members of a number of BME groups (Sass et al., 2009). Working with these voluntary organizations to assist staff to upgrade their skills can be a helpful investment by psychiatrists and all mental health workers. It may also help in developing knowledge and trust about mainstream mental health services as well as establish referral pathways and potential partnerships (Manthorpe, et al., 2009). The role of the third sector in providing health and care services is increasing (Dickinson et al., 2012; Rees et al., 2014). This is related to varied modelling, budgets restraints and varying pressures on resources within mainstream services (Mental Health Task Force, 2015; Warren and Garthwaite, 2015). The Mental Health Policy Group, (2014) states that 75 per cent of people with mental health problems receive no support at all. There may be debates about the exact figures, but it appears that some people are not getting the support they need. It has been argued that volunteers often do not receive an adequate amount of training for the tasks they undertake (Duncan et al., 2010) and their contribution is sometimes not recognized (Dickinson et al., 2012).

The task given to the authors was centred on building capability to help the staff scale up and develop their knowledge and skills in working and providing support to voluntary workers at the Tamil Community Centre (TCC), a refugee community group, and registered charity. The TCC were approached on a daily basis by a wider range of people about mental health issues. The psychological intervention arose as a result of one of the authors being approached by a colleague from Race on the Agenda (ROTA; 2016) a charity, about running somthing for them to improve their skills, knowledge and understanding of referral pathways. The author invited colleagues from another charity – the UK Sri Lanka Trauma Group (UKSLTG, 2014) – to join her in this work. This group is comprised of mental health professionals from the Sri Lankan diaspora and other interested mental health professionals, who have a cultural understanding and commitment to working in partnership with organizations to improve mental health knowledge and understanding.

The Tamil Community Centre (TCC) runs a drop in and advice centre, as well as providing a hot meal every day, English and homework classes and a place for people to meet. The Tamil Community Centre is a voluntary organization and opened in response to high levels of unmet need within the Sri Lankan Tamil community. Many Tamils had been exposed to war, conflict and trauma and faced difficulties around resettlement in the UK (UKSLTG, 2014). The TCC supports Sri Lankan Tamils with health and social care needs and promotes community integration. Background about the TCC and the mental health issues many of their members face can be located in a short DVD online at (ROTA; 2016). (For a summary of the historical context see the section on Humanitarian Psychological Intervention.)

The TCC's philosophy is that all services are provided whenever possible by them acting as a one stop shop, but where they can refer people needing specialist help on to other resources. The staff report that attending the community centre does not carry the connotations or fear which may be associated with attending a psychiatric clinic or hospital and it is viewed as accessible and culturally appropriate and sensitive. In 2015, TCC assisted between 4,000 and 5,000 people. In addition to seeing people of Tamil heritage, they have visitors from a range of other communities and they offer a free hot meal every day. They run on a small budget (receiving a small amount of external funding but also holding fundraising events). All the staff are volunteers with Tamil heritage. A 10-week training programme was co-produced by TCC and the UKSLTG after a series of discussions, and is detailed below. The team offering the training included psychiatrists, psychologists, a priest (who was also trained as a psychologist) and a GP. Most of the training was conducted in English, though the team were happy to offer sessions either in Tamil (which a number of them spoke) or with an interpreter. The team were all volunteers. After meeting the project coordinator and her senior staff, a curriculum of training was developed as follows.

Healthy Minds: The Needs of the Tamil Diaspora:

1. Traumatic experiences and surviving as an asylum seeker, refugee or migrant (including self care)
2. Children and families overview including gang awareness
3. Parenting I
4. Negotiating the NHS effectively
5. Domestic violence
6. Parenting II
7. Somatization
8. Adapting to cultural change and a different country
9. Postnatal depression
10. Addiction
11. Tree of life (nurturing resilience and strengths)
12. Using available services and appropriate referrals to other agencies and review of the programme.

An audit of the work was conducted by a trainee psychologist with Tamil heritage (Angeline S. Dharmaindra, who was independent of the team and TCC, and we are very grateful for her input). A battery of measures was administered to the volunteers who had undertaken the training at three time points: t1 (baseline), t2 (post-training) and t3 (1 month follow up). Each participant completed a five point Likert scale for each session with seven questions and the options of writing further text. The measures included the Attitudes to Mental Illness Questionnaire (AMIQ; Luty et al., 2006), the Mental Health Knowledge Scale (MAKS; Evans-Lacko et al., 2010) and a brief measure of knowledge, and skills developed by the researcher specifically for the audit. A training evaluation form was also completed at t2 and t3. In addition, interviews were conducted with key informants. The aim of the evaluation was to explore whether the mental health literacy of volunteers increased as a result of the training programme. Mental health literacy referred to stigmatizing attitudes, knowledge, skills and confidence in this context. The volunteers were also asked to complete a consent form and demographics form.

The median scores for the subjective measure of knowledge and skills indicated an increase in knowledge from pre-training to post-training which was maintained at 1 month follow up. The frequency data for this measure indicated the frequency of volunteers who thought medication and psychotherapy could be helpful to people with mental health problems increased following training. The frequency data also showed that training increased the identification of mental health problems, particularly grief, stress and anxiety related to trauma. Friedman's ANOVA was used to compare the scores at t1, t2 and t3. The statistical test indicated that the mental health knowledge of the participants did not significantly change over the 10 week training programme or at follow up. One of the outcomes of this training that appeared to be particularly useful was the final session with a range of local mental health professionals who were invited to talk about their services, to establish links and open communication channels and referral pathways. Twelve months later, many of these mental health professionals remain in touch and the TCC staff report improved communication and feeling better prepared to deal with mental health issues.

The findings from this evaluation lend some support to the value of mental health training programmes for non-clinical staff working with people with mental health problems, however, further research is required. Future evaluation studies should involve larger samples and utilize or develop culturally specific tools which measure change. Future studies may also want to include qualitative or mixed data collection methods to explore people's experiences of the training in more depth.

The Use of Sport in Conjunction with Therapeutic Group Support: Football for Facilitating Therapeutic Intervention Among a Group of Refugees and Asylum Seekers

The ideas developed in this example of a psychological intervention, could be used with most team sports and with a range of potential service user groups or communities (Tribe, 2002). It discusses sport as part of a psychological intervention which contained three facets, weekly competitive football matches, training sessions for the football team and group meetings/talking therapy for the team members. It could be argued that the fourth facet of the intervention was the psychological benefits of the team supporters who were almost exclusively asylum seekers and refugees, many of whom turned out every week at matches. It appeared that being part of a welcoming, cohesive and supportive group and seeing their team win appeared to offer a range of therapeutic benefits. The regular supporters often took time to talk to the clinical workers at matches and at other activities we organized around the team. This intervention was based at a specialist organization working for survivors of organized violence or torture, located in a central London hospital. Almost all of the service users were asylum seekers and refugees. There are 141 countries that are reported to use torture (Amnesty International, 2014), despite it being outlawed by the Universal Declaration of Human Rights Article 5, Article 7 of the International Covenant on Civil and Political Rights and other international legislation.

The thinking behind this psychological intervention came from one of the service users (here called Simon, although that is not his real name). He drew on his personal experience to suggest that something which might have aided his recovery and that of other service users was a team sport that could be played regardless of language or nationality and alongside others who had shared experiences of surviving organized violence. John had been suffering from depression, had active suicidal ideation and met the diagnostic criteria for post-traumatic stress disorder, as well as a range of physical complaints when we started work together. He also felt that his body had been violated and was damaged by his experience of organized violence. When reviewing our work, John suggested establishing a sports team. He felt that this would enable him to regain a sense of his own physicality as well as his sense of self, identity and place in a community or group. Having a sports team which was comprised of people who had experienced torture and organized violence in a supportive team environment, where this experience was shared but was not the main focus would, he felt, be therapeutic. Much has been written on the psychological benefits of sport including intrinsic pleasure, affiliation and a sense of belonging (Gauron, 1984). For this team it appeared that the team provided social support and a normalizing function as well. In addition, refugees are often viewed as unwelcome or as other by the host society and many report trying to remain 'invisible' or to blend in with the wider society (Human Rights Watch, 2016: Refugee Council, 2016), and so meeting others as equals on the football pitch was an added benefit that we believed might pay psychological and physical health dividends.

Many of the service users attending this organization reported feeling that their bodies had been damaged irreparably by the torture and abuse they had experienced in their countries of origin, this is sadly a common pattern for survivors of such abuse (Schlapobersky, 1990). The exact relationship between body and mind is still being investigated and Cartesian dualism may not be as distinct or discrete as was once thought (Hargreaves, 1982; Biddle, 1995; Kim, 2000). In addition, culture and explanatory health beliefs may also play a mediating role in how this body–mind relationship is understood and experienced by the individual. Whilst the people in the countries practising torture are frequently only too aware of how the physical and psychological are entwined and use this to their advantage, therefore most of our service users also had a range of mental health issues to contend with. People's perception of their own physicality may have been damaged or changed by the violence or torture they have survived. Not to have control of one's own body is a harrowing and potentially life-changing experience, as is the anticipatory anxiety of not knowing what may happen to one next (Blackwell, 2005). Some of the players had been told that they would be killed. Many of the service users reported not being able to talk about these experiences except to close family members, and not always then. This was because it was thought by many to be protective to keep family members from knowing what had happened, for fear of this knowledge being used against them in their country of origin, as well as to protect family members psychologically. In countries which use organized state violence and torture, people often learn that secrecy is a functional strategy to keep them and their families safe. Issues of trust can become problematized (Tribe 1998). Once they had fled to the UK it was difficult to talk about their experiences of torture and organized violence and its after effects, as this was so outside the experience of the people they encountered in the UK (Blackwell, 2005).

This legacy of the torture combined with separation from their families and culture were immensely challenging. This was in addition to trying to make sense of the enormous losses they had experienced, which frequently included family, culture, language, friends, profession and work. Additional losses included an imagined future as well as an apparent inability to impact upon the asylum system in Britain, these losses and difficulties were reported to feel almost insurmountable on occasions. These were in addition to attempting to build a new life in the UK (many of the service users, who had not had their asylum claims dealt with, were facing constant uncertainty and the daily fear of their asylum claim being rejected and possible deportation/forcible removal to their country of origin). They also felt impotent to deal with an asylum system which they felt was unresponsive to them. Thus, life was extremely challenging and for most of the players and supporters their psychological health was extremely fragile. Many of the team also felt immense anger and rage about what had happened to them, with no recourse to do anything about it and few avenues to deal with this, except in talking to their psychiatrist, psychologist or other professional. In addition the loss of an anticipated future and the continuity of life was broken for many of the service users and trying to reconnect the different parts of it was perplexing and to imagine a future almost impossible. Defrin *et al.* (2013) found that ex-prisoners of war continued to suffer from dysfunctional pain perception 40 years after being tortured. Having said that, these survivors had shown immense resilience and strength in having not only survived but having managed to flee and seek asylum and to now try and carve out an entirely new life for themselves in the UK. Our work tried to help the team strengthen these skills as well as process some of the experiences they had lived through, with others in a safe therapeutic group.

All of the different aspects were important parts of this psychological intervention. Two members of the mental health team facilitated these group meetings where players met to discuss issues relating to their previous and current lives, as well as issues relating to the football team. This group enabled many of the players to talk about issues in a context where they might have chosen not to attend if the group had been labelled a therapy group. All of the team were refugees or asylum seekers and most had survived torture or organized violence in their countries of origin. In addition this intervention reached some other service users at the organization, as they regularly came to games to support the team. The regular matches also provided an opportunity to interact with a number of other people in a range of capacities. The therapeutic effects of sport have been noted by a number of writers including Ang and Gomez-Pinilla (2007), Weir (2011) and Blumenthal (2007), and the physical benefits of sport are well established in any number of domains (Biddle, 1995).

We were fortunate in that the team contained a service user who had been a national player in his country of origin and several others had previously played at high levels. We were interviewed by the Football Association (FA) and were able to join a local league, where the team played once a week. We were able to obtain the services of a coach for the team, who was also a filmmaker who wanted to make a film about the team and the support of a professional club coach, who all volunteered their time.

The team quickly developed a sense of camaraderie, belonging and support for one another both on and off the pitch. The team assisted the players in developing a sense of control/mastery of their own bodies and the establishment of a routine and reason to develop both their fitness and resilience. Having said that, there were a number of issues when the players' rage about what had happened to them in their countries of origin exploded on to the football field and the team had a poor disciplinary record (we received a lot of yellow and red cards). We were called to discuss this with a member of the league's management on several occasions, as the league wanted to suspend them at one point. At the end of the first season the team won the league they were playing in, which gave them all a sense of mastery and achievement at the individual and group level. Research shows that taking part in sport combined with winning may contribute to positive feelings of self-identity and achievement (Plante, 1993).

After some time, we obtained some funding for the team and German television made a programme about the team. All of these combined with regular wins on the field, and improved relationships with league officials all helped the team develop a sense of achievement, pride and mastery on the field which the players began to see could be reproduced off the field. We collected narrative accounts of the players' experiences and we also had some hard data in terms of outcomes which showed that 57 per cent of the team took up courses at college and 19 per cent obtained jobs. All reported that being part of the team had been a positive experience for their sense of well-being both physically and psychologically.

A Humanitarian Psychological Intervention with Academics Working in a Civil War Zone Background

Sri Lanka had a civil war of 26 years' duration, which started in 1983 and was won militarily by the Sri Lankan army in May, 2009. In summary, the Liberation Tigers of Tamil Eelam (LTTE), known more colloquially as the Tamil Tigers, were fighting against the Sri Lankan army for control of the north and east of the country, where Tamil people form the majority of the population, with the aim of creating an autonomous Tamil state within Sri Lanka. During the civil war 70,000 men, women and children from all the ethnic groups lost their lives (Reuters, 2009) and 1.8 million people were uprooted by the civil war (UNHCR, 2009). Throughout the period of the civil war, human rights violations were recorded by both sides in the conflict (European Commission, 2009; Amnesty International, 2009; Human Rights Watch, 2013). There are 20,000–40,000 people still reported missing or disappeared, although the exact number is contested (International Committee of the Red Cross, 2016). The psychological intervention (PI) the authors undertook took place in September 2008, after many months of planning, the clarifying of objectives and seeking of funds. Although the civil war is now over, it was taking place when this psychological intervention took place. Even now, many people are still dealing with the physical, psychological, social and community legacies of the conflict. (A presidential investigatory committee to investigate complaints about missing persons was set up in 2013 and has received approximately 20,000 complaints to date including 5,000 from the armed forces.) The civil war was a time of tremendous fear and anxiety for people whose homes and places of work were located within the theatre of war (Somasundaram, 2014).

Participants, Context and the Issue Being Addressed

The participants were a group of university academics working and living within the theatre of war in the north of the country; they were not combatants. At this time, travel was very restricted and a number of items were banned, including batteries (Somasundaram, 2014). The context to this intervention is that we were approached by a Sri Lankan psychiatrist with whom one of the authors had worked intermittently for over 20 years. The 'problem' that was presented was that many university academics (who were living and working in the theatre of the civil war) had spoken to him about constantly meeting very distressed and traumatized students who were requesting emotional support and help from them. They felt unable to assist as they would like, believing they lacked the necessary training and skills for this work, as well as having to deal with issues relating to their own ongoing struggles for survival, traumatic experiences and anxiety related to living in a war zone and concerns about the future. People were living on a daily basis with the possibility of bombs dropping or other military weaponry being used. In addition, issues of trust and the sharing of views about the civil war became problematic with many people living in fear of being anonymously denounced to the authorities as having links or sympathies to one of the militant groups including the Sri Lankan army, as people would sometimes give names to protect themselves (Doney, 1998).

We managed to secure funding from the World Bank for five days' residential training away from the war zone. The team consisted of a psychiatrist based in Sri Lanka and four psychologists with links of heritage or interest to Sri Lanka but who normally resided elsewhere. We were also supported by two academics from within the group who were training/trained in psychiatry or mental health. The academics came from a range of disciplines, including medicine, arts, agriculture, business and commerce, and Siddha medicine (which is a form of traditional medicine practised in Sri Lanka).

The psychological intervention mixed experiential small group work with intensive training on mental health, psychological well-being, trauma and counselling skills using a range of training methods including role plays and multi-media. In addition we worked with the participants to develop a support group outside the training which would act as a supportive network once the training was over. We also conducted three follow-up programmes, six months and approximately 1 and 2 years after the training. A follow up was to take place later in 2016. We also collected data on each session within the training which rated the participants' pre-training knowledge, at post-training and at 6 months and at 1 year. The measures showed an improvement on a range of measures. A number of extracts from the first evaluation point are given by the participants here to give a flavour of their experience of the training.

> I was able to understand 'what is trauma?', the effects of trauma, consequences of trauma/'phobia', symptoms and aims of trauma interventions. I learned about how to respond after a trauma, common responses after trauma in children and adults. I was given an opportunity to understand the 'scared mind'. Trauma is about fear of death. I understand well about 'trauma' and its reactions after this training.
>
> Through this I can able to understand other problems, their bad experiences and these effects. Owing to that I started to make empathy to others. But I had some bad experiences in my life. Sometime it may disturb me. So I feel like some more training in this field.
>
> We are living in a very stressful condition. After the training my stress management skills and awareness about stress improve drastically.
>
> All the skills [relating to mental health] are very useful to identify the problem of the students as well as us.
>
> Communication types and the effective communication skills were elaborately exhibited through examples. I understand the listening and communication skills still I need to know more on this. Such training program could be repeated in future to strengthen on knowledge and skills.
>
> (Participants of the Sri Lankan psychological intervention)

When the war finished in 2009, some of the academics relocated, but the team are still involved in ongoing work with the group.

In summary, the range of psychological interventions discussed briefly here, all show how knowledge and skills from within cultural psychiatry and psychology can helpfully be used in a range of contexts. A number of psychological interventions have been described in a variety of contexts with very diverse populations in the UK and abroad. Psychological interventions can be innovative and dynamic and make a difference to people's lives. They may be used to promote mental health and well-being, to develop and provide both internal and external resources (including but not limited to knowledge, skills and support) as well as to develop confidence and maximize resilience and coping strategies for individuals as well as groups and communities. The interventions were all designed to benefit not only the people participating in them but to assist (in different ways) the wider communities of which they are a part.

Acknowledgement

We would like to thank all the people whom we worked with on all these projects in the UK and Sri Lanka. They are too many to thank individually, but you know who you are. We learned so much from you and hope that we have done justice to our work together here.

References

Amnesty International (2009). World must not abandon Sri Lanka's victims, available online at www.amnesty.org .uk/world-must-not-abandon-sri-lankas-victims-after-commonwealth-heads-government-meeting.

Amnesty International (2014). Torture in 2014, available online at www.amnestyusa.org/files/act400042014en.pdf.

Amnesty International (2015). Sri Lanka: UN war crimes resolution marks a turning point for victims. Available online at www.amnesty.org/en/latest/news/2015/10/sri-lanka-un-war-crimes-resolution-marks-a-turning-point-for-victims/.

Ang, E. T. and Gomez-Pinilla, F. (2007). Potential therapeutic effects of exercise to the brain. *Current Medicinal Chemistry*, **14**(24), 2564–2571.

Bhugra, D. and Bhui, K. (eds) (2007). *Textbook of Cultural Psychiatry*. Cambridge: Cambridge University Press.

Bhugra, D. and Gupta, S. (eds) (2011). *Migration and Mental Health*. Cambridge: Cambridge University Press, p. 263.

Biddle, S. J. H. (1995). Exercise and psychosocial health. *Research Quarterly for Exercise and Sport.* **66**, 292–297.

Blackwell, D. (2005). *Counselling and Psychotherapy with Refugees*. London: Jessica Kingsley.

Blumenthal, J. A., Babyak, M. A., Doriswamy, P. M. *et al.* (2007). Exercise and pharmacotherapy in the treatment of major depressive disorder. *Psychosomatic Medicine*, **69**(7), 587–596.

Boniwell, I. and Tunariu, A. D. (2010). *Face Up: Emotional Resilience Programme for Young People. A Trainer's Guide and Materials*. London: Commissioned by London Metropolitan Police in association with the Young Foundation.

Boniwell, I. and Tunariu, A. D. (2018). *Positive Psychology: Theory, Research and Applications*, 2nd edn. London: Open University Press/McGraw-Hill Education.

Bromberg, P. M. (1983). The mirror and the mask: on narcissism and psychoanalytic growth. *Contemporary Psychoanalysis*, **19**, 359–387.

Chatterjee, D. and Dasroy, S. (2016). Iswar Sankalpa: experience with the homeless persons with mental illness. In *The Palgrave Handbook for Global Mental Health: Socio-cultural Perspectives*, ed. R. White, S. Jain, D. Orr and U. Read. Basingstoke: Palgrave Macmillan.

Condor, S. (1991). Sexism in psychological research: a brief note. *Feminism and Psychology*, **1**(3), 430–434.

Corey, G. and Corey, S. M. (2014). *I Never Knew I Had a Choice. Explorations in Personal Growth*, international edition. Belmont, CA: Brooks/Cole, Cengage Learning.

de Antiss, H., Ziaian, T., Proctor, N., Warland, J. and Baghurst, P. (2009). Help-seeking for mental health problems in young refugees: a review of the literature. *Transcultural Psychiatry*, **46**, 584–607.

Defrin, R., Ginzburg, K., Mikulincer, M. and Solomon, Z. (2013). The long term impact of tissue injury on pain processing and modulation: a study on ex-prisoners of war who underwent torture. *European Journal of Pain*, **18**(4), 548–558.

Dickinson, H., Allen, K., Alcock, P., Macmillan, R. and Glasby, J. (2012). *The Role of the Third Sector in Delivering Social Care. Scoping Review*. London: NIHR School for Social Care Research.

Doney, A. (1998). A survey of Sri Lankan ex-detainees. In *Scarred Minds: The Psychological Impact of the War on Sri Lankan Tamils*, ed. D. Somasundaram. Colombo: Vijitha Yapa, pp. 256–287.

Duncan, G., Shepherd, M. and Symonds, J. (2010). Working with refugees: a manual for caseworkers and volunteers. *Rural and Remote Health*, **10**(4), 1–12.

European Commission (2009). www.trade.ec.europa.eu/do clib/press/index.cfm?id=515.

Evans-Lacko, S., Little, K., Meltzer, H. *et al.* (2010). Development and psychometric properties of the mental health knowledge schedule. *Canadian Journal of Psychiatry*, **55**(7), 440–448.

Fernando, S. (2014). *Mental Health Worldwide: Culture, Globalization and Development*. Basingstoke: Palgrave Macmillan.

Gauron, E. (1984) *Mental Training for Peak Performance*. Lansing, New York: Sport Science Associates.

Hall, C., Baillie. D., Basangwa. D. and Atukunda. J. (2016). Brain gain in Uganda: a case study of peer working as an adjunct to statutory mental health care in a low income country. In *The Palgrave Handbook for Global Mental Health: Socio-cultural Perspectives*, ed. R. White, S. Jain, D. Orr and U. Read. Basingstoke: Palgrave Macmillan.

Hargreaves, J. (1982) Theorising sport: an introduction. In *Sport, Culture and Ideology*, ed. J. Hargreaves. London: Routledge, pp. 1–30.

Hickling, F. (2016) Taking the psychiatrist to school: the development of a Dream-A-World Cultural Therapy program for behaviorally disturbed and academically underperforming primary school children in Jamaica. In *Handbook of Global Mental Health: Socio-cultural Perspectives*, ed. R. White, *et al.* Basingstoke: Palgrave-Macmillan.

Human Rights Watch (2013). World Report 2013, available online at www.hrw.org/world-report/2013/country-cha pters/sri-lanka.

Human Rights Watch (2016). The Human Rights of Refugees and Asylum Seekers, available online at www.hrw.org/legacy/.

International Committee of the Red Cross (2016). Sri Lanka: Report released on needs of families of missing persons, available online at www.icrc.org/en/document/ sri-lanka-families-missing-persons

Jones, D. and Gill, P. S. (1998). Refugees and primary care: tackling the inequalities. *British Medical Journal*, **317**, 7170.

Kim, J. (2000). *Mind in a Physical World*. Cambridge, MA: MIT Press.

Kohut, H. (1972). Thoughts on narcissism and narcissistic rage. *The Psychoanalytic Study of the Child*, **27**, 360–400.

Lindert, J., Heinz, A. and Priebe, S. (2012). Mental health care utilisation of migrants in Europe. *European Psychiatry*, **23**, 14–20.

Luty, J., Fekadu, D., Umoh, O. and Gallagher, J. (2006). Validation of a short instrument to measure stigmatised attitudes towards mental illness. *The Psychiatrist*, **30**, 257–260.

MacConville, R. and Rae, T. (2012). *Building Happiness, Resilience and Motivation in Adolescence. A Positive Psychology Curriculum for Well-Being*. London: Jessica Kingsley Publishers.

Manthorpe, J., Illife, S., Moriarty, J., Cones, M., Clough, R., Bright, T. and Rapaport, J. (2009). 'We are not blaming anyone, but if we don't know about amenities, we can't see them out.' Black and minority older people's views on the quality of local health and personal social services in England. *Ageing and Society*, **29**, 93–113.

Mental Health Policy Group (2014). A Manifesto for Better Mental Health, available online at www.mind.org.uk/m edia/1113989/a-manifesto-for-better-mental-health.pdf.

Mental Health Task Force, (2015). The Five Year Forward View Mental Health Task Force: Public Engagement Finding. A report from the independent Mental Health Taskforce to the NHS in England, available online at www.england.nhs.uk/mentalhealth/wp-content/upload s/sites/29/2015/09/fyfv-mental-hlth-taskforce.pdf.

Miettinen, R. (2000). The concept of experiential learning and John Dewey's theory of reflective thought and action. *International Journal of Lifelong Education*, **19**(1), 54–72.

Miller, K. (1999). Rethinking a familiar model, psychotherapy and the mental health of refugees. *Journal of Contemporary Psychology*, **29**, 283–306.

Mind (2013). Improving mental health support for refugee communities: an advocacy approach. London: Mind,

available online at www.mind.org.uk/media/192447/Ref ugee_Report_1.pdf.

Mind (2015). Commissioning mental health services for vulnerable adult migrants: guidance for commissioners, available online at www.mind.org.uk/media/3168649/ vulnerable-migrants_2015_mindweb.pdf.

Parks, A. C. and Schueller, S. (eds) (2014). *The Wiley-Blackwell Handbook of Positive Psychological Interventions*. Chichester: Wiley-Blackwell.

Plante, T. G. (1993). Aerobic exercises in prevention and treatment of psychopathology. In *Exercise Psychology*, ed. P. Seraganian. London: Wiley-Interscience, pp. 358–379.

Prashanth, N. S., Sridharan V. S., Seshadri, T. *et al.* (2016). Mental health in primary health care: the Karuna Trust experience. In *The Palgrave Handbook for Global Mental Health: Socio-cultural Perspectives*, ed. R. White, S. Jain, D. Orr and U. Read. Basingstoke: Palgrave-Macmillan.

Race on the Agenda (2016). DVD available online at: www.rota.org.uk/category/our-work/healthy-mobi lised-and-bame.

Rees, J., Miller, R. and Buckingham, H. (2014). *Public Sector Commissioning of Local Mental Health Services from the Third Sector*. Birmingham: University of Birmingham, Third Sector Research Centre.

Refugee Council (2016). Website available online at www.refugeecouncil.org.uk.

Reuters (2009). www.reuters.com/article/2009/./us-sri lanka-waridUSTRE54DGR200905.

Sashidharan, S. P. (2001). Institutional Racism in British Psychiatry. *Psychiatric Bulletin*, **25**, 244–247.

Sass, B., Moffat, J., Bhui, K. and McKenzie, K. (2009) Enhancing pathways to care for black and minority ethnic populations: a systematic review. *International Review of Psychiatry*, **21**(5), 430–438.

Schimmenti, A. (2012). Unveiling the hidden self: developmental trauma and psychological shame. *Psychodynamic Practice*, **18**(2), 193–211.

Schlapobersky, J. (1990). Torture as the perversion of a healing relationship. In *Health Services for the Treatment of Torture and Trauma Survivors*, ed. J. Gruschow and K. Hannibal. Washington DC: American Association for the Advancement of Science, pp. 51–72.

Sedikides, C., Gaertner, L., Luke, M. A., O'Mara, E. M. and Gebauer, J. E. (2013). A three-tier hierarchy of self-potency: individual self, relational self, collective self. *Advances in Experimental Social Psychology*, **48**, 235–295.

Somasundaram, D. (2014). *Scarred Communities. Psychological Impact of Man-Made and Natural Disasters on Sri Lankan Society*. Delhi: Sage.

Spencer-Oatey, H. (2012). *What Is Culture? A Compilation of Quotations*. GlobalPAD/University of Warwick, available online at http://wrap.warwick.ac.uk/id/eprint/ 74260.

Third Sector Commissioning Task Force (2016). *No Excuses: Embrace Partnership Now: Step Towards Change*. London: Department of Health, available online at www.dh/gov.uk/en/publicationsandstatistics/DH_4137144.

Tribe, R. (1998). What can psychological theory and the counselling psychologist offer in situations of civil conflict and war overseas? *Counselling Psychology Quarterly* **11**(1), 109–115.

Tribe, R. (2002). Football for facilitating therapeutic interventions among a group of refugees. In *Solutions in Sport Psychology*, ed. I. Cockerill. London: Thomson, pp. 173–183.

Tribe, R. (2007). Health pluralism: a more appropriate alternative to Western models of therapy in the context of the conflict and natural disaster in Sri Lanka? *Journal of Refugee Studies*, **20**(1), 21–36.

Tunariu, A. D. (2015). *The iNEAR Psychological Intervention. A Resilience Curriculum Programme for Children and Young People. Teacher and Student Guides.* London: University of East London.

Tunariu, A. D. (2017). Coaching for resilience within an Islamic context: a case study. In *Coaching in Islamic Culture: The Principles and Practice of Ershad*, ed. C. Van Nieuwerburgh and R. Allaho. London: Karnac Publishers.

Tunariu, A. D., Tribe, R., Frings, D. and Albery, I. P. (2017). The iNEAR programme: an existential positive psychology intervention for resilience and emotional wellbeing. *International Review of Psychiatry*, **29**(4), 362–372.

UK Sri Lanka Trauma Group (2014). Charity working towards increasing awareness of mental health issues, more information available online at www.uksrilankatrauma.org.uk/.

UNHCR (2009). 2009 Global Trends, available online at www.unhcr.org/4c11f0be9.pdf.

UNHCR (2010). Refugee statistics, available online at www.unhcr.org/statistics.html and www.unhcr.org/uk/publications/fundraising/4c08f2d99/unhcr-global-report-2009-sri-lanka.html.

van der Geest, R. (2016) A family-based intervention for people with a psychotic disorder in Nicaragua. In *The Palgrave Handbook for Global Mental Health: Sociocultural Perspectives*, ed. R. White, S. Jain, D. Orr and U. Read. Basingstoke: Palgrave-Macmillan.

Warren, J. and Garthwaite, K. (2015). 'We are volunteers and that sometimes gets forgotten': exploring the motivations and needs of volunteers at a healthy living resource centre in the north east of England. *Perspectives in Public Health*, **135**(2), 102–107.

Weir, K. (2011). The exercise effect. *Monitor on Psychology*, **42**(11), 48.

Winnicott, D. (1958). The capacity to be alone. In *The Maturational Process and the Facilitating Environment*, ed. D. Winnicott. London: Hogarth.

Spiritual Aspects of Management

Christopher C. H. Cook and Andrew Sims

Editors' Introduction

An integral part of many cultures is the role religion and spirituality play. Migrants often carry with them these rituals and taboos and values wherever they go. However, until recently psychiatry did not pay sufficient attention to the role religion plays both as a resilience factor but also as contributing to stress especially if it interferes with the process of acculturation. Cook and Sims point out that this interest is beginning to change. In this chapter they describe spiritual aspects of psychiatric management especially in the context of cultural psychiatry, demonstrating how spirituality is integral to the practice of psychiatry. They remind us of the meaning of spirituality and religion, and how these are relevant not only to the practice of clinical psychiatry but also to research. They illustrate that there is now much evidence linking religious/spiritual belief and practice to better mental health outcomes. Spiritual assessment is a critical clinical skill and mental health professionals should pay more attention to the spiritual needs of patients, irrespective of their own personal religious values. Cook and Sims go on to illustrate that contributions to spiritual management are also made by hospital and community chaplains, service users and carers. Spiritual management should be seen as complementary to other methods of psychiatric treatment and it needs to be recognized that such an approach benefits the whole person. Good clinical practice demands that imposing the world view of the psychiatrist upon the patient is not acceptable no matter what the circumstances. Professional boundaries must remain clear. Each psychiatric condition requires different management. Cook and Sims argue that spiritual management is not another addition to the menu of possible treatment regimens, it is an attribute of the physician that is all pervasive and affects every part of practice.

Introduction

The significance given to the religious or spiritual concerns of the patient reflects the culture of psychiatry in that place, and time. In Europe and North America, it is a product of the long-term ideological conflict within psychiatry between reductionist tendencies and a philosophy of assessment and treatment that aspires to help the whole person. Both of these extreme positions have made contributions to the effective treatment of patients, and probably some degree of dynamic tension has been beneficial to the academic discipline of psychiatry. Most practitioners have learnt from both schools of thought, and apply an amalgam in their clinical practice. In recent years there has been much more interest in spirituality by psychiatrists throughout the world, and this has been recognized by the World Psychiatric Association as well as at national level (Leon *et al.*, 2000).

There have been major changes within psychiatry towards the concepts of spirituality and religion over the last half-century. For example, in the standard British textbook of psychiatry in the 1950s through to the 1970s,[1] there are only two references to religion in the index: '"Religiosity" in deteriorated epileptic', and 'Religious belief, neurotic search for' (Slater and Roth, 1979). The latter was aimed as an attack upon psychoanalysis but assumed religion is for 'the hesitant, the guilt-ridden, the excessively timid, those lacking clear convictions with which to face life'. The attitudes of those influential in psychiatry tended to regard

---

[1] This appeared in the first, second and third editions of *Clinical Psychiatry* by Meyer-Gross, Slater and Roth in 1954, 1960 and 1969. See, for example, the third revised edition by Slater and Roth (1979). Insofar as the standard textbooks are concerned, it would appear that little has changed. In the second edition of the *New Oxford Textbook of Psychiatry* (Gelder *et al.*, 2012), there are still only two entries for 'religious', respectively for 'religious delusions' and 'religious healing ceremonies'.

religious belief in patients as 'neurotic' and in doctors as unscientific. By contrast, in the early twenty-first century, the Spirituality and Psychiatry Special Interest Group is one of the largest and most active special interest groups in the Royal College of Psychiatrists (Powell and Cook, 2006), and the College has published two books devoted to spirituality and psychiatry (Cook *et al.*, 2009, Cook *et al.*, 2016).

This chapter aims to put spiritual aspects of psychiatric management into the context of other types of psychiatric management and cultural psychiatry. The intention is to demonstrate how spirituality should be included as part of the theory and practice of the management of psychiatric disorders and how it fits into the complete picture of the treatment of patients.

Case examples are given to demonstrate what spiritual aspects of management mean in clinical practice. What is meant by spirituality and how it is relevant to the practice of psychiatry are discussed. How spiritual aspects of management complement other conventional methods of psychiatric treatment to benefit the whole person, both with the alleviation of symptoms and an improved ability to function appropriately, is also covered. There is brief description of some of the vast range of specific techniques used in spiritual healing. Mental illness subsumes a number of different psychiatric conditions and the relevance of spiritual aspects for these different diagnostic entities is considered. Pastoral care and user initiatives are explored and conclusions are drawn for the relevance of spiritual attitudes in the treatment of psychiatric patients.

Definitions

'Spirituality' is a useful, very imprecise word; perhaps useful because it does have varied meanings for different people. Dictionary definitions are not particularly helpful, and numerous definitions abound in the academic literature.[2] According to the Dalai Lama:

> Spirituality [is] concerned with those qualities of the human spirit – such as love and compassion, patience, tolerance, forgiveness, contentment, a sense of responsibility, a sense of harmony – which bring happiness to both self and others.
>
> (Gyatso, 1999: 23)

More comprehensively, spirituality may be defined as:

> a distinctive, potentially creative, and universal dimension of human experience arising both within the inner subjective awareness of individuals and within communities, social groups and traditions. It may be experienced as a relationship with that which is intimately 'inner' immanent and personal, within the self and others, and/or as a relationship with that which is wholly 'other', transcendent and beyond the self. It is experienced as being of fundamental or ultimate importance and is thus concerned with matters of meaning and purpose in life, truth, and values.
>
> (Cook, 2004: 548–549)

It is sometimes suggested that religion is easier to define, but in fact religion is also a complex concept not susceptible to simple or uncontested definition (Bowker, 1999: 15–24). Similarly, it is often compared unfavourably with spirituality, the former being represented as more individual, subjective and 'authentic', the latter as more collective, institutional and rule bound. In fact the relationships between spirituality and religion are complex, the two concepts being inseparable for some people and representing contrasting opposites to others. The tendency to adopt a position of being 'spiritual but not religious' (Casey, 2013) is a relatively recent Western phenomenon and would not make any sense at all historically, or in many parts of the world today (e.g. in Islamic countries or in India). However, it represents a separation of spirituality from religion which is an important consideration in psychiatric practice. A patient may not consider herself to be 'religious' in any traditional sense, and may not affiliate with any faith community, but may yet consider spirituality to be at the heart of her priorities, values and purpose in life.

Spirituality and Mental Health

There is now considerable research evidence for the effects of religious belief, or spirituality, upon health and disease. This has been systematically collated by Koenig *et al.* in two editions (better seen as Volume 1, reviewing studies up to 2000, and Volume 2, reviewing subsequent studies) of the *Handbook of Religion and Health* (Koenig *et al.*, 2001, Koenig *et al.*, 2012).

The first edition of the *Handbook* reviews and discusses research that has examined the relationships between the patient's religious beliefs and a variety of mental and physical health conditions. It covers the whole of medicine, and is based on 1,200 research studies and 400 reviews. Research on religion and mental health occupies ten chapters. Under *research and*

---

[2] Some of these are reviewed – mainly in relation to addiction psychiatry – in Cook (2004).

mental health are discussed: religion and well-being, depression, suicide, anxiety disorders, schizophrenia and other psychoses, alcohol and drug use, delinquency, marital instability, personality, and a summarizing chapter on understanding religion's effects upon mental health. The authors are cautious in drawing conclusions but the results are overwhelming. To quote:

> In the majority of studies, religious involvement is correlated with:
> - Well-being, happiness and life satisfaction;
> - Hope and optimism;
> - Purpose and meaning in life;
> - Higher self-esteem;
> - Adaptation to bereavement;
> - Greater social support and less loneliness;
> - Lower rates of depression and faster recovery from depression;
> - Lower rates of suicide and fewer positive attitudes towards suicide;
> - Less anxiety;
> - Less psychosis and fewer psychotic tendencies;
> - Lower rates of alcohol and drug use and abuse;
> - Less delinquency and criminal activity;
> - Greater marital stability and satisfaction
>
> ... We concluded that, for the vast majority of people, the apparent benefit of devout religious belief and practice probably outweigh the risks.
>
> (Koenig *et al.*, 2001: 228)

Correlations between religious belief and greater well-being 'typically equal or exceed correlations between well-being and other psychosocial variables, such as social support' (Koenig *et al.*, 2001: 215). That is a considerable assertion, comprehensively attested to by a large volume of evidence, for example, in Brown and Harris's (1978) studies on the social origins of depression, various types of social support were the most powerful protective factors against depression.

Eighty per cent or more of the studies reported an association between 'religiousness' and greater hope or optimism about the future; 15 out of 16 studies reported a statistically significant association between 'greater religious involvement' and a greater sense of purpose or meaning in life; 19 out of 20 studies reported at least one statistically significant relationship between a religious variable and greater social support. Of 93 cross-sectional or prospective studies of the relationship between religious involvement and depression, 60 (65%)

reported a significant positive relationship between a measure of religious involvement and lower rates of depression; 13 studies reported no association; 4 reported greater depression among the more religious; and 16 studies gave mixed findings. With all the 13 factors, religious belief proved beneficial in more than 80 per cent of mental health studies. This is despite very few of these studies having been initially designed to examine the effect of religious involvement on health.

The authors develop a model for how and why religious belief and practice might influence mental health. There are direct beneficial effects upon mental health, such as better cognitive appraisal and coping behaviour in response to stressful life experiences. There are also indirect effects, such as developmental factors and even genetic and biological factors.

Most of the studies were carried out in the USA and most subjects have belonged to the Judeo-Christian tradition. There is some work from other countries and other religions, and the results are similar. At our present state of knowledge it is important to have more sophisticated measures of religious and spiritual belief for psychiatric research.[3]

The second edition of the *Handbook* largely supported the overall findings of the first edition (Cook, 2012). Disappointingly, the authors found that there had been no overall improvement in the methodological quality of research published in this field, but this should not be allowed to distract from the many high quality studies that are now being published, and the authors found that the better quality studies were more likely to report positive relationships between spirituality/religion and health. Overall, at least two-thirds of studies reviewed were found to demonstrate positive relationships between spirituality/religion and emotional and social well-being and healthier lifestyle.

Religious belief and practice are associated with decreased rates for suicide (Cook, 2014), with decreased rates of delinquency (Benson and Donahue, 1989), with higher rates of marital stability (Call and Heaton, 1997), lower rates for hostility (Kark *et al.*, 1996), more hope and optimism (Mickley *et al.*, 1992), and an internalized locus of control (Jackson and Coursey, 1988). As an

---

[3] See, for example, King *et al.* (2001). However, it is interesting that use of their instrument in UK and European samples has produced somewhat different results than those most commonly seen in US studies (e.g. King *et al.*, 2013).

example of the association with well-being, a questionnaire was administered to 474 students in the United Kingdom enquiring about religious orientation, frequency of personal prayer and church attendance, alongside measures of depressive symptoms, trait anxiety and self-esteem (Maltby *et al.*, 1999). Frequency of personal prayer was the dominant factor in a positive relationship between religiosity and psychological well-being.

Whilst there continues to be debate about the strength and interpretation of the evidence, there is now sufficient recognition of the link between spirituality/religion and mental health that various national and international professional bodies, including the Royal College of Psychiatrists (Cook, 2013b) and the World Psychiatric Association (Moreira-Almeida *et al.*, 2016) have implemented policies concerning the part played by spirituality/religion in psychiatric training, professional development, and clinical practice.

Assessment of Spirituality

As part of clinical assessment it is recommended that the doctor take a spiritual/religious history, perhaps employing questions such as those illustrated in Box 36.1.

Patients are more likely to have confidence in their psychiatrist if he or she demonstrates a sympathetic attitude toward their beliefs. Ascertaining spiritual belief is also a vital ingredient of the mental state examination of the patient and gives valuable information for assessment and treatment. The

---

BOX 36.1 Questions that may be used in the assessment of spirituality/religion in clinical practice[4]

- Is religion or spirituality important to you?
- Do your religious or spiritual beliefs influence the way you look at your medical problems and the way you think about your health?
- Would you like me to address your religious or spiritual beliefs and practices with you?

---

[4] Matthews and Clark (1998: 274). For a more extended discussion of the assessment of spiritual needs, see Culliford and Eagger (2009).

psychiatrist therefore needs to give validity to the patient's beliefs. This will imply being able to discuss belief with the patient in the context of their psychiatric symptoms. It may mean a preparedness to confer, at the patient's request, with a designated religious leader or chaplain. It will mean acknowledging the value of prayer to the patient and of the benefits of a faith community such as a church, synagogue or mosque.

Spirituality in the Management of Psychiatric Disorder

Spirituality and religion are often neglected in clinical practice when planning the management of psychiatric disorders. We, as psychiatrists, purport to deal with the whole person, and psychiatrists have sometimes criticized the orthopaedic surgeon who treats 'a knee' in isolation, or the renal physician who cannot see beyond the deranged physiology of the kidney.

> We psychiatrists complain when our medical colleagues cannot get beyond the physical, even when evidence for psychosocial aetiology is quite blatant, but we may be guilty of an equivalent error in almost totally excluding spiritual considerations from the way we understand our patients. (Sims, 1994)

That was written more than 20 years ago, but it is still to some extent true.

A robust comment on the need of mental health professionals to take spiritual aspects of their patients into account is made by Swinton (2001). Our patients are apprehensive because of the hostility psychiatrists have shown in the past towards their religious beliefs. They want psychiatrists to acknowledge these beliefs and integrate them into treatment. There is a 'religiosity gap' between patients, who are more likely to be religious, and psychiatrists, who are more likely to be atheist or agnostic (Cook, 2011). Mental health practitioners show consistently lower rates for religious beliefs and practice than either their patients or the general population.

There is much encouragement for psychiatrists to work with other disciplines in the care of their patients, both practising in a team and collaborating with other, external, multidisciplinary agencies. Religious people and organizations are often very helpful, sometimes providing the only spiritual support for psychiatric patients, and optimum care should therefore, at least on occasion, involve working more closely with them. This point was made cogently by Lord Carey, when Archbishop of Canterbury, in an address jointly to the Association of European Psychiatrists and the Royal College of Psychiatrists (Carey, 1997).

The onset, course, outcome and treatment for the various psychiatric disorders are markedly different, and therefore so should be the spiritual aspects of their management. Little attention has been paid to this in the past. For those with mental disorder there is, in general, a better outcome if the patient has religious belief; this is true for most individual psychiatric conditions (Koenig *et al.*, 2001, Koenig *et al.*, 2012). It pertains, for example, for schizophrenia (Verghese *et al.*, 1989), depression (Kendler *et al.*, 1997), anxiety disorders (Koenig *et al.*, 1993), and substance use disorders (Cook, 2009).

It would therefore appear helpful both for mental health professionals to pay more attention to the specific spiritual needs of different types of patients, and for religious leaders, such as hospital chaplains, to take psychiatric diagnosis into account to a greater extent in their pastoral work. Spirituality and religion are also important factors to be taken into account by carers and mental health service users themselves.

Mental Health Professionals

Spirituality and religion impact upon the management of different psychiatric disorders in different ways.

Patients with *dementia* may have specific spiritual needs. These result from loss of awareness and relatedness to God's transcendence, loss of sense of meaning, hopelessness, loss of meaning, purpose and value; and, apparent disinterest in the spiritual dimension (Lawrence and Raji, 2005).

Depressed patients may have all-pervasive feelings of guilt and self-blame; they may believe that they have committed the unforgivable sin or will be consigned to eternal punishment. On occasions such religiously inspired beliefs have been dispelled with antidepressant medication and/or electroconvulsive therapy. On the other hand, depressed people with firm religious convictions, and their relatives, are frequently terrified of psychiatric treatment because they anticipate psychiatric staff being antagonistic to religion and challenging their beliefs. Sadly, there has been justification for their fears in the past (see page 475).

Religious delusions are not infrequent with *schizophrenia* and whilst it has been argued that they more often occurred in the past (Klaf and Hamilton, 1961), worldwide the frequency of religious delusions may not be declining (Cook, 2015b). The frequency of this association does not imply that religion causes delusions but rather that delusions tend to take on the content of the sufferer's prevailing interests and concerns. A skilful clinician will find the middle ground between appearing to accept the delusional ideas and diminishing the patient's self-respect and confidence in the doctor by rejecting them – avoiding collusion and confrontation.

Cognitive-behavioural therapy (CBT) and other forms of psychological treatment can work with the grain of religious belief in the treatment of *anxiety disorders*. Using the patient's own beliefs, the patient debates within himself to correct his own negative thinking. Religiously and/or spiritually integrated CBT is now being developed and studied in application to anxiety disorders (Rosmarin *et al.*, 2010, Williams *et al.*, 2002), obsessive–compulsive disorder (Akuchekian *et al.*, 2011), affective disorders (Koenig *et al.*, 2015), and substance use disorders (Hodge and Lietz, 2014).

Faith, and religious conversion, has proved of great benefit to some people trying to recover from their *addiction to alcohol or other drugs* (Cook, 2009). The spiritual programme of the Twelve Step organizations (Alcoholics Anonymous, Narcotics Anonymous, and the other related 'Anonymous' groups) has been particularly important in the recovery of many people from substance use disorders and is accessible to people from all faiths and none. The so-called 'higher power' does not have to be religiously interpreted and many agnostics and atheists report having found these programmes helpful (Dossett, 2013).

A more extended account of the spiritual aspects of different psychiatric conditions is to be found in Swinton (2001). Some of the questions concerning the ethical implications and the nature of good professional practice are addressed by Cook (2013a, 2015a). In particular, it is important to recognize here that addressing spiritual/religious concerns in the assessment and treatment of psychiatric disorders should be a patient-centred exercise, and that this does not allow any place for proselytizing or imposing the world view of the psychiatrist upon the patient (whether that be an atheistic, traditionally religious or spiritual belief system).

It was not infrequent in the past for some psychiatrists, not realizing that they were expressing their own religious opinions, to disparage and denigrate their patient's religious beliefs. This is vividly described by Jean Davison (2009) in her book, *The Dark Threads*. Jean was a Christian teenager treated as an inpatient in a mental hospital in the 1970s. She describes how different psychiatrists repeatedly belittled her faith – until, sadly, she abandoned it:

> If they wanted me to relinquish all thoughts of God, why didn't they try to help me see that life could be bearable, even happy, without a God to believe in? Instead they kept on subjecting me to 'treatment' which made me cry out in desperation to this remote, perhaps fictitious, 'God' to help me. More than ever before I wanted and needed Him now.
>
> (Davison, 2009: 138)

When Jean was first admitted to hospital, her doctor said to her:

> 'Hell doesn't exist. The Bible isn't meant to be taken literally: it's full of metaphors ... Heaven doesn't exist either. The world's moved on from fairy tales to science.' The doctor sighed, 'But really, love, you ought to have had more sense than to try to believe things like that in the first place, don't you think?'
>
> (Davison, 2009: 62–63)

In 2013, the General Medical Council published an updated version of its guidance on *Personal Beliefs and Medical Practice* (General Medical Council, 2013). This guidance does acknowledge a positive place for taking into account religious and spiritual beliefs in clinical practice, but emphasizes that 'you must not put pressure on a patient to discuss or justify their beliefs, or absence of them' (ibid. para. 29). It further indicates that a doctor should not discuss their own beliefs with a patient unless this is initiated by the patient, or the patient clearly indicates that they would welcome such a discussion. Imposing beliefs on a patient, or causing distress by insensitive expression of them, is clearly warned against (ibid. para. 31).

Frequently, patients have said that they were disturbed by their treating psychiatrist, during the course of psychiatric interview, attacking their religious beliefs, recommending that they discontinue their religious practice and disassociate themselves from their church or other affiliation. This has, of course, caused them enormous distress, and has often been an expression of the psychiatrist's atheist, secular views; it has certainly been an imposition of the psychiatrist's belief upon the patient. Belittling of patients' Christian beliefs by psychiatrists has been frequent to the extent that many church leaders discouraged their members from consulting a psychiatrist, sometimes to the considerable detriment of the potential patient. Such 'proselytizing' is clearly as much a problem (if not more), and equally unacceptable, as proselytizing on behalf of particular religious beliefs or traditions.

Chaplaincy

Within the National Health Service in the United Kingdom, hospital or community mental health chaplains are often employed. They are valuable in many ways, and often contribute to the treatment of patients. Another clinical case history illustrates this issue.

A 14-year-old girl of Pakistani origin was referred to a child psychiatrist for school refusal, disturbed behaviour and vivid descriptions of frightening visual perceptions. The general practitioner thought that she might be psychotic. She and her parents were most concerned about her 'visions'. They had wanted to consult the imam but had discovered that he was out of the country. The child psychiatrist reassured them that she was not psychotic and, with the family's permission, arranged for her to discuss her strange experiences with the hospital chaplain. This seemed to work, as spiritual guidance was given and accepted.

Service Users and Carers

Psychiatrists, and other mental health workers, sometimes fail to realize that they are not the only people trying to help those with mental illnesses to cope better, feel some relief from symptoms and relate in a mutually rewarding way to others in the community. Identified mentally ill people, *service users* in conventional jargon, make an increasing contribution in identifying the sort of services they require. Their close relatives and friends, *carers*, have over the last couple of decades shaped the provision of services and individual patient contact in a beneficial manner. Religious organizations, in the British context especially churches, have always had involvement with the mentally ill, and over recent years have approached their working with such people in a more systematic and knowledgeable manner.

An example of spiritual management in the contribution that users and carers themselves make to the care of those with mental illnesses is the Association for Pastoral Care in Mental Health. In a newsletter, the Chairman queried:

> [How] might we . . . reduce the gap between the most traumatised and the normal person whoever that might be? Perhaps all we can share is what we have and who we are, our time and our love, that which is given freely and received freely – all God's gifts. Resolutions without the recognition of God's provision are empty resolutions, like works without faith are empty. We spend millions striving for the perfect manifesto but fail to provide that one essential ingredient that the whole nation is yearning for. 'Love', without which as St Paul says, 'We are nothing'. By listening, ministering, nurturing, valuing and responding to the needs of the spirit, the journey begins – when we begin to walk, that's where the road starts.
>
> (Heneghan, 2005)

This is certainly a most important area of discourse. What is the significance of love in the management of the mentally ill? What does *love* mean in this context and how can this be provided by the individual mental health professional, the National Health Service, users and carers? This is too big a subject to embark on in this chapter but requires ongoing discussion (Sims, 2006).

Another example of user initiative in this area is the report *Knowing Our Minds*, published by the Mental Health Foundation (1997), which surveyed 401 people's experience of mental health services and treatments. The sufferers are considered to be the 'primary experts' on their own mental health. Those surveyed recommended very strongly that mental health professionals recognize and take into account the spiritual aspects of mental health and its problems.

Churches in Britain have taken a positive position towards the treatment of the mentally ill in recent years and have taken steps to help such people and co-operate with statutory mental health services. Addressing psychiatrists, senior clergy have recommended collaboration between psychiatrists and clergy for the benefit of sufferers (Carey, 1997), and have, noting the move away from a mechanistic view of humankind, recommended psychiatrists to take more care of their own spiritual and mental state (Hope, 2004). This does not imply any blurring of role between psychiatrists and priests. Rowan Williams, when Archbishop of Canterbury, recommended empathic and informed listening to patients (Williams, 2005). The Church of England has also produced a significant report on healing, which deals with the whole subject from a more theological perspective (Working Party on Healing, 2000).

Spiritual Healing

Spiritual healing is a specific type of intervention involving acknowledgment of the importance of the spiritual dimension in the treatment of human illness and malaise.

> Spiritual healing in the form of prayer, healing meditation, or the laying on of hands has been practised in virtually every known culture. Prayers and rituals for healing are a part of most religions. Reports of folk-healers are familiar from legend, the Bible, anthropological studies of traditional cultures, the popular press, and more recently from scientific research.
>
> (Benor, 2001: 3)

Spiritual healing was recognized as a form of complementary therapy by the House of Lords Select Committee on Science and Technology. In their classification it was placed in 'Group 2' of therapies used to complement conventional medicine without purporting to embrace diagnostic skills (House of Lords Select Committee on Science and Technology, 2000). Here, healing was defined as: 'a system of spiritual healing, sometimes based on prayer and religious beliefs, that attempts to tackle illness through non-physical means, usually by directing thoughts towards an individual. Often involves "the laying on of hands".' Conventional medicine is not universally effective, for all people, for all illnesses and conditions, and at all times. That truism being immediately accepted by patients and doctors alike, patients will search for alternative and complementary therapies, sometimes those that conform better with their world view, and it behoves doctors to be open-minded, certainly to give cautious warnings when appropriate, but also to be humble in their claims. On occasions they should cooperate and collaborate for the benefit of patients.

The range of different types of spiritual healing is immense, and beyond the scope of this chapter to describe, or even list. Healing may take place at a distance or by laying on of hands. It may involve meditation and prayer by the subject. According to Fulder (1984), the patient is encouraged to see healing as an enterprise towards health and self-discovery, rather than a cure for a specific illness. Benor (2001) lists the following 12 systems of healing, which he has encountered and whose practitioners he has generally found reliable. He gives strengths and limitations for each:

- Spiritual healing in religious settings
- Qigong healing
- Medical dowsing
- Reiki healing
- LeShan healing
- Therapeutic Touch
- Craniosacral therapy
- The Bowen technique
- Barbara Brennan healing
- Polarity therapy
- SHEN healing
- Healing Touch.

These are all available in the USA, whatever their country of origin. Rees (2003) lists techniques of healing from all over the world, including his own country of Wales. The similarities between some of these methods from places far distant from each other are remarkable.

Overall, the evidence for efficacy of spiritual healing is positive, but only weakly so, not as strong, nor as unidirectional as the evidence for health benefits from religious belief and practice. Positive results are reported. For example, significant effects of healing on AIDS were demonstrated in a report of 40 sufferers randomly allocated to treatment and control groups with distant healing for 10 weeks from 40 experienced healers (Sicher et al., 1998). After six months the treatment group had significantly fewer AIDS-related illnesses and lower severity of illness with fewer visits to doctors, hospitalizations and days in hospital. However, although there are a large number of accounts of healing for human physical problems, overall the results are equivocal and many of the strongly positive studies have not been published in peer reviewed medical journals, nor replicated.

Conclusions

Spiritual management is not another addition to the overburdened menu of possible regimens with which to treat patients, or to the ever-increasing curriculum for hard-pressed psychiatric trainees. It is more an attribute of the physician that is all pervasive and affects every part of practice. It is particularly reflected in the capacity for insightful listening. Shooter (2005) has categorized this as: 'listening with the ears, listening with the eyes, listening with the heart and listening with the hands, the latter perhaps what takes place in some types of spiritual healing'.

Spiritual management is something which should happen as part of the investigations and interventions of conventional medicine, in the same way that the general physician should take a drinking history and reckon to treat the patient taking behaviour into consideration, and the psychiatrist should pay attention to the physical state of the patient. There is also a set of therapeutic techniques outside but complementary to medicine. Finally, spiritual management occurs in the work of other professionals, such as the clergy, with whom the doctor cooperates and collaborates for the benefit of their mutual patient. It is, therefore, an integral and essential part of cultural psychiatry.

References

Akuchekian, S. H., Almasi, A., Meracy, M. R. and Jamshidian, Z. (2011). Effect of religious cognitive-behavior therapy on religious content obsessive compulsive disorder. *Procedia – Social and Behavioral Sciences*, **30**, 1647–1651.

Benor, D. J. (2001). *Spiritual Healing: Scientific Validation of a Healing Revolution*. Southfield, MI: Vision Publications.

Benson, P. L. and Donahue, M. J. (1989). Ten year trends in at-risk behaviors: a national study of black adolescents. *Journal of Adolescent Research*, **4**, 125–139.

Bowker, J. (1999). *The Oxford Dictionary of World Religions*. Oxford: Oxford University Press.

Brown, G. W. and Harris, T. O. (1978). *Social Origins of Depression*. London: Tavistock.

Call, V. R. A. and Heaton, T. B. (1997). Religious influence on marital stability. *Journal for the Scientific Study of Religion*, **36**, 382–392.

Carey, G. (1997). Towards wholeness: transcending the barriers between religion and psychiatry. *British Journal of Psychiatry*, **170**, 396–397.

Casey, P. (2013). 'I'm spiritual but not religious' – implications for research and practice. In *Spirituality, Theology and Mental Health*, ed. C. C. H. Cook. London: SCM, pp. 20–39.

Cook, C. C. H. (2004). Addiction and spirituality. *Addiction*, **99**, 539–551.

Cook, C. C. H. (2009). Substance misuse. In *Spirituality and Psychiatry*, ed. C. Cook, A. Powell and A. Sims. London: Royal College of Psychiatrists Press, pp. 139–168.

Cook, C. C. H. (2011). The faith of the psychiatrist. *Mental Health, Religion and Culture*, **14**, 9–17.

Cook, C. C. H. (2012). Keynote 4: spirituality and health. *Journal for the Study of Spirituality*, **12**, 150–162.

Cook, C. C. H. (2013a). Controversies on the place of spirituality and religion in psychiatric practice. In *Spirituality, Theology and Mental Health*, ed. C. C. H. Cook, London: SCM, pp. 1–19.

Cook, C. C. H. (2013b). *Recommendations for Psychiatrists on Spirituality and Religion*. London: Royal College of Psychiatrists.

Cook, C. C. H. (2014). Suicide and religion. *The British Journal of Psychiatry*, **204**, 254–255.

Cook, C. C. H. (2015a). Religion and spirituality in clinical practice. *Advances in Psychiatric Treatment*, **21**, 42–50.

Cook, C. C. H. (2015b). Religious psychopathology: the prevalence of religious content of delusions and hallucinations in mental disorder. *International Journal of Social Psychiatry*, **61**(4), 404–425.

Cook, C., Powell, A. and Sims, A. (eds) (2009). *Spirituality and Psychiatry*. London: Royal College of Psychiatrists Press.

Cook, C. C. H., Powell, A. and Sims, A. (eds) (2016). *Spirituality and Narrative in Psychiatric Practice: Stories of Mind and Soul*, London: Royal College of Psychiatrists Press.

Culliford, L. and Eagger, S. (2009). Assessing spiritual needs. In *Spirituality and Psychiatry*, ed. C. Cook, A. Powell and A. Sims. London: Royal College of Psychiatrists Press, pp. 16–38.

Davison, J. (2009). *The Dark Threads*. Bedlinog, Mid-Glamorgan: Accent Press.

Dossett, W. (2013). Addiction, spirituality and 12-step programmes. *International Social Work*, **56**, 369–383.

Fulder, S. (1984). *The Handbook of Complementary Medicine*. London: Hodder and Stoughton.

Gelder, M. G., Andreasen, N. C., López-Ibor, J. J. and Geddes, J. R. (eds) (2012). *New Oxford Textbook of Psychiatry*. Oxford: Oxford University Press.

General Medical Council (2013). *Personal Beliefs and Medical Practice*. London: General Medical Council.

Gyatso, T. (1999). *Ancient Wisdom, Modern World*. London: Little Brown.

Heneghan, S. (2005). The road to being alongside. *Association for Pastoral Care in Mental Health Newsletter*, 1–2.

Hodge, D. R. and Lietz, C. A. (2014). Using spiritually modified cognitive-behavioral therapy in substance dependence treatment: therapists' and clients' perceptions of the presumed benefits and limitations. *Health and Social Work*, **39**, 200–210.

Hope, D. (2004). *Spiritual Aspects of Caring*. London: Spirituality and Psychiatry Special Interest Group, Royal College of Psychiatrists.

House of Lords Select Committee on Science and Technology (2000). *Complementary and Alternative Medicine*. London: The Stationery Office.

Jackson, L. E. and Coursey, R. D. (1988). The relationship of god control and internal locus of control to intrinsic religious motivation, coping and purpose in life. *Journal for the Scientific Study of Religion*, **27**, 399–410.

Kark, J. D., Carmel, S., Sinnreich, R., Goldberger, N. and Friedlander, Y. (1996). Psychosocial factors among members of religious and secular Kibbutzim. *Israel Journal of Medical Science*, **32**, 185–194.

Kendler, K. S., Gardner, C. O. and Prescott, C. A. (1997). Religion, psychopathology, and substance use and abuse: a multimeasure, genetic-epidemiologic study. *American Journal of Psychiatry*, **154**, 322–329.

King, M., Speck, P. and Thomas, A. (2001). The Royal Free Interview for Spiritual and Religious Beliefs: Development and Validation of a Self-Report Version. *Psychological Medicine*, **31**, 1015–1023.

King, M., Marston, L., McManus, S., Brugha, T., Meltzer, H. and Bebbington, P. (2013). Religion, spirituality, and mental health: results from a national study of English households. *British Journal of Psychiatry*, **202**, 68–73.

Klaf, F. S. and Hamilton, J. G. (1961). Schizophrenia: a hundred years ago and today. *Journal of Mental Science*, **107**, 819–827.

Koenig, H. G., Ford, S., George, L. K., Blazer, D. G., Pritchett, J. and Meador, K. G. (1993). Religion and anxiety disorder: an examination and comparison of associations in young, middle-aged and elderly adults. *Journal of Anxiety Disorders*, 7, 321–342.

Koenig, H. G., McCullough, M. E. and Larson, D. B. (2001) *Handbook of Religion and Health*. New York: Oxford University Press.

Koenig, H. G., King, D. E. and Carson, V. B. (2012). *Handbook of Religion and Health*, 2nd edn. New York: Oxford University Press.

Koenig, H. G., Pearce, M. J., Nelson, B. and Daher, N. (2015). Effects of religious versus standard cognitive-behavioral therapy on optimism in persons with major depression and chronic medical illness. *Depression and Anxiety*, **32**, 835–42.

Lawrence, R. M. and Raji, O. (2005). Introduction to spirituality, health care and mental health. Available online at www.rcpsych.ac.uk/pdf/LawrenceOyepejuIntroSpirituality.pdf.

Leon, C. E., Tasman, A., Lopez-Ibor, J. J. *et al.* (2000). Culture, spirituality and psychiatry: comment. *Current Opinion in Psychiatry*, **13**, 531–543.

Maltby, J., Lewis, C. A. and Day, L. (1999). Religious orientation and psychological well-being: the role of personal prayer. *British Journal of Health Psychology*, **4**, 363–378.

Matthews, D. A. and Clark, C. (1998). *The Faith Factor: Proof of the Healing Power of Prayer.* New York: Viking.

Mental Health Foundation (1997). *Knowing Our Own Minds: A Survey of How People in Emotional Distress Take Control of Their Lives.* London: Mental Health Foundation.

Mickley, J. R., Soeken, K. and Belcher, A. (1992). Spiritual well-being, religiousness and hope among women with breast cancer. *IMAGE: Journal of Nursing Scholarship*, **24**, 267–272.

Moreira-Almeida, A., Sharma, A., Van Rensburg, B. J., Verhagen, P. J. and Cook, C. C. H. (2016). WPA position statement on spirituality and religion in psychiatry. *World Psychiatry*, **15**, 87–88.

Powell, A. and Cook, C. C. H. (2006). Spirituality and Psychiatry Special Interest Group of the Royal College of Psychiatrists. Reaching the Spirit: Social Perspectives Network Study Day, Paper 9. London, Social Perspectives Network, 33.

Rees, D. (2003) *Healing in Perspective.* London: Whurr.

Rosmarin, D. H., Pargament, K. I., Pirutinsky, S. and Mahoney, A. (2010). A randomized controlled evaluation of a spiritually integrated treatment for subclinical anxiety in the Jewish community, delivered via the Internet. *Journal of Anxiety Disorders*, **24**, 799–808.

Shooter, M. (2005). The soul of caring. *Advances in Psychiatric Treatment*, **11**, 239–240.

Sicher, F., Targ, E., Moore, D. and Smith, H. S. (1998). A randomised, double-blind study of the effects of distant healing in a population with advanced AIDS. *Western Journal of Medicine*, **169**, 356–363.

Sims, A. (1994). 'Psyche': spirit as well as mind? *British Journal of Psychiatry*, **165**, 441–446.

Sims, A. (2006). Neuroscience and belief: a Christian perspective. In *Medicine for the Person: Faith, Values and Science in Health Care Provision*, ed. J. Cox, A. Campbell and W. Fulford. London: Jessica Kingsley.

Slater, E. and Roth, M. (1979). *Clinical Psychiatry.* London: Bailliere Tindall.

Swinton, J. (2001). *Spirituality and Mental Health Care.* London: Jessica Kingsley.

Verghese, A., John, J. K., Rajkumar, S., Richard, J., Sethi, B. B. and Trivedi, J. K. (1989). Factors associated with the course and outcome of schizophrenia in India: results of a two-year multicentre follow-up study. *British Journal of Psychiatry*, **154**, 499–503.

Williams, C. J., Richards, P. and Whitton, I. (2002). *I'm Not Supposed to Feel Like This: A Christian Self-Help Approach to Depression and Anxiety.* London: Hodder and Stoughton.

Williams, R. (2005). The care of souls. *Advances in Psychiatric Treatment*, **11**, 4–5.

Working Party on Healing (2000). *A Time to Heal: A Contribution Towards the Ministry of Healing.* London: Church House.

Cultural Aspects of Suicide

Heidi Hjelmeland

Editors' Introduction

Suicide and suicidal acts are a major concern globally. In many countries the act of suicide is illegal thereby not allowing accurate data collection. It has also been shown that self-harm is practised in many religions. This chapter by Hjelmeland should be read in conjunction with the chapter by Fortune and Hawton. Hjelmeland reminds us that according to the WHO figures and policy, suicide is a major public health problem in every country of the world. Although the data vary across countries and regions, the reasons for such variation can be both biological and social and cultural. Hjelmeland reminds us that suicide research has for decades been dominated by the biomedical model with the inherent focus on quantitative risk factor research. This has resulted in a dominant understanding of suicide as a consequence of mental disorders. As qualitative suicide research has started to make its mark in recent times this has led to more contextualized and indeed more nuanced understandings of suicide and its impact on cultures and societies. Such approaches, argues Hjelmeland have led to better understanding of varying sociocultural and political contexts around the world with different and culture-specific meanings of suicide. Remarkable similarities across contexts have, however, also been found and are described in this chapter. Consequences of hegemonic masculinity seem important in many suicides in different sociocultural contexts for both men and women, albeit in different ways. Suicide seems to be a relational communicative act that can be interpreted as, for instance, escape from unbearable circumstances or expectations, or as a desperate protest or rebellion against family and/or societal oppression and abuse. Both the act and the chosen method seem to communicate something. Hjelmeland recommends that it might be fruitful across contexts to interpret suicidal behaviour within the framework of communication theory.

Introduction

The WHO (2014) declares suicide to be a major public health problem in every country of the world. However, suicide rates vary enormously across regions, countries, communities, and cultures, as well as by, for instance, age, sex, ethnicity, and religion (e.g. Canetto, 2015; Mars et al., 2014; Vijayakumar et al., 2005a, b; WHO, 2014).

Epidemiology

Suicide

The WHO (2014) estimated that 804,000 people worldwide took their own lives in 2012. This represents an annual global age-standardized suicide rate of 11.4/100,000 population (15.0 for males and 8.0 for females). However, there are numerous reasons to assume that suicide is under-reported. Many countries do not have reliable registration systems, and a number of factors may influence definitions and recording practices. For a detailed overview of suicide rates in each of WHO's 172 member states, see the report *Preventing Suicide. A Global Imperative* (WHO, 2014).

The WHO (2014) estimates the average suicide rate to be a little higher in high-income countries (12.7/100,000 population) compared to low-income countries (LMICs; 11.2/100,000). However, the average suicide rate per 100,000 population in LMICs varies greatly across the globe and is estimated to be highest in Southeast Asia (17.7), followed by Europe (12.0), Africa (10.0), western Pacific (7.5), eastern Mediterranean (6.4) and the Americas (6.1). Three quarters (76%) of all global suicides occur in LMICs with almost half (47%) of the global number of suicides occurring in China and India only (WHO, 2014).

Within-Country Variations in Suicide Rates

Suicide rates also vary greatly between groups or regions within countries. For instance, rates are higher in some minority groups compared to the majority population. One example is that the suicide rate among the Inuit of Arctic Canada is ten times higher than for the rest of Canada (Kral, 2012).

Europe has over the past decades become increasingly multicultural due to immigration, and currently immigrants and ethnic minorities make up more than 10 per cent of the population in many European countries (van Bergen *et al.*, 2015). At the time of writing, the proportion of immigrants is likely to increase substantially in many European countries due to the ongoing influx of refugees from countries in the Middle East and Africa. In their meta-analysis of associations between immigrant and country of birth suicide rates, Voracek and Loibl (2008) found a positive correlation for 45 nationalities in seven host countries. This indicates that immigrants carry their risk of suicide to their new countries. This might, however, vary across sub-groups.

With regard to within-country *regional* variation, Patel *et al.* (2012) found that in India, for example, suicide rates varied substantially between the states, and in general were nearly ten times higher in the states in the south compared to some of the states in the north. There are also urban–rural differences in suicide rates. In high-income countries urban–rural differences are in general relatively small and vary by location, whereas the rural suicide rates in India and China are more than double the urban rates (Phillips and Cheng, 2012). Based on all this, suicide rates at national level may be relatively uninformative.

Suicide Rates by Sex and Age

Three times as many men take their lives compared to women in high-income countries, whereas 1.5 men to each woman take their lives in LMICs (WHO, 2014). The male:female ratio of age-standardized suicide rates varies from 3.5 in high-income countries to 1.6 in LMICs. Among LMICs, the male:female ratio is highest in Europe (4.1) followed by the Americas (3.6), Africa (2.5), Southeast Asia (1.6), and eastern Mediterranean (1.4), with western Pacific countries having an inverse gender ratio (0.9; WHO, 2014). Although the male suicide rates are higher than the female rates in general, there are some exceptions. Also, some community studies in Muslim-majority countries, for example, Bangladesh, Iran, Iraqi Kurdistan, Pakistan and Turkey, have found the suicide rate to be higher for women (particularly for young women) than for men (see Canetto, 2015, for references). In China, the female suicide rate was previously higher than the male rate, but the sex difference has gradually decreased and from 2006 on the male rate has exceeded the female rate, although the difference is not statistically significant (Zhang *et al.*, 2014). Marecek and Senadheera (2012) found that the national male:female ratio of 3.47:1 in Sri Lanka (a predominantly Buddhist country) concealed a striking interaction between gender and age in that the male:female ratio for people 20 years and under was 0.76:1, that is, a reversal of the overall gender difference. This might also be the case elsewhere.

In general, the suicide rate is lowest among children (< 15 years of age) and highest among the elderly (70+). However, this varies across regions and in some countries the suicide rate is highest among the young. The suicide rates in elderly women and young adults are much higher in LMICs compared to their counterparts in high-income countries, whereas the suicide rates in middle-aged men are much higher in high-income countries compared to what they are in LMICs (WHO, 2014). Globally, suicide is the *second* leading cause of death in people 15–29 years old. However, suicide is *the leading cause of death* among 15–29-year-olds of both sexes in high-income countries as well as in LMICs in Southeast Asia (WHO, 2014).

Suicide Rates by Religion

The suicide rate is estimated to be lower in Muslim-majority countries compared to non-Muslim-majority countries, and is also typically low among Muslims in non-Muslim-majority countries (Canetto, 2015). In a cross-national study, Shah and Chandia (2010) found a negative correlation between the suicide rate and the proportion of Muslims in a country.

Reported Suicide Rates Should Be Treated with Caution

All estimates reported here should be treated with caution bearing in mind the many potential reasons for under-reporting, which is also likely to vary by, for instance, religion and gender. For instance, suicide rates are likely to be under-reported in Muslim societies because of Islam's strong condemnation of suicide, but the size of the under-reporting may vary by gender (Canetto, 2015). The agency implicit in a Muslim woman's suicide is challenging the authority of both God (only God has the right to take life) and men (who are supposed to control women) (Billaud, 2012; Dabbagh, 2012; Rasool and Payton, 2014), and might therefore be disguised to avoid making public men's failure to control women. Hence, women's suicides may be camouflaged as an accident, for instance, accidently falling down a well. However, there are also indications of over-reporting of women's suicide in that some of them actually are disguised homicides (see Canetto, 2015 for examples).

Also in India (a predominantly Hindu country), the number of suicides for married women is likely to be under-reported because the husband or his family may be held responsible if the suicide occurs within 7 years of marriage (Patel *et al.*, 2012). Several studies of women's death by self-burning from countries in Asia and Africa point to political and cultural issues in practices of registering causes of death (Canetto, 2008). Such deaths usually result from having caught fire while working near a household open stove or kerosene lamps. Since they typically involve young, recently married women following dowry or other disputes with in-laws, the lines separating suicide from accidents and homicides may be blurred (Canetto, 2008).

Non-Fatal Suicidal Behaviour

There is no consensus with regard to concepts, definitions, or how to classify self-injurious behaviours and there are no internationally accepted methods for standardization of recording non-fatal suicidal acts. It is commonly estimated that the number of attempted suicides is 10–20 times higher than the number of suicides. These estimates are, however, based on hospital-based data on *medically treated* acts of self-harm. There are hardly any national, or nationally representative, registrations of non-fatal suicidal behaviour (WHO, 2014), and many do not contact the health services after harming themselves. Some reports have suggested that there are 50–300 times as many non-fatal suicidal acts as there are suicides (Tatz, 2005/2012).

Willingness to report or record suicidal acts may vary by age, sex, religion, culture, etc. For instance, in some Muslim or patriarchal societies women's suicidal behaviour is likely to be under-reported either to protect women from social and/or legal consequences of the suicidal act, or to protect male family members from the public embarrassment connected to women's suicidal behaviour (Canetto, 2015). Moreover, attempted suicide still is illegal in 25 countries. In addition, 20 countries following Islamic or Sharia law may also punish people who attempt suicide without having a specific

statute. Penalties range from a small fine to imprisonment for a few years or for life (Mishara and Weisstub, 2016). This is likely to affect the reliability of registration practices in terms of under-registration.

Based on the above, it seems difficult both to assess and compare rates of non-fatal suicidal behaviour across regions, countries and local communities. In general, however, females are found to engage in non-fatal suicidal behaviour more often than males, but there are a number of exceptions in different regions of the world (Canetto, 2008).

Methods of Suicide

Choice of suicide method varies between population groups, but the most common methods worldwide are ingestion of pesticides, hanging and use of firearms (WHO, 2014). Self-poisoning by means of substances other than pesticides, jumping from heights, self-immolation, drowning, sharp objects and moving objects are other common suicide methods used to varying degrees in different population groups.

Choice of method is commonly assumed to depend on access, but emerging research suggests that cultural acceptability (Canetto, 2008) and cultural meanings (message value) of the method may be more important than mere availability (Canetto, 2015). For example, in the Kurdistan region of Iraq, Rasool and Payton (2014) found that self-burning should be interpreted as 'a communicative act with an indigenous semiology which functions as an expression of subordinated agency within a male-dominated society' (p. 237). In a society where women are denied control over their bodies, their choice of self-burning as the suicide method can be interpreted as reclaiming disputed territory, by means of completely destroying the body (Rasool and Payton, 2014). Another example is that hanging has culture-specific symbolic meanings of martyrdom, injustice and pathos for Aborigines in Australia (Tatz, 2005/2012).

Risk Factors for Suicide

The most common risk factors for suicide are previous self-harm, mental disorders (particularly depression), alcohol or drug abuse, somatic illness, unemployment, relationship break-up, family history of suicidal behaviour, exposure to suicidal behaviour by others and in the media, lack of social network, and availability of means (Hawton and van Heeringen,

2009). Although most of the evidence base for this is from high-income countries, some studies in LMICs have indicated that risk factors for suicide may be universal (e.g. Vijayakumar and Rajkumar, 1999). However, as research from LMICs has emerged to an increasing degree, conventional beliefs about suicide are seriously challenged. Risk factors for suicidal behaviour are indeed found to be culture specific, which means we 'cannot make inferences about the suicidogenic potential of an adversity without considering its meaning for particular individuals, given their sex, age, culture, and other social factors' (Canetto, 2008: 263).

Negative/stressful life events are considered to increase the risk for suicide everywhere, but their nature differs between high-income countries and LMICs (Vijayakumar et al., 2005a). Vijayakumar et al. mention social change as an example of a risk factor that may have more influence in LMICs than in high-income countries. However, this has also been found in minority groups in some high-income countries (e.g. Kral, 2012). Risk factors also vary considerably between immigrants and the majority population. For example, whereas many of the common risk factors, such as psychiatric disorders and previous self-harm, have a lower impact on suicidality, family problems, social isolation, acculturation difficulties, discrimination, and racism are commonly reported as risk factors among immigrants (Heredia Montesinos, 2015).

What is a *risk* factor in some communities/cultures may in fact be a *protective* factor in others. For instance, research from high-income countries has found being married a *protective factor*. However, being married was found to be a *risk factor* for suicidal behaviour among Muslim women in community studies in Bangladesh, Iran, the Kurdistan region of Iraq and Pakistan (see Canetto, 2015, for references). Also in India, a predominantly Hindu country, being widowed, divorced or separated correlated with a decreased suicide risk for women (Patel et al., 2012). Similar findings have also been reported in some studies from China (Phillips and Cheng, 2012).

What is found to be risk or protective factors also seem to vary by research method. For example, quantitative studies commonly find religion/religiosity to be a protective factor (Mars et al., 2014), whereas a qualitative study from Ghana, a highly religious (predominantly Christian) society, found that some attempted suicide because they were disappointed with God. They felt they had fulfilled their religious obligations and could therefore not understand why God still allowed them to suffer (Akotia et al., 2014).

Mental disorder as a risk factor for suicide deserves special attention. Based mainly on psychological autopsy studies (PA-studies hereafter) conducted mostly in high-income countries, one of the most established 'truths' in suicidology is that at least 90 per cent of suicides are preceded by a mental disorder, and a causal link between the two is implied (Cavanagh et al., 2003). This conventional belief has been challenged by research in LMICs as well as by qualitative research in high-income countries. A study from India found mental disorder in only 23% of the suicide cases (Rao et al., 1989), whereas studies in China found mental disorder in between 48% (Zhang et al., 2010) and 63% (Yang et al., 2005) of suicides. Yang et al. (2005) found mental disorder among only 39 per cent of young rural women. Chan et al. (2001) emphasized that a high suicide rate combined with a low prevalence of psychiatric disorders in China challenge the conventional view of a strong relationship between the two as found in 'the West'. All this prompted Phillips (2010) to ask whether it was time to rethink the role of mental disorder in suicide. Also studies in African countries have found low proportions of mental health problems in suicides (Mars et al., 2014).

The main evidence base for the 90 per cent statistic is PA-studies, which in fact are methodologically flawed as a diagnostic tool (Hjelmeland et al., 2012). In such studies, psychiatric diagnoses of the deceased are made based on interviews with a few of the bereaved, often many years after the suicide. However, many of the diagnostic questions asked in such interviews cannot be *reliably* answered by anyone other than the person to be diagnosed. And, if the questions cannot be answered *reliably*, the diagnoses made simply cannot be *valid*. In other words, even in 'the West' we do not have a *valid* evidence base for the common belief that almost all those who die by suicide suffer from one or more mental disorders, with the inherent causal implications (Hjelmeland et al., 2012). Also, a register-based study from Australia found that less than half of those who had died by suicide had a diagnosis of mental disorder (Judd et al., 2012). Several recent *qualitative* PA-studies from high-income countries as well as LMICs are also challenging the presumed important/causal role of mental disorder in suicide (Kizza, 2012 in Uganda; Kjølseth,

2010 in Norway; Owens and Lambert, 2012 in the UK; and Rasmussen, 2013 in Norway).

Problems with Risk Factor Research

Suicide research has for decades been dominated by quantitative risk factor research, despite all the inherent problems in such research (Hjelmeland, 2016). 'Cultural' suicide studies have traditionally been in the form of cross-national comparisons with the huge cultural differences within the countries compared ignored (Hjelmeland, 2010). When researchers find differences across the groups (or nations) compared, they state that 'cultural factors' have influenced the suicide rate (e.g. Portzky and van Heeringen, 2007). Thus, culture is viewed in an essentialist form that is rendered explanatory power. That is, the differences are described as *caused* by culture. This is problematic (Berliner, 2001).

First, 'culture' is not a measurable variable (Jenkins, 1994). Therefore, culture cannot be included in quantitative analysis in any meaningful way. Second, even though some argue that culture can be *represented* by a number of measurable 'cultural factors', it is difficult to 'decide which variables represent "culture" and should therefore not be controlled, and which variables do not, and should be controlled' (Medin *et al.*, 2007: 620). In other words, it is difficult to determine what 'cultural factors' actually are. Berliner (2001) maintains that when culture is granted explanatory/causal power, peoples' social and/or political life circumstances are erased. To contextualize peoples' life situation, we should talk about oppression, marginalization, racism, unemployment, stigmatization, etc., rather than culture.

Furthermore, there is hardly any limit as to what we can find to *be* a risk factor, if we go looking for it in correlational studies (Hjelmeland and Knizek, 2016a). However, what *all* risk factors have in common is that the vast majority displaying them does not take their life (Hjelmeland, 2016). According to Tatz (2005/2012: xxv), 'masses of statistics and catalogues of "at risk" factors provide neither insight nor comprehension'. Thus, risk factor research contributes little to our *understanding* of what suicidal behaviour *means* for those who are suicidal. For that, we need contextualized research; research taking the socio-cultural context into consideration in the analysis (Hjelmeland, 2010; Kral, 2012). Here, qualitative research comes to the fore (Hjelmeland and Knizek, 2010). Also, comprehensive reviews summarizing and contextualizing

findings from a large number of studies are of value here. Some examples from studies in different socio-cultural contexts are outlined in the following.

Meanings of Suicidal Behaviour in Different Socio-Cultural Contexts

'All cultures have canonical narratives of suicide, that is, taken-for-granted storylines that provide members of the culture with meaning systems for understanding suicides' (Marecek and Senaheera, 2012: 59). As outlined earlier, suicide in 'the West' is considered closely connected to, even caused by, mental disorder. Such attempts at mono-causal explanations of suicide have, however, been challenged by researchers in LMICs (e.g. Marecek and Senadheera, 2012) as well as in 'the West' (e.g., Hjelmeland *et al.*, 2012). Suicide should not be studied, since it cannot be understood, apart from the cultural, social and political contexts that provide its patterns and meanings. As qualitative research contextualizing the suicidal behaviour has emerged, this critique gains support (Hjelmeland and Knizek, 2016b). A number of examples are presented in the following, but first it should be emphasized that with the limited space available it is impossible to do full justice to the different contexts where each of the studies are conducted; contexts that are crucial in order to *understand* suicide in the respective study sites. For this, I therefore refer to the original sources.

First, an illustrative example from northern Uganda where we perhaps can say that social change played a central role for at least some suicides, and where the qualitative nature of the study allowed a deeper insight into contextualized details. This was a qualitative PA-study conducted among the Acholi (predominant ethnic group in the area) in internally displaced peoples' camps (IDP camps). There, suicide was found to be connected to the changes in gender roles and responsibilities enforced by a two decades long civil conflict between the Lord's Resistance Army and the Ugandan government. Because of this conflict, two million people had been forced to live in IDP camps under horrific conditions for about 10 years (Kizza, 2012).

Before the conflict, traditional gender roles prevailed in this area. That is, the husband was the breadwinner and head of the household with the right to make all decisions for the family, whereas the wife was to be humble, submissive and responsible for taking care of the husband and children. For a number of reasons, these traditional gender roles were changed in the camps. Because the men could not leave the camps to tend to their cattle (their source of income and wealth), women had to take over the role as breadwinners. However, the husband kept his role as head of the household. In this context, suicide in both men (Kizza *et al.*, 2012a) and women (Kizza *et al.*, 2012b) could be connected to men's 'loss of masculinity' (Kizza, 2012). The changes in context meant that men could no longer live up to the ideal masculine expectations, which meant they were no longer regarded as *real* men. This 'loss of masculinity' seems to have led to a fatal loss of dignity/self-worth and social value for some men (Kizza *et al.*, 2012a).

In a review contextualizing findings from all the research conducted to date on male suicide in Uganda, Knizek *et al.* (2014) concluded that what seems to drive some Ugandan men to suicide is when their aspiration towards normative masculinity is hindered by insurmountable obstacles, for instance, in the form of poverty, disease, lack of education, the colonial history and globalization. The reality on the ground (life circumstances) is changing faster than are the socialization practices. During all their lives, boys and men are socialized into aspiring to the traditional ideal role of masculinity. The gender roles and responsibilities are changing, but the psychological ability or willingness to adjust, seems to develop at a much slower pace (Knizek *et al.*, 2014).

Men's 'loss of masculinity' was also found to be significant for women's suicide in northern Uganda (Kizza *et al.*, 2012b). Whereas the men seemed to have lost their power as breadwinners, the women had gained power in that they had taken over this role. This made them unwilling to continue in their expected submissive role. However, challenging the traditional cultural norms led to violence and abuse from their husbands. This was aggravated by the men's increasing alcohol abuse, perhaps in an attempt to restore their lost masculinity (Kizza, 2012). The husbands had resorted to spending the wife's hard earned money on drinking and womanizing, and in the end they had even taken on a second wife explicitly against the first wife's will. Thus, men's quest for their 'lost masculinity', and women's attempt to fight for their rights being perceived as a cultural transgression, contributed to women's suicides (Kizza, 2012).

In this northern Ugandan context, young men's suicide seemed to be related to not being *able* to live up to the socio-cultural norms and expectations, whereas young women's suicide seemed to be related to not *wanting* to live up to these expectations (Hjelmeland and Knizek, 2016b; Kizza *et al.*, 2012a, 2012b). Thus, these women's suicides can be interpreted as a *protest* against the worst excesses of masculine domination.

The findings from Uganda are in keeping with what was found in many of the studies included in the 2012 special issue on suicide of the journal *Culture, Medicine and Psychiatry*. The studies therein were from India (Kerala), Mexico (among the Chol Mayan indigenous people), Sri Lanka (Madampe Division), Afghanistan (Kabul), Palestine (Ramallah region of the West Bank), Canada (among the Inuit of Arctic Canada), South Africa (Lowveld), UK (England) and Singapore (for references, see Staples and Widger, 2012). The socio-cultural and political contexts around the suicides described in these different studies are indeed very different, as are the various *meanings* of suicide. Still, there are some remarkable similarities in terms of how suicide can be interpreted or understood across many of the contexts (Staples and Widger, 2012).

Importantly, gender roles and responsibilities stood out as important in terms of understanding suicide in that consequences of *hegemonic masculinity* seemed to play an important role in the suicides of both men and women, albeit in different ways. Across different contexts, suicide in men could be interpreted as a means to *escape* when they were unable to live up to the traditional ideals of masculinity, or to escape from the constraints of masculine expectations (Staples and Widger, 2012). This has been found, for instance, in Uganda (Kizza *et al.*, 2012a; Knizek *et al.*, 2014), Ghana (Adinkrah, 2012), South Africa (Niehaus, 2012), Ireland (Cleary, 2012), and Australia (Alston, 2012). Suicide in women, on the other hand, could be interpreted as a *protest* against the worst excesses of masculine domination (Staples and Widger 2012), like, for instance, violence, drinking and womanizing (Kizza *et al.*, 2012b).

The Ugandan women's suicides can, however, also be interpreted as *escape*. When challenging the traditional cultural norms of submission, their husbands responded with severe violence. They could, however, not leave their husbands since that would entail their parents having to pay back the dowry, which was impossible due to abject poverty. They found themselves trapped in an intolerable situation, and their only way out, literally, was suicide (Kizza *et al.*, 2012b). Thus, women's suicides in this context could be interpreted both as a *desperate protest* and *escape*.

The Ugandan Acholi are predominantly Christian, but this finding is also in keeping with what was found in Canetto's (2015) comprehensive review of suicidal behaviour among Muslim women. This review included studies of suicidality in Muslim-majority countries (studies from 25 countries in Asia, Africa and the Middle East) as well as Muslim communities in non-Muslim-majority countries (the Netherlands, France and Israel). Canetto (2015) found a unique script of Muslim women's suicidality as a *desperate rebellion against*, or *escape from*, the suffocating restrictions and abuse women have to endure within their families and societies.

Family problems (e.g. quarrels with family members or marital conflict) are commonly found to be a risk factor for women's suicidality in Muslim countries and communities. One can then, erroneously, get the impression that the suicidal act is an over-reaction to ordinary family conflicts (Canetto, 2015). This is definitely a danger in risk factor studies, where researchers, at best, *speculate* as to *how* the risk factors found are related to suicide (Hjelmeland, 2016). However, such problems can actually be quite severe, difficult or impossible to escape from, and common among young women who are poor, uneducated or undereducated, and/or live in rural areas. Examples of such severe and inescapable family problems are:

> forced juvenile marriage, often to much older men; being forbidden to marry men of their own choosing; polygamy; early withdrawal from school; being prohibited the pursuit of paid work; close surveillance of their every behaviour; confinement to the house; bearing and raising a large number of children; family and social harassment for giving birth to girls only or for not producing children; having to serve the husband's extended family; addiction of the husband; difficulties in obtaining divorce; discrimination following a divorce; as well as emotional, physical, and/or sexual abuse by family members.
> (Canetto, 2015: 450–451)

When suicidal behaviour is contextualized like in the examples above, it becomes evident how limited is the common emphasis on the importance of mental disorders for suicidal behaviour (Hjelmeland and Knizek, 2016b). In case of severe oppression, it makes little sense to focus on the role of mental disorders in suicidal behaviour. Some of the women may,

of course, have a mental disorder, but even in those cases it may be triggered or made worse by the oppression they suffer, and the focus should therefore be on the oppression rather than on a potential disorder. And the mental disorder per se may have little or nothing to do with the suicide (Hjelmeland and Knizek, 2016b). Canetto (2015) maintains that rather than medicalizing Muslim women's suicidality, that is, reducing it to a mental disorder in keeping with the biomedical model, it should be viewed through a *human rights lens*.

For some, suicide may in fact be the *only way out* of family and/or social oppression and abuse. This has now been found across a multitude of socio-cultural contexts, as shown in the examples here, and also, for example, in rural China where married women's suicide is considered an act of *rebellion and revenge*, particularly against abusive husbands and/or in-laws (e.g. Meng, 2002). In the absence of other means of influence and self-determination, suicidal behaviour may be a culturally scripted way for women 'to speak out against and escape the suffocating restrictions and abuse they experience in their families and societies' (Canetto, 2015: 451).

Some suicide studies among ethnic minority groups point to social change as an important factor and also here qualitative studies have contributed more contextualized knowledge. The main example outlined below is a study by Kral (2012) among the Inuit of Arctic Canada, but many of the findings are similar to what Tatz (2005/2012) found in his studies of suicide among Aborigines in Australia and Māoris in New Zealand. Tatz (2005/2012: xxii) maintains that 'To understand Aboriginal suicide, one has to understand Aboriginal history: their way of life has been destroyed, resulting in loss of structure, cohesion and meaning.' The same goes for suicide among the Inuit in Canada.

The suicide rate among the Inuit of Arctic Canada is among the highest in the world and ten times higher than the suicide rate in the rest of Canada (Kral, 2012). Kral found that suicide was related to the colonial social changes induced in Inuit communities by the Canadian government in the 1950s and 1960s. Inuit were then relocated to aggregated settlements run by government workers. Children were taken away to schools, some of which were run by Catholic missionaries, who abused many of the children sexually. Many of those who were taken away from their parents to attend residential schools, later developed problems with alcohol and domestic violence. Kral (2012) refers to these schools as 'assimilation factories' that created gaps between the children and their parents, and further maintains that the colonialism dramatically changed parenting among the Inuit. Traditionally, parents learned parenting skills from the older generation. This is, however, not the case for today's middle-aged adults, who were raised in residential schools.

Colonialism not only affected the relationship between children and their parents, but also romantic relationships. Kral (2012) describes suicidal young men not only feeling rejected by their parents, but also by their girlfriends. They developed possessiveness previously unknown in this context and became controlling and jealous. Kral wonders whether the young men perceive rejection by a girlfriend as a loss of masculine control and describes suicide in this context as 'communication of anger, a protest, and a form of revenge' (Kral, 2012: 318).

Concluding Remarks

It is evident how important for the development and meaning(s) of suicidality are the relational and socio-cultural and structural contexts in which people live. Suicide research in 'the West' has for decades been dominated by the biomedical model, where the search for risk factors in general, and mental disorders in particular, is central (Hjelmeland, 2016). The result has been a dominant understanding of suicide as a consequence of or caused by mental disorder (Cavanagh *et al.*, 2003; Goldney, 2015). Qualitative research contextualizing suicide has shown the limitations of such a perspective, and not only in 'non-Western' socio-cultural contexts. In traditional PA-studies, psychiatric diagnoses are based on a few of the bereaved's speculations about diagnostic questions which in many cases they cannot possibly answer with certainty on behalf of the deceased (Hjelmeland *et al.*, 2012). However, if the bereaved are allowed to speak freely about what *they* think was central to the suicide, as is the case in *qualitative* PA-studies, the picture becomes entirely different.

A clear example of this is a PA-study from England. In the first part of this study the informants answered diagnostic questions and 68 per cent of the deceased were assigned a psychiatric diagnosis (Owens *et al.*, 2003). When the narrative part of the interviews with the same informants was analysed qualitatively, however, it transpired that few spoke of psychiatric

disorders as being central to suicide (Owens and Lambert, 2012). Also in two qualitative PA-studies from Norway, one on suicide among young men (Rasmussen, 2013) and one on suicide among elderly people (Kjølseth *et al.*, 2010), the researchers found that the informants placed little emphasis on mental disorders in their narratives about what was central to the deceased's suicide. Few informants had seen signs of serious mental illness (Rasmussen, 2013), and many explicitly stated that the deceased had *not* been depressed (Rasmussen, 2013; Kjølseth, 2010). In her qualitative PA-study on suicide in northern Uganda, Kizza (2012) found mental disorder in only 1 of the 20 cases. This is in stark contrast to the conclusion drawn in most quantitative PA-studies and therefore challenges the established notion that suicide is mainly a consequence of mental disorder.

As emphasized by Staples and Widger (2012: 199), 'suicidal behaviour does not begin with the "precipitating factor" and end with the "suicidal act", but extends deep into individual and collective pasts and futures'. Hence, to increase our understanding of a suicide, we have to take the whole contextualized life history of the deceased into consideration in the analysis, which is not done in mainstream risk factor research. When the life history is taken into consideration in the analysis, suicide seems to a large extent to have more to do with existential issues than mental ill health (Hjelmeland and Knizek, 2016b).

Tatz (2005/2012) called his book *Aboriginal Suicide Is Different*. This was in order to dissociate Aboriginal suicide from the dominant biomedical understanding in 'the West'. He maintained that the medical model was inappropriate for Aboriginal suicide, which should rather be understood in the context of historical colonial relations. Aborigines have their own unique 'origins, backgrounds, histories, socialization, cultural milieu, family structures, experiences of racial discrimination, and alienation' (Tatz, 2005/2012: 145); a context crucial within which to understand Aboriginal suicide. The examples above, however, indicate that it is the narrow focus on quantitative risk factor research in 'the West', research that completely disregards the context that has lead to the monolithic understanding of suicide related to mental disorders. When qualitative suicide studies now are emerging, the importance of *context* for the understanding of suicide *everywhere*, including in 'the West', becomes obvious (Hjelmeland and Knizek, 2016b).

Contextualized suicide research across a number of very different socio-cultural and political contexts around the world finds different and culture-specific *meanings* of suicide. Some remarkable similarities across contexts have, however, also been found. Consequences of hegemonic masculinity seem important in many suicides for both men and women, albeit in different ways (Andinkrah, 2012; Alston, 2012; Cleary, 2012; Kizza *et al.*, 2012a, 2012b, Knizek *et al.*, 2014; Niehaus, 2012). Suicide clearly is a relational communicative act that can be interpreted as, for instance, *escape* from unbearable circumstances or expectations, or as a *desperate protest* or *rebellion* against family and/or societal oppression and abuse (Canetto, 2015; Staples and Widger, 2012). Since both the act and the chosen method seem to communicate something, it would be fruitful across contexts to interpret suicidal behaviour within the framework of communication theory; theory sensitive to cultural context (Knizek and Hjelmeland, 2007).

Culture is a complex concept with numerous different definitions beyond the scope of this chapter to discuss (for such a discussion, see Hjelmeland, 2010). Here, cultural aspects of suicide have been discussed by looking at it in different socio-cultural contexts, which then has illuminated various contextual understandings of suicide. However, we should perhaps talk about oppression, abuse, violence, racism, marginalization, etc., rather than culture or 'cultural factors' as contributors to suicide, although some of what is leading to, for instance, oppression, might be embedded in particular cultural norms.

References

Adinkrah, M. (2012). Better dead than dishonored: masculinity and male suicidal behavior in contemporary Ghana. *Social Science and Medicine*, **74**, 474–481.

Akotia, C. S., Knizek, B. L., Kinyanda, E. and Hjelmeland, H. (2014). 'I have sinned': understanding the role of religion in the experiences of suicide attempters in Ghana. *Mental Health, Religion and Culture*, **17**(5), 437–448.

Alston, M. (2012). Rural male suicide in Australia. *Social Science and Medicine*, **74**, 515–522.

Berliner, P. (2001). Transkulturel psykologi. Fra tværkulturel psykologi til community psykologi. [Transcultural psychology. From cross-cultural psychology to community psychology]. *Psyke and Logos*, **22**, 91–112.

Billaud, J. (2012). Suicidal performances: voicing discontent in a girl's dormitory in Kabul. *Culture, Medicine and Psychiatry*, **36**, 264–285.

Canetto, S. S. (2008). Women and suicidal behavior: a cultural analysis. *American Journal of Orthopsychiatry*, **78**(2), 259–266.

Canetto, S. S. (2015). Suicidal behaviors among Muslim women: patterns, pathways, meanings, and prevention. *Crisis*, **36**(6), 447–458.

Cavanagh, J. T. O., Carson, A. J., Sharpe, M. and Lawrie, S. M. (2003). Psychological autopsy studies of suicide: a systematic review. *Psychological Medicine*, **33**, 395–405.

Chan, K. P. M., Hung, S. F. and Yip, P. S. F. (2001). Suicide in response to changing societies. *Child and Adolescent Psychiatric Clinics of North America*, **10**(4), 777–795.

Cleary, A. (2012). Suicidal action, emotional expression, and the performance of masculinities. *Social Science and Medicine*, **74**, 498–505.

Dabbagh, N. (2012). Behind the statistics: the ethnography of suicide in Palestine. *Culture, Medicine, and Psychiatry*, **36**, 286–305.

Goldney, R. D. (2015). The importance of mental disorders in suicide. *Australian and New Zealand Journal of Psychiatry*, **49**(1), 21–23.

Hawton, K. and van Heeringen, K. (2009). Suicide. *The Lancet*, **373**, 1372–1381.

Heredia Montesinos, A. (2015). Precipitating and risk factors for suicidal behavior among immigrants and ethnic minorities in Europe: a review of the literature. In *Suicidal Behaviour of Immigrants and Ethnic Minorities in Europe*, ed. D. D. Van Bergen, A. Heredia Montesinos and M. Schouler-Ocak. Göttingen: Hogrefe, pp. 27–43.

Hjelmeland, H. (2010). Cultural research in suicidology: challenges and opportunities. *Suicidology Online*, **1**, 34–52.

Hjelmeland, H. (2016). A critical look at current suicide research. In *Critical Suicidology. Transforming Suicide Research and Prevention for the 21st Century*, ed. J. White, I. Marsh, M. J. Kral and J. Morris. Vancouver: UBC Press, pp. 31–55.

Hjelmeland, H. and Knizek, B. L. (2010). Why we need qualitative research in suicidology. *Suicide and Life-Threatening Behavior*, **40**(1), 74–80.

Hjelmeland, H. and Knizek, B. L. (2016a). Going in circles, getting nowhere? A critical look at current suicide research. Paper presented at 'Suicidology's Cultural Turn, and Beyond', Prague, 19–20 April.

Hjelmeland, H. and Knizek, B. L. (2016b). Qualitative evidence in suicide: findings from qualitative psychological autopsy studies. In *Handbook of Qualitative Health Research for Evidence-Based Practice*, ed. K. Olson, R. A. Young, I. Z. Schultz. New York: Springer Science+Business Media, pp. 355–371.

Hjelmeland, H., Dieserud, G., Dyregrov, K., Knizek, B. L. and Leenaars, A. A. (2012). Psychological autopsy studies as diagnostic tools: are they methodologically flawed? *Death Studies*, **36**, 605–626.

Jenkins, J. H. (1994). Culture, emotion, and psychopathology. In *Emotion and Culture*, ed. S. Kitayama and H. R. Markus. Washington DC: American Psychological Association, pp. 307–335.

Judd, F., Jackson, H., Komiti, A., Bell., R., Fraser, C. (2012). The profile of suicide: changing or changeable? *Social Psychiatry and Psychiatric Epidemiology*, **47**, 1–9.

Kizza, D. (2012). Suicide in post-conflict Northern Uganda. A qualitative psychological autopsy study. PhD thesis. Trondheim: Faculty of Social Sciences and Technology Management, Norwegian University of Science and Technology.

Kizza, D., Knizek, B. L., Kinyanda, E. and Hjelmeland, H. (2012a). Men in despair: a qualitative psychological autopsy study of suicide in northern Uganda. *Transcultural Psychiatry*, **49**(5), 696–717.

Kizza, D., Knizek, B. L., Kinyanda, E. and Hjelmeland, H. (2012b). An escape from agony: a qualitative psychological autopsy study of women's suicide in a post-conflict Northern Uganda. *International Journal of Qualitative Studies in Health and Well-Being*, dx.doi.org/10.3402/qhw.v7i0.18463.

Kjølseth, I. (2010). Control in life – and in death. An understanding of suicide among the elderly. PhD thesis. Oslo: Faculty of Medicine, University of Oslo.

Knizek, B. L. and Hjelmeland, H. (2007). A theoretical model for interpreting suicidal behaviour as communication. *Theory and Psychology*, **17**(5), 697–720.

Knizek, B. L., Kinyanda, E., Hjelmeland, H. (2014) Suicidal behavior in Ugandan men. In *Suicide in Men. How Men Differ from Women in Expressing their Distress*, ed. D. Lester, J. F. Gunn III, and P. Quinnett. Springfield, IL: Charles C. Thomas Publisher, Ltd.

Kral, M. (2012). Postcolonial suicide among Inuit in Arctic Canada. *Culture, Medicine, and Psychiatry*, **36**, 183–203.

Marecek, J. and Senadheera, C. (2012). 'I drank it to put an end to me': narrating girls' suicide and self-harm in Sri Lanka. *Contributions to Indian Sociology*, **46** (1&2), 53–82.

Mars, B., Burrows, S., Hjelmeland, H., and Gunnell, D. (2014). Suicidal behaviour across the African continent: a review of the literature. *BMC Public Health*, **14**, 606.

Medin, D. L., Unsworth, S. J. and Hirschfeld, L. (2007). Culture, categorization, and reasoning. In *Handbook of Cultural Psychology*, ed. S. Kitayama and D. Cohen. New York: Guilford Press, pp. 615–644.

Meng, L. (2002). Rebellion and revenge: the meaning of suicide of women in rural China. *International Journal of Social Welfare*, **11**, 300–309.

Mishara, B. L. and Weisstub, D. N. (2016). The legal status of suicide: a global review. *International Journal of Law and Psychiatry*, **44**, 54–74.

Niehaus, I. (2012). Gendered endings: narratives of male and female suicides in the South Africa Lowveld. *Culture, Medicine and Psychiatry*, **36**, 327–347.

Owens, C. and Lambert, H. (2012). Mad, bad or heroic? Gender, identity and accountability in lay portrayals of suicide in late twentieth-century England. *Culture, Medicine and Psychiatry*, **36**, 348–371.

Owens, C., Booth, N., Briscoe, M., Lawrence, C. and Lloyd, K. (2003). Suicide outside the care of mental health services: a case-control psychological autopsy study. *Crisis*, **24**(3), 113–121.

Patel, V., Ramasunarahettige, C., Vijayakumar, L., *et al.* (2012). Suicide mortality in India: a nationally representative survey. *The Lancet*, **379**, 2343–2351.

Phillips, M. R. (2010). Rethinking the role of mental illness in suicide (Editorial). *American Journal of Psychiatry*, **167**, 731–733.

Phillips, M. R. and Cheng, H. G. (2012). The changing global face of suicide. *The Lancet*, **379**, 2318–2319.

Portzky, G. and van Heeringen, K. (2007). Cultural aspects of suicide. In *Textbook of Cultural Psychiatry*, ed. D. Bhugra and K. Bhui, Cambridge: Cambridge University Press, pp. 445–458.

Rao, A. V., Mahendran, N., Gopalakrishnan, C., *et al.* (1989). One hundred female burn cases: a study in suicidology. *Indian Journal of Psychiatry*, **7**, 330–333.

Rasmussen, M. L. (2013). Suicide among young men: self-esteem regulation in transition to adult life. PhD thesis. Oslo: Faculty of Social Sciences, University of Oslo.

Rasool, I. A. and Payton, J. L. (2014). Tongues of fire: women's suicide and self-injury by burns in the Kurdistan region of Iraq. *The Sociological Review*, **62**, 237–254.

Shah, A. and Chandia, M. (2010). The relationship between suicide and Islam: a cross-national study. *Journal of Injury and Violence Research*, **2**, 93–97.

Staples, J. and Widger, T. (2012). Situating suicide as an anthropological problem: ethnographic approaches to understanding self-harm and self-inflicted death. *Culture, Medicine and Psychiatry*, **36**, 183–203.

Tatz, C. (2005/2012). *Aboriginal Suicide Is Different. A Portrait of Life and Self-Destruction.* Canberra: Aboriginal Studies Press.

Van Bergen, D. D., Heredia Montesinos, A. and Schouler-Ocak, M. (2015). Introduction. In *Suicidal Behaviour of Immigrants and Ethnic Minorities in Europe*, ed. D. D. Van Bergen, A. Heredia Montesinos and M. Schouler-Ocak. Göttingen: Hogrefe, pp. 1–10.

Vijayakumar, L. and Rajkumar, S. (1999). Are risk factors for suicide universal? *Acta Psychiatrica Scandinavica*, **99**, 407–411.

Vijayakumar, L., John, S., Pirkis, J. and Whiteford, H. (2005a). Suicide in developing countries. Risk factors. *Crisis*, **26**(3), 112–119.

Vijayakumar, L., Nagaraj, K., Pirkis, J. and Whiteford, H. (2005b). Suicide in developing countries. Frequency, distribution, and association with socio-economic indicators. *Crisis*, **26**(3), 112–119.

Voracek, M. and Loibl, L. M. (2008). Consistency of immigrant and country of birth suicide rates: a meta-analysis. *Acta Psychiatrica Scandinavica*, **118**, 259–271.

WHO (2014). *Preventing Suicide. A Global Imperative.* Luxembourg: WHO Press.

Yang, G.-H., Phillips, M. R., Zhou, M. G., *et al.* (2005). Understanding the unique characteristics of suicide in China: national psychological autopsy study. *Biomedical and Environmental Sciences*, **18**, 379–389.

Zhang, J., Xiao, S. and Zhou, L. (2010). Mental disorders and suicide among young rural Chinese: a case-control psychological autopsy study. *American Journal of Psychiatry*, **167**, 773–781.

Zhang, J., Sun, L., Liu, Y., Zhang, J. (2014). The change in suicide rates between 2002 and 2011 in China. *Suicide and Life-Threatening Behavior*, **44**(5), 560–568.

Chapter

38

Intellectual Disabilities across Cultures

Sabyasachi Bhaumik, Rohit Gumber, Shweta Gangavati
and Satheesh Kumar Gangadharan

Editors' Introduction

Intellectual disability has been known by different names in different countries, some commonly used terminologies are: mental retardation, learning disability, intellectual disability, mental handicap/disability, developmental disability and mental deficiency/subnormality. However, of late the preferred term has been intellectual disability which is described as a condition of arrested or incomplete development of the mind. It is characterized by impairment of skills manifested during the development period, which contribute to the overall level of intelligence i.e. cognitive, language, motor and social abilities. Bhaumik *et al.* in this chapter remind us that in epidemiological research, severity of intellectual disability is mostly defined on the basis of cognitive skills and International Classification of Diseases (ICD-10). However, this is historically based on statistical distribution of IQ scores. There is no doubt that intellectual disability is perhaps the most common developmental disorder. Inevitably it has major impact on not only the individual who has an intellectual disability but also on their carers and families and broadly on the society as well. This affects intellectual functioning and different cultures see it in different ways. Bhaumik *et al.* in this chapter go on to describe three areas of adaptive functioning which impact a person's ability to perform: (i) the ability to conceptualize which includes the ability to use language, read and write, mathematical skills, general knowledge, memory and reasoning; (ii) the ability to socialize which is demonstrated by the person being able to empathize with others, make social judgements, make appropriate interpersonal communication, make and keep friendships; (iii) the ability to perform practical tasks and to manage oneself in areas such as money, finding and holding a job, taking part in recreational activities, caring for personal appearance and hygiene and being able to organize school or work related activities. Cultures

have different attitudes to people with intellectual disability and also different sets of aetiological factors as well as management strategies.

Historical Perspective

> A nation's culture resides in the hearts and in the souls of its people.   (Mahatma Gandhi)

Historical perspectives were aptly described in detail in the previous edition of this chapter written by Jean O'Hara and Nick Bouras (2007). We have summarized this in the following section with the addition of other materials.

The earliest reference to intellectual disability dates back to the Egyptian Papyrus of Thebes in 1552 BCE (Harris, 2005). Hippocrates, in the late fifth century BCE proposed that intellectual disability was caused by an imbalance in the four humours of the brain (blood, yellow bile, black bile and phlegm) and may present as slow mental state. Greeks, on the other hand, believed that the birth of the child with an intellectual disability was God's way of punishing the parents. In Sparta, if the child were to be born deformed then it was supposed to be left to perish on a mountainside or in a chasm. The Romans also believed that people with intellectual disabilities should neither be granted Greek or Roman citizenship nor have any political rights.

With the advent of Christianity, the beliefs around human life began to change, especially in the light of the philosophy that any life is precious. This was particularly influenced by a strong view against infanticide but at the same time the main reason behind this was the concern for the parents' souls rather than the infant itself. This resulted in the setting up of hospitals and orphanages in Rome. St Nicholas, the Bishop of Myra was particularly known to be kind towards children with intellectual disability. However, contrary views existed; Martin Luther, who was the founder of Protestantism in the sixteenth century, is said to have stated 'take the changeling child to the river and drown it' (Shorter, 2000). The concept of 'changeling child' around that time was based on a folklore belief that a fairy child had been left in place of a human child stolen by the fairies.

Islamic society in the seventh century took the view that people with intellectual disability had their minds in heaven while their body moved around amongst ordinary mortals which resulted in people with intellectual disability being treated with respect and therefore being protected as well. However, Aminidav and Weller (1995) stated that Middle Eastern cultures regarded disability as a punishment from heaven, emanating from the spirits and caused by an evil eye.

Cheng and Tang (1995) describe that the Chinese traditions of praying to ancestors, seeking supernatural powers and having forbearance helped in dealing with the fate of having an intellectually disabled child.

Gabel's (2004) transcultural study concluded that the Hindus believed intellectual disability was God's gift. Similarly, the philosophy of 'Karma' is based on the belief that intellectual disability is a result of past life and may be described as 'suffering through' which is ordered by God as an opportunity to be released from the bond of rebirth. For the majority of people living in the Indian subcontinent, disabilities are believed to be of supernatural causation (Agrawal, 1994).

It was frequently assumed that Asian parents did not have a positive encouraging attitude towards disability because of their religious or superstitious beliefs (Shah, 1992) which resulted in under-use of resources that are available. This is further emphasized by a study by Channabasavanna *et al.* (1970) who found that Asian parents have the notion of curability and also the concept that marriage of the person with intellectual disability may cure the condition. Hence, it is not uncommon for Asian parents to disengage with professionals after the initial consultation which may not offer solutions that the parents were expecting.

As reflected in the historical perspectives, approaches to people with intellectual disability vary across different cultures in modern society as well. This is evidenced in a number of studies that looked at the cultural variations in societies' outlook towards this condition.

Table 38.1 Differences in attitude and beliefs of Asian and white British families

Asian British families
Had more contact with a 'holy' person ($p < 0.05$)
Were less aware of what their child's problem is called ($p < 0.01$)
Believed in a spiritual explanation/cause for their child's intellectual disability ($p < 0.05$)
Fifty per cent said that they did not know the cause of their child's intellectual disability
Believed that religion had something particular to say about intellectual disability ($p < 0.05$)
Their faith helped them to cope but offered little social or practical support
Wanted care to be provided by a relative when they were no longer able to provide it themselves ($p < 0.01$)

White British families
Most received a medical explanation for their child's disability
None offered a spiritual explanation for their child's disability
Only one felt that they did not know the cause of the child's intellectual disability
Religion/faith offered social support
Most wanted their child to be cared for in a community home provided by statutory/voluntary services ($p < 0.05$)

A study by Fatimilehin and Nadirshaw (1994) compared differences in attitudes and beliefs of white British and Asian families, and emphasized a finding that white British families were more accepting of a medical explanation of their child's disability (see Table 38.1).

Socio-Cultural Influence on the Presentation of Intellectual Disability

A significant proportion of those with moderate to profound intellectual disability suffer from underlying genetic conditions. However, the majority of people with intellectual disability have multifactorial causation. Down's syndrome is a genetic condition seen across all cultures and is easily recognizable due to its specific morphological features. Historically, this condition has been recognized in earlier civilizations with the first reference to it from the Neolithic period.

The term intellectual disability includes a heterogeneous group with wide ranging abilities and the main confusion comes in distinguishing those who have borderline and mild intellectual disability. The former may be reflective of an underperformance which has resulted from socio-cultural and educational disadvantages. People with intellectual disability have a higher risk of comorbidities including physical health condition such as epilepsy, and mental health problems. The latter are reported to be three to four times more common in those with intellectual disability (Cooper et al., 2007).

Race, ethnicity and culture influence the presentation of mental illness in all, but especially in those with intellectual disability (Hassiotis, 1996). Mental illness has been extensively studied in different cultures and societies, however, presentation of mental illness in those with intellectual disability in different cultures has not been explored through research processes to the same extent. Ethnic and cultural issues determine the use of health and mental health services in different countries and unless the issues of cultural diversity and historical perspectives are understood well by practising clinicians, the uptake of services may remain less than optimal. In addition, migration has brought in a different dimension and the complex relationship between migration and mental illness may or may not apply in the same way for those with intellectual disability.

For Western countries, with a higher educated population and better understanding of intellectual disability, parents seek support and help early whereas in low- and middle-income countries (LMIC), despite significant increase in the number of educated citizens, there is still reliance on traditional approaches to cure and care for these individuals. Some educated parents approach faith healers, religious leaders or seek herbal remedies in addition to seeking help from health professionals. The most recent trend has been linked with parents seeking help for educational underachievement of their child in urban areas whereas the pattern of seeking help through faith healers etc. remains the main approach with most of the rural population.

Influence of Culture on the Epidemiological Aspect of Intellectual Disability

Conceptual and practical difficulties with the definition make prevalence data for intellectual disabilities between ethnic groups and from communities around the world difficult to establish. Gabel (2004) describes difficulties when there is no Hindu word for the concept; 'disabled means without a limb, so "learning disabled" would mean without learning'. Other Hindi terms have slightly different meanings, such as 'weak brain' (dimaagi se kamzori), 'sick mind or intellect' (dimaagi bimaari) and 'slow intellect' (mundh buddhi). Mundh buddhi literally translated applies to a person who has bad desires (buddhi) of the heart (mundh). Bad desires means that the person has wanted and pursued something that is unhealthy, sinful or dangerous. Clearly, this is not what is meant by intellectual disabilities or mental retardation. Therefore, we may use similar words, but understand them differently; or we may use different words to talk about the same things without recognizing that we are doing so.

Intellectual disability prevalence rates vary according to the definitions, meanings and classification systems used. Harris (2005) reported the prevalence of intellectual disability to vary between 1 and 3 per cent, globally. A large meta-analysis of population-based studies was carried out by Maulik et al. (2011). The review included studies published between 1980 and 2009 and included data from populations throughout the globe, including a range of low-, middle- and high-income countries. The meta-analysis estimated the global prevalence to be 10.37/1,000 population, a figure similar to previous studies conducted. The rates vary according to the income of the country, with highest prevalence seen in low-income (16.41/1,000) and middle-income (19.94/1,000) countries, where the rate was most twice that in high-income countries (9.21/1,000). Emerson (2012) conducted a cross-sectional survey to identify an association between ethnicity (amongst other factors) and identification of intellectual and developmental disability using data that was extracted from a school census from England. The results showed a marked difference in the association between ethnicity and intellectual disability depending on the severity of the disorder. Less severe forms of intellectual disability were identified at much lower rates within ethnic minority groups, except for the Gypsy/Romany and Irish Traveller groups. In contrast to international studies, lower rates of milder intellectual disability were found in all of the other groups including African, Asian, South Asian and mixed heritage living within England. The rates of more severe intellectual disability were similar throughout the ethnic groups with very few statistically significant differences. The exceptions were children of Pakistani and Bangladeshi heritage, who were more likely to have severe and profound intellectual disability, and similarly the Gypsy/Romany and Irish Traveller groups who were more likely to have severe disability. These results took into account the effects of household social economic status, and area-level deprivation.

Epidemiological rates of severe intellectual disability are not dissimilar amongst most ethnic groups. Variations in the rates in international population-based studies may be explained by difference in diagnostic practices and tools used and differences in recruitment of cases to studies (Bakel et al., 2014). Religious and legal systems within a country may impact on rates, for example abortion is illegal in Ireland and many Islamic countries (except for medical reasons) and the religious views of Christians and Muslims within the Gypsy/Romany and Irish Traveller and Pakistani and Bangladeshi communities, respectively may also impact rates of termination and therefore affect rates of intellectual disability. But this does not fully account for the variation found globally. A number of factors are associated with an increased risk of intellectual disability, including prenatal causes such as genetic and congenital malformations and exposure to toxins, postnatal causes such as those related to childhood infections and the physical and psychological growth of the child and perinatal factors such as those related to infections and delivery-related causes (Maulik and Harbour, 2010). Higher rates in LMIC can be explained by low resources impacting on all of the causes highlighted earlier. There may be more births and higher hereditary illness due to lack of antenatal screening methods. This may also lead to lack of early diagnosis and treatment of conditions such as phenylketonuria. Low rates of antenatal consumption of vitamins, iodine and folic acid also contribute to higher rates of conditions such as neural tube defects and congenital hypothyroidism. Children under five in developing countries are exposed to multiple risks, including poverty and malnutrition, poor health and unstimulating home environments, which can impair cognitive, motor and socio-emotional development (WHO, 2011). Sanitation, malnutrition and lack of access to healthcare are all highly variable around the world, for example WHO (2011) estimated that only 36 per cent of people in Bangladesh had access to adequate sanitation, and only 63 per cent of those in Thailand were consuming iodine. Poor maternal and child healthcare services and lack of immunization programmes contribute to intrauterine growth retardation, higher birth-related infections and injuries, infectious disease and vitamin and mineral deficiencies in children (Maulik et al., 2011). Infectious diseases account for a significant burden of disease in LMIC (Mercadante et al., 2009) and these include diseases with neurological consequences such as meningitis, encephalitis, and childhood cluster diseases – such as measles, mumps and poliomyelitis. Furthermore, non-communicable chronic diseases such as diabetes, cardiovascular disorders and respiratory illness have a profound effect on disability and may also impact on intrauterine child development. Increased use of tobacco and alcohol in rapidly developing countries may also account for some of the burden of intellectual disability (WHO, 2011). Major environmental changes, such as those caused by natural disasters or conflict situations affect the prevalence and outcome of intellectual disability. Inadequate provision of health and social services to identify and support those with intellectual disability leads to poor outcomes like poor health, low educational achievement and high rates of poverty.

Identification of Intellectual Disability and Access to Services across Cultures

The assessment and the recognition of intellectual disability are primarily based on measures of IQ. However, in LMIC with lack of access to professional resources it may be extremely difficult to get an IQ assessment carried out. As a result, generally there is a move towards assessment through measuring adaptive functioning. Some international scales to measure adaptive functioning exist including Vineland Adaptive Behaviour Scales (Vineland™) and Adaptive Behaviour Assessment System (ABAS®). These scales are reliable and valid and have been used in large numbers of populations with intellectual disability.

However, they may falsely record under-performance due to underlying differences in cultural practice. Such scales therefore usually need modifications in relation to the prevailing culture of the country, and some of these initiatives have already been started globally. Owing to the general lack of healthcare resources and personnel, the primary port of call for help-seeking behaviours in these populations in LMIC are medical officers or the health visitors of health centres. These busy clinicians often do not have the opportunity or time to carry out a detailed assessment, hence there is a need for the development of a shorter scale, which is culturally fair and can be administered within a short period of time. One such scale (GLAD) is currently being piloted through the Royal College of Psychiatrists (RCPsych) Faculty of Psychiatry of Intellectual Disability in conjunction with some LMIC like Sri Lanka, India and Pakistan. The scale has already been piloted in some European countries such as Austria and Poland.

Intellectual disabilities of severe to profound degree can always be easily identified through their manifestations. Problems may arise in identifying those with mild/borderline intellectual disability (emergent intellectual disability). The help-seeking behaviour that currently prevails in different cultures may indicate a call for help in relation to physical health issues i.e. epilepsy, mobility problems or incontinence. Help is also often sought for behavioural issues which pose a challenge to the care-givers, but the main pattern of help-seeking behaviours in urban areas of LMIC is for educational underachievement of the child concerned.

For the vast majority of the population who live in rural areas of LMIC there appear to be fewer proactive approaches from the health professionals to recognize and support the management of intellectual disability, primarily due to the fact that many such professionals have not been trained in this area at all. Another key issue is to recognize the atypical presentations of underlying mental health problems for children and adults with ID, which quite often get missed. These individuals may not be provided with the opportunity for the management of underlying treatable conditions. Medical officers, health visitors, community practitioners and psychiatrists therefore need to be aware of how mental health problems may present in people with intellectual disability and what treatment approaches are available. Failure to recognize common conditions like depressive illness and anxiety disorder can lead to significant health morbidities which are reversible.

The lack of appropriate training and education for health professions is a pattern that has been noticeable in almost all LMIC and may sadly reflect a lack of socio-cultural priority for this area. However, in Western and developed countries, the socio-political environment assures strong support for children and adults with intellectual disability through development of government policies which lead to protection of these vulnerable individuals and set it as a social priority. The concerns are for those with intellectual disability living in LMIC, whose rights can be easily ignored and who may be deprived of receiving the right support and treatment for treatable conditions causing significant suffering (which many go through in silence). Many LMIC also lack in social effort to empower family carers and their suffering remains largely unaddressed, despite the best efforts of some NGOs.

Another issue which often is not addressed, related to sexually inappropriate behaviours due to lack of social understanding and boundaries in the person with intellectual disability. Help-seeking for such problems often takes the route of advice from religious and community leaders and support from broader organizations like the churches. Unfortunately many end up facing the criminal justice system for these behaviours. A number of individuals with mild/borderline intellectual disability who display unprovoked aggression may end up being incarcerated in prisons for years. There is some evidence that prisons throughout the world host a significant number of individuals with mild/borderline intellectual disability (Hellenbach *et al.*, 2017). In some countries steps have been taken to support and treat mental health problems amongst prisoners. However, many health professionals providing this support lack adequate training in dealing with intellectual disability and mental health problems. A solution to the problems may exist by providing mental health (mh) GAP training in intellectual disability for prison medical staff and eventually rolling out to all prison staff.

The WHO, the World Psychiatric Association (WPA) and RCPsych have developed training modules in intellectual disability (ID) (mhGAP-ID) for health professionals in LMIC, which aims to support the scaling up of services for intellectual disability. Modules are taught on key areas such as identification of intellectual disability, issues of diagnostic overshadowing when symptoms of mental health problems may be attributed to underlying intellectual disability and vice versa, and mental health problems in intellectual disability. This training has been successfully delivered by frontline staff in some areas of Sri Lanka, India and Pakistan. The hope is, that with 'training the trainers' modules these skills can be cascaded down to other frontline staff, especially within rural areas. Such training has been evaluated and has been found to be highly appreciated by its recipients (Gumber *et al.*, 2015).

Signposting to the appropriate professionals and seeking the right help for treatment will be crucial not only for this population but also for others who live in rural areas where there are no psychiatrists. The model for such care has been aptly described in a recent chapter by Bhaumik *et al.* (2016) for the book *Psychiatry in Practice*.

Services for ID across Cultures

Services vary widely across the globe with clearly delineated service support in Western countries to almost non-existent or rudimentary support in the majority of the LMIC. People with intellectual disability and their carers in most of the LMIC rely on the mainstream services which are themselves under-resourced. Professionals working in the mainstream services have very limited or no training to assess and manage health problems in people with intellectual disability, resulting in misdiagnoses and inadequate treatment. For the vast majority of the population in LMIC lack of professional support and training can be compensated through the provision of mhGAP training in intellectual disability in a systematic manner making the necessary cultural adjustments to the modules depending on the spiritual and belief system in the country. The service model is a pyramid of care where the frontline assessment and signposting can take place in primary and subsidiary health centres with a clear link with secondary care services (see Figure 38.1).

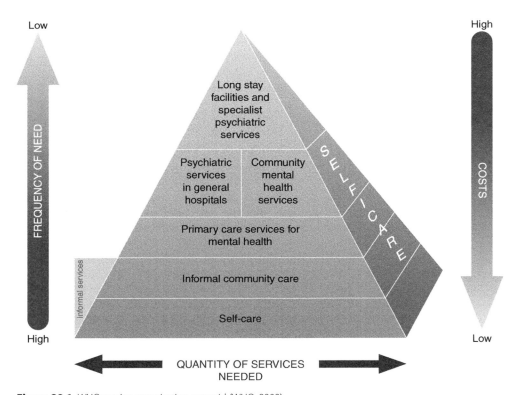

Figure 38.1 WHO service organization pyramid (WHO, 2009)

The link to secondary care services can happen through a process of referral or through the arrangement of weekly mobile clinics. The access to services can only be improved through the creation of a system of support for different levels of complexities. Educational establishments are becoming more aware of the need for recognition and support for those with intellectual disability in addition to the recognition of co-existing developmental disorders such as ADHD and/or ASD. Schools in LMIC always encourage input from professionals to improve recognition and treatment for such individuals, and health visitors and community practitioners can effectively link themselves with educational establishments to ensure support for the school children.

Due to lack of sufficient support through the public sector, LMIC rely on parents/carer initiatives as well as non-governmental organizations (NGOs). Active engagement with NGOs can be helpful for both healthcare services and family carers. Many NGOs are taking proactive steps of going out to the places where provision of health service is lacking. This, however, needs wider publicity and support from the healthcare staff to bring about a system change for a positive impact. There are seldom any respite care facilities which exist for individuals with intellectual disability in LMIC, however day-care centres and residential homes are beginning to be established mainly in response to the urban population demands and therefore these facilities are primarily located in the big cities only. The sociocultural perception determines the use of such facilities and it is unlikely that a mixed sex accommodation, whether for residential care or respite care, in LMIC will be accessed by many including offspring of some highly educated parents. Intellectual disability is still considered to be a social issue in many countries and therefore is more often linked to the policies produced by the department of social services which largely ignore the key health and mental health issues these individuals suffer from.

Cultural beliefs and expectations especially in the vast rural populations in LMIC across the globe vary widely as highlighted in the previous section of this chapter. The religious and cultural beliefs can be supportive for a person with intellectual disability in terms of social acceptance and social role valorization (Wig *et al.*, 1981). Through this, many gain supported employment but many still remain subject to possible abuse by others on occasions. The beliefs and stigma,

on the other hand might incarcerate a person who may be kept confined largely to the family care home with few opportunities to receive education, skills development support and integration. Abuse may occur in such situations, and may encompass physical, emotional and sexual areas which are reported fairly widely, with examples of individuals being chained, not being fed properly and lacking in basic resources including that of access to clothes and basic rights. Such abuses often go unrecognized and are kept confined within the family setting. Resolving these significant issues may not be easy, however, one good approach might be to make health professionals aware of how to recognize the signs and symptoms that would suggest underlying abuse. Such competencies can be acquired through training and there is also a useful WPA document on child sexual, physical and emotional abuse and intellectual disability which is likely to be published this year with needed core competencies identified (WPA Action Plan).

Carers

In the first national UK survey of adults with intellectual disabilities, those from black and Asian communities reported they were more likely to be unemployed, poor, see their friends less often, have poor health and be sad or worried. In addition, adults with intellectual disabilities from the Asian community had less privacy, felt less confident and felt left out (DoH, 2005). Whilst there are, of course, ethnicity factors per se, such as different culturally sanctioned behaviours and belief systems, gender and family expectations, there are other factors linked to ethnicity, which may impact on the ability of families from BME communities to cope or engage with services. This can broadly be described as the 'minority experience' and includes aspects of everyday life such as living in poorer circumstances, the 'minority status', clashing cultures, dealing with loss and migration/immigration uncertainties, social and language barriers (Sue and Sue, 1999). The double discrimination of racism and stigma are pervasive in the lives of people with intellectual disabilities from these communities, yet there exists a strong sense of ethnic and racial identities amongst them (Azmi *et al.*, 1997).

Family carers play a central role for the person with intellectual disability and this is evident in all the cultures across the globe. The reaction of family carers after having a child with intellectual disability can range from being extremely supportive or over-protective to total rejection and isolation. More often than not, one of the parents restores the balance in these difficult situations. Families need to recognize that over-protective approaches may hinder the skills development and independence of the person. However, at the other extreme, rejection and stigmatization will damage the person significantly in all areas. The mainstay of support for people with intellectual disability especially in LMIC across the globe comes from the family carers and extended family members, in addition to the support which can be gained from NGOs and government initiatives. If we are to make any difference in the quality of care individuals with intellectual disability receive, we need our main thrust of initiatives focused and directed towards supporting family carers in order to reduce their burden of care and supporting life's journey for their children with intellectual disability. We mentioned before the importance of providing training to the frontline healthcare staff. One cannot minimize the major impact that can be created by providing the right training and support to the parents. Parental awareness of the underlying conditions and the best ways of managing health, mental health issues and developing skills for the individual should be the key focus for health professionals, if they wish to make any difference in the quality of care that the person with intellectual disability receives. Establishing parental support groups has been known to be very helpful and may create a platform for sharing views and learning from each other. Setting up parental support groups may not be seen as a priority initiative for many healthcare professionals but this may result in reduced demand on services in the long run. NGOs can be approached to make this happen.

Policy Development

With the context of community accessibility and fundamental rights, we need to refer to the foundations of health promotion laid out in the Ottawa Charter (Mahler et al., 1986). The key issues within these include, amongst others, enabling people with intellectual disability to make positive lifestyle changes, health screening for people with intellectual disability and making the lives of people with intellectual disability safer. Many countries have now accepted and adapted acts similar to that of the Disability Discrimination Act (UK) thereby empowering the

rights of individuals with intellectual disability and those with other disabilities. However, health promotion has not been seen as a priority in many LMIC, especially those lacking baseline services to manage underlying health and mental health problems for people with intellectual disability. The treatment gaps are significant in LMIC but initiatives around addressing the health inequalities for individuals with intellectual disability should not be ignored or forgotten. The main way of delivering this might be to develop global strategies that promote health amongst this population as a public health priority.

Achieving Cultural Competence

Addressing the needs of people with intellectual disabilities from black and minority ethnic (BME) communities has to be carefully planned due to the influence of socio-cultural factors in addition to the needs related to the presence of intellectual disability. People with intellectual disability from BME communities are often under-represented in the uptake of intellectual disability services. The government's 3 year strategy for people with an intellectual disability, Valuing People Now (DoH, 2009), emphasizes the need to make specific changes to ensure that the needs of people with intellectual disability are met, including those from BME backgrounds and emerging communities. It is reported that intellectual disability services are perceived in different ways by different communities, and that people with intellectual disability from BME groups experience stigma, prejudice, and often exclusion from their community. There is also a problem of trust, where potential BME service users and their carers fear engaging with services (Tonkiss and Staite, 2012). This may arise for many reasons, including that of a lack of culturally sensitive service provision. Some useful strategies for practice are outlined in Table 38.2.

In order to remove the barriers that prevent people with intellectual disability and their carers accessing appropriate support, it is important for them to have access to the right information which should be provided from the very beginning (when a child with disability is born). The process of informing the family of the child's disability, the immediate support provided as well as the ongoing provision of right information and support (both formal and informal support) enables or disables the support network around the individual with disability. People with intellectual disabilities often need lifelong contact

Table 38.2 Strategies for practitioners

Recognize the socially constructed nature of intellectual disability – without denying the biological reality of impairment

Recognize how different understandings and beliefs influence how people live their lives, the decisions they make for themselves and their children, and the outcomes they hope to see

Recognize that the individual, parents and families are already living with the reality of disability. An additional 'diagnosis', e.g. of a mental illness or epilepsy, may compromise already fragile coping strategies and informal support networks

Dialogue – to elicit not only assessment information but the family's cultural orientation

Use of professional interpreters

Use of cultural interpreters

Take care to avoid stereotyped or 'colour-blind' approaches

Address cultural tensions sensitively. They often involve basic ethics – keeping safe from physical, emotional and mental harm; living dignified lives; living with respect

Planning and approach to care in a person-centred way

Partnership with community groups

Develop skills in cross-cultural communication – one of the best skills to have is never to assume anything about cross-cultural beliefs until they are learned first-hand

Source: adapted from Gabel (2004); Raghavan and O'Hara (2005)

with services. Culturally sensitive service supports (O'Hara, 2003) reinforce collaborative relationships between parents and professionals, allowing a partnership to develop that will see the individual through the family life cycle, whilst helping to reduce the burden of care and consequent parental ill health.

References

Agrawal, R. (1994). India. In *Comparative Studies in Special Education*, ed. K. Mazurel and M. Winzer. Washington DC: Gallaudet University Press.

Aminidav, C. and Weller, L. (1995). Effects of country of origin, sex, religiosity and social class on breadth of knowledge of mental retardation. *British Journal of Developmental Disabilities*, **40**(80), 48–56.

Azmi, S., Hatton, C., Emerson, E. *et al.* (1997). Listening to adolescents and adults with intellectual disability in South Asian communities. *Journal of Applied Research in Intellectual Disability*, **10**, 250–263.

Bakel, M., Einarsson, I., Arnaud, C. *et al.* (2014). Monitoring the prevalence of severe intellectual disability in children across Europe: feasibility of a common database. *Developmental Medicine and Child Neurology*, **56**(4), 361–369.

Bhaumik, S., Kiani, R., Gangavati, S. *et al.* (2016). Management of intellectual disability. In *Psychiatry in Practice: Education, Experience and Expertise*, ed. A. Fiorillo, U. Volpe and D. Bhugra. Oxford: Oxford University Press, pp. 359–376.

Channabasavanna, S. M., Bhatti, R. S. and Prabhu, L. R. (1970). A study of attitudes of parents towards the management of mentally retarded children. *Child Psychiatry Quarterly*, **18**, 44–47.

Cheng, P. and So-Kum Tang, C. (1995). Coping and psychological distress of Chinese parents of children with Down's Syndrome. *Mental Retardation*, **33**(1), 10–20.

Cooper, S. A., Smiley, E., Morrison, J. *et al.* (2007). Mental ill-health in adults with intellectual disabilities: prevalence and associated factors. *The British Journal of Psychiatry*, **190**(1), 27–35.

Department of Health (2005). Adults with Learning Difficulties in England 2003/4. Full survey report. London: HMSO.

Department of Health (2009). Valuing People Now: a new three year strategy for people with learning disabilities. London: HMSO.

Emerson, E. (2012). Deprivation, ethnicity and the prevalence of intellectual and developmental disabilities. *Journal of Epidemiology and Community Health*, **66**(3), 218–224.

Fatimilehin, I. A. and Nadirshaw, Z. (1994). A cross-cultural study of parental attitudes and beliefs about learning disability (mental handicap). *Mental Handicap Research*, 7(3), 202–227.

Gabel, S. (2004). South Asian Indian cultural orientations toward mental retardation. *Mental Retardation*, **42**, 12–25.

Gumber, R., Gangavati, S., Cooray, S. and Bhaumik, S. (2015). mhGAP (mental health gap) Programme on People with Disorders of Intellectual Development (PWDID) (The Sri Lanka experience). *BJPsych International*, **12**, S19–22.

Harris, James C. (2005). *Intellectual Disability: Understanding its Development, Causes, Classification, Evaluation, and Treatment.* Oxford: Oxford University Press.

Hassiotis, A. (1996). Clinical examples of cross-cultural work in a community learning disability service. *International Journal of Social Psychiatry*, **42** (4), 318–327.

Hellenbach, M., Karatzias, T. and Brown, M. (2017). Intellectual disabilities among prisoners: prevalence and mental and physical health comorbidities. *Journal of Applied Research in Intellectual Disabilities*, **30**(2), 230–241.

Mahler, H., Epp, J., Franklin, W. and Kickbusch, I. (1986). Ottawa Charter for health promotion. *Health Promotion International*, **1**(4), 405.

Maulik, P. K. and Harbour, C. K. (2010). Epidemiology of intellectual disability. In International Encyclopaedia of Rehabilitation available online at http://sphhp.buffalo .edu/rehabilitation-science/research-and-facilities/fun ded-research-archive/center-for-international-rehab-res earch-info-exchange.html (accessed 25 May 2016).

Maulik, P. K., Mascarenhas, M. N., Mathers, C. D. *et al.* (2011). Prevalence of intellectual disability: a meta-analysis of population-based studies. *Research in Developmental Disabilities*, **32**(2), 419–436.

Mercadante, M. T., Evans-Lacko, S. and Paula, C. S. (2009). Perspectives of intellectual disability in Latin American countries: epidemiology, policy, and services for children and adults. *Current Opinion in Psychiatry*, **22**(5), 469–474.

O'Hara, J. (2003). Learning disabilities and ethnicity: achieving cultural competence. *Advances in Psychiatric Treatment*, **9**, 166–176.

O'Hara. J. and Bouras, N. (2007). Intellectual disabilities across cultures. In *Textbook of Cultural Psychiatry*, ed. D. Bhugra and K. Bhui. Cambridge: Cambridge University Press.

Raghavan, R. and O'Hara, J. (2005). Cultural diversity, mental health and learning disabilities. Chapter 18 and Training Module 18. In *Mental Health in Learning Disabilities*, ed. G. Holt, S. Hardy and N. Bouras. Brighton, UK: Pavilion.

Shah, R. (1992). *The Silent Minority: Children with Disabilities in Asian Families*. London: National Children's Bureau.

Shorter, E. (2000). *The Kennedy Family and the Story of Mental Retardation*. Philadelphia, PA: Temple University Press.

Sue, D. W. and Sue, D. (1999). *Counselling the Culturally Different: Theory and Practice*, 3rd edn. New York: John Wiley.

Tonkiss, K. and Staite, C. (2012). *Learning Disabilities and BME Communities: Principles for Best Practice*. Birmingham: University of Birmingham.

Wig, N. N., Murthy, R. S. and Harding, T. W. (1981). A model for rural psychiatric services: Raipur Rani experience. *Indian Journal of Psychiatry*, **23**(4), 275.

World Health Organization (2009). *Improving Health Systems and Services for Mental Health*. Geneva: WHO.

World Health Organization (2011). *World Report on Disability*. Geneva: WHO

Child Psychiatry across Cultures

Angela Glover, Niranjan Karnik, Nisha Dogra and Panos Vostanis

Editors' Introduction

Child rearing is very strongly influenced by cultures and these cultural patterns also define what is seen as normal or abnormal in childhood behaviours. Therefore clinical practice of child psychiatry will also be influenced by cultural factors which will include the development and funding of services. The childhood behaviours occur in the context of families and cultures, and balancing respect for variation and the need for universality is a key challenge. In many cultures and societies child psychiatry services focus up to a certain age range depending upon what age children finish school. The needs of children from different cultures will vary as will the parental and social expectations. However, it must also be recognized that there are individual cultural variations within each broad culture. The earlier chapter by Dogra and her colleagues set the scene in clinical matters related to child psychiatry across cultures. This chapter by Glover and colleagues provides an overview on management. These authors point out that good clinical practice in the West would involve valuing the child's perspective and ensuring their views were heard and accommodated, but how far this would work in other cultures remains questionable. Cultural values must be taken into account when planning any intervention, especially psychotherapies or family therapy. Ethnic and cultural variations be they biological or diet related will affect the impact of pharmacotherapy. Using attachment theory as an example, Glover *et al.* propose that addressing the child's attachment may take different forms across cultures and this too will depend upon the cultural and social context. Children's social networks will differ across cultures and the role of peers must be taken into account as this is significant in the development of a child's self-esteem and subsequent (adult) identity. Special attention must be paid to vulnerable and at risk children so that appropriate cultural interventions can be instituted.

The Management of Children in Cross-Cultural Context: Introduction

Practising child psychiatry across cultures is one of the most challenging and yet potentially gratifying areas of professional practice. The challenge comes from the fact that children are dynamic beings, whose developmental trajectory causes them to have a large degree of variability of behaviours; and these occur in the context of families with a seemingly endless degree of composition, structure and cultural context. The attentive clinician must, therefore, not only be careful to observe the child, but also to have a view of the family and the degree to which it is a part of a broader cultural milieu.

Accounting for cultural variation could potentially result in a specific approach to each cultural context for each psychiatric condition. Such an approach may be seen as daunting, because the amount of information that needs to be learned far exceeds anything that a single practitioner could absorb. Balancing respect for variation and the need for universality is, therefore, the core challenge for child psychiatry across cultures. In order to contend with this dilemma, we have favoured a cultural sensibility approach in our teaching and research (Dogra and Karnik, 2003; Karnik and Dogra, 2010). The stance of cultural sensibility attempts to place the practitioner in a position of learning about the cultural situation of the child and his or her family, and trying to use the clinical space for gaining the important information that will help guide culturally sensitive treatment. A great deal of additional information about the life of the child can also be gained by looking at the artefacts, toys and the nature of play that the child engages with in his or her everyday life (Mukherji, 1997).

Child psychiatry in its existence and approach varies across cultures. In North America and

Europe, specialist providers in child psychiatry are available, but continue to constitute a relatively limited group. The vast majority of behavioural problems faced by children are addressed by paediatricians, family and general practitioners, social workers and the non-statutory agencies. These structural differences in the professional disciplines providing care for children with psychiatric problems result in a wide variety of approaches.

In considering the management of childhood psychiatric disorders, it is important to emphasize resources. By developing world standards the Western world is embarrassed by therapeutic riches. However, there is the question of whether these are effectively utilized and whether the interventions are as cost-effective as they could be. In developing countries, pharmaceutical interventions may be the most cost-effective and socially acceptable treatments for mental health problems.

Good clinical practice in child psychiatry in much of North America, the UK and Europe would involve valuing the child's perspective and ensuring their views were heard and accommodated when planning the management. It is debatable how acceptable this would be in other parts of the world, where cultural contexts and the views of children differ as discussed in Chapter 26.

In another context, such respect for the child's views, especially if they differ from parental views, may be seen as undermining. Again, the issue of the role that children play in society is essential to consider when thinking about management.

In working with families of diverse backgrounds, Sue *et al.* (1996) suggest the following:

- Different theoretical models may need to be applied and integrated for different contexts.
- There is recognition that therapist and client identities are formed and embedded in multiple levels of life experiences and contexts, and understandably in cultures, therefore treatment needs to take into account the young person's experience in relation to their context.
- Multicultural therapy is enhanced when the therapist uses modalities and defines goals consistent with the life experiences and cultural values of the client.

Of course, the latter may be more difficult if young people hold values that are different from those held by their parents and grandparents. Garland *et al.* (2004) interviewed 170 adolescents, their care-givers

and their therapists to identify three desired outcomes for each stakeholder. The most commonly reported desired outcome across all three stakeholder groups was to reduce anger and aggression on an aggregate level. Almost two-thirds of the triads did not agree on even one of the desired outcomes for the adolescent's treatment when desired outcomes for individual cases were compared. Youths and therapists were each more likely than parents to report desired outcomes that related to the family environment; youths were the least likely to report desired outcomes that were related to youth symptom reduction. Essentially, there was a lack of agreement of the desired outcome among key stakeholders or desired outcome priorities for adolescent services. This lack of consensus may limit engagement in treatment and the effectiveness of care (Ronzoni and Dogra, 2012).

This chapter does not aim to review all of the available approaches, but instead focuses on the different domains available by the broad systems that children can encounter and the various perspectives that provide a way to understand childhood development and child psychiatry. The divisions between biological, individual, family and social modalities are artificial. Ideally, a combination of these approaches should be employed in order to maximize the potential benefits and outcomes.

Biological and Pharmacological Approaches

A biological perspective toward child psychiatric disorders is often a good starting point for considering the presentation of symptoms. Many psychiatric disorders have been shown to have strong biological transmission, including bipolar affective disorder (Duffy *et al.*, 2012) and schizophrenia (Hameed and Lewis, 2016). Even those that lack strong evidence for familial transmission are thought to have a biological component. In most instances, a risk accumulation model seems to provide the best explanatory system wherein biological risk factors add to social and individual risk factors to produce psychiatric morbidity (Steiner, 2004).

Children are in the midst of continuous and substantial biological change. The neurobiology of development is complex and has been detailed in a few thoughtful reviews (Post and Post, 2004; Rubenstein and Puelles, 2004). It is clear that there is a complex relationship between biology and environment.

Grossman and his colleagues have shown the powerful impacts that environmental factors play on the pruning of neural systems in animal models, and have presented very powerful arguments on the ways that environment and biology interact to produce psychopathology (Grossman *et al.*, 2003). As the neurobiology of development becomes clearer, the picture that emerges is one of complex systems of interaction, with neurodevelopment continuing well into the early twenties, and growth and loss of cells possibly occurring even later in life through systems of gene regulation and expression.

The range of biological interventions available to child psychiatrists is currently limited. The most accessible forms of interventions are pharmacological strategies. For children, the use of medication always requires a significantly higher level of consideration than in adults. Not only must the risks and benefits to the child be considered, but the views of the family and their beliefs about medications must also be taken into account. Far from being simply medication management, the approach must be one of pharmacotherapy, where medications are used within a broader therapeutic framework.

Among the most widely used agents for treatment of childhood psychiatric problems are selective serotonin reuptake inhibitors (SSRIs). These agents as a class have been widely used for the treatment of depression and anxiety disorders in adults. In the US, drugs from this class were approved for the treatment of childhood depression and obsessive–compulsive disorder. In 2004, the US Food and Drug Administration (FDA) followed the lead of the British Medicine and Healthcare Products Regulatory Agency a year earlier, in warning about increased suicidal ideation among children and adolescents taking SSRIs (Vitiello and Swedo, 2004; Wessely and Kerwin, 2004).

The availability of these medications outside North America and Europe is not as controlled. The costs of treatment for many people make the routine use of these medications difficult. The only antidepressants currently listed on the World Health Organization's *Model List of Essential Medicines* (2015) are an SSRI, fluoxetine, and a tricyclic antidepressant, amitriptyline. Tricyclic antidepressants, while efficacious, are also known to have side effects that are problematic to manage in children, and can be lethal in overdose.

The lack of data using cultural factors to study medication effects in children limits our ability to examine this issue fully and we now need to look to the adult literature to some degree. For bipolar affective disorder and schizophrenia in adults, biological interventions work very well and have significantly beneficial effects. Lithium has been the mainstay of treatment for bipolar affective disorder, and is relatively inexpensive and accessible. In addition to listing lithium, the *WHO Model List of Essential Medicines* (2015) also recommends valproate and carbamazepine as medications that countries should make available in their national formularies. Among antipsychotics, haloperidol, chlorpromazine, risperidone and fluphenazine are all listed. Interestingly, recent data showed that, while newer atypical antipsychotics have fewer side effects and may be safer than typical antipsychotics, adherence to pharmacotherapy was poor across all groups with olanzapine, with risperidone groups having slightly better adherence (Lieberman *et al.*, 2005). In the use of antipsychotics, one predictor of adherence that has been demonstrated in small-scale trials has been if the provider is of the same ethnicity as the patient (Ziguras *et al.*, 2001). In another study, schizophrenia patients who were black, female or over the age of 65 were at a higher risk of not adhering to their pharmacotherapy recommendations (Leslie and Rosenheck, 2004). These two findings may strengthen the argument that culture is an important variable in helping enable pharmacotherapy.

Cultural values need to be considered when employing any intervention strategy on behalf of children, but may be especially important when considering pharmacotherapy. While medications may be routine to prescribe for some practitioners, their use is likely to be a new experience for the child and his or her family. In addition, just as some families view medications as toxic (and indeed other professionals such as teachers), other families may perceive medications as not only necessary but somehow mystical or magical as well. The variety of views of medications and their role in treatment are likely to be affected by a number of factors in cultures that employ such practices, and as such it is important for the provider to gain some idea of how the family and child understand the medication and its role, including the risks and benefits.

Family Therapy

We begin by discussing family therapy because it is among the most established and the research in this domain has given the most attention to cultural factors, and hence why we devote significant space to this modality. There are different models of family therapy, which have developed over time. These have taken into account the changing roles of families and the changing structure of families within particular societies. It is important to acknowledge that many of the developments in family therapy work have come from Western perspectives. However, more recently, family therapy has been influenced by constructivism and social constructionism. These two are related but different concepts, and their links to post-modern theories have recently begun to challenge some of the orthodox thinking and techniques of systemic and psycho-dynamic practice.

The post-modern theories reject the notion that there is a single fixed truth or reality about individual or family process that needs to be developed or established. It suggests that each individual constructs his or her personalized views and interpretations of what the family might be experiencing together. This approach enables the importance of cultural diversity, and the multiple realities and acceptance of a wide range of belief systems to be considered. Constructivism stems from the biology of cognition, which argues that individuals have unique nervous systems that permit different assumptions to be made about the same situation. The argument is that our unique biology means that we respond differently to the same context. Social constructionism is similar in that it argues that there is no such thing as objective reality, but that what we do is constructed from what we observe; and arises from the language system, relations and cultures we share with others. This means that there is a more collaborative style of working. The focus is on helping the child or young person examine and reassess the assumptions individuals make about their lives, rather than focusing on specific patterns of family communication or roles. Using these approaches, therapists take the position of uncertainty and not knowing, and join the family to find workable solutions on an equal basis. Because this approach recognizes different values and perspectives that all individuals in the room may hold, it should be applicable to a wider range of contexts. However, if the family expects the therapist to take an expert position, they may be rather disconcerted when the therapist claims to have little expertise.

Family therapy can have a place in the treatment of many child mental health disorders and has been shown to be a very effective treatment modality (Stratton, 2005). In major psychiatric disorders it may be complementary to pharmaceutical interventions. It can also help in chronic conditions, helping families to understand how they can find workable solutions to make the best of whatever situation their lives are in. Canino and Inclan (2001) argued that clinicians often find the cultural dissonance between the culture of the families they see, and their own culture and theoretical approaches as potential obstacles for appropriate assessment and management. Hampson and Beavers (1996) indicated that functional rather than demographic variables, including ethnicity, were more important in predicting therapy outcome.

Kumpfer *et al.* (2002) argued that few family interventions have been adapted to be culturally sensitive for different ethnic groups. They reviewed five research studies that tested the effectiveness of the generic version of the Strengthening Families Program (SFP) compared to culturally adapted versions. Cultural adaptations that reduced dosage (that is the number of sessions), or eliminated critical core content to try and be culturally accommodating, increased retention of minority families up to 40 per cent but reduced positive outcomes. However, from this study it is unclear on what basis therapists made these adaptations, thus the authors concluded that additional research is required. Family therapy has been shown to be effective in helping families from as far apart as South America and Cambodia (Mitrani *et al.*, 2004; Rousseau *et al.*, 2004).

Brief strategic family therapy was found to be effective in Hispanic adolescents with conduct disorders and substance use (Santisteban *et al.*, 2003; Szapocznik and Williams, 2000), whilst multidimensional family therapy was found to be efficacious with unmarried African American mothers with adolescents with similar problems (Becker and Liddle, 2001). Jung (1984) argued that structural family therapy offers an appropriate treatment model for dysfunctional Chinese families as it enables the cultural emphasis on the family unit to be recognized. It also allows a problem orientated approach as opposed to one in which values are questioned. This was also reported for Puerto Rican families (Bird and Canino, 1982). Tamura and Lau (1992) emphasize that Japanese families might prefer a process of integration, that is, how a person can be effectively integrated into the given system, rather than a process of differentiation.

Individual Therapeutic Approaches

One of the most common approaches to child psychiatric problems is to engage in individual therapy with the child. For children, one-to-one therapy is rarely done exclusively with the child. Families need to be involved, regardless of whether the child is seen primarily alone or with parents present. The following sections briefly review a few of the many therapeutic approaches that are available and the ways that these interact with cultural factors.

Attachment-Focused Therapies

John Bowlby pioneered the study of early attachment in childhood. His studies are one of the anchors of modern child psychiatry. He posited that the reciprocal relationship between parent and child forms the basis of sound development for the child (Bowlby, 1979, 1988). Mary Ainsworth built on this work and expanded it to include the development of a series of typologies of childhood based on the nature of the attachment and early relationship between parent and child (Ainsworth, 1978). Interestingly, Ainsworth developed many of her theories by studying child-rearing practices in Uganda, and drew from these observations to form her theory of attachment (Ainsworth, 1967). For an excellent review of attachment theory and its implications, see the paper by Fonagy (1999).

When considering attachment theory through the lens of cultural psychiatry, it would be easy to hold with Ainsworth that this process is somehow universal. The post-modern turn has brought about a reconsideration of all theories that make this assumption. While it is likely that aspects of the attachment process are universal, there are likely to be cultural variants. In some cultures, child-rearing is a more community and kinship-based process that may have a small handful of parents caring for all of the children of the community. Attachment, in such contexts, is likely to take a different trajectory from that which happens in the Western dyad of mother and child.

Therefore, addressing the attachment of the child might take different forms, depending on the context. From a therapeutic standpoint, healing disordered attachment can be a challenging experience for the therapist. To do so in the context of cultural variables makes it even more challenging, but at this point employing a cultural sensibility model can help to ensure that therapy is provided in a sensitive and productive way, especially if that is consistent with the individual family's world view.

Play Therapy

The history of play therapy is long and complex, dating back to Anna Freud, who made specific comments about the meaning of play. Later Melanie Klein, Jean Piaget and D. W. Winnicott all expanded on notions of play and helped to establish traditions for interpretation of play in a therapeutic perspective. Children often spontaneously play when they find themselves in a group, but this is not the frame through which play therapy takes place. Cultural meanings of play may differ, and the types and natures of games can also vary. This is why it is important to make the objects, rules, artefacts and systems of play an object of scrutiny as a few scholars have argued (Hinman, 2003; Mukherji, 1997). Hinman asserts that even the decoration of the therapy room is important, as it could reflect individualist Western ideals or more interdependent ideals. The experience should be as natural as possible to the child, from the room decoration, to the material of toys, to the ethnicity of dolls.

Cognitive-Behavioural and Psychodynamic Therapies

Individual therapy with children can take many forms, including cognitive-behavioural and psychodynamic. The range and types of techniques available are manifold, and the two that we highlight here are simply examples of techniques that are popular in child mental health services. Cognitive-behavioural therapy (CBT) has good empirical support for its use in children and young people. The cornerstone of this technique lies in identifying disordered patterns of thought that are leading to affective dysfunction, and then showing the child how to reorient his or her thinking to achieve a more functional affective state. Many protocols exist for CBT, and there are versions that have a manualized form that can be completed in between 6 and 12 sessions. The literature surrounding CBT techniques for children and adolescents highlights their utility for treating obsessive–compulsive disorder, anxiety (Hudson *et al.*, 2015, Peris *et al.*, 2015), depression, and disorders of conduct (Erickson and Achilles, 2004).

Psychodynamic therapy for children and adolescents has a long history dating to its genesis with Sigmund Freud. Until the emergence of pharmacological treatments, this modality was the dominant school of treatment in the field of child psychiatry. It continues to exert a strong influence on the field, but the interest in it has fallen as the neurosciences and empirically based therapies have gained ascendancy. This has also evolved to a range of psychodynamic approaches. Nevertheless, this school of treatment continues to have valuable lessons to teach, especially the ways that therapists and patients interact in the encounter. These have relevance for the study of children (Fonagy, 2004; Loughran, 2004) by enabling children to openly express themselves and learn ways to reflect on their emotions as they emerged. This approach diverges significantly from the more structured approaches.

Globally, psychodynamic psychotherapy is likely to be one of the basic theoretical perspectives that all psychiatrists have had some exposure to during their training, even though its implications are culturally bound. Practitioners in this field will be far fewer, and for many providers outside Europe and North America, the applicability of psychodynamic theories may seem limited due to a lack of attention to specific cultural matters. Posed as another universal theory, psychodynamic psychotherapy has been revisited in light of culture, race and ethnicity and its implications have been explored in the context of many psychotherapeutic approaches (Tseng and Streltzer, 2001).

Children's Social Networks and Communities

Children grow and develop in a context of family, peers, community and broader social networks (Karnik, 2004). These networks are linked to family and group processes, and any attempt to intervene using these approaches must be cognizant of the connections among these levels of intervention (see Figure 39.1). They are not connected in the linear progression as depicted, but rather in complex and often overlapping ways.

Urie Bronfenbrenner is among the most widely known of theorists of the social environment that have been recognized within medicine and psychiatry. He divided the social environment into three spheres (Bronfenbrenner, 1979). The microsystem includes the immediate family, peers and local social institutions. A step further out from this level leads to the mesosystem in which he placed larger social institutions and broader cultural influences. Finally, there is the macrosystem which includes the global and international culture, as well as geopolitical events. Bronfenbrenner recognized that many social forces move between and among these levels and he was quite cognisant of the limitations of such a theory. Along related lines of thought, Lev Vygotsky proposed the idea of the zone of proximal development which he theorized as a time period during which children could be socialized given adequate social interactions (Vygotsky, 1978). Both these theorists conceptualized children as situated in multiple spheres of influence, with family being closer than other social institutions. In children's social development and in the development of their identity, peers play a crucial role. In cultural identity development, schools, universities and other institutions contribute to the way the individuals see themselves.

When considering community factors and social systems, some analysts have chosen to look at example programmes. Felton Earls, in his review of this area of child–community interaction, uses the Project on Human Development in Chicago Neighborhoods as an example of community-level analysis and intervention (Earls, 2001). Earls found that there was a series of links between 'neighborhood social organization, children's exposure to violence, and maladaptive aggression' (Earls, 2001: 701). He argued for two major pathways to address the needs of communities. One is to extend clinical interventions into the community using schools and other community-based organizations as a base from which to reach children in need of psychiatric care. The second involves a more grass-roots approach, whereby the capacities of communities to provide for children's needs on an ongoing basis are built and sustained.

Both of these approaches translate well into the complex needs of children across the globe. Cultural differences make it difficult to generate specific recommendations, but the general thesis that there

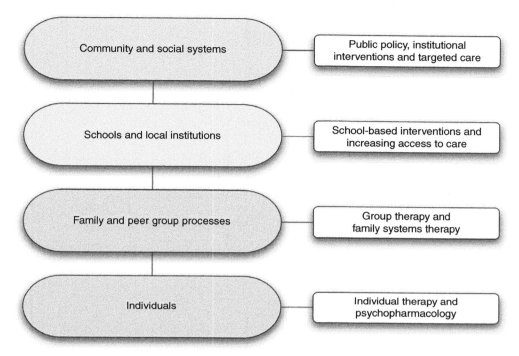

Figure 39.1 Levels of care and intervention for children

are two paths to helping communities and children continue to hold relevance (see Figure 39.2). Depending on the community, the relevant grass-roots providers may be teachers or clergy, or even shamans and local healers. In an urban, formerly homeless population, important community sectors-of-care could include domestic violence shelters or even supportive housing organizations. Though challenges exist because many grass-roots organizations simply do not have access to children's mental health resources (Shonkoff and Phillips 2000), Gewirtz and August (2008) explored the efficacy of an evidence-based mental health prevention programme in this population, focusing on supportive housing agencies to champion mental health prevention. Communities differ, and sectors that could be trained in child and adolescent mental health (CAMH) prevention are always changing. It is important keep in mind the rate of employee turnover in targeted grass-roots community sectors-of-care, as this can be a factor in the sustainability of implemented programmes (Glisson *et al.*, 2012). Urbanization, industrialization and globalization have changed roles and functions and the everyday geography of life, and thus

community-based interventions need to be geared to the local context.

In parallel, child mental health service providers need to be working to support people in the community who work with children by providing education and specialist knowledge. The range of providers who may be responsible for child mental health will vary by locale. There are difficulties in ensuring that there are enough appropriately trained clinical staff to meet the mental health needs of children given the increasing prevalence rates. In some countries (for example, Ethiopia), primary care staff allied to medicine are often trained to deliver this care as there are so few psychiatrists to do so. In these situations, child psychiatry may have a greater role in consultation and supporting staff rather than providing direct care. Increasingly, child mental health specialists are finding success by working in school based settings (Patel and Rahman 2015) as we discuss later.

In situations where there is no direct access to a child psychiatrist or a severe shortage, provision of services requires other staff such as general practitioners, pediatricians, or adult psychiatrists to develop special interests to ensure the mental health needs of

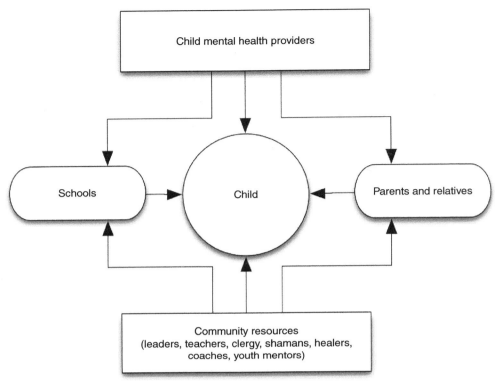

Figure 39.2 Pathways to supporting children

children are met. Another option may be to train up nursing staff or other staff (for example, teachers) who have access to families for other reasons such as delivering maternity or educational services, respectively. Training should allow staff to deliver care to the problems most encountered in their context. This requires applying the principles described in the following section. Clearly, it is important for staff to be supported and this may be done through links with centres that have child psychiatrists who are able and willing to provide consultation and support. There are examples of modern technology being used to provide support to those delivering frontline services and the potential of this in child mental health has yet to be fully realized.

Contextual or School-Based Approaches

The school is by far the most important institution outside the family that shapes the development of children. Globally, organizations like the United

Nations Children's Fund (UNICEF) have placed education at the top of their priority list of action areas because education has broad impacts on child health.

Earlier studies of school-based services documented their wide-scale efficacy and accessibility (Anglin *et al.*, 1996; Kaplan *et al.*, 1999; Kisker and Brown, 1996; Santelli *et al.*, 1996a; Walter *et al.*, 1995). Students generally support the notion of school-based services and reported that they found the level of care to be excellent (Santelli *et al.*, 1996b). With regard to child mental health, Flaherty and colleagues studied the history of the development of school-based mental health services and found that these programmes can have positive effects on both mental health outcomes as well as educational achievement (Flaherty *et al.*, 1996; Weist *et al.*, 1996). In one study, students that enrolled in a school-based mental health programme tended to be suspended for fewer days per month and be promoted to the next grade at a higher rate (Kang-Yi *et al.*, 2013). Interestingly, Farahmand *et al.* (2011) also found that school-based approaches targeting internalizing problems such as depression and other broad mental health tended to be more effective than those targeting externalizing problems. Schools have been used as the key point for the provision of services around the globe. UN agencies, governmental departments, and non-governmental organizations (NGOs) have all adapted and created programmes to provide services through the school systems. Child psychiatrists have increasingly embraced the school-based care model in recent years in the US (Joshi, 2004). The practicality of extending this model to other regions will be dependent on the extent of local resources, since these models do take the professional away from other sites of care. At the same time, efficient collaboration between schools and child mental health services can result in more efficient use of resources by avoiding duplication (Vostanis *et al.*, 2013).

Child Mental Health Service Models: Similarities and Differences across Cultures and Societies

In trying to establish commonalities in planning and developing service models, one needs to take into account the characteristics of different cultural groups, the structures and strengths of different societies, and the context of their welfare and health systems, including resource constraints (Vostanis *et al.*, 2015). There is also the need to take a multi-dimensional view of culture to be able to deliver services to meet the needs of individuals within systems developed using public health data. But can child mental health service models apply across different population groups and countries?

The four-level (tier) CAMHS model, which has been widely adopted in the UK during the last decade (Health Advisory Service, 1995), is a good example. This defines CAMHS at four levels. Level 1 is usually the first point of service contact for children with mental health problems and their families. It consists of health professionals such as school nurses, health visitors and general practitioners, social workers, teachers and youth workers or other non-statutory agencies. In other words, level 1 is a broader service concept than primary care within the health service. Level 2 includes individual child mental health professionals, who may also be members of a local mental health service, but working at level 1 (e.g. schools or health centres –

usually primary mental health workers). Level 3 consists of specialist outpatient multidisciplinary teams for a defined locality (geographical area). Level 4 services provide treatment for specific, complex and severe disorders. They include day and in-patient units covering a larger geographical area.

At first look, such a model may be considered prohibitive for developing countries, or indeed for health systems without primary care. To a large extent, the achievement of standards such as access and quick response will rely on available resources (Kelvin, 2005). However, there are more parallels than first meet the eye. Schools in India (Sinha *et al.*, 2003) or Pakistan (Rahman *et al.*, 1998) or paediatric departments in Nigerian hospitals (Tunde-Ayinmode, 2012) are examples of primary-care-level services that can be equally supported to manage mild child mental health problems. The effectiveness of such health structures should be maximized in recognizing and managing less complex child mental health problems as much as possible.

In developing countries, non-governmental organizations have a major role to play in working across statutory services. For example, they are the key agencies to respond to natural disasters or political conflict (Thabet *et al.*, 2008). Limited specialist time can be used sparingly and effectively, through consultation, joint work with primary care staff and brief therapeutic interventions. Training also has an important role to play (Dogra *et al.*, 2005). Specialized (tier 3 or 4) services often overlap with existing paediatric (for children with autism and learning disability) or adult mental health services (for older adolescents with severe mental disorders). The child mental health service at Aga Khan University Hospital in Pakistan started from the private psychiatry services where there was only one part-time child psychiatrist (Syed *et al.*, 2007). Even if the autonomous development of mental health services for children and adolescents is not realistic for some countries in the near future, the above principles can be applied by sharing expertise with key professionals from the paediatric and adult mental health sectors.

All such initiatives should be developed taking into consideration the socio-cultural beliefs of children, young people and families (Abera *et al.*, 2015; Dogra 2015); their understanding of mental health (Thabet *et al.*, 2006); their perceived barriers to services; and the characteristics of their communities which could facilitate access and engagement with CAMHS (Barry *et al.*, 2013; Owens *et al.*, 2002; Patel *et al.*, 2008). It is also important to consider socio-economic factors that may contribute to poor service use through their link with ethnic status (Alegria *et al.*, 2001; Pumariega *et al.*, 1998). Research on families' perceptions of mental health and mental illness, help-seeking attitudes (Abera *et al.*, 2015; Cauce *et al.*, 2002; Eapen and Ghubash, 2004), and patterns and reasons of service utilization (Sourander *et al.*, 2004), is essential in planning service models based on evidence rather than assumptions. For example, although it is widely established that, even in Western societies, ethnic-minority groups have limited access to child mental health services (Burns *et al.*, 2004; Zwaanswijk *et al.*, 2003), there is neither supportive evidence nor policy consensus on how these needs should be best met.

Reduction of stigma of mental illness and stigmatization (Venkatesh *et al.*, 2015) is important across all cultural and ethnic groups, although the process may differ to involve local communities, schools, community and religious leaders and groups, as well as the media. Finally, although it is beyond the remit of this chapter to discuss the needs of specific client groups in detail, particular attention should be given to vulnerable and at-risk children such as those exposed to violence and trauma, refugees and asylum seekers, homeless children and children in public care. These needy groups of children and young people offer an additional challenge to the generic service requirements and previously discussed cultural needs, as these children and young people are mobile, lack advocacy and stability, and have multiple and interrelated social, developmental and educational difficulties (Vostanis, 2014). For this reason, services for these groups of children require clearly laid out international and national policies, joint commissioning between health and social-care organizations, an active role for the voluntary sector, and designated and accessible services and applied interventions.

Developing universal recommendations for child psychiatry and mental health prevention is a difficult task when various cultures enter the equation. It is important to acknowledge what the child's and family's perception of mental illness might be, and what say the child should have in their own health management. This differs vastly between cultures. While the economic status of a country plays a large part in the quality and accessibility of CAMH resources, successful programmes have been put in place in schools, primary care clinics, and other more accessible community sectors.

References

Abera, M., Robbins, J. M. and Tesfaye, M. (2015). Parents' perception of child and adolescent mental health problems and their choice of treatment option in southwest Ethiopia. *Child and Adolescent Psychiatry and Mental Health*, **9**, 40

Ainsworth, M. (1967). *Infancy in Uganda: Infant Care and the Growth of Love*. Baltimore: Johns Hopkins Press.

Ainsworth, M. (1978). *Patterns of Attachment: A Psychological Study of the Strange Situation*. New York: Lawrence Erlbaum Associates; distributed by Halsted Press Division of Wiley.

Alegria, M., McGuire, T., Vera, M., Canino, G., Matias, L. and Calderon, J. (2001). Changes in access to mental health care among the poor and nonpoor: results from the health care reform in Puerto Rico. *American Journal of Public Health*, **9**, 1431–1434.

Anglin, T., Naylor, K. and Kaplan, D. (1996). Comprehensive school-based health care: high school students' use of medical, mental health and substance abuse services. *Pediatrics*, **97**, 318–330.

Barry, M. M., Clarke, A. M., Jenkins, R. and Patel, V. (2013). A systematic review of the effectiveness of mental health promotion interventions for young people in low and middle income countries. *BMC Public Health*, **13**, 835.

Becker, D. and Liddle, H. (2001). Family therapy with unmarried African American mothers and their adolescents. *Family Process*, **40**, 413–427.

Bird, H. and Canino, G. (1982). The Puerto Rico family: cultural factors and family intervention strategies. *Journal of the American Academy of Psychoanalysis*, **10**, 257–268.

Bowlby, J. (1979). *The Making and Breaking of Affectional Bonds*. London: Tavistock Publications.

Bowlby, J. (1988). *A Secure Base: Parent–Child Attachment and Healthy Human Development*. New York: Basic Books.

Bronfenbrenner, U. (1979). *The Ecology of Human Development: Experiments by Nature and Design*. Cambridge, MA: Harvard University Press.

Burns, B., Phillips, S., Wagner, R. *et al.* (2004). Mental health need and access to mental health services by youths involved with child welfare: a national survey. *Journal of the American Academy of Child and Adolescent Psychiatry*, **43**, 960–970.

Canino, I. and Inclan, J. (2001). Culture and family therapy. *Child and Adolescent Psychiatric Clinics of North America*, **10**, 601–612.

Cauce, A., Domenech-Rodriguez, M., Paradise, M. *et al.* (2002). Cultural and contextual influences in mental health help seeking: a focus on ethnic minority youth. *Journal of Consulting and Clinical Psychology*, **70**, 44–55.

Dogra, N. (2015). Principles of Child and Adolescent Psychiatry. In *International Encyclopedia of Social and Behavioral Sciences*, 2nd edn. Oxford: Elsevier Limited.

Dogra, N. and Karnik, N. (2003). First-year medical students' attitudes toward diversity and its teaching: an investigation at one US medical school. *Academic Medicine*, **78**(11), 1–10.

Dogra, N., Frake, C., Bretherton, K., Dwivedi, K. and Sharma, I. (2005). Training CAMHS professionals in developing countries: an Indian case study. *Child and Adolescent Mental Health*, **10**, 74–79.

Duffy, A., Lewitzka, U., Doucette, S., Andreazza, A. and Grof, P. (2012). Biological indicators of illness risk in offspring of bipolar parents: targeting the hypothalamic-pituitary-adrenal axis and immune system. *Early Intervention in Psychiatry*, **6**(2), 128–137.

Eapen, V. and Ghubash, R. (2004). Help-seeking for mental health problems of children: preferences and attitudes in the United Arab Emirates. *Psychological Reports*, **94**, 663–667.

Earls, F. (2001). Community factors supporting child mental health. *Child and Adolescent Psychiatric Clinics of North America*, **10**, 693–709.

Erikson, S. and Achilles, G. (2004). Cognitive behavioral therapy with children and adolescents. In *Handbook of Mental Health Interventions in Children and Adolescents: An Integrated Developmental Perspective*, ed. H. Steiner. San Francisco: Jossey-Bass.

Farahmand, F. K., Grant, K. E., Polo, A. J. and Duffy, S. N. (2011). School-based mental health and behavioral programs for low-income, urban youth: a systematic and meta-analytic review. *Clinical Psychology: Science and Practice*, **18**(4), 372–390.

Flaherty, L., Weist, M. and Warner, B. (1996). School-based mental health services in the United States: history, current models and needs. *Community Mental Health Journal*, **32**, 341–352.

Fonagy, P. (1999). *Transgenerational Consistencies of Attachment: A New Theory*. Washington DC: American Psychoanalytic Association Meeting.

Fonagy, P. (2004). Psychodynamic therapy with children. In *Handbook of Mental Health Interventions in Children and Adolescents: An Integrated Developmental Perspective*, ed. H. Steiner. San Francisco: Jossey-Bass.

Garland, A., Lewczyk-Boxmeyer, C., Gabayan, E. and Hawley, K. (2004). Multiple stakeholder agreement on desired outcomes for adolescents' mental health services. *Psychiatric Services*, **55**, 671–676.

Gewirtz, A. and August, G. (2008). Incorporating multifaceted mental health prevention services in community sectors-of-care. *Clinical Child and Family Psychology Review*, **11**, 1–11.

Glissen, C., Hemmelgarn, A., Green, P. *et al.* (2012). Randomized trial of the Availability, Responsiveness, and Continuity (ARC) organizational intervention with community-based mental health programs and clinicians serving youth. *Journal of the American Academy of Child and Adolescent Psychiatry*, **51**(8), 780–787.

Grossman, A., Churchill, J., McKinney, B., Kodish, I., Otte, S. and Greenough, W. (2003). Experience effects on brain development: possible contributions to psychopathology. *Journal of Child Psychology and Psychiatry*, **44**, 33–63.

Hameed, M. A. and Lewis, A. J. (2016). Offspring of parents with schizophrenia: a systematic review of developmental features across childhood. *Harvard Review of Psychiatry*, **24**(2), 104–117.

Hampson, R. and Beavers, W. (1996). Measuring family therapy outcome in a clinical setting: families that do better or do worse in therapy. *Family Process*, **35**, 347–361.

Health Advisory Service (1995). *Child and Adolescent Mental Health Services: Together We Stand*. London: HMSO.

Hinman, C. (2003). Multicultural considerations in the delivery of play therapy services. *International Journal of Play Therapy*, **12**(2), 107–122.

Hudson, J. L., Rapee, R., Lyneham, H. J. *et al.* (2015). Comparing outcomes for children with different anxiety disorders following cognitive behavioural therapy. *Behaviour Research and Therapy*, **72**, 30–37.

Joshi, S. V. (2004). School consultation and intervention. In *Handbook of Mental Health Interventions in Children and Adolescents: An Integrated Developmental Perspective*, ed. H. Steiner. San Francisco: Jossey-Bass.

Jung, M. (1984). Structural family therapy: its applications to Chinese families. *Family Process*, **23**, 365–374.

Kang-Yi, C. D., Mandell, D. S. and Hadley, T. (2013). School-based mental health program evaluation: children's school outcomes and acute mental health service use. *Journal of School Health*, **83**, 463–472.

Kaplan, D., Brindis, C., Phibbs, S., Melinkovich, P., Naylor, K. and Ahlstraud, K. (1999). A comparison study of an elementary school-based health center: effects on health care access and use. *Archives of Pediatrics and Adolescent Medicine*, **153**, 235–243.

Karnik, N. S. (2004). The social environment. In *Handbook of Mental Health Interventions in Children and Adolescents: An Integrated Developmental Perspective*, ed. H. Steiner. San Francisco: Jossey-Bass.

Karnik, N. and Dogra, N. (2010). The cultural sensibility model for children and adolescents: a process oriented approach. *Child and Adolescent Psychiatric Clinics of North America*, **19**(4), 719–738.

Kelvin, R. (2005). Capacity of tier 2/3 CAMH and service specification: a model to enable evidence-based service development. *Child and Adolescent Mental Health*, **10**, 63–73.

Kisker, E. and Brown, R. (1996). Do school-based health centers improve adolescents' access to health care, health status, and risk-taking behavior? *Journal of Adolescent Health*, **18**, 335–343.

Kumpfer, K., Alvarado, R., Smith, P. and Bellamy, N. (2002). Cultural sensitivity and adaptation in family-based interventions. *Preventive Sciences*, **3**, 241–246.

Leslie, D. L. and Rosenheck, R. A (2004). Adherence of schizophrenia pharmacotherapy to published treatment recommendations: patient, facility, and provider predictors. *Schizophrenia Bulletin*, **30**(3), 649–658.

Lieberman, J., Stroup, T., McEvoy, J. *et al.* and the Clinical Antipsychotic Trials of Intervention Effectiveness (2005). Effectiveness of antipsychotic drugs in patients with chronic schizophrenia. *New England Journal of Medicine*, **353**, 1209–1223.

Loughran, M. (2004). Psychodynamic therapy with adolescents. In *Handbook of Mental Health Interventions in Children and Adolescents: An Integrated Developmental Perspective*, ed. H. Steiner. San Francisco: Jossey-Bass.

Mitrani, V., Santisteban, M. and Muir, J. (2004). Addressing immigration-related separations in Hispanic families with a behaviour-problem adolescent. *American Journal of Orthopsychiatry*, **74**, 219–229.

Mukherji, C. (1997). Monsters and muppets: the history of childhood and techniques of cultural analysis. In *From Sociology to Cultural Studies*, ed. E. Long. Malden, MA: Blackwell Publishers.

Owens, P., Hoagwood, K., Horwitz, S. *et al.* (2002). Barriers to children's mental health services. *Journal of the American Academy of Child and Adolescent Psychiatry*, **41**, 731–738.

Patel, V. and Rahman, A. (2015). Editorial Commentary: an agenda for global child mental health. *Child and Adolescent Mental Health*, **20**, 3–4, doi:10.1111/camh.12083.

Patel, V., Flisher, A., Nikapota, A., Malhotra, S. (2008). Promoting child and adolescent mental health in low and middle income countries. *Journal of Child Psychology and Psychiatry* **49**(3), 313–334.

Peris, T., Compton, Scott N., Kendall, Philip C. *et al.* (2015). Trajectories of change in youth anxiety during cognitive-behavior therapy. *Journal of Consulting and Clinical Psychology*, **83**(2), 239–252.

Post, R. and Post, S. (2004). Molecular and cellular developmental vulnerabilities to the onset of affective disorders in children and adolescents: some implications for therapeutics. In *Handbook of Mental Health Interventions in Children and Adolescents: An Integrated Developmental Perspective*, ed. H. Steiner. San Francisco: Jossey-Bass.

Pumariega, A., Glover, S., Holzer, C. and Nguyen, H. (1998). Utilization of mental health services in a tri-ethnic sample of adolescents. *Community Mental Health Journal*, **34**, 145–156.

Rahman, A., Mubbashar, M., Gater, R. and Goldberg, D. (1998). Randomised trial of impact of school mental health programme in rural Rawalphindi, Pakistan. *The Lancet*, **352**, 1022–1025.

Ronzoni, P. and Dogra, N. (2012). Children, adolescents and their carers' expectations of child and adolescent mental health services (CAMHS). *International Journal of Social Psychiatry*, **58**(3), 328–336, doi:10.1177/0020764010397093.

Rousseau, C., Drapeau, A. and Platt, R. (2004). Family environment and emotional and behavioural symptoms in adolescent Cambodian refugees: influence of time, gender, and acculturation. *Medical Conflict and Survival*, **20**, 151–165.

Rubenstein, J. and Puelles, L. (2004). Survey of brain development. In *Handbook of Mental Health Interventions in Children and Adolescents: An Integrated Developmental Perspective*, ed. H. Steiner. San Francisco: Jossey-Bass.

Santelli, J., Kouzis, A. and Newcomer, S. (1996a). School-based health centers and adolescent use of primary care and hospital care. *Journal of Adolescent Health*, **19**, 267–275.

Santelli, J., Kouzis, A. and Newcomer, S. (1996b). Student attitudes toward school-based health centers. *Journal of Adolescent Health*, **18**, 349–356.

Santisteban, D., Coatsworth, J., Perez-Vidal, A. *et al.* (2003). Efficacy of brief strategies family therapy in modifying Hispanic adolescent behaviour problems and substance use. *Journal of Family Psychology*, **17**, 121–133.

Shonkoff, J. P. and Phillips, D. A. (2000). *From Neurons to Neighborhoods: The Science of Early Childhood Development*. Washington DC: National Academy Press.

Sinha, V., Kishore, T. and Thakur, A. (2003). A school mental health program in India. *Journal of the American Academy of Child and Adolescent Psychiatry*, **42**, 624.

Sourander, A., Santalahti, P., Haavisto, A., Piha, J. and Ikaheimo, K. (2004). Have there been changes in children's psychiatric symptoms and mental health service use? A 10-year comparison from Finland. *Journal of the American Academy of Child and Adolescent Psychiatry*, **43**, 1134–1145.

Steiner, H. (2004). The scientific basis of mental health interventions in children and adolescents: an overview. In *Handbook of Mental Health Interventions in Children and Adolescents: An Integrated Developmental Perspective*, ed. H. Steiner. San Francisco: Jossey-Bass.

Stratton, P. (2005). *Report on the Evidence Base of Systemic Family Therapy on Behalf of the Academic and Research Committee of the Association for Family Therapy.* London: Association for Family Therapy.

Sue, D., Ivey, A. and Penderson, P. (1996). *A Theory of Multicultural Counseling and Therapy.* New York: Brooks/Cole Publishing.

Syed, E. U., Hussein, S. A., Yousafzai, A. W. (2007). Developing services with limited resources: establishing a CAMHS in Pakistan. *Child and Adolescent Mental Health*, **12**(3), 121–124.

Szapocznik, J. and Williams, R. (2000). Brief strategic therapy: 25 years of interplay among theory, research and practice in adolescent behaviour problems and drug abuse. *Clinical Child Family Psychology Review*, **3**, 117–134.

Tamura, T. and Lau, A. (1992). Connectedness versus separateness: applicability of family therapy to Japanese families. *Family Process*, **31**, 319–340.

Thabet, A. A., El Gammal, H. and Vostanis, P. (2006). Palestinian mothers' perceptions of child mental health problems and services. *World Psychiatry*, **5**(2), 108–112.

Thabet, A. A., Tawahina, A., El Sarraj, E. and Vostanis, P. (2008) Children exposed to political conflict: implications for health policy. *Harvard Health Policy Review*, **8**, 158–165.

Tseng, W. S. and Streltzer, J. (2001). *Culture and Psychotherapy: A Guide to Clinical Practice.* Washington DC: American Psychiatric Press.

Tunde-Ayinmode, M., Adegunloye, O., Ayinmode, B. and Abiodun, O. (2012). Psychiatric disorders in children attending a Nigerian primary care unit: functional impairment and risk factors. *Child and Adolescent Psychiatry and Mental Health* **6**, 28.

Venkatesh, B. T., Andrews, T., Mayya, S. S., Singh, M. M., Parsekar, S. S. (2015). Perception of stigma toward mental illness in South India. *Journal of Family Medicine and Primary Care*, **4**, 449–453.

Vitiello, B. and Swedo, S. (2004). Antidepressant medications in children. *New England Journal of Medicine*, **350**, 1489–1491.

Vostanis, P. (2014). *Helping Children and Young People who Experience Trauma: Children of Despair, Children of Hope.* London: Radcliffe Publishing.

Vostanis, P., Humphrey, N., Fitzgerald, N., Deighton, J. and Wolpert, M. (2013). How do schools promote emotional well-being among their pupils? Findings from a national survey of mental health provision in English schools. *Child and Adolescent Mental Health*, **18**, 151–157.

Vygotsky, L. (1978). *Mind in Society: the Development of Higher Psychological Processes.* Cambridge, MA: Harvard University Press.

Walter, H., Vaughan, R., Armstrong, B., Krakoff, R., Tiezzi, L. and McCarty, J. (1995). School-based health care for urban minority junior high school students. *Archives of Pediatrics and Adolescent Medicine*, **149**, 1221–1225.

Weist, M., Paskewitz, D., Warner, S. and Flaherty, L. (1996). Treatment outcome of school-based mental health services for urban teenagers. *Community Mental Health Journal*, **32**, 149–157.

Wessely, S. and Kerwin, R. (2004). Suicide risk and the SSRIs. *Journal of the American Medical Association*, **292**, 379–381.

World Health Organization (2015). *WHO Model List of Essential Medicines*, 19th edn. Geneva: World Health Organization.

Ziguras, S., Klimidis, S., Lambert, T. and Jackson, A. (2001). Determinants of anti-psychotic medication compliance in a multicultural population. *Community Mental Health Journal*, **37**, 273.

Zwaanswijk, M., Van der Ende, J., Verhaak, P., Bensing, J. and Verhulst, F. (2003). Factors associated with adolescent mental health service need and utilization. *Journal of the American Academy of Child and Adolescent Psychiatry*, **42**, 692–700.

Chapter

40

Management of Sexual Dysfunction across Cultures

Dinesh Bhugra, Antonio Ventriglio and Gurvinder Kalra

Editors' Introduction

As mentioned in the earlier chapter on sexual dysfunction, cultures affect presentation and help-seeking. The many factors which influence this include explanatory models and accessibility of the healthcare systems. In planning and delivering interventions and clinical management of sexual dysfunction in patients from different cultures a number of factors must be recognized. Some of these are general whereas others are more specific. These interventions, especially if the therapist is from another culture, raise interesting questions about the role of perceived and real power embedded in the therapist. Furthermore, the perceptions and expectations of the therapeutic encounter and functions of therapy have to be taken into account. Recognition and understanding of social and cultural factors and their inherent complexities are a useful generic first step in building blocks of therapeutic alliance between couples and therapists. While individual therapy and couple therapy have many common principles and overlaps, couple therapy brings with it at least two sets of clear expectations (others' expectations, e.g. children's, which may be hiding behind those of the couple) and challenges. Knowing a couple's type of marriage (arranged/love/open) may allow the therapist to explore potential therapeutic obstacles. Satisfaction with marriage is related to the type of marriage amongst other factors. In this chapter, Bhugra *et al.* recommend some strategies in assessment and management of sexual dysfunction. Culturally influenced components of therapies may not easily be acceptable to all individuals, especially if their cultures differ from those where these therapies have been developed. The nature of mixed-race couples has to be addressed differently. They argue that ethnicity and personality of the partner, along with the couple's willingness to communicate on other unrelated issues, will allow the therapist to deal with and potentially to reduce conflict and increase satisfaction within the relationship.

Introduction

The management of sexual dysfunctions is as complex as its aetiology. As the rates of prevalence of sexual dysfunction across cultures remain controversial, its management is influenced by a number of factors including cultural perception of sexual dysfunctions, perceived purpose of the sexual act, explanatory models of the dysfunction as well as availability and accessibility of therapies.

With demographic shifts, impact of rapid urbanization, industrialization and globalization, the attitudes towards sex, sexual dysfunctions and help-seeking are beginning to shift, often very rapidly, thereby creating tensions across generations which can have major implications in terms of whether the sexual act is seen as a procreative or pleasurable activity. Apps such as Grindr and Tindr and others in many countries are rapidly accessible to young especially urban people changing the nature and expectations of intimacy.

There is no doubt that there indeed are biases in treatment availability and healthcare systems across the globe. Many insurers do not allow treatment for sexual dysfunction. Access is also influenced by age, gender, and prevalent economic and political factors. Various types of therapies are available for managing sexual dysfunction but the evidence base for some of them is seriously lacking. In addition, different culturally influenced therapies may be used for managing sexual dysfunction – the knowledge base and therapeutic outcome for those may not be clear either.

There has been a question over whether the therapies developed in one culture for one set of patients are suitable for or can be used for patients in other cultures. For example, psychoanalytic theory and therapies were the product of nineteenth-century Europe and America; can these be applied universally and, indeed, if so who should apply them? Hodes (1989) points out that there appear to be two extreme positions at opposite ends of the spectrum. At one end is the universalist position, which dictates that since all human suffering is universal, the application of such therapies is acceptable as there are more similarities than differences in terms of individual development, although social and cultural rules may change. The other end of the spectrum holds the position of cultural relativism, which argues that each culture is unique and cannot be embraced by a single universal theory. It is evident that these two positions both entail ideological as well as practical considerations, which have to be understood in terms of the historical and political contexts within which psychotherapies have evolved (Lloyd and Bhugra, 1993). We illustrate some of these key issues with examples from different cultures as applied to management of sexual dysfunction. As has already been described (see Bhugra *et al.* in Chapter 30 in this volume), we do not propose to go through the basic levels of cross-cultural differences in psychosexual dysfunction. It is fair to say that both psychiatry and psychoanalysis have been criticized from a number of perspectives for their collaboration in the domination of a sub-junction of groups within Western societies and in other cultures colonized by the West (see Doermer, 1981; Foucault, 1967; Eichenbaum and Orbach, 1982; Porter, 1987 for social histories of psychiatry in the West especially in regards to gender and social class; and see Bhugra and Littlewood, 2000; Littlewood and Lipsedge, 1999; Sabshin *et al.*, 1970; Thomas and Sillen 1972 for commentaries on psychiatry's position and relationship with colonialism and racism). Some commentators have argued forcefully that racial differences have an inhibiting effect on psychotherapy (Griffith, 1977) and others have played down these ideological concerns and attempted to obtain a severe sense of scientific objectivism which may be superficially attractive and indeed seductive to the medical audience but does not represent the full picture (Leff, 1988).

Principles

Assessing a case of sexual dysfunction will involve assessing the couple if possible, with detailed history and appropriate investigations; but the most important question is why here and why now. This has to be clarified especially in context of motivation and degree of commitment to the relationship and consequently to the treatment. In addition, it is always helpful to exclude any underlying physical causations and carry out suitable physical investigations if needed. Furthermore, the distinction between primary and secondary sexual dysfunctions and underlying physical or psychiatric conditions must be explored thoroughly. Alcoholism may contribute to sexual dysfunctions and cultural responses to alcohol and alcoholism need to be understood and taken into account for part of the assessment. For detailed assessment strategies, see Bancroft (2008), Hawton (1985), Leiblum (2007, 2010), Balon (2008) and others.

Assessment across Cultures

In addition to normal clinical assessment, detailed information may be required of the patient in respect of their cultural values and norms, acculturations and cultural expectations of the sexual behaviour. As noted in Chapter 30, if the basic cultural value of the sex act is procreative and lack of privacy a major issue, then giving the couple sensate focus or body exploration exercises and setting time aside for these is likely to prove counterproductive.

Often cultures are blamed for creating sexual problems. As Hall and Graham (2013) go on to highlight, a culturally sensitive perspective goes beyond blaming a fault in the culture (e.g. placing a premium on semen or on virginity) for sexual problems. The cultural assessment and cultural formulation have been described by Bhugra and Bhui (1997). These assessments, although originally developed to assess patients from black and minority ethnic groups within the UK, can easily be modified for use elsewhere. If the therapist and the patient are from the same culture, this may still create a conflict because, for their therapeutic interaction, they may bring different expectations, experiences and values to the encounter. However, one could also hypothesize that therapists from the same culture as the clients may be better able to communicate and understand the clients than therapists from other cultures. All therapeutic interactions have been thus noted as 'intercultural' because no two people will have identical internalized constructions of their own cultural worlds (Wohl, 1989). Culturally transmitted concerns about sex can affect an individual's sexual functioning. Sometimes these may present with what is seen as culture-bound syndromes (see Bhugra *et al.*, Chapter 14 in this volume) but more often the individual's overall beliefs and attitudes to sex cause or contribute to more generalized difficulties, and the same variables can also affect the attitude and response (as well as the acceptance of the treatment modality) to therapy (Bhugra and de Silva, 1993). The role of women, fecundity, need for a son and other similar factors must be explored further in any assessment.

Special Issues

Irrespective of specific culture issues, additional factors that may play a role in the acceptance of any treatment include single male, gay and lesbian single individuals or couples and polyamorous individuals. Sexual fluidity depends upon sexual behaviour and not on the actual sexual orientation. The therapist would need to modify the clinical approach in the context of the patients' cultural values and norms. It has to be a collaborative process between the therapist and the client (Peavy and Li, 2003).

Gender Differences

Guirguis (1995) notes that the single male can present in any one of the following three clinical conditions: primary impotence, secondary impotence and the widower's impotence. Each of these groups has a different set of problems and expectations. As Anson (1995) points out, in terms of type of complaint and duration of complaint, there were no differences for single men presenting for treatment. To help men presenting with sexual problems alone, therapists can help them by educating them and introducing them to healthier sexual habits (Kleinplatz, 2013). Being single plays a major role in whether help is sought and where it is sought from. As Catalan *et al.* (1991) found, amongst their female patients seeking help alone, orgasmic dysfunction was more likely and low sexual interest less likely when compared with women presenting with their partners. Around 40 per cent of women attending a family planning clinic (who also had a sexual dysfunction) believed that their partners would not attend for couple treatment.

Cultural Factors

For people originating from non-Western cultures, the potential of non-couple therapy will relate to a number of factors including beliefs about the causes of the dysfunction, the prevalence of various types of dysfunction and issues related to attendance of a spouse or partner (Anson, 1995). The beliefs about the notion of physical causation of the dysfunction being masturbation, nocturnal emissions and semen loss in men pose problems for treatment and poor compliance for behavioural

therapy (de Silva, 1982). De Silva (1982) also noted a reluctance to bring spouses to the clinic in Sri Lanka as well as an unwillingness of women to come to the clinic to discuss sexual problems. Additional factors of sexual taboos, social expectations, poor levels of education and information have already been touched upon.

Gay and Lesbians

Homophobia, societal attitudes to homosexuality and long-term same-sex partnerships will all play a role in acceptance of treatment. Gordon (1986) noted that gay men were more likely to present without partners and Reece (1985) used group therapy as a potential treatment. Malyon (1982) observed that homophobia can play a very strong role in rejection of treatment. The stages of coming out especially in a couple may not be synchronous and the therapist may need to vary treatment options accordingly. The sexual dysfunctions among lesbians are likely to be similar to those in heterosexual females, but their experience of homophobia, societal attitudes and importance of orientation are likely to be similar to those experienced by gay men (Bhugra and Wright, 1995). The therapist must use psychosexual objectivity because homosexuality and heterosexuality have far more similarities than differences (Masters and Johnson, 1979), though Gordon (1986) criticizes this approach and, like the debate on ethnic matching between therapist and patient, a skilled sympathetic therapist is seen as more important that one with a similar orientation (Anthony, 1982). Levounis and Drescher (2012) and Cabaj and Stein (2013) offer helpful overviews on the subject.

Couple Therapy

In addition to individual factors, relationship factors play a key role in the genesis and maintenance of sexual dysfunctions. They will be moulded by the reactions of the partners in the context of circular causations, i.e. the actions of one become the 'cause' of the actions of the other and so on (Crowe, 1995). Thinking systematically in this way has distinct advantages as the sexual relationship is the microcosm of the general relationship. The degree of trust, overprotection, dependency, jealousy and variation in sexual interest may all contribute to the genesis and maintenance of the problem. The type of marriage i.e. love or arranged marriage may have a role to play in these issues as the manner in which spouses are selected varies across cultures (Regan *et al.*, 2012). If the couple are part of an 'arranged marriage' then their expectations of each other, their relationship with each other and the extended kinship will be quite different, and consequently the systems structure will be quite different. However, as Sandhya (2009) points out, globalization may result in barometers of happiness such as intimacy in a relationship assuming a critical role in the quality and longevity of marriage even for arranged marriages. Couples' experience and expression of intimacy predicts levels of happiness in marriage (Sandhya, 2009); however it is worth noting that this experience may differ for the two partners. In a heterosexual marital relationship for instance, wives may be generally less satisfied than their husbands with their marital and sexual relationships (Zhang *et al.*, 2012).

The principles of behavioural systems couple therapy are beyond the scope of this chapter and interested readers are referred to Crowe (1995) and Crowe and Ridley (2000). A hierarchy of alternative levels of interventions can be used by reciprocity negotiation, communication training, role play, tasks and timetabling, paradox and adjustment to the symptom approaches.

In dealing with couples where one individual is from one culture and the other individual from a different culture, different strategies may be indicated, especially if the therapist is of a culture that matches one or the other. This raises questions in managing the sexual dysfunction if the therapist is from one or the other culture (see Figure 40.1). The focus in this chapter is on heterosexual relationships.

Couple Relationships

In assessing couples and their needs for psychological treatments, it is helpful for the therapist to consider not only the relationship patterns but also the childhood developmental patterns, especially attachment. Mikulincer *et al.* (2002) propose that sense of attachment security has been identified as a major variable explaining variations in the quality of dating and marital relationships. They build on the observation that every meaningful interaction with significant others throughout adult life is influenced by childhood attachment experiences. Those who have a sense of attachment security are more likely to react to stressful events with lower levels of stress compared with those who score high on avoidance or anxiety domains. The former (i.e. those with secure attachments) are also more likely to cope with stress by seeking support, and are also likely to have more positive expectations about relationship partners than those who score high on avoidance domination. Those more secure in their attachments, not surprisingly, also hold more positive self-views than those who score high on anxiety dimension. Perhaps more intriguingly, this group of individuals is also likely to engage in exploration and affiliation activities and is more sensitive and responsive to their partner's needs. There is indeed a causal relationship between an individual's experiences with his/her parents and their capacity to make affectional bonds in later life. Mikulincer *et al.* (2002) raise methodological issues in both the assessment of attachment as well as marital quality. It is not surprising that patterns of attachment will determine the quality of dating relationships as well as of long-term romantic relationships. These authors conclude that the sense of attachment security is associated with:

1. positive beliefs about couple relationships;

2. formation of more stable couple relationships;

3. satisfaction with dating relationships and marriage;

4. high levels of intimacy, commitment and emotional involvement within the relationship;

5. positive patterns of communication and interactions in both dating and married couples.

They postulate that the affective consequences of secure attachment interaction with distress alleviation, positive mental representations of the self and others and secure attachment facilitates the satisfaction of other basic psychological needs (e.g. exploration, affiliation, care-giving) within the couple relationship, which in turn will further increase relationship satisfaction.

Using a systematic theoretical framework, they suggest that in their model, marital interactions are patterned along intra-psychic and interpersonal regularities, and the structure of the intra-psychic and interpersonal elements in the whole system affects how one element acts with another. Partners, too, influence one another in complex reciprocal and cross-construct ways. These intra-psychic and interpersonal influences are circular rather than linear. Of course, systems are also self-regulating. Mikulincer *et al.* (2002) propose that self-representations are extremely useful and important in contributing to the formation and maintenance of stable and

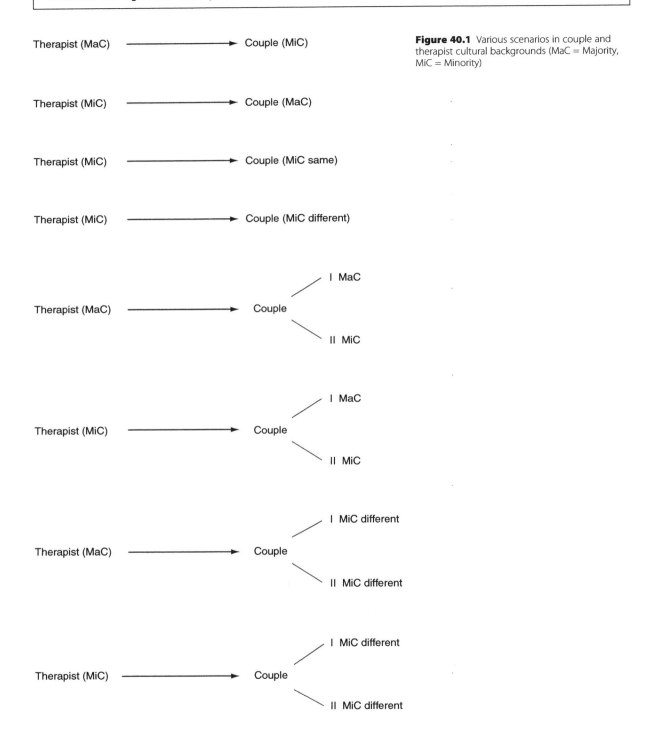

Figure 40.1 Various scenarios in couple and therapist cultural backgrounds (MaC = Majority, MiC = Minority)

satisfying couple relationships. Securely attached persons, therefore, will feel accepted and valued and this will encourage them to reciprocate this love and further strengthen their willingness to care for their partner in times of need. In addition, these positive representations include a sense of self-efficiency in dealing with threats and life problems, which may lead to the adoption of a more confident attitude towards their relationship obstacles and to the adoption of more constructive interpersonal problem-solving strategies. The models of representations of others may similarly influence the care-giving and maturing of each other. Thus inner resources and previous experiences will play an important role in the dynamic relational process, which categorizes different stages of marriage and family development.

From a practical point of understanding, couple relationships and satisfaction within the relationship, attachment has a role to play. As Mikulincer et al. (2002) themselves note, the interplay between different factors and the directional nature of this interplay is very difficult to ascertain. Furthermore, integration of research data and family dynamic processes is worth exploring. It will also be helpful both for therapists and couples to ascertain the attachment in later stages of marriage and as the family develops.

Huston (2000) analyses marital relations and suggests that marriage be studied at three levels: that of society, that of the individual and that of the process itself. This translates as the macrosocial context, with the spouse's ecological niche, at a 'lower' level the spouse's beliefs and attitudes and, third, marital behaviour in the dyad context. Such an approach obviously allows and encourages the therapist to analyse the relationship at a more inclusive level rather than simply relying on two individuals. Nwoye (2000; see below) confirms this in a different culture.

De Maris (2000) reported from a survey of 3,508 married couples on a 5–7-year follow-up that male violence significantly elevated the risk of disruption and that its impact did not appear to differ according to the female partner's socio-economic resources. Verbal conflict was not reported to be a significant predictor of disruption of the relationship, but the style of conflict resolution was. Violence, by men especially, may well have influenced relationship quality for both partners. Co-habitees would be seen as unusual and, therefore, either very conventional in their commitment or very unconventional. Interestingly, the role of violence in dissolution of the relationship did not differ between those who were married and those who were co-habiting.

Wang and Amoto (2000) suggest that post-divorce adjustment in couples is related to income, remarriage, favourable attitudes to dissolution of the marriage before divorce and being the initiator of the divorce. Older individuals appeared to adjust worse than younger ones. The progression of marriage to divorce

can occur at different levels and different stages. Hostile and distancing behaviours have been predicted as contributing to marital stress. Using a sample of 97 couples, Roberts (2000) reported that, on assessing marital distress and withdrawal behaviour, spouses' responses were directly related to the level of hostility expressed in the relationship. The primary predictor of marital outcomes for wives was a partner's hostile responsiveness, whereas for husbands it was partner withdrawal. The study highlights some of the key problems in understanding the context in which marital distress occurs. Although these are all newly married couples (first marriage) and perhaps relatively inexperienced, it is important for couple therapists to be aware of these findings too, and include some questions on hostility and distance in their assessments. Marital satisfaction also depends on the partners' experiences of various relational factors. Zhang et al. (2012) demonstrated in a study in Hong Kong Chinese couples that husbands were more likely to be satisfied with their marriages when they were 2 to 4 years older than their wives than when they were of similar age to their wives. Wives on the other hand were more likely to be sexually satisfied with their husbands if the husbands were older than them.

In an interesting paper, Nwoye (2000) presents the indigenous theory and marriage therapy in contemporary East and West Africa. It is argued in this paper that, in these areas, marriage is based on a theoretical framework, which suggests that obligations/expectations and privileges are taken as being linked to the occupancy of social positions. Harmony and peace result when people occupying such positions perform their expected roles credibly and disharmony and distress occur when these obligations are not met. The traditional model of family therapy in Africa follows the mediatorial session, which involves the presence of a mediating team of elders as the jury, with the couple being litigants. The elders listen to arguments, identify the faults and pronounce judgements, which may well include damages. Thus the elders are not only detectives but allies and advocates as well as judges to uphold the traditions and values of the kinship. They are not neutral observers. Nwoye suggests that marital therapists follow this model where changes in the number of therapists in each session may be required. The process of marriage therapy has the social stage, where the husband presents his side without the wife. The initial hearing again has two components – the first one where the man gives his side and a second where the wife does. The length of the sessions is not dictated by the clock. In the second hearing, which follows one or two days after the initial hearing, the wife's 'accusations' are presented to the man and this gives the therapist the opportunity to confront the husband and identify misperceptions and expectations about the marriage and the relationship. The wife then has a second meeting with the therapist and the response to her complaints is shared. Faulty logic, unwarranted conclusions and generalizations are all things that the therapist may well be able to uncover. After these meetings, reconciliation is suggested, with a conclusive verdict. This is followed by a re-enactment of unity, where the spouses reflect on their current decision, and prescription of and opportunity for sharing a drink. This follows a ritual where the therapist blesses the couple. Nwoye goes on to acknowledge the patriarchal nature of such therapy, but it would be interesting to have some empirical data on the success of such an approach.

Helmeke and Sprenkle (2000) suggest that clients' perceptions of pivotal moments in the couple therapy are: (a) identifiable from the transcripts of sessions and (b) useful in getting couples to think about disclosure and its impact on the relationship. There is little doubt from the research data and from individual experiences that these moments are highly individualized and highly emotional ones, and that the individuals place varying degrees of significance upon them. These pivotal moments are closely related to presenting problems as well. The changes achieved in the sessions are also linked to clearly identifiable events. Although these findings are based on only three cases and on one therapist, these are interesting developments for the therapist to be aware of.

Marital and family therapy can influence pathways into care and will also affect help-seeking from various professional and non-professional sources. Law and Crane (2000) report from their case-note study data that usage of healthcare services dropped by one-fifth after the individuals had received couple, marital or family therapy.

Couples and the Therapist

The interaction between the therapist and the couple can be affected in a number of ways. These include, for the couple: race, class, level of education and culture, which can be broadly termed 'external' factors; and self-concept, religious belief and language, which may be termed 'internal' factors. They also include various

key factors in the therapist: race, class, gender, language as general background factors, and professional training, experience and preconceptions in the therapeutic setting. Needless to say, in each partner as well as in the therapist, these factors constantly interact. And they also influence, separately and in combination, the therapeutic relationship. However 'objective' a therapist claims to be, the operation of these factors in the therapeutic relationship is inevitable and needs to be acknowledged.

Within such an interaction, there are several scenarios, all of which have implications for the planning and implementation of therapy. First, the therapist might come from the majority culture and the couple from a minority culture. Second, the therapist might come from a minority culture and the couple from a majority culture. The first is very common in present-day therapeutic settings in Britain and Australia, and the second is an increasingly common situation. Third, the therapist and the couple could both be from the same minority culture. Fourth, the therapist might be from one minority culture, and the couple from a different minority culture. In today's Britain, with several groups of minorities, this is not a rare situation. Then there are those scenarios where the partners come from different cultures, either the majority culture and a minority culture, or different minority cultures. In each of these situations, the therapist might be from the majority culture or from the minority culture as discussed earlier. In addition, there are situations where the therapist will be of the same minority culture as one of the partners.

Each of these combinations will create a set of expectations and problems, which need to be considered by the therapist while assessing the couple and planning any intervention. Within such a combination, there are three key components which need to be emphasized. The first is the ethnocentrism of the couple, of each partner, of the therapist and of the wider culture surrounding them. Second, with the therapeutic interaction, there will be an imbalance of power related to various domains, including communication, both verbal and non-verbal, and the subjective experience of coercion or oppression. The third component is the therapeutic relationship where the therapist and the couple forge an alliance in order to move forward. This alliance is influenced by the presenting problem itself and by the shared world view of the parties, as well as by their different cultural background.

The power relationship between the therapist and the two partners is, in many ways, a microcosm of the society they live in. Power has been given to the therapist by virtue of professional experience and the role they play in the interaction. Asking questions to probe details is something that the therapists do but at the same time they can refuse questions from the clients or avoid and evade them. This helps in creating and maintaining the power differential by creating a hierarchy between the therapist and client (Zur, 2015). However, this is also affected by other factors. In commenting on this subject, d'Ardenne (1991) says:

> All therapists have some power over their clients, but the situation between clients from a minority culture and a therapist from the majority culture compounds this power imbalance further. The clients' perception of your age, social class, professional background and cultural skills will also affect your status, and how your clients see it.

As noted earlier, the past experience of the therapist with the clients may influence interactions in such a way that makes therapeutic progress difficult. This is further complicated in the setting of couple therapy where the two individuals come with their separate or different expectations, roles and power relationships. If the couple are from the same cultural background, then the interactions between the couple and the therapist may raise different issues from those that arise if all three members come from different ethnic and cultural backgrounds.

Some additional comments are in order at this point about mixed-race or intercultural couples, as this area has not been widely discussed in the literature. Intercultural couples have two additional sources of difficulty, which other couples do not have. One is society's overall attitude to such relationships, which varies from curiosity to open prejudice, including in the extreme case non-acceptance of the partners by each other's families and cultures. The second stems from the differences in habits, beliefs, values and customs that the two partners have. A greater adjustment is needed by such couples when compared with same-culture couples. Communication difficulties are common, not just verbal but non-verbal as well. The expression of moods may be non-congruent and often misunderstood. The way one partner relates to other males (or other females) may be seen by the other as unacceptable, simply because that is the way one's own culture considers such behaviour. There may also be discrepancies with regard to child-rearing practices and the role of the extended family. These mismatches can cause much couple disharmony and lead to the couple having to seek help. The couple may not always articulate these culturally based difficulties as their problem, but may complain of general incompatibility, one partner's unreasonableness or simply stress. The therapist needs to probe more deeply when such couples come for help, and to do this sensitively and without allowing him/her to be perceived as allying herself/himself with one of the partners. In the scenarios noted earlier, where the therapist and one of the partners belong to the same culture, this is particularly important. The other partner is very likely to feel alienated in such a situation. He/she may perceive a 'coalition' between the therapist and his/her partner. The effects of such a perception are therapeutically negative. The therapist needs to be fully aware of these potential difficulties, and to make every effort to minimize them.

Depending upon the culture and society from which the couple emerges, the notions of self and self-esteem will play an important role, not only in the relationship but also in the help-seeking, as well as in the acceptance of any therapeutic interventions. Cross-cultural definitions of family may well differ. Some couples may be in nuclear family set-ups. Others may be in extended or joint living arrangements. Even in these, the couple may have separate cooking and other arrangements, thereby making 'individuation as a couple' possible. Thus there are varied and complex ways in which a couple operates and functions. The therapist needs to have knowledge and sensitivity about these aspects. This requires study of the cultures of the couples one is dealing with, and training programmes for couple therapists need to include such study in their curriculum (see de Silva, 1999). In addition, practising therapists have their own responsibility to acquire such knowledge as part of their ongoing professional education. We believe that regular discussion among peers, including peer supervision, is a useful component in this kind of education.

Theoretically, the systems approach is the most appropriate strategy for assessment and treatment in these complex settings. The style and content of assessment and treatment have to reflect appropriate components of the culture in question, and the systems approach enables a therapist to do this effectively. The reason for this is that cultural factors, both within the couple and in relation to their interactions with the extended families and wider society or sub-culture, play an important role within the 'system' that one has to assess and try to modify. The systems approach also enables the therapist to look at his/her own relationship with the two partners in the thera-peutic triad that couple therapy inevitably is, and at how it affects the couple's interaction, and vice versa. No other therapeutic approach enables the therapist to conceptualize and handle these issues as effectively as the systems approach does (see Crowe and Ridley, 2000).

Couple therapy may not easily be accepted by vari-ous cultural and ethnic groups, and the therapist must recognize that, in some situations, it is not the couple but the whole family which may be the best 'target' for therapeutic intervention. Sometimes, while the couple brings an apparent specific problem for help, the wider family has a powerful presence in the background. The key aim is to try to be aware of these factors and to adjust one's strategy accordingly. In order to function effectively in these situations, the therapist needs to be aware of his/her own strengths and weaknesses, includ-ing a possible lack, or deficiency, of knowledge of the cultural factors surrounding the couple.

Issues in Assessment

Assessment in psychotherapy in general, and in couple therapy in particular, relies on a number of factors. For the sake of completeness, the following is a list of some of the key factors that need to be assessed. They include:

- presenting problems;
- how the problem is defined by the couple/each partner;
- why they are seeking help now;
- expectations, as a couple and as individual partners;
- the nature of the relationship, including roles in home management, finance, children, etc.;
- external sources of stress;
- role of families of origin;
- strength of the relationship;
- past marriages or relationships;
- areas of conflict;
- fidelity;
- physical and mental health.

There are many excellent sources in the literature on the subject of the areas of enquiry (e.g. Crowe and Ridley, 2000).

Table 40.1 Assessment in couple therapy across cultures

- Normative age for marriage
- Why that age?
- Do men have to achieve certain things before getting married?
- When are men/women considered eligible?
- How much free will do they have?
- History of arranged marriage?
  - Definition of arranged marriage
  - Whose responsibility?
- Do these patterns continue with migration?
- Other basis for mate selection
  - If so, how different?
  - How is it accepted by the culture?
- Role of common interest, mutual attraction, love or lust
- Expected duties of husband/wife
- Gender roles
- Self-concepts
- Division of responsibilities
- Power, alteration of power equation
- Role of families of origin
- Conception of sexual relations
- Dos and don'ts in interactions with outsiders

In the assessment of couples from minority cul-tures or mixed cultural origins, cultural norms for the couple are particularly important and must be assessed. This assessment includes questions about norms for marriage and expected roles and responsi-bilities within the relationship. Some of these are listed in Table 40.1.

The assessment in couple therapy generally focuses on the quality of the relationship because that is primarily where the problem lies. Yet add-itional problems such as sexual dysfunction may underlie or confound the relationship difficulties. The therapist must be aware of, and sensitive to, these in order to elicit details of such problems, which may indeed be the main cause of the relation-ship dysfunction, or at least a complicating factor. The therapist must be able to ascertain the quality, strengths and weaknesses of the relationship so that appropriate interventions can be put in place. It is imperative that assessment is value free and culturally sensitive so that it paves the way for appropriate treatment to occur. In intercultural unions, often the strength of the relationship may result from factors like more thorough preparation for marriage and greater commitment to the relationship. But, as noted earlier, there are also problems and disadvantages. Some of these are highlighted in Table 40.2.

These possible advantages and disadvantages need to be explored by the therapist as part of the assessment. One often finds in these situations that there is a mismatch in the views of the two partners with regard to these. One partner might, for example, highlight the exposure of the children to two cultural backgrounds as an essentially positive factor, while the other may be more concerned about the difficulties that the exposure to divergent cultural norms has brought about. In the early stages of intercultural marriage the couple tends to be idealistic and very positive about the advantages of such a union. With passing time, and with the experience of difficulties, they tend to become more realistic and even negative in their appraisal of the marriage. This transformation rarely happens at the same rate for both partners.

In the early stages of assessment, the therapist should make an effort to find out the reasons for referral and expectations of therapy. While this is an obvious requirement in all couple therapy, these

Table 40.2 Intercultural marriages: some advantages and disadvantages

Advantages	Disadvantages
More thorough preparation for marriage	Less common ground in relationship
Greater degree of commitment	Differences causing doubts
Greater degree of self–other • differentiation • tolerance • respect • acceptance	Sense of loss of self
Broader opportunity for learning and growth	Learning and growth interfered with
Greater opportunities for children	Social stigma and non-acceptance
More accepting of differences	Institutional racism

matters have particular significance when dealing with a couple from a different culture. The threshold for help-seeking, and thus referral, may be higher for some cultures than in the majority culture. This may be because of greater tolerance of disharmony, or a greater reluctance to turn to the established agents of help. Sometimes, the culture may provide the couple with other help/resolution options, such as through the extended family or a key religious figure, so that their eventual referral to a conventional therapy setting may be considerably delayed.

Therapy Strategies

Two key strategies in the therapeutic intervention are the educational and the psychological. This suggests that the therapist is primarily an agent with both educative and psychological functions. These strategies are not mutually exclusive; they can and should be used in combination, and in conjunction with other therapeutic approaches. The method of implementing these needs to take into account the couple's, and each partner's, sensitivities and expectations.

In some situations, the members of a minority culture may have their own indigenous therapies and use these along with the therapist's instructions. This has already been noted in the discussion of the threshold for referral and help-seeking. Indigenous therapies have been used in original form, as well as in modified forms. To cite an example from a different area, working with Indo-Trinidadian clients with alcohol problems, Maharajh and Bhugra (1993) found that brief family therapy with an emphasis on cultural meanings and expectations was successful. Neki's (1973) notion of the *guru–chela* (parent–teacher) roles in psychotherapy also seems appropriate for some cultural groups. There is scope for similar work in couple therapy. Therapies developed in one culture may of course be used in other settings as well (see Lloyd and Bhugra, 1993; Bhugra and Bhui, 1998). Combining different types of therapies is not necessarily contraindicated in couple work, but therapists must be aware that not enough evaluation research data are available at present with regard to this. While using such additional culture-related strategies, the therapist must therefore try to evaluate the contribution of these to the outcome of therapy.

Pitfalls

Some of the key problems in psychotherapy in general, and couple therapy in particular, are related to issues

525

like 'missionary racism' – there the clinician rather patronizingly conveys to patients that his/her role and goal is to 'save them from their plight', or to take care of these 'poor' people who are unable to look after themselves. Therapists either end up being too controlling or identify too closely with the client. In couple therapy, such a problem is further compounded, so that, if therapists are not aware of their own feelings towards race and ethnicity, they may over-identify with one member of the couple and become too controlling towards the other. Some of the pitfalls are illustrated in Table 40.3. This is more likely to happen in some scenarios than others, e.g. when the therapist and one partner are from the majority culture, and the other partner is from a minority culture.

These pitfalls are easy to fall into, and many inexperienced therapists often do so (Bhugra and Bhui, 1998). Therapists need to be constantly alert to these dangers, and an examination of one's own responses and attitudes needs to be undertaken. Again, it is necessary to emphasize the need to discuss pitfalls, and how to avoid them, as part of the curriculum in training programmes for therapists. Equally, regular supervision – at least peer supervision – that keeps

these issues on the agenda will help the therapist to avoid these pitfalls.

Marriage across Cultures

Patterns of marriage vary across cultures. For example, models of marriage in African American culture, as in any other group, are strongly influenced by larger social trends such as increased economic pressures, greater participation of females in the workplace and diminished stigma for marital discussion.

Previous research (Fowers and Olson, 1992) indicated that four types of marriages (according to relational levels) existed: vitalized, harmonious, traditional and conflicted. There was also a suggestion that the type of marriage affected the outcome. Those with vitalized marriages indicated most satisfaction with their relationships, whereas conflicted marriages, not surprisingly, reflected low satisfaction and high marital discord. There is little doubt that culture and ethnicity play critical roles in shaping the relationship experience, even more so if the individuals come from minority backgrounds. Ethnicity can be linked to individual as well as to group identity, mate selection, parent–child relationships and social support networks. African American marriages exhibit much of the economic and social diversity of couples from other ethnic groups.

Allen and Olson (2001) found that there was convincing evidence of five types of African American marriage, based on an analysis of 415 couples, and that these types were strongly associated with marital satisfaction both at individual and dyadic levels. The five types were similar to those previously observed, namely vitalized, harmonious, traditional, conflicted and devitalized. Harmonious and vitalized couples reported high marital satisfaction and high positive couple agreement on most relationship domains. Age and ethnicity per se were not associated with types, but number of children and education were.

Rosenfeld (2002) studied the patterns of marriage of Mexican Americans and attempted to link these with segmented assimilation. The process of segmented assimilation is related to the fact that assimilation with whites is no longer the only, or even the nodal, type of assimilation. This suggests that, although integration into middle class white Americans is still a viable option for some

Table 40.3 Some common pitfalls

Colour blindness:	Assumption that minority-culture client is the same as majority-culture client
Colour consciousness:	All problems result from the minority status
Colour transference:	Client's feelings result from therapist's race
Cultural counter-transference:	Therapist's feelings towards client result from their race
Cultural ambivalence:	Therapist wishes to help but needs to control to maintain power
Over-identification:	Minority therapist over-identifies everything in terms of racism and defines problems as racially based (same as colour consciousness)
Identification with oppressor:	Minority therapist denies his/her status by virtue of power and because it is painful

immigrant groups, for others, especially those who are non-white, urbanization in many countries, usually means joining the inner-city underclass who work in the most menial jobs, live in the heart of central cities, go to school and work with black Americans who have learnt to reject what they see as the values and ideals of middle-class white America, and poverty along with blocked mobility can lead to an oppositional subculture. Rosenfeld (2002) reported on the specific assimilation of Mexican Americans with non-Hispanic white, specific assimilation of Mexican Americans with non-Hispanic blacks and generalized assimilation of Mexican Americans. When groups migrate, in the initial stages endogamous marriages take place. The group slowly de-emphasizes the customs associated with their ancestry but this in itself may not be good enough for purposes of being accepted by the larger society. Using the data from the census on marital status, Rosenfeld (2002), with the most basic measure of general assimilation, percentage endogamy, reported that this percentage had declined from 77 per cent in 1970 to 66 per cent in 1990. However, this measurement has a limitation in that it does not account for group size. It is apparent that smaller groups are likely to out-marry more, which is a reflection of lack of opportunity and increased exposure rather than a measure of assimilation. However, when odds ratios take into account not only the odds of marrying within the group, but by controlling for group size, it would appear that some groups remain endogamous. Rosenfeld (2002) concludes that measures of assimilation for the Mexican Americans are different compared with the blacks. The social distance between the Mexican Americans and non-Hispanic blacks is greater than the social distance between Mexican Americans and non-Hispanic whites. Thus, the idea of solidarity between the minority groups is not upheld and neither is the evidence for segmented assimilation for Mexican Americans upheld. This study provides a critical overview of assessing cultural assimilation at a broader group level rather than at an individual level. The social distance model provides an unusual insight into the process of assimilation as well.

For Arab Americans, a similar study was conducted by Kulczycki and Lobo (2002). They too studied levels of intermarriage among Arab Americans using the 1990 census data and observed that 80 per cent of Arab Americans were married to non-Arab spouses. Logistic regression revealed that, for both sexes, those with past Arab ancestry, the US born, those with strong English-language ability and those who were highly educated were more likely to marry out, as were Arabs of Lebanese ancestry. These authors used a number of variables in their analysis. They propose that many Arab immigrants who may not be initially acculturated are still able to be structurally assimilated into the US economy, given their levels of education and skills. In their sample only 3 per cent of Arabs were married within the same Arab ancestry. Rates of intermarriage among the native born and those with strong English proficiency (two indicators of assimilation) demonstrate that marriage outside the group is more likely. Both men and women who are well educated and have higher incomes are also more likely to marry out and this too may be seen as a measure of assimilation. The authors conclude that Arab Americans are conforming to the patterns of assimilation of migrant groups. The data do not suggest whether any specific factors such as numbers, education, religion or income are more important than the others.

Management across Cultures

The therapists must be sensitive to the patient's difficulties in reporting openly about their problems. Men may be embarrassed, particularly as an open acknowledgement of their sexual problem may be seen as an aspersion on their masculinity and male gender role, which may vary somewhat across cultures. Such individuals may present with embarrassment, anxiety or depression. Although notions and preconceptions of masculinity remain similar across societies, subtle differences in the context of patriarchal hierarchy may further contribute to stress and stigma. Similarly, female gender roles may determine who the primary patient is. Anecdotal evidence suggests that South Asian women in the UK with sexual dysfunctions are likely to be referred by gynaecologists for failure to conceive. In addition, women may not wish to discuss sexual matters openly, especially with a male therapist. It is sometimes seen that the male does not wish his wife or partner to discuss intimate matters (which may be seen to reflect badly on him) to outsiders even in therapy (de Silva,

1982; Gillan, 1987). This may well further change in the twenty-first century. The therapist has to be sensitive to gender-related issues and take appropriate actions, e.g. using a co-therapist to balance the gender issue and to allow a safe environment for discussions and exploration of sexual and relationship matters. The therapist should reach a robust therapeutic formulation, which will provide the basis for appropriate and successful intervention. To do this in a suitable fashion, information is needed on predisposing, precipitating and perpetuating factors. Cultural factors will play an important role in all of these and ignoring these facts may lead to an inaccurate and misleading formulation. Additionally lack of understanding and acknowledgment of each other's culture could lead to difficulties and misunderstandings in non-sexual areas of the relationship, especially in an intercultural relationship which may have an impact on the sexual area of the relationship (Tseng and Streltzer, 2008). Tseng and Streltzer (2008) also suggest that the therapist can help such a couple be curious about each other's culture by acting as a cultural 'broker'.

Therapeutic techniques used for psychosexual dysfunction must be appropriate. Treatment methods evolved in one culture need to be modified for application in another cultural setting. The use of suitably modified approaches among Bangladeshis in the UK and Bengalis in India has been shown to be successful by d'Ardenne (1986) and Gupta *et al.* (1989), respectively. Bourne (1985) notes that traditional healers may do better with some types of individuals because they may have more time and patience to listen, which may be core to their therapeutic efficiency in contrast with general practitioners or others. In the intimate area of sex, patient listening and spending time with the patient appear to be important factors, which enhance the patient's trust in the therapist, which in turn will improve compliance with the therapeutic instructions. The acceptability of these instructions by the patient is a vital part of the therapeutic interaction. Gillan (1987) noted the difficulties that couples from some non-Western cultures may experience in carrying out some aspects of Masters and Johnson's (1970) type of intervention. As mentioned earlier, certain expectations and inhibitions may create problems. For example, in some cultures, encouraging the female to take the initiative may

well be a major disincentive. If there are cultural inhibitions to any part of the treatment package, suitable modifications must be made along with encouragement to the couple to overcome their hesitations.

The myths and taboos, especially in the field of sex, have a very strong presence and may well be further complicated by a lack of proper knowledge; therapy packages must include components of education. When attitude change is considered to be important, cognitive techniques may be indicated (Baker and de Silva, 1988). We shall illustrate some of these issues by presenting some data from different parts of the world.

The Indian Subcontinent

There are reasonable data on management and outcome of sexual dysfunction in the Indian Subcontinent. Bagadia *et al.* (1959) noted that, in their sample, ignorance of sexual matters, superstition, fear and guilt played an important role. Using group approaches they reported that 50–60 per cent of their patients improved remarkably. The primary sources of knowledge about sex, most of which are informal such as peer groups, may have an important role to play in the initiation and maintenance of these superstitions (Kalra *et al.*, 2015). In a case note-based study Singh (1985) reported on 96 patients and found that masturbation was seen as an important and common cause of sexual dysfunction, and a large majority of cases had improved with education and supportive psychotherapy with physical treatment such as minor tranquillizers. It is difficult to disentangle from this data which component of intervention produced the improvement. When Bagadia *et al.* (1972) studied 258 males attending their clinic, they found that 87 had presented with nocturnal emissions, 32 with masturbation, 91 with passage of semen in the urine, 32 with watery semen and 33 were preoccupied with the size and the shape of their penis. These complaints were accompanied by vague aches and pains, weakness, palpitations, poor appetite, poor concentration and irritability. Their concepts of semen, nocturnal emissions and masturbation were incorrect and contrasted with socially imposed values of abstinence. Thus, for young adults who have masturbated and get married at an early age with pressure to procreate, it produces not only conflict but anxiety, tension, guilt and shame. The sex act may be seen as pleasurable, but pressure to procreate becomes anxiety provoking. This ambivalence therefore puts pressure on the male to prove his manliness by procreating soon after marriage. The pressure on the newly married female is even worse and she may respond with irritation, withdrawal, anorgasmia and dyspareunia.

Agarwal (1970) treated 11 married males who had presented with premature ejaculation and found that, if the therapist contradicted their views on the role of semen, the therapeutic relationship did not work. He would use comments like, 'maybe energy is lost in emission, but the body has got a self-regulatory mechanism which recoups this loss quickly' and found that this seemed to work. The need for physical treatment and explanation cannot be underestimated as is diagnosing and treating depressive and anxiety symptoms which are common comorbidities (Udina et al., 2013). A lack of acceptance of behaviour therapy among Hindus in India (Kuruvilla 1984) and among South Asians in the UK (Bhugra and Cordle, 1986, 1988) led to high dropout rates from both centres. In a case note-based study over an 8-year period, Bhugra and Cordle (1986) found 32 patients of South Asian origin of whom 14 (44%) dropped out at some point before completion of treatment. The symptoms had been present much longer in men (longer than 5 years) in comparison with women. Of the 14, four dropped out because their partner had returned to India or had gone on a long holiday. Christopher (1982) noted that, among non-Western couples presenting to her clinic, Indian men were more likely to present at an average older age and three out of four Asian women were referred because of premature ejaculation of their husbands. She noted that Asians missed more appointments, did not inform the clinic of their intended absence and dropped out more often. However, d'Ardenne (1986, 1988, 1991) and d'Ardenne and Crown (1986) present a more optimistic picture for treating Bangladeshi couples. Drawings and pictures were used for educating them and other members of the family became involved and took a more authoritarian role in therapy.

Gupta et al. (1989) reported success in 76 per cent of their male sample presenting with erectile dysfunction and premature ejaculation. In addition to relaxation, they used sensate focus and education and encouraged patients to keep a diary. In the second stage of sensate focus they were given psychoanalytic interpretations. They note that themes of parental dominance and fears of damaging the male organ during sexual intercourse were common. They observe that, where abstinence is glorified as a precondition to the salvation of the spirit, carnal pleasure must be at a discount and marital sex becomes a duty rather than a pleasure. Hindu ideals of purity and contamination may further complicate explanations.

In Sri Lanka, in several studies, de Silva (1982), de Silva and Samarasinghe (1985) and Rodrigo (1992) found that males who presented to their clinics believed very strongly that their problems were due to physical causes, especially loss of semen, and they sought physical treatments. They also showed poor response to behavioural therapy and were reluctant to bring their partners. In addition, lack of privacy and shortage of space made carrying out of home assignments very difficult. These researchers overcame some of the problems by recruiting female therapists, using medication and public education.

Among females, sex may be seen as a chore or gift rather than a right and their own attitudes may be ambivalent. Ambivalent attitudes were seen among the females in a clinic sample with 25 per cent females reporting in-law problems, and those who had married against their parental choice were under greater stress (Agarwal, 1977), although the numbers are small.

Some common themes of male role, female gender role and gender-role expectations, search for physical causes and physical treatments and difficulties in therapeutic engagement emerge from the Indian subcontinent sample.

The Middle East

Although limited information is available from the Middle East, studies indicate that there are similarities with the Indian subcontinent. Of 70 cases of sexual dysfunction reported from Jordan, only six came with their partners, but the therapist gave recorded information on audiotape for the absent partners and in general outcome was poor (Takriti, 1987). Takriti also reported that tremendous pressure for quick improvement, poor education and low social class were additional factors. A very high level of performance anxiety was noted in that, in one case, a young man developed panic when approaching his nude wife. This intense anxiety leads to avoidance but social and familial pressures to deflower the bride and consummate the marriage put additional pressure on the male. Basoglu *et al.* (1986) allocated Turkish males with sexual dysfunction to psychotherapy or drug treatment and found that low socio-economic status, erectile failure, shorter duration and higher levels of dysfunction were associated with premature termination of psychotherapy. Demerdash and colleagues (1977, 1978) have identified various factors contributing to sexual dysfunction and their psychosocial correlates, which are not dissimilar to the factors elsewhere.

Cognitive and Behavioural Therapies

Cognitive therapy offers a potentially useful intervention provided the normative data from the population on cognitions is available and understood by the therapists. Techniques used in cognitive therapy to explore and verify assumptions, which lead to generating alternative explanations, solutions and strategies, are potentially very attractive. For example, the cognitive triad of depression as described and used in the West is not directly applicable across cultures as the definitions of the self differ across cultures. However, it should be relatively straightforward to explore cognitions and work with them. Cognitive-behavioural and cognitive-analytic therapies can be easily used across cultures.

Although behavioural therapies focus on objections and observable behaviour, cultures do play a significant role in identifying what is normal behaviour and how behaviour is modified. Attempts to use social skills assessment, assertiveness training, dating behaviour and attitudes to sexual education are all areas that can be potentially problematic and produce discord between the patient and the therapist. Any attempts to modify sexual behaviour in the therapist's direction may be deeply offensive or threatening to the patient, and the therapist may risk being offended by culturally determined sexual stereotypes which may contrast with his/her own beliefs (McCarthy, 1988). Under the circumstances, a careful preliminary negotiation of treatment targets and working within the same set of expectations may work better.

Physical Therapies

From availability of intracavernosal injections to external devices such as vacuum pumps and surgical interventions such as implants and revascularizations to oral medication such as yohimbine, sildenafil, tadalafil, various physical therapies have been used. However, virtually no data are available on their usage elsewhere in other cultures. It is imperative that therapists are aware of specific cultural issues related to pharmacodynamics and pharmacokinetics (see Bhugra and Bhui, 1999; and Ng and Bousman in this volume, see Chapter 33). Physical treatments of erectile dysfunction may place too much emphasis on erection, thereby equating it with sexual intercourse. Physical treatments must be offered only after detailed discussion and proper and thorough assessment of the patient and the couple.

The aetiology and management of sexual dysfunction is a complex matter; the clinician must place both these into the context of the patient's and his/her partner's culture and any outcomes also should take these crucial factors into account. It is possible that, prior to commencing any treatment, the therapist and the patient can agree on a set of ground rules and agreed outcomes. 'Cultural demand for effectiveness of sexual performance' as identified by Masters and Johnson (1970) to focus on erections being sufficient for intercourse is a clear indication regarding the role social factors play in seeking, providing and accepting treatments. A combination of physical and psychological therapies may prove to be successful and effective (Kaplan, 1993).

Conclusions

The challenge for any therapist in dealing with patients with sexual dysfunction is to be aware of the potential pitfalls and to understand the problem in all its cultural complexity. Even if such an understanding is not possible, a clear nod to the patient to state that would be helpful. In discussion with the patients and other significant individuals from that culture and community, it should be possible to gather enough information on cultural aspects of sexual dysfunction. It requires a willingness on the part of the therapist to acknowledge lacunae in his/her knowledge of cultural factors and an element of sensitivity in exploring these is necessary. It also requires ingenuity, as illustrated above, by combining different modalities of treatment from using audiotapes for educating the partner to broader public education. The therapist has to show a willingness to be flexible in applying therapeutic modalities.

References

Agarwal, A. K. (1970). Treatment of impotence. *Indian Journal of Psychiatry*, **12**, 88–96.

Agarwal, A. K. (1977). Frigidity: a clinical study. *Indian Journal of Psychiatry*, **19**, 31–37.

Allen, W. D. and Olson, D. H. (2001). Five types of African-American marriages. *Journal of Marital and Family Therapy*, **27**, 301–314.

Anson, M. (1995). Non-couple therapy for sexual dysfunction. *International Review of Psychiatry*, **7**, 205–216.

Anthony, B. (1982). Lesbian client: lesbian therapist. In *Homosexuality and Psychotherapy*, ed. J. C. Gonsiorek. New York: Haworth.

Bagadia, V. N., Vardhachari, K. S., Mehta, B. C. and Vahia, N. S. (1959). Education group psychotherapy for certain minor sex disorders of males. *Indian Journal of Psychiatry*, **1**, 237–240.

Bagadia, V. N., Dave, K. P., Pradham, P. V. and Shah, L. P. (1972). A study of 258 male patients with sexual problems. *Indian Journal of Psychiatry*, **14**, 143–151.

Baker, C. and de Silva, P. (1988). The relationship between male sexual dysfunction and belief in Zilbergeld's myths: an empirical investigation. *Sexual and Marital Therapy*, **3**, 229–238.

Balon, R. (2008). *Sexual Dysfunction: The Brain-Body Connection*. Basel: Karger.

Bancroft, J. (2008). *Human Sexuality and its Problems*, 3rd edn. Edinburgh: Churchill Livingstone.

Basoglu, M., Yerkin, N., Sercan, M. and Karraduman, B. (1986). Patterns of attention for psychological and pharmacological treatment of male sexual dysfunction. *Sexual and Marital Therapy*, **1**, 69–75.

Bhugra, D. and Bhui, K. S. (1997). Issues in assessment in cross-cultural psychiatry. *Advances in Psychiatric Treatment*, **3**, 103–110.

Bhugra, D. and Bhui, K. S. (1998). Psychotherapy for ethnic minorities: issues, context and practice. *British Journal of Psychotherapy*, **14**, 310–326.

Bhugra, D. and Bhui, K. S. (1999). Ethnic and cultural factors in psychopharmacology. *Advances in Psychiatric Treatment*, **5**, 89–95.

Bhugra, D. and Cordle, C. (1986). Sexual dysfunction in Asian couples. *British Medical Journal*, **92**, 111–112.

Bhugra, D. and Cordle, C. (1988). Sexual dysfunction in Asian couples: a case control study. *Sexual and Marital Therapy*, **3**, 69–75.

Bhugra, D. and de Silva, P. (1993). Sexual dysfunction across cultures. *International Review of Psychiatry*, **5**, 143–252.

Bhugra, D. and Littlewood, R. (2000). *Colonialism and Psychiatry*. New Delhi: Oxford University Press.

Bhugra, D. and Wright, B. (1995). Sexual dysfunction in gay men: diagnosis and management. *International Review of Psychiatry*, **7**, 247–252.

Bourne, S. (1985). Traditional remedies or health issues. *The Listener*, **23** November, 8–10.

Cabaj, R. and Stein, T. (2013). *Textbook of Homosexuality and Mental Health*. Washington DC: APA Press.

Catalan, J., Hawton, K. and Day, A. (1991). Individuals presenting without partners at a sexual dysfunction clinic: psychological and physical morbidity and treatment offered. *Sexual and Marital Therapy*, **6**, 15–23.

Christopher, E. (1982). Psychosexual medicine in a mixed racial community. *British Journal of Family Planning*, **7**, 115–119.

Crowe, M. (1995). Couple therapy and sexual dysfunctions. *International Review of Psychiatry*, **7**, 195–204.

Crowe, M. and Ridley, J. (2000). *Therapy with Couples*, 2nd edn. Oxford: Blackwell.

d'Ardenne, P. (1986). Sexual dysfunction in a transcultural setting: assessment, treatment and research. *Sexual and Marital Therapy*, **1**, 23–34.

d'Ardenne, P. (1988). Sexual dysfunction in a transcultural setting. In *Sex Therapy in Britain*, ed. M. Cole and W. Dryden. Milton Keynes: Open University Press.

d'Ardenne, P. (1991). Transcultural issues in couple therapy. In *Couple Therapy: A Handbook*, ed. D. Hooper and W. Dryden. Milton Keynes: Open University Press.

d'Ardenne, P. and Crown, S. (1986). Sexual dysfunction in Asian couples. *British Medical Journal*, **292**, 1078–1979.

De Maris, A. (2000). Till discord do us part. *Journal of Marriage and the Family*, **62**, 683–692.

de Silva, P. (1982). Cultural problems in sexual dysfunction therapy. Paper presented at 6th International Congress of the International Association for Cross-cultural Psychology, Aberdeen.

de Silva, P. (1999). Leading comment: culture and sex therapy. *Sexual and Marital Therapy*, **14**, 105–107.

de Silva, P. and Samarasinghe, D. (1985). Behaviour therapy in Sri Lanka. *Journal of Behaviour Therapy and Experimental Psychiatry*, **16**, 95–100.

Demerdash, A. (1977). The early life of Arab patients suffering from psychogenic sexual inadequacy. *Acta Psychiatrica Scandanavica*, **56**, 61–68.

Demerdash, A., Lotaif, E., Bishry, Z., Ashour, A. and Okash, A. (1978). A cross-cultural study of cases of functional sexual disorders among Arabs. *Egyptian Journal of Psychiatry*, **1**, 51–56.

Doermer, K. (1981). *Mad Men and the Bourgeoisie*. Oxford: Basil Blackwell.

Eichenbaum, I. and Orbach, S. (1982). *Outside in, Inside out Women's Psychology: A Feminist Psychoanalytic Perspective*. Harmondsworth: Penguin.

Foucault, M. (1967). *Madness and Civilisation*. New York: Basic Books.

Fowers, F. and Olson, D. (1992). Four types of premarital couples. *Journal of Family Psychology*, **6**, 10–30.

Gillan, P. (1987). *Sex Therapy Manual*. Oxford: Blackwell.

Gordon, P. (1986). Sex therapy with gay men: a review. *Sexual and Marital Therapy*, **1**, 221–226.

Griffith, M. S. (1977). The influence of race on the psychotherapeutic relationship. *Psychiatry*, **40**, 27–40.

Guirguis, W. R. (1995). The problem of the single impotent man. *International Review of Psychiatry*, **7**, 191–194.

Gupta, P., Bannerjee, G. and Nandi, D. N. (1989). Modified Masters and Johnson technique in the treatment of sexual inadequacy in males. *Indian Journal of Psychiatry*, **31**, 63–69.

Hall, K. S. K. and Graham, C. (2013). *The Cultural Context of Sexual Pleasure and Problems*. New York: Routledge.

Hawton, K. (1985). *Sex Therapy: A Practical Guide*. Oxford: Oxford University Press.

Helmeke, K. B. and Sprenkle, D. H. (2000). Clients' perception of pivotal moments in couples therapy. *Journal of Marital and Family Therapy*, **26**, 469–484.

Hodes, M. (1989). Annotation: culture and family therapy. *Journal of Family Therapy*, **11**, 116–128.

Huston, T. L. (2000). The social ecology of marriage and other intimate unions. *Journal of Marriage and the Family*, **62**, 298–321.

Kalra, G., Kamath, R., Subramanyam, A., and Shah, H. (2015). Psychosocial profile of male patients presenting with sexual dysfunction in a psychiatric outpatients department in Mumbai, India. *Indian Journal of Psychiatry*, **57**, 51–58.

Kaplan, H. S. (1993). The psychiatric aspects of injection treatment. In *The New Injection Treatment for Impotence*, ed. G. Wagner and H. S. Kaplan. New York: Brunner/Mazel.

Kleinplatz, P. J. (2013). *New Directions in Sex Therapy: Innovations and Alternatives*. Philadelphia: Routledge.

Kulczycki, A. and Lobo, A. P. (2002). Patterns, determinants and implications of intermarriage among Arab Americans. *Journal of Marriage and Family*, **64**, 202–210.

Kuruvilla, K. (1984). Treatment of single impotent males. *Indian Journal of Psychiatry*, **26**, 160–163.

Law, D. D. and Crane, D. R. (2000). The influence of marital and family therapy on care utilisation in a health-maintenance organisation. *Journal of Marital and Family Therapy*, **26**, 281–292.

Leff, J. (1988). *Psychiatry around the Globe*. London: Gaskell.

Leiblum, S. (2007). *Principles and Practice of Sex Therapy*, 4th edn. New York: Guilford.

Leiblum, S. (2010). *Treating Sexual Desire Disorders*. New York: Guilford.

Levounis, P. and Drescher, J. (2012). *The LGBT Casebook*. Washington DC: APA Press.

Littlewood, R. and Lipsedge, M. (1999). *Aliens and Alienists*, 2nd edn. London: Routledge.

Lloyd, K. and Bhugra, D. (1993). Cross cultural aspects of psychotherapy. *International Review of Psychiatry*, **5**, 291–304.

McCarthy, B. (1988). Working with ethnic minorities. In *New Developments in Clinical Psychology*, ed. F. N. Watts. Chichester, UK: Wiley, pp. 122–139.

Maharajh, H. and Bhugra, D. (1993). Brief family therapy with alcohol-dependent men in Trinidad and Tobago. *Acta Psychiatrica Scandinavica*, **87**, 422–426.

Malyon, A. K. (1982). Psychotherapeutic implications of internalized homophobia in gay men. In *Homosexuality and Psychotherapy*, ed. J. C. Gonsiorek. New York: Haworth.

Masters, W. and Johnson, V. (1970). *Human Sexual Inadequacy*. Boston: Little Brown.

Masters, W. and Johnson, V. (1979). *Homosexuality in Perspective*. Boston: Little Brown.

Mikulincer, M., Florian, V., Cowan, P. A. and Cowan, P. C. (2002). Attachment security in couple relationships. *Family Process*, **41**, 405–434.

Neki, J. S. (1973). *Guru chela* relationship: the possibility of a therapeutic paradigm. *American Journal of Orthopsychiatry*, **3**, 755–766.

Nwoye, A. (2000). Building in the indigenous: theory and method of marriage therapy in contemporary Eastern and Western Africa. *Journal of Family Therapy*, **22**, 347–359.

Peavy, R.V., and Li, H.Z. (2003). Social and cultural context of intercultural counselling. *Canadian Journal of Counseling*, **37**, 186–196.

Porter, R. (1987). *Mind Forg'd Manacles: A History of Madmen in England*. London: Athlone Press.

Reece, R. (1985). Group treatment of sexual dysfunction in gay men. In *A Guide to Psychotherapy with Gay and Lesbian Clients*, ed. J. C. Gonsiorek. New York: Haworth, pp. 113–129.

Regan, P. C., Lakhanpal, S., and Anquiano, C. (2012). Relationship outcomes in Indian-American love-based and arranged marriages. *Psychological Reports*, **110**, 915–924.

Roberts, L. J. (2000). Fire and ice in marital communication. *Journal of Marriage and the Family*, **62**, 693–707.

Rodrigo, E. K. (1992). Personal Communication.

Rosenfeld, M. J. (2002). Measures of assimilation in the marriage market: Mexican Americans 1970–1990. *Journal of Marriage and Family*, **64**, 152–162.

Sabshin, M., Diesenhaus, H. and Wilkerson, R. (1970). Dimensions of institutional racism in psychiatry. *American Journal of Psychiatry*, **127**, 787–793.

Sandhya, S. (2009). The social context of marital happiness in urban Indian couples: interplay of intimacy and conflict. *Journal of Marital and Family Therapy*, **35**, 74–96.

Singh, K. (1985). Dhat syndrome revisited. *Indian Journal of Psychiatry*, **27**, 119–122.

Takriti, A. (1987). Sexual dysfunction in Jordan (unpublished paper) cited in Bhugra, D. and de Silva, P. (1993): Sexual dysfunction across cultures. *International Review of Psychiatry*, **5**, 243–252.

Thomas, A. and Sillen, S. (1972). *Racism and Psychiatry*. New York: Brunner/Mazel.

Tseng, W.S., and Streltzer, J. (2008). *Culture and Psychotherapy: A Guide to Clinical Practice*. Washington DC: American Psychiatric Press.

Udina, M., Foulon, H., Valdés, M., Bhattacharyya, S., and Martin-Santos, R. (2013). Dhat syndrome: a systematic review. *Psychosomatics*, **54**, 212–218.

Wang, H. and Amoto, P. (2000). Predictors of divorce adjustment. *Journal of Marriage and the Family*, **62**, 655–668.

Wohl, J. (1989). Integration of cultural awareness into psychotherapy. *American Journal of Psychotherapy*, **43**, 343–355.

Zhang, H., Ho, P.S., and Yip, P.S. (2012). Does similarity breed marital and sexual satisfaction? *Journal of Sex Research*, **49**, 583–593.

Zur, O. (2015). Power in psychotherapy and counseling. Online publication by the Zur Institute, available at www.zurinstitute.com/power_in_therapy.html (accessed 9 October 2016).

Transgenderism
Cross-Cultural Perspectives

Gurvinder Kalra

Editors' Introduction

Sex and gender carry different connotations across cultures. It is recognized that gender roles and gender role expectations are strongly influenced by cultural factors and values. Certain behaviours related to sexual preference and sexual identity may be more easily accepted in some cultures in comparison with others. Kalra in this chapter emphasizes that that is because culture is a very strong factor that determines how we experience and express ourselves in terms of our own identity. He points out that transgenderism is a universal phenomenon and is well recognized across various societies and cultures. In some cultures such as Hindu cultures (third sex has been recognized as a separate category in India), *hijras* are an integral part of the society and are expected to participate in specific joyous occasions such as marriages and births. Historically, there have been many alternatives to male or female gender in different cultures with some of them being seen as the third gender, often with male/female as the two points of reference. Increasingly in many countries, a non-binary approach to gender and sex has developed. In clinical settings it is important that clinicians are aware of social norms but also individual variations also confirming the dynamic nature of cultures around the globe. Kalra states that transgender individuals tend to go through a complex process of coming to terms with their sexuality which comprises their biological sex, gender identity, gender expression, gender role and sexual orientation. This may well be much more complex than gay/lesbian/bisexual individuals who tend to come to terms with their sexual orientation and associated issues along a relatively different pathway but perhaps similar stages. Gender affirmation is the interpersonal process by which gender variant individuals' self-identified gender identity is affirmed through the means of social interactions.

Introduction

Recognition of the rights of the lesbian, gay, bisexual, transgender, intersex and queer (LGBTIQ) population has received considerable attention over the last few decades across the globe. Grouping the transgender and intersex identities with the lesbian, gay and bisexual acronym would give a sense of them belonging to a community. However, they (i.e. transgender and intersex individuals) are often the most ignored and least recognized of all the other groups. This is despite the fact that they are equally vulnerable and are the victims of discrimination, violence and persecution like other identities under the umbrella term of LGBTIQ. Often referred to as gender minority, transgender individuals have diverse sexual orientation, identities and behaviours.

Not surprisingly, the exact estimated prevalence of transgenderism globally is difficult to predict. A number of factors affect this estimation including willingness of individuals to come forward, as well as the definition of transgender used in different studies. While trans-activism has been present in the Western world for quite some time now, it is not universal. Furthermore, it is interesting to note that transgenderism has been a culturally accepted phenomenon in various other cultures across the world for a long time.

Culture and Sexuality

Before understanding the interface of culture and sexuality, one needs to understand various terms that are often used interchangeably in day to day life without much thought as to what they actually mean. These terms and the meanings attached to them have gained significant importance in recent times with better biopsychosocio-cultural understandings of these terms.

The term *sex* refers to the objectively measurable anatomical structures (sex organs), hormones and chromosomes that make an individual a man (if he has a penis and testicles with XY chromosomes and testosterone), a woman (if she has a vagina, ovaries and uterus with XX chromosomes and oestrogen/progesterone) or an intersex person (various combinations of male/female sex characteristics). Biological sex is thus used to assign gender at birth. *Gender identity* is an individual's internal sense of being a man, woman or as someone anywhere along the gender continuum. Contrary to sex which is objective, gender identity is more subjective, internal and can often be dynamic. *Gender expression* is the way an individual expresses the felt gender identity to others and may include how the person acts, behaves, dresses and interacts with others. Gender expression could be masculine, feminine or androgynous. *Gender role* on the other hand refers to the behaviours that are designated as appropriate to one's given gender and are deemed so by the society/culture that one lives in. Thus, a woman engaging in household chores, staying at home and caring for the children is the gender role that is 'expected' from her given her female gender. The term gender expression and gender role, although appearing somewhat similar are not so. Gender expression on one hand appears more intrinsically driven while gender role is something that appears externally imposed on an individual by the set of rules that the society governs. *Sexual orientation* refers to the sex of those to whom an individual is emotionally, sexually and romantically attracted. An individual's sexual orientation could be homosexual, heterosexual or bisexual. It is important to note that all the above described concepts *may* affect one another but they are independent of one another. For most people biological sex and gender identity are usually congruent with each other (cis-gender), which leads to a congruent gender expression. However, for some the biological sex and gender identity may be incongruent with each other. For example, a person assigned male by birth may feel a woman on the inside and may come across as quite feminine in gender expression. Such individuals who seem to have transcended the gender identity 'boundaries' are transgender individuals. A transgender person may self-identify as a woman born in a man's body (trans-woman) or a man born in a woman's body (trans-man). Most of these concepts, except for sex, appear fairly dynamic and people may move from one end of the continuum to the other depending on various factors, most of which are internal. However, all these are highly likely

to be influenced by external factors, most important of which is the immediate surroundings of the individual, the socio-cultural milieu where the individual lives. Gender has been described as fluid, something that is not limited within restrictive boundaries of the stereotypical definitions of a man and a woman. Non-binary thus refers to having a transgender identity that does not use female or male dichotomies as reference points, often identified as the third gender in some cultures. Another term that blurs these rigid gender stereotypes is *genderqueer*, individuals who may not identify as male or female, but as both, neither or a blend. A simpler term, gender variance or gender non-conforming is sometimes used to refer to the entire gamut of variances that are seen within the gender identity spectrum. Another often used neologism (Ryan, 2014), 'trans*' is an umbrella term that refers to all identities within the gender identity spectrum. This term was popularized by Killerman (2012) via various online blogs to refer to individuals who do not identify themselves as cis-gendered. The asterisk (*) after the word 'trans' emerged from the computer codes for searching databases to help be inclusive of the entire range of gender variant identities without the risk of limiting it to just trans-men or trans-women. Throughout this chapter, I will be using both the terms transgender and trans* interchangeably at different points.

Transgender individuals tend to go through a complex process of coming to terms with their sexuality which comprises their biological sex, gender identity, gender expression, gender role and sexual orientation. This is more complex than gay/lesbian/bisexual individuals who tend to come to terms with their sexual orientation and associated issues along a relatively different pathway. Gender affirmation is the interpersonal process by which gender variant individuals' gender identity is affirmed through social interactions as and when they are acknowledged, recognized and supported for their gender identity and expression. One could hypothesize four core facets or stages in the gender affirmation process of trans* individuals (Nuttbrock *et al.*, 2009; Sevelius, 2013; Reisner *et al.*, 2016): *social* (e.g. gender appropriate name, pronoun, dressing, etc.), *psychological* (e.g. internal, felt self within the context of one's gender), *medical* (e.g. hormone replacement therapy, sex reassignment surgery), and *legal* (e.g. change in name and gender on birth certificate). These stages are not necessarily linear and can occur

535

at various times in one's life. Various identities within the trans* spectrum may choose to go ahead with any of these stages in their transition. The dynamic nature of gender identity/expression (gender fluidity) may affect this process and an individual may travel across the gender spectrum depending on various factors. It seems likely that during development, a trans* individual initially faces the social and psychological struggles followed by medical and legal if transition occurs. However, all these four can continue throughout their lives at different points and different pace. Arguably socio-cultural factors could dominate the entire gender affirming process and be the deciding factor whether or not a trans* individual comes out and transitions.

This is because culture is a very strong factor that determines how we experience and express ourselves in terms of our own identity. This would then also include our experience of our gender and how we express the same. For example, most cultures expect men to behave more masculinely and engage in more dominant, competitive and autonomous behaviours (Ashmore *et al.*, 1986). Different cultures attach meanings to these behaviours that increase their significance to those who are involved in the behaviours (role players). We thus tend to live within cultures that lay out the norms and rules of how we live and express ourselves. These norms are usually unwritten and are passed on intergenerationally (vertical transmission) as well as within generations (horizontal transmission). Any variations from these norms are seen as deviations or abnormalities and may be seen as taboo, often generating a sense of secrecy around them. One can examine transgenderism from this perspective in different cultures and understand how it is perceived variously in these cultures ranging from normalcy to deviancy to a taboo issue. The aim of this chapter is to take a combined overview (etic and emic) of transgenderism across various cultures and highlight the importance of the same within the context of mental health.

Transgenderism across Cultures

Transgenderism is a universal phenomenon that has existed in various societies and cultures for ages and is thus easy to view from an etic perspective. There have been many alternatives to male or female gender in different cultures with some of them being seen as the third gender, often with male/female as the two points of reference. Emically (arising from emic meaning

from within) these alternative gender/gender roles are seen as perfect fits within the culture in which they are present. One could argue that since culture is dynamic, it has flexibly accommodated gender variant individuals assigning them with accepted roles, for example *hijras* in India are known to sing and dance to congratulate newlyweds and hence are socio-culturally accepted, although marginalized and stigmatized. Cultures thus could be seen as flexible, dynamic and generally accepting and accommodating of uncertainties in life including that of gender variations.

Some authors have also examined transgenderism in various cultures from an androphilic point of view. Androphilia is sexual attraction to physically mature males. In the Western context, gay men would be called androphilic since they experience and express their attraction to other men (Murray, 2000). They do not have to take on different roles to experience or express this attraction but can enter into a relationship as 'men'. However in some cultures, androphilia occurs between a male who is gender-atypical (trans*) and another male who is gender-typical (cis-gender). This is referred to as transgendered male androphilia and the partners involved tend to take on 'alternative' gender and social roles (Herdt, 1996). This is especially true for the male partner who allows himself to be anally penetrated and may thus be seen as 'less of a man' and more of a woman (Kulick, 1997). Cultural undertones beneath such transgendered male androphilia tend to be similar between most cultures. For instance, transgender individuals such as *hijra* of India, *kathoey* of Thailand, and *fa'afafine* of Samoa are known to include mostly trans-women but also accommodate many other sexual and gender identities. From a more biological perspective, one could look at the fraternal birth order effect or older brother effect theory (Blanchard, 2004). Researchers have suggested that the existence of older brothers increases the odds of androphilia in later born males. Each additional older brother increases the odds of homosexuality/androphilia by approximately 33 per cent (Blanchard and Klassen, 1997). This is hypothesized due to progressive immunization of some mothers to the male-specific antigens produced during gestation of each successive male fetus. As a result the antibodies that are produced affect the sexual differentiation of the developing male fetus's brain (maternal immune hypothesis) (Blanchard and Klassen, 1997). The older brother effect has been noted in transgender individuals in different Western countries including the US, England, Italy, the Netherlands, Canada (Blanchard, 2004) as also in some non-Western cultures such as the *fa'afafine* in Samoa (VanderLaan and Vasey, 2011).

For in-depth emic accounts of transgenderism in various cultures, the reader is referred to other sources such as Bolich (2007).

In this chapter, I focus on trans* identities within the Asia–Pacific context with passing references to trans* identities in other cultures.

Asia

South Asia

In the South Asian context, the *hijra* is an institutionalized third gender role (Nanda, 1985) that may lie closest to the Western transgender identity (Kalra, 2012). However, *hijra* groups may be constituted by individuals who may include effeminate gay men, transsexual men (pre/post-emasculation), transvestites and rarely true hermaphrodites. Men who have sex with men (MSM) are known to have more gender non-conforming behaviours or appearance and may sometimes join the *hijra* communities to allow for better gender affirmation in the context of social exclusion and marginalization (Tomori *et al.*, 2016). Kalra (2012) thus argues that the best way to understand the *hijra* identity would be to look at how the individual defines self within the context of own gender identity, thus giving it a more individual-centric approach. Most *hijra* individuals would agree that they are a third gender. Because this identity stands separate from the male and female genders, it is able to challenge the stereotypes of masculinity and femininity. *Hijras* are thus able to behave in a less inhibited manner than either men or women who are expected to be reserved and inhibited in the traditional sense.

Transgender individuals across the subcontinent including India, Pakistan and Bangladesh are mostly referred to as *hijras*. In Pakistan, a more polite term is *khwaja sara* or *khwaja sira* (Khan, 2016) and the *hijra* may comprise of *khusra* and *zanana*. The *khusras* are apparently hermaphrodite *hijras* who have a guru who is a true hermaphrodite. They do not indulge in either begging or sex work as means of their livelihood but depend on earnings through alms given by people in return for their prayers and blessings. *Zananas* on the other hand are those *hijras* who are men by birth but feel like women or in other words, are trans-women.

The *zananas* earn their livelihood through commercial sex or begging (Abdullah *et al.*, 2012).

Hijras have an important socio-cultural significance especially in the Indian society. They are known to dance at homes for newlyweds and childbirths congratulating the family, a tradition that is called '*badhai*' and signifies the special powers that *hijras* are supposed to have (Kalra, 2012). Apparently these blessings bring luck, fertility and riches. The host families in return are obligated to pay *hijras* in money, grain or other things (Duthel, 2013). *Hijras* are also known to engage in commercial sex work as a means of earning their livelihood. Some consider it as survival sex work to support themselves after being rejected by their families of origin. They are often the passive partners in these acts (Kalra and Shah, 2013), and this receptivity during sexual intercourse is often experienced by them as a gender affirming behaviour (Bockting *et al.*, 1998).

In terms of the gender affirmation process, *hijras* in India undergo simple social transition and live within their defined *gharanas* with other *hijra* individuals. In some areas in northern India and Pakistan, *hijra* groups can be very territorial (Duthel, 2013). It is likely that this structured living arrangement provides them with both security and psychological transition since each of them seems to understand the other and provide for gender affirmation through gender appropriate names, pronouns and clothing. One could argue that this could reduce the felt need for medical and legal transition to achieve gender affirmation in the *hijras* and this could have been the reason for them not accessing medical transition in addition to various other barriers. However with emerging trans* activism within the subcontinent, a greater number of *hijras* are accessing medical transition and legal recognition.

Meti in Nepal refers to a transgender woman but tends to include a range of gender identities (Wilson *et al.*, 2011). In the neighbouring small country of Myanmar (Burma), men with cross-gender behaviours are called *acaults* and usually are seen in roles such as shamans and seers, which tends to give them a revered position in society (Coleman *et al.*, 1992). Interestingly, in the island country of Sri Lanka there are no structured or culturally accepted trans-communities. There is possibly a lack of understanding of the trans* identity. Effeminate men are sometimes considered transgender in a more commonplace way and are referred to as *nachchis* or *pons*.

Southeast Asia

Among the Southeast Asian countries, Thailand has been quite tolerant to alternate sexualities for a very long time (Ocha, 2012). The term *kathoey* (pronounced *kateuyee*) has been historically used to refer to gender non-conforming males in Thailand and has been extended to include gay men as well. However, authors have argued that *kathoey* have to be seen as women (Brummelhuis, 1999) since many of them see and identify themselves as *phuying* (woman) or *phuying prophet song* (a second kind of woman) (Winter, 2006). The term *kathoey*, or ladyboys as they are also called, is almost exclusively used to refer to biological males or trans-women (Jackson and Sullivan, 1999) and other terms including transvestite, gay or crossdresser have been seen as inappropriate (Totman, 2011). Today they exist as part of the wider Thai society and engage in various occupations including sex work, cabarets and the entertainment industry.

In the Phillipines, the terms *bakla* or *bayot* are used to refer to trans-women but can end up being used quite loosely to describe gays and effeminate men. Although used and perceived pejoratively in the past, the term has been more positively adopted in contemporary times just like the word 'queer' has been in the West (Manalansan, 2015). In both these countries, trans* individuals within their locally accepted identities form an important part of social life but continue to experience marginalization like the *hijras* in the subcontinent.

In Malaysia, transgender women (MtF) are referred to as *mak nyah*, a term that is argued to have evolved to distinguish trans-women from other sexual identities, including gay men, transvestites, cross dressers, and drag queens (The and Koon, 2003). *Mak nyahs* have struggled for a long time just like the trans* identities in other countries (Slamah, 2005). This is specifically true for the *mak nyahs* who also identify themselves as Muslims and as a result face the most religious and cultural resistance, often being rejected by both religious and legal officials for having changed their sex, if they do (Juergensmeyer and Roof, 2011; Goh, 2012).

Oceania

French Polynesia

The Polynesian society has been quite tolerant of gender variations especially in the pre-colonial times; colonization having resulted in stigmatization of such variations. *Mâhû* or *raerae* is a sociological and anthropological trans* identity in French Polynesian islands, and includes people considered neither men nor women but half-men/half-women or the third Polynesian gender (Stip, 2015). Both *mâhû* or *raerae* have a cultural meaning. A *mâhû* is a man who publicly takes on feminine roles and activities such as child-care and dresses like a woman and in modern-day Hawai'i would mostly refer to male to female transgendered people, although in old Hawai'i, this meant 'hermaphrodite' and would refer to both feminine men and masculine women (Matzner, 2001). They may engage in fellatio with other men and thus may be seen as homosexual (Bullough and Bullough, 1993). A *raerae* refers to more feminized *mâhû* (Elliston, 2014). Being exclusively male-bodied, a *raerae* is actually closer to a trans* identity with some of them having had sex-change operations, whilst others take female hormones (Lewin *et al.*, 2002). *Mâhû* on the other hand can be male-bodied or female-bodied. Interestingly both *raerae* or *mâhû* are not rigid 'identities' in a fixed sense as essentially one can move in and out of their identities as *raerae* or *mâhû* (Elliston, 2014).

Raerae and *mâhû* are known to engage in commercial sex work (and may also earn money by stealing from prospective and actual clients) but also work for the households where they may live in exchange for being looked after. Both these identities appear to have an accepted sociocultural significance within the Polynesian society both in the pre-European and the current times. They were valued members of their families and male to female *mâhû* were especially respected as dance teachers (Matzner, 2001). They are also involved in child-rearing practices within families (Zanghellini, 2010).

Another culturally accepted trans* Polynesian identity, the Samoan *fa'afafine* are male at birth but self-identify as women thus making up a large proportion of this population (Poasa, 1992). The word *fa'afafine* literally means 'in the way of a woman' (Poasa, 1992), however, the group comprises of a range of individuals who can be very feminine at one end of the spectrum or be very masculine at the other. They are known to engage in women's chores in addition to dressing up and behaving as women. Today, *fa'afafine* are known to also work in the entertainment industry including drag shows and fashion parades.

Americas

The Native North American *berdache* can be seen as a morphological male who has non-masculine character, often stereotyped as effeminate. *Berdache* has a clearly recognized social status, often fulfilling special ceremonial roles. They occupy an alternative gender role that is seen as a blend of both male and female gender. They are not only seen as a mediator between men and women but also between the physical and the spiritual and are hence also sometimes referred to as *two-spirit* individuals. The acceptance of these terms varies with some individuals considering *berdache* inappropriate and insulting, while others reject the latter (Thomas and Jacobs, 1999). Traditionally *two-spirit* individuals have had various roles including medicine, healing and religious roles.

Travesti are trans* prostitute individuals from Latin America, especially from Brazil. The word *travesti* means 'cross-dress'. However, this only represents a minutiae of their lives as the *travesti*, in addition to cross-dressing, also adopt feminine names and pronouns, take female hormones and also resort to some sort of semi-permanent cosmetic surgeries (silicone implants for wider hips/bigger breasts) to give them a more feminine appearance (Kulick, 1998). It is interesting to note that *travestis* may still not self-identify as a woman meaning that they do not wish to transition into a woman and do not want to give up some male characteristics, like their genitals. To this effect, Kulick (1998) also notes that *travestis* consider any male who claims to be a woman is psychologically unbalanced and in need of psychological help. This identity thus appears an interface of feminine morphology with androphilic psychological feeling. One could argue that this is akin to the Western concept of homosexuality since the *travesti* participants in the relationship do not necessarily feel like a woman. However, Kulick (1997) clarifies that the Latin American configurations of sex, gender and sexuality are slightly different and consist not of men and women, but of men and not-men. Brazilian *travestis*, like their ally trans* individuals from other cultures, are equally marginalized and discriminated against. Violence is an integral dimension of daily life in Brazil (Kulick, 2009), but is more so for a *travesti* who has to tolerate both verbal and physical abuse and harassment (Kulick, 2009: 31–32).

Others

In Oman, effeminate men who participate in homosexual acts as the passive partner are called *xanith* (pronounced: *hanith*). The active partner who performs the role of a 'man' in such relationships is not seen as a *xanith* but as a man. It is thus interesting to see that the sexual behaviour and not the sexual organs determine what would be an individual's gender expression and/or role. They usually see themselves as women often dressing in a way that lies intermediate to the appearance of men and women, called the *dishdasha* (Bolich, 2007). Socio-culturally, they are identified with women and are free to move among women. They are also known to marry a woman sometimes, which is when they lose this freedom of being with women but instead would be treated as any other man. With such marriages between a *xanith* and a woman, the *xanith* ceases to be a *xanith* and instead is seen as a man having provided evidence of successful consummation with a blood-stained cloth (Denny, 2013). Interestingly, they could move in and out of the *xanith* and male identities of their own accord and have been seen as neither man nor woman but as third gender (Wikan, 1991). Many *xaniths* work as prostitutes offering men in Oman an alternative to inexpensive paid sex with women (Wikan, 2015).

Significance of the Issue

Trans* individuals are known to be negatively impacted in terms of various health outcomes across cultures and in different income settings (low-, middle- and high-income settings) (Reisner *et al.*, 2016). Globally, trans* individuals are highly vulnerable to stigmatization, marginalization, discrimination and violence in various forms. The recent update of the Trans Murder Monitoring Project (Transgender Europe, 2016) shows a significant rise in reported killings of trans* people over the last few years with about 2016 reported killings in 65 countries worldwide from 1 January 2008 to 31 December 2015. Unfortunately this figure only includes reported cases of murders of trans* individuals through Internet research and those reported with the help of trans organizations and activists. Worth noting is also the fact that majority of the murdered individuals were in the most productive years of their lives, between 20 and 29 years of age and 65 per cent of all murdered individuals whose profession was known were sex workers (Transgender Europe, 2015). Sex work as we have seen earlier is a known profession in various trans* individuals across different countries and cultures. Human rights of these individuals are violated leading to ongoing abuse, stigmatization, victimization and discrimination in all societies including India (Shaikh *et al.*, 2016), Pakistan (Alizai *et al.*, 2016) and others.

Trans* individuals may use different coping mechanisms to deal with such negative experiences. They may form subcultures as in the case of the *hijra* in India and exist side-by-side with the wider society. They may migrate from their place of birth for a variety of reasons. This may include, for instance, migration of the Brazilian *travesti* to Europe for greater social, symbolic and economic well-being (Vartabedian, 2014) or migration in the Indian *hijras* to escape familial pressures and start their lives afresh in places with established *hijra* subculture (Kalra and Shah, 2013). Migration may then bring its own set of stresses and have an impact on these individuals in terms of both mental and physical health. This combined with poor healthcare access across countries and cultures including Indian *hijras* (Kalra and Shah, 2013), Nepali *metis* (Wilson *et al.*, 2011), and Thai *kathoeys* (Nemoto *et al.*, 2012), leads to double jeopardy. We thus stand to lose individuals who could otherwise contribute significantly to the society, socio-economically, thus leading to a lose–lose situation.

To deal with this Reisner *et al.*, (2016) recommend inclusion of transgender populations in health surveillances along with integrating health and human rights approaches. They also suggest engaging transgender individuals, thus asking for a more collaborative healthcare model. One could look at the recovery model in mental healthcare for inspirations to improve transgender healthcare access. Having trans* peer support workers as consumer consultants is likely to send out a message to the trans* population about the health service being trans-friendly. Although possibly a step in the right direction, this would require extensive discussions within the stakeholders of health services who could further this process. This would be a highly challenging endeavour since it would mean breaking all the existing stereotypes regarding the transgender identity that may exist in that particular culture.

Conclusions

Transgender identities are known to exist in various cultures globally and tend to share many similarities. They mostly comprise of trans-women but also accommodate other sexual and gender identities. Such identities seem to have emerged to safely accommodate alternative gender expressions and roles to the male and female gender identities and are thus most likely seen as the third gender. Although such identities seem to have culturally been accommodated, they are still marginalized and stigmatized, often remaining excluded from the wider society. They are thus vulnerable in a variety of ways across cultures. Although terminologies continue to evolve with time, one common underlying facet of this gender minority is the exposure to the stress of social exclusion leading to economic and healthcare burdens. A suggested starting point to help deal with this 'chronic crisis' is to encourage more research in the area of transgenderism across different cultures to gain further understanding of the existing and evolving identities from a biopsychosocio-cultural-economic perspective.

References

Abdullah, M. A., Basharat, Z., Kamal, B., Sattar, N. Y., Hassan, Z. F., Jan, A. D. and Shafqat, A. (2012). Is social exclusion pushing the Pakistani hijras (transgenders) towards commercial sex work? A qualitative study. *BMC International Health and Human Rights*, **12**, 32.

Alizai, A., Doneys, P. and Doane, D. L. (2016). Impact of gender binarism on hijras' life course and their access to fundamental human rights in Pakistan. *Journal of Homosexuality*, **64**(9), 1214–1240.

Ashmore, R. D., Frances, K. D. B and Arthur, J. W. (1986). Gender stereotypes. In *The Social Psychology of Female–Male Relations: A Critical Analysis of Central Concepts*, ed. R. D. Ashmore and K. D. B. Frances. New York, Academic Press, pp. 69–119.

Blanchard, R. (2004). Quantitative and theoretical analyses of the relation between older brothers and homosexuality in men. *Journal of Theoretical Biology*, **230**, 173–187.

Bockting, W., Robinson, B. and Rosser, B. (1998). Transgender HIV prevention: a qualitative needs assessment. *AIDS Care*, **10**, 505–526.

Bolich, G. G. (2007). *Transgender History and Geography: Crossdressing in Context*, vol. 3. Raleigh, NC: Psyche's Press.

Brummelhuis, H. (1999). Transformations of transgender. *Journal of Gay and Lesbian Social Services*, **9**, 121–139.

Bullough, V. L. and Bullough, B. (1993). *Cross Dressing, Sex and Gender*. Philadelphia: University of Pennsylvania Press.

Coleman, E., Colgan, P. and Gooren, L. (1992). Male cross-gender behavior in Myanmar (Burma): a description of the acault. *Archives of Sexual Behavior*, **21**, 313–321.

Denny, D. (2013). *Current Concepts in Transgender Identity*. Abingdon, Oxon: Routledge.

Duthel, H. (2013). *Kathoey Ladyboy: Thailand's Got Talent*. Norderstedt: Books on Demand.

Elliston, D. (2014). Queer history and its discontent at Tahiti: the contested politics of modernity and sexual subjectivity. In *Gender on the Edge: Transgender, Gay, and Other Pacific Islanders*, ed. N. Besnier and K. Alexeyeff. Hong Kong: Hong Kong University Press.

Goh, J. N. (2012). Mah Nyah bodies as sacred sites: uncovering the queer body-sacramentality of Malaysian male-to-female transsexuals. *Cross Currents*, **62**, 512–521.

Herdt, G. (1996). *Third Sex, Third Gender: Beyond Sexual Dimorphism in Culture and History*. New York, NY: Zone Books.

Jackson, P. A. and Sullivan, G. (1999). *Lady Boys, Tom Boys, Rent Boys: Male and Female Homosexualities in Contemporary Thailand, Issues 2–3*. New York: Haworth Press.

Juergensmeyer, M. and Roof, W. C. (2011). *Encyclopedia of Global Religion*. London: SAGE Publications.

Kalra, G. (2012). Hijras: the unique transgender culture of India. *International Journal of Culture and Mental Health*, **5**, 121–126.

Kalra, G. and Shah, N. (2013). The cultural, psychiatric and sexuality aspects of hijras in India. *International Journal of Transgenderism*, **14**, 171–181.

Khan, F. A. (2016). Khwaja Sira activism: the politics of gender ambiguity in Pakistan. *Transgender Studies Quarterly*, **3**, 158–164.

Killerman, S. (2012). What does the asterisk in 'trans*' stand for? (blog). Available online at http://itspronouncedme trosexual.com/2012/05/what-does-the-asterisk-in-trans-stand-for/ (accessed 22 October 2016).

Kulick, D. (1997). The gender of Brazilian transgendered prostitutes. *American Anthropologist*, **99**, 574–585.

Kulick, D. (1998). *Travesti: Sex, Gender, and Culture among Brazilian Transgendered Prostitutes*. Chicago: University of Chicago Press.

Kulick, D. (2009). *Travesti: Sex, Gender, and Culture among Brazilian Transgendered Prostitutes*. Chicago: University of Chicago Press.

Lewin, E., Leap, W. and Leap, W. L. (2002). *Out in Theory: The Emergence of Lesbian and Gay Anthropology*. Chicago: University of Illinois Press.

Manalansan, M. F. (2015). Bakla (Phillipines). *The International Encyclopedia of Human Sexuality*. Chichester: Wiley Blackwell, pp. 113–196.

Matzner, A. (2001). *O Au No Keia: Voices from Hawai'i's Mahu and Transgender Communities*. Bloomington, IN: Xlibris Corporation.

Murray, S. O. (2000). *Homosexualities*. Chicago, IL: University of Chicago Press.

Nanda, S. (1985). The hijras of India: cultural and individual dimensions of an institutionalized third gender role. *Journal of Homosexuality*, **11**, 35–54.

Nemoto, T., Iwamoto, M., Perngparn, U., Areesantichai, C., Kamitani, E. and Sakata, M. (2012). HIV-related risk behaviors among kathoey (male-to-female transgender) sex workers in Bangkok, Thailand. *AIDS Care*, **24**, 210–219.

Nuttbrock, L. A., Bockting, W. O., Hwahng, S., Rosenblum, A., Mason, M., Macri, M. and Becker, J. (2009). Gender identity affirmation among male-to-female transgender persons: a life course analysis across types of relationships and cultural/lifestyle factors. *Sexual and Relationship Therapy*, **24**, 108–125.

Ocha, W. (2012). Transsexual emergence: gender variant identities in Thailand. *Culture, Health and Sexuality*, **14**, 563–575.

Poasa, K. (1992). The Samoan Fa'afafine: one case study and discussion of transsexualism. *Journal of Psychology and Human Sexuality*, **5**, 39–51.

Reisner, S. L., Poteat, T., Keatley, J., Cabral, M., Mothopeng, T., Dunham, E., Holland, C. E., Max, R., and Baral, S. D. (2016). Global health burden and needs of transgender populations: a review. *The Lancet*, **388**, 412–436.

Ryan, H. (2014). What does trans* mean and where did it come from? Slate Online Magazine, 10 January. Available online at www.slate.com/blogs/outward/2014/01/10/trans_what_does_it_mean_and_where_did_it_come_from.html (accessed 22 October 2016).

Sevelius, J. M. (2013). Gender affirmation: a framework for conceptualizing risk behavior among transgender women of color. *Sex Roles*, **68**, 675–689.

Shaikh, S., Mburu, G., Arumugam, V., Mattipalli, N., Aher, A., Mehta, S. and Robertson, J. (2016). Empowering communities and strengthening systems to improve transgender health: outcomes from the Pehchan programme in India. *Journal of the International AIDS Society*, **19**, 20809.

Slamah, K. (2005). The struggle to be ourselves, neither men nor women: Mak nyahs in Malaysia. In *Sexuality, Gender and Rights: Exploring Theory and Practice in South and South East Asia*, ed. G. Misra and R. Chandiramani. London: SAGE Publications, p. 99.

Stip, E. (2015). RaeRae and Mahu: third Polynesian gender. *Sante Mentale au Quebec*, **40**, 193–208.

541

The, Y. K. and Koon, T. Y. (2003). *The Mak Nyahs: Malaysian Male to Female Transsexuals* (Gender Studies). Singapore: Marshall Cavendish Academic.

Thomas, W. and Jacobs, S. (1999). '. . . And we are still here': from Berdache to two-spirit people. *American Indian Culture and Research Journal*, **23**, 91–107.

Tomori, C., Srikrishnan, A. K., Ridgeway, K., Solomon, S. S., Mehta, S. H., Solomon, S. and Celentano, D. D. (2016). Perspectives on sexual identity formation, identity practices, and identity transitions among men who have sex with men in India. *Archives of Sexual Behavior*, 1–10.

Totman, R. (2011). *The Third Sex: Kathoey: Thailand's Ladyboys*. London: Souvenir Press.

Transgender Europe (2015). Trans Murder Monitoring Update. Available online at http://transrespect.org/wp-content/uploads/2015/11/TvT-TMM-Tables_2008–2015_EN.pdf (accessed 22 October 2016).

Transgender Europe (2016). Trans Murder Monitoring Update. Over 2000 trans people killed in the last 8 years. Available online at http://transrespect.org/wp-content/uploads/2016/03/TvT_TMM_TDoV2016_PR_EN.pdf (accessed 22 October 2016).

VanderLaan, D. P. and Vasey, P. L. (2011). Male sexual orientation in independent Samoa: evidence for fraternal birth order and maternal fecundity effects. *Archives of Sexual Behavior*, **40**, 495–503.

Vartabedian, J. (2014). Trans migrations: Brazilian travesti migrant sex workers in Europe. *Cadernos Pagu*, **42**, 275–312.

Wikan, U. (1991). *Behind the Veil in Arabia: Women in Oman*. Chicago: University of Chicago Press.

Wikan, U. (2015). Xanith (Oman). *The International Encyclopedia of Human Sexuality*. Chichester: Wiley Blackwell, pp. 1445–1446.

Wilson, E., Pant, S. B., Comfort, M. and Ekstrand, M. (2011). Stigma and HIV risk among Metis in Nepal. *Culture, Health and Sexuality*, **13**, 253–266.

Winter, S. (2006). Thai transgenders in focus: demographics, transitions and identities. *International Journal of Transgenderism*, **9**, 15–27.

Zanghellini, A. (2010). Queer kinship practices in non-Western contexts: French Polynesia's gender-variant parents and the law of La Republique. *Journal of Law and Society*, **37**, 651–677.

Chapter

42

Refugee Mental Health
A Problem for the World to Solve?

Albert Persaud, Kamaldeep Bhui, Antonio Ventriglio
and Dinesh Bhugra

Editors' Introduction

People have always sought refuge in safe places when they have faced persecution for religious or political reasons. This has led to a global movement of people which of late has become more striking and perhaps more serious. Changes in geopolitics have led to further opprobrium on refugees and those who may seek asylum. People migrate for short-term or long-term and often migrate for all sorts of reasons. The most difficult reasons for migration are political when people are either persecuted for their religious beliefs, for their political beliefs or for their sexual orientation. Both push and pull factors play a role in this situation. People may be expelled or pushed out or be attracted towards safety for their own and their families' sake. Persaud *et al.* in this chapter focus on mental health needs of refugees and asylum seekers. They place these needs in the context of major geopolitical conflicts and reasons for the movement of people. They argue that even within the legal context and international obligations, countries often treat refugees and asylum seekers in very negative ways which further contribute to mental ill-health creating further long-term problems. These authors highlight that not all refugees and asylum seekers have mental illness and in some cases they may well be more sturdy. In both clinical and research needs a major challenge is to explore the cultural impact on expression of distress, illness perceptions, on the diagnostic process and the clinical processes of assessment and decision-making about healthcare. Persaud *et al.* propose that this issue is both controversial and politicized, even while refugees continue to experience discrimination shaped by asylum policies and practices, and then the reception in the host country. Clinical services should provide adequate treatment in the context of harsh political realities facing refugees.

Introduction

In recent times, there has been a massively recognized increase in refugees and asylum seekers in the world. Although the numbers are huge most of the burden is often borne by low- and middle-income countries. The mental health needs of refugees and asylum seekers need to be recognized as a number of factors can impact upon this. The psychological trauma often experienced by refugees can contribute to mental ill health and their psychiatric needs therefore, are further complicated by poor nutritional levels and physical ill health. In this chapter we provide an overview of the geopolitical factors which play a major role in the settlement of refugees and make some suggestions for clinical interventions. There are, of course, many international agreements under the aegis of the United Nations but countries often either ignore these wilfully or bypass these due to a lack of resources.

Definitions

An 'asylum seeker' is a person who has applied for asylum in another country and whose asylum application is still under consideration by the relevant authorities and who is in the process of waiting for it to be accepted or rejected. An asylum seeker becomes a refugee if he or she is granted refugee status by the host country.

Stateless people are not considered as a national by any state ('de jure') or don't enjoy fundamental rights in their homeland ('de facto') (UNHCR, 2000).

Almost all refugees are primarily asylum seekers unless they are admitted to the host countries through refugee resettlement programmes. Refugee status is normally granted on the basis of fulfilling the 1951 United Nations Convention on the Status of Refugees and the following 1967 Protocol.

Within the 1951 Convention, 'refugee' is defined as:

a person who owing to well-founded fear of being persecuted for reasons of race, religion, nationality, memberships of a particular social group or political opinion, is outside the country of his nationality and is unable, or owing to such fear, is unwilling to avail himself of the protection of that country; or who, not having a nationality and being outside the country of his former habitual residence . . . is unable, or owing to such fear, is unwilling to return to it . . .

(UNHCR, 2010)

Thus, a refugee is someone who has been forced to flee his or her home country and is unable or unwilling to return due to fear of persecution. The 1951 UN Convention relating to the status of refugees gives refugees legal protection under the international refugee law. The United Nations High Commissioner for Refugees (UNHCR) is mandated to respond to refugee needs.

An internally displaced person (IDP) is someone who is forced to flee his/her home but who did not cross an actual state border. All IDPs benefit from the legal protection of international human rights law and, in armed conflict, international humanitarian law.

Almost all countries are among the signatory nations of both the 1951 Convention and the 1967 Protocol related to the status of refugees. This means that an asylum seeker who meets the UNHCR criteria is recognized as a refugee, with the same legal, social, education and other welfare rights as that of the host citizen. Such rights are protected by the UNHCR. However, this rule is not often followed in many countries for a number of political imperatives.

Global Conflict

The year 2014 marked the centenary of the start of the First (ironically 'Great') World War (1914–1918), one of the largest wars in history – 70 million military personnel, 9 million combatants with over 7 million civilian deaths. Then there was the Second World War (1939–1945), a global war involving 100 million people and 30 countries, 60 million deaths including the Holocaust in which there were approximately 11 million deaths; the deadliest war in history. Armed conflict in the world has continued, for example Vietnam, Falklands, Bosnia, the Syrian civil war, also Iraq, Myanmar, Kashmir, and Sudan to name a few. However, a defining moment in the history of conflict at the beginning of the twenty-first century was the attacks on 11 September in New York and Washington.

Also referred to as 9/11, this was a series of four coordinated attacks by al-Qaeda, killing 3,000 people and injuring over 6,000 people. This was a major attack on the mainland of the United States of America, which until then had been unthinkable. The United States responded to this attack by launching the so-called 'War on Terror', invading Afghanistan to defeat the Taliban which sheltered al-Qaeda and subsequently invading Iraq to find the 'weapons of mass destruction' (WMD).

The Arab Spring began in Tunisia in December 2010. It was the start of a series of non-violent and violent demonstrations and protests that spread across the Middle East, mostly by young people seeking a new dawn of democracy, freedom and choice. Many had hoped that the Arab Spring would bring changes in Arab governments; instead, it brought a violent crackdown by oppressive governments on those who dared to speak and protest. Conflict has subsequently escalated, visibly so in Egypt and Libya, and was indeed the precursor to the current Syrian conflict. The vacuum created from the chaos in Iraq, Egypt, Libya and Syria has allowed terrorist organizations like Daesh (also known as ISIS or IS), to build, recruit, flourish and impose their barbaric brand of brutality and export their vile doctrine across the globe, for which Europe has been targeted.

War and conflict, along with major natural disasters – in Nepal, Haiti, Italy, earthquakes; tsunamis in Sri Lanka and Japan; public health crises like Ebola and Zika; and climate change – carry with them largely invisible, often crippling, mental scars that have an impact on millions of lives and often create large numbers of refugees, asylum seekers and internally displaced people.

Refugees, Asylum Seekers and Internally Displaced People

In 2015, the global number of refugees, asylum seekers and internally displaced people reached 65.3 million – equivalent to the population size of either France or the United Kingdom (World Bank, 2016). Many were fleeing the brutality of their own government and/or terrorist groups like Daesh, the Taliban, Boko Haram and al-Qaeda (34,000 people a day forced to flee their homes because of conflict and persecution). There were 21.3 million refugees, of whom 51 per cent were under the age of 18 years, and 10 million stateless people. Fifty-four per cent of refugees come from three countries – Somalia 1.1 million, Afghanistan 2.7 million and Syria 4.9 million. World displaced people are hosted by some of the poorest countries – 39% in the Middle East and North Africa, 29% in Africa, 14% in Asia and the Pacific, 12% in the Americas and 6% in Europe. The United Nations Refugee Council (UNHCR, 2015a) reported a record 98,400 asylum requests from unaccompanied or separate minors and 32,000 refugees gaining citizenship from 28 countries.

While the current crisis is severe, over the past 25 years the majority of both refugees and internally displaced persons under the UNHCR's mandate can be traced to just a few conflicts in the following areas: Afghanistan, Iraq, Syria, Burundi, the Democratic Republic of Congo, Somalia, Sudan, Colombia, former Yugoslavia, and the regions between Asia and Europe known as the Caucasus (UNHCR, 2015a,b).

People have historically fled to the neighbours of their country of origin; however, the responsibility for hosting has not been shared evenly across continents. About 15 countries have consistently been hosting the majority of refugees. At the end of 2015, Turkey, Lebanon and Jordan, Syria's neighbours, hosted 27% of all refugees worldwide; Pakistan and Iran, Afghanistan's neighbours, hosted 16%; and Ethiopia and Kenya, Somalia and South Sudan's neighbours, hosted 7%.

European Migrant Crisis

Europe is struggling to cope with the large-scale arrival of migrants making their way across the Mediterranean to Europe, the biggest since the aftermath of the Second World War – sparking a humanitarian crisis, as countries struggle to cope with this influx. This has created division in the European Union (EU) over how best to deal with the crisis and resettle people. With tensions running high, Europe's leaders remain divided and challenged on how best to respond; a disproportionate burden continues to be faced by some countries, particularly Greece and Italy. Ruiz and Bhugra (2010) point out that ambivalent feelings which exist in many countries are related to statistics and feeling overwhelmed by the number of refugees, creating tensions with the majority community who may feel that their values and cultures are being eroded. They also cite problems in the USA and attitudes to refugees which are hardening rapidly.

Squalid conditions in makeshift refugee camps and a heartbreaking photograph of a drowned Syrian toddler and that of the child covered in dust in a hospital in Aleppo have all helped bring Europe's refugee crisis into the global spotlight. Many refugee camps are running short of food, lack basic healthcare, and women and children have become victims of human trafficking, rape and other abuses. This has not stopped people making desperate bids to reach Europe. In 2015 more than a million migrants crossed the Mediterranean Sea to Europe, many fleeing the war in Syria. Most had travelled the short route between Turkey and Greece, which is about 5 miles long at its closest point; however, this route was closed in March 2016 when the EU signed a 3 billion Euro ($3.3 bn; £2.3 bn) deal with Turkey to control and stop the movement of migrants to Europe. This has merely moved the movement of migrants to Libya from where the crossing to Europe is much more hazardous and dangerous, because it is longer and the water current much more unpredictable. Though this route is dangerous, International Organization for Migration (IOM) figures to August 2016 report in excess of 107,000 refugees arriving in Italy, more than 11,000 being intercepted by the Libyan coast guard and more than 3,000 dying en route, many of whom were children and unaccompanied young people. However, the true number of migrant deaths will never be known, because tracking or monitoring is minimal at best, or non-existent. The only mode of protection for migrants facing almost certain death with this crossing are European nations' navies, rescue ships commissioned by humanitarian organizations and commercial vessels operating under the code of maritime law for assisting boats in distress.

The reaction to the influx of migrants into Europe has challenged its liberal stance against an increasingly tense nationalist reaction. There have been over 300 deaths on mainland Europe associated with terrorism. Though very few of these deaths are linked to migrants fleeing conflict, the majority are nationals of the country affected by terrorism, mainly France, Belgium and Germany. Migrants have experienced violent attacks across the EU; hate speech, arson and violence are commonly reported, along with the resurgence of some unpleasant right wing anti-immigrant sentiments. This has been further fuelled by many EU politicians' rhetoric on keeping 'Europe Christian'. Too often, politicians use anti-refugee, xenophobic, racist rhetoric to chase approval ratings, unfortunately this fuelling of emotions has led to a rise of violence against ethnic minority nationals, including a serious rise in anti-Semitic attacks and recent polls have reflected these feelings.

Terrorism fears in Europe have led to punitive crackdowns on garments worn by women: in France the full face veil, like the burka, is banned; conservatives in Germany want a ban on the full face veil as a security measure; in Bulgaria the national assembly has approved the first reading to ban the veil that partially covers the face; in Denmark the populist party cited security in proposing a burka ban and in Austria the far right party has promised a burka ban if it wins the election.

The EU proposed a scheme to relocate 160,000 migrants to be distributed among EU nations, with binding quotas to ease the burden on those countries most affected. However, this proposal was not fully supported by EU governments, with eastern European countries opposing the scheme for two reasons: because (1) many of their voters are virulently opposed to Muslim immigration and (2) refugee admissions should be a sovereign national decision. Britain is exempt due to its historic opt-out on justice matters. Ironically, the testimony of aid workers and EU officials show the scheme has flopped as migrants have no desire to be 'relocated' to poor eastern European states when they would rather go to Germany or Sweden.

Interestingly, a recent Amnesty International Global Survey (2016) found the vast majority of people (80%) would welcome refugees with open arms, with many even prepared to take them into their own homes, with Germany and the UK being top of the EU list.

Geopolitics, the UK and EU

The United Kingdom (UK) has been an active partner in the changing face of geopolitics and shaping foreign policy in different regions of the world. In 2016, two defining events happened that now reset the UK relationship with Europe and the global arena.

First, the people of the United Kingdom voted in an EU referendum on whether to stay in or leave the EU. More than 33 million UK citizens voted in this referendum on 23 June, 2016; the turnout was 72% and the result was 52% to 48% in favour of the UK leaving the EU (known as Brexit). The result unleashed a range of emotions, a media frenzy and, importantly, an array of political calculations around

deals and predictions. But this result goes beyond UK citizens' desire to 'take back control' – the successful slogan of those who campaigned to leave. Control of migration, the UK's ultimate right of sovereignty for its Parliament (subsidiarity on legislation) and a desire to stop an ever-increasing financial contribution – £10 billion per year, the second largest contributor to the EU budget, which is seen as spent by unaccountable bureaucrats – were the defining considerations in the referendum.

Both the UK and EU seem to have sleep-walked into Brexit; they did not expect the vote to go this way, neither was there any planning to anticipate this result. The withdrawal of one of the EU's largest member states loses one of its two permanent members on the UN Security Council (France being the other). The Brexit implications could also have a wider knock-on effect for the North Atlantic Treaty Organization (NATO), through its trans-Atlantic relationship, leaving France as the sole large and capable military force in the EU, weakening wider European political stability and Europe's position in the international world. Brexit is likely to add to Europe's divisions and security weaknesses and could turn it further inwards, which would be of serious concern to Washington, in particular at a time when Russia is repositioning its military strength in eastern Europe, with the annexation of Crimea and hostilities with Ukraine, and its profound military and political backing of Assad's Syrian regime. Brexit could not have happened at a better time for Russia as it counters the effects of UN sanctions for the Crimean annexation.

Second, the Chilcot Report (2016) also known as the Iraq Inquiry, published 7 years after the inquiry was announced, contained 2.6 million words (four times the length of *War and Peace*), and comprised 12 volumes plus a summary of costs at £10 million. It spans almost a decade of UK government policy decisions between 2001 and 2009. The UK chose to join the invasion of Iraq before peaceful options for disarmament had been exhausted, and military action at that time was not a last resort; the threat posed by the Iraqi regime was deliberately exaggerated. Judgements about the severity of the threat posed by Iraq's 'weapons of mass destruction' (WMD), were presented with a certainty that was not justified. The prime minister sought to make the case for military action to members of Parliament (MPs) and the public in the build-up to the invasion in 2002 and 2003.

Invasion and regime change seemed to be the only objectives, with no evidence of a post-war strategy for Iraq, rebuilding, civil society, security and economic reconstruction.

The UK government, like the public, is 'battle fatigued' and this was vividly demonstrated during the House of Commons debate on Syria and the use of chemical weapons (House of Commons, 2013) on whether to intervene militarily in Syria. Parliament decided not to intervene. There were concerns about the chemical weapon attacks in Syria, but MPs wanted things to be done in the right way, to learn the lessons of Iraq and work with the international community to find a solution to the conflict. With time, the situation in Syria has got worse with more interventions by 'a coalition force' to tackle terrorist groups: Aleppo is a poignant testament to the brutality which many blame the Russian bombings for. The British public is sensitive yet politically astute regarding the various conflicts its military have participated in. They have witnessed interventions in Iraq, with occupation that has left Iraq in chaos; for Libya there was intervention, no occupation but yet resulted in a Libya in chaos; and with Syria, no intervention, no occupation, yet Syria is now one of the most chaotic, violent and destructive places on Earth. They have seen the regular repatriation of British soldiers from Iraq and Afghanistan and want no further participation in foreign conflicts. In spite of this Britain remains one of the most compassionate nations, readily giving aid to countries in need and the UK government provides the world's second largest aid budget of £12.2 billion (Department for International Development, 2017), equivalent to 0.7 per cent of gross national income.

Ongoing Global Conflict

Deadly conflict was in decline after the end of the cold war. Fifteen years ago, there were fewer conflicts, thus fewer deaths, but since then, there has been a serious escalation, with worsening humanitarian consequences, spreading across Afghanistan, Syria, Iraq, South Sudan, Yemen, Chad, Libya, Burundi, Turkey, Ukraine, Myanmar, Columbia, Mali, Republic of Congo (see the Center for Preventive Action (CPA) Global Conflict Tracker, CPA, 2016). Conflict, violence, death and misery show no abating and with the diplomatic stand-off between the United States and Russia on agreeing a way forward on the carnage in Syria, in particular Aleppo, the picture is truly grim.

The majority of conflict involves brutal dictators and extremist groups like Daesh and other similar jihadist groups, whose doctrine and ideology are based on sectarianism, legitimacy and influence, delivered through the means of brutality and violence. Interestingly, some dictators find favour amongst Western and other global leaders, giving them legitimacy: this was profoundly evident with Saddam Hussein, Colonel Gaddafi, Robert Mugabe, Kim Jong-un, to name a few. The consequence is an ever greater flow of refugees heading for safety – including towards Europe.

A New World Order

The United Nations was established in 1945 to replace the previous, ineffective, League of Nations. Its purpose was basically to do good and promote cooperation; unfortunately in the last few years the effectiveness and competence of the UN has been diminishing. It has become an organization that protests and calls for action, with very few countries listening. This can be borne out by the number of resolutions that go unheeded, decision-making remains vested in the five permanent members of the Security Council (USA, France, UK, Russia, China), the poor response to crises like Ebola, a peace-keeping force that is short of personnel and an ever increasing bureaucracy that is costly. It is time that the UN principles and functions were modernized so as to reflect the changing geopolitical and globalized world, making more countries strategic decision-makers and enhancing regional cooperation in areas of security, population mobility and economic and environment stability.

Globalization has brought benefits to many, prosperity and a rebalancing of the global economy resulting in a powerful G-20 group of nations; improvements in health resulting in many parts of the world in people living longer. But for many, globalization has not been the panacea for survival: climate change has brought chaos to many lives through flooding, droughts, crop failure. There is no doubt that some of the negative effects of neo-liberalism and globalization have led to major political upheavals in the UK and the USA where significant numbers of people feel left behind. This competitiveness and an untrammelled market economy have increased poverty in some parts of the world. Many in the Western countries view globalization as a threat to their heritage and culture, fearing it will replace local economies, traditions and languages. It is time for the world economy to be rebalanced so as to invest in the many who seek a better life, and share the rewards more fairly.

Sectarianism has fuelled the flames of conflict for hundreds of years. Religious, ethnic, political, cultural and racial divides will continue to fester with no meaningful resolution acceptable, as can be seen in places like Iraq where there is still Sunni and Shia conflict. Indeed there is no clear understanding what a post-Assad Syria might look like. Even in areas where there is no conflict, like Scotland and Catalonia, the people there are seeking more self-rule and self-determination, with the belief that people have the right to choose their own political status and to determine their form of economic, cultural and social development. It is time for international laws on self-determination and diplomacy to be modernized and for the international community to accept that in the interest of stability, more countries will evolve, similar to the former Yugoslavia.

It is saddening to think that, despite the terrible losses and suffering caused by these conflicts and disasters, humankind continues to resort to brutality to settle disputes and ideological differences; in the twenty-first century we find ourselves still caught up in these global conflagrations. They are often triggered by romantic, idealized views of the past, or fuelled by skewed interpretations of sacred religious or philosophical texts and teachings.

The Scale of a New World Problem

The UNHCR data for 2015 suggest there are 65.3 million people who have been forcibly displaced worldwide (UNHCR, 2015a, b). Of 21.3 million refugees, half are under 18 years of age, and 16.1 million are under the UNHCR mandate, with 5.2 million Palestinians registered under UNWRA. Over half the refugees worldwide come either from Somalia, Syria or Afghanistan, and the countries hosting most refugees are Turkey, Pakistan, Lebanon, Iran, Ethiopia and Jordan. There are 10 million stateless people without provisions of state protections for citizens, with no entitlement to health, education or welfare. On a daily basis 34,000 people are forcibly displaced. A recent crisis that has been in the new media around the world is sea arrivals through the Mediterranean, predominantly via Greece and Italy, for which, in 2016, Syria, Iraq, Nigeria and Afghanistan were the most significant sources (UNHCR, 2016). Of 336,000 arrivals in 2016 (a fall from more than a million in 2015), 4,233 are dead or missing.

In Latin America, it is noted that over 16 million migrants and refugees have been moving across countries. Nearly half a million migrants from Cuba are currently present in Costa Rica awaiting entry to Mexico from where they wish to migrate to the USA. Costa Rica also experiences regular entry of temporary migrants from Nicaragua to help harvest coffee crops. This seasonal migration further adds to the stretched resources. This ebb and flow of migrant workers and refugees in Latin America is often not recognized or talked about. Their status in Latin America does not appear to have the same sense of urgency and need as in Europe. However, poverty, disasters – both natural and man-made – also play a key role in mass migration of people as has been shown recently in Haiti where people have started moving to neighbouring Dominican Republic. Stress and mental illness consequent upon migration and settling down under such circumstances are often complicated by infectious and other physical illnesses.

Mental Health and Illness

Being an asylum seeker or refugee is not necessarily linked to mental illness; indeed, the rates of psychosis and depression may not be dissimilar to those of host populations (WHO, 2015). However, pre-, peri- and post-migration risk factors (Bhui et al., 2003; Stompe et al., 2010; Beiser and Hou, 2016; and further details in Bhugra et al., 2010), such as exposure to war and conflict, material deprivation, trauma and torture, loss and bereavements of people and place, can all contribute to greater risks of post-traumatic stress disorder (PTSD) that have been reported in both children and adults. These losses and cultural bereavement can further complicate matters and must be taken into account during any clinical assessment (Wojcik and Bhugra, 2010). Children may be especially vulnerable to the powerful emotions associated with trauma, injustice and loss events (McGuinness and Durand, 2015; Zamani and Zarghani, 2016). School-based programmes are helpful and preferred by children who worry about their uncertain plight and who suffer traumatic refugee journeys (Fazel et al., 2016). Clearly, opportunities for employment and having adequate material resources (housing, income, food and safety) play an important part in protecting the mental health of vulnerable individuals and groups. Geographical mobility even after migration remains an issue, especially if forced (Warfa et al., 2006). Indeed, employment following asylum may be an important determinant of good mental health, perhaps more so than provision of formal mental health services after someone has developed a mental illness (Warfa *et al.*, 2012). Furthermore, the experience of those in receiving countries is often that mental health is the priority (Colborne, 2015). In fact, complexity of need may be what gives the impression of insurmountable obstacles to health and well-being (Bhui *et al.*, 2006), not to mention asylum policies that prohibit work or involve prolonged periods in detention centres (Steel *et al.*, 2004; Silove *et al.*, 2007).

Cultural Complexities in Decision-Making and Diagnostic Practice

One of the challenges of all research on refugee and asylum seekers is the cultural impact on expression of distress, illness perceptions, on the diagnostic process and the clinical process of assessment and decision-making about care (Bhui *et al.*, 2006). Other chapters in this volume attend to issues such as explanatory models determining the care pathways taken, stigma associated with mental illness, discrimination both individual and institutional, and the allocation of resources for those perceived to be less worthy or those perceived by the political system to draw on the nation's resources. These sentiments have been most prominent in the recent debates in the UK about sovereignty and border controls, with migration into the UK and asylum seeker claims being presented as political reasons to leave the EU. As controversial and politicized as this issue is, the reality is that refugees do suffer the plight that is shaped by asylum policies and practices, and then the reception in the host country. Many studies fail to account fully for both the cultural factors in the expression and recognition of mental illness, and then the provision of adequate treatment; the harsh political realities facing refugees, and the lack of opportunity some will face, often resorting to jobs in which their skills from their home country are not valued or permitted expression. Cultural competence is one form of intervention that seeks to remedy inequalities and better understand cultural expressions of distress, and enable public servants to better appreciate the mental health, health and social care needs, and also the value of asylum seekers and refugees to the future economy of host nations, especially at a time when most high-income countries need net in-migration to ensure there are sufficient people of working age to sustain the economy and provide resources through taxation for the care of their growing numbers of elderly people.

The controversy that is still rarely aired is why diagnostic and related research confusion prevails, when considering asylum seekers and refugees. For example, much attention is paid to PTSD, but not to resilience (Stevens and Walsh, 2016), or to comorbid depression (Bhui *et al.*; 2003; Fazel *et al.*, 2005), which is far more common and perhaps disabling, and yet is amenable to treatment. Furthermore, trauma exposure may lead to PTS symptoms, which then mediate the impact on mental health leading to depression (Kim, 2016).

Public Health and Prevention

Given the lack of resources to provide direct treatments for refugees with multiple and complex problems in the receiving countries (most of them being low-income countries), prevention needs more attention. This means primary prevention of conflict and anticipation of the mental health casualties of war and conflict, as well as early recognition and intervention where possible. However, mental health intervention in the midst of a conflict or seeking asylum is not likely to be helpful or an immediate priority for many; rather if people are escaping war and conflict and persecution, supporting humanitarian rights and accepting responsibilities of those countries signed up to the UNHCR provisions is a priority. An understanding of the role of international clinical and practice organizations, and governments, to work together in order to prevent and minimize conflict is certainly in the best interests of all. However, as is witnessed in Syria and historically in Iraq and Afghanistan, there are no easy and linear ways of resolving war, not least if terrorism is invoked and there are conflicting global priorities and alliances. The role of the UN and organizations such as WHO, World Psychiatric Association (WPA) and World Association of Cultural Psychiatry (WACP) needs careful marshalling for the greater good. It is with this in mind that WPA and WACP have both issued position statements on migration and the migrant crisis, in order to set out shared responsibilities (WPA, 2016; WACP, 2015). Bhugra *et al.* (2010) urge that clinicians are not only clinicians but also as members of the society have a role to advocate for refugees and asylum seekers so that they get the best treatments available and are not discriminated against.

Conclusions

Refugees and asylum seekers, in addition to their experiences of loss and potential culture shock, face major discrimination if they develop mental ill-health. This double jeopardy can get further complicated due to gender, sexual orientation and religion. However, the impact of changing geopolitics and the shift of global health bodies also reflect a growing awareness among practitioners that prevention means being involved early in the chain of events, and that healthcare practitioners have a role to play in disaster prevention and management, war and conflict being one of those harrowing scenarios facing the world.

References

Amnesty International (2016). Amnesty International Global Survey: Refugees Welcome Index. Available online at www.amnesty.org/en/latest/news/2016/05/refugees-welcome-survey-results-2016/.

Beiser, M. and Hou, F. (2016). Mental health effects of premigration trauma and postmigration discrimination on refugee youth in Canada. *Journal of Nervous and Mental Disorders*, **204**, 64–70.

Bhugra, D., Craig, T. and Bhui, K. (2010). Conclusions: what next? In *Mental Health of Refugees and Asylum Seekers*, ed. D. Bhugra, T. Craig and K. Bhui. Oxford: Oxford University Press, pp. 299–302.

Bhui, K., Abdi, A., Abdi, M. *et al.* (2003). Traumatic events, migration characteristics and psychiatric symptoms among Somali refugees: preliminary communication. *Social Psychiatry and Psychiatric Epidemiology*, **38**, 35–43.

Bhui, K., Craig. T., Mohamud, S. *et al.* (2006). Mental disorders among Somali refugees: developing culturally appropriate measures and assessing socio-cultural risk factors. *Social Psychiatry and Psychiatric Epidemiology*, **41**, 400–408.

Center for Preventive Action (CPA) (2016). Global Conflict Tracker available online at www.cfr.org/global/global-conflict-tracker/p32137#!/.

Chilcot Report (2016). The Report of the Iraq Inquiry; 'The Chilcot Inquiry'. Available online at www.iraqinquiry.org.uk/.

Colborne, M. (2015). Syrian refugees' mental health is top priority. *Canadian Medical Association Journal*, **187**, 1347.

Department for International Development (DFID) (2017). Statistics available online at www.gov.uk/government/organisations/department-for-international-development.

Fazel, M., Wheeler, J. and Danesh, J. (2005). Prevalence of serious mental disorder in 7000 refugees resettled in Western countries: a systematic review. *The Lancet* **365**(9467), 309–314.

Fazel, M., Garcia, J. and Stein, A. (2016). The right location? Experiences of refugee adolescents seen by school-based mental health services. *Clinical Child Psychology and Psychiatry*, **21**, 368–380.

House of Commons (2013). Syria and the Use of Chemical Weapons. Available online at www.publications.parliament.uk/pa/cm201314/cmhansrd/cm130829/debtext/130829-0001.htm.

Kim, Y. J. (2016). Posttraumatic stress disorder as a mediator between trauma exposure and comorbid mental health conditions in North Korean refugee youth resettled in South Korea. *Journal of Interpersonal Violence*, **31**, 425–443.

McGuinness, T. M. and Durand, S. C. (2015). Mental health of young refugees. *Journal of Psychosocial Nursing and Mental Health Services*, **53**, 16–18.

Ruiz, P. and Bhugra, D. (2010). Refugees and asylum seekers: conceptual issues. In *Mental Health of Refugees and Asylum Seekers*, ed. D. Bhugra, T. Craig and K. Bhui. Oxford: Oxford University Press, pp. 1–8.

Silove, D., Steel, Z., Susljik, I. *et al.* (2007). The impact of the refugee decision on the trajectory of PTSD, anxiety, and depressive symptoms among asylum seekers: a longitudinal study. *American Journal of Disaster Medicine*, **2**, 321–329.

Steel, Z., Frommer, N. and Silove, D. (2004). Part I: The mental health impacts of migration: the law and its effects failing to understand: refugee determination and the traumatized applicant. *International Journal of Law and Psychiatry*, **27**, 511–528.

Stevens, G. W. and Walsh, S. D.(2016). Deepening our understanding of risk and resilience factors for mental health problems in refugee youth: a plea for scientific research. *Journal of Adolescent Health*, **58**, 582–583.

Stompe, T., Holzer, D. and Friedman, A. (2010). Pre-migration and mental health of refugees. In *Mental Health of Refugees and Asylum Seekers*, ed. D. Bhugra, T. Craig and K. Bhui. Oxford: Oxford University Press, pp. 23–38.

United Nation Refugee Agency (UNHCR) (2000). See www.unhcr.org/uk/aboutus.html.

United Nation Refugee Agency (UNHCR) (2010). Convention and Protocol Relating to the Status of Refugees, available online at www.refugeelegalaidinformation.org/sites/default/files/uploads/1951%20convention%20and%201967%20protocol.pdf.

United Nation Refugee Agency (UNHCR) (2015a). Global Trends Forced Displacement in 2015, available online at www.unhcr.org/uk/statistics/unhcrstats/576408cd7/unhcr-global-trends-2015.html?

United Nations Refugee Agency (UNHCR) (2015b). Figures at a Glance, statistical yearbooks available online at www.unhcr.org/uk/figures-at-a-glance.html.

United Nations Refugee Agency (UNHCR) (2016). Operational Portal, refugee situations available online at http://data.unhcr.org/mediterranean/regional.php.

Warfa, N., Bhui, K., Craig, T. *et al.* (2006). Post-migration geographical mobility, mental health and health service utilisation among Somali refugees in the UK: a qualitative study. *Health Place*, **12**, 503–515.

Warfa, N., Curtis, S., Watters, C. *et al.* (2012). Migration experiences, employment status and psychological distress among Somali immigrants: a mixed-method international study. *BMC Public Health*, **12**, 749.

Wojcik, W. and Bhugra, D. (2010). Loss and cultural bereavement. In *Mental Health of Refugees and Asylum Seekers*, ed. D. Bhugra, T. Craig and K. Bhui. Oxford: Oxford University Press, pp. 211–223.

World Association of Cultural Psychiatry (2015). Position Statement on the Migrant Crisis around the World, available online at www.wcprr.org/wp-content/uploads/2015/12/WACP-Declaration-nov-2015-Final-copy.pdf.

World Bank (2016). *Forcibly Displaced: Toward a Development Approach Supporting Refugees, the Internally Displaced, and their Hosts*. Washington DC: World Bank, available online at https://openknowledge.worldbank.org/handle/10986/25016.

World Health Organization (2015). WHO Europe Policy Brief on Migration and Health: Mental Health Care for Refugees, available online at www.euro.who.int/__data/assets/pdf_file/0006/293271/Policy-Brief-Migration-Health-Mental-Health-Care-Refugees.pdf?ua=1.

World Psychiatric Association (WPA) (2016). Position Statement Migrant Crisis, available online at www.wpanet.org/detail.php?section_id=7&content_id=1772.

Zamani, M. and Zarghami, A. (2016). The refugee and immigration crisis in Europe: urgent action to protect the mental health of children and adolescents. *Journal of Adolescent Health*, **58**, 582.

Chapter 43

Working with Elderly Persons across Cultures

Carl I. Cohen, Mehdi Elmouchtari and Iqbal Ahmed

Editors' Introduction

As the world population grows older the complexity of ageing and comorbidities between physical and mental illnesses become clearer. Rates of dementia are rising globally but more so in some countries and cultures. Cultures see changes in behaviours due to ageing in very different ways. Many cultures use different terms from psychiatry of old age or psychiatry of older adults or geriatric psychiatry or psychogeriatrics but all these terms refer to psychiatric practice related to older adults. Cohen *et al.* in this chapter use various perspectives: (1) the comparative cross-cultural studies of psychiatric disorders; (2) the study of migrant populations and cultural variations in illness within ethnically diverse nations; (3) the cultural critique of psychiatric theory and practice; and (4) therapeutic strategies. As the global population is beginning to live longer, with the impact of globalization, urbanization and industrialization bringing changes in family structures in their wake, there is an urgent need for more multidisciplinary research. It is also more interesting to note that more and more people are growing old outside their countries of birth. This, coupled with negative population growth in many countries, has brought with it specific issues related to financial resources and physical support. Cohen *et al.* remind us that by 2050, all major areas of the world except Africa will have nearly a quarter or more of their populations aged 60 or over. They point out that cross-cultural studies of ageing populations between and within countries have suggested that there are differences in the prevalence of dementia, depression, anxiety, suicidality, and psychoses. Obviously physical health, social stressors and community transitions, migration, belief systems, cohort effects, and socio-cultural effects of role and identity often influence these differences.

Introduction

There are compelling reasons to examine transcultural issues among older adults. In 2015, there were 901 million people aged 60 or over comprising 12 per cent of the global population (United Nations, 2015). The population aged 60 or above is growing at a rate of 3.26 per cent annually. Currently, among the continents, Europe has the greatest percentage of its population aged 60 or over (24%), but rapid ageing is occurring elsewhere. Among the developed countries, Japan has the oldest population with 33 per cent of the population being over age 60. By 2050, all major areas of the world except Africa will have nearly a quarter or more of their populations aged 60 or over. The number of older persons in the world is projected to be 1.4 billion by 2030 and 2.1 billion by 2050, and as much as 3.2 billion in 2100. In 2025, 72 per cent of persons aged 60 and over will be living in developing countries (Levkoff *et al.*, 1995). However, even within developed nations there will be marked demographic shifts. For example, in the United States, the proportion of elderly persons who are non-Hispanic whites will decline from 79 per cent in 2010 to 61 per cent in 2050 (Ortman *et al.*, 2014). Ethnic elders aged 85 and over are the fastest growing segment of the American population.

Worldwide, over 20 per cent of adults aged 60 and over suffer from a mental or neurological disorder (excluding headache disorders) and 6.6 per cent of all disability (disability adjusted life years, DALYs) among persons over 60 is attributed to neurological and mental disorders (WHO, 2016). Mental health problems are under-identified by healthcare professionals and older people themselves, and the stigma surrounding mental illness makes people reluctant to seek help. In this chapter, we will present an overview of the key concepts that are critical to understanding transcultural issues in the mental health of ageing individuals. We will not undertake an in-depth review of general conceptual and methodological issues that will be covered in other chapters in this volume. Rather, we have endeavoured to focus primarily on the interplay of ageing, culture and psychiatry.

Basic Concepts

It is important to distinguish between 'cross-national' and 'cross-cultural' studies (Sokolovsky, 2009a). The former refers to the nation state as a unit and compares whole countries on various measures. In recent years, there has been considerable growth in cross-national geropsychiatric studies, many of which will be described in this chapter. By contrast, cross-cultural studies focus on small-scale societies or individual communities of industrial states. 'Culture' and 'ethnicity' are often used interchangeably, although most of the ageing literature on transcultural psychiatry deals with ethnic differences. Culture refers to a system of values, beliefs and learned behaviours shared across whole populations or sub-groups of people, whereas ethnicity refers to a group identification based on a common heritage, customs, place of origin, religion, diet, language, dress, self-concept and normative expectations. Neither culture nor ethnicity is a fixed trait. Rather, they are fluid processes that interact with a variety of social factors such as modernization, immigration, assimilation, minority issues, socio-economic status, gender, and period-cohort and intergenerational issues (Ahmed, 1997).

There are a variety of ways to define ageing: biological, psychological and social. Typically, we identify ageing with chronological age. In Western societies, age 65 is used commonly as the cut-off for old age. However, this cut-off has been lowered to some extent based on declining legal ages of retirement. Age 60 has also been used in world demographic data on ageing (United Nations, 2015). A review by Glascock and Feinman (1981) found that in non-Western traditional societies there are three ways to identify old age: change in social or economic role, chronology, and change in physical characteristics. Changes in social and economic roles had been the most common way to demarcate old age. However, most societies have multiple definitions of old age that add complexity and some ambiguity to any categorization. Biological ageing cannot be precisely defined. However, based on markers of disease, disability and functional decline, Hazzard (2001)

defined true old age as 'above 75 years'. Dramatic demographic changes occurring worldwide have resulted in many societies having to redefine old age. For example, in many Western societies, persons are taking longer to reach various adult life stages (e.g. marriage, parenthood) and living longer. Indeed, some gerontologists are conceptualizing age based on life expectancy (Sanderson and Scherbov, 2008); thus, with increases in lifespan, '65' can be viewed as the 'new 50'.

'Life course' is another important concept for understanding ageing in diverse cultures. Life course refers to a sequence of age-graded events and social roles that are embedded in social structure, culture and historical change (Elder, 2001). Much of what are considered age effects in individuals and groups may not be related to the ageing process, but rather to the experiences of the cohort group to which they belong. Individual trajectories interact with socio-cultural processes. In societies undergoing rapid change, historical effects may take the form of a cohort effect so that social change distinguishes the life experiences of successive cohorts (Elder, 2001). Thus, coming of age in a time of prosperity will have a different effect on a life trajectory than coming of age during a depression. Cohort effects may impact on all persons in a society or they may impact on certain ethnic sub-groups. Each ethnic group has unique historical experiences. For example, Baker and Lightfoot (1993) describe how various events of twentieth century America – e.g. northern migration from the south, the Klu Klux Klan, the Great Depression, the desegregation of the military in the Korean war, the Civil Rights movement – had a differential effect on African Americans born in the first quarter of the twentieth century versus those born later in the century. Levkoff and colleagues (1995), in discussing the potential cumulative psychological impact of social change and upheaval, cite the example of elderly Chinese who have lived through the Imperial Era, the warlord years, the occupation by the Japanese during World War II, the Communist Revolution, the Great Leap Forward and the ensuing famine, the Cultural Revolution, and the opening of the economy and market reform.

Another important aspect to the life course perspective concerns the variations in social roles by age, e.g. parenting, grandparenting, retirement and so forth. However, the timing of these social roles is influenced by the interplay of historical events (i.e.

cohort effects). Baker and Lightfoot (1993) contend that historical experience and cultural context can have appreciable influence on elders' definitions of medical and psychiatric illness, their expectation of the healthcare delivery system, the time at which a decision is made to enter the treatment system, and the persons and/or systems from which treatment is sought.

Finally, the 'survivor' effects must also be considered when comparing older persons in different groups. Although all older persons are survivors, there is considerable difference between the 75-year-old person in a developed nation, where half the population lives to that age, and a 75-year-old in a developing nation where the life expectancy is age 60. The latter individual may have exceptional physical and psychological traits versus their fellow citizens or versus persons in the developed world. Unfortunately, the impact of survivor effects is rarely considered in comparisons between elderly groups, both cross-nationally and within countries.

Aging, Culture and Psychopathology: General Principles

There has been increased interest in trying to understand cross-cultural psychological differences in the context of age-based attitudes (North and Fiske, 2015). It has been long recognized that societies differ in their levels of appreciation for the aged; e.g. Eastern cultures that emphasize Confucian expectations to respect one's elders tend to hold older adults in high regard. Also supporting these traditional East–West distinctions are psychological research paradigms comparing the two regions on perceptual and cognitive tasks. In Western tradition, there is a focus on individuals over the context that surrounds them versus the Eastern tendency to view each person as part of a collective whole. However, over the past few decades societal changes have begun to impinge on these cultural differences, and industrialization may be eroding such expectations. Consequently, modernized societies may come to devalue their elders in the traditional roles of storytelling and wisdom sharing, and as these decrease in importance, the aged lose control over means of production (Nelson, 2005; Schoenberg and Lewis, 2005). Moreover, the ageing of the population has placed enormous pressure on societies to accommodate their elders, presenting potential burdens in healthcare and labour (Börsch-

Supan, 2003; UN, 2013). Thus, older people may face negative images in industrialized, ageing societies, regardless of eastern or western geography, or presumed cultural expectations.

From an empirical standpoint, whether Eastern and Western cultures differ in their respect for older adults remains surprisingly unclear. A study by Löckenhoff and coauthors (2009) provided support for a revised modernization framework based on societal and cultural shifts in the notion that older persons deserve respect and authority solely because of their age (hierarchical), but rather that they now garner respect based on their experiences and knowledge (wisdom) as well as a concern for their well-being. A recent meta-analysis of articles from 23 countries on attitudes towards older adults found that, contrary to conventional wisdom, evaluations tend to be more *negative* in the east overall with the strongest levels of senior derogation emerging in East Asia (compared with South and Southeast Asia) and non-Anglophone Europe (compared with North American and Anglophone western regions); however, there was considerable heterogeneity with some western countries scoring more poorly than eastern countries (North and Fiske, 2015). Notably, the speed of increase in the ageing population in a country significantly predicted negative elder attitudes, controlling for industrialization. More surprisingly, the authors found that cultural *individualism* significantly predicted relative *positivity* – suggesting that, for generating elder respect within rapidly ageing societies, collectivist traditions may backfire. The findings provide tantalizing data with respect to the importance of demographic challenges in shaping modern attitudes toward elders and how these forces may affect their psychological well-being.

There are a variety of ways that culture may affect the development and course of psychiatric conditions in older persons. These factors are not mutually exclusive and there is often interplay of these elements. First, there may be the direct physical or biological impact of the ecosystem or of the lifestyle patterns engendered by the culture. For example, older persons may be more vulnerable to air pollution that can impair respiratory capacity and diminish physical vigour. Similarly, cultures that promote smoking or unhealthy diets result in greater health problems as people grow older. It is well-established that health problems are associated with increased rates of psychiatric symptoms such as depression and anxiety, and may predispose to dementia.

A second way culture influences mental health is through the impact of various social forces on mental well-being. For example, in our discussion of the impact of globalization and urbanization that follows, we describe how changes in social structures may affect mental health of older adults. A third way in which culture may affect psychiatric symptoms is through the fostering of certain personality patterns that may become dysfunctional in later life. For example, a person may grow up in a culture that allows for a higher level of suspiciousness, but this may be inappropriate should this person move to a country where this is not acceptable. This is illustrated in a discussion that follows regarding paranoid ideation, especially in the African Caribbean population in the United States. Likewise, in Western countries, the so-called Type A personality configuration – the hard-driving, perfectionistic individual – is socially rewarded, although it may lead to cardiovascular disease and unhappiness as the person grows older. Finally, culture may play a role in the recognition, treatment and the consequences of displaying and experiencing psychiatric problems (Estroff, 1981).

Several theories of ageing and psychopathology may be relevant to our understanding this relationship from a transcultural perspective. One such theoretical model is the 'double jeopardy' hypothesis. In some Western societies and many transitional societies, the status of older persons is relatively low versus other age groups; being old and a member of a minority group is a double disadvantage (Dowd and Bengston, 1978). Older women may be subject to triple jeopardy because they are typically accorded lower status than men. An additional jeopardy would be the stigma of mental illness, and therefore ethnic minority elderly mentally ill women will face quadruple jeopardy.

Another useful theoretical perspective is the 'acculturation stress hypothesis' (Markides *et al.*, 1990). It is postulated that acculturation of younger generations may have a negative impact on the psychological well-being of their parents. For example, the latter may have come from cultures in which younger persons were expected to care for their ageing parents, and if necessary, to live together with them. In their new environment, this may no longer be possible. Ahmed's (1997) review concluded that acculturation stress interacts with age, race and gender discrimination, language

barriers, lower socio-economic status and diminished physical and psychological resources. However, Ahmed further points out that there are also protective factors for ethnic elders. Thus, ethnic identity may compensate for the identity loss that often occurs with ageing. Moreover, intergenerational solidarity and continued family closeness can enhance life satisfaction and decrease levels of depression.

Factors Affecting Well-Being of Older Persons in Developed Countries

Virtually all groups' traditional lifestyles and values have been altered by the immigration experience. While the negative and disorienting features of immigration have been the focus of much research, for some groups, migration may be part of successful ageing (Sokolovsky, 2009b). For example, coming to the United States and owning a home, is considered an important achievement for many older immigrants. Our understanding of cultural diversity of older immigrant ethnic minority persons within developed nations has become increasingly more rigorous. Immigrants from any country may be from different socio-economic, ethnic-cultural, religious, urban versus rural, and other backgrounds that may impact their adaptation to the host country. In addition, several immigration factors may affect adaptation to the host culture. These include age at immigration, historical events leading to immigration, degree of familiarity with cultural norms, laws, the institutions in the host country, presence of family, cultural and religious institutions from the immigrant's background, and how many generations have passed since immigration.

Sakauye (2004) identified four subcategories of ethnic elders based on distance from immigration and level of assimilation. First, there are immigrants who have arrived within the past 10 years, often preceded by their children. They commonly have language barriers, experience social isolation and cultural shock. Their mental health problems may include adjustment disorders or even post-traumatic stress disorders, and they may be more apt to display culture-bound syndromes. A second group of immigrants are those who have been in the country for a decade or more. Many arrived when they were young adults and their language skills are better. They may focus more on social and health-related issues. Among native-born ethnic elders there are also two categories. The first native-born group, poorly assimilated elderly persons, may encounter problems due to language barriers, poverty, fear of the majority group, social stressors, poor health, and inadequate healthcare. They also may present with culture-bound syndromes. A second native-born group consists of those older adults who are generally well assimilated but who still feel the socio-cultural impact of prejudice, discrimination and even overt racism. Such individuals may have problems with self-esteem, difficulties concerning their racial or ethnic identity, or feel socially isolated, depending upon the demographics of their neighborhood.

Language and culture congruity can substantially affect mental health of immigrants. For example, a study in Canada found those immigrants from non-English or non-French speaking countries were more likely to report loneliness than those persons who spoke languages similar to the Canadians (Gierveld et al., 2015). Paradoxically, having a social network comprising predominantly speakers from their country of origin was associated with greater loneliness, perhaps because it limited the possibilities for broadening social contacts. On the other hand, a study in Hawaii found that the least culturally assimilated men of Japanese ancestry (95 per cent US born) had the lowest prevalence of depressive symptoms, which might reflect cultural norms about reporting depressive symptoms or it may be that individuals who identify as more Japanese may have a network of extended families typically seen in Japan, which can ameliorate the development of depression (Harada et al., 2012).

Collectivism and individualism are the two most widely used concepts in cross-cultural studies of stress and coping (Lee and Mason, 2014). It is theorized that in more individualistic societies, such as western Europe and the United States, that place more weight on individual rights, people are likely to control or change their environment to fit their own personal needs. By contrast, in more collectivistic societies that emphasize interdependence, such as those in eastern Asia, people are likely to cope by adjusting to group needs. However, among immigrant groups, these hypothesized differences may be modified by enculturation factors (Lee and Mason, 2014).

Sokolovsky (2009c) has described how traditional ethnic responses can sometimes exacerbate difficulties.

For example, in Latino cultures, differences in male–female perspectives often places a heavier burden on women to provide care. Another problem is that new elderly immigrants may lose access to the cultural fabric of easy engagement within socially enmeshed neighbourhoods that they had in their native country, and they may be faced with social isolation and loneliness. This may be more acute in women, since among some immigrant populations, men will spend more time than women outside the ethnic family, and consequently, they typically have more extensive linkages to the broader community. As a result, the older men have better mental health. Moreover, some social networks that emphasize too much reciprocity and obligations with children and other kin may not be satisfying. Thus, in Asian groups, there may be guilt in elderly persons because they could not materially help their children. While preferring independence, they are often trapped in dependent isolated social situations by linguistic limitations, lack of culture and social capital, and little control over their lives. Others feel trapped into child-caring roles, that may create guilt and sadness, especially as the older person becomes more physically impaired and unable to assist.

Living alone is not the same as feeling lonely or socially isolated. In Nordic countries there are high rates of living alone but low rates of loneliness. In the southern European countries, living alone is associated with higher rates of loneliness (Gusmano, 2009). Sokolovsky (2009c) provides several illustrations of how merely assaying the frequency or number of kin contacts may not be helpful. In San Diego, older Latinos living alone reported four times more extended kin than older whites, but many were less likely to turn to kin in times of need, i.e. they preferred to 'suffer in silence'. Asians in England were found to depend heavily on very narrow support kin sources in contrast to African Caribbeans who developed a more flexible construct of support from non-kin and church members. Kinship in black American families has flexible boundaries that allow for absorption of young grandchildren and other relatives. Many older black women live with a relative under 18. Increasingly, in developed countries, many ethnic elders live in 'granfamilies' (Sokolovsky, 2009d). In the United States, one in ten grandparents will have primary responsibility for a grandchild. Worldwide there have been increases in granfamilies, especially in Africa because of the AIDs epidemic.

Factors Affecting Well-Being of Older Persons in Developing Countries

Several writers (Desjarlais *et al.*, 1995; Levkoff *et al.*, 1995; Sokolovsky, 1997) have noted that while there has been considerable romanticizing of the role of older persons in non-industrial, non-Western societies, a more realistic appraisal of ageing is needed. Thus, it is important to recognize that:

1. A single cultural system may provide highly successful solutions for some problems of ageing but do poorly with respect to others.
2. Not all non-Western, non-industrial cultural systems provide a better milieu for ageing than is found in the West.
3. Modernization does not invariably result in a diminished quality of life for elders, but can have a positive impact on well-being. Some countries may provide pensions and healthcare resources that enhance the older person's ability to live independently.
4. A single cultural system may offer vastly different opportunities for successful ageing depending on class, gender, ethnicity and rural–urban variation.
5. Security and life quality are enhanced for older persons when cultures promote both community and kin roles for elders.
6. There are no geriatric utopias where older persons are free of diseases of ageing such as dementia.
7. Multi-generational families were actually less common in traditional societies because of diminished life expectancy; hence, multi-generational families may be more likely to exist in industrialized nations.
8. Gerontocracy may reflect economic and demographic factors rather than purely cultural ones. Thus, co-residence with other family members may reflect housing shortages, or decreased economic dependence on inheritances may reduce the amount of care that families provide to their older kin.

The power and status of elderly people in developing countries often vary based on the following dichotomies: ill versus healthy, very old versus older, rich versus poor, male versus female. In short, there is inter-and intra-societal variability in the care of the aged.

Desjarlais and his coauthors (1995) and Levkoff and colleagues (1995) have identified several ways in which the economic and structural changes of modernization can potentially affect the mental health of elderly persons in developing nations:

1. Life expectancy is increasing and fertility rates are declining. Several consequences of this trend are apparent. First, this results in a greater number of older persons, and consequently, an increase in age-related diseases such as dementia. Second, there are also fewer children to care for their ageing parents. Third, because men whose wives die often remarry, and women live longer and marry men older than themselves, the number of widows will continue to increase. In developing countries, unmarried women are economically vulnerable.
2. Economic changes cause the price of agricultural products to decline relative to manufactured goods. The means by which traditional social structures guaranteed that elderly persons would be cared for through the inheritance of land and livestock have become attenuated. Consequently, older persons have become less valuable, lose respect, and face isolation or even abandonment. The psychiatric consequences might include low self-esteem, worthlessness, depression, suicidality, or substance abuse.
3. Rural to urban migration continues to increase. Although urban living per se may not be associated with higher rates of mental disorders, older persons who move to cities or who have grown old there, live frequently in substandard housing without basic sanitation and with the constant threat of eviction. Such a lifestyle increases stress and results in anxiety, depression, substance abuse and suicidality. Other persons who have migrated to cities in their youth may now return to their villages in later life. They find inadequate care for older persons, feel isolated and experience low self-esteem.
4. Increased education of the young. This may result in younger persons devaluing their elders along with their customs and traditions. Among the elders, this may decrease feelings of self-worth and result in depression or anxiety.
5. Increased education of the elderly persons. As the ageing population becomes better educated, they are able to obtain better jobs and more

effectively cope with social change. Their increased financial well-being and self-esteem will help buffer against depression and anxiety.

6. Per capita income rises and healthcare improves in some countries. This reduces mortality, especially among men, and consequently results in a smaller proportion of women becoming widowed at younger ages, although their absolute number may rise with increased longevity and number of older women in general. Thus, it diminishes loneliness and buffers against depression and anxiety.

7. War and displacement have occurred in many countries as a consequence of ethnic conflicts and factional fighting. Older people are thought to have lower psychological resilience to rapid social changes.

8. Identity systems are changing. There is increasing pull between modernization forces that create multiple and flexible identities, multi-ethnic communities, long-distance networks and reactions by communities to reassert their ethnic identities. Bhugra and Mastrogianni (2004) note that ethnic identity has a role in individuals' self-esteem and it can affect the social causes and courses of psychiatric disorders. The consequences of the new pluralist context of multicultural societies for individuals' psychological well-being are largely unknown. However, it is likely to have a more negative impact on older members of society who will experience an attenuation of their traditional ethnic identity without fully participating in the positive aspects of the new multi-identity community.

9. Older adults are 'expected' to be more productive and are even being asked to contribute more to their family and/or community as a consequence of the shift from agrarian to urban manufacturing economies (Yasamy *et al.*, 2013), and this can make disabled or unskilled elders feel guilty and worthless.

10. Retirement incomes are inadequate. In the developing world, half of workers earn US$2 or less per day (Fry, 2009). The World Bank found 70 per cent of the world's elders rely solely on their own labour or that of family for support. There is little or no opportunity to obtain retirement pensions. Thus, the economic strains on older adults are enormous.

Specific Psychiatric Disorders

Dementia

It is estimated that 47.5 million people worldwide are living with dementia. The total number of people with dementia is projected to increase to 75.6 million in 2030 and 135.5 million in 2050, with the majority of sufferers living in low- and middle-income countries (WHO, 2016). Dementia, which is a disorder primarily of older adults, provides an excellent illustration of how culture and ethnic origin interplay with biological forces. First, prevalence rates of dementia vary between countries, and within countries, among various ethnic groups. For example, Rizzi and colleagues' (2014) review of the literature found cross-national prevalence rates ranging from 2 to 21 per cent. In general, the highest rates occurred among the poor and uneducated elderly populations, although in some countries healthier diets and greater physical activity seemed to mitigate the negative impact of low education by diminishing risk factors such as hypertension, diabetes, obesity and dyslipidemia. In addition, other factors accounting for cross-national differences in prevalence of dementia include the low number of very old persons in developing countries, the stigma of psychiatric disorder so that it goes unreported, and difficulties in identifying dementia, especially among populations with low education and income.

The prevalence rates of the two principal types of dementia, Alzheimer's disease (AD) and vascular dementia (VaD), vary across the world. Thus, AD is more common than VaD in North America and Europe whereas the obverse is true in China (Desjarlais *et al.*, 1995). A recent trend among Asians has been a diminution in the prevalence of vascular dementia and an increase in the prevalence of Alzheimer's disease; in Japan, the ratio of the two types of dementia is now roughly equal (Rizzi *et al.*, 2014). Within the United States, most studies have found the prevalence of AD to be greater among African Americans and Latinos than among Caucasians.

Differences in medical conditions have been thought to contribute to these differences. For example, the higher rates of hypertension, hyperlipidemia and diabetes, all of which may be considered risk factors for both AD and VaD, are found more commonly among African American elders and may explain their higher rates of dementia versus US whites and Nigerians (Hendrie *et al.*, 2001). This possibility is heightened by the fact that the presence of the e4 allele of APOE, which is a strong genetic risk factor for late onset AD in Caucasians, does not seem to play as a prominent role among African Americans, and it plays essentially no role among Nigerians (Hendrie *et al.*, 2001).

Several recent epidemiological studies have suggested that the incidence of dementia may be declining in many countries. Studies from the United States (Satizabal *et al.*, 2016) and western Europe, viz., Sweden, the Netherlands, the United Kingdom, Spain (Wu *et al.*, 2016), and France (Grasset *et al.*, 2015) have found declining incidences of the disorder, although the prevalence of the disorder has continued to increase as the population of elderly persons rises. By contrast, studies in Japan (Dodge *et al.*, 2012), China (Chan *et al.*, 2013), and very old persons (age 85 and over) in Sweden (Mathilias *et al.*, 2011) found increasing incidences of dementia. Declining rates in the United States and some countries in western Europe are thought to be due to improvements in modifiable risk factors such as higher educational levels and reduction in vascular risk factors.

Racial differences have been reported in the types of neuropsychiatric symptoms seen in dementia. For example, Cohen (2000) found higher rates of delusions and hallucinations among black dementia patients, and higher rates of depression among white dementia patients, even after controlling for various sociodemographic, various health variables, and estimated length of illness. However, a more recent study from the same group found that these differences in neuropsychiatric symptoms and dementia stage at time of presentation have disappeared (Cohen *et al.*, 2012), thereby suggesting that the differences in neuropsychiatric symptoms primarily reflected the stage in their illness that persons were brought for evaluation.

There are considerable differences in the way dementia is handled among the world's societies. Desjarlais and coauthors (1995) note that in some societies dementia is treated as an understandable and expected part of ageing. These so called 'folk' explanations of dementia rather than 'biological' explanations of dementia may persist in certain ethnic minority immigrant groups and may delay appropriate care of patients with dementia (Suzuki *et al.*, 2015). Consequently, families may respond to it as they might to other aspects of ageing such as physical

illness and disability. Nevertheless, despite the transcultural differences in the interpretation of dementia, it still is an incapacitating illness in its later stages and requires considerable personal care.

The informal care system is the dominant mode for caring for older persons throughout the world, and women generally assume the care-giver role (Desjarlais *et al.*, 1995). Although informal care is the predominant form in developed countries, there has been increasing reliance on formal systems. Socio-cultural changes – e.g. migration of younger persons to urban areas, lower birth rates and the increase of women in the workforce – in countries such as China, Japan, and sub-Saharan Africa and parts of India are resulting in a decline in the family care of elderly persons. Nevertheless, formal care systems in developing nations are woefully inadequate in both the breadth of care and its quality. For example, there are 17 million elderly persons (15 per cent of the total) in China who are in need of daily assistance (Lou and Giu, 2012), but only 1.5 to 2.5 per cent of elderly persons are in institutional care (Feng *et al.*, 2012).

A fairly consistent finding in the North American literature has been the differential impact of caregiving on persons from diverse ethnic backgrounds. A review by Pinquart and Sorenson (2005) found that in comparison to Caucasian care-givers, ethnic minority care-givers in the United States had lower socioeconomic status, were younger, were less likely to be a spouse, and more likely to use informal rather than formal support services. They provided more care and had stronger filial obligations beliefs than white care-givers. Asian American care-givers, but not African American and Hispanic care-givers, used less formal support than white care-givers. While African American care-givers had lower levels of burden and depression than white care-givers, Hispanic and Asian American care-givers were more depressed than white care-givers. All groups of ethnic minority care-givers reported worse physical health than whites. For the Asian American care-givers, the more normative nature of care-giving in Eastern cultures may be protective against distress just as it may be in African American cultures; however, this was vitiated by a greater likelihood of being cared for by a daughter-in-law and that dementia symptoms may sometimes be a source of shame in Asian or Asian American cultures, and consequently, increase care-giver depression (Janevic and Connell, 2001).

Shahly and coauthors' (2013) 20-nation study of family care-giving found that burden in low/lower-middle income countries was two to three-fold higher than in higher income countries and is consistent with previous evidence of greater 'familism' in developing countries, i.e. the relationships with adult children and siblings are not as attenuated as in developed countries. A higher burden was reported by women than men. Moreover, the much higher magnitude of reported financial burden in low/lower-middle income countries than richer ones presumably reflected the fact that government resources and supports for family care-givers are relatively low in these countries, although strong social norms encouraging intra-familial financial support could also play a role in increased burdens.

In the United States there have been some interesting trends that portend trends elsewhere. Hispanics and Asians are the fastest-growing minority groups among nursing home residents, followed by blacks. All groups have outpaced whites. These findings reflect the changing face of the nursing home population and they signal an important shift in the use of long-term care options among racial and ethnic groups in the US population (Feng et al., 2011). The growing number of minority elders is one driver of these changes but it also reflects the likelihood that white elders may have more varied choices of care in their communities and may be better able to afford alternatives to nursing homes such as assisted living facilities, home care, or retirement communities. Minority elders may well face greater barriers than white elders in access to home and community-based alternatives to nursing home care .

Depression and Suicide

Unipolar depression occurs in approximately 7 per cent of the general elderly population worldwide (WHO, 2016). A cross-national study of the prevalence of late-life depression in nine countries in Asia, Africa and Latin America varied across sites according to diagnostic criteria (Guerra et al., 2015). Lower prevalence was observed for ICD-10 depressive episodes (0.3–13.8%); however, when using the EURO-D depression scale, the prevalence was higher and ranged from 1.0 to 38.6 per cent. The crude prevalence was particularly high in the Dominican Republic and in rural India. ICD-10 depression was also associated with increased age and being female. Both rural and

urban China had very low prevalence rates of 1 and 2.5 per cent, respectively, perhaps reflecting the fact that Western nosology does not match well with Chinese expressions of distress. A large community study conducted in ten European countries in persons aged 55 and above using the EURO-D measure reported prevalence rates of between 19 and 33 per cent (Castro-Costa et al., 2007). The findings of the two studies were generally consistent although there were some methodological differences between studies and there was more variability in prevalence rates among sites in the Guerra group's study, mainly arising from the low prevalence found in China.

Bhugra and Mastrogianni's (2004) review of transcultural aspects of depression found that somatic symptoms are common presenting features of depression throughout the world. Moreover, there is evidence that older persons are more apt to express depression and anxiety in somatic terms. For example, Bhugra and coworkers (1997) found that Punjabi women participating in a focus group in London recognized the English word 'depression', but the older women used terms such as 'weight on my heart/mind', or 'pressure on the mind'. A study of ethnic elders in London by Lawrence and colleagues (2006) underscored the importance of being sensitive to the 'language of depression' used by different groups, e.g. 'excessive thinking' in South Asians and excessive worrying in Caribbeans. Bhugra and Mastrogianni (2004) note that somatization is a concept that reflects the dualism inherent in Western biomedical practice, whereas in most forms of traditional medicine (e.g. Chinese or Ayurveda medicine), there are no sharp distinction between the mental and the physical. Consequently, persons from traditional cultures may not differentiate among the emotions of anxiety, irritability and depression, since they typically express distress in somatic terms, and their concepts of depression are different from those in the West. Bhugra and Mastrogianni (2004) speculate that globalization and urbanization will likely alter these metaphors and different idioms of distress will be used. It is probable that there will be an increase in medicalization of depressive symptoms.

In addition, work by Lawrence and associates (2006) in Britain suggest that in Western countries ethnic elders are somewhat more apt than whites to view depression within a social rather than a medical model, although the model used by all groups was more akin to a social than biological one. There were ethnic differences in the attribution of depression. For example, Caribbeans were more likely to attribute depression to loneliness whereas South Asians attributed depression to difficult home environments, and whites focused on lack of support and contact with family.

Like younger persons, older persons subject to higher levels of stressors exhibit higher rates of depression. For example, the high rates of depression found among elders in Sao Paolo, Brazil were attributed to stressors associated with rapid acculturation, poverty, difficult housing conditions, and inadequate retirement benefits (Blay et al., 1991). In addition to the factors that affect younger adults, the high rates and severity of medical disorders among older persons are noteworthy, since physical illness correlates closely with depression. Thus, like older persons in Western countries, rates of depression in primary care settings in northern India were found in two-fifths to three-fifths of patients (Gupta et al., 1991). Moreover, older persons in developing countries often suffer from malnutrition that may mimic or exacerbate symptoms of depression.

Although global migration, especially to Western nations, has increased dramatically, there is surprisingly little written about the impact of such migration on older adults. One of the more comprehensive studies by Aichberger and colleagues (2010) studied persons aged 50 and over in 11 European countries. First generation migrants in northern and western Europe had higher rates of depression than their indigenous age peers. Although migrants in southern Europe had higher rates of depression, they did not differ significantly from their indigenous age peers. Rates were increased with age and being women. The authors pointed out that lower income and physical illness contributed to depression. Van der Wurff and colleagues (2004) postulated that depression risk for immigrants likely depends on interplay of ethnicity, social class, and health factors.

Shah (2010) examined the World Health Organization's 1-year average of suicide rates for persons aged 65 and found that there were wide cross-national variations in elderly suicide rates. Elderly suicide rates were the lowest in Caribbean and Arabic/Islamic countries, and the highest in central and eastern European countries emerging from the former Soviet Union, some Asian, and some western European countries. In Western countries suicide rates increased with age, at least until age 75, whereas

the trend is more variable in developing countries. Globally, suicide rates among men are greater than women, but there are some notable exceptions, e.g. in China rates among older women may exceed men (Li and Baker, 1991). Within countries, there are also marked differences in suicide rates (Sakauye, 2004). In the United States, suicide rates for African Americans and Latino American elders have been lower than whites, whereas rates among Japanese, Chinese and Korean American elders are comparable to whites. Sakauye (2004) theorized that the lower rates of suicide found among some older ethnic minorities, despite their poverty or immigrant status, may reflect stronger family ties, the greater importance of elders in the minority family, and more powerful cultural or religious attitudes against suicide.

With respect to anxiety disorders in older adults, a cross-national study of anxiety disorders in seven Asian and Latin American countries found prevalence rates ranging from 0.1% in rural China to 9.6% in urban Peru (Prina et al., 2011). Two previous studies conducted in Europe of reported anxiety using the GMS/AGECAT diagnostic system found prevalence estimates of 3.2% and 4.0% in the Dutch and British populations respectively (Kvaal et al. 2008; Schoevers et al., 2003) and prevalence rates in the United States have ranged from 1.9% to 12% (Cohen et al., 2006; Byers et al., 2010). Overall, rates in urban Latin America equalled or exceeded European and North American rates of anxiety.

Several cross-national studies described above have found extremely low prevalence of various mental disorders in China and that this may be attributable to the stigmatization of mental illnesses that has been described in this Asian culture or that mental disorders are expressed differently, especially among older people living in rural areas.

Psychoses and Paranoid Ideation

In an 18-country study of psychotic experiences, McGrath and colleagues (2016) found that there were significant differences across three income strata in lifetime prevalence of any psychotic experiences, any hallucinatory experiences, or any delusional experiences. In each comparison, the prevalence estimates were significantly higher among respondents in middle- and high-income countries than among those in low-income countries. Moreover, the oldest strata (age 60 and over) had fewer delusional experiences than the youngest age strata (18–29), and there were no differences in hallucinatory experiences. Lifetime prevalence of a psychotic experience ranged from 1.2% (Iraq) to 14.9% (Brazil), and the mean was 5.8% across all sites.

There is an extensive literature documenting the cultural differences in the diagnostic interpretation of psychotic symptoms. In the United States, African Americans have been found to have higher rates of psychotic disorders such as schizophrenia (Keith et al., 1991). Most of the research has focused on younger populations or a broad age sample. A small retrospective study by Coleman and Baker (1994) found that misdiagnosis of older African American patients with schizophrenia was common. They identified four factors that contributed to the misdiagnoses: clinician bias, misinterpretation of psychotic symptoms, biased diagnostic instruments, and patient–clinician cultural distance.

Because older persons are more apt than younger persons to ascribe to traditional beliefs and superstitions (Yeo, 2001), it is likely that the prevalence of paranoid or psychotic ideation (i.e. hallucinations and psychotic delusions) would be greater among the former. A study in New York City documented very high levels of paranoid ideation or psychotic symptoms among blacks aged 55 and over, particularly among persons born in the Caribbean (Cohen et al., 2004). As compared to whites, the investigators found blacks were more than twice as likely to experience paranoid ideation: 21% vs 9%; three times more likely to report psychoses: 7% vs 2%; and twice as likely to experience either paranoid ideation or psychoses: 24% vs 10%. These differences were all statistically significant. Within the black population, there were appreciable, but statistically non-significant differences in the expression of paranoid ideation or psychotic symptoms: US-born blacks, French Caribbeans and English Caribbeans reporting rates of 18%, 38% and 18%, respectively. Although there was no association of paranoid ideation and/or psychotic symptoms with impaired daily functioning, there was a significant association with depressive symptoms. This suggested that experiencing paranoid ideation and/or psychotic symptoms was not totally benign but may represent an expression of dysphoria or distress, or alternately, it may lead to depression. A study by Cohen and Marino (2013) using a large US sample of adults found that the association between psychotic experiences and distress held across all ethnic groups except Asians, indicating that the psychotic experiences were not a cultural idiom of distress but common to most ethnic groups.

Diagnostic Instruments

One of the critical issues affecting the assessment of older adults is the validity of the diagnostic instruments. Content and construct validity are two forms of validity that are especially important in older adults (Edelstein et al., 2009). With respect to content validity, experience and symptoms of older persons differ from those of younger persons. Construct validity refers to how well the instrument assesses the construct of interest and must be demonstrated in elderly samples because age-related changes in psychological constructs may occur. Age norms, also adjusted for race and education, must be available for each measure. Because older adults may be mentally or physically slower, timed measures need to be normed for ageing effects. Older adults, especially in developing countries, have higher rates of illiteracy and innumeracy, and tests need to be adjusted to reflect problems with reading, writing and calculations. Instruments need to take into account cultural idioms of psychological distress, which may have greater expression in older persons who are typically less westernized than their children. Likewise, instruments translated into another language must be back-translated to ensure the fidelity of the translation. Finally, administration of instruments must take into account physical and sensory problems such as visual, hearing and arthritic changes that may affect various components of the test.

It was well known that many of the diagnostic scales and instruments have poor sensitivity and specificity across cultural groups. The World Health Organization has attempted to develop diagnostic instruments that are harmonious and consistent with the cultural, linguistic and educational norms of the subject population. However, instruments such as the Composite International Diagnostic Instrument have not been validated sufficiently in older adults, who may present differently, e.g. older depressed persons may present with more somatic complaints than younger persons, or have their symptoms attributed to physical disorders.

Jiang and Lee (2016) developed a state-of-the-art list of single and multidimensional instruments that can be used to comprehensively assess older adults. For example, the Comprehensive Geriatric Assessment provides detailed information on clinical, functional, and cognitive domains of older patients. Many of these measures have been used internationally or in cross-national comparisons. On the other hand, despite widespread translations into other languages, cognitive tests such as the Mini-Mental State Examination and the Montreal Cognitive Assessment are still prone to cultural and educational biases. Some gerontologists have proposed utilizing assessments of instrumental activities of daily living and everyday memory as a means to overcome cultural biases, although it is difficult to determine what 'everyday' is for older men and women within each culture (Sakauye, 2004).

Ethnicity and Pharmacology

Lin and Smith (2000) observed that a history of racist misinterpretation and/or fabrication of scientific data have made it difficult to discuss biological diversity among people. Moreover, because there are considerable within group differences, there is potential for over-simplification and stereotyping. Lin and Smith further note that the genetic factors involved in the response to drugs are substantially influenced by culture and ethnicity. They identify a variety of factors that influence medication response that depend on socio-cultural influences: diet and nutrition, smoking, drugs and alcohol, caffeine, exercise, disease and herbs. In addition, culture has non-biological effects on medication response that are due to factors such as patient compliance and placebo effects of medications. The intervening variables on these non-biological effects are related to the patient, the doctor and the patient–doctor relationship, as well as cultural beliefs about illness and medication, and the actual process of giving and receiving medications (Ahmed, 2001).

Pharmacokinetics, or how a drug moves through the body, becomes increasingly important with advancing age. Age affects the absorption, distribution, metabolism and elimination of medications to varying degrees (Jacobson et al., 2002). Oxidative liver metabolism utilizing the cytochrome P450 enzymes is the only pharmacokinetic process that is affected by ageing and ethnicity. Both CYP1A2 and CYP3A4 enzymes decline meaningfully with ageing, and all enzyme systems are affected by the interactions of various drugs on this metabolism; thus, older people who are typically on multiple medications are at increased risk for experiencing drug–drug interactions on liver metabolism. There is considerable biodiversity involving the enzymes of the P450 system. Thus, due to genetic polymorphisms involving the CYP2D6 enzymes, 5–9 per cent of Caucasians show no activity in the CYP2D6, while more than half of Asians and approximately one-fourth to two-fifths of blacks have slower metabolism involving these enzymes. The CYP2D6 metabolism also is influenced by ethnicity. Mexicans tend to have a more rapid metabolism, while rates of ultrarapid metabolism of 20–30% have been noted among Arabs and Ethiopians, far more than the 1–5% rate among Europeans (Lin and Elwyn, 2004). Similarly, due to allele differences, 20% of East Asians (Chinese, Japanese and Koreans), but only 3–5% of Caucasians show poor metabolism involving the CYP1A2 enzyme.

Pharmacodynamics, which is the end-organ responsiveness to medications, may be affected by ageing, although sensitivity varies with the type of drug and comorbid medical conditions. Ethnic differences in psychodynamics have been not been adequately studied. Preliminary work involving serotonin transport proteins found that Caucasians respond better to selective serotonin reuptake inhibitors (SSRIs) if they have a long allele variant in the gene controlling transport whereas Asians seem to have a better response if they have the short allele variant (Gerretson et al., 2009). How this interacts with ageing effects is unclear.

Finally, culture and ethnicity play an important role with respect to the adverse effects of antipsychotics, such as the development of the 'metabolic syndrome' that includes obesity, diabetes and hyperlipidemia. There are wide variations in the prevalence of metabolic syndromes throughout the world, with substantial group differences found within continents (Grundy, 2008). In the United States, the baseline risk of metabolic syndrome is substantially higher among all minorities, except for Alaskan natives, versus white populations (REACH, 2010). The risk further rises with lower socio-economic status and increased age, affecting more than 40 per cent of people in their 60s and 70s in the United States (Ford et al., 2002). These baseline risk factors increase the likelihood that minorities will develop metabolic syndrome secondary to anti-psychotic agents (Henderson, 2005).

Psychotherapy

Yeo (2001) has delineated four ways in which culture may affect the explanation of diseases and their treatment. They are all relevant to the care of older people:

1. 'Western' biomedicine has its own culture (e.g. knowledge, beliefs, skills, values) based on scientific assumptions and processes, producing definitions and explanations of disease. Older patients, familiar with other health traditions, may rely more on factors such as nature, balance or spiritual interventions to explain physical states.

2. People may identify conditions that do not match those found in biomedical references, yet these conditions can have a direct impact on healthcare, adherence to recommended treatment, and full communication between patient and provider.

3. Culturally defined somatic disorders and culture-bound syndromes with their own beliefs about treatment may make the practice of culturally appropriate geriatric care more complex.

4. Contrasting values of independence versus community/family may result in conflicting expectation of the involvement of others in the provision of care.

Sakauye (2004) has identified a variety of factors that may arise in the therapeutic session with older ethnic elders:

1. There may be issues related to authority figures.

2. Patients may be overly deferential, inhibited or ashamed of revealing personal feelings, or they may be hostile and suspicious.

3. Persons who have not worked or who had lived in rural settings may have difficulties adhering to strict time appointments.

4. For new immigrants, their primary psychological issues may revolve around adjustment issues, and they may be more apt to present with culture-bound syndromes whereas more established immigrants may present with more social and health related issues.

5. There is often a need for bilingual therapists, and even established elderly immigrants may say that they cannot fully express their emotional state in English, and that they can best express their

thoughts when they revert to their language of origin (Sadavoy and Lazarus, 2004). Language issues may become more pronounced among persons with dementia, since language abilities typically decline during the course of the illness.

6. Therapists must ensure that patients do not take refuge in cultural differences in order to explain away all emotional reactions and behaviours.

Transference issues are more complex when working with different cultural groups. Therapists often find that their elderly patients may experience transference at different generational levels: sometimes the therapist is the parent, sometimes it is the sibling or spouse, and at other times the therapist may be a child or even grandchild. In some ethnic groups with wider family relationships, transference towards the therapist may include aunts and uncles, cousins and other kin. Likewise, counter-transference issues (i.e. negative feelings toward the patient) may be expressed as ageism or lack of empathy toward the older person (Sakauye, 2008). In some therapists, negative feelings may be the expression of their own parental conflicts or their fears of ageing, fears of the patient dying, or that they are wasting their time. When treating ethnic elders, these negative feelings can be further compounded by racial stereotypes.

Crowther and colleagues (2006) have provided a few suggestions for conducting psychotherapy with ethnic elders:

1. Therapists should minimize note taking in order to reduce suspicions and mistrust of professionals.

2. Persons need to be socialized into therapy and it is better to start with exploring current problems rather than childhood issues.

3. Clinicians should emphasize that receiving psychotherapy does not mean that the older person is 'crazy'.

4. Taking a more active role is common, such as assisting elders to negotiate the medical and social service system.

5. Involving family is often beneficial, especially among immigrants whose family may be their only social and emotional support.

6. Clinicians should inquire about the use of indigenous healers, herbal remedies and inquire as to the role that faith, religion and/or spirituality play in helping the patient with the symptoms (Mintzer and Faison, 2009).

It is important to heed Sue and Sue's (1990) admonition that the reason minority group individuals underutilize and prematurely terminate therapy is often because of the services themselves. Such services are typically antagonistic or inappropriate to belief systems and life experiences of culturally different clients.

Summary and Conclusions

The worldwide growth in the ageing population in tandem with dramatic economic transitions has made cross-cultural geropsychiatric research more compelling. Increasingly more people are growing old both within and outside their countries of birth; in 2015, 244 million people, or 3.3 per cent of the world's population, lived outside their country of origin (UNFPA, 2015). Studies of ageing populations both between and within countries have suggested that there are differences in the prevalence of dementia, depression, anxiety, suicidality and psychoses. Research suggests that physical health, social stressors and community transitions, migration, belief systems, cohort effects and socio-cultural effects of role and identity often influence these differences. Moreover, the therapeutic response to these conditions reflects socio-economic and cultural forces. Levkoff and her colleagues (1995) theorize that family support plays a unique role in acting as both a stress-buffering mediator – i.e. acting on the structural forces delineated in this chapter – as well as having a direct bearing on mental well-being. Informal support is the mainstay of care in both industrialized and traditional societies because moral norms of assisting elderly persons persist even after modernization. Providing additional support to families makes sense for developing nations, since it is usually the most effective and least costly approach. The judicious development of formal systems to supplement informal care should fall within the economic capability of most developing countries.

Western nosology has not adequately captured the array of symptom presentation or provided the most reasonable conceptualization of symptoms among various cultures, and there have been additional difficulties in reconciling diagnostic criteria for ageing individuals. On the other hand, globalization is now subtly shaping the dissemination of psychiatric knowledge through the increased movement of people, communication, and products throughout the globe, and there is likely to be a gradual hybridization of the theories of psychopathology and treatment, and within such theories, an increased sensitivity to the burgeoning geriatric population.

Regardless of where on the globe an elderly patient resides, a more culturally informed and culturally sensitive approach can lead to more competent care of the individual elderly patient (Takeshita and Ahmed, 2004). Indeed, in the ageing field, cultural competence has been included as one of the cardinal principles of the 'patient-centred care' model of older persons in which clinicians are encouraged to explore, empathize and be responsive to patients' needs, values and preferences, and to strive to avoid stereotyping and oversimplification (Weissman et al., 2005). Metzl and Hanson (2014) have extended this concept to what they call, 'structural competency'. Thus, to be successful, clinicians must apprehend the impact of globalization and urbanization on older persons in developing countries and the interplay of culture and family on immigrants in developed nations; and in both settings, the role of gender, social class and educational background must be appreciated.

The progress in ageing geropsychiatric research in documenting the worldwide prevalence of mental disorders, understanding associated risk factors, and developing an array of treatment strategies is being eclipsed by a looming global crisis in the care of older adults with psychiatric disorders created by demographic and economic pressures. Approximately 180 million persons aged 60 and over suffer from a mental or neurological disorder and this will grow to 420 million persons by 2050. Concurrently, there is an historic low in the number of younger persons available to support their elders. This will create a paradoxical situation in which public funds available to support mental health, medical and social services for older adults will invariably shrink due to diminished tax bases caused by proportionately fewer workers, while the need for services will continue to grow. Moreover, in the developed countries pensions are shrinking, whereas in the developing countries, pensions are minimal or non-existent. Consequently, considerable strain will be placed on fewer family members to assist their elders. The implications for mental and physical well-being are enormous. As Fry (2009) ruefully concluded, 'it is fairly certain that in the 21st century it will be much scarier to grow old'. Thus, like climate change, a grey tsunami is approaching that requires broad policy interventions to forestall a future disaster.

References

Ahmed, I. (1997). Geriatric psychopathology. In *Culture and Psychopathology*, ed. W.-S. Tseng and J. Streltzer. New York: Brunner/Mazel, pp. 223–240.

Ahmed, I. (2001). Psychological aspects of giving and receiving medications. In *Culture and Psychotherapy: A Guide to Clinical Practice*, ed. W.-S. Tseng and J. Strelzer. Washington DC: American Psychiatric Press Inc., pp. 123–134.

Aichberger, M. C., Schouler-Ocak, M., Mundt, A. *et al.* (2010). Depression in middle-aged and older first generation migrants in Europe: results from the Survey of Health, Ageing and Retirement in Europe (SHARE). *European Psychiatry*, **25**(8), 468–475.

Baker, F. M., and Lightfoot, O.B. (1993). Psychiatric care of ethnic elders. In *Culture, Ethnicity, and Mental Illness*, ed. A. C. Gaw. Washington DC: American Psychiatric Press, pp. 517–552.

Bhugra, D. and Mastrogianni, A. (2004). Globalisation and mental disorders. *British Journal of Psychiatry*, **184**, 10–20.

Bhugra, D., Gupta, K. R. and Wright, B. (1997). Depression in north India: comparison of symptoms and life events with other patient groups. *International Journal of Psychiatry in Clinical Practice*, **1**(2), 83–87.

Blay, S. L., Bickel, H. and Cooper, B. (1991). Mental illness in a cross-national perspective. Results from a Brazilian and a German community survey among the elderly. *Society of Psychiatric Epidemiology*, **26**, 245–251.

Börsch-Supan, A. (2003). Labor market effects of population aging. *Labour*, **17**(1), 5–44.

Byers, A. L., Yaffe, K., Covinsky K. E. *et al.* (2010). High occurrence of mood and anxiety disorders among older adults: the National Comorbidity Survey Replication. *Archives of General Psychiatry*, **67**(5), 489–496.

Castro-Costa, E., Dewey, M., Stewart, R. *et al.* (2007). Prevalence of depressive symptoms and syndromes in later life in ten European countries. *British Journal of Psychiatry*, **191**(5), 393–401.

Chan, K. Y., Wang, W., Wu, J. J. *et al.* (2013). Epidemiology of Alzheimer's disease and other forms of dementia in China, 1990–2010: a systematic review and analysis. *The Lancet*, **381**(9882), 2016–2023.

Cohen, C. I. (2000). Racial differences in neuropsychiatric symptoms among dementia patients: a comparison of African Americans and whites. *International Psychogeriatrics*, **12**, 395–402.

Cohen, C. I., and Marino, L. (2013). Racial and ethnic differences in the prevalence of psychotic symptoms in the general population. *Psychiatric Services*, **64**, 1103–1109.

Cohen, C. I., Magai, C., Yaffee, R. and Walcott-Brown, L. (2004). Racial differences in paranoid ideation and psychoses in an older urban population. *American Journal of Psychiatry*, **161**, 864–871.

Cohen, C. I., Magai, C., Yaffee, R. and Walcott-Brown, L. M. S. (2006). The prevalence of anxiety and associated factors in a multiracial sample of older adults. *Psychiatric Services*, **57**, 1719–1725.

Cohen, C. I., McKenzie, S. E., Rahmani, M. *et al.* (2012). Historical changes in the severity of dementia and accompanying neuropsychiatric symptoms in persons presenting for evaluation in a multiracial urban dementia center. *Alzheimer Disease and Associated Disorders*, **26**(4), 352–357.

Coleman, D. and Baker, F. M. (1994). Misdiagnosis of schizophrenia in older, black veterans. *Journal of Nervous Mental Diseases*, **182**, 527–528.

Crowther, M. R., Shurgot, G. R., Perkins, M. and Rodriguez, R. (2006). The social and cultural context of psychotherapy with older adults. In *Psychotherapy for Depression in Older Adults*, ed. S. H. Qualls and B. G. Knight. Hoboken, NJ: John Wiley, pp. 179–200.

Desjarlais, R., Eisenberg, L., Good, B. and Kleinman A. (1995). *World Mental Health Problems and Priorities in Low Income Countries*. Oxford: Oxford University Press.

Dodge, H. H., Buracchio, T. J., Fisher, G. G. *et al.* (2012). Trends in the prevalence of dementia in Japan. *International Journal of Alzheimer's Disease*, **12**, 956354, doi: 10.1155/2012/956354.

Dowd. J. and Bengston, V. L. (1978). Aging in minority populations: an examination of the double jeopardy hypothesis. *Journal of Gerontology*, **33**, 427–436.

Edelstein, B. A., Heisel, M. J., McKee, D. R. *et al.* (2009). Development and psychometric evaluation of the reasons for living: older adults scale: a suicide risk assessment inventory. *The Gerontologist*, **49**(6), 735–745.

Elder, G. H. (2001). Life course. In *The Encyclopedia of Aging*, 3rd edn, ed. G. L. Maddox. New York: Springer Publishing, pp. 593–596.

Estroff, S. (1981). *Making It Crazy*. Berkeley: University of California Press.

Feng, Z., Fennell, M. L., Tyler, D. A. *et al.* (2011). Growth of racial and ethnic minorities in US nursing homes driven by demographics and possible disparities in options. *Health Affairs*, **30**(7), 1358–1365.

Feng, Z., Liu, C., Guan, X. and Mor, V. (2012). China's rapidly aging population creates policy challenges in shaping a viable long-term care system. *Health Affairs*, **31**(12), 2764–2773.

Ford, E. S., Giles, W. H. and Dietz, W. H. (2002). Prevalence of the metabolic syndrome among US adults: findings from the third National Health and Nutrition Examination Survey. *Journal of the American Medical Association*, **287**, 356–359.

Fry. C. L.(2009). Globalization and the risks of aging. In *The Cultural Context of Aging: Worldwide Perspectives*, 3rd edn, ed. J. Sokolovsky. Westport, CT: Praeger Publishers, pp. 185–195.

Gerretsen, P., Müller, D. J., Tiwari, A. *et al.* (2009). The intersection of pharmacology, imaging, and genetics in the development of personalized medicine. *Dialogues in Clinical Neuroscience*, **11**(4), 363–376.

Gierveld, J. D. J., Van der Pas, S. and Keating, N. (2015). Loneliness of older immigrant groups in Canada: effects of ethnic-cultural background. *Journal of Cross-Cultural Gerontology*, **30**(3), 251–268.

Glascock, A. P. and Feinman, S. L. (1981). Social assets or social burden: treatment of the aged in non-industrial societies. In *Dimensions: Aging, Culture, and Health*, ed. C. Fry. South Hadley, MA: Bergin and Garvey.

Grasset, L., Brayne, C., Joly, P. *et al.* (2015). Trends in dementia incidence: Evolution over a 10-year period in France. *Alzheimer's and Dementia*, **12**(3), 272–280.

Grundy, S. M. (2008). Metabolic syndrome pandemic. *Arteriosclerosis, Thrombosis, and Vascular Biology*, **28**(4), 629–636.

Guerra, M., Ferri, C., Llibre, J., *et al.* (2015). Psychometric properties of EURO-D, a geriatric depression scale: a cross-cultural validation study. *BMC Psychiatry*, **15**(1), 1.

Gupta, R., Singh, P., Verma, S. and Garg, D. (1991). Standardized assessment of depressive disorders: a replicated study from northern India. *Acta Psychiatrica Scandinavica*, **84**, 310–312.

Gusmano, M. K.(2009) Growing older in world cities: benefits and burdens. In *The Cultural Context of Aging: Worldwide Perspectives*, 3rd edn, ed. J. Sokolovsky. Westport, CT: Praeger Publishers, pp. 395–417.

Harada, N., Takeshita, J., Ahmed, I. *et al.* (2012). Does cultural assimilation influence prevalence and presentation of depressive symptoms in older Japanese American men? The Honolulu–Asia Aging Study. *The American Journal of Geriatric Psychiatry*, **20**(4), 337–345.

Hazzard, W. R. (2001). Aging, health, longevity, and the promise of biomedical research: the perspective of the gerontologist and geriatrician. In *Handbook of the Biology of Aging*, ed. E. J. Masoro and S. N. Austad. San Diego: Academic Press.

Henderson, D. C., Nguyen, D. D., Copeland, P. M. *et al.* (2005). Clozapine, diabetes mellitus, hyperlipidemia, and cardiovascular risk and mortality: results of a 10 year naturalistic study. *Journal of Clinical Psychiatry*, **66**, 1116–1121.

Hendrie, H. C., Ogunniyi, A., Hall, K. S. *et al.* (2001). Incidence of dementia and Alzheimer disease in 2 communities: Yoruba residing in Ibadan, Nigeria, and African Americans residing in Indianapolis, Indiana. *Journal of the American Medical Association*, **285**, 739–747.

Jacobson, S. A., Pies, R. W. and Greenblatt, D. J. (2002). *Handbook of Geriatric Psychiatry*. Washington DC: American Psychiatric Publishing.

Janevic, M. R., and Connell, C. M. (2001). Racial, ethnic, and cultural differences in the dementia caregiving experience: recent findings. *The Gerontologist*, **41**(3), 334–347.

Jiang, S. and Li, P. (2016). Current development in elderly comprehensive assessment and research methods. *BioMed research international*, **2016**, 3528248, doi: 10.1155/2016/3528248.

Keith, S. J., Regier, D. A., and Rae, D. S. (1991). Schizophrenic disorders. In *Psychiatric Disorders in America*, ed. D. A. Regier and L. N. Robins. New York, Free Press, pp. 33–52.

Kvaal, K., McDougall, F. A., Brayne, C. *et al.* (2008). Co-occurrence of anxiety and depressive disorders in a community sample of older people: results from the MRC CFAS (Medical Research Council Cognitive Function and Ageing Study). *International Journal of Geriatric Psychiatry*, **23**(3), 229–237.

Lawrence, V., Murray, J., Banerjee, S. *et al.* (2006). Concepts and causation of depression: a cross-cultural study of the beliefs of older adults. *The Gerontologist*, **46**(1), 23–32.

Lee, H. and Mason, D. (2014). Cultural and gender differences in coping strategies between Caucasian American and Korean American older people. *Journal of Cross-Cultural Gerontology*, **29**(4), 429–446.

Levkoff, S. E., Macarthur, I. W. and Bucknail, J. (1995). Elderly mental health in the developing world. *Social Science and Medicine*, **41**, 983–1003.

Li, G. and Baker, S. P. (1991). A comparison of injury rates in China and the United States, 1986. *American Journal of Public Health*, **81**, 605–609.

Lin, K.-M. and Elwyn, T. S. (2004). Culture and drug therapy. In *Cultural Competence in Clinical Psychiatry*, ed. W.-S. Tseng and J. Streltzer. Washington DC: American Psychiatric Press, pp. 163–180.

Lin, K.-M. and Smith, M. W. (2000). Psychopharmacotherapy in the context of culture and ethnicity. In *Ethnicity and Psychopharmacology*, ed. P. Ruiz. Washington DC: American Psychiatric Press, pp. 1–36.

Löckenhoff, C. E., De Fruyt, F., Terracciano, A. *et al.* (2009). Perceptions of aging across 26 cultures and their culture-level associates. *Psychology and Aging*, **24**(4), 941–954.

Lou, V. W. Q. and Gui, S. (2012). Family caregivers and impact on caregiving mental health. A study in Shanghai. In *Aging in China. Implications to Social Policy of a Changing Economic State*, ed. S. Chen and J. L. Powell. New York: Springer, pp. 187–208.

Markides, K. S., Liang, J. and Jackson, J. S. (1990). Race, ethnicity, and aging: conceptual and methodological issues. In *Handbook of Aging and the Social Sciences*, 3rd edn, ed. R. H. Binstock and L. K. George. San Diego: Academic Press, pp. 112–125.

Mathillas, J., Lövheim, H. and Gustafson, Y. (2011). Increasing prevalence of dementia among very old people. *Age and Ageing*, **40**(2), 243–249.

McGrath, J. J., Saha, S., Al-Hamzawi, A. O. *et al.* (2016). Age of onset and lifetime projected risk of psychotic experiences: Cross-national data from the World Mental Health Survey. *Schizophrenia Bulletin*, **42**(4), 933–941.

Metzl, J. M. and Hansen, H. (2014). Structural competency: theorizing a new medical engagement with stigma and inequality. *Social Science and Medicine*, **103**, 126–133.

Mintzer, J. and Faison, W. (2009). Minority and sociocultural issues. In *Kaplan and Sadock's Comprehensive Textbook of Psychiatry*, ed. B. J. Sadock, V. A. Sadock, and P. Ruiz. Philadelphia: Lippincott Williams and Wilkins, pp. 4214–4224.

Nelson, T. D. (2005). Ageism: prejudice against our feared future self. *Journal of Social Issues*, **61**(2), 207–221.

North, M. S. and Fiske, S. T. (2015). Modern attitudes toward older adults in the aging world: a cross-cultural meta-analysis. *Psychological Bulletin*, **141**(5), 993–1021.

Ortman, J. M., Velkof, V. A., and Hogan, H. (2014). *An Aging Nation: The Older Population in the United States*. Washington DC: US Department of Commerce, US Census Bureau.

Pinquart, M. and Sörensen, S. (2005). Ethnic differences in stressors, resources, and psychological outcomes of family caregiving: a meta-analysis. *The Gerontologist*, **45**(1), 90–106.

Prina, A. M., Ferri, C. P., Guerra, M., Brayne, C. and Prince, M. (2011). Prevalence of anxiety and its correlates among older adults in Latin America, India and China: cross-cultural study. *The British Journal of Psychiatry*, **199**(6), 485–491.

REACH 2010 (2004). Surveillance for health status in minority communities: United States, 2001–2002. *MMWR Surveillance Summary*, **53**(6), 1–36.

Rizzi, L., Rosset, I., and Roriz-Cruz, M. (2014). Global epidemiology of dementia: Alzheimer's and vascular types. *BioMed Research International*, **2014**, 908915.

Sadavoy, J. and Lazarus L. W. (2004). Individual therapy. In *Comprehensive Textbook of Geriatric Psychiatry*, 3rd edn, ed. J. Sadavoy, L. F. Jarvik, G. T. Grossberg and B. S. Meyers. New York: W. W. Norton, pp. 993–1022.

Sakauye, K. (2004). Ethnocultural aspects of aging in mental health. In *Comprehensive Textbook of Geriatric Psychiatry*, 3rd edn, ed. J. Sadavoy, L. F. Jarvik, G. T. Grossberg and B. S. Meyers. New York: W. W. Norton, pp. 225–250.

Sakauye, K. (2008). *Geriatric Psychiatry Basics*. New York: W.W. Norton.

Sanderson, W. and Scherbov, S. (2008). *Rethinking Age and Aging*. Washington DC: Population Reference Bureau.

Satizabal, C. L., Beiser, A. S., Chouraki, V. *et al.* (2016). Incidence of dementia over three decades in the Framingham Heart Study. *New England Journal of Medicine*, **374**(6), 523–532.

Schoenberg, N. E. and Lewis, D. (2005). Cross-cultural ageism. In *Encyclopedia of Aging*, ed. E. Palmore, L. Branch and D. Harris. Binghamton, NY: Haworth Press, pp. 87–91.

Schoevers, R. A., Beekman, A. T. F., Deeg, D. *et al.* (2003). Comorbidity and risk-patterns of depression, generalised anxiety disorder and mixed anxiety-depression in later life: results from the AMSTEL study. *International Journal of Geriatric Psychiatry*, **18**(11), 994–1001.

Shah, A. (2010). Elderly suicide rates: a replication of cross-national comparisons and association with sex and elderly age-bands using five year suicide data. *Journal of Injury and Violence Research*, **3**(2), 80–84.

Shahly, V., Chatterji, S., Gruber, M. J. *et al.* (2013). Cross-national differences in the prevalence and correlates of burden among older family caregivers in the World Health Organization World Mental Health (WMH) Surveys. *Psychological Medicine*, **43**(04), 865–879.

Sokolovsky, J. (1997). Starting points: a global, cross-cultural view of aging. In *The Cultural Context of Aging*, 2nd edn, ed. J. Sokolovsky. Westport, CN: Bergin and Garvey, pp. xiii–xxxi.

Sokolovsky, J. (2009a). Introduction: human maturity and global aging in cultural context. In *The Cultural Context of Aging: Worldwide Perspectives*, 3rd edn, ed. J. Sokolovsky. Westport, CT: Praeger Publishers, pp. 1–12.

Sokolovsky, J. (ed.) (2009b). *The Cultural Context of Aging: Worldwide Perspectives*, 3rd edn. Westport, CT: Praeger Publishers.

Sokolovsky, J. (2009c). Ethnic elders and the limits of family support in a globalizing world. In *The Cultural Context of Aging: Worldwide Perspectives*, 3rd edn, ed. J. Sokolovsky. Westport, CT: Praeger Publishers, pp. 289–301.

Sokolovsky, J. (2009d). The ethnic dimension in aging: culture, context, and creativity. In *The Cultural Context of Aging: Worldwide Perspectives*, 3rd edn, ed. J. Sokolovsky. Westport, CT: Praeger Publishers, pp. 277–287.

Sue, D. W. and Sue, D. (1990). *Counseling the Culturally Different: Theory and Practice*, 2nd edn. New York: Wiley.

Suzuki, R., Goebart, D., Ahmed, I. and Lu, B. (2015). Folk and biological perceptions of dementia among Asian minorities in Hawaii. *The American Journal of Geriatric Psychiatry*, **23**(6), 589–595.

Takeshita, J. and Ahmed, I. (2004). Culture and geriatric psychiatry. In *Cultural Competence in Clinical Psychiatry*, ed. W.-S. Tseng and J. Streltzer. Washington DC: American Psychiatric Publishing, pp. 147–161.

United Nations Department of Economic and Social Affairs, Population Division (2013). World Population Ageing 2013, available online at www.un.org/en/development/desa/population/publications/pdf/ageing/WorldPopulationAgeing2013.pdf.

United Nations Department of Economic and Social Affairs, Population Division (2015). World Population Prospects: the 2015 Revision, Key Findings and Advance Tables. Working Paper No. ESA/P/WP.241.

United Nations Population Fund (UNFPA) (2015). Migration, available online at www.unfpa.org/migration.

Van der Wurff, F. B., Beekman, A. T., Dijkshoorn, H. et al. (2004). Prevalence and risk-factors for depression in elderly Turkish and Moroccan migrants in the Netherlands. *Journal of Affective Disorders*, **83**, 33–41.

Weissman, J. S., Betancourt, J. and Campbell, E. G. (2005). Resident physicians' preparedness to provide cross cultural care. *Journal of the American Medical Association*, **294**, 1058–1067.

World Health Organization (2016). Mental Health and Older Adults [Fact sheet]. Available online at www.who.int/mediacentre/factsheets/fs381/en</occ>.

Wu, Y. T., Fratiglioni, L., Matthews, F. E., et al. (2016). Dementia in western Europe: epidemiological evidence and implications for policy making. *The Lancet Neurology*, **15**(1), 116–124.

Yasamy, M. T., Dua, T., Harper, M. and Saxena, S. (2013). Mental health of older adults, addressing a growing concern. World Health Organization, Department of Mental Health and Substance Abuse.

Yeo, G. (ed.) (2001). *Core Curriculum in Ethnogeriatrics*. Stanford: Stanford University Press.

Cultural Overlays in Consultation–Liaison Psychiatry

Santosh K. Chaturvedi, Gayatri Saraf and Geetha Desai

Editors' Introduction

Psychiatrists are primarily physicians but the task of interlinking physical and mental health needs of patients can be complex. There is considerable research evidence to suggest that people with mental illness are likely to have higher levels of physical illness and are also more prone to die prematurely compared with those who do not have mental illness. It is also well known that people with physical illness are more prone to develop mental illness as a result of which it becomes very difficult to treat both illnesses. Consultation–liaison psychiatry (CLP) is a clinical discipline, which deals with biological, psychological and social factors in the causation and management of any disorder, particularly the psychiatric manifestations. In many countries this specialty of psychiatry is much better developed in comparison with other countries depending upon financial and human resources. Over the years, the field of CLP has seen tremendous growth and has evolved into a specialty in its own right. However, while working in a consultation–liaison (C–L) setting entails dealing with a varied repertoire of patients, doctors and different cultural settings the results can be particularly gratifying. Chaturvedi *et al.* in this chapter highlight that as the modern societies become increasingly multiethnic and multicultural, psychiatrists find themselves increasingly in situations where they are required to evaluate and treat patients from different cultural settings. These authors provide an overview for assessing and managing patients accordingly and point out that there are several varying models of delivering services within the consultation–liaison psychiatry model. They emphasize that clinicians must deal with the interview process, communication, clinical management and modes of intervention in C–L settings with special emphasis on cultural factors. The role of consultation–liaison psychiatry in some medical specialties is better developed in comparison with others. These ideas and lessons need to be shared.

Introduction

Consultation–liaison psychiatry (CLP) is a clinical discipline, which deals with biological, psychological and social factors in the causation and management of any disorder, particularly the psychiatric manifestations. The field has its origins in the early nineteenth century, when medicine sought to explain all illnesses as the result of a specific biological cause. Parallel to this was the trend in psychiatry to view the major psychiatric disorders as resulting from biological disturbances. This left those illnesses wherein no specific biological cause was as yet elucidated and the 'neurotic' disorders in which somatic symptoms predominated, without any explanation or means of management. The nascent psychoanalytic movement attempted to provide answers in the form of psychodynamic explanations. At the same time, internists began to view physical illnesses in a holistic manner by integrating psychosocial factors into the management of every patient. Thus, the gap in services to medically ill patients with psychiatric symptoms was filled by the convergence of these two professional streams. Over the years, the developments in the field have resulted in distinctions being made between consultation psychiatry, liaison psychiatry and psychosomatic medicine.

Consultation psychiatry refers to individuals trained as psychiatrists providing consultations to colleagues from other medical specialties upon receiving a specific referral. Occurring both in inpatient and outpatient settings, the consultation is limited to evaluating the referred patient for psychiatric symptoms and suggesting a plan of management. It involves limited interaction with the referring physician. The psychiatrist is usually not involved in the day-to-day care of the patient.

Liaison psychiatry is a much closer integration of psychiatric services with the medical services. Typically occurring in the inpatient setting, it involves a physician or psychiatrist (the consultation–liaison or C–L psychiatrist) being a part of the medical team and seeing all patients under their care irrespective of presence of psychiatric symptoms or referral.

Consultation–Liaison Psychiatry: Concept, Models and Contributions

'A consultation service is a rescue squad like a volunteer fire fighter; a consultant puts out the blaze and then returns home. Liaison, however, also includes setting up fire-prevention programmes and educating citizens about fire proofing' (Hackett and Cassem, 1978). Lipowski (1986) had described different developmental phases in consultation–liaison psychiatry up to the 1980s.

Consultation–liaison psychiatry's growth continued as a specialization in cancer units, ICUs, burns, dialysis, obstetrics and gynaecology, paediatrics, cardiology, neurology units, reaching non-referred populations by screening and triage methods. Liaison psychiatry encompasses clinical, teaching and research activities of psychiatrists in the non-psychiatric divisions of general hospitals. The liaison psychiatrist seeks to enhance the psychological status of all the medical patients, aims to participate in case detection rather than waiting for referral and provides educational programmes.

Many studies have shown the substantial size of psychological problems in the medically ill. First, around one-quarter of those with major physical disorders suffer from psychiatric disorder or other psychologically determined but 'medically unnecessary' complications, which include adverse effects on quality of life, poor compliance with effective medical treatments and possibly some effects on long-term physical morbidity and mortality. Second, 'medically unexplained' symptoms are extremely common in primary and hospital care. Third, there is a wide range of behavioural problems including deliberate self-harm, substance misuse, sexual difficulties and eating disorders. Many of these result in persistent distress and disability, are often difficult to treat and are associated with huge use of medical resources. There is consistent and compelling evidence that psychiatric, psychological and educational interventions can be highly effective in improving outcome of clinical problems such as psychological status, quality of life, usage of medical care facilities and mortality.

Models of Consultation–Liaison Programmes

Consultation Model

Patients are referred to the psychiatrist for management. Usually consultation is a one-time service or a couple of follow-ups and does not involve any formal, structured teaching methods to medical specialists. By this model, primarily psychiatric morbidity in the general hospital is identified and referred by the non-specialist physicians.

Liaison Model

In addition to consultation, structured teaching, e.g. psychosomatic rounds involving psychiatrist and respective medical specialists, the psychiatrist–teacher often becomes a part of the medical/surgical unit helping in case detection.

Bridge Model

The psychiatrist is connected with a formal department of psychiatry, but assigned a primary-care site and participates in structured teaching.

Hybrid Model

Psychosocial teaching is provided by a psychiatrist, psychologist, social worker or primary-care staff.

Autonomous Model

The psychiatrist is hired by the primary-care physician, and has no formal connection with the department of psychiatry.

Integrative Model

This is a theoretical model based on the aim of C–L psychiatrists for the inclusion of psychological care as a component of patient care as the right of every sick person. The five major components include open-access psychiatric consultation, high-risk evaluation and care, early identification of stress problems, system of triage and quality-assurance monitoring. Psychiatric consultation has opened the door for the delivery of mental healthcare to the medically ill. High frequency of psychiatric morbidity in certain medico-surgical settings, e.g. geriatric units, ICUs, cancer units, HIV/ AIDS units required extension of these services to every patient in these units.

Virtual Model

This is already in practice in different centres, but would soon become a modern technological based consultation method.

Irrespective of the model used, psychiatric consultation and psychological care of the medically ill reduces the total healthcare cost by reducing hospital stay. Consultation–liaison psychiatry also results in increased recognition of psychosocial factors in physical disorders. The C–L psychiatrist's role in educating medical specialists has helped in better care of the medically ill. The common psychiatric disorders noted in the medically ill during the referral, liaison or consultation services are depression, anxiety, delirium, behavioural problems and somatization.

The late 1990s saw a controversy over what constitutes consultation–liaison psychiatry as applied to general practice. While some were of the view that the integration of psychiatric services with general practice and liaison with the general practitioner constituted C–L psychiatry (Carr *et al.*, 1997), others were of the opinion that such a practice should be termed 'shared care' as the majority of patients seen were not suffering from any physical illness nor from somatization (Gribble, 1998). The underlying debate was once again of funding: whether this particular service should be funded through community psychiatry or CLP.

Cultural Factors in Consultation–Liaison Psychiatry

Culture has a phenomenal influence on ways of living, traditional and family values, ways of relating to the world, and ways in which illness or trauma is perceived and processed. Culture shapes, modulates and defines beliefs about health, illness, death and dying; expectations concerning disclosure of diagnosis and prognosis; family decision-making roles; symptom expression; and perspectives concerning complementary and alternative medicine (Chaturvedi *et al.*, 2014). The impact of culture on the practice of consultation–liaison psychiatry is manifold. The immediate and obvious effect is on the presentation and management of the Axis I and Axis II psychiatric disorders. The patient's perception about physical disease and means of coping with it are subject to cultural influence in a significant way. The treating team's relationship with the patient, the dominance of autonomy or dependence, the role of the family,

religious and spiritual factors are all culturally determined. These issues could be the source of friction and discontent in the treating team and the patient and lead to a referral to the mental health team. The C–L psychiatrist is therefore entrusted with the task of not only understanding the patient, his/her cultural background, the disorders and treatments, but also the cultural variance between the referring team and the patient.

Working in a consultation–liaison setting entails dealing with a varied repertoire of patients, doctors and different cultural settings. As the modern society becomes increasingly multi-ethnic and multicultural, psychiatrists find themselves increasingly in situations where they are required to evaluate and treat patients from different cultural settings. Healthcare providers must be attentive and responsive to cultural factors that shape world view, values and ethos. Communication between healthcare providers and patients/families in different sociological and institutional environments is also shaped by the varied multicultural societies within and across these environments. It requires an innate sensitivity and responsibility on the part of the C–L psychiatrist towards cultural, racial and ethnic differences. Cultural aspects of C–L psychiatry therefore would not only include the nature of problems in different cultural settings, but also the interview, the referral process and the clinical management.

Interview Process in Consultation–Liaison Psychiatry Settings

The Physician–Patient Relationship

In most traditional cultures, physicians are held in high esteem and given god-like status, where the patient respects the physicians for their skills and knowledge, the relationship being hierarchical. Patients or families may hesitate to discuss options and alternatives with the doctor, out of deference and awe. In Western culture, the physician is more of a service provider and the doctor–patient relationship is based on a respect for mutual needs, autonomy and individuality. Lawsuits are common in cases where the physician errs or is found to be negligent. In culturally diverse settings where one is required to see patients from various diverse backgrounds, going back and forth between these two diametrically opposite attitudes to oneself and one's profession is something a psychiatrist must take in their stride. Additionally, in C–L settings, since the referral has been initiated by the treating team, it is important to establish a good rapport in order to facilitate the interview process.

Respecting Cultural Norms of Privacy and Confidentiality

The construct of confidentiality varies greatly among different cultures. In individualistic cultures, the patient's rights to privacy and confidentiality assume paramount importance and a breach of diagnosis without consent can even result in litigation. However, in more traditional cultures, where family systems play a major role in the treatment process, clinicians frequently walk the tightrope of respecting the care-giver's wishes vis-à-vis the patient's right to confidentiality.

History Taking

Eliciting history in a manner that is culturally appropriate, yet sufficient and detailed enough to reach a diagnosis is an art. The process of history taking starts by establishing an adequate rapport, which might seem difficult if the patient does not speak the doctor's language or comes from a completely different ethnocultural group from that of the doctor. When it is warranted, the use of an interpreter to ensure adequate communication might be considered. When in spite of ensuring the patient's comfort, one does not seem to make any headway or when a sensitive area is being explored, it is prudent to check with the patient if the information being asked for during the interview conflicts with their culture or background.

Especially in mental health, culture has a lot of bearing on what and how much is being disclosed. In some cultures, psychiatric illnesses are seen as arising out of lack of self-control or willpower and disclosure is not done for the fear of being considered 'weak' or lacking in self-control. Family pathology or conflict may not be discussed for the fear of spoiling family's reputation. Eliciting sexual history is challenging in situations where discussing sexual matters is considered as shameful. Assessments of previous treatments and help-seeking should include traditional systems of medicine such as Ayurveda, Unani or Chinese systems of medicine and also folk remedies.

Clinicians need to be mindful of the fact that religion and spirituality are often used by patients to respond to mental illness and give meaning to the illness experience (Whitley, 2012). Religion as a method of coping, especially in palliative care and serious medical illnesses needs to be explored. Cultural assessments should include an enquiry into how religion has been used to make sense of the illness experience, and help-seeking from religious support groups needs to be looked into (Whitley, 2012).

Mental Status Examination

Manner of dressing and grooming may vary in various cultures and it is important for a clinician not to let their own cultural bias come into play while commenting on general appearance and behaviour. Expression of affect might vary between and within communities. Matsumoto *et al.* (2009) observed that athletes from relatively urban, individualistic cultures expressed their emotions more, whereas athletes from less urban, collectivistic cultures were more likely to mask their emotions. Difficulties with language and communication might be construed as a thought disorder (Streltzer and Tseng, 2015). The interpretation of proverbs and general fund of information are heavily moderated by cultural influences (Streltzer and Tseng, 2015).

Communication in a Cultural Milieu

Non-Verbal Behaviours

Culture has a major role in understanding and interpreting non-verbal behaviours, hence it is important for the health professionals to be aware of the non-verbal behaviours and their interpretations. Non-verbal behaviours are cornerstones of effective communication. This again may vary across cultures and thus be misinterpreted by patient and/or provider, further contributing to communication barriers. Patients belonging to particular cultural groups may perceive the healthcare team to be acting with an unfamiliar set of norms that breach culturally influenced ideas of behaviour expected from a doctor, while the health team professionals might be unaware of the meaning of a patient's peculiar behaviour. Hence, there is a need to find an acceptable approach to care, keeping in mind cultural factors, which can be particularly challenging. A handshake might be appropriate in one culture but might be misinterpreted in another culture.

In terms of cultural attitudes toward pain, people from one culture may exercise stoic self-control, those from another may wail and moan with the same pain stimulus, and those from a third culture may first say how terrible it is and then face it nevertheless (Chaturvedi *et al.*, 2014). A healthcare professional's interpretation of these expressions of pain may influence the frequency and type of pain management offered. Authors studying patient perspectives in communication have developed an interesting typology of errors in communication: 'occasional misses' are errors within an overall appropriate communication and can be prevented by a discussion between patient and clinician and communication skills training; 'systemic misunderstandings' refer to departures from appropriate patterns of communication, such as giving excessive information, or withholding information, excessive use of numbers and statistics to convey possibilities and likelihoods; whereas 'repeat offenders' are clinicians whose communication patterns become a constant source of distress to the patients concerned (Thorne *et al.*, 2013).

Communication Skills

Physicians ofter find it stressful to deal with difficult questions raised by the patient or the family members. Disclosing diagnosis or breaking bad news is another delicate and sensitive area where the C–L psychiatrist is frequently called upon by the medical team to break the news of a serious diagnosis to the patient and family. In Western cultures such as Europe and North America, failure to communicate the gravity of patient's diagnosis is often considered as a serious omission, often resulting in malpractice suits. Whereas in most Asian societies, it is a common practice to conceal the diagnosis from the patient at the family's request, a phenomenon referred to as collusion. In fact, doing otherwise can lead to resentment from the family. In such situations, the C–L team needs to handle collusion keeping in mind cultural, individual and ethical considerations (Chaturvedi, 2010).

Collusion

Collusion implies any information (about the diagnosis, prognosis, and medical details about the person who is ill) being withheld or not shared among individuals involved. Collusion also means that relevant and complete medical information is selectively disclosed or not disclosed at all to patients and/or relatives. Cultural collusion is one of the types of collusion.

A study by Holland *et al.* (1987) documented that 40 per cent of oncologists revealed the cancer diagnosis to patients in Africa, Japan, France, Spain and Italy, whereas 80 per cent revealed it in Austria, Denmark and other European countries. In the US, in keeping with patient's right movement, all patients are informed. In a study done in Taiwan that looked at nurses' truth telling experiences, 70 per cent responded that they had told the truth to patients about their diagnosis (Huang *et al.*, 2014). In the remainder, the reasons cited for not doing so were collusion, considering it to not be part of one's duty, and perceiving it as difficult.

The decision-making by the key family decision-maker is generally supportive, but at times may be perceived as interference in management by the healthcare professionals and the patient themselves. Although collusion may impair the communication between the health professionals and family, its primary purpose is to protect the patient. On the negative side, collusion comes in the way of an individual's autonomy, and may deprive him/her of the benefits of health services and care. The decision-making by the key family decision-maker is generally supportive, but at times may be perceived as interference in management by the healthcare professionals and the patient themselves. This interference may adversely influence the treatment and outcome of the disease. Although collusion may impair the communication between the health professionals and family, its primary purpose is to protect the patient. On the negative side, collusion comes in the way of an individual's autonomy, and may deprive him/her of the benefits of health services and care. The C–L psychiatrist needs to be aware of collusion in various medical settings and handle it effectively in order to facilitate and ensure smooth communication between the treating team, patient and family.

Communication about Death and Dying

Culture and religion play a major role in attitudes towards death and bereavement. In end-of-life care, the health professional must be informed about the rituals related to death and bereavement in various religious groups: the construct of transmigration of soul in Hindus, concepts of heaven and hell in Christianity and Islam and a high degree of involvement with death in Hispanics (Mazanec and Tyler,

2003). Different societies place varying emphasis on different issues related to death and dying and this can have profound effects on their psychosocial care needs during this time. Barriers to providing satisfying and culturally appropriate end-of-life care may arise from cultural and/or religious differences between staff and cancer patients. For example, in traditional societies, decisions regarding where and how the patient dies, at home or in hospital, and when resuscitation and life support measures are withdrawn, are made by the family. In some countries, however, advanced directives such as do not resuscitate (DNR) allow the patient to pre-empt these issues and make an informed choice about matters related to death and life support.

The health professionals need to be aware of the religious rituals and sentiments of the individual, family and society to be able to appropriately and sensitively address the patient's and family's concerns during end-of-life care. The meaning of dying and fears around various issues related to death and dying must also be explored and addressed by healthcare providers. This may be facilitated by creating opportunities for open communication about the beliefs and rituals that are important to the patient and family.

The Cultural Formulation in C–L Psychiatry Settings

The growing cultural pluralism in most urban settings calls for a systematic approach to evaluate and assess the impact of cultural issues in clinical practice. One such approach is the cultural formulation, the guidelines for which also find a place in appendix 1 of DSM-IV.

Mental disorders are more frequently misdiagnosed among patients from ethnic minorities and immigrants as compared to their native counterparts (Good, 1992). Misdiagnosis includes failing to recognize the presence of a mental health condition (non-recognition or underdiagnosis), identifying a disorder when none is present (overdiagnosis), or mistaking a disorder for another one (misidentification) (Adeponle et al., 2012). Insufficient attention to socio-cultural and contextual factors that modify illness behaviour and symptom expression may account for misdiagnosis and consequently, wrong treatment.

Standardizing assessment procedures assumes a very important role in order to avoid misdiagnosis or clinician bias. Several studies have found that cultural and ethnic differences influence psychiatric diagnosis.

For instance, African American and Hispanic patients had a higher likelihood of being diagnosed with schizophrenia than their Caucasian counterparts (Strakowski et al., 1996; Choi et al., 2012). Culturally influenced experiences of illness often do not fit into mainstream psychiatric diagnostic systems. For example, disorders such as neurasthenia found in Chinese Americans and *ataque de nervois* (attack of nerves) in Latinos, that do not fit into existing nosological categories, highlight the need to consider culture as a significant variable that colours and modifies psychiatric illness. Encouragingly, interventions aimed at bridging the cultural barrier between the clinician and the patient lead to increased patient participation in the interview, a better interpersonal rapport and higher levels of patient satisfaction.

The cultural formulation (CF) consists of five components, including cultural identity, cultural explanation of the illness, cultural factors related to the psychosocial environment and levels of functioning, cultural elements of the clinician–patient relationship, and the overall impact of culture on diagnosis and care. The goal of the CF is to help clinicians identify the cultural factors associated with diagnosis and treatment. Some studies have indicated that CF increases the participation of non-medical professionals in a multidisciplinary team (Dinh et al., 2012).

However, the use of cultural formulation has been inconsistent, due to application, training and implementation in diverse settings being a major challenge. The applicability of CF has been criticized on several counts. It is not clear as to why, in which settings and what kind of patients the CF needs to be used (Cuéllar and Paniagua, 2000). It may also duplicate the information already obtained during the course of the clinical interview (Martinez, 2009). The time constraints of various clinical settings make it difficult to assess all the four domains of CF (Lewis-Fernandez, 2009). It is also unclear as to which domains of CF are relevant for treatment planning (Mezzich et al., 2009). To address this, the DSM-5 introduced the cultural formulation interview (CFI), that operationalizes the process of data collection for CF. The CFI is semi-structured, and was tested in APA supported field trials at 12 clinical sites in six countries. The sample interview questions in CFI are accompanied by guidelines elaborating the rationale behind each item, potentially rendering it useful for training purposes (Lewis-Fernandez et al., 2014).

Modes of Intervention

Cultural beliefs about methods of treatment both for medical illness and psychiatric conditions influence the treatment choices and compliance. Utilization of indigenous and traditional remedies might be used simultaneously during the treatment without disclosing it to the clinicians. Hence, it is pertinent to be open and non-dismissive about indigenous treatments while protecting patients' safety.

Psychotherapy as treatment modality in CLP settings is challenging and often needs modification to the CLP settings. Many patients are admitted for shorter periods of time compared to mental health admissions. Hence, many patients are unlikely to be attending many sessions of psychotherapy. Single session psychotherapy has been used in this context where in patients were seen only for one session and was found to be more acceptable (Desai *et al.*, 2015). There is limited work on cultural aspects of medical psychotherapy.

Unexplained Bodily Symptoms in Medical Clinics

Not all patients presenting with bodily complaints to physicians have physical disease. In fact, a sizeable proportion of the medical practices of most physicians consist of patients for whom no objective evidence of a pathophysiological process can be established and are diagnosed to have somatoform disorders. The reported prevalence of somatoform disorders varies from 5 to 40 per cent of patients in various specialties. Somatization is defined as 'a tendency to experience and communicate somatic distress in response to psychosocial stress and to seek medical help for it' (Lipowski, 1986). The prevalence of somatizing behaviour is highest when the type of medical practice studied includes patients who complain of vague, poorly differentiated or non-specific symptoms.

The process of somatization is influenced by a variety of personal and socio-cultural factors. Personality type, cognitive style and difficulty or inability to verbalize feelings (alexithymia) are some factors that may influence somatization. *Somatic cognition* is a concept that could explain the various cognitive, emotional and perceptual elements in unexplained bodily symptoms (Desai

and Chaturvedi, 2015). Cultures that facilitate somatization are those that accept physical disease as an excuse for disability but which reject psychological symptoms as a valid reason for assuming a sick role. Somatizing patients characteristically present their histories in an emotional manner, often dramatically exaggerating symptoms, and they are usually imprecise as to details such as dates, progress of illness, specific treatments, etc. Most somatizing patients visit several doctors for different complaints at different times and will have been hospitalized multiple times. In retrospect, the indication for hospitalization and surgical interventions often seems vague and poorly defined. Substance abuse or history of psychiatric disturbances is common. They may have received a wide variety of psychotropic medications, and abuse of sleep medications, pain medications or minor tranquillizers is a common finding. Somatizing behaviours are much more common in women than in men. They especially occur in middle-aged females from low socio-economic status with chaotic homes, which are often characterized by divorce, physical abuse and alcoholism.

The concept of the management of somatization disorder is more useful than considering curing it. The most effective management can be achieved by having one primary physician or psychiatrist responsible for the patient's medical care. This reduces the opportunities for manipulation by the patient, and having one physician who knows the patient well is an effective way of evaluating new symptoms. Regularly scheduled office visits for the patient are useful. The focus of these visits should not be on the patient's physical symptoms but rather enquiry should be on life situations and interpersonal relationships. There is often a close relationship between these life events and the patient's development of physical symptoms. The physician can employ a technique of behavioural modification during the office visit by selectively paying more attention to the more important and genuine psychosocial stressors that are being experienced than to the somatic complaints.

It is often useful for the physician to take an active role in providing advice and other supportive care to both patient and family at times of crisis. Supportive psychotherapy aimed at strengthening healthy coping strategies and healthy interpersonal relationships can improve the severity of distress in persistent somatizers.

Folk Illnesses

There are instances when no biomedical explanation or category can be ascribed to the cluster of symptoms described by the patient. These are known as 'folk illnesses', or illnesses which are commonly recognized and specific to a particular cultural group, and cannot be explained biomedically. Even in culturally pluralistic settings, patients may frequently present in hospital settings for relief of symptoms, in addition to seeking help from faith healers. Parallel utilization patterns such as these are frequently observed among African American, Indian and Puerto Rican patients and also in other traditional societies. In traditional societies, mental illness may be attributed to moral transgressions towards ancestors, wrath of gods, possession by spirits and demons, lack of willpower, witchcraft, magic, bad blood, astrology, karma (atonement for past sins), etc. (Ng, 1997). Some folk remedies such as branding and exorcism may be potentially hazardous for the mental health of a patient. Folk illnesses also have a bearing on the communication between the C–L psychiatrist and the patient's family. The C–L psychiatrist needs to be aware of the explanatory models of illness that the patient subscribes to, pathways to care including faith healers and traditional systems of medicine, and parallel utilization of other traditional treatment modalities.

Idioms of Distress

Idioms of distress are socially and culturally influenced experiences and expressions of distress (Nichter, 2010). Much has been written about the fact that in various cultures, ways of expressing psychological distress might vary and might not fit into standard Western descriptions of illness. Idioms of distress may take on different forms such as somatizing, self-medication or non-adherence (Nichter and Thompson, 2006), seeking multiple investigations and tests (Nichter, 2002), cultural reinterpretations of an existing biomedical disease (Strahl, 2003), and help-seeking (Nichter and Nordstrom, 1989). Recognizing idioms of distress not only helps one gain a unique perspective of a patient's illness, but also helps establish a good rapport, appreciate meta-communication, and make socially and culturally informed decisions about management (Nichter, 2010). In liaison settings it becomes important for the C–L team to understand and appreciate idioms and metaphors of distress in order to make a thorough assessment and management.

Spirituality in C–L Settings

Spiritual methods of coping assume a very important role in C–L psychiatry, more so in palliative care settings and end-of-life care. The need to pay attention to patients' spiritual needs and concerns is now being increasingly recognized. In C–L settings where patients battle intractable and terminal medical illnesses, it becomes essential for the C–L team to understand their spiritual distress and concerns.

As a coping mechanism, spirituality can lead to both adaptive or positive coping and maladaptive or negative coping. For example, positive coping can entail feelings of divine support, while negative coping can include feeling abandoned by God (Wachholtz et al., 2007). Such mechanisms can have very different impacts on the way patients perceive and process their pain and existential angst (Bhatnagar et al., 2016). Also important is the way patients bond with their care-givers and staff, which in turn can be impacted by patients' spiritual beliefs. For instance, it was observed that spiritual domain and social support from family and friends were correlated in Indian HIV/AIDS patients (Peter et al., 2014). The search for meaning and attempts to answer the 'why me' question are important spiritual concerns which might evolve into an acceptance of the illness and deriving meaning out of the illness experience (Chaturvedi et al., 2014). Chacko et al. (2014) observed that as many as 83.6 per cent of advanced cancer patients felt that it was very important to have their spiritual needs met. In addition, according to a study by Williams et al. (2011), patients who felt that religious/spiritual concerns had been discussed during the course of their hospital stay were more likely to be satisfied with their care. The interplay of ethnicity and spirituality and the way they influence patients' preferences and beliefs around the end of life needs to be taken into account. This can also have an impact on preferences for resuscitation and can influence treatment and ethical decisions. For instance, African American patients were more likely to report using spirituality to cope with their cancer as compared to their white counterparts and were more likely to desire life-sustaining measures (True et al., 2005). Hindu cancer patients may refuse treatment aimed at pain relief as they believe they may miss an opportunity to purify their karma (Bauer-Wu et al., 2007).

End-of-Life Care

End-of-life care or palliative care is care of individuals who are terminally ill. The prospect of death brings in a myriad of feelings in individuals. The person's attitudes towards end-of-life care including pain treatments and life support are influenced by the cultural factors. Health professionals need to understand and discuss end-of-life care with patients and families keeping in mind their cultural beliefs and background.

Future of Consultation–Liaison Psychiatry

Consultation–liaison psychiatry will assume greater importance in the field of psychiatry and in the field of health in general. This is due to the recognition of the large bi-directional overlap between psychiatric and physical illnesses, the trend of integration of psychiatric services with other health services and the inadequacy of general psychiatry. It is also recognized that, in the context of the rapid globalization of the majority of countries, C–L psychiatrists will inevitably be called upon to treat patients from various cultural backgrounds. At the same time, the replication of models of C–L services across countries with different cultural backgrounds would be unsuccessful. Thus, on one hand, the C–L psychiatrist will have to be sensitive to the explanatory models and cultural aspects of the individual case; on the other hand the C–L service will have to incorporate the cultural requirements of the population it serves. Greater emphasis on C–L issues during training is appropriate and is the need of the hour, as the vast majority of current and future psychiatry trainees will work in general hospital and community settings. Training in CLP as a part of residency programmes and emphasis on key cultural issues in CLP are essential. Joint case conferences and psychosomatic rounds might be utilized for training.

Research on cultural aspects in CLP is limited compared to individual psychiatric conditions. The future research needs to focus on cultural aspects in assessments, unique challenges in CLP settings and not limiting oneself to a mere psychiatric label.

The use of technology in healthcare will enlarge the scope of CLP as physicians will be able to consult specialists.

References

Adeponle, A. B., Thombs, B. D., Groleau, D. *et al.* (2012). Using the cultural formulation to resolve uncertainty in diagnoses of psychosis among ethnoculturally diverse patients. *Psychiatric Services*, **63**, 147–153.

Bauer-Wu, S., Barrett, R. and Yeager, K. (2007). Spiritual perspectives and practices at the end of life: a review of the major world religions and application to palliative care. *Indian Journal of Palliative Care*, **13**, 53–58.

Bhatnagar, S., Noble, S., Chaturvedi, S. K. *et al.* (2016). Development and psychometric assessment of a spirituality questionnaire for Indian palliative care patients. *Indian Journal of Palliative Care*, **22**, 9–18.

Brockington, I. F. (1997). Liaison psychiatry: focus on psycho-gynaecology. *Current Opinion in Psychiatry*, **10**, 466–469.

Carr, V. J., Lewin, T. J., Walton, J. M. *et al.* (1997). Consultation–liaison psychiatry in general practice. *Australian and New Zealand Journal of Psychiatry*, **31**, 85–94.

Cathol, R. G. (1994). Medical psychiatry units: the wave of the future. *General Hospital Psychiatry*, **16**, 1–3.

Chacko, R., Anand, J. R., Rajan, A. *et al.* (2014). End-of-life care perspectives of patients and health professionals in an Indian health-care setting. *International Journal of Palliative Nursing*, **20**, 557–564.

Chaturvedi, S. K. and Chandra, P. S. (2010). Breaking bad news: issues critical for psychiatrists. *Medical Education Corner. Asian Journal of Psychiatry*, **3**, 87–89.

Chaturvedi, S. K. and Tipirneni, S. K. (2005). General hospital and liaison psychiatry. In *Handbook of Psychiatry: A South Asian Perspective*, ed. Dinesh Bhugra, Ranjith Gopinath, Vikram Patel, N. C. Jagan. New Delhi: Byvord Viva Publishers.

Chaturvedi, S. K. and Uchitomi, Y. (2012). Psychosocial and psychiatric disorders. In *Clinical Psycho Oncology: An International Perspective*, ed. L. Grassi and M. Riba. Chichester, UK: John Wiley & Sons, Ltd, pp. 55–70.

Chaturvedi, S. K., Strohschein, F. J., Saraf, G. *et al.* (2014). Communication in cancer care: psychosocial, interactional, and cultural issues. A general overview and the example of India. *Frontiers in Psychology*, **5**, 1332.

Choi, M. R., Eun, H. J., Yoo, T. P., *et al.* (2012). The effects of sociodemographic factors on psychiatric diagnosis. *Psychiatry Investigation*, **9**, 199–208.

Cuéllar, I. and Paniagua, F. A. (2000). *Handbook of Multicultural Mental Health: Assessment and Treatment of Diverse Populations*. Orlando, FL: Academic Press.

Desai, G. and Chaturvedi, S. K. (2015). Somatic cognition: body talk and body language. *Medical Hypotheses*, **85**, 1034.

Desai, G., Thanapal, S., Gandhi, S. *et al.* (2015). Single session rehabilitation counseling. *Journal of Psychosocial Rehabilitation and Mental Health*, **2**, 75–77.

Dinh, N. M., Groleau, D., Kirmayer, L. J. *et al.* (2012). Influence of the DSM-IV Outline for Cultural Formulation on multidisciplinary case conferences in mental health. *Anthropology and Medicine*, **19**, 261–276.

Freyberger, H., Kohle, K. and Speidel, H. (1983). Consultation–liaison activities in West Germany: introduction. *Advances in Psychosomatic Medicine Consultation Liaison throughout the World*, **11**, 164–165.

Friedman, R. S. and Moray, F. (1994). A history of psychiatric consultation in America. *Psychiatric Clinics of North America*, **17**, 667–681.

Gelder, M., Gath, D., Mayou, R. and Cowen, P. (eds) (1996). Psychiatry and medicine. *Oxford Textbook of Psychiatry*. Oxford: Oxford University Press.

Good, B. J. (1992). Culture, diagnosis and comorbidity. *Culture, Medicine and Psychiatry*, **16**, 427–446.

Gribble, R. (1998). Shared care but not consultation–liaison psychiatry. *Australian and New Zealand Journal of Psychiatry*, **32**, 311–313.

Hackett, T. P. and Cassem, N. H. (1978). *Handbook of General Hospital Psychiatry*. St. Louis, MO: CV Mosby.

Holland, J. C., Geary, N., Marchini, A. *et al.* (1987). An international survey of physician attitudes and practice in regard to revealing the diagnosis of cancer. *Cancer Investigation*, **5**, 151–154.

Huang, S. H., Tang, F. I., Liu, C. Y. *et al.* (2014). Truth-telling to patients' terminal illness: what makes oncology nurses act individually? *European Journal of Oncology Nursing*, **18**, 492–498.

Huyse, F. J., Herzog, T. and Malt, U. F. (2002). International perspectives on consultation–liaison psychiatry. In *The American Psychiatric Publishing Textbook of Consultation–Liaison Psychiatry*, ed. M. G. Wise, J. R. Rundell. Washington DC: American Psychiatric Publishing.

Kurosawa, H. and Hosaka, T. (2001). General concepts of consultation–liaison psychiatry in Japan. *Advances in Psychosomatic Medicine: Consultation–Liaison Psychiatry in Japan*, **23**, 1–16.

Leigh, H. (1983). The evolution of psychosomatic medicine and consultation–liaison psychiatry. *Advances in Psychosomatic Medicine: Consultation Liaison throughout the World*, **11**, 1–22.

Lesse, S. (1968). The multivariant masks of depression. *American Journal of Psychiatry*, **124** (Suppl.), 35–40.

Lewis-Fernandez, R. (2009). The cultural formulation. *Transcultural Psychiatry*, **46**, 379–382.

Lewis-Fernandez, R., Aggarwal, N. K., Bäärnhielm, S. *et al.* (2014). Culture and psychiatric evaluation: operationalizing cultural formulation for DSM-5. *Psychiatry*, **77**, 130–154.

Lipowski, Z. J. (1986). Consultation–liaison psychiatry: the first-half century. *General Hospital Psychiatry*, **8**, 305–315.

Lipowski, Z. J. and Wise, T. N. (2002). History of consultation–liaison psychiatry. In *The American Psychiatric Publishing Textbook of Consultation–Liaison Psychiatry*, ed. M. G. Wise, J. R. Rundell. Washington DC: American Psychiatric Association.

Lopez-Ibor, J. J. (1972). Masked depression. *British Journal of Psychiatry*, **120**, 245–258.

Maguire, P. and Faulkner, A. (1988a). Communication with cancer patients. 1. Handling bad news and difficult questions. *British Medical Journal*, **297**, 907–909.

Maguire, P. and Faulkner, A. (1988b). Communicating with cancer patients. 2. Handling uncertainty, collusion and denial. *British Medical Journal*, **297**, 972–974.

Martinez, L. C. (2009). DSM-IV-TR cultural formulation of psychiatric cases: two proposals for clinicians. *Transcultural Psychiatry*, **46**, 506–523.

Matsumoto, D., Willingham, B. and Olide, A. (2009). Sequential dynamics of culturally moderated facial expressions of emotion. *Psychological Science*, **20**, 1269–1275.

Mayou, R. (1997). Psychiatry, medicine and consultation–liaison. *British Journal of Psychiatry*, **171**, 203–204.

Mayou, R. A., Simkin, S. and Cobb, A. (1994). Use of psychiatric services by patients referred to a consultation unit. *General Hospital Psychiatry*, **16**, 354–357.

Mazanec, P. and Tyler, M. K. (2003). Cultural considerations in end-of-life care: how ethnicity, age, and spirituality affect decisions when death is imminent. *American Journal of Nursing*, **103**, 50–58; quiz 59.

Mezzich, J. E., Caracci, G., Fabrega, H. *et al.* (2009). Cultural formulation guidelines. *Transcultural Psychiatry*, **46**, 383–405.

Ng, C. H. (1997). The stigma of mental illness in Asian cultures. *Australian and New Zealand Journal of Psychiatry*, **31**, 382–390.

Nichter, M. (2002). The social relations of therapy management. In *New Horizons in Medical Anthropology*, ed. Mark Nichter and Margaret Lock. London: Taylor and Francis.

Nichter, M. (2010). Idioms of distress revisited. *Culture, Medicine and Psychiatry*, **34**, 401–416.

Nichter, M. and Nordstrom, C. (1989). A question of medicine answering. Health commodification and the social relations of healing in Sri Lanka. *Culture, Medicine and Psychiatry*, **13**, 367–390.

Nichter, M. and Thompson, J. J. (2006). For my wellness, not just my illness: North Americans' use of dietary supplements. *Culture, Medicine and Psychiatry*, **30**, 175–222.

Oken, D. (1983). Liaison psychiatry (liaison medicine). *Advances in Psychosomatic Medicine, Consultation Liaison throughout the World*, **11**, 23–51.

Peter, E., Kamath, R., Andrews, T. *et al.* (2014). Psychosocial determinants of health-related quality of life of people living with HIV/AIDS on antiretroviral therapy at Udupi district, southern India. *International Journal of Preventive Medicine*, **5**, 203–209.

Schubert, D. S. P. (1983). Practical distinctions between consultative psychiatry and liaison medicine. *Advances in Psychosomatic Medicine: Consultation Liaison throughout the World*, **11**, 52–61.

Sollner, W., Deifenbacher, A. and Creed, F. (2005). Future developments in consultation–liaison psychiatry and psychosomatics. *Journal of Psychosomatic Research*, **58**, 111–112.

Strahl, H. (2003). Cultural interpretations of an emerging health problem: blood pressure in Dar es Salaam, Tanzania. *Anthropology and Medicine*, **10**, 309–324.

Strakowski, S. M., Flaum, M., Amador, X. *et al.* (1996). Racial differences in the diagnosis of psychosis. *Schizophrenia Research*, **21**, 117–124.

Streltzer, J. and Tseng, W. S. (2015). Cultural aspects of consultation–liaison psychiatry. In *Handbook of Consultation–Liaison Psychiatry*, ed. H. Leigh and J. Streltzer. Cham: Springer.

Summerglad, P. (1994). Medical psychiatry units and the roles of the inpatient psychiatric service in the general hospital. *General Hospital Psychiatry*, **16**, 20–30.

Thorne, S., Oliffe, J. L., Stajduhar, K. I. *et al.* (2013). Poor communication in cancer care: patient perspectives on what it is and what to do about it. *Cancer Nursing*, **36**, 445–453.

True, G., Phipps, E. J., Braitman, L. E., *et al.* (2005). Treatment preferences and advance care planning at end of life: the role of ethnicity and spiritual coping in cancer patients. *Annals of Behavioural Medicine*, **30**, 174–179.

Wachholtz, A. B., Pearce, M. J. and Koenig, H. (2007). Exploring the relationship between spirituality, coping, and pain. *Journal of Behavioural Medicine*, **30**, 311–318.

Whitley, R. (2012). Religious competence as cultural competence. *Transcultural Psychiatry*, **49**, 245–260.

Williams, J. A., Meltzer, D., Arora, V. *et al.* (2011). Attention to inpatients' religious and spiritual concerns: predictors and association with patient satisfaction. *Journal of General Internal Medicine*, **26**, 1265–1271.

Chapter

45

Psychiatric and Medical Conditions
Cultural Signatures and Evolutionary Framework

Horacio Fabrega Jr

Editors' Introduction

Cultures influence how people express psychological distress. It is well recognized that distress symptoms and help-seeking are strongly influenced by cultural values which also affect other behaviours. Fabrega in this chapter reminds us that cultural factors should be seen as 'signatures' of conditions of psychiatric interest (CPI). Keeping the role of culture in mind in influencing human conditions, Fabrega provides an overview on the role of symbols and their meanings (i.e. culture) in influencing the constitution, formulation, expression and interpersonal and societal consequences of psychiatric conditions. He recognizes and reminds us that there are differences between psychiatric conditions and medical conditions in diagnostic criteria, social consequences, treatment approaches, etc. In this chapter Fabrega focuses on both medical and psychiatric conditions to highlight similarities and differences. He examines and compares the biological and social–cultural nature of both types of medical conditions and does so with respect to their distinct differences when examined naturalistically from an evolutionary standpoint. He argues that both medical and psychiatric conditions share a long history that comprehends biological evolution and cultural evolution (e.g. standard individual gene selection, dual inheritance theory (DIT) or gene-culture selection, niche-constructing phenotypes). On the one hand, and viewed abstractly, the evolutionary history of medical and psychiatric conditions determines their common, shared biological nature. Fabrega observes that on the other hand, and viewed in concrete behavioural terms 'on the ground', the shared biology and ancestral history of both types of conditions are responsible for imprinting different types of changes in bodily functions. These in turn crucially elicit different interpretations, valuations, and responses. Such differences underscore the unique tie of psychiatric

conditions with brain changes and the effect of these on behaviours which exemplify different meanings and responses as a consequence.

Introduction

Persons who in their everyday behaviour exhibit *conditions of psychiatric interest* (CPI), for example, what we today in the clinic refer to as anxiety disorder, mood disorder, eating disorder, addiction disorder, psychotic disorder, or personality disorder, all exemplify and manifest a condition whose manifest social behavioural features are *different in kind and character* from those which today we refer to as *conditions of general medical interest* (CMI), for example, diabetes, cancer, heart disease, rheumatoid arthritis, ulcerative colitis and bacterial pneumonia. The word 'persons' at the beginning of the previous sentence indicates that the conventional theoretical and predominantly practical vantage point in any analysis of medical condition writ large is understandably centred squarely on modern human populations, namely, representatives of *Homo sapiens*. It is representatives of this species which in their long history have in effect *deliberatively* created (i.e. described and explained) medical conditions so as to control their adverse consequences (Fabrega, 1974, 1975, 1976a, 1997).

Scope and Overview

The theme of this book underscores cultural factors or 'signatures' of conditions of psychiatric interest (CPI). Its principal focus remains modern human populations. It discusses in detail the role of symbols and their meanings (i.e. culture) in influencing the constitution, formulation, expression and interpersonal and societal consequences of CPI in human populations. In effect, this book offers a compendium of how and why aspects of CPI (e.g. diagnostic criteria, social consequences, treatment approaches) differ compared to CMI. The focus of this chapter addresses both CPI and CMI but strays well beyond the domain of *Homo sapiens*. Specifically, this chapter examines and compares biological and social cultural natures of both types of medical conditions and does so with respect to their distinct differences when examined naturalistically from an evolutionary standpoint.

This chapter argues that both CMI and CPI, as attributes of human populations, share a long history that comprehends biological evolution and cultural evolution (e.g. standard individual gene selection, dual inheritance theory (DIT) or gene-culture selection, niche-constructing phenotypes). On one hand, and viewed abstractly, the evolutionary history of CMI and CPI determines their common, shared biological nature. On the other hand, and viewed in concrete behavioural terms 'on the ground', the shared biology and ancestral history of both types of medical condition are responsible for imprinting *different types* of changes in bodily functions whose behavioural manifestations crucially elicit different interpretations, valuations and responses. Such differences underscore the unique tie of CPI with brain changes and the effect of these on behaviours which exemplify different meanings and responses as a consequence of social symbols and their meanings (i.e. culture).

The principal focus of this chapter involves explaining the nature of, reasons for, and implications of the distinctive tie a CPI compared to CMI has with processes and outcomes determined by biological and cultural evolutionary factors. Writ large, evolution is responsible for the distinctive changes in character of behaviour of *evolutionary creatures* which devolve from adverse perturbations and strains of their underlying anatomy and physiology which in turn manifest in behaviours which are labeled and dealt with in highly contrastive ways. ('Evolutionary creatures' refers to sentient, animate, and adaptive organisms (i.e. human and non-human beings) shaped by and enmeshed in mechanisms and processes of natural selection (Dennett, 1995).)

To fully comprehend the distinctive evolutionary attributes (e.g. biological, anatomical, cultural) of CPI one must discuss several questions. One is when such conditions emerged in human evolutionary and recorded history; and in relation to this, what characterized their descriptive properties? This raises the question of why in the first place a CPI compared to CMI has and always has had a distinctive tie to

cultural factors *in light of and because the effects these two types of conditions have on* the physiological functions of the organic systems of the body bring about different parameters of behaviour. Pure and simple, the evolutionary biology of CPI determines changes in experience and behaviour different from CMI. Finally, while both CPI and CMI undermine and dysregulate biological, organic systems, a question arises as to how and why human societies and populations have responded so differently to these conditions as a consequence of the symbols and meanings devolving from their distinctive biological and cultural signatures.

Answering such questions of necessity requires that one adopt a comprehensive evolutionary framework about anatomy and physiology which embodies the types of medical conditions that evolutionary creatures can exhibit. It includes bread and butter individual genetic selection across the spectrum of life (Williams, 1966) which is responsible for organic characteristics and functions of the body and its organs; and broader aspects of evolutionary theory which include cultural and social selection and which have special consequences on human behaviour; for example, gene-culture co-evolution or dual inheritance theory (Boyd and Richerson, 1985; Richerson and Boyd, 2005) and the theory about niche-constructing phenotypes (Odling-Smee *et al.*, 2003).

Comprehending the special tie a CPI has with human evolution and culture requires that one compare it to its siblings, namely, conditions of general medical interest (CMI). Comparison here translates into several puzzles: when in the history of life of sentient beings on planet Earth did physical environments emerge that rendered medical conditions not only possible but inevitable, when and how did medical conditions emerge during *human* evolutionary history, and what about the emerging biology and psychology of representatives of species pre-dating the genus *Homo sapiens* is responsible for the distinctive behavioural attributes of CPI contra CMI?

This line of argument has a practical implication as per CPI: its different nature is a necessary consideration for understanding the unique cultural meanings and implications not just of psychiatric disorders per se but for understanding the unique consequences of the social role clinical psychologists, psychiatrists and mental health social workers of modern societies have as a consequence of their focus on CPI compared to related medical personnel whose focus is CMI simply because the former enter into the private, moral lives of persons exhibiting CPI in special ways compared to health workers addressing CMI (taken up later).

Topics and Specifics

In an anthropological and evolutionary frame of reference, conditions of medical interest (CMI) embody and exhibit general properties and characteristics that are common to conditions of psychiatric interest (CPI). As suggested earlier, however, the latter constitute a qualitatively separate and distinct class of medical entities. From an empirical biological standpoint, a philosophical standpoint (i.e. ontology and epistemology), from a social, psychological, cultural, and political standpoint, and from a standpoint of providing clinical and therapeutic care, CPI is transparently different in kind and character compared to CMI (Fabrega, 2006a, 2007, 2009, 2013). Yet, despite their essential tie to the biology of *Homo sapiens*, manifestations of both types of medical conditions must be presumed to a have phylogeny that extends far beyond and deeper than that of the last common ancestor (LCA) of man and apes (i.e. *earlier than* 5–6 million years ago).

The principal focus of this chapter is on evolutionary changes which took place in the human line following LCA (i.e. after 5–6 million years ago). Changes in the character of adaptive behaviour, its environmental demands and consequences, essentially sculpted CMI differently from CPI. Evolutionary behavioural changes which took place involved early hominins, later archaic humans (e.g. *Homo erectus, Homo neanderthalensis*), and the most recent history involving anatomically modern humans starting approximately 200,000 years ago. It is during this comparatively recent history of *Homo sapiens* that the different character of CMI and CPI has become visibly evident (Fabrega, 1997, 2002, 2007, 2009, 2013) and it is this history which serves as principal focus of this chapter. However, given our present knowledge of the biological validity of animal models of CPI and CMI (Conn, 2013) and, in light of Darwinian tenets and principles regarding animal–human continuity in areas of genetic factors, physiology, anatomy, and behaviour, one must presume that basic genotypes as well as precursor varieties (phenotypes) of both types of medical conditions were indwelling, existent during the history of *evolutionary creatures* on planet

Earth. Ultimately, this generalization and its conceptual ramifications present themselves as philosophically and metaphysically compelling yet challenging and vexatious because of the logically exigent and 'dangerousness of Darwin's idea' (Dennett, 1995).

As discussed later, the genetic and physiological materiality and natural history of CPI and CMI indicate that early in evolutionary history, biologically 'raw' (if culturally non-existent or at least 'very lean') precursor forms and varieties of these conditions were strewn across the phylogenetic landscapes of non-human animals (discussed elsewhere, Fabrega, unpublished a and b). The phrase 'evolution of medical conditions' covers the aforementioned ultimately complete, ancestral history of both types of medical conditions. However, comparatively late human evolutionary history involving the evolution of representatives of the genus *Homo*, the focus of this chapter, demarcates the crucial, determinative temporal landscape during which developments involving thought, experience and adaptive behaviour emerged and came to elucidate differences in the nature and impact of CPI compared to CMI, all of which are covered in what follows.

What is this difference that sets CPI apart from CMI? Differences special to a CPI devolve from the special relation it has with origin, nature, manifestations and consequences of mental activities. A discussion of the evolutionary origins and cultural evolutionary aspects of mental phenomena (i.e. mentalization) will be taken up later. For present purposes, it signifies mental states (e.g. awareness, cognition, experience, voluntariness), their special ties to language and neuro-cognition, and the natural consequences that devolve from functions of this special *psycholinguistic nexus* or amalgam with respect to behaviour generally and behaviours characteristic of CPI compared to CMI specifically.

Psycholinguistic nexus is responsible for the perception of, and sense and feeling about self, other and of reality itself which when dysregulated eventuate in distinctive behavioural parameters of CPI compared to CMI. Mentalization is exemplified in the sheer correlates of neuropsychological factors (Kandel, 2005; Kandel and Hudspeth, 2013), tied to and descriptive of the neurobiology of CPI (altered perceptions, thought patterns and contents, tonality of mood and its regulatory control, personality disorders) *and to the social behavioural consequences of such factors*, including in particular mental dispositions, attitudes, and socially nuanced and skewed interpersonal relationships. Aspects of personal and social identity of persons exhibiting CPI (compared to CMI) also devolve from negative social and cultural labels which uniquely attach to their condition which are prevalent in any and all societies (Fabrega, 1997, 2002, 2006a, 2009, 2013). Such labels devolve from the distinctive character of *biological and social attributes and behavioural effects* of CPI compared to CMI. Such differences contribute to distinctive personal and social experiences as well as identity of persons exhibiting CPI compared to CMI (and of course, to other persons who do not exhibit medical conditions).

It is a truism that signs and symptoms which CMI *share with* CPI can and often do involve alternative ways of seeing, understanding and experiencing the world. A victim of CMI can have their experiences tied to self and other changed as a consequence of the general effects of disease and these can influence the conduct of social relations and affect a victim's social standing and sense of integrity as a person. However, psychological and social consequences of CPI tack on a qualitative different set of mental and behavioural considerations from those associated with pure CMI which, by definition, neither predispose nor bring about structural, organic changes in the neuropsychology undergirding and responsible for definition of self, social perception of others and interpersonal behaviour (e.g. 'sense of reality', cognition, affect, behavioural attitudes and disposition, self-appraisal and identity, and social conduct) (Fabrega, 2006a, 2013).

Background: A General Anthropology of Medical and Psychiatric Conditions

Ethnomedicine and ethnopsychiatry are terms which traditionally have been used in cultural anthropology to describe the role played by symbols and their meanings in the psychology, world views (i.e. ideas, values) and social practices which through human history have come to be formulated, set apart and dealt with (acted upon) in ways construed as 'medical' (Fabrega, 1974, 1975, 1976a) in different types of society. While anthropology has high interest in the significance and meaning of the word segment 'ethno' *across human societies* so does the branch of sociology which focuses on the role of meanings, symbols and social labels on behaviours, this time, however, *within contemporary and usually modern societies*. Symbolic interactionism, for example, describes the work of eminent sociologists (e.g. Herbert Blumer, Erving Goffman, Howard Becker, Harold Garfinkel, Donald Black) whose focus is on the role of (cultural) *meanings of social labels* that are used to set apart members of groups negatively (e.g. as disvalued, deviants, minorities) within contemporary societies. Principles of symbolic interactionism are relevant to virtually all and any type of social relationship within a society, affect persons exhibiting CPI (social devaluation of the mentally ill) and CMI (e.g. leprosy, HIV, the terminally ill). Such principles can be applied to groups studied by cultural and symbolic anthropologists who, however, generally employ different terminological systems (e.g. Mary Douglas, Clifford Geertz, Edmund Leach, Sherry Ortner, Victor Turner) and study different types of societies.

The terms ethnomedicine and ethnopsychiatry are here formulated as involving a people's, group's or culture's conceptual understandings and social institutional approaches to CMI and CPI respectively ('sickness and healing behaviours' writ large). The 'ethno' approach to science in general and to medical phenomena in particular was an outgrowth of interest in the language, concepts and mental or cognitive organization of knowledge and meaning of different peoples around the world which was especially regnant in the 1950s, 1960s and immediately thereafter in cultural anthropology (Goodenough, 1956, 1957; Wallace, 1962; Berlin *et al.*, 1968; Metzger and Williams, 1966; Fabrega, 1974, 1975, 1976a, b, c; D'Andrade, 1981, 1987, 1995). During the late 1950s and 1960s, an 'ethno' emphasis on interpretations, responses and social practices surrounding all types of sickness and healing (the 'culture of and/or social labels tagged on to medical ideas, beliefs and actions') were salient concerns in the study of anthropology and sociology of medicine (see Fabrega, 1971, 1974, 1975) for early reviews and emphases). Resonance of cultural orientation, ethno affiliation, and social labelling of persons exhibiting CPI and CMI impact on their identity and cannot but impact also on attitudes and dispositions of clinical and professional medical practitioners as well as on medical educators, but dicta of medical objectivism and impersonality explicitly demand that they be excluded and negated.

With respect to general medicine and CMI, the emphasis placed on the role of cultural meaning systems on understanding the nature, manifestations and social movement of persons afflicted by them in societies at large and into and through clinics has lessened in the wake of the ascendancy of sheer biological factors (and for CPI, neurobiological ones or clinical neuroscience – all discussed later). Evolutionary medicine, for example, a relatively recent focus in modern study of disease (Gluckman *et al.*, 2009), concentrates on parameters of human pathologies which are situated squarely 'in the innate although plastic biology of *Homo sapiens*' and which play a central role in the modern understandings and approaches to human disease. In general, in the biological sciences, cultural meanings surrounding people's understandings and responses to CMI and CPI have given way to social and evolutionary aspects of medical problems encompassing demography, history of human populations, social structure and epidemiology (Cohen, 1989; Armelagos, 1990; Armelagos and Barnes, 1999; Strassmann and Dunbar, 1999; Stanford *et al.*, 2006). Social cultural factors which through behaviour (i.e. mating relationships, social preferences, actions, diet, levels of physical activity) influence the causes and shape (at least the expression of) the organic pathology of disease are addressed in biological medical anthropology and in human biological and cultural evolution. Together, such approaches have to answer to the exigencies which encompass individual selection, gene-culture selection, group selection, and theory of niche-construction phenotypes. In other words, a pocketful of genetic and environmental interactions which impact on and influence prevalence, responses to, and consequences of behavioural genotypes and phenotypes of medical conditions (Richerson and Boyd, 2005; Boyd and Richerson, 1985; Williams, 1966; Odling-Smee *et al.*, 2003; Parsons, 1951a, b; Fried, 1967; Service 1975; Sanderson 1999 and 2001) exemplify both commonalities as well as differences involving CPI and CMI.

Behaviours of sickness and healing from a meanings centred viewpoint and a people's ethnomedicine and ethnopsychiatry as embodiment of ideas, structures or institutional organizations of a group or society are topics of general intellectual, anthropological interest. However, far from representing contrastive and self-contained exotic perspectives which address and elucidate narrow, specialized social science disciplinary and purely symbolic questions, ethno approaches to medical conditions writ large are germane to diverse scholars across many disciplines

of evolutionary behavioural sciences and medicine. They are relevant to social, cultural, biological and evolutionary anthropologists. They are particularly relevant to psychiatrists and clinical psychologists who practice in complex, poly-ethnic societies and/or faraway places and who should know and internalize more than the current dominant, practical, powerful and yet restricted (and reductionist) emphasis devolving from the neurobiological and clinical neuroscience determinism which has come to grip the official establishment of psychiatry.

A proviso is appropriate here. Principal topics of this chapter include philosophical and scientific implications of differences between CPI and CMI. The differences devolve from the condition's evolutionary history (biological and cultural) and from ramifications of their effects on interpersonal relationships and social institutions all of which are taken up later. Putting aside such considerations for now, emphasis should be directed to matters which are not explicitly addressed in this chapter but which are central to its thesis nonetheless and especially to readers of this book. These involve characteristics of social role, clinical activities and goals of health personnel who provide help to individuals who exhibit the two types of conditions.

Put directly and succinctly: dialogues during therapy with clients exhibiting CPI *necessarily* ('by definition') involve practitioners in discussions of the former's attitudes, values, dispositions, motivations, and actions embedded in their conduct in any and all areas of social life. Clinically relevant discussions spotlight questions of competence and responsibility, matters freighted with moral, ethical, legal and political overtones. On the one hand, a mental health professional client's personal understanding of self and their grip of social happenings which involve their actions (e.g. their accuracy, validity, distortion) shed light on their motivations (i.e. reasons for acting) and, on the other hand, social consequences of the client's actions (and the client's reactions to them) bear equally on matters of the client's sense of social responsibility and possible culpability.

Matters central to morals, ethics and politics of self and behaviour are very frequently 'on the radar screen' of therapeutic exchanges with clients exhibiting CPI. This is so because the ontology, epistemology, pathology and morality of behaviours constituting CPI resonate with personal values and social ramifications different from those tied to CMI. And, for reasons discussed later, such differences are outcomes of the evolutionary foundations of such conditions. All such value laden overtones and ramifications of clinically relevant dialogues ('personal stuff') cannot easily be avoided and should ideally be pointed out and examined (hopefully sorted out) in therapeutic exchanges which, ironically, are presumed to reflect official, 'objective and impersonal' professional concerns of therapists administering to the needs of subjects exhibiting all types of medical conditions.

Such matters involving the distinctive character of CPI need emphasis today because they can easily be glossed over in the urgency and rush to clinical neuroscience reductive emphases which have sought to 'impersonalize' special nature and therapeutic implications and obligations of practitioners of subjects exhibiting CPI.

In summary, considerations integral to ethnomedicine and ethnopsychiatry are important because they remind and underscore the point that social and medical institutions and practices are first and foremost meaning centred, culturally laden social constructions and labels whose conceptual and practical/instrumental features and directives are embedded (as programmes) in templates and structures of the brain/minds of subjects served by those institutions. It is sobering to appreciate that contemporary disciplines of medicine and especially psychiatry and clinical psychology, namely, *our ethnomedicine and ethnopsychiatry of today*, involve comparatively recent modernist developments involving science and medical practice which are grafted on to and imposed on groups whose representatives exemplify different, evolutionarily and historically contingent attitudes, conceptions, values and dispositions regarding not just the nature and play of CMI and CPI but of basic conceptions of personal and social identity (i.e. personhood) and responsibility.

Evolutionary Affirmative Perspective on Medical and Psychiatric Conditions

Introductory Comment

In this perspective sickness and healing behaviours are framed primarily if not exclusively in the language of evolutionary behavioural sciences and organic pathology and physiology of disease. In an ultimate sense, effects and manifestations of CMI and CPI ('medical conditions' when writ large), exemplify potential loss of reproduction and function posed by the sheer genetic, physiological, organic pathology ('biological nature') of medical conditions. Such costs include evolutionarily selected mechanisms at microscopic level and in organ system functions and responses designed to cope and surmount medical threats to health and life itself. Responses to medical conditions (CMI and CPI) include social and behavioural responses and routines of evolutionary creatures generally (Hart, 1988, 1990), and among representatives of the species *Homo sapiens* in particular, deliberative, conscious efforts embodied in social transactions in medical institutions. Sickness involves patent breakdown and/or disrupted, stress-influenced adaptive responses of injured, lesioned or toxically/infectiously harmed biological systems of the organism or person (genotype and phenotype) which constitute a threat to evolutionary imperatives inherent in meeting milestones of life history and ultimately reproduction. In this perspective, interpretation of sickness and healing behaviours of CMI and CPI metaphorically echo the collective efforts of genes to survive. In contemporary *Homo sapiens*, this is realized in measures taken by the individual, family and significant group members to restore the integrity and functionality of the individual and enable them to reproduce and care for family.

Defining an Evolutionary Perspective on Medical and Psychiatric Phenomena

The significance of medicine as a system of behaviour, practice and regulation promotes enhancement of capacity of phenotypes to transfer genes to future generations so as to maximize inclusive fitness. Sickness endangers survival and reproduction of an individual who is sick and also the health of kin who share genes with the individual. Hence, an evolutionary perspective on sickness and healing (i.e. correlates of CMI and CPI) among representatives of a species would face problems such as balancing (1) threat of harming kin through pathogen stress, transmitting infectious agents (or pathological avoidance), (2) harmful influence not just on the family but on the social group devolving from, on the one hand, compromised resources and capabilities related to instrumental behaviour and, on the other, social, interpersonal, and psychological (including moral) consequences of manifestations and interpretations of behaviour tied to CMI and CPI in particular, and (3) enhancing survival of the sick individual by providing support, resources and healing.

Stated differently, an evolutionarily affirmative slant on medical and psychiatric problems (posed by and CMI and CPI, respectively) puts emphasis on the idea that individual and kin have to negotiate a balance between behaviours directly aimed at cutting costs by avoiding sickness altogether; and the possibility of preserving genetic material by confronting sickness and obtaining benefits through support and healing from kin and genetically unrelated group mates so as to enable the sick phenotype to survive. The latter scenario requires participation in processes of social exchange with kin (who have genetic stakes in supporting the sick family member), non-kin as through reciprocal altruism (which is based on implicit and/or explicit assurance of return favours and requires stable, durable social relations within the group), or non-kin through establishment of social bonds of mutual support and friendship (Tooby and Cosmides, 1996, 2005).

From a general anthropological perspective, then, social and biological correlates of CMI and CPI (sickness and healing behaviours writ large) reflect ultimate, distal genetic vulnerability factors and more proximally neurobiological and physiological perturbations and learning influences saliently exhibited among *Homo sapiens*. Correlates of such conditions answer to evolutionary imperatives and influence and manifest in what are termed psychological adaptations and behavioural strategies in evolutionary psychology and human behavioural ecology, respectively, two major divisions in the study of behaviour from an evolutionary standpoint. Dual inheritance theory (Richerson and Boyd, 2005; Boyd and Richerson, 1985) and niche-constructing phenotypes (Odling-Smee *et al.*, 2003) would represent an additional explanation of the role of evolutionary processes involved in conditioning, promoting and establishing sickness/healing related behaviours in an evolutionarily affirmative way. This involves genetic and cultural information interacting in biological and cultural co-evolutionary processes involving natural selection at individual level and cultural selection at group level.

Is the Nature and Response to Medical Conditions Unique to *Homo Sapiens*?

It is clear that higher primates, especially chimpanzees and bonobos, communicate emotions and respond to the emotional displays of other group mates in direct and varied ways. Depending on circumstances, they exhibit behavioural responses to group mates which have been described as fear, anger, jealousy, happiness, kindness, consolation, empathy and general caring. They generally display an emotional awareness and general appreciation of the plight of kin, unrelated group mates and even other species which are injured (Goodall, 1986a, b; de Waal, 1996, 2016), but all (according to strict reading of evolutionary ideas) in context of inclusive fitness of genes of individual and kin (i.e. reciprocal altruism). None the less, putting these observations together suggests that higher apes appear to exhibit a mental disposition for understanding the plight of others. By extension, the last common ancestor of pongids and hominins (approximately 5–6 million years ago) may have exhibited the same disposition. One can propose that higher apes and the last common ancestor (LCA) of man and apes exhibited a cognitive template involving emotional awareness and disposition that may have included special understandings and responses to the suffering of sickness (Fabrega, 1975, 1976a, 1997, 2006b, 2011, 2013).

Higher apes also exhibit behaviours described as 'self-medication' when they are sick (Wrangham, 1995; Huffman, 1997, 2006; Fabrega, 2010). When suffering from intestinal parasite infestation they resort to plants that have a positive effect on their health. These plants are not the usual items members of a group ingest as food when they are well. On a provisional basis, one can term such behaviours 'self-healing'. Chimpanzee groups also display what have been described as special *behavioural traditions* that are confined to a more or less ecologically isolated population (McGrew, 2004). For example, some groups exhibit special gestures (e.g. forms of hand holding while mating) or subsistence routines (e.g. techniques of termite fishing and nut cracking, washing potatoes soiled with dirt and sand) that are not found in other populations which exhibit other traditions. The use of specific plants and procedures while sick (i.e. self-medication) appears to correspond to a behavioural tradition as different plants are used by ecologically separated populations of chimpanzees. This raises the question of the cognitive processes involved in self-healing and other-healing; for example, the extent to which self-care and care of kin involves non-conscious behaviour, is a product of associative, conditioned learning compared to, for example, awareness of sickness in self and others, and corresponding needs for medical care exemplify intentional consciously motivated behaviour (Fabrega, 1993, 1997, 2002, 2006a, b, 2007, 2011).

Sick chimpanzees fail to keep up with group mates in daily rounds and sometimes this elicits a slowing down of subsistence rounds by group mates. Higher apes have also been described as helping, supporting and providing help to those suffering disability and sickness (Fabrega, 1997, 2002). These observations have mainly involved a parent's licking of wounds and bleeding of lacerations of offspring and providing general comfort in context of suffering. Monkeys also have been described as supporting visually and cognitively impaired younger group mates (Berkson, 1970, 1973; de Waal et al., 1996). It is assumed that behaviours of providing comfort, support and aid to handicapped group mates is a feature of their social life made possible when ecological and predator challenges are not major threats. However, and in general, information involving the responses of non-human primates to conditions of sickness, trauma and lesions in kin or non-kin group mates is not plentiful (see Fabrega, 2013, for a review of literature on psychiatric phenomena).

When severely sick, chimpanzees essentially desist from interacting and withdraw. The motivation of behaviours surrounding sickness on the part of a sick individual may represent sheer physiological limitation of effort (Hart, 1988, 1990; Lozano, 1998; Revusky, 1984; Huffman, 1997, 2006). Behaviour of an individual when sick and of group mates may represent an avoidance of pathology and pathogen stress, an innate response pattern or adaptation to limit spread of disease which diminishes inclusive fitness (Low, 1988, 1990). In general, the cognitive and motivational bases for providing other healing raises questions such as investment in parenting, kinship and friendship (Tooby and Cosmides, 1996; Sugiyama, 1996, 2004; Sugiyama and Chacon, 2000), the biological problem of altruism, and selected programmes influencing parasite avoidance and pathogen stress (Low, 1988, 1990).

Fitted onto chimpanzees, then, sickness and healing behaviours stemming from CMI and CPI, like their social behaviour in general, exemplify alternative varieties of intentionality, deliberation, calculation and empathy (de Waal, 1996, 2016). They are consistent with some of the features of the culturally affirmative view of general medical phenomena (discussed later) which construes sickness and healing as exemplifying existential sensitivity to the plight of self and others. However, and in general, it has proven difficult to support the claim that higher apes exhibit a conceptual understanding of their world which would include awareness of self, other and of states of health which are essential aspects of a cultural approach to medicine. In chimpanzees, sickness/healing behaviours can be explained as partly innate, ecologically tweaked, and a product of conditioned association (Hart, 1988, 1990; Lozano, 1998; Revusky, 1984; Rozin et al., 2000).

Cognitive capacities involved in awareness and understanding of self, other, wellness, sickness in self and others, and motivations and behaviours to remedy suffering of sickness (in either self or others) represent foundational building blocks of a medical tradition, system or institution (the 'ethno' approach discussed earlier). Members of a species which exhibited these traits would suggest a capacity for precursor variety or form of a cultural, psychological slant of medical problems. Such cognitive capacities set a baseline which would then lead to trial and error learning of routines of medical caring, healing, uses of resources and behavioural adjustments to help the sick individual through its sickness. The basic template for this would involve a biological adaptation for cognition and cultural learning (Tomasello, 1999).

Viewed in cognitive neuroscience terms, templates which exemplify adaptive and intentional responses to medical and psychiatric conditions rest on deliberative involvement of executive functions in the space of working memory, behaviour patterns that meet requirements of culture, cognition and communication which emerged following the pongid hominid split (Fabrega, 1997, 2002, 2013; Rossano, 2003, 2007; Wynn and Coolidge, 2005, 2012). As discussed later, in a culturally affirmative position respecting medicine, how such a cognitive capacity and associated behaviours surmounted biological problems posed by evolutionary imperatives (e.g. altruism, pathogen stress and avoidance of pathology) would need to be explained in terms of systems of social symbols and their meaning, perhaps involving behavioural contracting as formulated by Knight (1991, 1996, 1997, 1999) in context of cultural aspects of menstruation and gender relations (see also Dunbar, 1993, 1996a, b, 1999, 2003, 2004; Dunbar et al., 1999; Dunbar and Schultz, 2007).

Conditions of Psychiatric Interest in Higher Primates

In a formulation of how characteristics of CPI changed among hominins, archaic humans and then *Homo sapiens*, emphasis is understandably placed on aspects of mentalization which such species exhibited. This would include, for example, consciousness, experience, cognition, and language and culture ('linguistic and cultural psychology'). We are interested presently in situating analogues or early forms of CPI in such creatures about whom capabilities respecting such mental states and activities are contested and contestable. A secure baseline for inferring forms of CPI among species that preceded *Homo sapiens* (and beyond the last common ancestor of apes and man or LCA) is needed, nonetheless. What such conditions were like and how they were understood and dealt with prior to the advent of *Homo sapiens* can be gleaned from studies involving higher non-human primates with whom *Homo sapiens* shares common ancestors. Previous writings (Fabrega 2002, 2006a, b, 2009, 2011, 2013) have summarized the logic and relevant empirical data tracing origins of CPI in higher primates (e.g. behavioural anomalies of monkeys, syndromes indicating chimpanzee varieties of psychopathology). Work in progress (Fabrega, unpublished a, b) discusses findings in comparative psychology and cognitive ethology which address origins of animal mental capabilities which when dysregulated or disrupted are relevant to precursor varieties of CPI during earlier phases of biological evolution (see also Goddard et al., 2014).

A variety of ritualistic actions, rocking movements, behavioural stereotypes, bizarre actions toward body parts, coprophagy and other visible, seemingly nonsensical behaviour suggest a breakdown of normal routines. Some expressions of chimpanzee psychopathology are not marked by such aberrant anomalies but by social and biological antisocial behavioural differences that seem intrinsic to 'personality'

as well as biological and ecological contingencies (see Fabrega 2002: 143–341, chapters 7 and 8 for chimpanzees; Fabrega, 2013: 135–446, chapters III and IV).

Some of the syndromes have come to light vividly as a result of developmental interventions that have stressed mothers of infants whose behaviour is later examined and compared to that of 'normal' group mates. Behavioural anomalies and emotional breakdowns in higher primates have been linked to noxious, harmful and threatening social circumstances. The components of such conditions exhibit a measure of face validity of CPI and in fact are often qualified in these and semantically similar terms by field researchers who are neither psychologists nor psychiatrists. A detailed description of primate varieties of CPI is available in the recent work of Fabrega (2002, 2013). What is less than clear is how such manifestations fit in the overall (neural, social, ecological) psychology and social biology of the individual who displays them, and more specifically, their link to morbid effects of concurrent CMI and their functional consequences and implications. The correspondence of higher primate conditions of psychiatric interest to many indicators of descriptive psychopathology of humans (e.g. delusions, hallucinations, thought disorganization) is unclear because of obvious difficulty as to how non-linguistic higher primate cognitive capacities and states can be sampled and are best formulated to begin with, not to say how these might break down, and the effect the latter would have in undermining organization of behaviour among kinfolk and non-kin group mates, although observations by de Waal (1996, 2016) provide rich examples for chimpanzees.

A modern slant on CPI should not exclude the 'raw' behavioural phenomena visible in primate syndrome described by primatologists. A modernist's gaze is likely to be directed to material relevant to mental phenomena: concepts, symbolic meanings, attitudes, values and behaviours that reflect cultural understanding of social reality and the significance of behaviour. However, the psychological domain, as researchers of primate cognition make all too clear, is not accessible to the proverbial 'radar screen' that a clinician observer might use to make sense of the ape exemplars in indirect, implicit ways (recall dicta of critical anthropomorphism). Even if an individual primate had a mental, emotional representation of its situation that shaped its experience and consequent behavioural 'signs and symptoms' suggesting

CPI, validation of such phenomena simply could not be gotten to directly and has to be inferred through carefully designed studies (McGrew, 2004).

Moreover, even if one can observe aberrant, bizarre, nonsensical, avoidant, apathetic and seemingly purposeless behaviour in higher apes, victims exhibiting it cannot be expected to be experiencing mental phenomena which often represent modernist gold standards of CPI. In general, such things as auditory verbal hallucinations, delusions and obsessions, behaviours signalling depersonalization or derealization, worries, feelings of guilt and burdens about past actions and/or present impulses all communicate and symbolize changes in conception, perception and expression of 'human psyches' but their relevance to the life and especially mental experiences of chimpanzees is unknown (see Fabrega, 2002). Moreover, there is no evidence that chimpanzees have an awareness that such behaviours are abnormal or evidence of 'psycho' pathology. On the other hand, behaviours involving CMI such as evidence of swelling, inflammation, itching and scratching, pain, physical suffering, bleeding, coughing, vomiting, diarrhoea, slowing down of physical ambulation and sheer lassitude/weakness are responded to by conspecifics in ways that suggest perception ('a sense') of deviance, abnormality and suffering; and they elicit compassion and empathy and perhaps sympathy from group mates (Fabrega, 2002).

Nonetheless there is substantial evidence that, despite lacking direct, linguistic access to the mental radar screen of higher primates, expert observers of primate habitual dispositions, activities and social relationships have little difficulty in recognizing, identifying and labelling changes in behaviour of individuals as possible or candidate forms of conditions of psychiatric interest. For compelling descriptions of this and for good descriptions of the 'natural history' or expression of CPI in higher primates the reader is referred to work by Kummer (1995), Goodall (1986a, b), many publications by de Waal (1996, 2016), and the work of Brüne et al. (2006). In short, manifest changes of behaviour of non-human primates certainly can suggest misperceptions, distorted and aberrant programmes of behaviour, persistent fears and phobias, ritualistic and stereotyped behaviour routines, aggressive, destructive, 'antisocial' dispositions, and even personality abnormalities. Besides their obvious lack of disciplinary and professional training and experience in psychiatric matters, especially the psychosocial, psycho-cultural nature of CPI, and their reluctance to engage in (or reservations against 'undue') medicalization, psychologization, politicization or psychiatric labelling, biological anthropologists and cognitive ethologists keep using a psychiatric language when describing behaviour otherwise described as deviant, aberrant or anomalous and opaque (Fabrega 2002, 2006c, 2007, 2013).

In attempting to make sense of what conditions of behavioural irregularity and breakdown might mean when viewed from a general intellectual standpoint, one needs to keep separate the different frames of reference that are relevant. The syndromes of behavioural irregularity can be construed as:

1. based on intuitive notions of what is socially meaningful (e.g. making sense given the history of the group and its circumstances) and consequential (e.g. having an impact on the organization of group behaviour);

2. outright psychopathology (e.g. analogues of 'psychic' suffering, disordered cognition, distraught behaviour seen in humans);

3. phenomena related to CMI and CPI having a negative impact on fitness, survival and reproduction (i.e. devolving from breakdown of evolutionary imperatives involving adaptive behaviour);

4. as analogues of sickness and healing, namely, similar to how sickness and injury are expressed and 'read' by group mates and responded to inside the group (e.g. pain/suffering/weakness compared confused/disordered thinking and/or emotions; and

5. in a moral sense (e.g. phenomena that reflect suffering and elicit empathy and perhaps even sympathy or motivation to relieve).

Role of Mentalization in the Natural History of CMI and CPI

Human medical conditions share many properties which stretch backwards in time to include nonhumans. This includes, for example, their origin and eventuation in evolutionary creatures, their manifestations in sickness and healing behaviours writ large, and the play of the social and behavioural biology of (i.e. responses to) CMI and CPI in the life spaces of populations and groups. Previous discussion has also emphasized the special character and recent history of

CPI compared to CMI (see Fabrega, 2002, 2006a, b, c; 2007, 2011, 2013). Here I want to briefly underscore and make explicit that the origins and eventuation of the special character of CPI compared to CMI is crucially determined by its embodiment in neurocognitive templates responsible for activities I summarize as mentalization, a term which covers aspects of language, consciousness, awareness, cognition, voluntarism, affectivity and mental deliberation, all of which generally are thought of as exclusively human. In contemporary thought and research in evolutionary behavioural sciences the relevance and scope of mental activity has been expanded to include non-human animals through principles of critical anthropomorphism and exemplified in fields of cognitive ethology, experimental comparative psychology and consciousness studies (Ristau, 1991a, b; Burghardt, 1991, 1997, 1999, 2007, 2009; Griffin, 1981, 1992, 1998; Merker, 2007, 2010, 2012; de Waal, 1996, 2016; Hurley and Nudds, 2006; Safina, 2015).

A plausible case has been made that all animals embody biological templates which when dysregulated eventuate in stress related breakdowns in behaviour (including forms of CMI and CPI) which reflect, correlate with, and encompass mental activities (Fabrega, 2002). A theoretical position and general attitude respecting animal–human continuity in aspects of mentalization is reflected in work involving evolutionary semantics based on theory and method of natural semantic metalanguage for analyses of similarities and differences in the mental resources of groups of early human peoples (Goddard *et al.*, 2014) and, as discussed elsewhere (Fabrega, unpublished a, b) in recent literature involving evolutionary behavioural sciences underscoring the need for cross-species linguistics. The latter proposal extends and reformulates basic tenets of theory and method of natural semantic metalanguage or NSM as a language of thought paradigm. The raison d'etre of NSM is construed as a 'mini' lexicon and grammar which taps shared universal foundations of natural languages and cultures of *Homo sapiens*. First extension: a natural language expression analysed through NSM resources (e.g. semantic primes and their entailments), models inherited neurocognitive brain structures of *Homo sapiens* which have a natural history and describe and encompass activities of mentalization (what the linguistic expression evokes and stands for in the speaker's psychology). Second extension: the article proposes that when tenets, structures of

meaning and rationale of NSM are extended and integrated with data and tenets of evolutionary biology, cognitive ethology and comparative cognitive psychology including consciousness studies, it provides a framework which can be used to elucidate the nature of and role played by mental phenomena in biology of behaviour of animals generally and with respect to human evolution in particular. In the event, the NSM inventory of primates and their logical, linguistic connections function as an evolutionary behavioural science by providing a cross species linguistics for modelling aspects of mentalization as well as medical conditions in terms of Darwinian naturalism.

The line of argument under consideration presently underscores the natural Darwinian tie that connects evolution of mentalization functions with evolution of CPI compared to CMI. Put most directly: the special character of CPI in particular, underscores and exemplifies the influence of mentalization phenomena on conditions of medical interest writ large. Evolutionary processes governing change in manifestations and effects of CPI in social groups (i.e. among evolutionary creatures) will naturally reflect and correspond to changes in capabilities and resources associated with mentalization as played out in social relations of the respective species. In other words, the *psychology and social relations correlates of CPI compared to CMI*, specifically, not just definitional distinctions involving signs and symptoms as per modern clinical medicine but comprehending their origin and change in content during human evolution, reflect the centrality of mentalization processes and activities which became visibly manifest in the behaviour and social cultural accomplishments of human populations starting with *Homo erectus* approximately two million years ago (see Fabrega, 2013 and discussed in Fabrega unpublished a, b).

Mental phenomena are plausible correlates of evolutionary developments embracing size, organization and functions of brain networks and neurocognitive structures determined by natural selection which influence all non-human organisms and culminate in *Homo sapiens*. Individual genetic selection is modified by developments involving social environmental effects of animal behaviour and discussed as dual inheritance theory, geneculture selection and evolution, and the role played by niche constructing phenotypes. The special identity and character of CPI compared to CMI is determined by and an outcome of its special tie to phenomena involving mentalization, the component features of which embody a natural history that stretches into the phylogeny not only of humans and hominins but to species pre-dating the last common ancestor of apes and humans (Fabrega, 1997, 2002, 2007, 2009, 2013, unpublished a, b).

Elements of an Evolutionary Psychology of Medical Conditions

In evolutionary psychology it is not general mechanisms that hold sway in explanations of adaptive behaviour. Rather, it is *domain specific mechanisms or modules designed in ancestral environments* to cope with biological problems that in ultimate terms explain behaviours which are relevant to sickness and healing in any particular environment. While shaped for adaptive purposes a species' ecology may change and, thus, psychological adaptations may or not match contingencies of the contemporary environment and may thus not only prove salutary but can have harmful consequences (Tooby and Cosmides, 2005). On the other hand, in human behavioural ecology it is not psychological phenomena but *general behavioural strategies* determined by evolutionary imperatives which negotiate the potential costs of sickness *regardless of environment* (Alexander, 1987a, b, 1989, 1990; Cronk et al., 2000; Dunbar and Barrett, 2007). In both evolutionary psychology and behavioural biology, optimality theory and game theory exemplify principles on the basis of which one gauges the effectiveness of formulations, decisions, actual behaviours in response to local ecological contingencies involving disease, sickness and trauma. While the dicta of these two evolutionary social sciences respecting origins and functions of programmes of behaviour underscore different mechanisms and processes tied to their particular logic of explanation, they are obviously complementary when it comes to making sense of the social biology of sickness and human responses which aim at coping with, correcting and overcoming morbidity of pathology through healing dispositions, habitual behaviours and problem solving activities. Both explanatory models for sickness healing behaviours entail trade-offs between costs and benefits described earlier along with requirements of optimality theory.

Evolutionary Slant on Ontology and Epistemology of Medical Conditions

With respect to medicine, the function of evolved, naturally selected programmes of behaviour tied to medical conditions (i.e. sickness and healing responses) is to overcome impediments that block achievement of milestones dictated by life history theory, the architecture of which is determined by the play of genes and ecology. This is the raison d'etre of evolutionary imperatives enveloping sickness/healing behaviours and of medicine writ large (Fabrega, 1974, 1997, 2002, 2013). Such dicta exemplify important trade-offs in the allocation of finite amounts of energy and resources that spread across the lifetime of individuals and include mate selection, age at reproduction, fertility, parenting and providing for self and immediate family and more extended kin. Survival and caring for self and family represent basic costs posed by bacteria, viruses, parasites, trauma and toxins. Causes and effects of disease in impeding achievement of optimal and salutary life history milestones translate into routines that involve preservation of genetic material as per promotion of social relations of family and subsistence in relation to threat and challenge of sickness and disease.

Such an emphasis is a hallmark of an evolutionary perspective on phenomena conditioned by disease, sickness and healing responses among representatives of *Homo sapiens*. However, the significance and scope of an evolutionary slant of medical conditions (i.e. CMI and CPI) is broad: with due allowance for differences in size, organization of neural tissues and networks and behavioural resources conditioned by prevailing ecology, an evolutionary approach is applicable to many species not just non-linguistic higher primates and/or pre-linguistic hominins. When examined in general terms, 'evolutionarily affirmative' behaviours and responses to medical conditions encompass such things as dietary preferences, expenditure of energy, avoidance of toxins, trade-offs with commensal parasites, environmentally directed behaviours that promote and maintain health, prevent disease or provide support in the context of sickness or impaired biological functions more generally. All of the preceding, of course, are manifest and effectuated differently depending on resources and capabilities afforded by a species' form of organization of brain/mind activities at the level of cells, tissues, organ systems, neural networks and behavioural actions.

The philosophical underpinnings of the evolutionary perspective is that sickness *was* a risk to life and a killer and disabler when it *supervened* and healing *was* the behavioural response which *protected against and overcame* such harms in the service of survival, reproduction and fitness more generally. The past tense is highlighted in the previous sentence in order to underscore that the evolutionary perspective is concerned with origins, functions and reasons for the phylogenetic persistence of sickness and healing as evolutionary imperatives; specifically, as behavioural programmes geared to survival and reproduction that originated in ancestral environments.

The Stuff of Ideas, and Meanings in the Evolutionary Perspective

In contrast to the culturally affirmative slant on ethno conception of medical conditions (discussed later), in the evolutionary perspective, sickness and healing are not primarily about the existential and emotional plights of an individual and their immediate family nor about ideas, beliefs, values, myths or rituals which make of medicine a cultural enterprise writ large. It is about what sickness exemplifies about evolutionary imperatives and necessities determined by fitness as determined by natural selection; and its effects on biological processes which the sick individual happens to stand proof of. It is about how imperatives involving survival and inclusive fitness can be maintained in the context of the costs of disease, trauma and toxicity from inhabitants and products of the ecology.

In an ultimate sense, the stark reality about a medical condition is what it *caused* (and still causes) in the economy of survival and reproduction, how its costs were coped with, and which and how practices brought into play by disease and trauma came to be modulated and moulded in the ancestral past. Sickness and disease as instruments of natural selection shape adaptive behaviour routines that enabled balancing avoidance of pathology contra provision of healing despite the possibility of non-return of benefits conferred from maladapted healing routines.

Broader Implications of an Evolutionary Affirmation Perspective

In evolutionary terms, it is thwarted social routines of making a living and providing for self and family in the context of sickness, disease and trauma that are all important. In the context of impaired ability to solve basic biological functions and fulfil evolutionary imperatives it is how afflicted individuals and their dependents are able to surmount the crisis of disease and disability which is salient. Strict biological self-preservation and recourse to evolutionarily compatible forms of altruistic assistance are relevant for understanding the evolutionary formulation of sickness and healing. Tenets of inclusive fitness theory and reciprocal altruism are conservative self-interested routines typically invoked in neo-Darwinian synthesis as explanation for acts of helping of the type inherent in sickness and healing (Tooby and Cosmides, 1992, 2005; Sugiyama, 1996, 2004; Sugiyama and Chacon, 2000).

Supporting, comforting and providing healing to relatives (who share one's genes) and those one can be sure will reciprocate such costly favours or gifts represent *first order neo-Darwinian responses* to the risk and pathology of sickness. Here, sickness and healing behaviours boil down to doing for or favouring individuals who share one's genes and/or others are likely to reciprocate in a big way as insurance for obtaining their help in the event of sickness (Tooby and Cosmides, 1996; Sugiyama, 1996, 2004; Sugiyama and Chacon, 2000). Social exchange of benefits is viewed as centrally tied to the attachment and bonding following birth, during infancy and thereafter which privileges genetic relatives and attachment to others.

However, the evolutionary perspective on sickness and healing is not confined to dicta of inclusive fitness theory and reciprocal altruism. It acknowledges limitations and complications in the applicability of such directives in the case of early societies of *Homo sapiens* (and even in representatives of genus *Homo*) which evolved concepts, ideas, and social practices which differed in relation to their brain/mind resources and to the size, social organization, technology and practical biological problem solving capabilities (their 'science'), and cultural values. Progressive and continuous changes in size, complexity and scope of societies during prehistory and recorded history and especially modern societies have had a major impact on the types and levels of medical conditions, the understanding of such conditions, and on technologies and social practices designed to control and ameliorate their effects. This translates as degrees of understanding, avoidance, coping and controlling of sickness and healing phenomena. Social structures, group composition and the way individuals segregate and come to settle in groups (in small as well as large scale societies) do not always make directives of inclusive fitness theory and reciprocal altruism practical or realistic. For example, groups frequently break up, members often leave their natal group and migrants entering come with no ties, yet have to contend as possible helpers in the ordeals of group survival posed by recurring, inevitable conditions of disease and sickness.

To meet such contingencies, alternative *second order* mechanisms and motivations of behaviour have been formulated by evolutionary psychologists and human behavioural ecologists as a way of overcoming the limitations of sheer self-interest dictated by strictures constraining 'altruism' and 'morality' (Alexander, 1987a, b, 1989, 1990. The crisis of sickness/healing is a paradigm of need that calls into play programmes of behaviour designed to overcome challenges posed by disability and dependence (Fabrega, 1974, 1975). These involve 'adaptations' and 'strategies' aimed at building a network of support and help from unrelated group mates who are in a position to provide support and resources in cases of need (Tooby and Cosmides, 1996). Sickness and disability are a paradigm example of circumstances which give rise to a need for support and care and it is presumed that planning for this contingency is a factor motivating the conduct of social relations among genetically unrelated group mates in conformance to gene-culture selection necessities and contingencies. These considerations are presumed to motivate helping in work chores, giving of advice, sharing food resources, providing support to others in need of help, making friends likely to provide favours, building social standing and status as responsible and trustworthy.

Basically, an evolutionarily affirmative stance on medical conditions presumes that much of the stuff of social life expresses programmes of behaviour (i.e. adaptations) geared to ensuring social favours from others and through these a surmounting of the threat of extinction of phenotypes and genotypes (Tooby and Cosmides, 1992, 2005; Sugiyama, 1996, 2004; Sugiyama and Chacon, 2000). This underlies and helps explain programmes for effectively appraising who in one's circle of group mates can be benefactors to oneself and incur little in the way of costs to themselves for doing so. In other words, evolutionary costs and imperatives of sickness and healing are held to represent important motivating factors shaping an individual's appraisal of others as social beings and as potential sources of help through advice, lending resources, providing support and the like. Inevitable contingencies of need lead individuals to scour their social environment so as to identify, court and interpersonally bond with group mates who are in the position of providing help in various spheres of life (e.g. political, information, services of different types) and sickness represents an exemplar context of various needs required to meet evolutionary imperatives. It should be made clear that the present line of argument is framed in and exemplifies strict notions of evolutionary affirmation but that when the respective behaviours in question are unpacked and framed in terms of cultural affirmation an altogether different picture comes into view (discussed later).

The raison d'etre of 'adaptations' and strategies involving friendship and social helping and caring is that in ancestral and current environments social relations of this type countered and can still be expected to counter the risk to self and family in the event of sickness and disease. They are construed as an all important component of the glue that exemplifies sociality and keeps groups functionally organized towards shared goals. Social exchange mechanisms have as a corollary the detection and punishment of social cheaters; in the present focus, it would involve 'punishing' group mates who renege on social commitments to provide support and healing with respect to disease and healing.

In the evolutionary perspective, sickness was a universal eventuation (actual or potential) which threatened extinction in ancestral environments. It gave rise to a need for corrective action. Sickness does the same in chimpanzees and hence this perspective and the culturally affirmative one rest on innate basic biological imperatives on social behaviour. In the first it exemplifies the emotional responsiveness to suffering in others and the naturalness of commiseration and support realized in cultural meaning systems; whereas in the latter it buttresses the claim involving the innateness of practical routines of health maintenance as a naturally designed evolutionary imperative involving fitness, reproduction, and survival.

Summary Comment on Evolutionary Affirmative Conception

In the evolutionary perspective, it is not the meanings, dynamics, nor the drama of sickness and healing routines which count, as in the culturally affirmative tradition which is taken up later. In general, what counts are the practical exigencies brought into play that enabled and still enable individuals to overcome the threat to survival, reproduction and fitness. It follows from this line of argument that the stuff of a culturally affirmative stance (i.e. ethnomedicine and ethnopsychiatry) is not usually highlighted in a traditional biological evolutionary exposition. Little emphasis is given in conventional accounts of Darwinian tenets to existential implications and meanings inherent in culturally formulated harms and consternation to individuals and families. The social language and practices inherent in sickness, healing, world view, myth, ritual, cosmology, religion, politics and existential narratives are generally out of focus. Ethno conceptions and practices related to medical problems as socially learned and transmitted cultural knowledge involving sickness and healing are simply accorded little significance in an evolutionary affirmative conception of CPI. In pure and simple terms, not sickness/healing exegeses and scenarios but cold calculation about the energetics of survival and reproduction linked to a medical condition are what matter.

In evolutionary affirmation ideas, beliefs, and accounts are construed as variable phenomena, aspects of *evoked and transmitted culture* that exemplify universal behavioural vicissitudes brought into play in recurrent realities of disease and sickness (Tooby and Cosmides, 1992; but see their 1996). Ordinarily, symbols and meanings as emphasized in the culturally affirmative perspective are construed in evolutionary terms as mere epiphenomena of what are the more important underlying and universal adaptive perturbations to internal system functions, behavioural ecological concomitants and contingencies of sickness, and of the adaptive fitness calibrated responses linked to healing. Similarities within a group in the content of sickness and healing behaviours reflect results of the interaction between innate inherited mental mechanisms involving cognition and problem solving, effects of sickness on universal anatomical and physiological structures, and local contingencies of ecology which members of a group

share and which condition or tweak how and which universal response patterns happen to be activated (Tooby and Cosmides, 1992). In short, insofar as local ecological contingencies differ across societies an evolutionary slant on ethno conceptions of medical problems anticipates inter-group differences in ideas, beliefs and behaviours inherent in sickness and healing eventuation. But beyond its relation to fundamental and essential adaptive contingencies and consequences, the possible experiential, symbolic, political, and/or spiritual/cosmological significance of meanings brought into play in sickness/healing ensembles of behaviour appears to carry little theoretical weight in the evolutionarily affirmative conception of CMI and CPI.

Cultural Affirmation Perspective on Medical and Psychiatric Conditions

Introductory Comment

In contrast to an evolutionary affirmative slant, cultural affirmation position highlights the conceptual, meaning-centred perspective on personal identity and social behaviour which devolves from CPI as well as CMI. Cultural factors have and have had an important and persistent grip on medical phenomena; in particular, on the way sickness is understood and practices of healing formulated and played out in social relations and emotions across human societies. It has been language, ideas, beliefs, values, symbolic meanings, emotional dispositions and social practices based on and expressive of mental phenomena which have served as hallmarks of a culturally affirmative understanding of medical happenings in any and all societies (Fabrega, 2002, 2006a, c, 2013).

Cultural affirmation in the study of thought, experience, behaviour and social practices gained a solid grip in general anthropology and social science with new linguistic emphases and related perspectives on knowledge, classification and concepts about domains of human relevance (e.g. plants, animals, kinship, emotions, social relations, colours, spirituality). The traditional cultural slant in anthropology was sharpened and made more penetrating but also friendly so as to incorporate sickness and healing behaviours and experiences and elucidate variability and commonalities across societies (Turner, 1961, 1963, 1964; Fabrega, 1971, 1977, 1979; Good, 1977; Kleinman, 1980). With respect to medical conditions (CMI and CPI), cultural affirmation came to include larger questions of culture as burrowed into mind/brains and encased in social structures, medicine as institution, and sickness and healing behaviours viewed in universal biological, ecological and evolutionary terms as well as in tune with local, content-specific ideational concerns. Ethno conception of medical phenomena writ large can be said to live on with a central focus on ideas and beliefs of sickness and healing as explanatory models of behaviour relevant to the study of culture, medicine and psychiatry in modern societies. A primary emphasis in this approach is on how meanings influence and operate in any of a number of specific contexts of medical significance.

Characterizing the Cultural Approach to Medical Phenomena

A basic assumption of the *culturally affirmative* perspective on medical problems is that in a particular society sickness as ailment, impairment in health and associated interference in everyday activities is first and foremost an existential concern tapping into fundamental and emotionally charged questions of being, experience, personal identity and spiritual resonance. Sickness represents far more than somatic material and biological breakdown of processes or even sheer morbid behaviour, all of which were central features of disease as construed in the evolutionary affirmative position and indeed in conventional biomedicine where modern scientific ideas of disease predominate. An ethno stance affirms that being stopped in one's tracks by sickness, and coming to realize that one is afflicted by or said to exhibit a medical disorder of some type, involves pain and bodily disruptions for sure, but of equal importance it involves a sense of personal indisposition, a sense of aloneness, dependence and relative helplessness. Sickness is invariably an occurrence of disturbance, stress and worry that is causally problematic to the person and his or her family, far distant from matters involving survival of genes and fitness as per the evolutionary affirmative position.

If pushed as to what makes sickness and healing of surpassing significance to the economy of social identity and being of a person, a cultural meanings analyst would probably have to acknowledge that in the final analysis individuals want to stay alive and live to enjoy their life and family. This position comes close to that of the evolutionary affirmative colleague: it enunciates

what to an evolutionary behavioural scientist represents ultimate questions about fitness and reproduction as the *sine qua non* of medicine as a human area of concern and action (Fabrega, 1975, 1977, 1979). That in an ultimate sense individuals are impelled by evolutionary imperatives tied to fitness is a proposition that is not problematic to either cultural or biological medical clinicians, although allowances would have to be made for limitations devolving from the excesses of both biological and cultural reductionism. Concepts of person, self and society differ widely cross-culturally and regulate behaviour in different ways and directions and that they pertain to crises of disease and illness is hardly surprising. That individuals can be assumed to exhibit a measure of behavioural autonomy, and that they are self-aware, voluntary, cognizant of their mortality and motivated to get well so as to be able to resume their role in family and community, constitute human universals. Whether framed in terms of inclusive fitness or in terms of value laden cultural psychological resonance, the previous generalizations hold true.

Scope and Nuance of Cultural Affirmation

An ethno slant on medical problems (CMI and CPI) expresses the view that in ancestral environments and still today sickness was and is an existential crisis and healing a group-centred occurrence. In earlier phases of human pre- and recorded history, sickness involved sacred, spiritually laden phenomena; presently, it is more secular, impersonal and mechanical yet still coloured by ancestral overtones. It constitutes burden and worry and calls into play imperatives and necessities on the person, family, community and healers to restore the well-being of the individual and their family. This involves (involved) restoration of biological functions via administration of herbal preparations and medicines, of course; but in addition and especially, it entailed a working towards an existential alignment of the individual with or in tune with the workings of the world as the group construed it through its ideas, values, rituals, myths and cosmology. Thus, equally if not more important in calculating the burden of sickness and healing, and in calibrating the efficacy of an ethno medical intervention, social cultural conventions and standards entailed taking into effect the views and responses of family members and immediate group members who played an important role in coping with 'the drama and orchestration' of sickness and healing, helping to promote the integration of the individual, and coping with the effects of death should the intervention not be successful in reversing the course of the sickness (Turner, 1961, 1963, 1964; Kleinman, 1980; Good, 1977).

The cultural affirmation perspective of medicine exemplifies a content rich interpretation of sickness and healing as a meaning filled symbolically resonant phenomenon which happened to be backgrounded in disruptions involving somatic anatomy and physiology and its social behavioural consequences. In ancestral and traditional societies and cultures the symbolic dimension of medical scenarios would have been transparent, exposed and palpable and is still echoed, though faintly, in modern contemporary poly-ethnic societies. An individual when sick is construed as hurting, ailing and suffering but also as behaviourally, symbolically and implicitly communicating disability, plight, need, ambiguity and mystery regarding its beclouded and causally problematic origin and implication to person, immediate family, kinfolk and group. Regardless of society, a victim of a medical condition exemplifies and expresses their existential disarray morally and spiritually to an audience in a culturally meaningful vocabulary and idiom. Sickness also involves a potential and often real and significant breakdown in the architecture and mechanics of the family and immediate group of the individual. Ideas and beliefs about sickness, explanatory models of illness, the semantics of sickness, and disvalue of sickness and values tied in with healing as a social cultural practice are of central importance in establishing what a sickness exemplifies and symbolizes.

Virtually all of the above are intuitively, implicitly beclouded and not usually transparently compelling and obvious in a social circumstance of medical importance in any modern society. The point is that cultural resonance of a medical condition is generally off the conventional proverbial (objective, cut and dried, secularized) radar screen of participants of official medical transactions in the clinic or hospital. Secularization, objectivism, impersonality and somatic biological reductionism exemplify evolutionary affirmation about sickness and healing in general medicine whereas they pulsate, resonate and command focus and concern of highly personalized concerns in the cultural affirmation perspective.

How healers formulated (and still formulate) the problem of an individual's sickness and what they did (and still do), namely, their intellectual resources and rationales of practice, were (and still are) based on a system of meanings and values that was and is shared by and with the individual, family and group wherein sickness was and is situated. True, individuals are stricken with a biopsychosocial load that is personally problematic. But sickness in the culturally affirmative perspective on medical inquiries was not seen as something inert, sharply bounded, impersonal and mechanically altered. It was morally problematic, freighted with cultural renditions of worry, concern, danger and uncertainty.

This line of argument implies that systems of cultural meaning that configure a medical nexus resonate in the society and minds of the group well beyond phenomena of medical import. In contrast to the objective, mechanical, impersonal, reductionist evolutionary affirmative view now dominating official medicine transactions and in the social life of modern societies and advertising airwaves, ideas and beliefs of sickness and healing have generally directed and shaped a people's political, spiritual and practical economy of life. In this view sickness is something existentially troubling to the individual but its meanings are shared with other members of the group through ideas and values that encompass nonmedical concerns of surpassing social, cultural and existential relevance. Moreover, given that ideas, beliefs and values tied to sickness and healing are shared by group mates and integral to cultural phenomena writ large (e.g. politics, cosmology, spirituality), it follows that a correlate of the culturally affirmative perspective is its endorsement of the importance of medicine as a system or structure of knowledge and practice in the workings of a society or group.

An ethno slant and its grip on a medical system or tradition covers what an individual understands and does in the event of sickness *as well as what a group understands and does.* A medical tradition has functions, does things for society as well as its population, serves goals and can be said to exemplify cumulative cultural evolution (Henrich, 2001; Henrich and McElreath, 2007; Henrich and Henrich, 2007; Fabrega, 1997, 2002, 2009, 2013). An ethno perspective towards medical phenomena is consistent with a corporate interpretation of medicine as a culturally meaningful institution of society. A culturally affirmative view of ethno medical and ethno psychiatric problems is consistent with this for it reflects imperatives devolving from cultural and group selection and evolution.

Implications of Cultural Affirmation of a Medical Condition

The cultural affirmation perspective embodies and affirms distinctive evocations and directives. It presupposes that sickness and healing represent quintessential needs and expectations that individuals have universally been burdened with. Sickness crises are universal and recurring. In relation to them, peoples evolved and repeatedly turned to and elaborated cultural meaning systems for understanding and resolution of the sufferings, deficiencies and biological and social problems posed by sickness. In accepting the dictum of a social change or evolutionary perspective on medical knowledge and practice, the culturally affirmative thesis implies that sickness and healing represented a basic existential imperative the effect of which was to challenge human experience and cognitive resources during an extended phase governed by strict Darwinian tenets; and then prodded them into new directions and dimensions of medically practical ideas and practices which both influenced and were empowered by the group's ideology, myths and rituals. Sickness and healing in this view represents an important motivation and vehicle in the elaboration and evolution of culture akin to other basic biocultural considerations (Knight, 1996, 1997, 1999).

Stated baldly, in underscoring the biopsychosocial cum existential plight of sickness in matters of life and death, the culturally affirmative thesis can also be termed a 'culturally constructive thesis'. Given the ubiquitous and recurring practical and emotional significance that sickness and healing have had throughout human history, it can be presumed to have represented a motive force in the elaboration of cultural meaning systems not only in areas of medical thought and practice but also in matters of wider cultural traits and patterns in the process reinforcing human order, predictability and resourcefulness.

A key implication and worrisome consequence respecting the historical and cultural legacy that empowers urgency and personal concern with respect to medical conditions writ large and *especially with respect to psychiatry CPI* is: the rich, resonant, culturally laden psychosocial nature of CPI is in the process of being peeled away and scrubbed off in favour of political economic imperatives of the industrial, mechanistic, impersonal, medical/pharmaceutical approach which in psychiatry is played out through the melody and rhythm of clinical neuroscience reductionism.

The Culturally Affirmative Perspective and Psychiatric Conditions

As indicated earlier, factors germane to the comprehension of CMI are equally germane to the comprehension of conditions of psychiatric interest or CPI, insofar as all types of medical conditions exemplify genetic predispositions, environmental influences and organ disturbances involving breakdown of underlying mechanisms and processes responsible for social behaviour. Culturally and evolutionarily affirmative conceptions share this genetic biological background. However, what sets psychiatry apart from general medicine is that basic conceptual and philosophical (i.e. ontological and epistemological) differences obtain devolving from the essential and natural character of their respective medical conditions (CPI compared to CMI). To re-emphasize this point: signs and symptoms of CMI are embodied in behavioural manifestations of a victim, but the victim's psychological and social identity remains relatively unaffected through the unfolding of the primary pathology although secondary influences linked to prognosis, social labelling and stigma can be influential in how a victim of CMI responds to social implications of their condition. On the other hand, conditions of psychiatric interest or CPI are distinguished because their basic, primary pathology is entangled in and directly influential on parameters of perceiving, feeling, orienting, thinking and doing which constitute the nature of the victim's moral persona and social and personal identity.

A cultural approach to medical phenomena stipulates that when observed analytically and abstractly, the focus of human social cultural institutions about medical phenomena involves knowledge about the nature, cause and social practices of healing directed at recurrent varieties of CMI and CPI. The two 'ethnos' of medicine and psychiatry, in other words, are components of a general anthropological perspective on disease and medical problems which is a human universal (Fabrega, 1974, 1975, 1997, 2002, 2009,

2013, unpublished a, b). It is a fact that as one moves across geographic and population boundaries as well as within modern complex societies today, one encounters many differences in the ethos and tonality of peoples' mental and social lives. These are described, for example, as Eastern/Western, simple/complex, modern/traditional, and as involving prevailing religion/spirituality orientation contra secularization. The world of physical and social objects, of persons and selves, of the imagination of persons, and, with respect to present concerns, the signs and symptoms of medical problems (CMI and CPI), are seen as different, talked about in terms of different descriptors, and played out in different tunes and melodies in societies across the world and of course within the social territories of a modern society.

However, a culturally affirmative approach to CPI compared to CMI is of overpassing significance. The rich literature involving culture-bound disorders centres largely on CPI and the rich literature in cultural differences in the content, experiential and phenomenological characteristics of psychiatric disorders in contemporary modern societies underscores differences tied to ethnicity, cultural background, social class, educational level and language proficiency. In any human vehicle of CPI all such *social cultural phenomena shape and fashion each and every psychiatric disorder in a distinctive attire, disposition and expressive pattern of behaviour.* These are staple themes in cultural psychiatry that hardly need emphasis presently.

It goes without saying that the assumptive world of individual subjects is magnified greatly when matters of general interest including CMI and CPI are canvassed *across historical, pre-historical, and even evolutionary time lines* (Fabrega, 1974, 1975, 1997, 2002, 2007, 2009, 2013, unpublished a, b). In general, a useful orientation is that today, were one to be transported across geographic regions and populations wherein alternative cultural meaning systems prevailed (i.e. contents of concepts, perceptions, values and social actions), one would find theoretical and philosophical (i.e. as per ontology and epistemology) differences in the way CMI and CPI are perceived, ideas about them formulated and expressive behavioural patterns enacted. Put succinctly, when compared to persons exhibiting CMI, what one can describe as the phenomenology, content and frequently the structure and organization of thought and behaviour manifestations of persons exhibiting

CPI (i.e. their grip on self, psychology and social behaviour) differ qualitatively across social cultural groups and societies. On the one hand, synchronic geographic differences in manifestations of and social responses to CMI and CPI are human universals which, on the other hand, are determined by and inherent in diachronic differences in their natural history which stretch across evolutionary and historical time lines.

Comment

Studying aspects of sickness and healing linked to CPI as culturally organized behaviour flourishes as a topic in relation to any of a large number of facets of a people's participation in medical care and practice in complex societies (Kleinman, 1980; Good, 1977; Kirmayer, 1984, 2010) but is particularly salient and determinative with respect to simpler human societies (e.g. hunter-gatherers, tribal agricultural, historically ancient) where one finds emphasis on culture-bound syndromes and ethnically complex societies wherein one sees rich differences in the cultural psychology and phenomenology of CPI. An important matter in a cultural meanings approach to CMI and CPI is that, compared to evolutionarily affirmative conception, it rarely addresses larger questions involving the evolutionary, social biological and ecological aspects of medical conditions. The latter are addressed by evolutionary anthropologists and psychologists who, because of disciplinary conceits, often gloss over or ignore cultural meanings tied to the nitty-gritty of sickness and healing which exemplifies the cultural affirmation point of view. Furthermore, the idea that a group or society exemplifies a system or institution of medicine that can be described as a whole, analysed separately and compared to that of another system of society or across societies, and that these matters impact in a significant way on material aspects of disease, has not been a central focus in contemporary approaches in medical biological anthropology and much less in evolutionary behavioural sciences as discussed earlier.

Here, the evolutionary affirmative exponent makes a compelling demand of its culturally affirmative cousin for collaboration. Based on self-contained, contemporary social, cultural and geographic markers, CPI are not just synchronically (i.e. now and cross-sectionally) unique mental and expressive states of being (compared to CMI). The biological and evolutionary history of CPI imparts a distinctive diachronic trajectory and legacy to it. A comprehensive understanding of CPI requires taking into consideration that across evolutionary landscapes their nature, form and consequences (as the culturally affirmative scientist sees it) are a product of the special evolution of brain, mind, experience and culture. Evolutionary and culturally affirmative scientists and clinicians have to join their perspectives so as to specify why and how CPI acquired their special social, psychological and cultural character and nature because of developments involving the evolution of mental phenomena (mentalization as discussed earlier).

Summary and Conclusions

As traditionally construed in cultural anthropology, an 'ethno' approach to medical problems, a people's representation of sickness and healing in terms of their world view, involves a realization and affirmation of the power of beliefs, values and motivations that hold members of a society conceptually, morally, philosophically and spiritually together. However, cultural meaning frameworks seem hardly relevant in the evolutionary perspective. The latter construes ideational phenomena as evocations of secondary importance, fluffy stuff obscuring universal primal imperatives determined by practical, instrumental functions of having to survive and make a living. Through natural selection, and in the context of prevailing local ecological contingencies, evolutionary imperatives which shaped cognitive, social biological and physiological adaptations (human universals) figure as the effective players in an evolutionarily affirmative approach to medical conditions (CMI and CPI). Existential and morally resonant ramifications of symbols and values *about* phenomena, essential concerns of the culturally affirmative view, are simply bleached away in favour of material, practical contingencies of somatic pathology and of making a living and seeking genetic benefits through self-interested social relationships, the latter constituting the essential rationale of the evolutionary affirmative perspective.

Each perspective accords foundational importance to what the other appears to favour in contrary fashion. In light of the prevailing dominance and scope of science as a world view today, it is thus not surprising but somewhat ironic that the function of sickness and healing in the evolutionary perspective is to bring into play and reinforce what the culturally affirmative perspective expounds upon as central to its view of society, behaviour and medicine. It turns out that naturally selected mechanisms geared to coping with the imperative of reproduction, staying alive, overcoming 'pathology risk' and 'fitness costs of sickness', all central constructs of the evolutionary affirmative perspective, are played out on the ground through concepts and values undergirding culture; namely, caring, morality, spirituality, myths of origins and myths of collegiality, and rituals of expiation, gratitude and social obligation. Mental phenomena echo and play out practical material concerns. On the one hand, culturally affirmative imperatives and goals cannot but be met in other than social interpersonal and inter-group contexts involving negotiation and optimal coping with existential predicament and moral dilemmas involving sickness and healing. On the other hand, cultural ideas and strivings are brought into play as a consequence of organic factors which are conditioned by strict gene and gene-culture selection influences on brain structures which not only determine but shape biological imperatives and necessities of staying alive and negotiating benefits and costs – all salient themes of an evolutionary affirmative stance impacting on CPI and CMI in different ways. In other words, all of the former comprises the stuff of the culturally affirmative view whereas that of the latter represents underlying adaptive constraints of evolutionary dicta. Both perspectives share the same overarching drama, the processes of individual genetic selection and gene-culture co-evolution (Williams, 1966; Parsons, 1951a, b; Fried, 1967; Service 1975; Rappaport, 1979; Sanderson 1999, 2001; Boyd and Richerson, 1985; Richerson and Boyd, 2005).

The evolutionary perspective's critical rendition of a traditional cultural anthropological construal of medical problems all too often implies that the latter is merely descriptive and ideational. The content of ideas and beliefs are mere superficial and ideational distractions of what is really important, namely, universal reasoning heuristics applied to practical exigencies of biological problem solving and fitness imperatives as construed in evolutionary biology. In the evolutionary slant, cultural, symbolic and interpretive 'information' may be inventive, perhaps, but appears as of little intrinsic importance other than as records of the playing out of ecological contingencies, historical precedents and a person's capacity to think, imagine and seek coherence as a way of allaying and controlling emotions. Meanings of ideas and practices are acknowledged as significant in the closed envelope of social dynamics of healthcare practices but in this context what really count are developing, nurturing and servicing effective bonds that counteract and cope with potential risks of decreased fitness and potential death of genes and phenotypes due to disease. In an evolutionary affirmation perspective, the value of 'native' beliefs and values embodied in cultural healing routines and practices translate directly as physiological effects devolving from possible benefits of diets and plant products (ethno-pharmacology) as per gene-culture co-evolution, niche-constructing phenotypes, on the one hand, or indirectly through psychological expectations and influences that inspire hope and translate into beneficial effects of physiological well-being, on the other. The symbolic, existential and phenomenological character of myths, rituals, beliefs and practices are not centrally important in the evolutionary perspective.

It cannot be denied that sickness and healing represent deliberative, practical and exigent considerations with a long history in the human lineage. The power of existential dramas involving sickness and suffering, which a culturally affirmative 'ethno' medicine underscores as central and pervasive, gives expression to and helps validate central evolutionary biological concerns which, in the first place, undergird, shape and give validity to beliefs and practices of religion and moral philosophy as well as medicine. Traditional 'ethno' or ideational phenomena more and more are incorporated in explanatory models germane to evolutionary behavioural sciences (Rappaport, 1979, 1999; Boyd and Richerson, 1985; Boyer, 1994; Atran, 2002; Wilson, 2002; Pyysiainen, 2003; Richerson and Boyd, 2005). Looked at from a purely abstract and analytical standpoint, an exclusive dualist, deterministic view of the human condition such as problems linked to disease is unwarranted. Fundamental tenets which each perspective affirms are shared with those of the other. Each not only complements but needs the other. When writ large, an 'ethno' conception of medicine as organization and institution of society exemplifies a historical and ideational expression of evolutionarily patterned ideas, beliefs and practices that are adaptive in different ways and different levels. It underscores a limitation of adhering to one perspective at the expense of the other.

Coda

This chapter has argued that understanding the core nature of CMI necessitates untangling roles played by distal and ultimate evolutionary genetic factors (phylogenetic, natural selection) and proximal environmental, socio-cultural factors impacting on evolutionary developments which begin with archaic humans and become tangible during human pre-, recorded and contemporary history. The evolutionary biology of CMI is responsible for shaping behavioural expressions of the 'organic pathology' of CMI. Dysregulation and/or breakdown of organ-based chemical physiological systems compromise social functions and behaviour which in turn elicit social responses and labels that further shape and colour the trajectory of CMI in social and cultural settings.

To general physicians who are not psychiatrists, aspects of psychological or 'mental' phenomena enmeshed in and crucial to expression of CMI (e.g. differences involving meaning, values, thinking, feelings, attitudes) among diverse peoples in modern society around the globe are important, but in a secondary sense and thus differently from CPI. What is important in the strict biomedical evolutionary perspective involves mental phenomena (e.g. ideas, beliefs, emotional responses and habits) that influence (and sometimes determine) risk factors and basic physiological functions all of which can predispose to CMI, can influence its course positively, and embody its character. Furthermore, interpretations and meaning respecting CMI directly motivate and can delay presentation for care; and they influence whether and if so how medical therapies are understood, accepted and adhered to.

With respect to conditions of psychiatric interest (CPI), the factors relevant to general medical conditions (CMI) just reviewed are equally germane. From a purely medical standpoint, both types of conditions reflect and embody similar genetic, biological and socio-cultural considerations. However, compared to CMI, the relevance and influence of CPI tack on additional and *categorically distinct considerations*; namely, those stemming from its (i.e. CPI) distinct, 'internal' neurobiological nature which express as mentalization and especially from their 'external' cultural symbolic resonance which in turn determines their distinctive social identity and plays in behavioural contexts via meanings of social labels and especially their effects on identity and sense of worthiness.

In contemporary education and practice of medicine and psychiatry especially, the difference between CPI and CMI is ontologically and epistemically compelling yet all too often minimized, misunderstood and trivialized if not altogether forgotten in the necessity of having to respect dicta, imperatives and necessities of brain/mind reductionism and pharmaceutical imperatives ('clinical neuroscience') and associated political, economic and practical considerations tied to the system of modern medical professionalism which has come to involve strict medical scheduling, limited time allocation for services, competitive practices of compensation, and bread and butter routines of strict medicalization. Viewed from a standpoint not only of sheer cognition, subjectivity, phenomenology and content but on their crucial relevance to social, cultural and medical exigencies, CPI are played out differently compared to CMI yet in establishment clinics they are both administratively 'managed' in similarly reductive, practical ways.

When compared to CMI, CPI are not only qualitatively different entities: they pose a distinctly different class of scientific, theoretical, practical and *moral imperatives and responsibilities* on agents who have been selected and empowered or burdened with having to care and provide support for those who exhibit their manifestations precisely because the two conditions exemplify a similar yet different mix of values, constraints and vicissitudes (Fabrega, 2010). Conditions of psychiatric interest can hamper and constrain morale and social, instrumental functions just as much as CMI but their social and cultural identity as perceived and acted upon by social and institutional agents and gatekeepers of society influence and shape the psychologies of victims in very different ways and place different demands on their respective healers (Fabrega, 2006c).

The prevailing theoretical position in the academy and professional establishment of psychiatry, necessarily influenced by powerful exigencies and necessities tied to professional status and political and economic considerations, tend to gloss over and obscure the special nature of CPI (compared to CMI). It also tends to play down the special attributes of CPI in the education and training of medical students, physicians and psychiatrists. To accommodate economic exigencies, the administration of clinical care for CPI has required cost-effective appointment scheduling and time constraints on (duration of) clinical encounters that conform to those adopted for CMI. Similar directives and guidelines of treatment are enjoined for practitioners of CMI and CPI despite the fact that difference in the nature, social behavioural ramifications, methods of assessment, clinical consequences and moral imperatives exemplified in CPI impose qualitatively different approaches from health practitioners in the conduct of their care compared to CMI.

References

Alexander, R. D. (1987a). *The Biology of Moral Systems*. New York: Aldine DeGruyter.

Alexander, R. D. (1987b). The evolutionary approach to human behavior: what does the future hold? In *Human Reproductive Behavior: A Darwinian Perspective*, ed. L. L. Betzig, M. Borgerhoff Mulder and P. W. Turke. Cambridge: Cambridge University Press, pp. 317–341.

Alexander, R. D. (1989). Evolution of the human psyche. In *The Human Revolution: Behavioural and Biological Perspectives on the Origins of Modern Humans*, ed. P. Mellars and C. Stringer. Princeton, NJ: Princeton University Press, pp. 455–513.

Alexander, R. D. (1990). *How Did Humans Evolve? Reflections on the Uniquely Unique Species*. Ann Arbor: Museum of Zoology, University of Michigan.

Armelagos, G. J. (1990). Disease in Prehistoric Populations in Transition. In *Disease in Human Population in Transition*, ed. A. C. Swedlund and G. J. Armelagos. South Hadley: Bergin and Garvey, pp. 124–142.

Armelagos, G. J. and Barnes, K. (1999). The evolution of human disease and the rise of allergy: epidemiological transitions. *Medical Anthropology*, 18(2), 187–213.

Atran, S. (2002). *In Gods We Trust: The Evolutionary Landscape of Religion*. Oxford: Oxford University Press.

Berkson, G. (1970). Defective infants in a feral monkey group. *Folia Primatologica*, 12(4), 284–289.

Berkson, G. (1973). Social responses to abnormal infant monkeys. *American Journal of Physical Anthropology*, 38(2), 583–586.

Berlin, B., Breedlove, D. E. and Raven, P. H. (1968). Covert categories and folk taxonomies. *American Anthropologist*, 70, 290–299.

Boyd, R. and Richerson, P. J. (1985). *Culture and the Evolutionary Process*. Chicago: University of Chicago Press.

Boyer, P. (1994). *The Naturalness of Religious Ideas: A Cognitive Theory of Religion*. Berkeley: University of California Press.

Brune, M., Brune-Cohrs, U., McGrew, W. C. and Preuschoft, S. (2006). Psychopathology in great apes: concepts, treatment options, and possible homologies to human psychiatric disorders. *Neuroscience and Biobehavioral Reviews*, **30**, 1246–1259.

Burghardt, G. M. (1991). Cognitive ethology and critical anthropomorphism: a snake with two heads and hognose snakes that play dead. In *Cognitive Ethology: The Minds of Other Animals*, ed. C. A. Ristau. Hillsdale, NJ: Lawrence Erlbaum, pp. 53–90.

Burghardt, G. M. (1997). Amending Tinbergen: a fifth aim for ethology. In *Anthropomorphism, Anecdotes, and Animals*, ed. R. W. Mitchell, N. S. Thompson and H. L. Miles, Albany: State University of New York Press, pp. 254–276.

Burghardt, G. M. (1999). Conception of play and the evolution of animal minds. *Evolution and Cognition*, **5**(2), 114–122.

Burghardt, G. M. (2007). Critical anthropomorphism, uncritical anthropocentrism and naïve nominalism. *Comparative Cognition and Behavior Reviews*, **2**, 136–138.

Burghardt, G. M. (2009). Darwin's legacy to comparative psychology and ethology. *American Psychology*, **64**(2), 102–110.

Burkhardt, R. W., Jr (1997). The founders of ethology and the problem of animal subjective experience. In *Animal Consciousness and Animal Ethics: Perspectives from the Netherlands*, ed. M. Dol, S. Kasanmoentalib, S. Lijmbach, E. Rivers and R. van den Bos. Assen, the Netherlands: Van Gorcum, pp. 1–13.

Cohen, M. N. (1989). *Health and the Rise of Civilization*. New Haven, CT: Yale University Press.

Conn, P. M. (ed.) (2013). *Animal Models of Disease for the Study of Human Diseases*. San Diego, CA: Academic Press.

Cronk, L., Chagnon, N. and Irons, W. (eds) (2000). *Adaptation and Human Behavior: An Anthropological Perspective*. New York: Aldine de Gruyter.

D'Andrade, R. G. (1981). The cultural part of cognition. *Cognitive Science* **5**, 179–191.

D'Andrade, R. G. (1987). A folk model of the mind. In *Cultural Models in Language and Thought*, ed. D. Holland and N. Quinn. Cambridge: Cambridge University Press.

D'Andrade, R. G. (1995). *The Development of Cognitive Anthropology*. Cambridge: Cambridge University Press.

Dennett, D. C. (1995). *Darwin's Dangerous Idea: Evolution and the Meanings of Life*. New York: Simon and Schuster.

De Waal, F. B. M. (1996). *Good Natured. The Origins of Right and Wrong in Animals and Other Humans*. Cambridge, MA: Harvard University Press.

De Waal, F. B. (2005). *Our Inner Ape*. New York: Riverhead Books, Penguin.

De Waal, F. (2016). *Are We Smart Enough to Know How Smart Animals Are?* New York: W. W. Norton and Company.

De Waal, F. B. M., Uno, H., Luttrell, L., Meisner L. and Jeanotte, L. (1996). Behavioral retardation in a Macaque with autosomal trisomy and aging mothers. *American Journal of Mental Retardation*, **100**(4), 378–390.

Dunbar, R. (1993). Co-evolution of neocortex size, group size, and language in humans. *Behavioral and Brain Sciences*, **16**, 681–735.

Dunbar, R. I. M. (1996a). Determinants of group size in primates: a general model. In *Evolution of Social Behaviour Patterns in Primates and Man*, ed. W. G. Runciman, J. M. Smith and R. I. M. Dunbar. New York: Oxford University Press, pp. 33–57.

Dunbar, R. I. M. (1996b). On the evolution of language and kinship. In *The Archaeology of Human Ancestry: Power, Sex and Tradition*, ed. J. Steele and S. Shennan, New York: Routledge, pp. 380–396.

Dunbar, R. I. M. (2003). The social brain: mind, language, and society in evolutionary perspective. *Annual Review of Anthropology*, **32**, 163–181.

Dunbar, R. I. M. (2004). *Grooming, Gossip and Evolution of Language*, 2nd edn. London: Faber & Faber.

Dunbar, R.I.M. and Shultz, S. (2007) (September). Evolution in the social brain. *Science*, **317**, 1344–1347.

Dunbar, R. I. M., Knight, C. and Power, C. (eds) (1999). *The Evolution of Culture*. New Brunswick, NJ: Rutgers University Press.

Fabrega, H., Jr (1971). Medical anthropology. In *Biennial Review of Anthropology*, ed. B. Siegel. Stanford, CA: Stanford University Press, pp. 167–229.

Fabrega, H., Jr (1974). *Disease and Social Behavior: An Interdisciplinary Perspective*. Cambridge, MA: The MIT Press.

Fabrega, H., Jr (1975). The need for an ethnomedical science. *Science* **189**, 969–975.

Fabrega, H., Jr (1976a). The biological significance of taxonomies of disease. *Journal of Theoretical Biology*, **63**, 191–216.

Fabrega, H., Jr (1976b). Towards a theory of human disease. *Journal of Nervous and Mental Disease*, **162**, 299–312.

Fabrega, H., Jr (1976c). The function of medical-care systems: a logical analysis. *Perspectives in Biology and Medicine*, **20**, 108–119.

Fabrega, H., Jr (1977). Disease viewed as a symbolic category. In *Mental Health: Philosophical Perspectives*, ed. H. T. Engelhardt and S. F. Spicker, Boston: D. Reidel, pp. 79–106.

Fabrega, H., Jr (1979). The scientific usefulness of the idea of illness. *Perspectives in Biology and Medicine*, **22**, 545–558.

Fabrega, H., Jr (1993). A cultural analysis of human behavioral breakdowns: an approach to the ontology and epistemology of psychiatric phenomena. *Culture, Medicine and Psychiatry*, **17**(1), 99–132.

Fabrega, H., Jr (1997). *Evolution of Sickness and Healing*. Berkeley: University of California Press.

Fabrega, H., Jr (2002). *The Origins of Psychopathology: The Phylogenetic and Cultural Basis of Mental Illness*. New Brunswick, NJ: Rutgers University Press.

Fabrega, H., Jr (2006a). Why psychiatric conditions are special: an evolutionary and cross-cultural perspective. *Perspectives in Biology and Medicine*, **49**(4), (autumn), 586–601.

Fabrega, H., Jr (2006b). Making sense of behavioral irregularities in great apes. *Neuroscience and Biobehavioral Reviews*, **30**, 1260–1273.

Fabrega, H., Jr (2006c). Evils of psychiatric medicalization. *Psychiatry: Interpersonal and Biological Processes*, **69**(2), 167–182.

Fabrega, H., Jr (2007). How psychiatric conditions were made. *Psychiatry: Interpersonal and Biological Processes* **70**(2), 130–153.

Fabrega, H., Jr (2009). *History of Mental Illness in India: A Cultural Retrospective*. Delhi, India: Motilal Banarsidass.

Fabrega, H., Jr (2010). Understanding the evolution of medical traditions: brain/behavior influences, enculturation, and the study of sickness and healing. *Neuropsychoanalysis: An Interdisciplinary Journal for Psychoanalysis and the Neurosciences*. **12**(1), 21–27.

Fabrega, H., Jr (2011). Sickness and healing and the evolutionary foundations of mind and minding. In *International Seminar on Mind, Brain and Consciousness*, ed. A. R. Singh and S. A. Singh. Mumbai: Mens Sana Research Foundation and Medknow Publications, Mens Sana Monographs 9.1: pp. 159–182.

Fabrega, H., Jr (2013). *Conditions of Psychiatric Interest in Early Human History*. Lampeter, Ceredigion, Wales: Edwin Mellen Press.

Fabrega, H., Jr (n.d.). Unpublished a: Need for a cross-species linguistics: natural semantic metalanguage as resource for evolutionary behavioral sciences.

Fabrega, H. Jr. (n.d.). Unpublished b: A unified conception of mental phenomena is Darwinian natural: evolutionary behavioral sciences, mentalization, and natural semantic metalanguage.

Fried, M. H. (1967). *The Evolution of Political Society: An Essay in Political Anthropology*. New York: Random House.

Gluckman, P., Beedle, A. and Hanson, M. (2009). *Principles of Evolutionary Medicine*. Oxford: Oxford University Press.

Goddard, C., Wierzbicka, A. and Fabrega, H., Jr (2014). Evolutionary semantics: using NSM to model stages in human cognitive evolution. *Language Sciences*, **42**, 60–79.

Good, B. (1977). The heart of what is the matter: the semantics of illness in Iran. *Culture, Medicine, and Psychiatry* **1**, 25–58.

Goodall, J. (1986a). *The Chimpanzees of Gombe: Patterns of Behavior*. Cambridge, MA: Harvard University Press, Belknap Press.

Goodall, J. (1986b). Social rejection, exclusion and shunning among the Gombe chimpanzees. *Ethology and Sociobiology*, **7**, 227–236.

Goodenough, W. H. (1956). Componential analysis and the study of meaning, *Language*, **32**, 195–216.

Goodenough, W. H. (1957). Cultural anthropology and linguistics. In *Report of the Seventh Annual Round Table Meeting on Inguistics and Language Study*, ed. P. L. Garvin. Washington DC: Georgetown University Press, Monograph Series on Language and Linguistics, No. 9.

Griffin, D. R. (1981). *The Question of Animal Awareness*, 2nd edn, New York: Rockefeller University Press.

Griffin, D. R. (1992). *Animal Minds*. Chicago, IL: The University of Chicago Press.

Griffin, D. R. (1998). From cognition to consciousness. *Animal Cognition*, **1**, 3–16.

Hart, B. L. (1988). Biological basis of the behavior of sick animals. *Neuroscience and Biobehavioral Reviews*, **12**, 123–137.

Hart, B. L. (1990). Behavioral adaptations to pathogens and parasites: five strategies. *Neuroscience and Biobehavioral Reviews*, **14**, 273–294.

Henrich, J. (2001). Cultural transmission and the diffusion of innovations: adoption dynamics indicate that biased cultural transmission is the predominate force in behavioral change. *American Anthropologist*, **103**, 992–1013.

Henrich, N. and Henrich, J. (2007). *Why Humans Cooperate: A Cultural and Evolutionary Explanation*. Oxford: Oxford University Press.

Henrich, J. and McElreath, R. (2007). Dual-inheritance theory: the evolution of human cultural capacities and cultural evolution. In *The Oxford Handbook of Evolutionary Psychology*, ed. R. I. M Dunbar and L. Barrett. Oxford: Oxford University Press, pp. 555–570.

Huffman, M. A. (1997). Current evidence for self-medication in primates: a multidisciplinary perspective. *Yearbook of Physical Anthropology*, **40**, 171–200.

Huffman, M. A. (2006). Primate self-medication. In *Primates in Perspective*, ed. C. Campbell, A. Fuentes, K. MacKinnon, M. Panger and S. Bearer. Oxford: Oxford University Press, pp. 677–690.

Hurley, S. and Nudds, M. (eds) (2006). *Rational Animals?* Oxford: Oxford University Press.

Kandel, E. R. (2005). *Psychiatry, Psychoanaysis, and the New Biology of Mind*. Washington DC: American Psychiatric Publishing, Inc.

Kandel, E. R. and Hudspeth, A. J. (2013). The brain and behavior. In *Principles of Neural Science*, 5th edn, ed. E. R. Kandel, J. H. Schwartz, T.M. Jessell, S. A. Siegelbaum and A. J. Hudspeth, New York: McGraw-Hill Medical, pp. 5–20.

Kirmayer, L. J. (1984). Culture, affect and somatization. *Transcultural Psychiatry Research Review* **21**(3), 159–188.

Kirmayer, L. J. (2010). Unpacking the placebo response: insights from ethnographic studies of healing. *Journal of Mind Body Regulation*, **1**(3), 112–124.

Kleinman, A. (1980). *Patients and Healers in the Context of Culture: An Exploration of the Borderland between Anthropology, Medicine, and Psychiatry.* Berkeley: University of California Press.

Knight, C. D. (1991). *Blood Relations: Menstruation and the Origins of Culture.* New Haven: Yale University Press.

Knight, C. D. (1996). Darwinism and collective representations. In *The Archaeology of Human Ancestry: Power, Sex and Tradition*, ed. J. Steele and S. Shennan, New York: Routledge, pp. 331–346.

Knight, C. (1997). The wives of the sun and moon. *Journal of the Royal Anthropological Institute*, **3**, 133–153.

Knight, C. (1999). Sex and language as pretend-play. In *The evolution of culture*, ed. R. Dunbar, C. Knight and C. Power. New Brunswick, NJ: Rutgers University Press, pp. 228–247.

Kummer, H. (1995). *In Quest of the Sacred Baboon: A Scientist's Journey*, trans. M. A. Biederman-Thorson. Princeton, NJ: Princeton University Press.

Low, B. S. 1988. Pathogen stress and polygyny in humans. In *Human Reproductive Behaviour: A Darwinian Perspective*, ed. L. Betzig, M. B. Mulder and P. Turke. Cambridge: Cambridge University Press.

Low, B. S. (1990). Marriage systems and pathogen stress in human societies. *American Zoology*, **30**, 325–39.

Lozano, G. G. (1998). Parasitic stress and self-medication in wild animals. *Advances in the Study of Behavior*, **27**, 291–317.

McGrew, W. C. (2004). *The Cultured Chimpanzee: Reflections on Cultural Primatology.* Cambridge: Cambridge University Press.

Merker, B. (2007). Consciousness without a cerebral cortex: a challenge for neuroscience and medicine. *Behavioral and Brain Sciences*, **30**, 63–134.

Merker, B. (2010). Nested ontology and causal options: a paradigm for consciousness. Copyright manuscript supplied by Bjorn Merker.

Merker, B. (2012). The vocal learning constellation: Imitation, ritual culture, encephalization. In *Music, Language, and Human Evolution*, ed. N. Bannan. Oxford: Oxford University Press, pp. 215–260.

Metzger, D. and Williams, G. (1966). Some procedures and results in the study of native categories: Tzeltal 'firewood'. *American Anthropologist*, **68**, 389–407.

Odling-Smee, F. J., Laland, K. N. and Feldman, M. W. (2003). *Niche Constructions: The Neglected Process in Evolution.* Princeton, NJ: Princeton University Press.

Parsons, T. (1951a). Illness and the role of the physician. *American Journal of Orthopsychiatry*, **21**, 452–460.

Parsons, T. (1951b). *The Social System.* New York: The Free Press.

Pyysiainen, I. (2003). *How Religion Works: Towards a New Cognitive Science of Religion.* Leiden: Brill.

Rappaport, R. A. (1979). *Ecology, Meaning and Religion.* Berkeley, CA: North Atlantic Books.

Rappaport, R. A. (1999). *Ritual and Religion in the Making of Humanity.* Cambridge: Cambridge University Press.

Revusky, S. (1984). Associative predispositions. In *The Biology of Learning*, ed. P. Marler and H. Terrace, Berlin: Springer-Verlag, pp. 447–460.

Richerson, P. J. and Boyd, R. (2005). *Not by Genes Alone: How Culture Transformed Human Evolution.* Chicago: University of Chicago Press.

Ristau, C. A. (1991a). Aspects of the cognitive ethology of an injury-feigning bird, the Piping Plover. In *Cognitive Ethology: The Minds of Other Animals*, ed. C. A. Ristau. Hillsdale, NJ: Lawrence Erlbaum, pp. 91–126.

Ristau, C. A. (1991b). Cognitive ethology: an overview. In *Cognitive Ethology: The Minds of Other Animals*, ed. C. A. Ristau. Hillsdale, NJ: Lawrence Erlbaum, pp. 291–314.

Rossano, M. J. (2003). Expertise and the evolution of consciousness. *Cognition*, **89**, 207–236.

Rossano, M. J. (2007). Did meditating make us human? *Cambridge Archeological Journal*, **17**(1), 47–58.

Rozin, P., Haidt, J. and McCauley, C. R. (2000). Disgust. In *Handbook of Emotions*, 2nd edn, ed. M. Lewis and J. M. Haviland-Jones. New York: Guilford Press, pp. 637–653.

Safina, C. (2015). *Beyond Words: What Animals Think and Feel.* New York, NY: Picador.

Sanderson, S. K. (1999). *Social Transformation: A Theory of Historical Development* (expanded edition). New York: Rowman and Littlefield.

Sanderson, S. K. (2001). *The Evolution of Human Sociality: A Darwinian Conflict Perspective.* New York: Rowman and Littlefield.

Service, E. R. (1975). *Origins of the State and Civilization: The Process of Cultural Evolution.* New York: W. W. Norton.

Stanford, C., Allen, J. S. and Anton, S. C. (2006). *Biological Anthropology: The Natural History of Mankind.* Upper Saddle River, NJ: Pearson Prentice-Hall.

Strassmann, B. I. and Dunbar, R. (1999). Human evolution and disease: putting the Stone Age in perspective. In

Evolution in Health and Human Disease, ed. S. C. Stearns. New York: Oxford University Press, pp. 91–101.

Sugiyama, L. S. (1996). In search of the adapted mind: a study of human cognitive adaptations among the Shiwiar of Ecuador and Yora of Peru. (Dissertation) Ann Arbor, MI: UMI.

Sugiyama, L. S. (2004). Illness, injury, and disability among Shiwiar forager-horticulturalists: implications of health-risk buffering for the evolution of human life history. *American Journal of Physical Anthropology*, **123**, 371–389.

Sugiyama, L. S. and Chacon, R. (2000). Effects of illness and injury on foraging among the Yora and Shiwiar. In *Adaptation and Human Behavior: An Anthropological Perspective*, ed. L. Cronk, N. Changon and W. Irons. New York: Aldine de Gruyter, pp. 371–396.

Tomasello, M. (1999). *The Cultural Origins of Human Cognition.* Cambridge, MA: Harvard University Press.

Tooby, J. and Cosmides, L. (1992). The psychological foundations of culture. In *The Adapted Mind: Evolutionary Psychology and the Generation of Culture*, ed. J. H. Barkow, L. Cosmides and J. Tooby. New York: Oxford University Press, pp. 19–136.

Tooby, J. and Cosmides, L. (1996). Friendship and the banker's paradox: other pathways to the evolution of adaptations for altruism. In *Evolution of Social Behaviour Patterns in Primates and Man*, ed. W. G Runciman, J. M. Maynard Smith and R. I. M. Dunbar. Oxford: Oxford University Press, pp. 129–143.

Tooby, J. and Cosmides, L. (2005). Conceptual foundations of evolutionary psychology. In *The Handbook of Evolutionary Psychology*, ed. D. M. Buss. New York: John Wiley and Sons, pp. 5–67.

Turner, V. W. (1961). *Ndembu Divination: Its Symbolism and Techniques.* The Rhodes-Livingston Papers, #31. Manchester: Manchester University Press.

Turner, V. W. (1963). *Lunda Medicine and the Treatment of Disease.* Publication of the Rhodes Livingstone Museum (Livingstone Northern Rhodesia). Lusaka, Northern Rhodesia: Government Printer.

Turner, V. W. (1964). A Ndembu doctor in practice. In *Magic, Faith and Healing*, ed. A. Kiev, New York: The Free Press.

Wallace, A. F. C. (1962). Culture and cognition. *Science*, **135**, 351–357.

Williams, G. C. (1966). *Adaptation and Natural Selection: A Critique of Some Current Evolutionary Thought.* Princeton, NJ: Princeton University Press.

Wilson, D. S. (2002). *Darwin's Cathedral: Evolution Religions, and the Nature of Society.* Chicago, IL: University of Chicago Press.

Wrangham, R. W. (1995). Relationship of chimpanzee leaf-swawing to tape worm infection. *American Journal of Primatology*, **37**, 297–303.

Wynn, T. and Coolidge, F. L. (2005). Working memory, its executive functions, and the emergence of modern thinking. *Cambridge Archeological Journal*, **14**(1), 5–26.

Wynn, T. and Coolidge, F. L. (2012). *How to Think Like a Neandertal.* Oxford: Oxford University Press.

Chapter 46

Globalization, Social Stressors and Psychiatry

Brendan D. Kelly

Editors' Introduction

Globalization is the movement of people, goods and resources around the globe. Not only can migration by itself bring stress to individuals and their families but also changes in the new society and culture to which people move. Migration can be described as the process by which individuals move to another culture or geographical area on a more or less permanent basis. The experiences of migration are individualistic and are as important in the genesis and maintenance of psychiatric disorders as is the physical process of migration itself. The views of many researchers and opinion makers do not move beyond the notions of racism, where almost every experience is seen as caused by/influenced by/coloured by racism. Racism is not a recent phenomenon although race itself was identified in the eighteenth century to differentiate between the colonized and their masters.

Kelly updates and explores the challenges of racism and migration as potential and real stressors to patients, researchers and service providers. For patients, experiences of unwelcoming culture as well as a new healthcare system can contribute to stress. His argument follows from epidemiological studies which demonstrate variable rates of various psychiatric illnesses in different ethnic groups. He highlights the ethical and methodological challenges for researchers, especially the problem of definition and cultural adaptation of research tools along with interpretation of findings outside the social and cultural context without community consultation. He points out that there is a paucity of studies examining the precise interrelationship between biological factors and socio-political factors in the aetiology of specific psychiatric illnesses. Ethical issues in cultural psychiatry research deserve a wider discussion and agreement. The research base is necessary but the aim should be to build this appropriately and sensitively.

Introduction

The aim of this chapter is to explore the particular challenges that stressors such as migration present to mental health service users, service providers and, in particular, mental health researchers. For mental health service users, stressors such as racism and migration may perpetuate social problems, precipitate psychological symptoms or complicate pre-existing psychiatric disorders. For service providers, racism and migration present formidable challenges to the provision of effective mental healthcare that meets the increasingly diverse needs of service users. For mental health researchers, the study of stressors such as racism presents both methodological and ethical challenges that need to be addressed at all stages of research.

First, this chapter provides a brief overview of the effects of stressors such as racism and migration on mental health and mental health services, and establishes the importance of addressing methodological issues in this area. Second, I then look specifically at the methodological and ethical challenges that face mental health researchers working in the field of transcultural psychiatry. Lastly, I aim to provide suggestions for future work and developments in this field.

The Relevance of Social Stressors to Mental Health and Mental Health Services

Social Stressors and Mental Health

The association of socio-economic and political factors, including racial discrimination and migration, with physical and mental ill health is well documented (Kelly, 2003). Racism may operate at either an institutional or an individual level, leading to problems such as stereotyping, rejection, prejudice, devaluation of culture, threats and attacks (Bhugra and Ayonrinde, 2001). Such discrimination has been linked to physical health problems such as hypertension (Williams and Neighbors, 2001; Karlsen and Nazroo, 2002), respiratory illness (Karlsen and Nazroo, 2002) and low birthweight (Collins et al., 2004). Racism also affects mental health (McKenzie, 2003), with increasing evidence of associations between perceived discrimination and rates of common psychiatric disorders (Karlsen and Nazroo, 2002), as well as delusional ideation levels in the population (Janssen et al., 2003). In addition, parental responses to racism appear to have measurable effects on the mental health and behaviour of children (Caughy et al., 2004).

Migration has been consistently associated with increased rates of a range of physical disorders (Gleize et al., 2000) and mental disorders (Nazroo, 1997; Gavin et al., 2001). In the United Kingdom, individuals from Caribbean, Irish and Pakistani communities have significantly increased rates of deliberate self-harm (Nazroo, 1997), while those of Egyptian and Asian origin have increased rates of bulimia and anorexia nervosa (Bhugra and Jones, 2001). Schizophrenia is up to six times more common in African Caribbeans living in the UK compared to the native population (Harrison, 1990) and four times more common among migrants to the Netherlands (Selten et al., 1997). While the reasons for this are incompletely understood, one compelling piece of evidence is that the increase in risk of schizophrenia shows an inverse relation with the size of the migrant group within the general population (Boydell et al., 2001) – a finding that is more consistent with a social rather than a biological explanation. This finding, however, is not consistent across studies (Cochrane and Bal, 1988) and requires further examination.

Schizophrenia, indeed, provides a particularly good example of the interaction between biological factors and social factors in determining the clinical features of psychiatric illness. There is now clear evidence of a substantial biological basis to the aetiology of schizophrenia, involving combinations of genetic factors (Straub et al., 2002; Harrison and Owen, 2003), disturbances to prenatal development (Murray et al., 1992; Weinberger, 1996; Kelly et al., 2005), obstetric complications (Cannon et al., 2002) and various other factors, such as cannabis misuse (Arseneault et al., 2004). At the same time, there is a growing body of evidence indicating that social, economic and political factors

also help to shape the presentation, clinical features and prognosis of the illness (Kelly, 2005). For example, individuals from lower socio-economic groups present with schizophrenia at an earlier age (Mulvany, et al., 2001) and have longer durations of untreated psychosis (Clarke et al., 1999) compared to those from higher socio-economic groups. These are important associations because both early age at first presentation (Bellino et al., 2004) and long duration of untreated illness (Addington et al., 2004) are associated with more severe illness. Moreover, in addition to socio-economic group, various other socio-ecological factors may also have a significant effect on mental health: reduced social capital (Putnam, 2000), for example, is one possible explanation for the inverse relationship reported between size of migrant group and increased risk of schizophrenia amongst migrants in London (Boydell et al., 2001).

Despite these provocative findings, there is still a marked paucity of studies examining the inter-relationships between biological factors and social, economic and political factors in the aetiology, treatment and outcome of mental illness. While there is considerable research interest in specific areas (such as the relationship between migration and psychosis), other areas (such as racial discrimination in health services and the effects of globalization) receive considerably less attention.

Globalization, Racial Discrimination and Mental Health Services

The advent of 'globalization' has increased the importance of issues related to migration, racial discrimination, sexual discrimination and political discrimination in the context of mental health services. 'Globalization' refers to the dismantling or opening of social, cultural and political borders between countries, continents and peoples; examples of this trend include increased ease of travel, improved communication technologies and deregulation of commercial and economic activity (The Economist, 2001).

The effects of globalization on mental health services include the emergence of a wider range of attitudes and beliefs about mental illness, increased ethnic and cultural diversity amongst service users, and increased ethnic and cultural diversity amongst service providers, resulting in a broader range of approaches to mental healthcare (Kelly, 2003). In developed countries, increased rates of inward migration may also result in increased rates of certain mental illnesses associated with migration (see earlier), while in rapidly developing countries, there may be increased rates of mental illnesses associated with social change, economic change and life events. From the perspective of the service providers, it is likely that globalization of health services planning will result in a sustained emphasis on the implementation of international protocols, directives and recommendations in relation to psychiatric training, mental health policy and the protection of human rights (United Nations, 1991; Institute of Medicine, 2001; Lavikainen *et al.*, 2001; World Health Organization, 2001).

The advent of globalization emphasizes the effects that social factors (such as migration and racial discrimination) can have on mental health and highlights the multiplicity of challenges that increasingly face service providers and researchers in this area. Racial discrimination presents a particular problem in medicine (Bhopal, 2001), as evidenced by reports of significant racial discrimination against overseas doctors and medical students from ethnic minorities (Coker, 2001). In terms of patient care, there is evidence of poorer access to care, differences in service provision, and differences in treatment outcomes amongst patients from ethnic minorities (McKenzie, 1999). Racial issues are also relevant in the context of mental healthcare (Cope, 1990), as evidenced by reports of 'race thinking' amongst psychiatrists, which may lead to inappropriate diagnosis and management of mental illnesses (Lewis *et al.*, 1990). Racial issues may also have significant effects on service provision, with, for example, evidence of overrepresentation of black people in secure psychiatric facilities in the United Kingdom (Lelliot *et al.*, 2001; Bhui, 2001); this phenomenon may be related to non-engagement with treatment options in less secure environments or to a perception that black patients are more dangerous, despite lower ratings of psychopathology (Bhui, 2001).

The case of Ireland demonstrates the complexity of the issues involved. Traditionally, Ireland has been more accustomed to outward rather than inward migration but between 1995 and 2000 approximately 250,000 persons migrated into Ireland: the aggregate figure for immigrants over this 5-year period represented some 7 per cent of Ireland's entire population (MacÉinrí, 2001). But despite the fact that many

countries report increased rates of involuntary psychiatric admission among migrants and persons of minority ethnic groups (Lay *et al.*, 2011; Ng and Kelly, 2012; Kelly *et al.*, 2015), figures from Dublin suggest that rates of involuntary admission among persons not born in Ireland do not differ from those for persons born in Ireland.

Curley *et al.* (2016) performed a study in an inner-city Dublin area where 35.0% of residents were born outside Ireland (compared to 20.4% nationally) and found that just over one-third (34.2%) of involuntary psychiatric admissions were of individuals born outside Ireland, yielding a rate of 69.7 involuntary admissions per 100,000 population per year (53.5, when adjusted for the area's high deprivation) compared to 72.0 for individuals born in Ireland (deprivation-adjusted rate: 55.4). Even more strikingly, just 1 in 10 (10.3%) voluntary admissions were of individuals born outside Ireland, yielding a rate of 130.1 voluntary admissions per 100,000 population per year (deprivation-adjusted rate: 100.0) compared to 596.7 for individuals born in Ireland (deprivation-adjusted rate: 459.0). This indicates that migrants in Dublin experience real difficulty accessing voluntary mental healthcare. This is an important, growing issue (Wilson *et al.*, 2013; Kelly, 2015, 2016): in 2015 there were 3,271 applications for refugee status in Ireland, more than double the figure for 2014 and triple that for 2013 (O'Connell *et al.*, 2016).

In summary, migration, racism, discrimination and globalization present important issues for mental health service users, service providers and service planners. These social, economic and political factors present particularly urgent challenges to researchers who seek to enhance the evidence base for mental health interventions aimed at meeting the increasingly diverse needs of service users. The challenges are both methodological and ethical, and psychiatry's response to them is likely to have far-reaching effects on psychiatric practice and mental health research in the future.

Methodological and Ethical Challenges for Researchers

The Ethical Perspective

Medicine and medical research have a long history of engagement with the concepts of 'race' and 'ethnicity' (Kuper, 1975: Cruikshank and Beevers, 1989). A substantial proportion of this research is now considered to be unethical, racist and/or invalid (Kuper, 1975; Stepan, 1982). In recent years, therefore, there has been renewed interest in addressing the ethical issues inherent in studying ethnicity and race in relation to disease (Bhopal, 2001). One of the most prominent developments in this area is the use of self-described 'ethnicity' rather than externally defined 'race' for the identification of groups for study or comparison; this is a generally positive development, albeit that some confusion between terms still persists.

In terms of overall ethical standards, it is fundamentally important that research projects should be valid and useful, and designed so as to optimize the likelihood of producing a clinically significant result. As Bhopal (2001) points out, much research in health and ethnicity falls into the category of 'black box epidemiology', which means that the research may succeed in identifying a statistically significant association (e.g. associating a specific aspect or risk of disease with a specific 'ethnicity') but fail to identify the precise causal mechanism that links the disease to the ethnic group. This approach treats ethnicity as an unknown 'black box' and fails to dissect out the precise biological processes that account for the observed association. This approach is especially regrettable because certain studies of disease and ethnicity (e.g. migrant studies) offer unique opportunities to elucidate the causes of certain diseases (e.g. schizophrenia), but this potential will not be realized if ethnicity is simply regarded as a 'black box' and no attempt is made to identify precise causal mechanisms.

In addition to this central ethical consideration, the study of race and ethnicity also raises several other issues in relation to the established principles of medical ethics; i.e. autonomy, non-maleficence, beneficence and justice (Beauchamp and Childress, 2001). A full consideration of these issues is beyond the scope of the present chapter, but it should be noted that the history of research in this field provides considerable cause for concern (Kuper, 1975: Stepan, 1982; Cruikshank and Beevers, 1989). Central issues relate to participants' provision of informed consent for research; the obligation on researchers to avoid harm and promote health; the obligation on researchers to ensure that participants enjoy the benefits of research; and the obligation to ensure that the burdens and benefits of research are distributed in a manner that is equitable and just. Various accounts of the Tuskegee syphilis study in the United States provide an educational reminder of the need to

rigorously observe the centrality of ethical principles in the design, conduct and appraisal of research studies (Thomas and Quinn, 1991; Corbie-Smith, 1999; Reverby, 2000). For historical reasons, these issues are especially acute in relation to research attempting to examine relationships between health and ethnicity or race. An awareness of the likely dissemination pattern and public impact of results (e.g. in the popular media) is also important.

Methodological Challenges in Cultural Psychiatry Research

In addition to the 'black box' problem and various ethical issues, research into ethnicity and disease presents a range of important methodological challenges for researchers. These include: (1) providing appropriate training and supervision for researchers and psychiatrists; (2) defining terms such as 'ethnicity' and 'race' for research purposes; (3) cultural adaptation of research tools; (4) identifying and adjusting for confounding variables; and (5) interpreting findings and putting research into practice. These broad issues will each be considered in turn. Other more specific methodological issues include the selection of valid study samples, the selection of control groups, the balance between 'etic' approaches (from outside a system) and 'emic' approaches (from within a system), and the consideration of cultural 'equivalence'; these issues are discussed by Berry *et al.* (2002).

Training and Supervision in Transcultural Psychiatry and Research

The provision of training and supervision for researchers and workers in transcultural psychiatry presents a range of challenges that are, at once, formidable and urgent. Dogra and Karim (2005) emphasize that overall policy in this field needs to place a strong priority on education, and that training programmes should have a sound evidence base, appropriate evaluation programmes, and identifiable outcome measures. They also highlight two different models for teaching cultural competence: one based on cultural expertise and the other based on cultural sensibility (Dogra and Karim, 2005). Multicultural training in psychiatry is, however, a complex undertaking, and trainers may encounter resistance and emotional reactions that can take multiple forms, including passivity, avoidance and anger (Jackson, 1999). These responses may be related, at least in part, to individuals' previous experiences as mental health workers, their personal experiences of racial discrimination, or their lack of experience in these areas.

The lack of appropriately trained personnel to train both psychiatrists and researchers is a fundamental issue in this field. This problem will only be addressed in a systematic and lasting way when basic psychiatric training broadens its remit in response to the demographic realities of rapidly globalizing service user populations (Kelly, 2003). As part of this process, the World Psychiatric Association had developed a 'template for undergraduate and graduate psychiatric education' which places substantial emphasis on 'the centrality of cultural competencies in the teaching of medical students and residents' (see www.wpanet.org). There is a clear need for ongoing emphasis on transcultural issues, not only during basic training in psychiatry, but also throughout programmes of continuing professional development (CPD) and continuing medical education (CME) for more experienced practitioners.

Defining 'Ethnicity' or 'Race' for Research Purposes

The definition of 'ethnicity' or 'race' for research purposes requires careful consideration, especially in light of the history of medical research in this area (Kuper, 1975: Stepan, 1982; Cruikshank and Beevers, 1989). This issue has an important ethical dimension (as outlined previously), as well as important methodological dimensions. The term 'ethnic type' has been recommended to researchers in place of the previously used term 'race' (Stepan, 1982), although this suggestion has not been without controversy (Senior and Bhopal, 1994). Whichever term is used (e.g. ethnicity or ethnic group), the term needs to be clearly defined in order to optimize consistency and comparability both within and between studies. The terminology also needs to be non-discriminatory and acceptable to study participants, researchers and those who ultimately implement the research findings in clinical practice. In this light, the trend toward using self-defined 'ethnicity' is likely to be more acceptable to participants in research but may raise issues about consistency, especially if ethnic categories are not clearly defined in the research materials.

Given the 'black box' criticism of much research in this area, it may be more scientifically useful to investigate some health issues that may be related to ethnicity through prisms other than that of ethnicity itself.

For example, studies of the excess risk of schizophrenia in migrant populations have tended to focus on specific mechanisms that might mediate the excess risk, such as rates of schizophrenia in the country of origin (Hickling and Rodgers-Johnson, 1995), rates of obstetric complications (Hutchinson et al., 1997) and size of migrant groups (Boydell et al., 2001), rather than focusing on a broad and arbitrarily defined concept like 'ethnicity' as a possible explanation. In general terms, a more scientifically grounded approach is likely to optimize the scientific value of these kinds of studies and to maximize their relevance not only in terms of understanding the increased rates of illness amongst migrant populations, but also in terms of the overall aetiology of the given illness.

Cultural Adaptation of Research Tools

In order to achieve meaningful results from research, the measures used must be valid and culturally relevant. Some basic mental health concepts may not be applicable to certain migrant populations. For example, high expressed emotion has not been found to be a predictor of relapse in schizophrenia in Asian families living in the United Kingdom (Hashemi and Cochrane, 1999). Standard measures used to assess post-traumatic stress disorder have also found very widely varying prevalence rates among different migrant populations, thus calling into question the validity of the concept of post-traumatic stress disorder when applied to certain populations (Abeug and Chun, 1996; van Ommeren et al., 2001).

Research instruments in mental health generally take the form of questionnaires or structured interviews. It cannot be assumed that the validity and reliability of such instruments will be maintained across different populations. In psychiatry, gold standards for comparison purposes are generally the diagnoses made by clinicians who are trained in the use of semi-structured diagnostic interviews such as the Structured Clinical Interview for DSM-IV (SCID) (First et al., 1998). In order for such a standard to be applied to migrant populations, there needs to be evidence of measurement validity and reliability in the context of that particular population. For many instruments, this evidence is not available and, as a result, certain instruments used to conduct mental health research in migrant populations cannot be relied upon.

Where research instruments are employed, further problems may arise as a result of translation from the original language. Commonly used English terms such as 'the blues' or 'butterflies in the stomach' cannot be literally translated if the instrument is to retain content validity. Translators need to have an adequate understanding of how such concepts are expressed in the original language and in the language the instrument is being translated into.

Particular populations may also have quite different ideas about similar conditions. For example, an important component of panic disorder among Khmer refugees is catastrophic cognitions of 'wind overload' (Bhui et al., 2003). Again, mental health researchers need to have access to detailed local knowledge regarding the population they wish to study if they are to achieve meaningful results.

In summary, research instruments to be used must have cross-cultural equivalence, and local knowledge needs to be employed in the development of such instruments; and such instruments need to be administered by clinicians who are trained in their use. These tasks may prove both expensive and time-consuming, but without such a considered, methodological approach, research results will lack validity.

Identifying and Adjusting for Confounding Variables

Research in cultural psychiatry is commonly complicated by multiple cross-cultural challenges to understanding; by personal, institutional and methodological biases; and by a particularly broad range of confounding factors. Studies of racism, for example, can be confounded not only by the usual confounders identified in epidemiological studies (age, gender, socio-economic group), but also by additional factors such as community size, ethnic sub-groupings and differing social and cultural arrangements (e.g. family structure, diet, etc.). Migration studies, too, are particularly prone to confounding by socio-economic group (McGrath et al., 2004).

In designing studies in this area, it is important to identify potential sources of bias and confounding prior to data collection. Rather than simply controlling for these factors from the very outset, however, it may be useful to examine and evaluate each factor not only as a potential confounder but also as a potential causal factor. For example, there is now substantial evidence that migration is associated with increased risk of schizophrenia (Harrison, 1990; Selten et al., 1997), but the causal mechanism for this association remains unclear (Hickling and Rodgers-Johnson,

1995; Hutchinson et al., 1997; Boydell et al., 2001). If researchers designing studies in this area indiscriminately 'control' for a large number of poorly understood 'confounding' factors, they run the risk of inadvertently controlling for the very factor they seek (the causal factor) and thus rendering their study incapable of producing a valid result. Some potential confounders, then, need to be evaluated not only in relation to the methodological criteria for confounding but also in relation to the epidemiological criteria for causation (van Reekum et al., 2001).

In addition to racially based biases, studies in cultural psychiatry may also be prone to other forms of bias, including cultural biases, selection bias, observer bias and various other methodological biases. Many of these problems can be overcome through rigorous design, execution and analysis of studies. Methodological pluralism has also been recommended as a form of overcoming some of these problems; Harrison et al. (1997), for example, argued that the link between migration and psychosis required support from multiple studies from multiple sites using various different methodologies, in order to produce a valid and reliable overall finding. Multilevel analysis can also help overcome some of these methodological challenges, especially in the context of research that addresses factors at both individual and group levels (Karlsen et al., 2002).

Interpreting Research Findings and Putting Research into Practice

Issues of race, culture and ethnicity are increasingly recognized as having a significant influence on psychiatric practice and mental healthcare (Schultz, 2004). The central aims of research in transcultural psychiatry are to bring an awareness of transcultural issues to the service-planning and service-delivery processes, and to help bring an end to racial discrimination in existing mental health services (Kmietowicz, 2005). The interpretation and implementation of findings from transcultural research is a critical step in this process.

Once research is completed, the effective interpretation and implementation of findings may prove challenging. These challenges may stem from a range of factors, including pre-existing organizational structures, inflexible organizational cultures or rigid decision-making styles (Berry et al., 2002). The prevailing political context is also relevant, especially if the motivation to address transcultural issues is derived chiefly from transient political concerns, rather than more substantive demographic or epidemiological realities. The interpretation and implementation of findings may also differ significantly across different ethnic and sub-ethnic contexts, especially as the emphasis placed on individual approaches and collective approaches to health varies across groups.

At the outset, it is essential to establish that research findings are truly appropriate to the social, political and medical contexts in which they are to be implemented. This process may be complicated by the fact that idioms, cognitions and expressions of distress are likely to vary significantly between different cultural groups (Bhugra, 2005). Nonetheless, these variations may provide opportunities to (1) develop a more fine-grained understanding of psychological distress in different groups; (2) identify commonalities as well as differences between groups; and (3) develop a greater understanding of opportunities for intervention. It is similarly important that the implementation of findings takes account of existing health beliefs and practices. In this context, the examination of the various pathways used to access mental healthcare (van Os and McKenzie, 2001) may help locate the precise relevance of novel findings in the specific contexts in which proposed interventions are to be developed.

Racial discrimination and other issues related to race may present particular difficulties when implementing the findings of transcultural research. Not only are there strong links between racism and physical illness (Williams and Neighbors, 2001; Karlsen and Nazroo, 2002; Collins *et al.*, 2004) and racism and mental illness (Karlsen and Nazroo, 2002; McKenzie, 2003; Janssen *et al.*, 2003), but there is also evidence that even being worried about being the victim of racial harassment can have a negative effect (Karlsen and Nazroo, 2004). This latter finding emphasizes the importance of addressing issues in the psychological environment that may have a critical influence on people's fear of racial discrimination and, in turn, a significant influence on their health. In addition, there is an ongoing need to address issues of racial discrimination in the fields of medical education and medical practice (Coker, 2001), in order to ensure that transcultural research findings are implemented, and transcultural services are developed, in a fashion that is non-discriminatory, equitable and acceptable to service users and service providers alike.

Future Work and Developments

Social and psychological stressors such as migration and racial discrimination present considerable challenges in the context of transcultural psychiatry. As outlined above, there is now strong evidence of increased rates of certain physical and mental illnesses (e.g. schizophrenia) amongst migrant populations and there is similarly strong evidence that racial discrimination has a significant and adverse effect on mental health. Despite these findings, there is still a marked paucity of studies examining the precise interrelationships between biological factors and socio-political factors (e.g. migration) in the aetiology of specific illnesses, and there is a similar paucity of studies examining the relationships between racial discrimination, mental health and mental health service uptake.

The advent of 'globalization' has added to the importance of many of these issues in recent years and has brought new urgency to researchers' efforts to enhance the evidence base for interventions aimed at meeting the increasingly diverse needs of mental health service users. It is, of course, important to note that existing mental health services can, on occasion, respond very well to these challenges, with some service users providing positive assessments of relevant aspects of services (Madhok *et al.*, 1998). Nonetheless, the process of globalization has highlighted a clear need to address cultural issues in a more systematic, explicit and evidence-based fashion in the future. The challenges are, at once, ethical and methodological.

In the first instance, there is an ongoing need to address the ethical issues presented by demographic, epidemiological and cultural changes, bearing in mind that ethical principles may vary between ethnic groups, especially as the emphasis placed on individual rights and collective rights varies across cultures. These differences point to the need for an ethical dialogue that is inclusive, respectful and pragmatic and is focused on the identification of explicit, agreed goals for mental health services.

In terms of methodology, both qualitative and quantitative approaches are needed, with qualitative studies playing a particularly important role in opening the 'black box' that can lie at the heart of some epidemiological studies. An increasing focus on causal and biological mechanisms, rather than arbitrarily defined concepts such as 'race', would also help develop a more fine-grained understanding of the interactions between overtly biological factors and socio-economic factors in the aetiology of specific illnesses. Other challenges include the provision of appropriate training and supervision for researchers and service providers; more consistent uses of terms such as 'ethnicity' and 'ethnic group' in both health research and policy spheres; cultural adaptation of research instruments; more systematic analysis of confounding variables from the perspectives of both confounding and causality; more careful interpretations of research findings; and more appropriate integration of research findings into existing models of service delivery. In this context, there are particular needs for the identification of the pathways to care currently used by different ethnic groups (van Os and McKenzie, 2001), and for the revision of existing models of service delivery to reflect these new cultural practices and demographic realities.

In terms of overall approach, there are a number of different overall measures that might help improve the standards of both research and clinical practice in transcultural psychiatry. Bhopal (2001) argues convincingly that increased participation of ethnic minorities in designing policy and conducting research is one way to improve the ethical standard of research into ethnicity and disease. A more explicit discussion of methodological issues is also needed, along with a closer examination of the extent to which current institutional structures may or may not act to discriminate against certain areas of research. In this light, discussions about possible or perceived editorial racism in psychiatry are both valuable and refreshing (Tyrer, 2005; Timimi, 2005).

Ultimately, social and political phenomena such as migration, racism and globalization present increasingly important challenges to mental health service users, service providers and mental health researchers alike. Psychiatry's response to these challenges is likely to have far-reaching effects on mental healthcare and mental health research in future years. A solid, pragmatic research base is essential to this response. If properly constructed, this research-base will help service providers and service users to build mental health services that are effective, equitable and appropriate to the needs of our increasingly diverse, increasingly globalized, societies.

References

Abeug, F. R. and Chun, K. M. (1996). Traumatization stress among Asians and Asian Americans. In *Ethnocultural Aspects of Posttraumatic Stress Disorder: Issues, Research and Clinical Applications*, ed. A. J. Marsella, M. J. Friedman, E. T. Gerrity *et al.* Washington DC: American Psychological Association.

Addington, J., Van Mastrigt, S. and Addington, D. (2004). Duration of untreated psychosis. *Psychological Medicine*, **34**, 277–284.

Arseneault, L., Cannon, M., Witton, J. and Murray, R. M. (2004). Causal association between cannabis and psychosis. *British Journal of Psychiatry*, **184**, 110–117.

Beauchamp, T. C. and Childress, J. F. (2001). *Principles of Biomedical Ethics*, 5th edn. Oxford: Oxford University Press.

Bellino, S., Rocca, P., Patria, L. *et al.* (2004). Relationships of age at onset with clinical features and cognitive functions in a sample of schizophrenia patients. *Journal of Clinical Psychiatry*, **65**, 908–914.

Berry, J. W., Poortinga, Y. H., Segall, M. H. and Dasen, P. R. (2002). *Cross-Cultural Psychology: Research and Applications*, 2nd edn. Cambridge: Cambridge University Press.

Bhopal, R. (2001). Racism in medicine. *British Medical Journal*, **322**, 1503–1504.

Bhugra, D. (2005). Cultural identities and cultural congruency: a new model for evaluating mental distress in immigrants. *Acta Psychiatrica Scandinavica*, **111**, 84–93.

Bhugra, D. and Ayonrinde, O. (2001). Racism, racial life events and mental ill health. *Advances in Psychiatric Treatment*, **7**, 343–349.

Bhugra, D. and Jones, P. (2001). Migration and mental illness. *Advances in Psychiatric Treatment*, **7**, 216–223.

Bhui, K. (2001). Over-representation of black people in secure psychiatric facilities. *British Journal of Psychiatry*, **178**, 575.

Bhui, K., Mohamud, S., Warfa, N., Craig, T. J. and Stansfeld, S. A. (2003). Cultural adaptation of mental health measures: improving the quality of clinical practice and research. *British Journal of Psychiatry*, **183**, 184–186.

Boydell, J., van Os, J., McKenzie, K. *et al.* (2001). Incidence of schizophrenia in ethnic minorities in London: ecological study into interactions with environment. *British Medical Journal*, **323**, 1336–1338.

Cannon, M., Jones, P. B. and Murray, R. M. (2002). Obstetric complications and schizophrenia. *American Journal of Psychiatry*, **159**, 1080–1092.

Caughy, M. O., O'Campo, P. J. and Muntaner, C. (2004). Experiences of racism among African American parents and the mental health of their preschool-aged children. *American Journal of Public Health*, **94**, 2118–2124.

Clarke, M., Brown, S., McTigue, O. *et al.* (1999). Duration of untreated psychosis in first episode schizophrenia and its relationship to premorbid functioning. *Schizophrenia Research*, **36**s, 38–39.

Cochrane, R. and Bal, S. S. (1988). Ethnic density is unrelated to incidence of schizophrenia. *British Journal of Psychiatry*, **153**, 363–366.

Coker, N. (ed.) (2001). *Racism in Medicine: An Agenda for Change*. London: King's Fund.

Collins, J. W., Jr, David, R. J., Handler, A., Wall, S. and Andes, S. (2004). Very low birthweight in African American infants: the role of maternal exposure to interpersonal racial discrimination. *American Journal of Public Health*, **94**, 2132–2138.

Cope, R. (1990). Psychiatry, ethnicity and crime. In *Forensic Psychiatry*, ed. R. Bluglass and P. Bowden. London: Churchill Livingstone.

Corbie-Smith, G. (1999). The continuing legacy of the Tuskegee Syphilis Study: considerations for clinical investigation. *American Journal of the Medical Sciences*, **317**, 5–8.

Cruikshank, J. K. and Beevers, D. G. (1989). *Ethnic Factors in Health and Disease*. Oxford: Butterworth-Heinemann.

Curley, A., Agada, E., Emechebe, A., Anamdi, C., Ng, X.T., Duffy, R. and Kelly, B. D. (2016). Exploring and explaining involuntary care: the relationship between psychiatric admission status, gender and other demographic and clinical variables. *International Journal of Law and Psychiatry*, **47**, 53–59.

Dogra, N. and Karim, K. (2005). Diversity training for psychiatrists. *Advances in Psychiatric Treatment*, **11**, 159–167.

Economist, The (2001). Globalisation. London: *Economist/Profile*.

First, M. B., Spitzer, R. L., Gibbon, M. and Williams, J. B. (1998). *Structured Clinical Interview for DSM-IV Axis I Disorder: Patient Edition (SCID-I/P)*. New York: New York State Psychiatric Institute.

Gavin, B. E., Kelly, B. D., Lane, A. and O'Callaghan, E. (2001). The mental health of migrants. *Irish Medical Journal*, **94**, 229–230.

Gleize, L., Laudon, F., Sun, L. Y., Challeton-de Vathaire, C., Le Vu, B. and de Vathaire, F. (2000). Cancer registry of French Polynesia: results for the 1900–1995 period among native and immigrant population. *European Journal of Epidemiology*, **16**, 661–667.

Harrison, G. (1990). Searching for the causes of schizophrenia: the role of migrant studies. *Schizophrenia Bulletin*, **16**, 663–671.

Harrison, G., Glazebrook, C., Brewin, J. *et al.* (1997). Increased incidence of psychotic disorders in migrants from the Caribbean to the United Kingdom. *Psychological Medicine*, **27**, 799–806.

Harrison, P. J. and Owen, M. J. (2003). Genes for schizophrenia? Recent findings and their pathophysiological implications. *The Lancet*, **361**, 417–419.

Hashemi, A. H. and Cochrane, R. (1999). Expressed emotion and schizophrenia: a review of studies across cultures. *International Review of Psychiatry*, **11**, 219–224.

Hickling, F. W. and Rodgers-Johnson, P. (1995). The incidence of first contact schizophrenia in Jamaica. *British Journal of Psychiatry*, **167**, 193–196.

Hutchinson, G., Takei, N., Bhugra, D. *et al.* (1997). Increased rate of psychosis among African-Caribbeans in Britain is not due to an excess of pregnancy and birth complications. *British Journal of Psychiatry*, **171**, 145–147.

Institute of Medicine. (2001). *Neurological, Psychiatric and Developmental Disorders: Meeting the Challenge in the Developing World*. Washington: National Academy Press.

Jackson, L. C. (1999). Ethnocultural resistance to multicultural training: students and faculty. *Cultural Diversity and Ethnic Minority Psychology*, **5**, 27–36.

Janssen, I., Hanssen, M., Bak, M. *et al.* (2003). Discrimination and delusional ideation. *British Journal of Psychiatry*, **182**, 71–76.

Karlsen, S. and Nazroo, J. Y. (2002). Relation between racial discrimination, social class, and health among ethnic minority groups. *American Journal of Public Health*, **92**, 624–631.

Karlsen, S. and Nazroo, J. Y. (2004). Fear of racism and health. *Journal of Epidemiology and Community Health*, **58**, 1017–1018.

Karlsen, S., Nazroo, J. Y. and Stephenson, R. (2002). Ethnicity, environment and health: putting ethnic inequalities in health in their place. *Social Science and Medicine*, **55**, 1647–1661.

Kelly, B. D. (2003). Globalisation and psychiatry. *Advances in Psychiatric Treatment*, **9**, 464–474.

Kelly, B. D. (2005). Structural violence and schizophrenia. *Social Science and Medicine*, **61**, 721–730.

Kelly, B. D. (2015). Migrants need support but they also need dignity. *Irish Times*, 16 September.

Kelly, B. D. (2016). Psychiatric admission in Ireland: the role of country of origin. In *Ethical and Legal Debates in Irish Healthcare: Confronting Complexities*, ed. M. Donnelly and C. Murray. Manchester: Manchester University Press, pp. 194–207

Kelly, B. D., Lane, A., Agartz, I., Henriksson, K. M. and McNeil, T. F. (2005). Craniofacial dysmorphology in Swedish schizophrenia patients. *Acta Psychiatrica Scandinavica*, **111**, 202–207.

Kelly, B. D., Emechebe, A., Anamdi, C., Duffy, R., Murphy, N. and Rock, C. (2015). Custody, care and country of origin: demographic and diagnostic admission statistics at an inner-city adult psychiatry unit. *International Journal of Law and Psychiatry*, **38**, 1–7.

Kmietowicz, Z. (2005). Plan aims to end discrimination in mental health services. *British Medical Journal*, **330**, 113.

Kuper, L. (ed.) (1975). *Race, Science and Society*. London: Allen and Unwin.

Lavikainen, J., Lahtinen, E. and Lahtinen, V. (2001). *Public Health Approach on Mental Health in Europe*. Helsinki: Stakes.

Lay, B., Nordt, C. and Rössler, W. (2011). Variation in use of coercive measures in psychiatric hospitals. *European Psychiatry*, **26**, 244–251.

Lelliott, P., Audini, B. and Duffett, R. (2001). Survey of patients from an inner-London health authority in medium secure psychiatric care. *British Journal of Psychiatry*, **178**, 62–66.

Lewis, G., Croft-Jeffreys, C. and David, A. (1990). Are British psychiatrists racist? *British Journal of Psychiatry*, **157**, 410–415.

MacÉinrí, P. (2001). *Immigration into Ireland*. Cork: Irish Centre for Migration Studies.

Madhok, R., Hameed, A. and Bhopal, R. (1998). Satisfaction with health services among the Pakistani population in Middlesbrough, England. *Journal of Public Health Medicine*, **20**, 295–301.

McGrath, J., Saha, S., Welham, J., El Saadi, O., MacCauley, C. and Chant, D. (2004). A systematic review of the incidence of schizophrenia: the distribution of rates and the influence of sex, urbanicity, migrant status and methodology. *BMC Medicine*, **2**, 13.

McKenzie, K. (1999). Something borrowed from the blues? *British Medical Journal*, **326**, 65–66.

McKenzie, K. (2003). Racism and health. *British Medical Journal*, **326**, 65–66.

Mulvany, F., O'Callaghan, E., Takei, N., Byrne, M., Fearon, P. and Larkin, C. (2001). Effect of social class at birth on risk and presentation of schizophrenia. *British Medical Journal*, **323**, 1398–1401.

Murray, R. M., O'Callaghan, E., Castle, D. J. and Lewis, S. W. (1992). A neurodevelopmental approach to the classification of schizophrenia. *Schizophrenia Bulletin*, **18**, 319–332.

Nazroo, J. (1997) *Ethnicity and Mental Health*. London: PSI.

Ng, X. T. and Kelly, B. D. (2012). Voluntary and involuntary care: three-year study of demographic and diagnostic admission statistics at an inner-city adult psychiatry unit. *International Journal of Law and Psychiatry*, **35**, 317–326.

O'Connell, M., Duffy, R. and Crumlish, N. (2016). Refugees, the asylum system and mental healthcare in Ireland. *BJPsych International*, **13**, 35–37.

Putnam, R. D. (2000). *Bowling Alone: The Collapse and Revival of American Community*. New York: Simon and Schuster.

Reverby, S. M. (ed.)(2000). *Tuskegee's Truths: Rethinking the Tuskegee Syphilis Study (Studies in Social Medicine)*. Chapel Hill, NC: University of North Carolina Press.

Schultz, D. (2004). Cultural competence in psychosocial and psychiatric care: a critical perspective with reference to research and clinical experiences in California, US and in Germany. *Social Work in Health Care*, **39**, 231–247.

Selten, J. P., Slaets, J. P. and Kahn, R. S. (1997). Schizophrenia in Surinamese and Dutch Antillean immigrants to the Netherlands: evidence of an increased incidence. *Psychological Medicine*, **27**, 807–811.

Senior, P. and Bhopal, R. S. (1994). Ethnicity as a variable in epidemiological research. *British Medical Journal*, **309**, 327–329.

Stepan, N. (1982). *The Idea of Race in Science*. London: Macmillan Press.

Straub, R. E., Jiang, Y., MacLean, C. J. *et al.* (2002). Genetic variation in the 6p22.3 gene DTNBP1, the human ortholog of the mouse dysbindin gene, is associated with schizophrenia. *American Journal of Human Genetics*, **71**, 337–348.

Thomas, S. B. and Quinn, S. C. (1991). The Tuskegee Syphilis Study, 1932 to 1972: implications for HIV education and AIDS risk education programs in the black community. *American Journal of Public Health*, **81**, 1498–1505.

Timimi, P. (2005). Racism in psychiatry. *British Journal of Psychiatry*, **186**, 540.

Tyrer, P. (2005). Combating editorial racism in psychiatric publications. *British Journal of Psychiatry*, **186**, 1–3.

United Nations (1991). *Principles for the Protection of Persons with Mental Illness and the Improvement of Mental Health Care*. New York: United Nations, Secretariat Centre for Human Rights.

Van Ommeren, M., de Jong, J. T. V. M., Sharma, B., Kompro, I., Thapa, S. B. and Cardena, E. (2001). Psychiatric disorders among tortured Bhutanese refugees in Nepal. *Archives of General Psychiatry*, **58**, 475–482.

Van Os, J. and McKenzie, K. (2001). Cultural differences in pathways to care, service use and outcome. In *New Oxford Textbook of Psychiatry*, ed. M. Gelder, J. Lopez-Ibor and N. Andreasen. Oxford: Oxford University Press.

Van Reekum, R., Steiner, D. L. and Conn, D. K. (2001). Applying Bradford Hill's criteria for causation to neuropsychiatry: challenges and opportunities. *Journal of Neuropsychiatry and Clinical Neuroscience*, **13**, 318–325.

Weinberger, D. R. (1996). On the plausibility of 'the neurodevelopmental hypothesis' of schizophrenia. *Neuropsychopharmacology*, **14**(3 Suppl.), 1S–11S.

Williams, D. R. and Neighbors, H. (2001). Racism, discrimination and hypertension: evidence and needed research. *Ethnicity and Disease*, **11**, 800–816.

Wilson, F. E., Hennessy, E., Dooley, D., Kelly, B. D. and Ryan, D. A. (2013) Trauma and PTSD rates in an Irish psychiatric population: a comparison of native and immigrant samples. *Disaster Health*, **1**, 74–83.

World Health Organization (2001). *The World Health Report 2001. Mental Health: New Understanding, New Hope*. Geneva: World Health Organization.

Chapter

47 Cultural Psychiatry
Past, Present and Future

Dinesh Bhugra and Kamaldeep Bhui

The revised contents of this volume highlight the changes that cultural psychiatry has gone through in the last decade. The DSM-5 (American Psychiatric Association, 2013) for the first time describes cultural formulation and the role it can play in the management of people from across cultures, especially if the cultural background of clinicians differs from that of the patients they are treating.

How individuals express what they are experiencing when distressed and the terms they use (also known as idioms of distress), and how they explain their distress (explanatory models) is not only at the heart of cultural psychiatry, but it is also at the core of good clinical practice. It is essential to recognize that cultures affect the way individuals are brought up, the manner in which they view their inner and outer worlds and the way they think. These shape the interactions between the individual and their proximal world (as reflected in the family, their employers) and their distal world (society and culture at large). Such an understanding is significant in ensuring that appropriate management strategies are put into place, especially the ones which patients and their family and carers are likely to accept and feel that their explanatory models are recognized, even if these are not accepted totally. In clinical settings, it is also important to recognize that cultures affect and mould the personality of the individual, as well as the social support system. Clinicians and researchers alike need to take cultural factors into account in the same way they take biological factors into account. Cultural factors include not only cultural values but also micro-identities related to religion, gender and sexual orientation. In addition, an awareness of religious practices, taboos and dietary preferences, along with permitted use of legal substances such as tobacco, alcohol, etc., is important. Taking an interest (during clinical assessment or interactions) in individuals' cultural values (including cultural identity) can improve therapeutic engagement and adherence.

Cultures are not static entities. They change for a number of reasons, and may well in turn change the individual's cultural identity and attitudes as well as behaviours. These factors are perhaps more important in understanding what individuals in distress are experiencing and whether their culture sees these as normal or deviant.

Cultural identities: No matter where individuals move or migrate to, they carry their core cultural values with them. Some cultural values are prone to change: for example, language, religious values and practices; but other values, such as the world view, remain reasonably consistent. This is evident in traditional attitudes or modern attitudes the individuals may have gathered in their childhood and growing up.

There is no doubt that with the movement of people or exposure to other cultures as a result of globalization and migration or social media, individuals' cultural identities will change. Many traditional cultures around the globe are in underground transition, and the tensions in many of these cultures – especially between the older and younger generations – are becoming evident. Recent outpourings of demonstrations in what has been called the Arab Spring can be seen as a manifestation of this tension. As cultures change (not many individuals or cultures would wish to be seen as forever traditional), the degree of change will be influenced by a number of factors, including individual personalities, social support networks and contacts, as well as broader social factors.

Hofstede (1980, 2000) has described that cultures have five dimensions. Although his work originated from his studies of multinational companies, there is something useful for broader cultural psychiatry. These dimensions are worth reiterating and include ego-centricism/socio-centricism, masculine/feminine, coping with uncertainty, avoidance, distance from the centre of power. There was a time when most cultures would have been traditional or socio-centric, but his has changed. Ego-centric societies are those where the ties between individuals are loose and everyone is expected to look after themselves and their immediate nuclear family. Socio-centric cultures, on the other hand, are where individuals have a specific place and the family members look after each other. In these collectivist societies, the individuals have a 'we-consciousness', emotional dependence and interdependence on each other, group solidarity, sharing duties and obligations which are performed within stable and pre-determined friendships and group decisions (Hofstede, 2000). These are respectively called idiocentrism (ego-centricism) and allocentricism by Triandis *et al.* (1985). Similarly, these are described as independent and dependent views of the self by Markus and Kitayama (1991). These may be simple and somewhat crude divisions as not all individuals born into a socio-centric society are likely to be socio-centric, and not all individuals in an ego-centric society are likely to be ego-centric. There is some evidence that ego-centric societies show high rates of crime, divorce and levels of common mental disorders, but this needs to be investigated further and in greater detail, especially now that cultures are changing and evolving. The ego-centric/socio-centric divisions continue in the same way as modernism/traditional dimensions pan out. Cultures are not homogeneous – even within the same cultures, local and perhaps regional cultures may vary from others. This variation also deserves further exploration.

Ethnic identities: Ethnic identity differs from cultural identity. It can rely upon the cultural and physical characteristics which a group may have. Often ethnic identity or ethnicity is self-ascribed. However, with inter-racial relationships and marriages this may change further. The ethnic group sets itself apart using physical characteristics as a measurement. This may be confused with race, which is physical and biological (see Helms, 1990; Thompson, 1989). Racial identity refers to a group or collective identity, depending upon the individual's perceptions that they share a heritage with a similar biological group. Such an approach can lead to easy and cheap stereotyping, leading in turn to a sense of entitlement, which may lead to racist attitudes and practices. This distinction between cultural identity, ethnic identity and racial identity deserves further exploration. Future research needs to take this distinction into account while developing measurement tools assessing cultural determinants. As mentioned in this volume, Berry recommends using the term ethnocultural identity (see Chapter 16).

Fluidity of some of the micro-identities needs to be borne in mind. Wachter *et al.* (2015) draw our attention to the fact that some micro-identities can be hidden, whereas others cannot. This selective exposure brings yet another variable to the clinical setting.

Ethnic Identity vs Ethnic Diversity

As a result of the movement of people, many cultures around the world have become multicultural and diverse. In many countries, industrialization and urbanization have meant that people have migrated within boundaries as well as to other countries. Notions of the self vary across cultures, and within diverse cultures two types of self – ego-centric and socio-centric – may be seen. Schwartz (1994) noted that in many countries certain characteristics such as mastery, hierarchy and conservatism, are distributed differently. His work on the type and character of cultures ensures that we look at both the individuals in the culture and also at the characteristics of the culture as a whole. Future research needs to explore such interactions in a more pragmatic manner. Within diverse cultures, there is also prevalent the notion of ethnic density. It can be argued that if ego-centric individuals (from a socio-centric or ego-centric society) migrate to ego-centric countries, they are more likely to settle down better, also because ego-centric individuals are more likely to move easily between in groups. If such individuals are socio-centric, they may have more difficulty in settling down. If they are ego-centric and are surrounded by socio-centric individuals in a broader ego-centric society, that may lead to further cultural conflict. Cultural congruity thus becomes important in settling down (Bhugra, 2005).

Globalization and Cultural Values

Globalization is a term that defines a cumulative set of processes which deal with the social, economic, political and cultural exchange of ideas. Seen as a purely productive process, it includes the transfer of resources from one part of the world to another which produce goods which are then moved to yet another (possibly different) part of the world. Definitions of globalization have tended to emphasize the material aspects of the development of goods, societies, cultures and people. There is no doubt that the process of globalization has led to major changes in people's longevity and health, especially mental health. Specifically affected is the mental health of those who migrate, of those who are left behind and of those who are faced with migrants. The social determinants and changing economic, social and political relations all affect individual, social and cultural mental health. Rapidly changing circumstances, residential settings and financial insecurities all cause specific mental health concerns which researchers and clinicians ignore at their peril.

Globalization and its sequelae are inherently related to normative processes of forming relationships which are influenced by individual ethnic and cultural identities. Research into so-called global mental health appears to be confirming Western disease models not taking into account cultural relativism and patient experiences and definitions of illness which can be understood in a narrative style. As shown in this volume, social media and immediacy of response and urgent expectations have meant that the sharing of ideas can be rapid. Explicit theoretical models in our understanding of these phenomena need further exploration and extrapolation into models of illness behaviour as well as help-seeking.

Given that globalization has a significant and major impact on human beings and their mental health, it is essential that researchers take into account what the macro, meso and micro impacts of globalization are on individuals and their communities. It is important that research uses multilevel frameworks and multifaceted models to look at population and public mental health. Health research must be framed within the institutional, economic, socio-cultural and environmental influences taking the biomedical model into account. Political, social, cultural and economic spheres need to have considerable overlap in ensuring that public mental health and the health of the general population are improved. A lifespan approach is needed in order to ensure that artificial age-based boundaries followed in many healthcare systems are not rigid and do not stop those in need from getting the healthcare they deserve. Evolving flow of people, ideas, resources, technologies and capital as a result of globalization are bound to affect healthcare systems and clinicians need to take these factors into account.

Historical Factors

As Kirmayer in this volume reminds us, cultural psychiatry stands at the crossroads of various disciplines, having emerged from a history of multiple and often complex contacts between people of different backgrounds. These encounters between us and 'the others' led to frankly colonial views, often treating natives as exotic and alien people. In contrast with social psychiatry, as Kirmayer argues, cultural psychiatry has a major clinical imperative. The subject has three important facets to it. These include an understanding of inherent cultural differences in a culturally relativist manner, healing practices and the need and delivery of services to diverse societies and, finally, the analysis of particular cultural history and globalization (see Kirmayer, Chapter 1, in this volume). He reminds us that originally the term culture meant cultivation, which subsequently gave way to collective identity, which is what this volume has been about. Of course, the anthropological understanding and definition of cultures carry with it the clear cause that it is a way of life.

From being part of social psychiatry in the last half century, cultural psychiatry has developed as a discipline. Benedict (1834) saw culture as personality writ large.

Changing Acculturative Values: In this volume, Berry describes acculturation as a process that occurs in response to two cultures coming together. As a result, groups change their identity in a way which may lead to a degree of comfort. Initially, the processes of acculturation were studied at a group level, but of late these are being explored at an individual level (Bhugra et al., 2009). This process of acculturation is intimately related to ethnic racial and cultural identity, and it is possible to measure this. However, whether these measures are equally applicable to all members of the same group is worthy of further research and exploration. The process of acculturation can be seen at psychological as well as cultural levels, and measurements are needed at both these levels – as well as at group and individual levels too. Deculturation, assimilation or the actual cultural adaptation need detailed exploration at individual clinical levels. It must also be recognized that among certain individuals cultural expansion and cultural contraction may be seen. We use cultural expansion to describe the expansion and gathering of certain skills, attitudes and behaviours from a new culture and giving up of certain cultural traits as cultural contraction. Gender, age, religion, educational and economic status – along with sexual and cultural orientation – can play a role in enabling or interfering with acculturation, and deserve further exploration.

National Characters: Often the notion of national character is used as a stereotype and a shortcut to describe various communities. There are major problems in this approach, which can lead to levels of racism and rejection. However, national character can also be looked at as a particular way of describing the coherence of culturally defined values or behaviour patterns. These are the patterns within the personality which are seen as common or standardized ways within a given society (Inkles, 1997). Therefore, national character deserves to be studied on the basis of collective policies and products, rituals, folklore, media, art, mass communication, etc., which can help describe the overall psychological characterization of society. Understanding these collective behaviours, child-rearing systems and collective adult phenomena (e.g. institutional practices, political behaviours, religious ideas and rituals) is key to explaining the relationship between culture and personality.

National character needs to be explored and understood within the context of the type of society in which the individuals live and work. Perhaps national character may be displaced by cultural characteristics and formulations which will allow researchers to place the epidemiological data within the social and cultural context. Therefore, we urge all researchers that epidemiological studies should be embedded within the cultural context for which specific qualitative methods be used.

Cultural Competency: Rather perversely, for the first couple of decades in cultural psychiatry in the UK it was assumed that ethnic minorities had a culture and white clinicians needed to learn about culture. It is evident that everyone has a culture, and cultural competency is about being competent in ascertaining cultural needs, values and cultural factors of all patients who need help. In a way, this should be seen as basic good clinical practice. There is no doubt that cultural psychiatry can provide valuable insights into the core principles of delivering healthcare to individuals from other cultures and societies.

A key aspect of cultural competency is about exploring an individual's cultural identity and cultural framework including attitudes and behaviours. At one level, it has to be done in a sensitive individual manner. On a different level, using culture brokers, culture mediators and cultural advocates can help clinical teams to work with wider groups and communities. These culture brokers, mediators and advocates can provide a two-way link between the healthcare system and the community. Cultural elements can change rapidly, but more often than not they change slowly.

In societies with a long traditional view and a long history of collectivism, elements of socio-centrism may continue to persist despite increased levels of ego-centrism. The changes in structures of culture, society and country as a result of migration or movement of people can bring with it new ideas, but both new entrants to the society and the new country may respond by reverting to even more rigid traditional positioning and posturing.

In order to be culturally competent, clinicians must not take a colour blind approach (meaning that they treat everyone in the same way), but be aware of their own prejudices whilst assessing patients. Furthermore, they should focus on the individual in front of them and the proximal factors (family, kinship, employers) as well as distal social and cultural factors. When clinical assessments are being carried out, clinicians must also explore ego-centric/socio-centric or individualist/collectivist dimensions. The formation of beliefs about the self as well as those about the illness experience are related to these and deserve further exploration.

Cultural competence training is to be embedded in curricula across all healthcare training. It will allow sensitive healthcare to be delivered with a clear focus on the individual who needs such care, in a culturally appropriate and sensitive manner. Cultural competence is essential for *all* healthcare professionals, even if it is of more relevance in the field of psychiatry. All clinicians need to be fully cognisant of cultural and social differences, as well as similarities with their patients. Knowing about one's own culture – its weaknesses and strengths – and prejudices is an important first step.

Conclusions

Cultural psychiatry as a discipline has come a long way in the last 50 years. From comparative psychiatry to cultural psychiatry, the discipline has developed. For the first time, there are clear and agreed components for cultural formulation. There is no doubt that in these times of rapid globalization (though as a result of recent political events this may be slowing down), the type of society we move from and move to and live in, both acculturative levels – at individual and at group levels – provide a connection to the stresses any individual feels and goes through. Understanding the cultural values, attitudes and biases of the patient is as important as the clinician being aware of their own values, attitudes, biases and prejudices. Cultural values are internalized in a way which is often unconscious. Cultural adaptation needs to be understood as to how individuals adapt and respond to cultural changes, but also how these changes contribute to the dynamics of cultures. Cultural identity is fluid, and a large number of internal and external factors will play a role in cultural identity formation and cultural adjustment. The heterogeneity of individuals, societies and cultures often interacts in unpredictable ways. Both clinicians and researchers need to take these into account to ensure that healthcare policies and healthcare systems are sensitive and appropriate to the needs of patients, no matter what their cultures are.

References

American Psychiatric Association (APA) (2013). *Diagnostic and Statistical Manual of Mental Disorders*, 5th edn. Washington DC: American Psychiatric Association.

Benedict, R. (1834). *Patterns of Culture*. Boston: Houghton Mifflin.

Bhugra, D. (2005). Cultural identities and cultural congruency: a new model for evaluating mental distress in immigrants. *Acta Psychiatrica Scandinavica*, **111**(2), 84–93.

Bhugra, D., Leff, J., Mallett, R., Morgan, C. and Zhao, J.-H. (2009). The culture and identity schedule: a measure of cultural affiliation: acculturation, marginalization and schizophrenia. *International Journal of Social Psychiatry*, **56**(5), 540–556.

Helms, J. E. (1990). Introduction: a review of racial identity terminology. In *Black and White Racial Identity: Theory, Research and Identity*, ed. J. E. Helms. Westport, CT: Greenwood Press, pp. 3–8.

Hofstede, G. (1980, 2000). *Culture's Consequences*. Beverley Hills, CA: Sage.

Inkles, A. (1997). *National Character: A Psychosocial Perspective*. New Brunswick, NJ: Transaction Publishers.

Markus, H. and Kitayama, S. (1991). Culture and self: implications for cognition, emotion and motivation. *Psychological Review*, **98**, 224–253.

Schwartz, S. (1994). Beyond individualism/collectivism: new cultural dimensions of values. In *Individualism and Collectivism: Theory, Method and Applications*, ed. U. Kim, H. Triandis, C. Kagitcibasi, S.-C. Choi and G. Yoon. Thousand Oaks, CA: Sage, pp. 85–119.

Thompson, R. H. (1989). *Theories of Ethnicity: A Critical Appraisal*. New York: Greenwood.

Triandis, H. C., Leung, K., Villareal, M. J. and Black, F. L. (1985). Allocentric versus idiocentric tendencies: convergent and discriminant validation. *Journal of Research in Personality*, **19**, 395–415.

Wachter, M., Ventriglio, A. and Bhugra, D. (2015), Micro-identities, adjustment and stigma. *International Journal of Social Psychiatry*, **61**(5), 436–437.

Index